Graft-vs.-Host Disease

Graft-vs.-Host Disease

Second Edition, Revised and Expanded

edited by

James L. M. Ferrara

Dana-Farber Cancer Institute, Children's Hospital,
and Harvard Medical School
Boston, Massachusetts

H. Joachim Deeg

Fred Hutchinson Cancer Research Center
and University of Washington
Seattle, Washington

Steven J. Burakoff

Dana-Farber Cancer Institute
and Harvard Medical School
Boston, Massachusetts

Marcel Dekker, Inc. New York • Basel • Hong Kong

Library of Congress Cataloging–in–Publication Data

Graft–vs.–host disease / edited by James L.M. Ferrara, H. Joachim
Deeg, Steven J. Burakoff.—2nd ed., rev. and expanded.
p. cm.
Includes index.
ISBN 0–8247–9728–0 (hardcover : alk. paper)
1. Graft versus host disease. I. Ferrara, James L.M.,
II. Deeg, H. Joachim. III. Burakoff, Steven J.
RD123.5.G73 1996
617.4'4—dc20

96–31581
CIP

The publisher offers discounts on this book when ordered in bulk quantities. For more information, write to Special Sales/Professional Marketing at the address below.

This book is printed on acid-free paper.

MARCEL DEKKER, INC.
270 Madison Avenue, New York, New York 10016

Current printing (last digit):
10 9 8 7 6 5 4 3 2 1

PRINTED IN THE UNITED STATES OF AMERICA

Foreword

The modern era of marrow transplantation spans about three decades. Some patients once thought to have "reached the end of the road" are now surviving more than 25 years as healthy "chimeras," that is, with hematopoiesis and an immune system derived from the graft provided by their marrow donor. However, despite considerable progress in many areas, problems remain. In part, this is related to success: As more and more patients were cured with a marrow transplant from a sibling who was matched with the patient for the major histocompatibility antigens (HLA), attempts were made at expanding the indications for transplantation to patients who did not have an HLA identical sibling. However, with the use of those "alternative" donors, HLA-nonidentical family members, and unrelated volunteers, problems were encountered. This is particularly true for graft-versus-host disease (GVHD), both in its acute and chronic form. GVHD is of central importance, since it accounts for considerable morbidity, and GVHD and its treatment represent major risk factors for the development of subsequent complications including infection, pulmonary, musculo-skeletal, ocular disease, and other problems.

Nevertheless, advances and gains made even since the publication of the first edition of this book are remarkable. Histocompatibility typing, so essential to the selection of compatible donors, has advanced to the point where single DNA base pair differences at an HLA locus between donor and patient can be identified, and in individual cases have been shown to affect graft outcome. Molecular typing for HLA class II genes has replaced almost completely the mixed leukocyte culture. Gene loci such as HLA-C, which were ignored in the past, have been shown to have an effect on transplant outcome. The same appears to be true for HLA-DQ (DQB1).

The availability of new immunosuppressive agents such as FK506, mycophenolate mofetil, rapamycin, and others has provided more flexibility in the design of GVHD prophylactic regimens. Preliminary results from prospective studies using a combination of FK506 and methotrexate are encouraging. Preclinical studies with combinations of methotrexate and mycophenolate mofetil, or cyclosporine plus rapamycin, suggest that the incidence and severity of GVHD can be further reduced.

T-cell depletion from the donor marrow continues to be explored as an approach to GVHD prevention, but so far has not provided the expected advantages. Recent investigations into the use of selective subset depletion (both CD4 and CD8 depletion has been reported to be beneficial) need to be further expanded before firm conclusions can be drawn. Another potentially exciting development is the infusion of donor lymphocytes that have been genetically marked by a "suicide gene." These altered cells are infused to provide their potential graft-enhancing and antileukemic effects. If GVHD develops, however, the patient can be treated with ganciclovir to trigger the "suicide" mechanism to eliminate the GVHD-inducing cells. A similar approach is being tested in patients who experience a post-transplant relapse. Although the infusion of donor lymphocytes induces remissions in many patients, a frequent complication is the occurrence of GVHD and myelosuppression. If cells are marked by a "suicide gene," they can be eliminated by appropriate treatment of the patient. The technology is rapidly evolving to select specific donor cell clones presumably reactive with minor antigens on patient leukemic cells.

Another area that has grown at a rapid pace is the "science of cytokines." While the network that governs the interactions of donor and host cells is rather complex, some interventions, e.g., those aimed at TNF-alpha, IL-4, IL-12, and others, may reduce toxicity and enhance the development of tolerance. Considerable work is still required to further characterize the various pathways that may be involved.

Recently, there has been a shift in interest from the use of marrow cells to the use of peripheral blood stem cells, generally after mobilization with cytokines (growth factors). When used in autologous transplantation, these stem cells resulted in extraordinarily fast hematopoietic recovery. With allogeneic transplants, however, there was a concern about the induction of GVHD, in part because of the increased number of T lymphocytes, and in part because of activation of those cells by cytokine mobilization. Surprisingly, early studies in matched sibling transplants have not shown an increase in GVHD despite a log increase in the number of T cells given. Further study is needed to determine whether the benefit (faster engraftment) justifies the potential risk (more GVHD).

Yet another source of hematopoietic stem cells, cord blood cells, has been introduced clinically, particularly for use in pediatric patients. One potential advantage might be a lower incidence of GVHD than seen with marrow cells due to the immaturity of the cells transplanted. Current data are still too limited to predict how this source of stem cells will be used in the future.

This volume brings together contributions by numerous experts summarizing what has been achieved and what we think may lie ahead.

E. Donnall Thomas, M.D.
Fred Hutchinson Cancer Research Center
Seattle, Washington

Preface to the Second Edition

We begin this preface to the second edition of *Graft-vs.-Host Disease* with gratitude to our readership for the overwhelmingly positive response to the first edition, which required a second printing even while the revised volume was in progress. We appreciate the many thoughtful reviews and constructive suggestions, several of which have been incorporated into this new volume.

Many of our readers have specialty training in the fields of hematology and oncology, but relatively limited backgrounds in basic immunology, an area of investigation that has exploded in the past decade. Yet nowhere is transplantation immunology more complex than in a graft-vs.-host reaction, where the immune system is both effector and target. As a result, detailed discussions of graft-vs.-host disease (GVHD) are often dense and sometimes impenetrable to the very readers for whom this book was intended. We have therefore included, as introduction, a series of chapters that review important aspects of immunobiology necessary to the understanding of GVHD pathophysiology as well as the current efforts used to control this disease.

The first chapter in Part I reviews thymic ontogeny and summarizes the complex process of T-cell maturation and differentiation. The appreciation of the thymus as a target organ of GVHD helps to explain how the disease can have such devastating effects on the reconstitution of the immune system. Chapters on MHC Class I and Class II antigens review the structure and function of these molecules, which are responsible for activating $CD8^+$ and $CD4^+$ T cells, respectively. Overviews are presented on T-cell costimulation and anergy, molecular mechanisms of immunosuppression, and adhesion molecules critical to T-cell migration and traffic. One entire chapter is devoted to a detailed discussion of cytokine networks, an area of intense investigation that is central to multiple aspects of GVHD. Finally, reviews of target cell death by both cytolytic T lymphocytes and natural killer cells provide a context for mechanisms of specific target organ pathology.

The middle part of the book has been reorganized to bring together research from experimental models and clinical protocols into single chapters. The classic triad of target organs—skin, liver, and intestinal tract—is reviewed first, followed by other, less "classic" target organs such as the immune system, the hematopoietic system, and the lung. Mechanisms of graft-vs.-leukemia effects are explored in extensive detail, with a thorough discussion of the different cellular populations that participate in this process. This part concludes with two chapters that summarize recent contributions to GVHD pathophysiology: the role of endotoxin and infections and the functional interactions between lymphocytes from the perspective of their cytokine profiles.

The third and final part concentrates on clinical GVHD, its prevention and treatment. The first three chapters review the clinical spectra of GVHD after both allogeneic and autologous bone marrow transplantation (BMT), as well as transfusion-associated GVHD. Current strategies for preventing GVHD are summarized next: the matching of donor and host at HLA loci, the depletion of T cells from the donor marrow, the nonspecific immunosuppression of the host, and the use of cytokine antagonists. The following chapter reviews the emerging role of IL-10 in the induction and maintenance of donor–host tolerance after BMT. Alternative approaches to reducing GVHD are summarized next, including the selection of stem cells, adoptive immunotherapy, and the increasing efforts at genetic modification of hematopoietic cells and T cells. The last chapter serves as a sort of coda to the entire book, with contributions from 21 investigators reviewing the most recent advances in GVHD research, many of them still in press at this time.

An endeavor of this size and complexity requires the generous efforts of many contributors, whom we gratefully acknowledge. We would like to dedicate this volume to two groups of individuals who remain the bedrock of both experimental and clinical GVHD research: first, the outstanding animal care technicians and veterinarians without whose care and diligence the exploration of animal models would be impossible, and second, the nurses, residents, and fellows whose superb skills and compassion continue to offer hope to our patients for a brighter tomorrow. If this book can contribute in some small way to that hope, our efforts in bringing it forth will be more than amply rewarded.

James L. M. Ferrara
H. Joachim Deeg
Steven J. Burakoff

Preface to the First Edition

There are two major reasons for producing a broad overview of graft-vs.-host disease (GVHD). From a clinical standpoint, GVHD can be a devastating complication of bone marrow transplantation. Significant progress has been made; however, several obstacles remain in overcoming this problem, particularly in patients given histoincompatible grafts. Multiple approaches, discussed in the clinical sections of this book, have been taken, each with advantages and disadvantages. Frequently, those approaches were based on experimental models. Thus, it is only logical that the clinical sections are preceded by a description of preclinical studies. It is these animal models that have been critical in advancing our understanding of the physiology of GVHD. Control of genetic variables as well as the ability to produce GVHD in a variety of models have permitted insights not possible in a strictly clinical context. In addition, these systems have also provided models for understanding lymphocyte development and function in vivo irrespective of GVHD. The increasing sophistication and precision of cellular and molecular probes have initiated an analysis of cellular mechanisms in physiological environments rather than in a petri dish or test tube. The abnormalities of GVHD thus provide a perspective from which to understand the complexities of normal lymphocyte differentiation and activation. The insights from these studies should lead to improved understanding of fundamental lymphocyte biology and thus to new therapeutic strategies, not only in bone marrow transplantation, but in other areas, such as autoimmune diseases. It is our hope that future editions of this book will reflect this increased understanding and will witness further movement from experimental models to clinical realms.

The production of a book this size is a long and complex undertaking, and we are grateful to the many people who have given generously of their time and effort. We would like to thank particularly Joshua Hauser and Michele Fox for their labors in the preparation of the index. We also wish to acknowledge the continued support of our colleagues and teachers who have encouraged us over many years, especially David G. Nathan, Fred S. Rosen, Baruj Benacerraf, Rainer Storb, and E. Donnall Thomas.

Steven J. Burakoff
H. Joachim Deeg
James L. M. Ferrara
Kerry Atkinson

Contents

III. CLINICAL GVHD: PREVENTION AND TREATMENT

Contributors

Kenneth C. Anderson, M.D. Medical Director, Blood Component Laboratory, Dana-Farber Cancer Institute, and Associate Professor, Department of Medicine, Harvard Medical School, Boston, Massachusetts

Joseph H. Antin, M.D. Director, Bone Marrow Transplant Program, Department of Hematology/Oncology, Brigham and Women's Hospital and Harvard Medical School, Boston, Massachusetts

Matthew Baker University of Miami School of Medicine, Miami, Florida

Patrick G. Beatty, M.D., Ph.D. Director, Blood and Marrow Transplant Program, and Professor, Department of Internal Medicine, University of Utah Health Sciences Center, Salt Lake City, Utah

Barbara E. Bierer, M.D. Director, Pediatric Bone Marrow Transplantation, Department of Pediatric Oncology, Dana-Farber Cancer Institute, Boston, Massachusetts

Bruce R. Blazar, M.D. Professor, Department of Pediatrics, and Associate Director, Division of Bone Marrow Transplantation, University of Minnesota, Minneapolis, Minnesota

Steven J. Burakoff, M.D. Chief, Division of Pediatric Oncology, Dana-Farber Cancer Institute, and Professor of Pediatrics, Harvard Medical School, Boston, Massachusetts

Nelson J. Chao, M.D. Assistant Professor, Department of Medicine/Bone Marrow Transplantation, Stanford University Medical Center, Stanford, California

Curt I. Civin, M.D. Professor, Departments of Oncology and Pediatrics, Johns Hopkins University School of Medicine, Baltimore, Maryland

Kenneth R. Cooke Dana-Farber Cancer Institute, and Children's Hospital, Boston, Massachusetts

James M. Crawford, M.D., Ph.D. Associate Professor, Department of Pathology, Brigham and Women's Hospital and Harvard Medical School, Boston, Massachusetts

Stephen W. Crawford, M.D. Critical Care Director and Associate Member, Department of Pulmonary and Critical Care Medicine, Fred Hutchinson Cancer Research Center, and Associate Professor, University of Washington, Seattle, Washington

Amy Crum Vander Woude, M.D. Research/Clinical Fellow in Medicine, Department of Pediatric Oncology, Dana-Farber Cancer Institute, Boston, Massachusetts

John M. Cunningham, M.B., M.Sc., M.R.C.P. Assistant Member, Division of Experimental Hematology, St. Jude Children's Research Hospital, Memphis, Tennessee

H. Joachim Deeg, M.D. Member, Fred Hutchinson Cancer Research Center, and Professor of Medicine, University of Washington, Seattle, Washington

Julie Desbarats, Ph.D. Postdoctoral Fellow, Department of Physiology, McGill University, Montreal, Quebec, Canada

Bimalangshu Dey Massachusetts General Hospital, Boston, Massachusetts

David B. Fearnley, M.B., Ch.B. Research-Fellow, Department of Hematology, Christchurch Hospital, Christchurch, New Zealand

James L. M. Ferrara, M.D. Staff Physician, Dana-Farber Cancer Institute and Children's Hospital, and Associate Professor of Pediatrics, Harvard Medical School, Boston, Massachusetts

Daniel H. Fowler, M.D. National Cancer Institute, National Institutes of Health, Bethesda, Maryland

Anita C. Gilliam, M.D., Ph.D. Assistant Professor, Department of Dermatology, Case Western Reserve University, Cleveland, Ohio

Ronald E. Gress, M.D. Head, Transplantation Therapy Section, Medical Oncology Branch, National Cancer Institute, National Institutes of Health, Bethesda, Maryland

Frances T. Hakim, M.D. Expert, Medicine Branch, National Cancer Institute, National Institutes of Health, Bethesda, Maryland

Derek N. J. Hart, M.B., Ch.B., D.Phil. Professor, Department of Hematology, Christchurch Hospital, Christchurch, New Zealand

Pierre A. Henkart Senior Investigator, Experimental Immunology Branch, National Cancer Institute, National Institutes of Health, Bethesda, Maryland

Helen E. Heslop, M.D., F.R.A.C.P., F.R.C.P.A. Associate Member, Division of Bone Marrow Transplantation, St. Jude Children's Research Hospital, and Associate Professor of Pediatrics, University of Tennessee, Memphis, Tennessee

Allan D. Hess, Ph.D. Professor of Oncology and Pathology, Department of Oncology, Johns Hopkins Oncology Center, Johns Hopkins University School of Medicine, Baltimore, Maryland

George A. Holländer, M.D. Assistant Professor of Pediatrics, Department of Pediatric Oncology, Dana-Farber Cancer Institute, Boston, Massachusetts, and Assistant Professor of Pediatrics, Division of Pediatric Immunology, Department of Research, Kantonsspital, and the University Children's Hospital, Basel, Switzerland

Ernst Holler, M.D. Medizinische Klinik III, Klinikum Grosshadern der Universitat, Munich, Germany

Stephen M. Jane, M.D., Ph.D. Rotary Bone Marrow Research Laboratory, Royal Melbourne Hospital, Parkville, Victoria, Australia

Bryon D. Johnson, Ph.D. Assistant Professor, Department of Pediatrics, Medical College of Wisconsin, Milwaukee, Wisconsin

Nancy A. Kernan, M.D. Associate Member, Department of Pediatrics, Memorial Sloan-Kettering Cancer Center, New York, New York

Krikor Kichian Department of Physiology, McGill University, Montreal, Quebec, Canada

Takashi Kei Kishimoto, Ph.D. Department of Immunological Diseases, Boehringer Ingelheim Pharmaceuticals, Inc., Ridgefield, Connecticut

Robert Korngold, Ph.D. Professor, Kimmel Cancer Institute, Jefferson Medical College, Philadelphia, Pennsylvania

Werner Krenger, Ph.D. David Abraham Fellow in Pediatric Oncology, Department of Pediatrics, Dana-Farber Cancer Institute, and Harvard Medical School, Boston, Massachusetts

Wayne S. Lapp, Ph.D. Professor, Department of Physiology, McGill University, Montreal, Quebec, Canada

Jeffrey A. Ledbetter, Ph.D. Distinguished Research Fellow, Department of Autoimmunity/Transplantation, Bristol-Myers Squibb Pharmaceutical Research Institute, Seattle, Washington

Robert B. Levy, Ph.D. Professor, Departments of Microbiology and Immunology, University of Miami School of Medicine, Miami, Florida

Andrew H. Lichtman, M.D., Ph.D. Associate Professor, Department of Pathology, Brigham and Women's Hospital and Harvard Medical School, Boston, Massachusetts

Peter S. Linsley, Ph.D. Senior Research Fellow and Department Chair, Department of Immunomodulators, Bristol-Myers Squibb Pharmaceutical Research Institute, Seattle, Washington

Eric O. Long, Ph.D. Senior Investigator, National Institute of Allergy and Infectious Diseases, National Institutes of Health, Rockville, Maryland

Crystal L. Mackall, M.D. Staff Fellow, Experimental Immunology Branch, National Cancer Institute, National Institutes of Health, Bethesda, Maryland

David K. Madtes, M.D. Associate Member, Department of Medicine, Fred Hutchinson Cancer Research Center, and Associate Professor, University of Washington, Seattle, Washington

David H. Margulies, M.D., Ph.D. Chief, Molecular Biology Section, Laboratory of Immunology, National Institute of Allergy and Infectious Diseases, National Institutes of Health, Bethesda, Maryland

Paul J. Martin, M.D. Member, Division of Clinical Research, Fred Hutchinson Cancer Research Center, and Professor of Medicine, University of Washington, Seattle, Washington

Cathleen M. McCabe, M.D. Department of Pediatrics, Medical College of Wisconsin, Milwaukee, Wisconsin

Allan Mowat, M.D., Ph.D., M.R.C.Path Reader and Honorary Consultant, Department of Immunology, University of Glasgow, Glasgow, Scotland

George F. Murphy, M.D. Herman Beerman Professor of Dermatology, Department of Dermatology, University of Pennsylvania School of Medicine, Philadelphia, Pennsylvania

Frederick Nestel, Ph.D. Postdoctoral Fellow, Department of Physiology, McGill University, Montreal, Quebec, Canada

Dietger Niederwieser University Hospital, Innsbruck, Austria

Stephen J. Noga, M.D., Ph.D. Assistant Professor of Oncology and Pathology, and Director, Graft Engineering Laboratory, Johns Hopkins Oncology Center, Johns Hopkins University School of Medicine, Baltimore, Maryland

Lu Ying Pan Dana-Farber Cancer Institute, and Children's Hospital, Boston, Massachusetts

Effie Petersdorf Fred Hutchinson Cancer Research Center, Seattle, Washington

Premysl Ponka, M.D., Ph.D. Professor of Physiology and Medicine, Lady Davis Institute for Medical Research, Sir Mortimer B. Davis–Jewish General Hospital, Montreal, Quebec, Canada

David L. Porter, M.D. Director, Allogeneic Bone Marrow Transplantation, Department of Hematology/Oncology, University of Pennsylvania School of Medicine, Philadelphia, Pennsylvania

Kursteen Price, M.D. Department of Physiology, McGill University, Montreal, Quebec, Canada

Olle Ringdén, M.D., Ph.D. Professor of Transplantation Immunology and Director, Bone Marrow Transplantation, Departments of Clinical Immunology and Transplantation Surgery, Karolinska Institute and Huddinge Hospital, Stockolm, Sweden

Maria-Grazia Roncarolo, M.D. Senior Staff Scientist, Department of Human Immunology, DNAX Research Institute of Molecular and Cellular Biology, Palo Alto, California

Robert Rothlein, Ph.D. Department of Immunological Diseases, Boehringer Ingelheim Pharmaceuticals, Inc., Ridgefield, Connecticut

Gary L. Schieven, Ph.D. Senior Research Investigator II, Department of Autoimmunity/Transplantation, Bristol-Myers Squibb Pharmaceutical Research Institute, Seattle, Washington

Thomas A. Seemayer, M.D., F.R.C.Path Professor, Departments of Pathology/Microbiology and Pediatrics, University of Nebraska Medical Center, Omaha, Nebraska

Michail V. Sitkovsky, Ph.D. Chief, Biochemistry and Immunopharmacology Section, Laboratory of Immunology, National Institute of Allergy and Infectious Diseases, National Institutes of Health, Bethesda, Maryland

Megan Sykes, M.D. Associate Professor of Surgery and Medicine (Immunology) and Immunologist, Bone Marrow Transplantation Section, Transplantation Biology Research Center, Massachusetts General Hospital and Harvard Medical School, Boston, Massachusetts

Robert M. Townsend, Ph.D. Kimmel Cancer Institute, Jefferson Medical College, Philadelphia, Pennsylvania

Giorgio Trinchieri, M.D. Professor, Wistar Institute, Philadelphia, Pennsylvania

Robert L. Truitt, Ph.D. Professor of Immunology in Pediatrics, Department of Pediatrics, Medical College of Wisconsin, Milwaukee, Wisconsin

Bruce Walcheck, Ph.D. Department of Immunological Diseases, Boehringer Ingelheim Pharmaceuticals, Inc., Ridgefield, Connecticut

Michael B. Weiler, M.D. Department of Pediatrics, Medical College of Wisconsin, Milwaukee, Wisconsin

Kong You-Ten, Ph.D. Postdoctoral Fellow, Department of Physiology, McGill University, Montreal, Quebec, Canada

Yong-Guang Yang Massachusetts General Hospital, Boston, Massachusetts

Graft-vs.-Host Disease

1

Thymic T-Cell Development

Georg A. Holländer
Dana-Farber Cancer Institute
Boston, Massachusetts
and Kantonsspital and University Children's Hospital
Basel, Switzerland

Steven J. Burakoff
Dana-Farber Cancer Institute
and Harvard Medical School
Boston, Massachusetts

I. INTRODUCTION

The thymus plays a central role in the development of a fully functional immune system. Its major purpose is to provide the appropriate milieu for the development and maturation of the majority of peripheral T cells. This is suggested by the observation that, in all vertebrate species studied, an identical structure is found. The mechanism for thymocyte development, expansion, maturation, and antigen receptor repertoire selection of thymocytes follows a common motif. Thus, an enormous wealth of information concerning the complex function of the thymus has been gained from animal studies and has allowed the beginning of a precise understanding of the thymus as a primary lymphoid organ.

Historically, a large number of different functions have been attributed to the thymus (reviewed in Refs. 1 and 2) including speculations that the thymus secretes "the elixir of life" or that this organ represents "the heart of good health" (3). Although modern biological studies could not confirm the existence of these functions, the fact that the thymus provides an important site of lymphopoiesis is generally compatible with these concepts. The role of the thymus as an organ of lymphocyte production was first suggested in the eighteenth century, as it was proposed that the thymus contained "numberless small solid particles, similar to those found in the lymphatic glands" and that "lymphatic vessels arising from the thymus convey this fluid to the blood" (2). Studies at the turn of this century dismissed an immunological role for the thymus, since it was demonstrated at that time that it did not produce antibodies and that its removal in adult animals bore no consequences for the well-being of the operated animal (as reviewed in Ref. 2). It was not until later that the increased incidence of thymomas in patients with agammaglobulinemia established a distinct link between the thymus and the immune system. In parallel, the critical role of the thymus for the generation of a normal immune response was established in experiments where the removal of the thymus from newborn mice resulted in animals with a severe immunodeficiency, unable to reject skin allografts or to produce specific antibodies in response to various antigens (4). What has followed over the course of the last 35 years, since these classic studies were reported, is a fascinating account of the molecular and cellular events that are responsible for the thymic ontogeny of T lymphocytes.

Hematopoietic stem cells seed continuously during the later stages of gestation from the fetal liver and after birth from the bone marrow via the circulation to the thymic lobes. In the milieu of the thymic microenvironment, these lymphoid precursor cells proceed in an orderly progression of differentiation from immature prothymocytes to fully functional, mature T cells enabled to recognize foreign antigen in the context of self–major histocompatibility complex (MHC) molecules but concurrently tolerant to self-peptides presented by the identical MHC molecules. The different stages of thymocyte development are characterized by the surface expression of a number of differentiation antigens. Both the presence and absence of the surface molecules CD4 and CD8 allows the separation of the $\alpha\beta$ T-cell receptor–positive (TcR^+) T-cell lineage into four developmentally discrete thymocyte subpopulations (Fig. 1). The earliest intrathymic precursors express neither CD4, CD8, nor the T-cell antigen receptor. This population of cells, commonly known as triple negative (TN) thymocytes, can further be differentiated into distinct transitional stages as identified by the expression of additional surface molecules such as CD44 or the α-chain of the interleukin-2 (IL-2) receptor (CD25). The simultaneous expression of CD4 and CD8 represents a next maturational stage. Somewhat later in development, these so-called double-positive (DP) thymocytes begin to express low to intermediate amounts of the $\alpha\beta$ TcR. During their further maturation, they become subject to mechanisms that aim collectively at shaping the TcR repertoire of mature T cells. The stringent thymic selection process results in the deletion of self-reactive cells (negative selection) and the selection of thymocytes with an antigen-specific TcR restricted by self-MHC molecules in association with foreign antigen (positive selection). These selective mechanisms result in the survival of a relatively small number of TcR^+ thymocytes that express either CD4 or CD8, a developmental stage referred to as single-positive (SP) thymocytes. Single CD4 positive (CD4SP) thymocytes bear a TcR that recognizes antigen in the context of MHC class II molecules, and CD8SP thymocytes express a TcR specific for the recognition of antigen presented by MHC class I molecules. These SP thymocytes represent the most mature stage, and they are poised to exit the thymus to the periphery.

The thymic microenvironment plays a key role in the development and selection of T cells. Extracellular matrix proteins as well as epithelial and bone marrow–derived cells collectively form a composite architecture of functionally distinct compartments. The bidirectional interaction of thymocytes and stromal cells is required for the normal differentiation of thymocytes as well as the normal composition of the stromal thymic microenvironment (5,6). Thymic stromal cells produce a number of cytokines important for the survival of early lymphoid cells and their differentiation to mature T cells. Based on histophysiological observations that different stromal cells form distinct areas in the thymus, various steps in T-cell differentiation may be assigned to discrete stromal microenvironments. In this context, epithelial

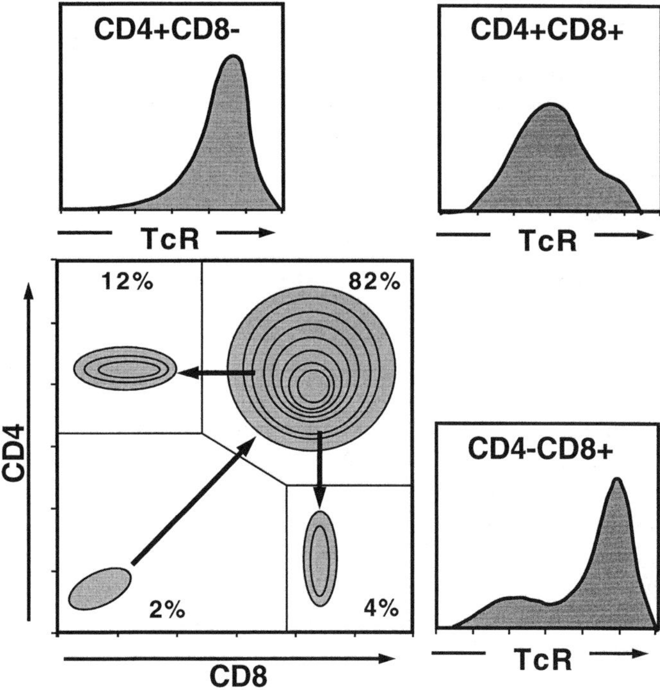

Figure 1 Phenotypic analysis of thymocytes. Four different subpopulations of thymocytes can be distinguished by surface staining for CD4 and CD8. The most immature cells lack CD4 and CD8 expression and represent the precursor population for the more mature thymocytes expressing simultaneously CD4 and CD8. Positively selected mature thymocytes are either $CD4^+$ or $CD8^+$ and express high surface levels of the TcR/CD3 complex (for details see text).

cells have been implicated in positive thymic selection while bone marrow-derived stromal cells appear to mediate efficient negative selection. The correlation of function with a particular type of stromal cells is, however, far from absolute, since both in vivo and in vitro experimental systems have demonstrated that, under certain conditions, positive as well as negative selection can be mediated by any of these stromal cells. The importance of stromal cells in T-cell differentiation is further emphasized by the finding that fetal lymphoid precursors enter the primordium only if the thymic stromal compartment is developed (7). Also, after sublethal irradiation, lymphoid reconstitution occurs only if the stromal compartment has been restored (8). Proliferation and selection of thymocytes is, moreover, dependent on the expression of MHC molecules on the surface of thymic stromal cells. In this context it is noteworthy that the expression of MHC class II molecules on thymic stromal cells is dependent on the presence of lymphoid cells, as suggested by studies in thymic rudiments of embryonic nude mice (9).

This chapter outlines the structure and function of the mammalian thymus as it pertains to the development of thymocytes and the selection of their $\alpha\beta$ T-cell antigen receptor repertoire. The physiological processes operative in the homing and maturation of lymphoid precursor cells to the thymus during fetal development are similar to those that occur after total body irradiation and subsequent bone marrow cell transplant. Thymic ontogeny after bone marrow transplantation may take place in the presence of graft-versus-host disease (GVHD), but allospecific recognition of the microenvironment affects thymic function and in particular the complex mechanisms of repertoire selection.

II. ANATOMY AND BASIC STRUCTURE OF THE THYMUS

The adult mammalian thymus is a pyramid-shaped organ formed of two structurally identical lobes that meet in the midline. The thymus is located in the upper mediastinum and the foundation of the organ rests on the pericardium, with both cervical extensions reaching to the base of the neck. Each thymic lobe is surrounded by a connective tissue capsule. Analysis of the thymic structure at the histological level allows the distinction of three separate areas: the thin subcapsular region, the lymphocyte-rich cortex, and the epithelial cell-dense medulla. Strands of connective tissue at irregular intervals extend from the surface of the thymus into the organ to form septa that carry nerve bundles, blood vessels, and efferent lymphatics which drain septa and capsule. These invaginations are rich in fibroblasts and type I collagen and reach to the level of the corticomedullary junction, where they widen and end. Adipocytes, neutrophil and eosinophil granulocytes, macrophages, mast cells, B lymphocytes, and plasma cells are found in the septa. Branching out from these connective tissue septa are perivascular spaces that extend into the thymus proper and serve as sites where cells and solvents are exchanged between the periphery and perithymic stroma. These perivascular spaces constitute the blood-thymus barrier and contain, like the septa, mature myeloid cells as well as B and T lymphocytes. B cells can form cell aggregates and occasionally active germinal centers.

The vascular supply of the thymus is achieved by three different sets of arterioles that enter the corticomedullary junction at the base of the septa. Two sets of vessels supply the subcapsular zone and the cortex, while the third set forms capillary loops that extend to the medulla. High endothelial venules, which are thought to be the site of lymphocyte traffic during the latter part of gestation and in the postnatal period, can be seen in the inner cortex and the corticomedullary junction. These anatomical structures also suggest that any circulation-derived cell or macromolecule may have access to the thymus, hence modifying the thymic microenvironment and influencing the maturation and selection of lymphocytes. This is illustrated by the observation that mature T cells can home to the thymus under physiological conditions as well as during the immunopathological changes of GVHD (6,10). The venous return is collected at the corticomedullary junction and exits through the septa to the thymic capsule. A basement membrane lies immediately below both capsule and septa and, in addition, also lines the thymic blood vessels. This basement membrane forms the first physical barrier between the perivascular space and the thymus proper, and it supports a specialized flattened epithelium (type 1 thymic epithelial cells, see below). This is of particular importance, since the influx of lymphoid precursor cells has to pass this structure to gain access to the epithelial compartment of the thymus.

III. CELLULAR COMPOSITION OF THE THYMUS

A. Lymphoid Cells

The most numerous cells in the thymus are lymphocytes at varying developmental stages. The subcapsular area contains approximately 5% of the lymphocytes. These cells are immature, stain negatively for CD4 and CD8, lack the expression of the T-cell antigen receptor complex, and are characterized by a blast-like appearance, reflecting their high mitotic activity. The majority of thymocytes (80 to 85%) are found below the subcapsular area of the cortex. Thymocytes of this subpopulation express CD4 and CD8 simultaneously, and approximately half of them also express low to intermediate amounts of TcR. Typically smaller than mature peripheral T cells, DP thymocytes are predominately nondividing (11) and are closely packed between the network of cortical epithelial cells, allowing for characteristic dark histological appearance on nuclear stains. The DP thymocytes are particularly sensitive to the influence of stress, as exposure to increased concentrations of glucocorticoids results in their depletion. Furthermore, 5×10^7 DP thymocytes are produced daily in young adult mice and as many as 98% will be eliminated in situ during the physiological selection of the TcR repertoire (12). The remaining 10% of total thymocytes are located in the medulla and are the progeny of cortical thymocytes. These cells are phenotypically and functionally similar but not identical to peripheral T cells (see below).

B. Thymic Epithelial Cells

Thymic lymphocytes develop in close physical contact with several types of stromal cells, i.e., thymic epithelial cells and cells of mesodermal origin. Thymic epithelial cells constitute the majority of this heterogeneous population of stromal cells. A classification of thymic epithelial cells based on their ultrastructural morphology has been developed (13). Four different types of thymic epithelial cells have been identified, which are located in either the subcortical zone or the cortex. In the medulla, two additional types of stromal cells can be distinguished (13,14). Using an extensive panel of monoclonal antibodies to novel antigenic surface determinants (reviewed in Refs. 15 through 18), these different types of epithelial cells were further defined (19). It was suggested that each stromal cell type may have a distinct function in the provision of a thymic microenvironment critical for different stages of T-cell maturation.

Type 1 epithelial cells are stellate, contain an irregularly shaped and heterochromatic nucleus, and contact each other by means of fine cytoplasmic ramifications, which are connected by desmosomes (13,17). It has been suggested that type 1 cells may secrete substances that form the basal membrane and/or factors that act as chemoattractants for circulating lymphoid precursor cells (20) or as growth factors for lineage-committed thymocytes (3,21).

Type 2 and 3 epithelial cells are located throughout the cortex and together with type 4 epithelial cells form the cortex proper. By appearance metabolically active, type 2 and 3 thymic epithelial cells also appear to have engulfed small islands of cortical thymocytes. This intimate interaction of epithelial cells with thymocytes is particularly prominent in the uppermost layer of the cortex and may represent the in vivo correlate of thymic nurse cells (TNC).

TNC have been described in the murine (22,23) and human thymus (13,24), and it has been suggested (25) that these lymphoepithelial complexes may characterize separate environments within the thymus. In vivo and in vitro experiments have provided evidence for a function of TNCs in both positive and negative thymic selection (Refs. 24 and 26 through 29) (see below).

Type 4 epithelial cells are located in the deep cortex, at the boundary to and within the medulla (13). By electron microscopy, the heterochromatic nucleus is irregularly shaped and the cytoplasm contains residual bodies and swollen mitochondria, giving it the typical morphology of dying cells. Hence, these cells may represent an end stage of the development of cortical epithelial cells.

The undifferentiated *type 5 epithelial cells* have a rounded nucleus with some heterochromatin and a relatively sparse and poorly organized cytoplasm forming short processes (13). *Type 6 epithelial cells,* also known as large medullary epithelial cells, form a loose cellular network. This cell type forms the Hassall's corpuscles, a small cluster (or "swirl") of keratinized epithelial cells. Hassall's corpuscles are prominent in human tissue but less conspicuous in the mouse. As embryonic development proceeds, Hassall's corpuscles gain progressively in size, with the most central concentric epithelial cells losing their nuclei and eventually dying. Macrophages may be located at the perimeter of and less frequently within the Hassall's corpuscles, consistent with the hypothesis that their major function is the scavenging of dead or dying cells (30).

Thymic epithelial cells may also play a critical part in the homing of lymphoid precursors to the thymus (20,31–36) and in the provision of a milieu competent to guarantee their viability, as detailed below. With regards to this latter point, thymic epithelial cells secrete a variety of cytokines, including IL-1, IL-6, IL-7, tumor necrosis factor alpha (TNF-α) and colony stimulating factor for macrophages (CSF-M), which may be necessary for the survival of intrathymic lymphoid precursors and the later development of thymocytes. Several lines of evidence have also suggested that thymic epithelial cells located in the subcapsular and medullary region produce a variety of polypeptides, collectively termed thymic hormones (reviewed in Refs. 2 and 3). Thymic subcapsular and medullary epithelial cells seem to provide the site of synthesis of factors such as thymopoietin, TP-5, thymosin $\alpha 1$, thymosin $\beta 4$, thymosin $\alpha 7$, thymic humoral factor (THF), and thymulin. Despite a plethora of alleged functions for the peripheral T-cell compartment (37,38) there is little evidence for a direct role of these hormones in the thymus, and their influence on T-cell development is unproven.

C. Thymic Dendritic Cells

A second important cell type, dendritic (or interdigitating) cells, constitute another important component of the thymic microenvironment (39). Dendritic cells are derived from the bone marrow and are competent to present antigens to naive T cells. Their long cytoplasmic projections give them a stellate appearance (40) and allow for close and extended contact with thymocytes (18). Thymic dendritic cells (DC) are restricted to the medulla and are typically located at the corticomedullary junction (41). The relative frequency of DC is comparable between mouse and human thymus; there is approximately 1 DC per 10^3 thymocytes (42), and kinetic studies suggest a turnover rate for DC of approximately 15% per day (43). DC stain abundantly for MHC class I and II molecules and demonstrate phenotypic characteristics of epidermal Langerhans cells (including the presence of Bierbeck granules). Murine and human DC express heat-stable antigen (HSA), and adhesion molecules CD40, CD44, LFA-1, LFA-3, ICAM-1, and the leukocyte common antigen CD45, but they lack the macrophage markers Fc receptor and F4/80 and the granulocyte marker Gr-1 (44,45). In addition, DC of the human thymus express high levels of CD4 but low levels of CD8, while the corresponding cell in the murine thymus stains strongly positive for CD8 but only weakly for CD4 (46,47).

Although of bone marrow origin, it has been suggested that thymic DC derive from a minute population of bipotential intrathymic precursors expressing, in addition to low levels of CD4, a phenotype similar to bone marrow hematopoietic stem cells (42,48). The notion of a common precursor for T cells and DC is also consistent with the histological observation that thymic DC can be detected in a human fetus as early as the seventh week of gestation—a time when the first hematopoietic cells seed to the thymic rudiment (49).

D. Thymic Macrophages

Macrophages are found throughout the thymus and become especially obvious during involution of the thymus, when they have a "starry sky" appearance on sections (3).

Functionally, thymic macrophages have been implicated in the induction of self-tolerance via clonal anergy but not via deletion of autoreactive thymocytes (50). This particular mechanism of thymic tolerance is further reflected by the insufficient capacity of thymic macrophages to function as antigen-presenting cells in vivo as well as in thymic organ cultures (50,51). Cytokine production and release by thymic macrophages may be another important function affecting thymocyte proliferation, maturation, and differentiation.

E. Thymic B Cells

Although the thymus is considered a "T-cell organ," immunohistochemical staining and functional analysis have revealed the presence of a low number of B cells in both human and murine thymic tissue. Mature B cells are present in the extrathymic perivascular space as well as within the medulla proper, where they are either diffusely distributed or concentrated around the Hassall's corpuscles (52).Their phenotype is consistent with that of activated B cells from peripheral lymphoid tissue in that they express markers such as CD19, CD20, CD22, CD37, CD72, and CD76 (53). Furthermore, thymic B cells also express immunoglobulins IgM, IgD, and IgG but only rarely IgA and never IgE (52), and thymic B lymphocytes are ontogenetically the first immunoglobulin-secreting cells in the mouse (54,55). The close topographic association of thymic B cells with T cells suggests a role in negative T-cell repertoire selection, a phenomenon described for the murine thymus (see below and Refs. 51 and 56). Such a mechanism is further suggested by the physical contact of thymic B lymphocytes with rosetting T cells, which demonstrate condensation of nuclear chromatin but lack segregation of nucleolar components, the structural hallmark of apoptotic cell death (52).

F. Thymic NK Cells

Natural killer (NK) cells are present in the thymus of mice and humans, albeit at a very low frequency (0.1% of all the cells). Thymic NK cells express in certain strains of mice the prototypic membrane phenotype $CD3^-NK1.1^+$ and in humans the $CD3^-CD56^+CD16^{+/-}$ phenotype (57). The functional role of NK cells in the thymus is not known.

G. Other Thymic Stromal Cells

Myoid cells are another cell type found among nonlymphoid cells in the thymus. Of mesenchymal origin, myoid cells are unevenly distributed in the thymus (mainly located in the medulla and frequently grouped in clusters) (18) and express actin and striate muscle myosin (58). Their function is not known. Fibroblasts also belong to the thymic stromal cells. Their physiological functions in T-cell development and selection have yet to be determined, although fibroblasts can participate in positive thymic selection despite their inability to process and present antigens efficiently (59).

H. Extracellular Matrix

The extracellular matrix (ECM) constitutes an important part of the overall thymic microenvironment. The distribution of ECM differs between fetal and adult thymic tissue and parallels changes associated with age and the physiological involution of the thymus (60). Among the defined components of the ECM are various collagens, reticulin fibers, glycosaminoglycans, and glycoproteins, which can support in vitro the attachment of a subpopulation of immature thymocytes (61). The extracellular matrix forms the basal membrane underlying the type 1 thymic epithelial cells and builds a fine network throughout the medulla and possibly also in certain areas of the cortex (i.e., around thymic nurse cells) (62). Thymic epithelial cells have been demonstrated to synthesize and secrete type IV collagen and basement membrane glycoproteins like laminin and fibronectin (60). Thymocytes express receptors for different ECM components: CD44, which is expressed by a small proportion of immature triple-negative thymocytes, binds to hyaluronic acid as well as to collagen. Other receptors on thymocytes and thymic epithelial cells are members of the integrin superfamily: VLA-2, -3, and -4 attach to fibronectin; VLA-2 and -3 bind both collagen and laminin; and VLA-6 recognizes laminin (63), which is also bound by $\alpha6\beta4$ integrins expressed on thymocytes (60). The proposed functions of the extracellular matrix include the homing of hematopoietic multipotential precursor cells to the thymic microenvironment, the support of thymocyte and epithelial cell growth and differentiation, the promotion of cell migration, and the binding of cytokines to achieve high local concentrations (reviewed in Ref. 62).

IV. EMBRYOGENESIS AND THE POSTNATAL INVOLUTION OF THE THYMUS

The thymus develops from a paired epithelial anlage in the neck during the sixth to the eighth week of gestation in humans and on day 10 of gestation in mice. By the end of the fetal period, the thymus has descended from the neck to the upper mediastinum, where it forms a broad, irregularly lobulated single organ. Although reaching its largest relative mass in relation to body size at the time of birth, the human thymus continues to grow until puberty, when it attains its maximum weight of 30 to 40 g (64).

Two separate growth periods can be distinguished that relate to cell proliferation and cell differentiation during murine thymus ontogeny (65). Approximately 1 day after the entry of the first lymphoid precursor cells into the murine fetal thymus anlage at day 11 of gestation, prothymocytes begin to proliferate. The following expansion of thymocytes is exponential, as shown by a 10-fold increase of these cells within the 24 hr of day 14 of gestation, suggesting nearly three cell cycles of 8 hr each. It has been demonstrated that stem cells colonizing the thymus before day 13 of fetal development are exclusively responsible for the generation of all maturing thymocytes until day 5 to 6 after birth, despite the continuous entry of stem cells during this time (66). Similar kinetics of cell proliferation have been observed in studies of irradiated and bone marrow–transplanted adult mice: hematopoietic stem cells seed to the thymus shortly after intravenous injection, but their capacity for self-renewal and proliferation lags behind for a substantial period of time (67). The human thymus gains maturity rather early during fetal life and can already be considered fully functional at the end of the 16th week of gestation, when SP T cells begin to seed from the thymus to peripheral lymphoid tissues. This early functional maturity is in sharp contrast to other vertebrate species, such as the mouse, where neonatal thymectomy inhibits T-cell colonization of peripheral lymphoid tissue (68).

During postnatal life, the thymus is subject to two different forms of involution: (1) stress-induced acute involution and (2) age-related involution. In response to increased serum concentrations of corticosteroids, triggered by various external influences (i.e., infections, malnutrition, surgery, and pregnancy), immature (cortical) thymocytes undergo structural changes that culminate in the blebbing of the cell membrane and the fragmentation of genomic DNA, ultimately leading to cell death (apoptosis). This form of involution is temporary and the thymus regenerates as soon as the noxious influence abates. In contrast, the age-related involution of the thymus is characterized by a reduction in size and weight as a consequence of a progressive loss of cells within the lymphoid and stromal cell compartments. The rate of involution is most rapid during the first 10 years of life and continues thereafter at a progressively decreasing rate, with replacement of lymphoid tissue, septa, and perivascular spaces by adipose tissue. Despite these structural changes, the thymus remains throughout life as a primary lymphoid organ with functional lymphostromal islands.

V. DYNAMICS OF THYMOCYTE DEVELOPMENT

A. The Hematopoietic Stem Cell

All T lymphocytes derive ultimately from hematopoietic stem cells (HSC) present in the fetal liver and after birth in the bone marrow. HSC are characterized by their ability for self-renewal and multilineage differentiation, and HSC of adult murine bone marrow cells reveal a number of distinct biological features (69): (1) permanent and continuous hematopoiesis can originate from only one stem cell; (2) HSC are always multipotent and contribute in vivo to all major myeloid and lymphoid cell populations, and, conversely, conclusive evidence for lineage-restricted reconstituting "stem cells" is missing; (3) although single HSC may frequently reconstitute only some but not all hematopoietic lineages early after bone marrow transplantation, this fluctuation will later change to stable hematopoiesis; and (4) the biological behavior of HSC from different hematopoietic sources is ultimately determined by the host environment.

The first time that commitment to hematopoiesis can be detected during mammalian embryogenesis is after implantation, when blood islands develop in the extraembryonic yolk sac. The yolk sac is formed on day 7 of murine embryogenesis, well before either the organization of the fetal liver (site of hematopoiesis; after day 8 to 9) or the establishment of blood circulation (day 9). Later during embryogenesis, lymphohematopoietic precursor cells of the yolk sac enter the bloodstream and reach, in the embryo proper, tissues with a supportive microenvironment for further growth and differentiation (i.e., fetal liver and thymus) (70). Murine yolk sac HSC express heat-stable antigen, CD45, and the *c-kit* receptor (71,72) and give rise to multiple lineages, including T cells, B cells, and myeloid cells as detected in transplantation experiments in vivo, in fetal thymic organ cultures (FTOCs), in in vitro cultures with bone marrow–derived stromal cells, or in methylcellulose cultures (71,72).

Murine HSC from fetal liver or bone marrow express concurrently the differentiation antigens Sca-1 (Ly-6-A/E), CD43, the *c-kit* receptor, low levels of Thy-1, and CD4, but they lack the expression of a panel of antigens expressed on mature and maturing myeloid and lymphoid cells (thus lineage negative, designated Lin^-) (73–79). Human pluripotent HSC are found within the $CD34^+$ $CD38^-$ $CD43^+$ fraction of bone marrow cells and express, like their murine counterpart, the *c-kit* receptor and MHC class II molecules as well as low levels of Thy-1 (80–88). Comparative analyses of human HSC in fetal liver, cord blood, and bone marrow reveal an increased staining profile for CD34 and Thy-1 expression among some but not all fetal liver HSC. Although Thy-1 expression on HSC is relatively low, purging of bone marrow cells with anti-Thy-1 antibodies to deplete T cells does not usually eliminate the hematopoietic precursor population. Commitment and differentiation of HSC to the various cell lineages results in a decrease of surface Thy-1 expression (89), which is, however, transient in the case of T-cell precursors.

Despite these surface markers, the relative frequency of functionally multipotent HSC is substantially lower ($\sim 10\%$) than the number of cells with the characteristic phenotype (90,91). It has therefore been estimated that HSC represent only 0.02 to 0.1% of all nucleated bone marrow cells in mice and humans (77,82).

The time point at which HSC development is confined to lymphopoiesis has not been unequivocally determined. Commitment to the T-cell lineage is understood to occur when human bone marrow progenitor cells begin to express CD2, CD5, and CD7 (92). However, this assumption has not been formally tested for fetal bone marrow cells (93). Moreover, these markers are not specific for the T-cell lineage: CD2 is also expressed on NK cells and thymic B cells; CD5 can be detected on the surface of a subpopulation of B cells; and CD7 is found on platelets as well as NK cells (57). However, this correlation between phenotype and lineage commitment is far from absolute, because $CD34^+CD7^{high+}$ fetal liver cells cannot develop into T cells and $CD34^+CD7^{dull}$ fetal cells may give rise to myeloid cells in addition to T cells (94).

Thymic precursors have been estimated to represent as may as 1 in 3.3×10^4 bone marrow cells (95,96), although the actual number of these cells that effectively home to the thymus to give rise to a measurable clonogenic progeny may be substantially lower. Only 1 in 20 to 25 T-cell-committed bone marrow–derived precursors will lodge in the thymus after intravenous injection when compared to direct intrathymic injection (95,97). For murine precursor cells, commitment to the T-cell lineage may occur either early, at extrathymic sites (31,96,98,99), or may take place after homing to the thymus (100). Prothymocytes (Thy-1 $^+$c-kit^{low}CD3$^-$) can already be detected in the fetal blood of 15.5-day embryos (99). These cells generate a single wave of mature $\alpha\beta$TcR$^+$ thymocytes after intrathymic injection but fail to reconstitute the B-cell compartment or myeloid and erythroid lineages after intravenous transfer. It remains to be determined, however, whether these prothmocytes can also give rise to extrathymic T-cell development and to intrathymic $\gamma\delta$TcR$^+$ T cells and NK cells (99). In contrast, intrathymic precursor cells have also been found with a developmental potential for B lymphocytes (101), NK cells (102) DC (39,42), and myeloid cells (103), although a clonal analysis is missing as proof that these different cell types derive from a common intrathymic precursor.

B. Homing of Hematopoietic Precursor Cells to the Thymus

As suggested by histological studies, access of extrathymic precursor cells to the thymus anlage may occur during the initial period of embryogenesis independent of the vasculature via migration through the capsule of the thymic anlage (70). After establishment of the blood circulation, high endothelial venules at the corticomedullary junction provide the site of entry for hematopoietic precursor cells throughout life (104). Based on the particular structure of the thymus, the phenomenon of homing can be separated into three different phases: (1) attachment of precursor cells to the vascular endothelium with subsequent extravasation; (2) migration through the perivascular space; and (3) entry to the thymus proper after crossing of the basal membrane. Cell-surface molecules and soluble factors with chemotactic and chemokinetic properties have been implicated in the regulation of each phase.

Adhesion of mature cells to the vascular endothelium of high endothelial venules has been extensively studied (105,106), although little is known about the interactions of lymphoid precursor cells with endothelial cells in primary lymphoid organs such as the thymus. It has, however, been established that the binding of a prothymocyte cell line to thymic endothelial cells is independent of P-selectin, E-selectin and ICAM-1 but mediated by $\alpha6\beta1$ and possibly $\alpha6\beta4$ integrins expressed on the surface of endothelial cells (35). Furthermore, the $\alpha6\beta4$ integrin has also been detected on immature murine thymocytes immediately after migration to the thymus (107), supporting a role of integrins in the process of thymus homing.

HSC and/or the earliest intrathymic precursor may express ligands that assist in the complex process of homing and may recognize tissue-specific surface molecules (i.e., addressins). CD44—phagocyte-glycoprotein-1 (Pgp-1)—which is expressed on very early HSC and on 80 to 90% of murine thymocytes on days 13 to 14 of gestation, may serve the purpose of a molecule stabilizing interactions between more specific homing receptors and their respective ligands (108). CD44 has been shown to bind collagen types I and VI, fibronectin, and hyaluronate (109,110), structures on the surface of high endothelial venules (HEV), and components of the extracellular matrix. Furthermore, anti-CD44 antibodies prevent the homing of bone marrow cells to the thymus (111,112).

The protooncogene *c-kit* is expressed on HSC (75,113), and *c-kit* ligands have been identified as soluble or transmembrane forms of the SC factor (SCF) (114). SCF transcripts are expressed in many different tissues, including thymic stromal cells (115,116). Mice deficient in the expression of *c-kit* (W/W) or SCF (SI/SI) have a significantly reduced number of the most immature intrathymic T-cell precursor population (117). Moreover, the expansion rate of early immature thymocytes in SCF-deficient thymic grafts is reduced by approximately 50% (117). In addition to this direct role of *c-kit*/SCF in the intrathymic expansion of recent thymic immigrants, *c-kit* may serve an extra function as an accessory molecule important in the homing of progenitor cells to the thymus. Indeed, *c-kit* is expressed on the immediate progeny of HSC, which have a potential to seed to and repopulate the thymus (100,118). SCF is expressed within the thymus in a membrane-bound form (119), thus providing an anchored structure for *c-kit*-mediated cell adhesion.

A role in cell-cell interactions has also been ascribed to Thy-1, a glycosylphosphatidylinositol (GPI)-linked surface glycoprotein with a primary structure resembling that of the Ig-V domain (120). Expressed at low levels on the surface of HSC and immature human and murine thymocytes, Thy-1 has been reported to play a role in the interaction with a yet unknown ligand expressed on the surface of a cloned epithelial cell line (121,122).

The binding of thymic precursors to HEV at the corticomedullary junction may further be regulated by soluble factors that either affect the expression of addressins on the luminal surface of HEV or that exert a direct influence on HSC. Increased efficiency of prothymocyte adhesion to endothelial cells has been observed in coculture experiments when thymic epithelial cells were present. Although the epithelial factors responsible for this increased cell-cell interaction in vivo are not known, cytokines such as interferon gamma (IFN-γ) regulate in vitro the expression of a HEV-specific antigen implicated in homing and increase the capacity of HEV to bind lymphocytes in vivo (123,124).

C. Early Intrathymic T-Cell Precursors

In the postnatal human thymus, the most immature precursor to give rise to T cells expresses CD34^{+} but lacks CD3, CD4, or CD8 (94,125,126). Interestingly, these CD34^{+} TN thymocytes have the potential to develop in vitro into myeloid cells upon exposure to cytokines derived from thymic epithelial cells (127). CD34^{+} TN thymocytes progress to a more mature developmental stage via an intermediate CD34^{low+} phenotype, which is paralleled by the acquisition of other surface markers such as CD1 and CD5 (126,128).

Phenotypically, early thymocytes in mice, as in humans, resemble bone marrow–derived HSC (101). This population represents 0.05% of all thymocytes and is characterized by the expression of Sca-1, *c-kit*, Thy-1^{low}, CD4^{low}, and Sca-2, a surface antigen of unknown function. Sca-2 is acquired only by early intrathymic progenitor cells after several cell divisions and several days of residence in the thymic microenvironment (129,130). Approximately 15% of these HSC-like cells are in cycle, and the majority are in a state of cellular activation, as suggested by staining with the fluorescent vital dye rhodamine 123 (48). Transfer of purified intrathymic precursor cells to irradiated syngeneic recipients delineates their developmental potential in that they reconstitute the $\alpha\beta TcR^+$ and $\gamma\delta TcR^+$ T cells, the B-cell lineage, and thymic dendritic cells (42,48). However, precursor cells expressing Sca-2$^+$ are at an advanced developmental stage, since their transition to single CD4$^+$ or CD8$^+$ mature T cells is accelerated when compared to the intrathymic injection of bone marrow–derived Sca-2$^-$ HSC (101).

D. Thymocyte Subsets

Classification of thymocytes using the surface expression of CD4 and CD8 has been most useful in defining the major phenotypic stages of thymocyte development within the $\alpha\beta$TcR lineage. The CD4$^-$CD8$^-$ negative cell population, which can be further defined using a number of additional surface markers, contains all cells with thymus-homing precursor potential. These early immature thymocytes develop in close contact with thymic epithelial cells and begin to express, for a short period of time, either CD4 or CD8 prior to becoming CD4$^+$CD8$^+$ cells, a population that constitutes the majority of thymocytes. DP thymocytes can be further divided into discrete subpopulations based on the level of surface CD3/TcR complex expressed. Only a minority of these cells are selected to reach the final stage of intrathymic maturation. Thymocytes with a TcR-recognizing antigen bound by MHC class II molecules will generally become CD4$^+$CD8$^-$ T cells, while thymocytes bearing a TcR restricted by MHC class I molecules will mature to CD4$^-$CD8$^+$ T cells.

1. CD3$^-$CD4$^-$CD8$^-$ Immature Thymocytes

Thymocytes lacking the expression of CD4 and CD8 have been termed initially double-negative and have been viewed to encompass only immature thymocytes (131). However, it became apparent that this subpopulation also contains mature cells that express CD3/$\alpha\beta$TcR, thus representing mature cells belonging to alternative pathways of T-cell development. The population of early thymocyte precursors is therefore more appropriately termed triple-negative (TN) thymocytes.

Using the surface expression of CD44, CD25, and *c-kit* receptor, TN thymocytes from adult mice can be subdivided into four distinct subsets, representing progressive stages of maturation strictly regulated by the thymic microenvironment (118,132,133): CD4^{low}CD44$^+$CD25$^-$c-kit$^+$ $\rightarrow$ CD4$^-$CD44$^+$CD25$^+$c-kit$^+$ $\rightarrow$ CD44$^-$-CD25$^+$c-kit^{low} $\rightarrow$ CD44$^-$CD25$^-$c-kit$^-$. During embryogenesis, there appears to be a somewhat different sequence in that the expression of CD44 and CD25 persist beyond the TN stages (134). The first stage of postnatal TN thymocytes, CD4^{low}-CD44$^+$CD25$^-$c-kit$^+$, is characterized on the molecular level by the lack of rearrangement of the TcR β- and γ-chain locus. On a cellular level, these thymocytes bear the developmental potential to repopulate the lymphoid compartment and thymic dendritic cells but have lost the capacity to differentiate to myeloid or erythroid cells.

Thymocytes at the next developmental stage are CD4$^-$CD44$^+$CD25$^+$c-kit$^+$ cells (129), but the signals necessary and sufficient for this phenotypic transition are not known. Although CD25 expression is well recognized as a developmental marker (135), IL-2 is not critical for thymic development (136). By contrast, a defect in the common γ chain for the cytokine receptors of IL-2, IL-4, IL-7, and IL-15 results in the failure of T-cell development and the clinical entity of the X-linked severe combined immunodeficiency (SCID) syndrome. CD44$^+$CD25$^+$c-kit$^+$ thymocytes are responsive to a combination of cytokines, including IL-7 and SCF, which appear to maintain their viability in vitro for a relatively extended period of time (129). The importance of the common γ chain in the IL-7 receptor complex has been demonstrated in FTOCs using an antibody specific for the common γ chain of the IL-7 receptor. Treatment of FTOCs with this blocking antibody inhibits completely the progression of CD44$^+$c-kit$^+$ TN thymocytes to the CD44$^-$c-kit$^-$ stage (137). When stimulated with phorbol myristate acetate (PMA) and ionomycin, CD44$^+$CD25$^+$c-kit$^+$ thymocytes produce IL-2, IFN-γ, and TNF-α (129). Cells at the CD44$^+$CD25$^+$c-kit$^+$ stage in thymic development represent the first population of thymocytes committed exclusively to the T-cell lineage, since they have lost their potential in transfer experiments to differentiate into B cells and dendritic cells.

The transition to the next developmental stage, CD44$^-$CD25$^+$c-kit^{low}, is controlled by as yet unidentified factors present in the thymic microenvironment (118) that allow for the rearrangement of the TcR β- and γ-chain loci (129,138). This maturation is paralleled by the downregulation of the *c-kit* receptor and diminished responsiveness to IL-7 (139,140). When stimulated concurrently with PMA, ionomycin, and IL-1, CD44$^-$CD25$^+$ thymocytes will produce IL-2, IFN-γ, and TNF-α, albeit at a much lower level than thymocytes at an earlier developmental stage (129). CD44$^-$CD25$^+$ thymocytes represent cells at an important control point because they are the last subset with the ability to differentiate into both the TcR $\alpha\beta^+$ and TcR $\gamma\delta^+$ T-cell lineages when transferred to fetal organ culture (129). The precise signals that influence this branching into either lineage have not been defined.

Mutations in either the RAG-1 or RAG-2 gene products will arrest thymic development at the CD44$^-$CD25$^+$ TN stage (138,141,142) because progression to the next developmental stage appears to be dependent on the surface expression of, and signaling through, a pre-TcR consisting of a productively rearranged TcR β chain and an invariant surrogate α chain (142–146). Neither the respective ligand(s) nor the necessary intracellular signals are presently known for the progression to the CD4$^-$CD44$^-$CD25$^-$c-kit$^-$ stage. However, cross-linking of CD3ϵ on the surface of early fetal thymocytes from normal mice and animals deficient in the expression of a TcR β chain [i.e., SCID and recombination-activating gene (RAG)-deficient mice] may mimic these signals. In vivo treatment of RAG-deficient mice with anti-CD3 antibodies induces (1) an accelerated progression of TN thymocytes to the CD4$^+$CD8$^+$ stage, (2) downregulation of intracellular production of TcR β chains, and (3) downregulation of IL-2Rα chains (147,148).

The transition of CD44$^-$CD25$^+$c-kit^{low} thymocytes to the CD44$^-$CD25$^-$c-kit$^-$ stage involves the induction of CD4 and CD8 expression, a process thought to occur over the course of 48 hr (133). Although termed TN thymocytes, a substantial number of these early thymocytes already express on their cell surface low levels of CD4 and CD8 (CD4^{lo}, CD8^{lo}) (149). CD44$^-$CD25$^-$c-kit$^-$ thymocytes fail to secrete detectable levels of cytokines upon mitogenic activation (129). The progression to CD4/CD8 expression is dependent on an intact thymic microenvironment and is paralleled by (but not dependent on) the rearrangement of the TcR α chain

(129,132,150–152). The transition of the least immature subpopulation of TN thymocytes to $CD4^-CD8^+/CD4^+CD8^-$ and later to $CD4^+CD8^+$ (DP) thymocytes can also occur spontaneously in vitro within 24 hr of culture (153). The phenomenon suggests that the $CD44^-CD25^-$c-kit$^-$ TN cells have already received in vivo the differentiation signals necessary to express high surface levels of CD4 and CD8 and that this phenotypic shift is independent of the thymic microenvironment.

2. $CD3^{-/lo}CD4^{lo}CD8^{lo}$ Thymocytes

Thymocytes with a $CD4^+CD8^+$ phenotype represent the major subpopulation in the cortex and in the entire thymus. Their generation from $CD44^-CD25^-$c-kit$^-$ TN precursor cells occurs via two alternative but not mutually exclusive intermediates, $CD4^-CD8^{lo}$ and $CD4^{lo}CD8^-$ (93,154–159) and is dependent on the enzymatic activity of protein tyrosine kinases, which have not been well characterized (160). Although these transitional stages are either $CD4^+$ or $CD8^+$ when analyzed by flow cytometry, very low amounts of the corresponding T-cell coreceptor are also expressed on the cell surface as determined by panning (149). Designated more precisely as $CD4^{lo}CD8^{lo}$, these cells are rapidly cycling, with more than 50% of the cells in S+G2+M phase (151,157), and develop in overnight cultures (153) or in vivo into $CD4^+CD8^+$ thymocytes (158).

3. $CD3^{lo/int}CD4^+CD8^+$ Thymocytes

The predominant residents of the tightly packed thymic cortex are thymocytes that express high levels of CD4 and CD8 simultaneously. DP cells (80 to 85% of all thymocytes) possess neither mature T-cell functions nor substantial repopulating capacity when they are transferred to irradiated recipients (154,161). The initially large $CD4^+CD8^+$ blast cells generate the small nondividing G_0 thymocytes, the vast majority of DP thymocytes. The 50-fold expansion during this stage in development corresponds in mice to the generation of approximately 5×10^7 cells per day (162). Progressive maturation within the DP thymocytes is paralleled by the differential expression of a number of surface molecules, including the upregulation of TcR/CD3 to an intermediate level. This increase in surface expression is an important prerequisite for positive and negative thymic selection (163–168) and is further characterized by the transition from rapidly dividing DP blasts to small DP cortical thymocytes (169). Interestingly, the life span of 2 to 3 days is the same for all DP thymocytes, whether they are subjected to programmed cell death or whether they will undergo positive selection (170).

Despite the controversy as to whether negative selection precedes (171) or follows positive selection (172), the large majority (approximately 97%) of DP thymocytes are negatively selected because they express either a TcR with an inadequate affinity for the MHC complex or a TcR that cannot bind to MHC molecules at all. The cell stages implicated in negative selection of T cells reactive with self- or superantigens are characterized by low, intermediate, or even high surface expression of the CD3/TcR complex (see below) (171,173,174). Apoptosis represents the morphological correlate to programmed cell death and is characterized by ruffling and blebbing of the cell membrane and the activation of endogenous nucleases with fragmentation of genomic DNA (175). This form of cell death ensues without signs of inflammation, although apoptotic cell death can be detected directly in situ (176) and apoptotic cell debris has been demonstrated within thymic macrophages.

The capacity of the thymic microenvironment to provide niches allowing for positive thymic selection appears to be limited in number (170). Positively selected DP thymocytes upregulate their TcR/CD3 surface expression and differentiate into $CD4^+CD8^-$ or $CD4^-CD8^+$ thymocytes even when placed in suspension cultures devoid of thymic stromal cells (177). Thymocytes that have been positively selected will also upregulate their MHC class I molecules on the cell surface; they begin to express CD69 and will downmodulate the surface expression of HSA (178–179). How the differential downregulation of either CD4 or CD8 in positively selected DP thymocytes is accomplished in order to avoid a mismatch of TcR-restriction and coreceptor expression is presently unclear, although different mechanistic models have been proposed to explain this phenomenon (see below).

4. $CD3^+CD4^+CD8^-$ and $CD3^+CD4^-CD8^+$ Thymocytes

The maturational transition from DP to SP thymocytes is gradual, contains various intermediate cell stages, and is paralleled by the physical translocation from the cortex to the medulla. Both CD4SP and CD8SP $CD3^{high}HSA^{lo/-}$ thymocytes are thought to represent end products of the intrathymic differentiation process within the $\alpha\beta$TcR lineage. DP thymocytes constitute the precursors to SP thymocytes, since intrathymic transfer of DP TcR^{lo} blasts will give rise to SP thymocytes (154) and since CD4-dependent recognition of specific self antigens expressed in the thymus will delete CD4SP as well as CD8SP thymocytes (167). Nevertheless, treatment of mice with anti-CD4 monoclonal antibodies blocks the maturation of CD4SP thymocytes from DP cells but has no influence on the differentiation of these immature cells to T cells with CD8SP $CD3^{high}$ phenotype (180).

The different kinetics in the generation of SP $CD3^{high}$ thymocytes, with CD8SP cells appearing later than CD4SP cells, suggests that the maturation of CD4SP and CD8SP may follow different pathways (154,161). Positive selection leads to the immediate downregulation of CD8 and the simultaneous upregulation of the TcR/CD3 complex, a process dependent on the complete expression of the CD3 complex (181). Thymocytes with $CD4^+CD8^+TcR^{high}$ phenotype and later with $CD4^+$-$CD8^{lo}TcR^{high}$ phenotype represent subsequent intermediate cell stages. Some of these thymocytes will become $CD4^{high}CD8^-$SP cells specific for the recognition of antigen presented by MHC class II molecules (182), while others will eventually develop into $SPCD8^+$ mature thymocytes with a MHC class I restricted TcR (183).

On the basis of size, buoyant density, surface marker expression, and functional competence, SP thymocytes can be distinguished from mature peripheral T cells. Analysis of $CD4^+CD8^-TcR^{high}$ reveals that the majority of these cells still express heat-stable antigen (HSA) but do not yet express the nonclassic MHC class I molecule Qa-2 (178). HSA is a heavily glycosylated protein of only 27 amino acids, which is anchored by a glycosyl phosphatidylinositol moiety to the cell membrane. Expressed by many hematopoietic cells including HSC and immature thymocytes (184), HSA expression does not seem to be important as a developmental regulator for the progression of DP to SP thymocytes (185). Qa-2 is a GPI-linked nonpolymorphic class I molecule expressed on all peripheral T cells (and to a lesser extent B cells) (186). $Qa\text{-}2^+$ thymocytes are large, nonmitotic cells in G_1 and typically express high levels of CD5 but decreased amounts of HSA (187,188). SP thymocytes that have not yet expressed the Qa-2 molecule are nonresponsive to many TcR-mediated stimuli (178,187), suggesting a developmental progression from immature Qa-2^{-}HSA^{high} thymocytes to Qa-2^{+}HSA$^{low/-}$ cells.

Analysis of recent thymic emigrants in peripheral lymphoid tissue demonstrates that these cells bear the identical physical and phenotypic properties of mature SP thymocytes and that they are slightly larger than mature peripheral T cells. While this size difference is lost after 24 hr, there is no change in the low surface expression of HSA (189). Lymph nodes of young mice (190) may contain recent thymic immigrants with a DP phenotype that express levels of CD3 and HSA similar to cortical thymocytes. These DP cells appear not to have been subjected to the stringent thymic selection process and may therefore be responsible for the increased frequency of autoreactive T cells observed in young thymectomized mice (191–195).

VI. THYMIC REPERTOIRE SELECTION

The T-cell repertoire is the complete set of TcR specificities expressed by T lymphocytes and is established by two basic events: (1) negative selection by mechanisms of deletion or anergy excludes potentially self-reactive thymocytes, while (2) positive selection results in the maturation of thymocytes to T cells that recognize foreign antigen in the context of self-MHC. Thymic repertoire selection has been explained by two alternative hypotheses. The first proposes that the affinity of the interaction between TcR and self-MHC molecules determines the fate of developing thymocytes. Cells expressing a TcR with either a high or a minimal affinity will undergo negative thymic selection, while thymocytes endowed with a TcR of moderate affinity escape the induction of programmed cell death and are positively selected (see below; reviewed in Ref. 196). The second hypothesis, called altered-ligand hypothesis, argues for a difference between the MHC/peptide complexes able to induce positive and negative selection, respectively. Moreover, it has been proposed that only thymocytes with a TcR of high affinity can be selected after recognition of these restriction elements (197). (This latter model has been further refined by proposing that distinct antigen-presenting cells are responsible for the discrimination between positive and negative thymic selection (198)). Finally, it has also been argued (199) that conformational changes of the TcR may play an equally decisive role in thymocyte selection that occurs with recognition of MHC/peptide. A number of experimental results in different systems have, however, made the affinity model the more likely one to account for the complex mechanism of thymic selection.

A. Positive Thymic Selection

1. Cell Stage

The factors known to determine whether a developing thymocyte is positively selected are (1) the expression and the specificity of the TcR and (2) the coexpression of the appropriate CD4 or CD8 accessory molecules. Positive selection is different from many other control points during thymic development where the presence of signals only determines progression to the next stage of differentiation but has no influence on the cell's function. Thymic selection occurs at the DP stage of cortical thymocytes that express high levels of RAG products and terminal denucleotide transferase (TdT) (200–203). These thymocytes have ceased to divide (161,204,205).

Thymocytes that are positively selected represent approximately 2% of all DP cortical cells. This relatively small number is contrasted by the very rapid rate of thymocyte production; approximately one-third of all thymocytes (i.e., about 60 $\times$ 10^6 cells in a typically young adult mouse thymus of 200 $\times$ 10^6 cells) are newly generated each day. The low rate for positive thymic selection is, however, in close agreement with the number of mature T cells being exported from the murine thymus, which has been estimated to be about 1 to 2 $\times$ 10^6 cells/day or 1 to 2% of all thymocytes in young adult mice (169,204). Labeling studies have further delineated as few as 2 but as many as 4 days until the DP cortical blasts give rise to positively selected $CD4^+TcR^{high}$ or $CD8^+TcR^{high}$ thymocytes (170,206). Since the formation of SP cells occurs in the absence of further cell divisions, a differentiation rather than a selective clonal expansion is suggested to follow positive thymic selection (204).

2. Cells That Effect Positive Thymic Selection

The cortex is the exclusive site for positive thymic selection (207,208,209). The cellular requirements for positive thymic selection are much more stringent than those for negative selection (see below). Cortical epithelial cells effect positive selection, as demonstrated by transgenic animal models (210,211), by bone marrow chimeras (212,213), and by selection with purified thymic epithelial cells and epithelial cell lines (212–215,217). Despite recent experiments demonstrating positive selection in vivo by fibroblasts and hematopoietic cells, juxtaposed epithelial cells may provide additional components (e.g., surface molecules) in situ that are essential for positive selection (218–221). The requirement for a costimulatory (second) signal in addition to the TcR recognition of the MHC/peptide complex (first signal) is reminiscent of the activation of peripheral T cells, where both signals are essential in order to evade the induction of tolerance.

3. The Role of the MHC/Peptide Complex in Positive Thymic Selection

Developing thymocytes are rescued from a default pathway of programmed cell death via active signaling through the TcR-mediated recognition of MHC molecules: intrathymic development to mature CD4SP thymocytes is limited to cells with a MHC class II–restricted TcR and CD8SP thymocytes conversely develop from DP thymocytes expressing a MHC class I–restricted TcR (168,208,222,223). Both MHC class I and class II antigens are expressed on thymic epithelial cells. A direct functional role in thymic maturation was initially suggested by experiments where mice treated in vivo with high doses of monoclonal antibodies against MHC class I or class II antigens lacked positive selection of CD4SP and CD8SP mature cells, respectively (224,225). This arrest in T-cell development is primarily due to the prevention of the physical interaction between TcR and MHC molecules and not a consequence of negative signaling (226–230). The surface density of MHC molecules has a profound influence on the efficiency by which (low-avidity) TcRs are positively selected, since a two- to threefold decrease in the surface MHC expression of thymic epithelial cells reduces the number of positively selected thymocytes (165,231,232). Moreover, mice deficient in one of the cellular components essential for the delivery of peptides from the cytosol to the endoplasmic reticulum (transporter associated with antigen processing 1, or TAP1) have a severely decreased surface expression of MHC class I molecules (233) and also have a marked reduction in the number of mature CD8SP thymocytes (234).

4. The Role of CD4 and CD8 in Positive Selection

Physical disruption of the ligand-receptor interaction between CD4 and MHC class II molecules and CD8α and MHC class I molecules results in the absence of single positive T cells restricted to MHC class II and class I molecules, respectively. For positive thymic selection of CD8SP to occur, TcR and CD8α have to bind to the same MHC protein, since mice transgenic for the expression of a MHC class I molecule with a mutation in the α3 domain necessary for CD8α interaction fail to generate mature T cells restricted by this altered MHC molecule despite the presence of functional MHC class I molecule expression of another haplotype (226).

CD4 and CD8 coreceptor molecules, at a minimum, increase the avidity of the interaction between thymocytes and MHC-presenting cortical epithelial cells. Whether both coreceptors also have to transduce distinctive signals to achieve positive selection has been a point of considerable controversy, since the presence of the cytoplasmic tail (and thus the ability to bind to Lck, the src-like protein tyrosine kinase) is not absolutely required for the generation of mature SP thymocytes (235,236). However, mice that express only a CD8α mutant transgene, unable to associate with Lck, have a sevenfold decrease in the number of peripheral CD8$^+$T cells and a fivefold reduced capacity to generate an antiviral cytotoxic response (237).

CD8 is a disulfide-linked heterodimer of two polypeptide chains, α and β, and most thymocytes express simultaneously CD8α and CD8β (reviewed in Ref. 238). CD8α has an extracellular domain that binds to MHC, while the cytoplasmic domain associates with Lck. By contrast, CD8β does not bind MHC nor Lck and its surface expression is dependent on the concomitant expression of CD8α. The role of CD8β in thymic development was studied in mice either lacking CD8β expression (239,240) or expressing only cytoplasmic-deficient CD8β molecules (241). Positive thymic selection appears to be affected by these changes, with the development of only 20 to 30% of the normal number of CD8SP thymocytes (239). In addition to positive thymic selection, the absence of CD8β may also influence negative thymic selection, as demonstrated in a TcR transgenic mouse model (239). However, those CD8$\alpha\alpha^+$ T cells that seed to the periphery display normal cytotoxic activity, although they may express a restricted repertoire of TcR specificities (239).

5. Signals Involved in Positive Thymic Selection

Two general models have evolved to account for receptor-mediated stimulation. The prevalent model predicts that cross-linking of the TcR and coaggregation of the T-cell coreceptors provide the focal concentration of receptor-associated kinases necessary to activate molecules located further downstream in the biochemical cascade—a process leading ultimately to full T-cell stimulation. An alternative model argues that agonistic ligands induce a conformational change of the TcR which, in turn, will allow signal transduction by (1) activating bound kinases, (2) encouraging the docking of other molecules to the CD3 complex, and (3) initiating the association with additional T-cell surface molecules. It remains to be determined whether the activation of tyrosine kinases in vivo depends on dimerization of the TcR/CD3 complex—analogous to receptor tyrosine kinases (242)—or whether monovalent serial engagement of the TcR independent of clustering is sufficient for T-cell activation (243). It is, however, also conceivable that both models of activation are correct and that the use of one over the other mechanism may depend on different conditions, such as the stage of T-cell development.

B. Negative Thymic Selection

Self-tolerance is established in the thymus by two operationally different events: clonal deletion and clonal unresponsiveness (anergy). Clonal deletion of thymocytes bearing a self-reactive TcR was suspected over 35 years ago as the mechanism of maintaining a state of self-tolerance (244) and has later been attributed to an active process during intrathymic T-cell development (245). Clonal deletion is not restricted to T cells with a self-reactive TcR specificity but also affects thymocytes that express a TcR that is non-MHC-restricted and thus fails to be positively selected (176). More recently, cellular unresponsiveness has been implicated as a nondeletional mechanism in the maintenance of self-tolerance.

1. Developmental Stage at Which Negative Thymic Selection Occurs

The first demonstrations of negative thymic selection were reported in mice expressing an endogenous viral superantigen called mammary tumor virus (Mtv). Recognition of these self-peptides results in the deletion of thymocytes expressing specific variable region gene segments of the TcR β chain (Vβ) (164,167). Immature $CD4^+CD8^+$ thymocytes are only minimally affected by superantigen-mediated negative selection. In contrast, thymocytes at the late DP stage (172,246,247) and SP mature cells (173,248) are particularly susceptible to this form of deletional thymic selection.

The developmental stage at which negative selection occurs for nominal non-Mtv-encoded self-peptides has been less clearly defined, for the nature of the antigen and the antigen-presenting cell type are of additional importance (165,223,249,250). Moreover, initial results obtained with FTOCs suggest that deletion of thymocytes can occur at the earliest stage of CD4, CD8, and TcR coexpression and that the avidity of thymocytes for their APC has little if any bearing on the maturational stage at which negative selection occurs (251). In contrast, other studies have concluded that TcR affinity determines the developmental stage of thymic selection, with a low TcR affinity directing deletion to a late stage within the DP compartment (252). Whether SP thymocytes are susceptible to non-superantigen-mediated negative selection also remains controversial (250,251).

2. Cells That Effect Thymic Clonal Deletion and Anergy

Despite some controversy (198,253,254), there is general agreement that negative selection takes place mainly in the thymic medulla. Experiments with radiation-induced bone marrow chimera [(A $\times$ B)F1 $\rightarrow$ B] first demonstrated that the antigen-presenting cell responsible for negative thymic selection is of hematopoietic origin. Repopulation of the murine thymic microenvironment with donor bone marrow–derived stromal cells occurs as early as 2 to 3 weeks after lethal irradiation and bone marrow reconstitution (255). The presence of donor-derived APC in allogeneic chimeras is first noted in the medulla and assures the deletion of host- and donor-reactive thymocytes. Interestingly, the size of the bone marrow inoculum determines the efficiency with which host-derived T cells are deleted early after transplantation (256).

The cell types operative in the induction of negative thymic selection have been characterized in vitro and in vivo and include dendritic cells (DC), macrophages, B cells, thymic epithelial cells, and thymocytes but also fibroblasts, melanoma cells, neuronal cells, and lymphoma cells (51,257–262). This broad spectrum of cells able to induce deletional thymic selection suggests that the nature of the antigen-presenting cell is as important as characteristics intrinsic to thymocytes—i.e., their developmental stage and TcR affinity. DC within the thymic microenvironment are primarily responsible for deletional selection (259), since they repopulate the thymus within a few weeks after lethal radiation and bone marrow transplantation and parallel the establishment of self-tolerance (263,264). Although DC from anatomical sites other than the thymus can mediate negative selection, their relative potency may be markedly diminished (260).

There is generally less agreement on the role of thymic epithelial cells in clonal deletion. Thymocytes have been shown to develop normally (265–268), to be deleted (269), or to be rendered unresponsive to an antigen-stimulation (269–275) if the cognate self-antigen is expressed on thymic epithelial cells.

B cells may also play a special role in negative thymic selection. Experiments with FTOCs have suggested a cooperation between dendritic cells and B cells for the deletion of superantigen-reactive thymocytes (51). Interestingly, the permissive MHC molecule and the superantigen do not necessarily have to be expressed on the same cell: B cells may provide the antigenic peptide that is taken up and presented efficiently by DC cells (276,277). The role of thymic macrophages in negative selection is unsettled. In vitro studies with FTOCs have not been able to demonstrate that macrophages delete viral superantigen–reactive thymocytes (51). The relatively low surface expression of MHC class II antigens on thymic macrophages and/or differences in accessory molecules may account for this observed lack of clonal deletion (278). However, murine thymic macrophages expressing an allogeneic MHC molecule transgenically can achieve self-tolerance by induction of clonal anergy (50).

3. The Fate of Negatively Selected Thymocytes

Only 2% of all thymocytes emigrate from the thymus, while the vast majority die at the immature DP stage (279). The fate of these latter cells has been an intriguing issue for some time. Conventional histology of thymus sections does not reveal a "cell graveyard," despite the very large number of thymocytes that are unable to mature into SP cells. Studies with radioactive nucleotides have proposed that immature cells die within the confines of the thymus (279). In view of the obvious discrepancy between the massive cell death and the inconspicuous thymic histology, it has been suggested that cortical thymocytes may leave the thymus and die elsewhere (280). Sensitive methods to detect early molecular changes in thymocytes undergoing programmed cell death (apoptosis) have provided direct evidence for cell death throughout the thymic cortex and local engulfment of dying cells by medullary macrophages (176). Approximately 1% of all cortical thymocytes undergo apoptosis in situ at any given time, as detected by DNA strand breaks. This relatively low percentage may reflect the rapidity of apoptotic changes (as detected by the method used) and may translate to as many as 25% of thymocytes undergoing programmed cell death each day (176)—a figure comparable to kinetic studies in vivo (170). Since the percentage of cells undergoing apoptosis is not reduced in MHC-deficient mice, T-cell death at an immature stage of intrathymic development appears to be regulated by a default process of nonselection: cells that have not been able to express a functional self-MHC–restricted TcR will undergo programmed cell death (176).

4. The Role of Costimulatory Molecules in Negative Thymic Selection

Different experimental models have ascertained a critical role for CD4 and CD8 in negative thymic selection despite the in vitro finding that antibody-mediated cross-linking of TcR on the surface of immature thymocytes is sufficient to induce programmed cell death (281). The pivotal function of CD4 in negative selection has been established in mice, where the expression of endogenous superantigens results in the deletion of T cells bearing a particular (i.e., reactive) TcR Vβ determinant. Syngeneic bone marrow transplantation followed by administration of anti-CD4 monoclonal antibodies blocks the deletion of DP thymocytes specific for a MHC class II/superantigen complex but allows for continuous positive selection of non-autoreactive CD8SP cells (167,180). Although not formally tested, it is generally accepted that negative thymic selection for conventional MHCII-restricted self-antigens is also dependent on CD4 binding. Mechanisms accounting for this action of anti-CD4 monoclonal antibodies include the possible disruption of the CD4/MHC class II interaction, blocking of the association of CD4 with the TcR, or the transmission of signals through CD4 (282). Several studies also provide evidence for the involvement of CD8 in negative thymic selection (226,283). The dependence on coreceptor function for negative thymic selection also seems to be controlled by TcR affinity, because negative selection of CD8α-deficient thymocytes will take place if the transgenic TcR is of high affinity (284). Conversely, overexpression of CD8 shifts the outcome of the interaction with APCs from positive selection to clonal deletion, due to the increased avidity of thymocytes for the cell APC (285,286). Thus, engagement of the TcR alone is sufficient for clonal deletion of some but not all thymocytes, implying that the affinity of the TcR determines coreceptor dependency (287).

A critical role for other costimulatory molecules important in negative thymic selection is presently unknown. While a coordinate stimulation via B7(-1 and -2)/CD28(CTLA-4) is required for optimal activation of peripheral T cells, similar restrictions for the negative selection of thymocytes are unlikely. This conclusion is based on two observations: (1) mice homogenous for the homologous disruption of the genes encoding CD28 or B7.1 display normal thymocyte development and selection (288,289), and (2) the use CTLA-4Ig fusion protein, which binds with higher affinity than CD28 to members of the B7 family, does not disturb negative thymic selection by endogenous superantigens (290,291). However, there is a developmentally regulated expression pattern of CD28, with expression first detected on DP thymocytes and downregulation on mature SP thymocytes (292). Moreover, B7 is expressed in the mouse at high levels on a subpopulation of thymic B cells and on DC. In humans DC stain positively for B7 in the fetal but not the adult thymus (290,293). By contrast, thymic epithelial cells do not express detectable amounts of B7 (290). This and the persistence of negative thymic selection after interruption of the CD28/B7 interaction may therefore mirror the lack of a costimulatory role for these molecules or, alternatively, may reflect the redundancy of the system, suggesting that other receptor-ligand pairs of costimulatory molecules are necessary and sufficient for the induction of negative selection (294,295). Recent data suggest that negative selection for some endogenously produced antigens is dependent on CD40 ligand expression on thymocytes (296). Moreover, deletion of antigen-specific immature thymocytes by dendritic cells requires the interaction of LFA-1 with ICAM-1 (297).

5. Mechanisms of Negative Selection

Programmed cell death is induced in immature thymocyte as the result of either active signal transduction (negative selection) or the failure to express a functional T-cell receptor (nonselection by default). In general, death by default occurs in most multicellular organisms and represents a fundamental mechanism for differentiation and development (298). To this end, programmed cell death can be initiated by a multitude of different induction events; the state of activation and the degree of differentiation influence susceptibility to programmed cell death (299). Apoptosis as a result of negative thymic selection or as a consequence of nonselection by default demonstrates identical morphological and biochemical changes typical of programmed cell death, suggesting a common final pathway. For negative thymic selection, binding of the TcR and coreceptors to their respective ligands is thought to initiate the transduction of signals operative in programmed cell death (300–303). It remains to be determined, however, whether thymocytes with low affinity or nonfunctional TcRs are destined to undergo apoptosis secondary to the lack of a survival signal or whether these cells succumb to programmed cell death via an active mechanism.

Programmed cell death is characterized by a series of morphological changes, termed *apoptosis*, which include plasma and nuclear membrane blebbing, dilatation of the endoplasmic reticulum, cytoskeletal reorganization, and shrinkage of cells arrested in the G1 phase of the cell cycle (304,305). Moreover, the structural changes in the nucleus are characterized by condensation, formation of chromatin caps under the nuclear membrane, dissociation of the nuclear fibrillar center, and finally the breakup of the nucleus into multiple fragments (306). After a lethal stimulus, the time to onset of these morphological and molecular changes is variable; once initiated, however, they occur rapidly. Apoptotic cells disintegrate into several membrane-bound bodies that prevent the release of intracellular contents and thus the generation of an inflammatory reaction. Neighboring phagocytic cells ingest apoptotic bodies. The rapidity of programmed cell death in the normal thymus and the efficient scavenger function of thymic phagocytes results in the infrequent detection of apoptotic cells (176). It has, therefore, been controversial in which subcellular compartment the commitment to apoptosis may first take place.

Cytosolic proteins may be involved in both cytoplasmic and nuclear changes associated with programmed cell death (307,308). However, nuclear signaling is sufficient to initiate chromatin condensation and DNA fragmentation, which is the result of the formation of high-molecular-weight DNA fragments of 300 kb (termed rosettes) and 50 kb (chromatin loops). These molecular changes may occur as early as 5 min after activation of programmed cell death (309) and may represent an irreversible commitment to apoptosis. The complete cleavage of DNA to oligonucleosomal fragments (multimers of 180-bp length termed a "DNA ladder") occurs within 90 min of stimulation.

The molecular events that influence programmed cell death and ultimately result in apoptosis can be conveniently grouped into three distinct entities: (1) triggering signals that initiate programmed cell death; (2) a common effector pathway; and (3) modulation of susceptibility to apoptosis (306). Triggers of apoptosis may be either physiological regulatory signals initiated at the cell surface (e.g., TcR/co-receptor–mediated signals, APO-1/Fas ligand binding, glucorticoid hormones, TNF-α or -β or physical and pharmacological events that cause DNA strand breakage (e.g., UV light, ionizing radiation, or DNA chelating agents) (250,310).

The downstream events of the apoptotic pathway, following TcR signaling and the engagement of other cell surface molecules, are not well characterized. However, an early rise in cytoplasmic calcium concentrations has been demonstrated in autoreactive thymocytes (309) and has been directly correlated to their deletion (311). Elevation of the intracellular calcium levels may promote apoptosis either by directly stimulating the enzymatic activity of proteases, phospholipases, and/or endonucleases or by indirectly activating signaling pathways involving protein kinases and/or phosphatases that regulate downstream effector molecules and gene transcription (309).

Bcl-2, a novel protooncogene, is a transmembrane protein localized to mitochondria, endoplasmic reticulum, and perinuclear membrane that appears to function in an antioxidant pathway to inhibit programmed cell death (308,312). Bcl-2 is also involved in the regulation of intracellular calcium (313). Mice deficient in Bcl-2 demonstrate involution of and massive apoptosis in the thymus, leading to profound depletion of thymocytes (314). In contrast, transgenic overexpression of Bcl-2 in immature thymocytes can counter cell death induced by a variety of apoptotic stimuli (315). Within the thymus, Bcl-2 is uniformly present in mature SP thymocytes in the medulla but is expressed only in scattered cells in the cortex (316). Bcl-2 may be critical in the progression of CD25$^+$ TN thymocytes to DP thymocytes, and Bcl-2 is upregulated at the DP stage under conditions of positive thymic selection (317).

VII. COMMITMENT OF DP THYMOCYTES TO CD4 AND CD8 T-CELL LINEAGES

The differentiation of DP thymocytes to SP T cells is controlled by a binary decision—namely, the exclusive expression of either CD4 or CD8 coreceptor molecules on the surface of mature T cells. This differentiation requires signals generated by the interaction with thymic stromal cells and is tied to the MHC restriction of the TcR for MHC class I or class II molecules. However, the mechanisms by which this process is regulated remain unclear. Two basic models, an instructive model and a selective model, have initially been put forth to explain the molecular changes associated with the differentiation of DP thymocytes to mature CD4 and CD8 T cells.

The instructive model proposes that the thymocytes are instructed in their choice by signals generated upon TcR engagement with MHC molecules expressed in the thymic microenvironment (318). CD4$^+$CD8$^+$ thymocytes with a MHC class II–restricted TcR will downregulate the superfluous CD8 molecule upon positive thymic selection. Conversely, DP thymocytes bearing a MHC class I-restricted TcR will receive signals that downregulate the unnecessary CD4 coreceptor.

The selective (or stochastic) model (319,320) postulates that DP thymocytes downregulate either CD4 or CD8 at random and that only those SP thymocytes will be selected positively which have by chance chosen the correct coreceptor to match the MHC restriction of their TcR. Thymocytes with an incorrect TcR/coreceptor pair will be negatively selected. Although it is not clear how the downmodulation of only one coreceptor is regulated, the selective model infers that the commitment to either lineage is first established at the DP stage and that positive thymic selection follows sequentially at the SP stage. Interestingly, this model foresees that there should be a transient population of SP thymocytes which express a mismatched TcR/coreceptor pair but which have not yet been positively selected. Indeed, elegant experiments could detect immature thymocytes with a mismatch between TcR restriction and coreceptor expression (228,321,322).

Using a different approach, another model (183) has recently been proposed based on the observation that the TcR recognition requirements are remarkably assymetrical for thymocyte commitment to either the CD4 or CD8 lineage: the decision to become a $CD8^+$ T cell requires MHC class I-dependent instruction signals, whereas thymocyte commitment to the $CD4^+$ lineage is MHC-independent and may occur by default. These findings—i.e., that instructional signals induce CD8 lineage commitment whereas the absence of instructional signals results in CD4 commitment—provide an attractive resolution for the discrepant experimental results that have been generated in support of either the stochastic or the instructional model.

VIII. CONCLUSION

Recent years have witnessed enormous progress in our understanding of the cellular and molecular mechanisms that direct multipotent stem cells to mature MHC-restricted thymocytes within the thymic microenvironment. The analysis of these complex processes involved in thymic T-cell maturation has been feasible due to refined molecular techniques and flow cytometry in conjunction with transgenic mice. Within the last decade, a precise phenotypic and functional description of the different developmental thymocyte stages has been obtained. Future experiments will now aim at the identification of the signals important for cell progression along this developmental pathway and at the description of the biochemical requirements necessary for thymic selection. A better understanding of the mechanisms governing T-cell ontogeny will significantly contribute to our knowledge of diseases associated with malfunctioning of the immune system and may provide the basis for novel therapeutic strategies.

REFERENCES

1. Davies AJ. The tale of T cells. Immunol. Today 1993; 14:137–140.
2. Ritter MA, Crisp IN. The Thymus. Oxford, U.K. IRL Press, 1992.
3. Kendall MD. Functional anatomy of the thymic microenvironment. J Anat 1991; 177: 1–29.
4. Miller JFAP. Immunological function of the thymus. Lancet 1961; 2:748–751.

5. Holländer GA, Simpson S, Mitzgouchi E, et al. Severe colitis in mice with aberrant thymic selection. Immunity 1995; 3:27–38.
6. Holländer GA, Wang B, Nichogiannopoulou A, et al. Developmental control point in induction of thymic cortex regulated by a subpopulation of prothymocytes. Nature 1995; 373:350–353.
7. van Vliet E, Jenkinson EJ, Owen JJT, van Ewijk W. Stroma cell types in the developing thymus of the normal and the nude mouse embryo. Eur J Immunol 1985; 15:675–681.
8. Huiskamp R, van Ewijk W. Repopulation of the mouse thymus after sublethal fission neutron irradiation. J Immunol 1985; 134:2161–2169.
9. Jenkinson EJ, van Ewijk W, Owen JJT. Major histocompatibility complex antigen expression on the epithelium of the developing thymus of normal and nude mice. J Exp Med 1981; 153:280–287.
10. Michie SA, Kirkpatrick EA, Rouse RV. Rare peripheral T cells migrate to and persist in normal mouse thymus. J Exp Med 1988; 168:1929–1934.
11. Penit C, Vasseur F. Sequential events in thymocyte differentiation and thymus regeneration revealed by a combination of bromodeoxyuridine DNA labeling and antimitotic drug treatment. J Immunol 1988; 140:3315–3323.
12. von Boehmer H. The developmental biology of T lymphocytes. Annu Rev Immunol 1988; 6:309–326.
13. van de Wijngaert FP, Kendall MD, Schuurman H-J, et al. Heterogeneity of epithelial cells in the human thymus. Cell Tissue Res 1984; 237:227–237.
14. Nabarra B, Andrianarison I. Ultrastructural studies of the thymic reticulum: I. The epithelial component. Thymus 1987; 9:95–121.
15. Brekelmans P, van Ewijk W. Phenotypic characterization of murine thymic microenvironments. Semin Immunol 1990; 2:13–24.
16. de Maaged RA, MacKenzie WA, Schuurman HJ, et al. The human thymus microenvironment: Heterogeneity detected by monoclonal anti-epithelial cell antibodies. Immunology 1985; 54:745–754.
17. van Ewijk W. T-cell differentiation is influenced by thymic microenvironments. Annu Rev Immunol 1991; 9:591–615.
18. von Gaudecker B. Functional histology of the human thymus. Anat Embryol 1991; 183:1–15.
19. van Ewijk W. Cell surface topography of thymic microenvironments. Lab Invest 1988; 59:579–590.
20. Dargemont C, Dunon D, Deugnier M-A, et al. Thymotaxin, a chemotactic protein, is identical to β_2-microglobulin. Science 1989; 246:803–806.
21. Schmitt D, Monier JC, Dardenne M, et al. Location of FTS (facteur thymique sérique) in the thymus of normal and auto-immune mice. Thymus 1982; 4:221–231.
22. Weckerle H, Ketelsen UP. Thymic nurse cells: IA-bearing epithelium involved in T-lymphocyte differentiation. Nature 1980; 238:402–405.
23. Weckerle H, Ketelsen UP, Ernst M. Thymic nurse cells: Lymphoepithelial cell complexes in murine thymuses: Morphological and serological characteristics. J Exp Med 1980; 151:925–944.
24. Ritter MA, Sauvage CA, Cotmore SF. The human thymus microenvironment: In vivo identification of thymic nurse cells and other antigenically distinct subpopulations of epithelial cells. Immunology 1981; 44:439–446.
25. Andrews P, Boyd RL. The murine thymic nurse cell: An isolated thymic microenvironment. Eur J Immunol 1985; 15:36–42.
26. Hiramine C, Hojo K, Koseto M, et al. Establishment of a murine thymic epithelial cell line capable of inducing both thymic nurse cell formation and thymocyte apoptosis. Lab Invest 1990; 62:41–54.

27. Kyewski BA. Seeding of the thymic microenevironments defined by distinct thymocyte-stromal cell interactions is developmentally controlled. J Exp Med 1987; 166:520-538.
28. Nishimura T, Takeuchi, Y, Ichimura Y, et. al. Thymic stromal cell clone with nursing activity supports the growth and differentiation of murine $CD4^+CD8^+$ thymocytes in vitro. J Immunol 1990; 145:412–417.
29. Wick G, Oberhuber G. Thymic nurse cells: A school for alloreactive and autoreactive cortical thymocytes? Eur J Immunol 1986; 16:855–858.
30. Izon DJ, Boyd RL. The cytoarchitecture of the human thymus detected by monoclonal antibodies. Hum Immunol 1990; 27:16–32.
31. Bauvois B, Ezine S, Imhof B, et. al. A role for the thymic epithelium in the selection of pre-T cell from murine bone marrow. J Immunol 1989; 143:1077–1086.
32. Deugnier MA, Imhof BA, Bauvois B, et al. Characterization of rat T cell precursors sorted by chemotactic migration toward thymotaxin. Cell 1989; 56:1073–1083.
33. Dunon D, Imhof BA. Mechanisms of thymus homing. Blood 1993; 81:1–8.
34. Dunon D, Kaufman J, Salomonsen J, et al. T cell precursor migration towards β_2-microglobulin is involved in thymus colonization of chicken embryos. EMBO J 1990; 9:3315–3322.
35. Dunon D, Ruiz P, Imhof BA. Pro-T cell homing to the thymus. Curr Top Microbiol Immunol 1993; 184:139–150.
36. Imhof BA, Deugnier MA, Girault JM, et al. Thymotaxin: A thymic epithelial peptide chemotactic for T-cell precursors. Proc Natl Acad Sci USA 1988; 85:7699–7703.
37. Bordigoni P, Faure G, Bene MC, et al. Improvement of cellular immunity and IgA production in immunodeficient children after treatment with synthetic serum thymic factor (STF). Lancet 1982; 2:293–297.
38. Dardenne M, Charriere J, Bach J-F. Alterations in thymocyte surface markers after in vivo treatment by serum thymic factor. Cell Immunol 1978; 39:47–54.
39. Ardavin C, Wu L, Ferrero I, Shortman K. Mouse thymic dendritic cell populations. Immunol Lett 1993; 38:19–25.
40. Crowley M, Inaba K, Witmer-Pack M, Steinman RM. The cell surface of mouse dendritic cells: FACS analysis of dendritic cells from different tissues including thymus. Cell Immunol 1989; 118:108–125.
41. Sprent J, Webb S. Function and specificity of T cell subsets in the mouse. Adv Immunol 1987; 41:39–133.
42. Ardavin C, Wu L, Li CL, Shortman K. Thymic dendritic cells and T cells develop simultaneously in the thymus from a common precursor population. Nature 1993; 362: 761–764.
43. Salomon B, Lores P, Pioche C, et al. Conditional ablation of dendritic cells in transgenic mice. J Immunol 1994; 152:537–548.
44. Ardavin C, Shortman K. Cell surface marker analysis of mouse thymic dendritic cells. Eur J Immunol 1992; 22:859–862.
45. Landry D, Donyon L, Poudrier J, et al. Accessory function of human thymic dendritic cells in ConA-induced proliferation of autologous thymocyte subsets. J Immunol 1990; 144:836–843.
46. Vremec D, Zorbas M, Scollay R, et al. The surface phenotype of dendritic cells from mouse thymus and spleen: Investigation of CD8 expression by a subpopulation of dendritic cells. J Exp Med 1992; 176:47–58.
47. Winkel K, Sotzik F, Vremec D, et al. CD4 and CD8 expression by human and mouse thymic dendritic cells. Immunol Lett 1994; 40:93–99.
48. Wu L, Antica M, Johnson GR, et al. Developmental potential of the earliest precursor cells from the adult mouse thymus. J Exp Med 1991; 174:1617–1627.
49. Haynes BF, Heinly CS. Early human T cell development: Analysis of the human

thymus at the time of initial entry of hematopoietic stem cells into the fetal thymic microenvironment. J Exp Med 1995; 181:1445–1458.
50. Miyazaki T, Suzuki G, Yamamura K. The role of macrophages in antigen presentation and T cell tolerance. Int Immunol 1993; 5:1023–1033.
51. Mazda O, Watanabe Y, Gyotoku J, Katsura Y. Requirement of dendritic cells and B cells in the clonal deletion of Mls-reactive T cells in the thymus. J Exp Med 1991; 173: 539–547.
52. Spencer J, Choy M, Hussell T, et al. Properties of human thymic B cells. Immunology 1992; 75:596–600.
53. Fend F, Nachbaur D, Oberwasserlechner F. Phenotype and topography of human thymic B cells: An immunohistologic study. Virchows Arch B-Cell Pathol Pathol 1991; 60:381–388.
54. Andreu-Sanchez JL, Faro J, Alonso JM, et al. Ontogenic characterization of thymic B lymphocytes: Analysis in different mouse strains. Eur J Immunol 1990; 20:1767–1773.
55. Nango K, Inaba M, Adachi Y, et al. Ontogeny of thymic B cells in normal mice. Cell Immunol 1991; 133:109–115.
56. Inaba M, Inaba K, Hosons M, et al. Distinct mechanisms of neonatal tolerance induced by dendritic cells and thymic B cells. J Exp Med 1991; 173:549–559.
57. Lanier LL, Spits H, Phillips JH. The developmental relationship between NK cells and T cells. Immunol Today 1992; 13:392–395.
58. Drenckhahn D, von Gaudecker B, Müller-Hermelink HK, et al. Myosin- and actin-containing cells in the human postnatal thymus: Ultrastructural and immunohistochemical findings in normal thymus and in myasthenia gravis. Virchows Arch B-Cell Pathol Mol Pathol 1979; 32:33–45.
59. Hugo P, Kappler JW, McCormack JE, Marrack P. Fibroblasts can induce thymocyte positive selection in vivo. Proc Natl Acad Sci USA 1993; 90:10335–10339.
60. Savino W, Villa-Verde DMS, Lannes-Vieira J. Extracellular matrix proteins in intrathymic T cell migration and differentiation? Immunol Today 1993; 14:158–161.
61. Utsumi K, Sawada M, Narumiya S, et al. Adhesion of immature thymocytes to thymic stromal cells through fibronectin molecules and its significance for the induction of thymocyte differentiation. Proc Natl Acad Sci USA 1991; 88:5685–5689.
62. Boyd RL, Tucek CL, Godfrey DI, et al. The thymic microenvironment. Immunol Today 1993; 14:445–459.
63. Watt S, Thomas JA, Edwards AJ, et al. Adhesion receptors are differentially expressed on developing thymocytes and epithelium in human thymus. Exp Hematol 1992; 20:1101–1111.
64. Steinmann GG. Changes in the human thymus during aging. Curr Top Pathol 1986; 75:43–88.
65. Penit C, Vasseur F. Cell proliferation and differentiation in the fetal and early postnatal mouse thymus. J Immunol 1989; 142:3369–3377.
66. Jotereau FV, Henze F, Salomon-Vie V, Gascan H. Cell kinetics in the fetal mouse thymus: Precursor cell input, proliferation and emigration. J Immunol 1987; 138: 1026–1034.
67. Scollay R, Smith J, Stauffer V. Dynamics of early T cells: Prothymocyte migration and proliferation in the adult mouse thymus. Immunol Rev 1986; 91:129–157.
68. Good RA, Dalmasso AP, Martinez C, et al. The role of the thymus in the development of immunological capacity in rabbits and mice. J Exp Med 1962; 116:773–796.
69. Lamischka I. Purification and properties of fetal hematopoietic stem cells. Semin Dev Biol 1993; 4:379–385.
70. Moore MAS, Owen JJT. Experimental studies on the development of the thymus. J Exp Med 1967; 126:715–726.
71. Huang H, Auerbach R. Identification and characterization of hematopoietic cells from

the yolk sac of the early mouse embryo. Proc Natl Acad Sci USA 1993; 90:10110-10114.
72. Palacios R, Imhof B. At day 8.-8.5 of mouse development the yolk sac, not the embryo proper, has lymphoid precursor potential in vivo and in vitro. Proc Natl Acad Sci USA 1993; 90:6581-6585.
73. Fredrickson GG, Basch RS. L3T4 antigen expression by hemopoietic precursor cells. J Exp Med 1989; 169:1473-1478.
74. Moore T, Huang S, Terstappen LWMM, et al. Expression of CD43 on murine and human pluripotent hematopoietic stem cells. J Immunol 1994; 153:4978-4987.
75. Ogawa M, Matsuzaki Y, Nishikawa S, et al. Expression and function of c-kit in hematopoietic progenitor cells. J Exp Med 1991; 174:63-71.
76. Okada S, Nakauchi H, Nagayoshi K, et al. Enrichment and characterization of hematopoietic stem cells that express c-kit molecule. Blood 1991; 78:1706-7612.
77. Spangrude GJ, Heimfeld S, Weissman IL. Purification and characterization of mouse hematopoietic stem cells. Science 1988; 241:58-62.
78. van de Rijn M, Heimfeld S, Spangrude GJ, Weissman IL. Mouse hematopoietic stem cell antigen Sca-1 is a member of the Ly-6 antigen family. Proc Natl Acad Sci USA 1989; 86:4634-4638.
79. Wineman JP, Gilmore GL, Torbett BE, Müller-Sieburg CE. CD4 is expressed on murine hematopoietic stem cells. Blood 1992; 80:1717-1724.
80. Andrews RG, Singer JW, Bernstein ID. Precursors of colony forming cells in humans can be distinguished from colony forming cells by expression of the CD33 and CD34 antigens and light scatter. J Exp Med 1989; 169:1721-1731.
81. Andrews RG, Singer JW, Bernstein ID. Human hematopoietic precursors in long-term culture: Single $CD34^+$ cells that lack detectable T cell, B cell and myeloid cell antigens produce multiple colony-forming cells when cultured with marrow stromal cells. J Exp Med 1990; 172:355-358.
82. Baum CM, Weissman IL, Tsukamoto A, Buckle AM. Isolation of a candidate human hematopoietic stem-cell population. Proc Natl Acad Sci USA 1992; 89:2804-2808.
83. Briddell RA, Broudy VC, Bruno E, et al. Further hemotypic characterization and isolation of human hematopoietic progenitor cells using a monoclonal antibody to the c-kit receptor. Blood 1992; 79:3159-3167.
84. Craig W, Kay R, Cutler R, Lansdorp P. Expression of Thy-1 on human hematopoietic progenitor cells. 1993; 177:1331-1342.
85. Huang S, Terstappen LWMM. Lymphoid and myeloid differentiation of single human CD34+, HLA-DR+, CD38- hematopoietic stem cells. Blood 1993; 83:1515-1526.
86. Lansdorp M, Dragowska W. Long-term erythropoiesis from constant numbers of CD34+ cells in serum-free cultures initiated with highly purified progenitor cells from human bone marrow. J Exp Med 1992; 175:1501-1509.
87. Terstappen LWMM, Huang S, Safford M, et al. Sequential generations of hematopoietic colonies derived from single non-lineage-committed CD34+CD38- progenitor cells. Blood 1991; 77:1218-1227.
88. Verfaillie C, Blakomer K, McGlave P. Purified primitive human hematopoietic progenitor cells with long-term in vivo repopulating capacity adhere selectively to irradiated bone marrow stroma. J Exp Med 1990; 172:509-512.
89. Williams DE, Boswell HS, Floyd AD, Broxmeyer HE. Pluripotential hematopoietic stem cells in post-5-fluorouracil murine bone marrow express the Thy-1 antigen. J Immunol 1985; 135:1004-1011.
90. Smith LG, Weissman IL, Heimfeld S. Clonal analysis of hematopoietic stem-cell differentiation in vivo. Proc Natl Acad Sci USA 1991; 88:2788-2792.
91. Spangrude G, Smith L, Uchida N, et al. Mouse hematopoietic stem cells. Blood 1991; 78:1395-1402.
92. Tjønnford GE, Veiby OP, Steen R, Egeland T. Lymphocyte differentiation in vitro

from adult human pre-thymic CD34+ bone marrow cells. J Exp Med 1993; 177:1531–1539.
93. Terstappen LWMM, Huang S, Picker LJ. Flow cytometric assessment of human T cell differentiation in thymus and bone marrow. Blood 1992; 79:666–677.
94. Barcena A, Muench MO, Galy A, et al. Phenotypic and functional analysis of T cell precursors in the human fetal liver and thymus. CD4 expression in the earliest stages of T- and myeloid-cell development. Blood 1993; 82:3401–3414.
95. Goldschneider I, Komschlies K, Greiner D. Studies of thymocytopoiesis in rats and mice: I. Kinetics of appearance of thymocytes using a direct intrathymic adoptive transfer assay for thymocyte precursors. J Exp Med 1986; 163:1–17.
96. Spangrude GJ, Weissman IL. Mature T cells generated from single thymic clones are phenotypically and functionally heterogenous. J Immunol 1988; 141:1877–1890.
97. Katsura Y, Lina T, Armagai T, et al. Limiting dilution analysis of the stem cells for T cell lineage. J Immunol 1986; 137:2434–2439.
98. Palacios R, Samaridis J, Thorpe D, Leu T. Identification and characterization of pro-T lymphocytes and lineage-uncommitted lymphocyte precursors from mice with three novel surface markers. J Exp Med 1990; 172:219–230.
99. Rodewald H-R, Kretschmar K, Takeda S, et al. Identification of pro-thymocytes in murine fetal blood: T lineage commitment can precede thymus colonization. EMBO J 1994; 13:4229–4240.
100. de Vries P, Brasel KA, McKenna HJ, et al. Thymus reconstitution by c-kit expressing hematopoietic cells purified from adult bone marrow cells. J Exp Med 1992; 176:1503–1510.
101. Wu L, Scollay R, Egerton M, et al. CD4 expressed on earliest T-lineage precursor cells in the adult murine thymus. Nature 1991; 349:71–74.
102. Rodewald H-R, Moingeon P, Lucich JL, et al. A population of early fetal thymocytes expressing FcγRII/III contains precursors of T lymphocytes and natural killer cells. Cell 1992; 69:139–150.
103. Papiernik M, Lepault F, Pontoux C. Synergistic effect of colony-stimulating factors and IL-2 on pro-thymocyte proliferation linked to maturation of macrophage/dendritic cells with L3T4-Lyt2-la-Mac-cells. J Immunol 1988; 140:1410–1434.
104. Donskoy E, Goldschneider I. Thymocytopoiesis is maintained by blood-borne precursors throughout postnatal life. J Immunol 1992; 148:1604–1612.
105. Carlos TM, Harlan JM. Leukocyte-endothelial adhesion molecules. Blood 1994; 84: 2068–2101.
106. Springer TA. Traffic signals for lymphocyte recirculation and leukocyte emigration: The multistep paradigm. Cell 1994; 76:301–314.
107. Wadsworth H, Halvorson MJ, Coligan JE. Developmentally regulated expression of the β4 integrin on immature mouse thymocytes. J Immunol 1992; 149:421–428.
108. Husmann LA, Shimonkeivitz RP, Crispe IN, Bevan MJ. Thymocyte subpopulations during early fetal development in the BALB/c mouse. J Immunol 1988; 141:736–740.
109. Aruffo A, Stamenkovic I, Melnick M, et al. CD44 is the principal cell surface receptor for hyaluronate. Cell 1990; 61:1303–1313.
110. Carter WG, Wayner EA. Characterization of the class III collagen receptor, a phosphorylated glycoprotein expressed in human nucleated cells. J Biol Chem 1988, 263: 4193–4201.
111. Horst E, Meijer CJLM, Duijvesteijn A, et al. The ontogeny of human lymphocyte recirculation: High endothelial cell antigen (HECA-452) and CD44 homing receptor expression in the development of the immune system. Eur J Immunol 1990; 20:1483–1489.
112. O'Neil HC. Antibody which can define a subset of bone marrow cells that migrate to the thymus. Immunology 1987; 68:59–64.
113. Ikuta K, Weissman IL. Evidence that hematopoietic stem cells express mouse c-kit but

do not depend on steel factor for their generation. Proc Natl Acad Sci USA 1992; 89: 1502–1506.
114. Galli SJ, Szabo KM, Geissler EN. The kit ligand, stem cell factor. Adv Immunol 1994; 55:1–96.
115. Moll J, Eibel H, Schmid P, et al. Thymic hyperplasia in transgenic mice caused by immortal epithelial cells expressing c-kit ligand. Eur J Immunol 1992; 22:1587–1594.
116. Szebo KM, Williams DA, Geissler EN, et al. Stem cell factor is encoded at the SI locus of the mouse and is the ligand for the c-kit tyrosine kinase receptor. Cell 1990; 63:213–224.
117. Rodewald H-R, Kretschmar K, Swat W, Takeda S. Intrathymically expressed c-kit ligand (stem cell factor) is a major factor driving expansion of very immature thymocytes in vivo. Immunity 1995; 3:313–320.
118. Godfrey DI, Zlotnik A. Control points in early T cell development. Immunol Today 1993; 14:547–553.
119. Wiles MV, Ruiz P, Imhof BA. Interleukin-7 expression during mouse thymus development. Eur J Immunol 1992; 22:1037–1042.
120. Williams AF, Gangnon J. Neuronal cell Thy-1 glycoprotein: Homology with immunoglobulin. Science 1982; 216:696–703.
121. He HT, Naquent P, Caillol D, Pierres M. Thy-1 supports adhesion of mouse thymocytes to thymic epithelial cells through a Ca^{2+} independent mechanism. J Exp Med 1991; 173:515–518.
122. Hueber AO, Pierres M, He HT. Sulfated glycans directly interact with mouse Thy-1 and negatively regulate Thy-1 mediated adhesion of thymocytes to thymic epithelial cells. J Immunol 1992; 148:3692–3699.
123. Duijvsteijn AM, Schreiber AB, Butcher EC. Interferon-gamma regulates an antigen specific for endothelial cells involved in lymphocyte traffic. Proc Natl Acad Sci USA 1986; 83:9114–9118.
124. Manolios B, Geczy C, Schieber L. Anti-la monoclonal antibody (10-2.16) inhibits lymphocyte high-endothelial venule (HEV) interaction. Cell Immunol 1988; 117:152–164.,
125. Barcena A, Galy AHM, Punnonen J, et al. Lymphoid and myeloid differentiation of fetal liver $CD34^+$ lineage cells in human thymic organ culture. J Exp Med 1994; 180: 123–132.
126. Galy A, Barcena A, Verma S, Spits H. Precursors of $CD3^+CD4^+CD8^+$ cells in the thymus are defined by expression of CD34: Delineation of early events in human thymic development. J Exp Med 1993; 178:391–401.
127. Kurtzberg J, Denning SM, Nycum LM, et al. Immature human thymocytes can be driven to differentiate into nonlymphoid lineages by cytokines from thymic epithelial cells. Proc Natl Acad Sci USA 1989; 86:7575–7579.
128. Spits H. Early stages in human and mouse T-cell development. Curr Opin Immunol 1994; 6:212–221.
129. Godfrey DI, Kennedy J, Suda T, Zlotnik A. A developmental pathway involving four phenotypically and functionally distinct subsets of $CD3^-CD4^-CD8^-$ triple-negative adult mouse thymocytes defined by CD44 and CD25 expression. J Immunol 1993; 150: 4244–4252.
130. Spangrude GJ, Scollay R. Differentiation of hematopoietic stem cells in irradiated mouse thymic lobes. J Immunol 1990; 145:3661–3668.
131. Fowlkes BJ, Edison L, Mathieson B, Chused T. Early T lymphocyte differentiation in vivo of adult intrathymic precursor cells. J Exp Med 1985; 162:802–822.
132. Pearse M, Wu L, Egerton M, et al. A murine early thymocyte developmental sequence is marked by transient expression of the interleukin 2 receptor. Proc Natl Acad Sci USA 1989; 86:1614–1618.
133. Petrie HT, Hugo P, Scollay R, Shortman K. Lineage relationships and developmental

kinetics of immature thymocytes: CD3, CD4, and CD8 acquisition in vivo and in vitro. J Exp Med 1990; 172:1583–1588.

134. Andjelic S, Jan N, Nikolic-Zugic J. Ontogeny of fetal $CD8^{lo}4^{lo}$ thymocytes: Expression of CD44, CD25 and early expression of TcRα mRNA. Eur J Immunol 1993; 23: 2109–2115.

135. Rothenberg E. The development of functionally responsive T cells. Adv Immunol 1992; 51:85–214.

136. Schorle H, Holtschke T, Hunig T, et al. Development and function of T cells in mice rendered interleukin-2 deficient by gene targeting. Nature 1991; 352:621–624.

137. Hozumi K, Kondo M, Nozaki H, et al. Implication of the common γ chain of the IL-7 receptor in intrathymic development of pro-T cells. Int Immunol 1994; 6:1451–1454.

138. Godfrey DI, Kennedy J, Mombaerts P, et al. Onset of TCR-β gene rearrangement and role of TCR-β expression during $CD3^-CD4^-CD8^-$ thymocyte differentiation. J Immunol 1994; 152:4783–4792.

139. Grabstein KH, Waldschmidt TJ, Finkelman FD, et al. Inhibition of murine B and T lymphopoiesis in vivo by an anti-interleukin 7 monoclonal antibody. J Exp M 1993; 178:257–264.

140. Sudo T, Nishikawa S, Ohno N, et al. Expression and function of the interleukin 7 receptor in murine lymphocytes. Proc Natl Acad Sci USA 1993; 90:9125–9129.

141. Mombaerts P, Iacomini J, Johnson RS, et al. Rag-1 deficient mice have no B and T lymphocytes. Cell 1992; 68:869–877.

142. Shinkai Y, Koyasu S, Nakayama K-i, et al. Restoration of T cell development in RAG-2 deficient mice by functional TCR transgenes. Science 1993; 259:822–825.

143. Groettrup M, Ungewiss K, Azogi A, et al. A novel disulfide-linked heterodimer on pre-T cells consists of the T cell receptor beta chain and a 33 kd glycoprotein. Cell 1993; 75:283–294.

144. Groettrup M, von Boehmer H. T cell receptor beta chain dimers on immature thymocytes from normal mice. Eur J Immunol 1993; 23:1393–1396.

145. Kishi H, Borgyula P, Scott B, et al. Surface expression of the beta T cell receptor (TcR) chain in the absence of other TcR or CD3 proteins in immature T cells. EMBO J 1991; 10:93–100.

146. Shores EW, Nakayama T, Wiest DL, et al. Structurally distinct T cell receptor complexes on developmentally distinct T cell populations in severe combined immunodeficiency mice expressing a TCRβ transgene. J Immunol 1993; 150:1263–1275.

147. Levelt CN, Ehrfeld A, Eichmann K. Regulation of thymocyte development through CD3ϵ: I. Timepoint of ligation of CD3ϵ determines clonal deletion or induction of developmental program. J Exp Med 1993; 177:707–716.

148. Levelt CN, Mombaerts P, Iglesias A, et al. Restoration of early thymocyte differentiation in T-cell receptor β-chain-deficient mutant mice by transmembrane signaling through CD3ϵ. Proc Natl Acad Sci USA 1993; 90:11401–11405.

149. Nikolic-Zugic J, Moore MW, Bevan MJ. Characterization of the subset of immature thymocytes which can undergo rapid in vitro differentiation. Eur J Immunol 1989; 19: 649–653.

150. Mombaerts P, Clarke AR, Rudnicki M, et al. Mutations in T-cell antigen receptor genes α and β block thymocyte development at different stages. Nature 1992; 360:225–231.

151. Nikolic-Zugic J, Moore MW. T cell receptor expression on immature thymocytes with in vivo and in vitro precursor potential. Eur J Immunol 1989; 19:1957–1960.

152. Petrie HT, Scollay R, Shortman K. Commitment to the T cell receptor-$\alpha\beta$ or -$\gamma\delta$ lineages can occur just prior to the onset of CD4 and CD8 expression among immature thymocytes. Eur J Immunol 1992: 22:2185–2188.

153. Wilson A, Petrie HT, Scollay R, Shortman K. The acquisition of CD4 ad CD8 during

the differentiation of early thymocytes in short-term culture. Int Immunol 1989; 6: 605–612.

154. Guidos CJ, Weissman IL, Adkins B. Intrathymic maturation of murine T lymphocytes from $CD8^+$ precursors. Proc Natl Acad Sci USA 1989; 86:7542–7546.

155. Hugo P, Waanders GA, Scollay R, et al. Ontogeny of a novel $CD4^+CD8^-CD3^-$ thymocyte subpopulation: A comparison with $CD4^-CD8^+CD3^-$ thymocytes. Proc Natl Acad Sci USA 1989; 86:210–218.

156. Hünig T. Cross-linking of the T cell antigen receptor interferes with the generation of $CD4^+8^+$ thymocytes from their immediate $CD4^-8^+$ precursors. Eur J Immunol 1988; 18:2089–2092.

157. MacDonald HR, Budd RC, Howe RC. A $CD3^-$ subset of $CD4^-8^+$ thymocytes: A rapidly cycling intermediate in the generation of $CD4^+8^+$ cells. Eur J Immunol 1988; 18:519–523.

158. Nikolic-Zugic J, Bevan MJ. Thymocytes expressing CD8 differentiate into $CD4^+$ cells following intrathymic injection. Proc Natl Acad Sci USA 1988; 85:8633–8637.

159. Paterson DJ, Williams AF. An intermediate cell in thymocyte differentiation that expresses CD8 but not CD4 antigen. J Exp Med 1987; 1987:1603–1608.

160. Takahama Y, Hasegawa T, Itohara S, et al. Entry of CD4-CD8- immature thymocytes into the CD4/CD8 developmental pathway is controlled by tyrosine kinase signals that can be provided through TcR components. Int Immunol 1994; 6:1505–1514.

161. Lundberg K, Shortman K. Small cortical thymocytes are subject to positive selection. J Exp Med 1994; 179:1475–1483.

162. Picker LJ, Siegelman MH. Lymphoid tissues and organs. In: Paul WE, ed. Fundamental Immunology, 3d ed. Raven Press, New York, 1993:146–197.

163. Havron WL, Plonie M, Kimura J, et al. Expression and function of CD3-antigen receptor on murine $CD4^+CD8^+$ thymocytes. Nature 1987; 300:170–173.

164. Kappler JW, Roehm N, Marrack P. T cell tolerance by clonal elimination in the thymus. Cell 1987; 49:273–280.

165. Kisielow P, Teh HS, Bluethmann H, von Boehmer H. Positive selection of antigen-specific T cells in the thymus by restricting MHC molecules. Nature 1988; 335:730–733.

166. MacDonald HR, Lees RK, Schneider R, et al. Positive selection of $CD4^+$ thymocytes controlled by MHC class II gene products. Nature 1988; 336:471–473.

167. MacDonald HR, Schneider R, Lees RK, et al. T cell receptor $V\beta$ use predicts reactivity and tolerance to Mls^a-encoded antigens. Nature 1988; 332:40–45.

168. Sha WC, Nelson CA, Newberry R, et al. Selective expression of antigen receptor on CD8-bearing T lymphocytes in transgenic mice. Nature 1988; 335:271–274.

169. Shortman K, Vremec D, Egerton M. The kinetics of T cell antigen receptor expression by subgroups of $CD4^+CD8^+$ thymocytes: Delineation of $CD4^+CD8^+TcR2^+$ thymocytes as post selection intermediates leading to mature T cells. J Exp Med 1991; 173: 323–332.

170. Huesmann M, Scott B, Kisielow P, von Boehmer H. Kinetics and efficacy of positive selection in the thymus of normal and T cell receptor transgenic mice. Cell 1991; 66: 533–540.

171. Kieselow P, Bluethmann H, Staerz UD, et al. Tolerance in T cell receptor transgenic mice involves deletion of nonmature thymocytes. Nature 1988; 333:742–746.

172. Guidos CJ, Danska JS, Fathman CG, Weissman IL. T cell receptor-mediated negative selection of autoreactive T lymphocyte precursors occurs after commitment to the CD4 or CD8 lineages. J Exp Med 1990; 172:835–845.

173. Aiba Y, Mazda O, Matsuzaki Y, et al. Clonal deletion of thymic mature T cells induced by staphylococcal enterotoxin B in murine fetal organ cultures. Eur J Immunol 1993; 23:815–819.

174. Crompton T, Ohashi P, Schneider SD, et al. A cortisone sensitive CD3low subset of $CD4^+CD8^-$ thymocytes represents an intermediate stage in intrathymic repertoire selection. Int Immunol 1992; 4:153–161.
175. Cohen JJ. Apoptosis. Immunol Today 1993; 14:126–130.
176. Surh CD, Sprent J. T-cell apoptosis detected in situ during positive and negative selection in the thymus. Nature 1994; 372:100–103.
177. Swat W, Dessing M, Baron A, et al. Phenotypic changes accompanying positive selection of $CD4^+CD8^+$ thymocytes. Eur J Immunol 1992; 22:2367–2372.
178. Ramsdell F, Jenkins M, Dinh Q, Fowlkes BJ. The majority of $CD4^+CD8^-$ thymocytes are functionally immature. J Immunol 1991; 147:1779–1785.
179. Yamashita I, Nagata T, Tada T, Nakayama T. CD69 cell surface expression identifies developing thymocytes which audition for T cell antigen receptor-mediated positive selection. Int Immunol 1993; 5:1139–1150.
180. Fowlkes BJ, Schwartz RH, Pardoll DM. Deletion of self-reactive thymocytes occurs at a $CD4^+8^+$ precursor stage. Nature 1988; 334:620–623.
181. Malissen M, Gillet A, Rocha B, et al. T cell development in mice lacking the CD3-ζ/η gene. EMBO J 1993; 12:4347–4355.
182. Marodon G, Rocha B. Generation of mature T cell populations in the thymus: CD4 and CD8 down-regulation occurs at different stages of thymocyte differentiation. Eur J Immunol 1994; 42:169–204.
183. Suzuki H, Punt JA, Granger LG, Singer A. Asymmetric signalling requirements for thymocyte commitment to the $CD4^+$ versus the $CD8^+$ cell lineages: A new perspective on thymic commitment and selection. Immunity 1995; 2:413–425.
184. Sammar M, Aigner S, Hubbe M, et al. Heat stable antigen (CD24) as a ligand for mouse P-selectin. Int Immunol 1994; 6:1027–1036.
185. Nielsen PJ, Eichmann K, Köhler G, Iglesias A. Constitutive expression of transgenic heat stable antigen (mCD24) in lymphocytes can augment a secondary antibody response. Int Immunol 1993; 5:1355–1364.
186. Stroynowski IM, Soloski MJ, Low M, Hood L. A single gene encodes soluble and membrane-bound forms of the major histocompatibility Qa-2 antigen: Anchoring of the product by a phospholipid tail. Cell 1987; 50:759–768.
187. Rabinowitz R, Sharrow SO, Chatterjee-Das S, et al. Qa alloantigen expression on functional T lymphocytes from spleen and thymus. Immunogenetics 1986; 24:391–341.
188. Vernachio J, Li M, Donnenberg AD, Soloski MJ. Qa-2 expression in adult murine thymus: A unique marker for a mature thymic subset. J Immunol 1989; 142:48–56.
189. Kelly KA, Scollay R. Analysis of recent thymic emigrants with subset- and maturity-related markers. Int Immunol 1990; 2:420–425.
190. Bonomo A, Kehn PJ, Shevach EM. Premature escape of double-positive thymocytes to the periphery of young mice. J Immunol 1994; 152:1509–1514.
191. Murakami K, Murayama H, Nishio A, et al. Effects of intrathymic injection of organ-specific autoantigens, parietal cells at the neonatal stage on autoreactive effector and suppressor T cell precursors. Eur J Immunol 1993; 23:809–814.
192. Preud'homme GD, Sandes R, Parfrey NA, Ste.-Croix H. T cell maturation and clonal deletion in cyclosporine-induced autoimmunity. J Autoimmun 1991; 4:357–368.
193. Preud'homme GJ, Parfrey NA, Vanier LE. Cyclosporine-induced autoimmunity and immune hyperreactivity. Autoimmunity 1991; 9:345–356.
194. Preud'homme GJ, Sanders R, Parfrey NA, Ste-Croix H. T cell maturation and clonal deletion in cyclosporine-induced autoimmunity. J Autoimmun 1991; 4:357–368.
195. von Boehmer H. Development biology of T cells in T cell-receptor transgenic mice. Annu Rev Immunol 1991; 8:531–556.
196. Hogquist KA, Jameson SC, Bevan MJ. The ligand of positive selection of T lymphocytes in the thymus. Curr Opin Immunol 1994; 6:273–278.

197. Marrack P, Kappler J. The T cell receptor. Science 1987; 238:1073–1079.
198. Speiser DE, Lees RK, Hengartner H, et al. Positive and negative selection of T cell receptor Vβ domains controlled by distinct cell populations in the thymus. J Exp Med 1989; 170:2165–2170.
199. Janeway CA. Ligands for the T cell receptor: Hard times for avidity models. Immunol Today 1995; 16:223–225.
200. Borgulya P, Kishi H, Uematsu Y, von Boehmer H. Exclusion and inclusion of α and β T cell receptor alleles. Cell 1992; 69:529–537.
201. Brändle D, Müller C, Rulicke T, et al. Engagement of the T-cell receptor during positive selection in the thymus down-regulates RAG-1 expression. Proc Natl Acad Sci USA 1992; 89:9529–9533.
202. Petrie HT, Livak F, Schatz DG, et al. Multiple rearrangements in T cell receptor α chain genes maximize the production of useful thymocytes. J Exp Med 1993; 178:615–622.
203. Turka L, Schatz D, Oettinger M, et al. Thymocyte expression of RAG-1 and RAG-2: Termination of T cell receptor cross-linking. Science 1991; 253:778–781.
204. Egerton M, Scollay R, Shortman K. The kinetics of mature T cell development in the thymus. Proc Natl Acad Sci USA 1990; 87:2529–2582.
205. Shortman K, Vremec D, Lees RK, MacDonald HR. Does negative selection involve accumulation of self-reactive thymocytes in thymic rosettes? Immunol Lett 1991; 28: 201–205.
206. Penit C. In vivo thymocyte maturation. BUdR labeling of cycling thymocytes and phenotypic analysis of their progeny support the single lineage model. J Immunol 1986; 137:2115–2121.
207. Benoist C, Mathis D. Positive selection of the T cell repertoire: Where and when does it occur? Cell 1989; 58:1027–1033.
208. Berg L, Pullen AM, Fazekas de St. Groth B, et al. Antigen/MHC specific T cells are preferentially exported from the thymus in the presence of their MHC ligand. Cell 1989; 58:1035–1046.
209. Bill J, Palmer E. Positive selection of $CD4^+$T cells mediated by MHC class II-bearing stromal cells in the thymic cortex. Nature 1989; 341:649–651.
210. LeMeur M, Gerlinger P, Benoist C, Mathis D. Correcting an immune response deficiency by creating Eα gene transgenic mice. Nature 1985; 316:38–42.
211. van Ewijk W, Ron Y, Monaco Y, et al. Compartmentalization of MHC class II gene expression in transgenic mice. Cell 1988; 53:357–370.
212. Ron Y, Lo D, Sprent J. T cell specificity in twice irradiated F1→parent bone marrow chimeras: Failure to detect a role for immigrant bone marrow-derived cells in imprinting intrathymic H-2 restriction. J Immunol 1986; 137:1764–1771.
213. Zinkernagel R, Callahan GN, Althage A, et al. On the thymus in the differentiation of "H-2 self-recognition" by T cells: Evidence for dual recognition. J Exp Med 1978; 147: 882–896.
214. Hugo P, Kappler J, Godfrey DI, Marrack PC. A cell line that can induce thymocyte positive selection. Nature 1992; 360:679–682.
215. Jenkinson EJ, Anderson G, Owen JJT. Studies on T cell maturation on defined thymic stromal cell population in vitro. J Exp Med 1992; 176:845–853.
216. Vukmanovic S, Grandea III AG, Faas SJ, et al. Positive selection of T-lymphocytes induced by intrathymic injection of a thymic epithelial cell line. Nature 1992; 359:729–731.
217. Vukmanovic S, Jameson SC, Bevan MJ. A thymic epithelial cell line induces both positive and negative selection in the thymus. Int Immunol 1994; 6:239–246.
218. Anderson G, Owen JJT, Moore NC, Jenkinson EJ. Thymic epithelial cells provide unique signals for positive selection of $CD4^+CD8^+$ thymocytes in vitro. J Exp Med 1994; 179:2027–2031.

219. Bix M, Raulet D. Inefficient positive selection of T cells directed by haematopoietic cells. Nature 1992; 359:330–333.
220. Markowitz JS, Auchincloss H, Grusby MJ, Glimcher LH. Class II positive hematopoietic cells cannot mediate positive selection of $CD4^+$ T-lymphocytes in class II deficient mice. Proc Natl Acad Sci USA 1993; 90:2779–2783.
221. Schönrich G, Strauss G, Müller K-P, et al. Distinct requirements for positive and negative selection for selecting cell type and CD8 interaction. J Immunol 1993; 151: 4098–4105.
222. Berg LJ, Groth BFdS, Pullen AM, Davis MM. Phenotypic differences between $\alpha\beta$ versus β T-cell receptor transgenic mice undergoing negative selection. Nature 1989; 340:559–562.
223. Sha WC, Nelson CA, Newberry RD, et al. Positive and negative selection of an antigen receptor on T cells in transgenic mice. Nature 1988; 336:73–76.
224. Kruisbeek AM, Mond JJ, Fowlkes BJ, et al. Absence of the $Lyt\text{-}2^-$, $L3T4^+$ lineage of T cells in mice treated neonatally with anti-I-A correlates with absence of intrathymic I-A-bearing antigen presenting function. J Exp Med 1985; 161:1029–1047.
225. Marusic-Galesic S, Stephany DA, Longo DL, Kruisbeek AM. Development of $CD4^-CD8^+$ cytotoxic T cells requires interaction with class I MHC determinants. Nature 1988; 333:180–183.
226. Aldrich CJ, Hammer RE, Jones-Youngblood S, et al. Negative and positive selection of antigen-specific cytotoxic T lymphocytes affected by the $\alpha3$ domain of MHC I molecules. Nature 1991; 352:718–723.
227. Killeen N, Moriarty A, Teh HS, Littman DR. Requirement for CD8-major histocompatibility complex class I interaction in positive and negative selection of developing T cells. J Exp Med 1992; 176:89–97.
228. Cosgrove D, Gray D, Dierich A, et al. Mice lacking MHC class II molecules. Cell 1991; 66:1051–1066.
229. Grusby MJ, Johnson RS, Papaioannou VE, Glimcher LH. Depletion of $CD4^+$ T cells in major histocompatibility complex class II-deficient mice. Science 1991; 253:1417–1420.
230. Zijlstra M, Bix M, Simister NE, et al. β_2-Microglobulin deficient mice lack $CD4^-8^+$ cytolytic T cells. Nature 1990; 344:742–746.
231. Berg L, Frank GD, Davis MM. The effects of MHC gene dosage effects and allelic variation on T cell receptor selection. Cell 1990; 60:1043–1053.
232. Kovac Z, Schwartz RH. The nature of the immune response (IR) gene defect for pigeon cytochrome c in [B10.A(4R) × B.10PL]F1 mice. Int Immunol 1989; 1:1–10.
233. Shepherd JC, Schumacher TN, Ashton-Rickardt PG, et al. TAP-1 dependent peptide translocation in vitro is ADP-dependent and peptide selective. Cell 1993; 74:577–584.
234. van Kaer L, Ashton-Rickardt PG, Ploegh HL, Tonegawa S. TAP-1 mutant mice are deficient in antigen presentation, surface class I molecules and $CD4^-CD8^+$ T cells. Cell 1992; 71:1205–1214.
235. Chan IT, Limmer A, Louie MC, et al. Thymic selection of cytotoxic T cells independent of CD8α-Lck association. Science 1993; 261:1581–1584.
236. Killeen N, Littman DR. Helper T-cell development in the absence of CD4-$p56^{lck}$ association. Nature 1993; 364:729–731.
237. Fung-Leung WP, Louie M, Limmer A, et al. The lack of CD8α cytoplasmic domain resulted in a dramatic decrease in efficiency in thymic maturation but only a moderate reduction in cytotoxic function of $CD8^+$ T cells. Eur J Immunol 1993; 23:2834–2840.
238. Zamoyska R. The CD8 coreceptor revisited: One chain good, two chains better. Immunity 1994; 1:243–246.
239. Crooks MEC, Littman DR. Disruption of lymphocyte positive and negative selection in mice lacking the CD8β chain. Immunity 1994; 1:277–285.

240. Nakayama K-I, Nakayama K, Negishi I, et al. Requirement for CD8 β chain in positive selection of CD8-lineage T cells. Science 1994; 263:1131–1133.
241. Itano A, Cado D, Chan FKM, Robey E. A role for the cytoplasmic domain of the β chain of CD8 in thymic selection. Immunity 1994; 1:287–290.
242. Fantl WJ, Johnson DE, Williams LT. Signalling by receptor tyrosine kinases. Annu Rev Biochem 1993; 62:453–482.
243. Valitutti S, Müller S, Cella M, et al. Serial triggering of many T cell receptors by a few peptide-MHC complexes. Nature 1995; 375:148–151.
244. Burnett FM. The Clonal Selection of Acquired Immunity. New York: Cambridge University Press, 1959.
245. Fry AM, Jones LA, Kruisbeek AM, Matis LA. Thymic requirement for clonal deletion during T cell development. Science 1989; 246:1044–1046.
246. Hugo P, Boyd RL, Waanders GA, et al. Timing of deletion of autoreactive $V\beta 6^+$ cells and down-modulation of either CD4 or CD8 on phenotypically distinct $CD4^+CD8^+$ subsets of thymocytes expressing intermediate or high levels of T cell receptor. Int Immunol 1990; 3:265–272.
247. White J, Herman A, Pullen AM, et al. The V beta-specific superantigen staphylococcal enterotoxin B: Stimulation of mature T cells on clonal deletion in neonatal mice. Cell 1989; 56:27–35.
248. D'Adamio L, Awad KM, Reinherz EL. Thymic and peripheral apoptosis of antigen-specific T cells might cooperate in establishing self tolerance. Eur J Immunol 1993; 23: 747–753.
249. Bluthmann H, Kisielow P, Uematsu Y, et al. T-cell specific deletion of T-cell receptor transgenes allows functional rearrangement of endogenous α- and β-genes. Nature 1988; 334:156–159.
250. Murphy K, Heimberger A, Loh DY. Induction by antigen of intrathymic apoptosis in $CD4^+CD8^+TcR^{lo}$ thymocytes in vivo. Science 1990; 250:1720–1724.
251. Spain LM, Berg LJ. Developmental regulation of thymocyte susceptibility to deletion by "self"-peptide. J Exp Med 1992; 176:213–223.
252. Vasquez NJ, Kaye J, Hedrick SM. In vivo and in vitro clonal deletion of double-positive thymocytes. J Exp Med 1992; 175:1307–1316.
253. Pircher H, Burki K, Lang R, et al. Tolerance induction in double specific T-cell receptor transgenic mice varies with antigen. Nature 1989; 342:559–561.
254. Sprent J, Lo D, Gao E-K, Ron Y. T cell selection in the thymus. Immunol Rev 1988; 101:173–190.
255. Fukushi N, Wang B, Arase H, et al. Cell components required for deletion of an autoreactive T cell repertoire. Eur J Immunol 1990; 20:1153–1160.
256. Yoshikai Y, Ogimoto M, Matsuzaki G, Nomoto K. Bone marrow derived cells are essential for intrathymic deletion of self-reactive T cells in both host- and donor-derived thymocytes of fully allogeneic bone marrow chimeras. J Immunol 1990; 145: 505–509.
257. Eynon EE, Parker DC. Small B cells as antigen presenting cells in the induction of tolerance to soluble protein antigens. J Exp Med 1992; 175:131–138.
258. Lo D, Ron Y, Sprent J. Induction of MHC restricted specificity and tolerance in the thymus. Immunol Res. 1986; 5:221–243.
259. Matzinger P, Guerder S. Does T-cell tolerance require a dedicated antigen-presenting cell? Nature 1989; 338:74–76.
260. Pircher H, Brudscha K, Steinhoff U, et al. Tolerance induction by clonal deletion of $CD4^+8^+$ thymocytes in vitro does not require dedicated antigen-presenting cells. Eur J Immunol 1993; 23:669–674.
261. Shimonkewitz RP, Bevan MJ. Split tolerance induced by the intrathymic adoptive transfer of thymocyte stem cells. J Exp Med 1988; 168:143–156.

262. Speiser DE, Chvatchko Y, Zinkernagel RM, MacDonald HR. Distinct fates of self-reactive T cells developing in irradiation bone marrow chimeras: Clonal deletion, clonal anergy, or in vitro responsiveness to self-Mls1[a] controlled by hematopoietic cells in the thymus. J Exp Med 1990; 172:1305–1314.
263. Kampinga J, Nieuwenhuis P, Roser B, Aspinall R. Differences in turnover between thymic medullary dendritic cells and a subset of cortical macrophages. J Immunol 1990; 145:1659–1663.
264. Kyewski BA, Rouse RV, Kaplan HS. Thymocyte rosettes: Multicellular complexes of lymphocytes and bone marrow derived stromal cells in the mouse thymus. Proc Natl Acad Sci USA 1982; 79:5646–5650.
265. Carlow DA, Teh S-J, Teh H-S. Altered thymocyte development resulting from expressing a deleting ligand on selecting thymic epithelium. J Immunol 1992; 148:2988–2995.
266. Ready AR, Jenkinson EJ, Kingston R, Owen JJT. Successful transplantation across major histocompatibility barrier of deoxyguanosine-treated embryonic thymus expressing class II antigens. Nature 1984; 310:231–233.
267. Von Boehmer H, Schubiger K. Thymocytes seem to ignore class I major histocompatibility complex antigens expressed on thymus epithelial cells. Eur J Immunol 1984; 14: 1048–1052.
268. Webb S, Sprent J. Tolerogenicity of thymic epithelium. Eur J Immunol 1990; 20:2525–2530.
269. Gao E-K, Lo D, Sprent J. Strong T cell tolerance in parent → F1 bone marrow chimeras prepared with supralethal irradiation. J Exp Med 1990; 171:1101–1109.
270. Arase H, Arase N, Ogasawara K, et al. Clonal elimination of self reactive $V\beta6+$ T cells induced by H-2 products expressed on thymic radioresistant components. Int Immunol 1992; 4:75–82.
271. Good MF, Pyke KW, Nossal GJV. Functional deletion of cytotoxic T-lymphocyte precursors in chimeric thymus produced in vitro from embryonic anlage. Proc Natl Acad Sci USA 1983; 80:3045–3049.
272. Ramsdell F, Lantz F, Fowlkes BJ. A non-deletional mechanism of thymic self-tolerance. Science 1989; 246:1038–1041.
273. Roberts JL, Sharrow SO, Singer A. Clonal deletion and clonal anergy in the thymus induced by different cellular elements with different radiation sensitivities. J Exp Med 1990; 171:935–943.
274. Salaün J, Bandeira A, Khazaal I, et al. Thymic epithelium tolerizes for histocompatibility antigens. Science 1990; 247:1471–1474.
275. Schönrich G, Momburg F, Hämmerling GJ, Arnold B. Anergy induced by thymic medullary epithelium. Eur J Immunol 1992; 22:1687–1691.
276. Pullen AM, Marrack P, Kappler JW. The T cell repertoire is heavily influenced by tolerance to polymorphic self-antigens. Nature 1988; 335:796–799.
277. Speiser DE, Kolb R, Schneider H, et al. Tolerance to Mls[a] by clonal deletion of $V\beta6^+$ T cells in bone marrow and thymus chimera. Thymus 1989; 13:27–35.
278. Jayaraman S, Luo Y, Dorf M. Tolerance induction in T helper (Th1) cells by thymic macrophages. J Immunol 1992; 148:2672–2681.
279. Shortman K, Scollay R. Death in the thymus. Nature 1994; 372:44–45.
280. Rothenberg E. Death and transfiguration of cortical thymocytes: A reconsideration. Immunol Today 1990; 11:116–120.
281. Yachelin P, Falk I, Eichmann K. Deviations in thymocyte development induced by divalent and monovalent ligation of the alpha/beta T cell receptor and by its cross-linking to CD8. J Immunol 1990; 145:1382–1389.
282. Miceli MC, Parnes JR. Role of CD4 and CD8 in T cell activation and differentiation. Adv Immunol 1993; 53:59–122.

283. Ingold AL, Landel C, Knall C, et al. Co-engagement of CD8 with the T cell receptor is required for negative selection. Nature 1991; 352:721–723.
284. Fung-Leung W-P, Schilham MW, Rahemtulla A, et al. CD8 is needed for development of cytotoxic T cells but not helper T cells. Cell 1991; 65:443–449.
285. Lee NA, Loh DY, Lacy E. CD8 surface levels alter the fate of α/β T cell receptor-expressing thymocytes in transgenic mice. J Exp Med 1992; 175:1013–1025.
286. Robey EA, Ramsdell F, Kioussis D, et al. The level of CD8 expression can determine the outcome of thymic selection. Cell 1992; 69:1089–1096.
287. Knobloch M, Schönrich G, Schenkel J, et al. T cell activation and thymic tolerance induction require different adhesion intensities of the CD8 co-receptor. Int Immunol 1992; 4:1169–1174.
288. Freeman GJ, Borriello F, Hodes RJ, et al. Uncovering a functional alternative CTLA-4 counter-receptor in B7-deficient mice. Science 1993; 262:907–909.
289. Shahinian A, Pfeffer K, Lee KP, et al. Differential T cell costimulatory requirements in CD28-deficient mice. Science 1993; 261:609–612.
290. Jones LA, Izon DJ, Nieland JD, et al. CD28-B7 interactions are not required for intrathymic clonal deletion. Int Immunol 1993; 5:503–512.
291. Tan R, Teh S-J, Ledbetter JA, et al. B7 costimulates proliferation of $CD4^-CD8^+$ T lymphocytes but is not required for the deletion of immature $CD4^+CD8^+$ thymocytes. J Immunol 1992; 149:3217–3224.
292. Gross JA, Callas E, Allison JP. Identification and distribution of the costimulatory receptor CD28 in the mouse. J Immunol 1992; 149:380–388.
293. Vandenberghe B, Delabie J, de Boer M, et al. In situ expression of B7/BB1 on antigen presenting cells and activated B cells. Int Immunol 1993; 5:317–321.
294. Aiba Y, Mazda O, Davis MM, et al. Requirement of a second signal from antigen presenting cells in the clonal deletion of immature T cells. Int Immunol 1994; 6:1475–1483.
295. Page DM, Kanel LP, Allison JP, Hedrick SM. Two signals are required for negative selection of $CD4^+CD8^+$ Thymocytes. J Immunol 1993; 151:1868–1880.
296. Foy TM, Page DM, Waldschmidt TJ, et al. An essential role for gp39, the ligand for CD40, in thymic selection. J Exp Med 1995; 182:1377–1388.
297. Carlow DA, van Oers NSC, Teh S-J, Teh H-S. Deletion of antigen-specific immature thymocytes by dendritic cells requires LFA-1-ICAM-1 interactions. J Immunol 1992; 148:1595–1603.
298. Raff MC. Social control on cell survival and cell death. Nature 1992; 356:397–400.
299. King LB, Ashwell JD. Signalling for death of lymphoid cells. Curr Opin Immunol 1993; 5:368–373.
300. Aguilar LK, Aguilar-Cordova E, Cartwright J, Belmont JW. Thymic nurse cells are sites of thymocyte apoptosis. J Immunol 1994; 152:2645–2651.
301. Degermann S, Surh CD, Glimcher LH, et al. B7 expression on thymic medullary epithelium correlates with epithlium mediated deletion of $V\beta5^+$ thymocytes. J Immunol 1994; 152:3254–3263.
302. Matsuyama T, Kimura T, Kitagawa M, et al. Targeted disruption of IRF-1 or IRF-2 results in abnormal type 1 IFN induction and aberrant lymphocyte development. Cell 1993; 75:83–97.
303. Vukmanovic S, Jameson SC, Bevan MJ. A thymic epithelial cell line induces both positive and negative selection in the thymus. Int Immunol 1994; 6:239–246.
304. Ashwell JD, Cunningham RE, Noguchi PD, Hernandez D. Cell growth cycle block of T cell hybridomas upon activation with antigen. J Exp Med 1987; 165:173–194.
305. Wyllie AH, Kerr JFR, Currie AR. Cell death: The significance of apoptosis. Int Rev Cytol 1980; 68:251–305.

306. Howie SEM, Harrison DJ, Wyllie AH. Lymphocyte apoptosis: Mechanisms and implications in disease. Immunol Rev 1994; 142:141–156.
307. Peitsch MC, Polzar B, Stephan H, et al. Characterization of the endogenous deoxyribribonuclease involved in nuclear DNA degradation during apoptosis (programmed cell death). EMBO J 1993; 12:371–377.
308. Vaux DL, Haecker G, Strasser A. An evolutionary perspective on apoptosis. Cell 1994; 76:777–779.
309. McConkey DJ, Nicotera P, Orrenius S. Signalling and chromatin fragmentation in thymocyte apoptosis. Immunol Rev 1994; 142:343–363.
310. MacDonald HR, Lees RK. Programmed death of autoreactive thymocytes. Nature 1990; 343:642–644.
311. Nakayama T, Ueda Y, Yamada H, et al. In vivo calcium elevations in thymocytes with T cell receptors that are specific for self ligands. Science 1992; 257:96–99.
312. Hockenbery DM, Oltavi ZN, Yin X-M, Milliam CL, Korsmeyer SJ. Bcl-2 functions in an antioxidant pathway to prevent apoptosis. Cell 1993; 75:241–251.
313. Lam M, Dubyak G, Chen L, et al. Evidence that bcl-2 represses apoptosis by regulating endoplasmic reticulum-associated Ca^{2+} fluxes. Proc Natl Acad Sci USA 1994; 91: 6569–6573.
314. Veis DJ, Sorensen CM, Shutter JR, Korsmeyer SJ. Bcl-2 deficient mice demonstrate fulminant lymphoid apoptosis, polycystic kidneys, and hypopigmented hair. Cell 1993; 75:229–240.
315. Sentman CL, Shutter JR, Hockenbery D, et al. Bcl-2 inhibits multiple forms of apoptosis but not negative selection in thymocytes. Cell 1991; 67:879–888.
316. Pezella F, Tse A, Cordell JL, et al. Expression of the bcl-2 oncogene is not specific for the 14;18 chromosomal translocation. Am J Pathol 1990; 137:2115–2120.
317. Linette GP, Grusby JM, Hedrick SM, et al. Bcl-2 is upregulated at the $CD4^+CD8^+$ stage during positive selection and promotes thymocyte differentiation at several control points. Immunity 1994; 1:197–205.
318. von Boehmer H. The selection of the alpha beta heterodimeric T cell receptor antigen. Immunol Today 1986; 7:333–336.
319. Janeway CA. T cell development: Accessories or coreceptors? Nature 1988; 335:208–210.
320. Robey EA, Fowlkes BJ, Pardoll DM. Molecular mechanisms for lineage commitment in T cell development. Semin Immunol 1990; 2:25–34.
321. Chan SH, Cosgrove D, Waltzinger C, et al. Another view of the selective model of thymocyte selection. Cell 1993; 73:225–236.
322. Koller BH, Marrack P, Kappler JW, Smithies O. Normal development of mice deficient in $\beta 2m$, MHC class I proteins and $CD8^+$ T cells. Science 1990; 248:1227–1231.

2

MHC Class I: Structure and Function

David H. Margulies
National Institute of Allergy and Infectious Diseases
National Institutes of Health
Bethesda, Maryland

I. INTRODUCTION

Immunological recognition occurs at many levels, in solution in the body fluids where soluble antibodies neutralize foreign molecular invaders such as toxins, at cell surfaces where soluble antibodies coat viral or bacterial intruders, or at the cell-cell interface where local signals are transmitted through surface receptors from accessory cells to effectors or from effectors to targets. Among the oldest recognized immunological rules is the requirement that both the donor and recipient of a tissue graft express genetically identical cell surface tissue antigens and thus exhibit "histocompatibility" to permit graft survival or to prevent the activation of cells of the graft against the host. This histocompatibility is determined in part by the elimination, during the development of T lymphocytes, of those that bear surface receptors with the strongest tendency to bind major histompability complex (MHC) molecules of the host. Thus, immunological tolerance for self derives from a cellular selection process that deletes or functionally eliminates T cells having a high degree of autoreactivity. Although the molecular and cellular mechanisms that control graft rejection and graft-versus-host disease are admittedly complex, the central cell/cell interaction that regulates tolerance and the immune response is that which occurs between T lymphocytes and antigen presenting cells (APC) or target cells. These cell/cell signals are delivered by MHC molecules expressed on the surface of the APC to the T cell through its T-cell receptor. T cells are classified by the spectrum of cell surface molecules they express, whether they bear $\alpha\beta$ or $\gamma\delta$ receptors, as well as by the display of the coreceptors CD4 or CD8 (1). Of the $\alpha\beta$ T cells, the presence of the CD4 or CD8 coreceptor molecules operationally defines the reactivity of the T cell with either class I molecules of the MHC (MHC-I), usually restricted to the CD8 T-cell set, or with class II molecules of the MHC (MHC-II), which primarily interact with T lymphocytes expressing CD4. In addition, T cells can be grouped into T_{H1} and T_{H2} cells according to the soluble mediators (lymphokines) they secrete on activation (2).

The MHC molecules are flags that permit roving T cells to recognize cells infected with cellular pathogens such as viruses, parasites, or bacteria in the case of MHC-I (3). Similarly, MHC-II molecules signal the presence of foreign proteins in the tissue fluid or serum. The MHC-I molecule samples the fragments of degraded components of newly synthesized structures during its intracellular biosynthetic journey and displays them at the cell surface as part of the MHC-I molecule itself. Mature peripheral T cells with $\alpha\beta$ T-cell receptors (TCR) specific for a particular MHC-I/antigen complex are activated upon encounter with the APC displaying the correct complex. This encounter might be manifest as lymphokine release and/or as the stimulation of cytolytic activity against the infected target cell. Such a function clearly evolved to protect the organism from infectious microorganisms, but the same phenomenon is also exploited in the recognition of tumor cells marked by the cell surface display of aberrantly expressed self peptides complexed with MHC-I.

A more recently recognized, but possibly equally important function of MHC-I is to modulate the signals determining lytic activity of the T-cell receptor negative NK cells. Thus, specific MHC-I molecules on NK targets may interact with receptors on NK cells to inhibit the lysis of the target (4). The precise nature of the structure recognized, whether it be native MHC-I complexed with peptides or an unfolded variant, as well as the kinds of signals (stimulatory or inhibitory) delivered through the NK/target cell interaction, is presently a subject of active investigation.

The MHC-II molecule, although its surface display function is similar to that of MHC-I, derives its antigens from extracellular proteins that have been ingested by the presenting cells rather than from an intracellular source (5). In a variation of the MHC-I theme, MHC-II-bearing cells collect their antigenic peptides in an intracellular acidic compartment where their proteolytic fragments encounter the MHC-II molecules directed there. In contrast to the MHC-I antigen presentation pathway, which samples the intracellular cytoplasmic environment, the MHC-II pathway serves to brandish antigens gathered from the extracellular milieu. This simple dichotomy, MHC-I—inside out, MHC-II—outside in, illustrates how molecular and cellular evolution have permitted the exploitation of very similar mechanisms to distinct functions (3,6,7). In addition, like most biological paradigms, there are notable exceptions indicative of the intersections of parallel cellular pathways (8).

The MHC-I molecule, represented by HLA-A, B, or C in the human, H-2K, -D, or -L in the mouse, is among the most polymorphic known. Polymorphism, a reflection of the number of alleles in the population and proportion of alleles represented by the most frequent, is a clue to the unique function of the MHC molecules. They must have the potential to bind a large selection of potentially pathogenic peptides yet to preserve the ability to interact with T-cell receptors and coreceptors. In the human, more than 15 alleles have been identified at the A locus, and more than 35 at the B; in the mouse, more than 90 alleles are recognized at the K locus and more than 69 at the D (9).

Although the practical understanding of the clinical phenomenon of graft-versus-host disease, the subject of this volume, requires a less complete appreciation of the molecular details of the MHC-I- and MHC-II-mediated signaling of T lymphocytes, a comprehension of the molecular structures involved and their cellular function can underscore the complexity and beauty of the normal immune response. The purpose of this chapter is to describe the structure, biosynthesis, and function of the MHC-I genes and their encoded proteins. This exposition will take us through many exciting areas of modern biology—molecular biology and genetics, cell biology, biochemistry, and x-ray crystallography—and should imbue the reader with a cellular and molecular view of the initiating reaction of the immune response.

II. STRUCTURE OF MHC CLASS I

A. Overview

The early characterization of the genes that encoded MHC-I molecules derived from their function in mediating graft rejection and their ability to elicit antibodies in genetically distinct (allogeneic) hosts (10). We now view the MHC-I molecule as a cell surface glycoprotein, designed to sample components of the cell on which it is expressed, and to display these smaller molecules as a noncovalent complex on the surface of the cell, where they may be available for recognition by specific T lymphocytes (11). The MHC-I molecule is a cell surface heterodimer consisting of a polymorphic plasma membrane-associated heavy-chain glycoprotein containing about 350 amino acid residues, noncovalently assembled with a nonpolymorphic protein light chain of 99 amino acids known as β2-microglobulin (β2-m) (Fig. 1). The prototype MHC-I molecule has four major extracellular protein domains, each of about 90 amino acids in length. The α1 and α2 domains mesh to form a binding site for peptide, and the α3 and β2-m domains, each immunoglobulinlike in both sequence and three-dimensional structure, form a foundation for this binding site. The α3 domain also provides the core for the interaction of the T-cell coreceptor, CD8, with the MHC-I (12,13). A transmembrane region of the heavy chain, consist-

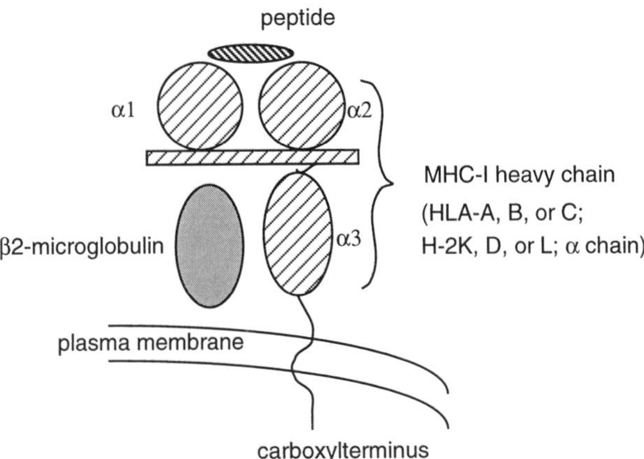

Figure 1 Schematic representation of a generic MHC-I molecule. A typical MHC-I molecule is illustrated, in which the membrane-bound, MHC-I heavy chain (α chain), lightly stippled, is anchored to the plasma membrane, the non-covalently attached β2-microglobulin (β2-m) (tightly stippled), and the peptide (stippled) are indicated.

ing of hydrophobic amino acids bounded by a series of basic residues to the carboxyl terminus, anchors the chain to the plasma membrane. The β2-m chain, the product of a gene unlinked to the human HLA or mouse H-2 locus, forms a necessary part of the MHC-I/peptide complex, since it is usually required for the cell surface expression of the MHC-I molecule. Peptide, representative of the degradation products of the cell that are transported from the cytoplasm to the endoplasmic reticulum via a mechanism dependent on the expression of the TAP-1/TAP-2 transporters, is bound by the MHC-I molecule in the endoplasmic reticulum, and allows the MHC/β2-m/peptide complex to achieve a native three-dimensional conformation that is permissive for the normal intracellular transport of the molecule, and its ultimate cell surface expression. On the cell surface, most assembled molecules are stable, although a small proportion may lose their β2-m and peptide and either be degraded, recycled into the cell, or remain available for the passive acquisition of peptides from the external milieu (14,15).

B. Primary Sequence

Because of the important antigen presentation function of the MHC-I molecule, the goal of correlating structure with function has been the focus of great interest and experimentation over the years. Early studies established the primary amino acid sequence of examples of MHC-I protein chains, a pursuit that advanced quickly with the cloning of both cDNA (16,17) and genomic fragments (18,19). Alignment of encoded amino acid sequences of a large number of MHC-I molecules indicated striking patterns: the membrane proximal α3 domains within a species are considerably more conserved than the membrane distal α1 and α2 domains (20). In addition, the disulfide loop of the α3 domain is immunoglobulinlike, while the disulfide loop of the α2 domain though conserved among MHC-I molecules, is not. The α1 domain lacks any disulfide. The four-domain structure of the MHC-I, two membrane proximal immunoglobulinlike domains (α3 and β2-m), and two distal (α1 and α2) that form the peptide binding site, is mimicked in the four-domain structure of the MHC-II which draws its membrane distal peptide binding site from the dimerization of the class II α1 and β1 domains. The primary amino acid sequence of a large number of MHC-I and MHC-II molecules of human and mouse provided a basis for understanding the polymorphisms of these molecules. Within the same species, MHC molecules appear to be a patchwork of all the other known related molecules. Thus it was proposed (19), and later confirmed (21), that the genes encoding the MHC molecules exploited genetic recombinational mechanism or "gene conversion" in the rapid diversification and evolution of this gene family. A more tangible understanding of the means by which the MHC-I molecule achieves its biological need to bind a wide diversity of self and antigenic peptides and to interact with the both T-cell receptors and the CD8 coreceptor, derives from a number of three-dimensional structural determinations based on the techniques of x-ray crystallography and molecular modeling.

C. Three-Dimensional Structure

The first three-dimensional structure of an MHC-I molecule was determined for the human HLA-A2 molecule, purified from tissue culture cells and containing in its binding cleft a heterogeneous repertoire of peptides derived from the cells of origin

(22–24). Subsequent studies have examined the three-dimensional structure of a number of human and murine MHC-I molecules, some complexed with homogeneous synthetic peptides (11,25–30) (see Fig. 2). The important features of the MHC-I high resolution three-dimensional structure are (a) the membrane proximal domains—i.e., the $\alpha3$ of the heavy chain and the noncovalently associated $\beta2$-m are immunoglobulinlike β barrel domains; (b) the membrane distal domains ($\alpha1$ and $\alpha2$) unite to form a cleft in which the peptide is bound; and (c) the peptide binding cleft is bounded by two antiparallel α helices, one from the $\alpha1$ and one from $\alpha2$ domain, and is supported by a floor of antiparallel β sheet. Half of this floor derives from the $\alpha1$ domain, half from the $\alpha2$. The membrane-proximal immunoglobulin-like domains, less polymorphic in primary amino acid sequence, provide structural support for the floor of the peptide binding cleft. The major site of interaction of the MHC-I molecule with the T-cell coreceptor CD8 is the $\alpha3$ immunoglobulinlike

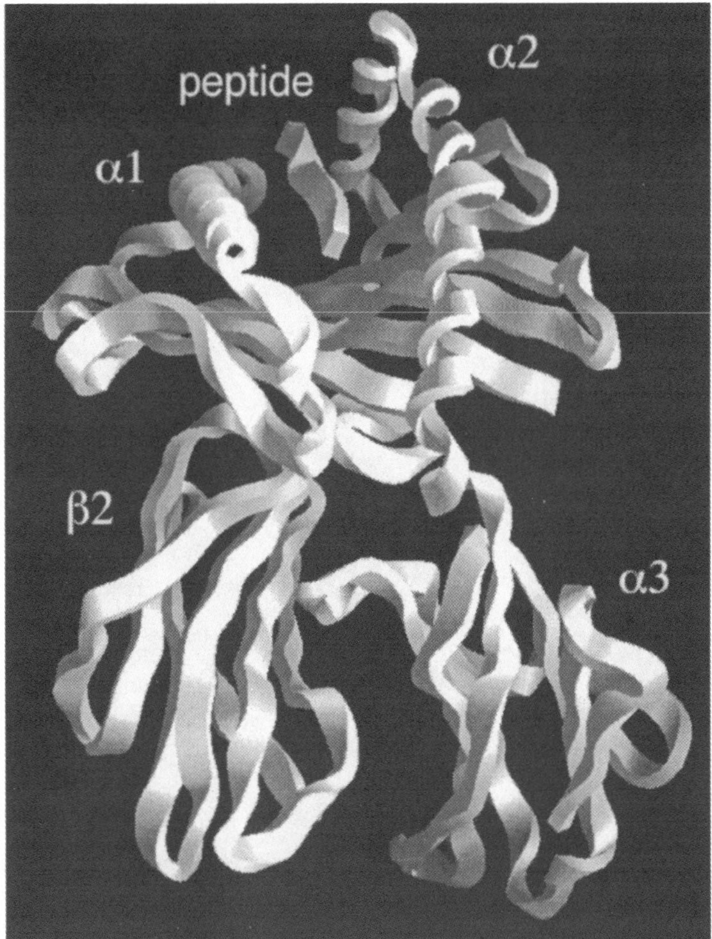

Figure 2 Diagram of the three-dimensional structure of the mouse H-2K^b molecule complexed with the antigenic peptide, VSV-8 (115).

domain (12,13). Amino acid polymorphism in parts of this domain has direct effects on the CD8 dependence of T-cell–MHC interactions and can be shown to influence the binding of CD8-expressing T cells to APCs.

The peptide-binding groove of the MHC-I molecule is about 30 Å long and 12 Å wide and lined by the most variable amino acid residues of the MHC-I heavy chain. Several regions of the cleft—particularly those that anchor the amino and carboxyl termini of the bound peptide—are highly conserved. The "standard" view of the peptide-binding cleft (see Fig. 3), has the α helix of the $\alpha 1$ domain at the top, running across the page, and the α helix of the $\alpha 2$ domain running antiparallel to this along the bottom. The orientation of the bound peptide is with the amino terminus of the peptide to the left and the carboxyl terminus to the right. Although some amino acid side chains are deeply buried in the MHC-I cleft and thus serve to anchor the peptide to the MHC-I, several amino acid side chains of the peptide are exposed to available solvent and thus may be available for T-cell receptor interaction.

Since the activation of an MHC-I–restricted peptide-specific T lymphocyte can be exquisitely sensitive and specific, capable of discriminating between peptides that differ by single amino acids or of mutant or polymorphic variant MHC-I molecules that differ at single positions, it is important to try to understand the structural

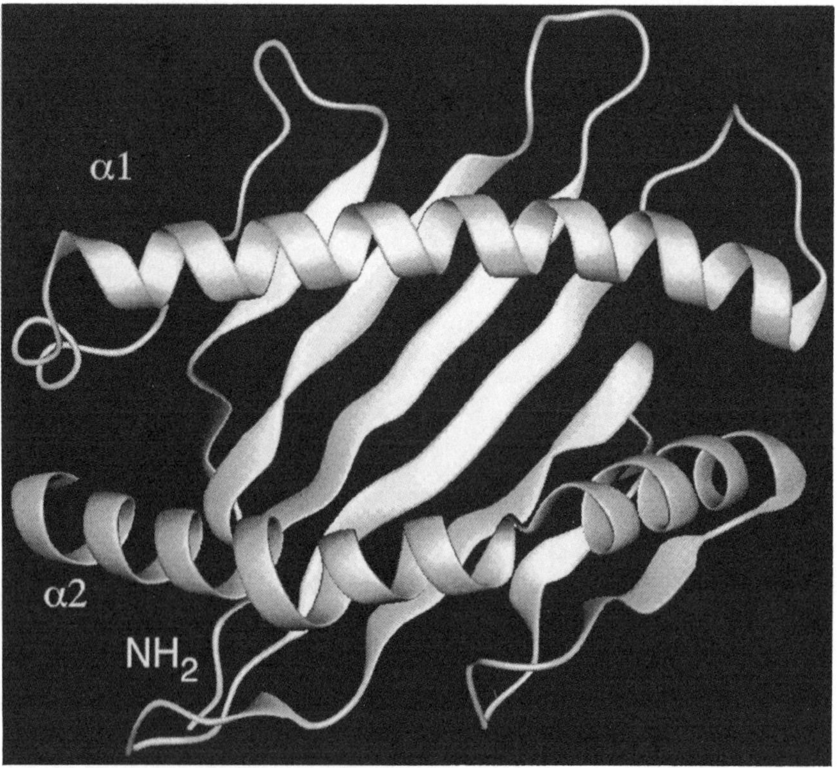

Figure 3 "Standard" view of the peptide binding cleft of an MHC molecule. A ribbon illustration of the $\alpha 1$ and $\alpha 2$ domains of H-2K^b (115) is shown.

differences between MHC/peptide complexes that have relatively few amino acid differences. One approach to this problem was to analyze the T-cell recognition of a panel of cytotoxic T lymphocytes of a set of somatic cells expressing mutations of the mouse class I molecules H-2K^{b} (31). By locating the sites of the mutations in a molecular model of the H-2K^{b} molecule, based on the then available HLA-A2 structure, and correlating the lack of recognition of a set of mutants by any of a number of given CTL clones, a crude estimate for the size of the surface of interaction of the T cell receptor on the MHC/peptide complex was established at about 600 Å^{2} (31). These dimensions are roughly equivalent in scale to those of the surface of interaction of antiprotein antibodies, such as antilysozyme antibodies, as determined from elucidation of the structure of the antibody-antigen cocrystal (32). The illustration in Fig. 4 provides some perspective of the way a T cell receptor might interact with an MHC-I molecule. Note that this picture is of an MHC-I molecule juxtaposed with an antibody Fab fragment, not with a T-cell receptor. Since the extracellular portion of T-cell receptor proteins is similar in length and size to that of antibody Fabs, this is a valid comparison for scale.

Another way of perceiving the kinds of structural differences detected by different T-cell receptors is to compare the structure of the same MHC complexed to several different peptide antigens. The crystallographic structures of the mouse MHC-I molecule, H-2K^{b} complexed with either of two viral peptides, that of the vesicular stomatitis virus (VSV) nucleoprotein octamer peptide, residues 52-59, RGYVYQGL, and that of the Sendai virus (SEV) nucleoprotein nonamer peptide, residues 324-332, FAPGNYPAL, were determined (26,33,34). Comparison of the structures of these two different H-2K^{b}/peptide complexes revealed that (a) the backbone of the MHC-I molecule was essentially identical in the two structures; (b) the side-chain orientation of a few MHC residues differed significantly between the two complexes, the greatest difference being the orientation of arginine 155 of the MHC-I molecule which partially covers the peptide in the complex with the VSV octomer but is twisted away and toward solvent in the SEV nonamer; and (c) the backbone tracing and the side-chain orientation of these two bound peptides is different, suggesting an ability of different peptide/MHC pairs to solve the specific binding problem differently.

Another comparison of structures, that made by Madden and colleagues (27), considered five different peptides bound to the MHC-I molecule HLA-A*0201. Here, the MHC-I molecule is itself quite constant, and although the four nonamer peptides and one decamer are fixed at position 2 and the carboxyl terminus, the side-chain orientation, and location of a bulge to allow accommodation of the different peptides show that there is great plasticity in the display of the bound peptides. Major differences in T-cell receptor interactions are likely due to the differences in the exposed peptidic residues.

D. Pockets for the Peptides

Although it was apparent from the early three-dimensional structural studies of HLA-A2 that the bound peptide was tightly engulfed by the binding site of the MHC-I mulecule, insight into the role of particular "pockets" of the MHC molecule derived primarily from a comparison of the structure of the MHC-I molecule HLA-A*0201 and the highly conserved HLA-A*6801 (24,35). A total of six putative

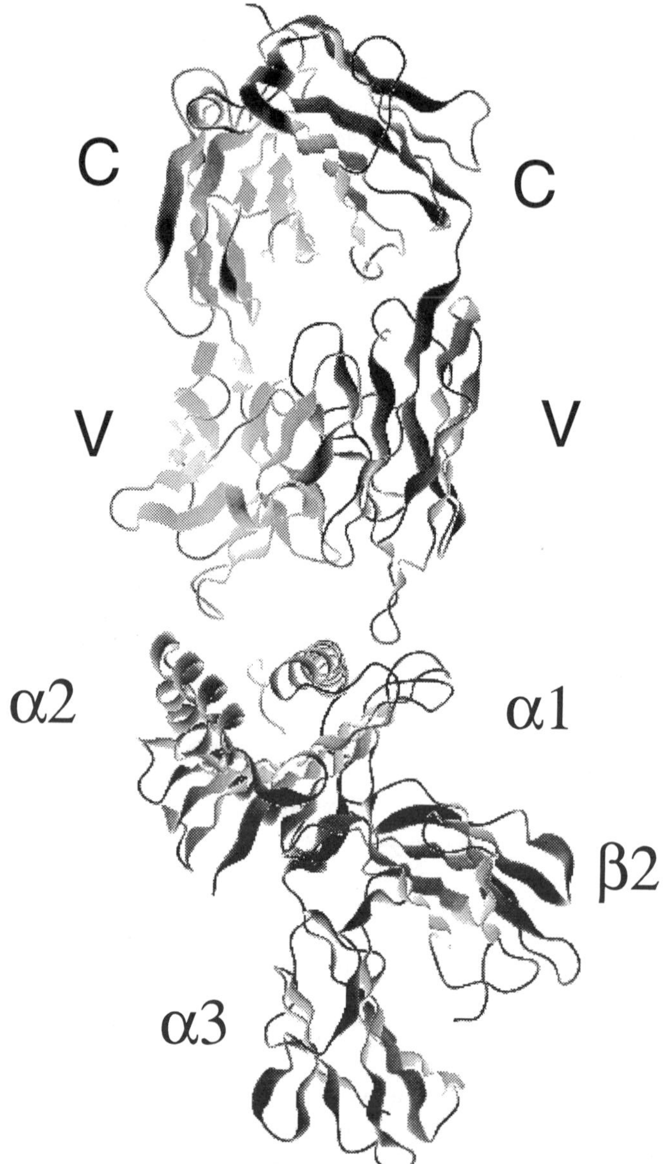

Figure 4 A model for the MHC-peptide/TCR interaction based on MHC and antibody Fab structures. Ribbon diagram of the antiphosphocholine antibody, MCP (116) is juxtaposed with the H-2K^b/VSV-8 complex (115). Such a model was suggested by Davis and Bjorkman (117).

binding pockets, named A through F, were identified and postulated to be available to accommodate the amino acid side chains of motif residues that might serve as anchors. Thus the overall view of the manner of peptide binding by MHC-I molecules is established: a general cleft formed by the $\alpha 1$ and $\alpha 2$ domains of the molecule serves as the peptide binding site; allelic differences in the size, charge, and hydrophobicity of pockets in this binding site contribute to the specificity of a particular MHC-I molecule for particular peptides. A number of studies—based on mouse MHC mutants, in vitro mutants, or polymorphic variants—have confirmed that the structure of particular pockets affects the self or presented peptide repertoire.

III. STRUCTURES AND MOTIFS OF BOUND PEPTIDES

The original description of the discrimination by T cells of MHC-I differences was based on recognition of allospecific target cells by cytolytic cells of distinct MHC types. Nevertheless, the most startling understanding of the function of CTL and MHC-I molecules in this cell-cell interaction derived from the seminal observations of Zinkernagel and Dougherty (36) that the recognition by MHC-I restricted, virus-specific CTL, required that the target (APC), infected with virus, and the effector (CTL) share MHC-I molecules. The same MHC restriction was observed for recognition even of target cells modified by chemical agents that covalently modify the target cells (37). Following the paradigms established by studies of the class II–restricted responses to protein antigens, in which it first was recognized that amino acid sequence differences in the antigens under study (such as myoglobin, cytochrome *c*, or hen egg lysozyme (see Ref. 38 for a comprehensive review)) governed the ability of T cells to discriminate different antigens. Subsequent studies indicated that MHC-I restricted T cells, raised against viruses, could be directed against synthetic peptides that represented specific stretches of amino acid sequences of the viral proteins (39,40). Using T-cell clones directed against the vesicular stomatitis virus protein as the assay, Van Bleek and Nathenson (41) purified the MHC-I molecule H-$2K^b$ from cells infected with the virus and determined the amino acid sequence of the peptide that copurified with the MHC-I molecule.

Rammensee and colleagues used acid elution and chemical degradative amino acid sequencing techniques and made the surprising finding that although the peptides that were eluted from the immunopurified MHC-I molecules were very heterogeneous in composition, they possessed specific amino acids (or only a limited representation) at particular positions in the peptide sequence—a specific footprint for the particular MHC-I molecule analyzed (42,43). Subsequently, isolation and sequencing methodologies have been significantly refined, including the introduction of mass spectroscopic techniques for the identification of the MHC-bound peptides (44). Thus, amino acid "motifs" characteristic of the bound peptides derived from many particular MHC-I molecules have been identified. An ever-expanding library of these motifs is being compiled (45).

Taking the primary amino acid sequence data of the bound peptides together with the known three-dimensional structure of the MHC-I molecules permits the formulation of a hypothesis that motif residues of MHC-binding peptides form the biochemical basis for the binding of peptides to the MHC-I in question. Thus, the "motif" serves as a guide to the "anchors," amino acid residues of the peptide that physically interact with the MHC molecule and contribute important binding energy. Table 1 offers an illustrative but noncomprehensive summary of several of the human and mouse MHC-I molecules and their binding motifs. The more common peptide motif is for there to be a preferred amino acid residue at position 2 of the peptide, and at position 9 (or the carboxyl terminus). The preferred carboxyl-terminal residue is usually a hydrophobic residue, although for several alleles this

Table 1 Examples of MHC Class I Peptide Motifs

	Peptide position									
	1	2	3	4	5	6	7	8	9	Reference
MHC molecule										
HLA-A1	E/D	P							Y	57
HLA-A2.1		L							V	42, 44
HLA-A3		L							Y.K	57
HLA-B27		R							R/K/Y	111
HLA-B53		P							Y	112
H-2K^b					F/Y				L	42, 45
H-2K^d		Y							L/I	42, 45
H-2D^b					N				M	42, 45
H-2D^d		G	P						I/L/M/F	113
H-2L^d		P							L/M/F/I	114

can be basic. No acidic carboxyl-terminal residues of self or antigenic peptides for any MHC-I molecule have yet been identified.

Using a variety of different binding assays and large panels of synthetic peptides, several laboratories have confirmed the observations that motif residues play an important role in the anchoring of peptides to their respective MHC molecules (46–49). However, it has also become clear that the quantitative interaction of a given peptide with a given MHC molecule is a sum of positive and negative contributions of each of the amino acids of the peptide (49,50), and a number of examples of peptides that either have the appropriate motifs but fail to bind or of those that lack the motif but bind respectably have been reported.

The peptides bound by the class I molecule are of limited length, most commonly 8 to 10 amino acid residues long (42–44), in contrast to the longer peptides bound by MHC II (44,51,52). This seems to be a direct consequence of the structure of the MHC class II molecule, which has open ends to its peptide-binding cleft and seems not to require interactions with amino- and carboxyl-terminal peptide groups for tight peptide binding (53). However, when care is taken to isolate MHC I molecules under gentle and nonbiased conditions (54,55), longer peptides can be identified. These may bind to the usually more restrictive MHC-I molecule by bulging in the middle, allowing the termini to still coordinate with the A and F pockets, or by extending past the pocket at the terminus. The structure of an HLA-A*0201/peptide complex which dangles a carboxyl-terminal glycine residue of the peptide beyond the binding cleft indicates that this is possible (56).

A. Predicting Antigenic Peptides by Motif Alignment

Knowledge of the motifs and length of peptides capable of binding to particular MHC-I molecules offers an alternative to screening of large numbers of synthetic peptides in the quest for peptides that might be used to prime against particular tumor antigens or intracellular pathogens. Exploiting such a strategy, one can take the amino acid sequence of a known antigenic protein, the known motif of the MHC-I–restricting element, and scan the antigen's sequence to identify candidate peptides that might bind the MHC of interest and thus would be expected to satisfy the first requirement for a peptide serving as an antigenic peptide: that it be presented by the MHC. Using this strategy, several laboratories have identified viral (57), parasite (58–60), and autoantigen MHC-I–restricted peptides (61). This is now a standard approach for identifying specific peptide antigens and is a baseline consideration in the development of vaccines directed against specific pathogens.

IV. BIOSYNTHESIS OF MHC-I

The class I MHC molecule, like other cell surface proteins, must proceed through a pathway of biosynthesis, disulfide bond formation, subunit assembly, core and terminal glycosylation, and transport from the rough endoplasmic reticulum, the site of initial translation, through the stacks of the *cis*, medial, and *trans* Golgi, to arrival of the mature molecule at the cell surface (62). The class I molecule should be considered a trimer, the heavy chain, β2-m, and peptide being the components of the fully assembled protein. Tissue culture cells defective in the production of β2-m fail to express the fully assembled protein at the cell surface, due to the failure of the MHC-I heavy chain to exit the endoplasmic reticulum (63,64). A similar phenotype is observed for "knockout" mice in which the β2-m gene has been rendered inactive by an engineered mutation (65,66).

The critical nature of the peptide's contribution to the native structure of the MHC-I molecule was emphasized by the observation that the phenotypic defect in some tumor cell lines could be corrected by exposure of the cells to high concentrations of synthetic peptides known to be capable of binding these MHC-I molecules (67,68). This cell surface–defective phenotype can also be remedied by cultivation of the cells at room temperature (69).

The MHC-I molecule accomplishes its sampling function along its biosynthetic route, and the pathway to its cell surface expression is distinct from that of the related MHC-II molecule (Fig. 5). The MHC-I heavy chain is synthesized on membrane-associated ribosomes and the nascent chain is vectorially delivered into the cisternae of the rough endoplasmic reticulum (ER), where the chain folds and assembles with the β2-microglobulin light chain and with one of a large number of peptides that have been delivered to the ER after being generated by proteolysis in the cytoplasm.

The peptides that provide the third subunit of the MHC-I molecule are generated in the cytoplasm, at least in part by proteolysis thought to be effected by the multisubunit proteasome complex (70,71). These peptide fragments must then be delivered to the endoplasmic reticulum by an active transport mechanism, which seems to be dependent on a dimeric structure composed of the TAP-1 and TAP-2 transporter proteins. These are endoplasmic reticulum membrane-bound molecules of the ATP-binding transporter molecules that are related structurally and perhaps functionally to the multidrug resistance proteins such as MDR (72).

Once in the cisternae of the endoplasmic reticulum, the peptides are quickly bound by nascent MHC-I molecules that have been cotranslationally delivered to the ER and are protected from β2-m and peptide engagement by a ER resident chaperonin molecule known as calnexin (73–79). The sequence of events now appears to be (a) cotranslational delivery of the nascent MHC-I molecule into the ER; (b) interaction of the nascent chain with calnexin, a resident ER chaperonin; (c)

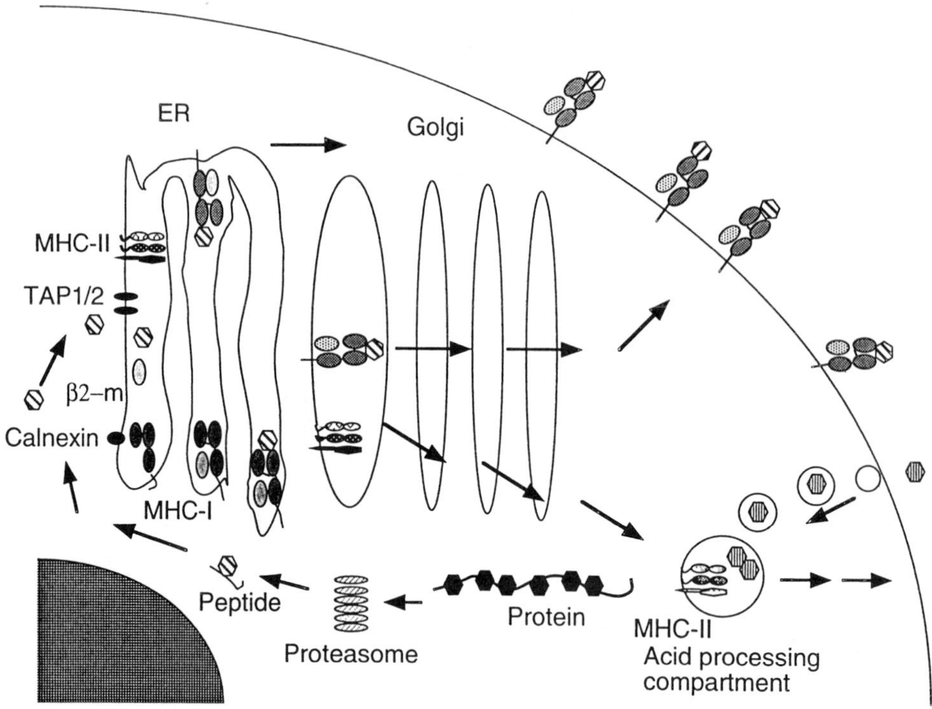

Figure 5 Pathways for antigen presentation.

release of MHC-I heavy chain by calnexin; (d) binding of β2-m; and (e) binding of peptides delivered into the ER from the cytoplasm via the TAP-1/TAP-2 transporter by the MHC-I β2-m complex. Core glycosylation takes place in the ER, and further carbohydrate maturation occurs with the transport of the MHC-I trimer through the *cis*, medial, and *trans* Golgi to the cell surface (see Fig. 5).

V. FUNCTION OF MHC-I

The true function of the MHC-I molecule can be viewed in several different cellular reactions: (a) as a recognition molecule for mature peripheral $\alpha\beta$ TCR bearing $CD8^+$ cytolytic T lymphocytes—MHC-I restricted and peptide specific as well as allospecific; (b) as the educating molecule on thymic antigen presenting cells that plays a critical role in the development of the MHC-I reactive T cells; and (c) in addition, MHC-I molecules have recently been shown to interact functionally with some receptors on NK cells, and a class of Fc receptors, though distinct in sequence, have the same protein fold as the MHC-I molecule.

A. MHC-I–Restricted, Peptide-Specific Recognition

Antigen-specific T lymphocytes that bear $\alpha\beta$ receptors can be primed by in vivo immunization by active infection with viruses or other intracellular parasites or with tumor cells (80). The $CD8^+$ cells elicited by such priming can then be shown to bear cytolytic activity against MHC-I–identical cells expressing the same viral antigen or tumor antigen. The crucial role of specific allelic forms of MHC-I molecules in the recognition by matched cytolytic effector cells was first demonstrated with transfectants of virus-infected target cells, and the amino terminal regions of the restricting MHC-I molecules were critical for the T-cell recognition (81). The current view of restricted recognition is that T-cell receptors, educated by passing through the thymus of the host, are negatively selected on self MHC, so that highly reactive cells are eliminated, and are positively selected on self MHC so that cells of moderate reactivity can enter the general peripheral circulation to patrol for cells expressing altered self. For infections by viruses or other intracellular parasites, the T cells bearing specific $\alpha\beta$ receptors that can engage novel MHC/peptide complexes can then be stimulated to effect cytolysis or lymphokine production. Thus, the host cells infected by the organism can be recognized and destroyed early in the life cycle of the infection, preventing the maturation of the infectious agent and arresting the infection.

This same theme is exploited in the immune surveillance role of MHC-I–restricted recognition (82). To elicit this phenomenon, the dysregulation of genes of the tumor cell leads to the aberrant expression of some self proteins, fragments of which associated with MHC-I are displayed in disproportionate amount on the surface of the tumor cell. In some cases, specific tumor-peptide antigens have been identified (83–85).

B. Allorecognition

Central to any discussion of MHC-I restricted T-cell recognition is the issue of allospecific interactions (86). The rejection of allografts is functionally related to the recognition of foreign MHC molecules on the graft by both MHC-I and MHC-II restricted T cells. MHC-II restricted T cells, activated by novel MHC-II/peptide complexes on the tumor provide lymphokine "help" for the MHC-I restricted cytolytic cells. These then are effector cells that dispense with the graft. This recognition is the "direct" allorecognition pathway and relies in part on the existence of MHC-II-expressing cells in the graft. In addition, processed antigens derived from the graft cells may also be displayed on host APCs in what has come to be called the "indirect" pathway. Thus, as the graft is infiltrated with host APCs, graft antigens are ingested, processed, and presented as modified self (self MHC-II/foreign antigen) for the activation of the host class II–restricted cell that then provides help for the MHC-I–restricted effectors. Direct pathway signals are due to recognition of non-self MHC-I and MHC-II in the CD8 and CD4-dependent responses respectively, while the indirect pathway is almost exclusively due to presentation of processed antigens via MHC-II.

The identification of peptides bound to MHC molecules has raised the question whether, in direct and cytotoxic recognition of MHC molecules on grafts, the donor T cells detect only MHC differences or whether the differences are partly or completely dependent on differences in the repertoire of peptides displayed by the allospecific MHC molecules. Current evidence (87,88) clearly indicates that the differences in peptides presented on MHC-I and conformational effects arising on the MHC-I peptide complex play a major role in the diversity and extent of allospecific recognition.

C. The MHC-I Molecule–A Role in NK Recognition

Natural killer (NK) cells were originally classified based on the apparent lack of MHC restriction in their recognition of target cells. Further experiments showed that differences in allelic MHC-I molecules controlled the apparent susceptibility of targets to NK lysis, and analysis of targets expressing parental and mutant MHC-I molecules indicated that the structure of the MHC-I was critical for the susceptibility or resistance to NK killing (89,90). Further evidence for MHC-I influence on NK recognition derived from the identification of a type II integral membrane glycoprotein, known in the mouse as Ly-49, that defined a subpopopulation of NK cells in the mouse (91). Remarkably, H-2D^d expressing targets are resistant to cytolysis by Ly-49$^+$ NK cells (92). In addition, NK cells (defined by the surface marker NK1.1) bearing the Ly-49 surface molecule, were not detected in mouse strains expressing H-2D^d, suggesting that the MHC-I molecule can play a role in the developmental expression of some NK markers. These and other data (91,93) are consistent with the view that the NK cell receptor Ly-49 receives a negative signal from cells bearing the MHC-I molecule H-2D^d. Other lines of evidence also point to other influences of MHC-I and their bound peptides on NK recognition (94).

D. H-2M3: A Different Kind of MHC-I Molecule

An intriguing tale of molecular detective work relates the characterization of the MHC-I–like molecule, H-2M3, encoded in the H-2T region of the mouse, that presents or serves as the restricting element for a maternally transmitted antigen, MTA. An antigen detected by CTL that was inherited via maternal transmission and was restricted by a gene that was linked to the MHC was finally characterized as being an antigen derived from the amino terminal peptide of the mitochondrial enzyme NADH dehydrogenase (95,96). As in bacteria, mitochondrial proteins are initiated by *N*-formyl methionine, which led to the postulate that the restricting element for the maternal, mitochondrial peptide antigen, had a preference for the binding of *N*-formyl peptides. This has been confirmed by synthetic peptide studies (97). In accord with this biochemical preference, the H-2M3 molecule has been shown to present a peptide antigen derived from the intracellular pathogen *Listeria monocytogenes* (98).

E. CD1: Paradigm Breaker

Another example of the diversity of MHC-related molecules that can be recognized with functional consequences by T lymphocytes is the CD1 molecule, originally described in the human and subsequently identified in the mouse as well. Recent evidence suggests that the CD1b molecule of the human can serve as the presentation element for a nonpeptidic antigen, namely a *Mycobacterium tuberculosis*–derived lipid (99). Thus, the paradigm that MHC-I molecules function in peptide binding and presentation of the complex to T cells is broken by the novel presentation function of this class I–related molecule. The T cells that recognize the lipid/CD1b complex in this example are $\alpha\beta^+$ but CD4 and CD8 negative. Further studies should clarify the breadth of the capacity of CD1 and related molecules to bind nonpeptide antigens, and the role that CD1-restricted T cells can play in normal immune responses, and T-cell selection.

F. The Rat Neonatal Fc Receptor: A Diverted MHC-I Structure?

Nature occasionally exploits the same fundamental protein fold to serve distinct functions. A relevant example is the rat neonatal Fc receptor, a molecule of the suckling rat, designed to transport maternal antibodies from the acidic lumen of the gut to the slightly basic bloodstream (100). Recently, the three-dimensional structure of this Fc receptor was shown to remarkably mimic that of the MHC-I molecule, although the site of the interaction with the immunoglobulin Fc takes advantage of other parts of the molecule than those used by the MHC-I for peptide or T-cell receptor binding (101,102). The molecule, unlike the MHC-I seems to have a closed peptide binding cleft, with no peptide occupying it. Other MHC-I related Fc receptors have recently been identified (103–105). The definition of their molecular physiology and possible cross-talk with classical MHC-I recognition remain to be determined.

VII. INTERACTIONS WITH T CELL RECEPTORS

Although the functional interaction of MHC molecules with T cell receptors has been appreciated for many years, the ability to use purified components to study the biochemistry of the binding reactions and the structure of the TCR has only been approached recently. In particular, engineered analogs of MHC molecules and T cell receptors have been used by several groups to evaluate the affinity and kinetics of binding of MHC peptide complexes to T-cell receptors, leading to the conclusion that these are moderate- to low-affinity interactions, characterized by rapid dissociation of the MHC–peptide complex from the T-cell receptor (106,107). In parallel with these physical chemical studies, recent progress has been made in the crystallization of T-cells receptor chains and domains (108,109), and the three-dimensional structure of a complete T-cell receptor β chain has recently been determined (110). This structure confirms the predictions that the TCR domains would be immunoglobulinlike but reveals a novel interaction of the V and C regions in this single chain structure. The location of superantigen binding sites appears to be contiguous with that of complementarity-determining regions (CDR) of this chain of the TCR. A future of precise understanding of TCR/MHC-peptide interactions awaits us.

VIII. SUMMARY

In this necessarily brief and superficial review of the MHC-I molecule and its function, I have attempted to convey some sense of the practical immunological importance of this family of molecules as well as a flavor for the molecular and cell biological aspects of its biology that we now understand. Little effort is needed to read beyond this and to realize that exciting experimental challenges lurk in all aspects of the immune system and that the complete understanding of the interactions of the MHC-I molecule with peptide, TCR, accessory molecules, and NK cell receptors is a microcosm of the molecular interactions in all complex biological processes. Not only will this knowledge be valid in its own right, but its implications for strategies for prevention and treatment of human disease will be evident.

ACKNOWLEDGMENTS

I thank Marie Jelonek for comments on the manuscript and the other members of my laboratory, Lisa Boyd, Charles Hoes, Sergei Khilko, Kannan Natarajan, Katarina Polakova, and Daniel Plaksin for their encouragement and forbearance.

REFERENCES

1. Sprent J. T Lymphocytes and the thymus. In: Paul WE, ed. Fundamental Immunology. New York: Raven Press, 1993:75–109.
2. Mossmann T, Coffman RL. Heterogeneity of cytokine secretion patterns and function of helper cells. Adv Immunol 1989; 46:111–147.
3. Germain RN, Margulies DH. The biochemistry and cell biology of antigen processing and presentation. Annu Rev Immunol 1993; 11:403–450.
4. Yokoyama WM. Natural killer cell receptors specific for major histocompatibility complex class I molecules. Proc Natl Acad Sci USA 1995; 92:3081–3085.
5. Cresswell P. Assembly, transport, and function of MHC class II molecules. Annu Rev Immunol 1994; 12:259–294.
6. Germain R. Immunology. The ins and outs of antigen processing and presentation. Nature 1986; 322:687–689.
7. Germain RN. MHC-dependent antigen processing and peptide presentation: providing ligands for T lymphocyte activation. Cell 1994; 76:287–299.
8. Malnati MS, Marti M, LaVaute T, et al. Processing pathways for presentation of cytosolic antigen to MHC class II-restricted T cells. Nature 1992; 357:702–704.
9. Klein J. Natural History of the Major Histocompatibility Complex. New York: Wiley-Interscience, 1986.
10. Gorer P. The detection of antigenic differences in mouse erythrocyte by the employment of immune sera. Br J Exp Pathol 1936; 17:42–50.
11. Madden DR. The three-dimensional structure of peptide-MHC complexes. Annu Rev Immunol 1995; 13:545–586.
12. Salter R, Norment A, Chen B, et al. Polymorphism in the alpha 3 domain of HLA-A molecules affects binding to CD8. Nature 1989; 338:345–347.
13. Potter T, Rajan T, Dick RD, Bluestone J. Substitution at residue 227 of H-2 class I molecules abrogates recognition by CD8-dependent, but not CD8-independent, cytotoxic T lymphocytes. Nature 1989; 337:73–75.
14. Rock K, Rothstein L, Gamble S, Benacerraf B. Reassociation with beta 2-microglobulin is necessary for Kb class I major histocompatibility complex binding of exogenous peptides. Proc Natl Acad Sci USA 1990; 87:7517–7521.
15. Otten GR, Bikoff E, Ribaudo RK, et al. Peptide and beta 2-microglobulin regulation of cell surface MHC class I conformation and expression. J Immunol 1992; 148:3723–3732.
16. Ploegh HL, Orr HT, Strominger JL. Molecular cloning of human histocompatibility antigen cDNA fragment. Proc Natl Acad Sci USA 1980; 77:6081–6085.
17. Sood AK, Pereira D, Weissman SM. Isolation and partial nucleotide sequence of a cDNA clone for human histocompatibility antigen HLA-B by use of an oligodeoxynucleotide primer. Proc Natl Acad Sci USA 1981; 78:616–620.
18. Moore K, Sher B, Sun Y, et al. DNA sequence of a gene encoding a BALB/c mouse Ld transplantation antigen. Science 1982; 215:679–682.
19. Evans G, Margulies D, Camerini-Otero R, et al. Structure and expression of a mouse major histocompatibility antigen gene, H-2Ld. Proc Natl Acad Sci USA 1982; 79:1994–1998.
20. Hood L, Steinmetz M, Goodenow R, et al. Genes of the major histocompatibility complex. Cold Spring Harb Symp Quant Biol 1983; 47(pt 2):1051–1065.

21. Schulze DH, Pease LR, Yokoyama K, et al. Diversity and polymorphism in the MHC appear to be generated by a copy mechanism. Transplant Proc 1983; 15:2009-2012.
22. Bjorkman PJ, Saper MA, Samraoui B, et al. Structure of the human class I histocompatibility antigen, HLA-A2. Nature 1987; 329:506–512.
23. Bjorkman PJ, Saper MA, Samraoui B, et al. The foreign antigen binding site and T cell recognition regions of class I histocompatibility antigens. Nature 1987; 329:512–518.
24. Saper MA, Bjorkman PJ, Wiley DC. Refined structure of the human histocompatibility antigen HLA-A2 at 2.6 A resolution. J Mol Biol 1991; 219:277–319.
25. Madden D, Gorga J, Strominger J, Wiley D. The structure of HLA-B27 reveals nonamer self-peptides bound in an extended conformation. Nature 1991; 353:321–325.
26. Fremont D, Matsumura M, Stura E, et al. Crystal structures of two viral peptides in complex with murine MHC class I H-2K^b. Science 1992; 257:919–927.
27. Madden DR, Garboczi DN, Wiley DC. The antigenic identity of peptide-MHC complexes: A comparison of the conformation of five viral peptides presented by HLA-A2. Cell 1994; 75.
28. Chang HC, Bao Z, Yao Y, et al. A general method for facilitating heterodimeric pairing between two proteins: Application to expression of alpha and beta T-cell receptor extracellular segments. Proc Natl Acad Sci USA 1994; 91:11408–11412.
29. Young AC, Nathenson SG, Sacchettini JC. Structural studies of class I major histocompatibility complex proteins: Insights into antigen presentation. FASEB J 1995; 9: 26–36.
30. Fremont DH, Stura EA, Matsumura M, et al. Crystal structure of an H-2K^b-ovalbumin peptide complex reveals the interplay of primary and secondary anchor positions in the major histocompatibility complex binding groove. Proc Natl Acad Sci USA 1995; 92:2479–2483.
31. Ajitkumar P, Geier SS, Kesari KV, et al. Evidence that multiple residues on both the alpha-helices of the class I MHC molecule are simultaneously recognized by the T cell receptor. Cell 1988; 54:47–56.
32. Padlan E, Silverton E, Sheriff S, et al. Structure of an antibody-antigen complex: Crystal structure of the HyHEL-10 Fab-lysozyme complex. Proc Natl Acad Sci USA 1989; 86:5938–5942.
33. Matsumura M, Fremont D, Peterson P, Wilson I. Emerging principles for the recognition of peptide antigens by MHC class I molecules. Science 1992; 257:927–934.
34. Zhang W, Young AC, Imarai M, et al. Crystal structure of the major histocompatibility complex class I H-2Kb molecule containing a single viral peptide: Implications for peptide binding and T-cell receptor recognition. Proc Natl Acad Sci USA 1992; 89: 8403–8407.
35. Garrett T, Saper M, Bjorkman P, et al. Specificity pockets for the side chains of peptide antigens in HLA-Aw68. Nature 1989; 342:692–696.
36. Zinkernagel R, Doherty P. Nature 1974; 248:701.
37. Shearer G. Cell mediated cytotoxicity to trinitrophenyl-modified syngeneic lymphocytes. Eur J Immunol 1974; 4:527–533.
38. Schwartz RH. Immune response (Ir) genes of the murine major histocompatibility complex. Adv Immunol 1986; 38:31–201.
39. Townsend A, Skehel J, Taylor P, Palese P. Recognition of influenza A virus nucleoprotein by an H-2 restricted cytotoxic T-cell clone. Virology 1984; 133:456–459.
40. Morrison L, Lukacher A, Braciale V, et al. Differences in antigen presentation to MHC class I- and class II-restricted influenza virus-specific cytolytic T lymphocyte clones. J Exp Med 1986; 163:903–921.
41. Van Bleek G, Nathenson S. Isolation of an endogenously processed immunodominant viral peptide from the class I H-2Kb molecule [see comments]. Nature 1990; 348:213–216.

42. Falk K, Rotzschke O, Rammensee H. Cellular peptide composition governed by major histocompatibility complex class I molecules. Nature 1990; 348:248–251.
43. Rotzschke O, Falk K, Deres K, et al. Isolation and analysis of naturally processed viral peptides as recognized by cytotoxic T cells. Nature 1990; 348:252–254.
44. Hunt D, Henderson R, Shabanowitz J, et al. Characterization of peptides bound to the class I MHC molecule HLA-A2.1 by mass spectrometry. Science 1992; 255:1261–1263.
45. Rammensee HG, Falk K, Rotzschke O. Peptides naturally presented by MHC class I molecules. Annu Rev Immunol 1993; 11:213–244.
46. Chen B, Parham P. Direct binding of influenza peptides to class I HLA molecules. Nature 1989; 337:743–745.
47. Boyd LF, Kozlowski S, Margulies DH. Solution binding of an antigenic peptide to a major histocompatibility complex class I molecule and the role of beta-2 microglobulin. Proc Natl Acad Sci USA 1992; 89:2242–2246.
48. Khilko SN, Corr M, Boyd LF, et al. Direct detection of major histocompatibility complex class-I binding to antigenic peptides using surface plasmon resonance–peptide immobilization and characterization of binding specificity. J Biol Chem 1993; 268: 15425–15434.
49. Ruppert J, Sidney J, Celis E, et al. Prominent role of secondary anchor residues in peptide binding to HLA-A2.1 molecules. Cell 1993; 74:929–937.
50. Parker KC, Bednarek MA, Coligan JE. Scheme for ranking potential HLA-A2 binding peptides based on independent binding of individual peptide side-chains. J Immunol 1994; 152:163–175.
51. Rudensky A, Preston-Hurlburt P, Hong S, et al. Sequence analysis of peptides bound to MHC class II molecules. Nature 1991; 353:622–627.
52. Chicz R, Urban R, Lane W, et al. Predominant naturally processed peptides bound to HLA-DR1 are derived from MHC-related molecules and are heterogeneous in size. Nature 1992; 358:764–768.
53. Stern LJ, Brown JH, Jardetzky TS, et al. Crystal structure of the human class II MHC protein HLA-DR1 complexed with an influenza virus peptide. Nature 1994; 368:215–221.
54. Urban RG, Chicz RM, Lane WS, et al. A subset of HLA-B27 molecules contains peptides much longer than nonamers. Proc Natl Acad Sci USA 1994; 91:1534–1538.
55. Joyce S, Kuzushima K, Kepecs G, et al. Characterization of an incompletely assembled major histocompatibility class I molecule ($H\text{-}2K^b$) associated with unusually long peptides: Implications for antigen processing and presentation. Proc Natl Acad Sci USA 1994; 91:4145–4149.
56. Collins EJ, Garboczi DN, Wiley DC. Three-dimensional structure of a peptide extending from one end of a class I MHC binding site. Nature 1994; 371:626–629.
57. DiBrino M, Tsuchida T, Turner RV, et al. HLA-A1 and HLA-A3 T cell epitopes derived from influenza virus proteins predicted from peptide binding motifs. J Immunol 1993; 151:5930–5935.
58. Lalvani A, Aidoo M, Allsopp CE, et al. An HLA-based approach to the design of a CTL-inducing vaccine against Plasmodium falciparum. Res Immunol 1994; 145:461–468.
59. Hill AV, Yates SN, Allsopp CE, et al. Human leukocyte antigens and natural selection by malaria. Philos Trans R Soc Lond B Biol Sci 1994; 346:379–385.
60. Hill AV, Elvin J, Willis AC, et al. Molecular analysis of the association of HLA-B53 and resistance to severe malaria. Nature 1992; 360:434–439.
61. Tsuchida T, Parker KC, Turner RV, et al. Autoreactive $CD8^+$ T-cell responses to human myelin protein-derived peptides. Proc Natl Acad Sci USA 1994; 91:10859–10863.

62. Krangel MS, Orr HT, Strominger JL. Assembly and maturation of HLA-A and HLA-B antigens in vivo. Cell 1979; 18:979.
63. Rosa F, Fellous M. Effect of interferon on human cell lines which do not express class I transplantation antigens: K562 and Daudi. Presence of a pseudo-messenger RNA of beta 2-microglobulin in Daudi cell line. CR Seances Acad Sci III 1982; 295:359.
64. Williams DB, Barber BH, Flavell RA, Allen H. Role of beta 2-microglobulin in the intracellular transport and surface expression of murine class I histocompatibility molecules. J Immunol 1989; 142:2796.
65. Zijlstra M, Li E, Sajjadi F, et al. Germ-line transmission of a disrupted beta 2-microglobulin gene produced by homologous recombination in embryonic stem cells. Nature 1989; 342:435–438.
66. Koller BH, Marrack P, Kappler JW, Smithies O. Normal development of mice deficient in beta 2W, MHC class I proteins, and $CD8^+$ T cells. Science 1990; 248:1227–1230.
67. Townsend A, Ohlen C, Foster L, et al. A mutant cell in which association of class I heavy and light chains is induced by viral peptides. Cold Spring Harb Symp Quant Biol 1989; 54(pt 1):299–308.
68. Townsend A, Ohlen C, Bastin J, et al. Association of class I major histocompatibility heavy and light chains induced by viral peptides. Nature 1989; 340:443–448.
69. Ljunggren H, Stam N, Ohlen C, et al. Empty MHC class I molecules come out in the cold. Nature 1990; 346:476–480.
70. Martinez C, Monaco J. Homology of proteasome subunits to a major histocompatibility complex-linked LMP gene. Nature 1991; 353:664–667.
71. Goldberg AL. Functions of the proteasome: The lysis at the end of the tunnel. Science 1995; 268:522–523.
72. Monaco JJ. Genes in the MHC that may affect antigen processing. Curr Opin Immunol 1992; 4:70–73.
73. Degen E, Williams D. Participation of a novel 88-kD protein in the biogenesis of murine class I histocompatibility molecules. J Cell Biol 1991; 112:1099–1115.
74. Degen E, Cohen-Doyle M, Williams D. Efficient dissociation of the p88 chaperone from major histocompatibility complex class I molecules requires both beta 2-microglobulin and peptide. J Exp Med 1992; 175:1653–1661.
75. Rajagopalan S, Brenner MB. Calnexin retains unassembled major histocompatibility complex class I free heavy chains in the endoplasmic reticulum. J Exp Med 1994; 180: 407–412.
76. Sugita M, Brenner MB. An unstable beta 2-microglobulin: Major histocompatibility complex class I heavy chain intermediate dissociates from calnexin and then is stabilized by binding peptide. J Exp Med 1994; 180:2163–2171.
77. Ware FE, Vassilakos A, Peterson PA, et al. The molecular chaperone calnexin binds Glc(1)Man(9)GlcNAc(2) oligosaccharide as an initial step in recognizing unfolded glycoproteins. J Biol Chem 1995; 270:4697–4704.
78. Jackson MR, Cohendoyle MF, Peterson PA, Williams DB. Regulation of MHC class-I transport by the molecular chaperone, calnexin (P88, IP90). Science 1994; 263:384–387.
79. Suk W-K, Cohen-Doyle MF, Fruh K, et al. Interaction of MHC class I molecules with the transporter associated with antigen processing. Science 1994; 264.
80. McMichael A, Klenerman P, Rowland-Jones S, et al. Recognition of viral antigens at the cell surface. Cancer Surv 1995; 22:51–62.
81. Reiss C, Evans G, Margulies D, et al. Allospecific and virus-specific cytolytic T lymphocytes are restricted to the N or C1 domain of H-2 antigens expressed on L cells after DNC-mediated gene transfer. Proc Natl Acad Sci USA 1983; 80:2709–2712.
82. Boon T, Cerottini JC, Van den Eynde B, et al. Tumor antigens recognized by T

lymphocytes genes coding for tumor rejection antigens: perspectives for specific immunotherapy. Annu Rev Immunol 1994; 12:337–365.
83. Wolfel T, Van Pel A, Brichard V, et al. Two tyrosinase nonapeptides recognized on HLA-A2 melanomas by autologous cytolytic T lymphocytes. Eur J Immunol 1994; 24: 759–764.
84. Szikora JP, Van Pel A, Boon T. Tum- mutation P35B generates the MHC-binding site of a new antigenic peptide. Immunogenetics 1993; 37:135–138.
85. Brasseur F, Marchand M, Vanwijck R, et al. Human gene MAGE-1, which codes for a tumor-rejection antigen, is expressed by some breast tumors. Int J Cancer 1992; 52: 839–841.
86. Auchincloss H, Sachs DH. Transplantation and graft rejection. In: Paul WE, ed. Fundamental Immunology. New York: Raven Press, 1993:1099–1141.
87. Chattopadhyay S, Theobald M, Biggs J, Sherman LA. Conformational differences in major histocompatibility complex-peptide complexes can result in alloreactivity. J Exp Med 1994; 179:213–219.
88. Sherman LA, Chattopadhyay S. The molecular basis of allorecognition. Annu Rev Immunol 1993; 11:385–402.
89. Storkus W, Alexander J, Payne J, et al. The alpha 1/alpha 2 domains of class I HLA molecules confer resistance to natural killing. J Immunol 1989; 143:3853–3857.
90. Storkus W, Alexander J, Payne J, et al. Reversal of natural killing susceptibility in target cells expressing transfected class I HLA genes. Proc Natl Acad Sci USA 1989; 86:2361–2364.
91. Yokoyama WM. Recognition structures on natural killer cells. Curr Opin Immunol 1993; 5:67–73.
92. Karlhofer FM, Ribaudo RK, Yokoyama WM. The interaction of Ly-49 with H-2Dd globally inactivates natural killer cell cytolytic activity. Trans Assoc Am Phys 1992; 105:72–85.
93. Kane KP. Ly-49 mediates EL4 lymphoma adhesion to isolated class I major histocompatibility complex molecules. J Exp Med 1994; 179:1011–1015.
94. Malnati MS, Peruzzi M, Parker KC, et al. Peptide specificity in the recognition of MHC class I by natural killer cell clones. Science 1995; 267:1016–1018.
95. Shawar SM, Cook RG, Rodgers JR, Rich RR. Specialized functions of MHC class I molecules: I. An N-formyl peptide receptor is required for construction of the class I antigen Mta. J Exp Med 1990; 171:897–912.
96. Lindahl KF, Hermel E, Loveland BE, Wang C-R. Maternally transmitted antigen of mice: A model transplantation antigen. Annu Rev Immunol 1991; 9:351–371.
97. Vyas JM, Shawar SM, Rodgers JR, et al. Biochemical specificity of H-2M3a. Stereospecificity and space-filling requirements at position 1 maintain N-formyl peptide binding. J Immunol 1992; 149:3605–3611.
98. Pamer EG, Wang CR, Flaherty L, et al. H-2M3 presents a Listeria monocytogenes peptide to cytotoxic T lymphocytes. Cell 1992; 70:215–223.
99. Beckman EM, Porcelli SA, Morita CT, et al. Recognition of a lipid antigen by CD1-restricted alpha beta$^+$ T cells. Nature 1994; 372:691–694.
100. Simister NE, Mostov KE. An Fc receptor structurally related to MHC class I antigens. Nature 1989; 337:184–187.
101. Burmeister WP, Gastinel LN, Simister NE, et al. Crystal structure at 2.2 angstrom resolution of the MHC- related neonatal Fc receptor. Nature 1994; 372:336–343.
102. Burmeister WP, Huber AH, Bjorkman PJ. Crystal structure of the complex of rat neonatal Fc receptor with Fc. Nature 1994; 372:379–383.
103. Blumberg RS, Koss T, Story CM, et al. A major histocompatibility complex class I-related Fc receptor for IgG on rat hepatocytes. J Clin Invest 1995; 95:2397–2402.
104. Story CM, Mikulska JE, Simister NE. A major histocompatibility complex class I-like

Fc receptor cloned from human placenta: possible role in transfer of immunoglobulin G from mother to fetus. J Exp Med 1994; 180:2377–2381.
105. Ahouse JJ, Hagerman CL, Mittal P, et al. Mouse MHC class I-like Fc receptor encoded outside the MHC. J Immunol 1993; 151:6076–6088.
106. Matsui K, Boniface JJ, Steffner P, et al. Kinetics of T-cell receptor binding to peptide/I-Ek complexes: Correlation of the dissociation rate with T-cell responsiveness. Proc Natl Acad Sci USA 1994; 91:12862–12866.
107. Corr M, Slanetz AE, Boyd LF, et al. T cell receptor-MHC class I peptide interactions: Affinity, kinetics, and specificity. Science 1994; 265:946–949.
108. Fields BA, Ysern X, Poljak RJ, et al. Crystallization and preliminary x-ray diffraction study of a bacterially produced T-cell receptor V alpha domain. J Mol Biol 1994; 239: 339–341.
109. Boulot G, Bentley GA, Karjalainen K, Mariuzza RA. Crystallization and preliminary x-ray diffraction analysis of the beta-chain of a T-cell antigen receptor. J Mol Biol 1994; 235:795–797.
110. Bentley GA, Boulot G, Karjalainen K, Mariuzza RA. Crystal structure of the beta chain of a T cell antigen receptor. Science 1995; 267:1984–1987.
111. Jardetzky TS, Lane WS, Robinson RA, et al. Identification of self peptides bound to purified HLA-B27. Nature 1991; 353:326–329.
112. Hill AVS, Elvin J, Willis AC, et al. Molecular analysis of the association of HLA-B53 and resistance to severe malaria. Nature 1992; 360:434–439.
113. Corr M, Boyd LF, Padlan EA, Margulies DH. H-2D^d exploits a four residue peptide binding motif. J Exp Med 1993; 178:1877–1892.
114. Corr M, Boyd LF, Frankel SR, et al. Endogenous peptides of a soluble major histocompatibility complex class I molecule, H-2L^{d}s: Sequence motif, quantitative binding, and molecular modeling of the complex. J Exp Med 1992; 176:1681–1692.
115. Fremont DH, Matsumura M, Stura EA, et al. Crystal structures of two viral peptides in complex with murine MHC class I H-2K^b. Science 1992; 257:919–927.
116. Satow Y, Cohen GH, Padlan EA, Davies DR. Phosphocholine binding immunoglobulin Fab McPC603: An x-ray diffraction study at 2.7 A. J Mol Biol 1986; 190:593–604.
117. Davis M, Bjorkman P. T-cell antigen receptor genes and T-cell recognition. Nature 1988; 334:395.

3

MHC Class II: Structure and Function

Eric O. Long
National Institute of Allergy and Infectious Diseases
National Institutes of Health
Rockville, Maryland

I. INTRODUCTION

The discovery of MHC class II molecules and of their critical function in immune responses has followed a long and arduous path, starting with genetic and serological studies that led to a biochemical characterization of these molecules and the cloning of their genes, culminating finally in the elucidation of atomic structures for class II molecules and in a detailed understanding of their function at the molecular level. Following the same path for a chapter on MHC class II may provide a historical perspective but would not result in the most coherent and straightforward story. Rather, the recently solved three-dimensional structure of a class II molecule and the molecular organization of the MHC class II gene complex provide a better background from which to understand MHC class II function. Such an approach will better illustrate how class II function is achieved through the biochemical properties and the extensive allelic polymorphism of class II molecules, even though it is the latter property that led to the initial discovery of MHC class II. The references cited in this chapter are review articles with the exception of a few recent or seminal papers.

MHC class II molecules, expressed primarily on specialized antigen-presenting cells, are crucial for most immune responses because they provide ligands for the activation of $CD4^+$ T cells, which, in turn, provide lymphokines that stimulate and regulate both humoral and cellular responses. $CD4^+$ T cells recognize peptides bound to MHC class II molecules (1). Most of these peptides are derived from the intracellular processing of antigens that have been delivered to acidic endosomal compartments where peptides load onto class II molecules. The peptide binding site is formed by the association of the two amino-terminal domains of the class II α and β chain heterodimer. At the cell surface, stable complexes of class II molecules with peptides can result in specific recognition by T cells through an elaborate interaction between the variable regions of the T-cell receptor (TCR) and the peptide/class II surface as well as additional conserved contacts between the CD4 coreceptor molecule and an exposed region on class II molecules. The genetic control of immune responses, discovered long before the biochemical identification of class II molecules, can now be beautifully explained by the position of polymorphic amino acid residues in the class II molecular structure. The majority of polymorphic residues affect the shape and chemical properties of the peptide binding site and thus control the repertoire of peptides that can be displayed at the cell surface. Alloreactivity is caused not only by differences between class II molecules from outbred individuals but also by the different peptides that bind to these class II molecules, even though these peptides are selected from the same set of mostly nonpolymorphic self proteins. The enormous strength of alloresponses is due to the vast array of different peptide sequences presented by different alleles of class II molecules.

It is very fortunate that such a clear picture of MHC class II function has been acquired, for it provides tools to study the mechanisms of antigen presentation and a firm basis on which to develop strategies to prevent autoimmunity and alloreactivities after transplantation.

II. STRUCTURE

A. Molecular Structure

Similarities in the function, domain organization, and biochemical properties of MHC class I and class II molecules led to the prediction that class II molecules would adopt a fold and overall structure similar to that of class I molecules. The elucidation of the crystal structure of an MHC class I molecule in 1987 revealed that the peptide binding site was formed by the pairing of the first two domains of the class I heavy chain into an eight-stranded β sheet over which two α helices extended. The peptide binds between the two helices and over the β sheet. A very similar structure for class II was elucidated in 1993, confirming the earlier structural predictions but revealing also interesting differences, particularly in the way peptides bind, a distinction made clear when the structure of a class II molecule bound to a single defined peptide was obtained (2). The major difference with class I molecules is that the peptide can extend outside of the binding cleft of class II molecules at either end. Whereas class I molecules bind peptides of defined length, mostly 8 to 10 residues long, class II molecules can accommodate a wider range of peptide sizes, including peptides with staggered ends.

The reason for this class I–class II dichotomy is that peptide binding to class I molecules occurs while protein folding is still taking place, whereas class II molecules acquire peptides much later in their biosynthetic life (1). To ensure that the cytotoxic response mediated by class I-restricted $CD8^+$ T cells is directed solely at cells expressing foreign or mutant proteins, a very stringent mechanism has evolved to load endogenous peptides onto class I molecules. Most of the hydrogen bonds between peptide and class I occur at the two ends of the peptide with nonpolymorphic (i.e. conserved) residues of the class I heavy chain. In contrast, most hydrogen bonds between peptide and class II molecules are distributed along the entire peptide and involve main-chain atoms rather than side chains of the peptide. Except for a single residue (Gln 9 on the β chain), all of the conserved residues involved in hydrogen bonding with the peptide are on the two α helices. The ability of class II molecules to bind peptides extending outside of the binding groove has two interesting implications. First, class II molecules have the ability to capture denatured proteins prior to their cleavage into shorter peptide fragments. Second, the invariant chain associated with newly synthesized class II molecules may occupy the peptide binding site. Both of these are discussed further below.

How is specificity of peptide binding achieved? The hydrogen bonds between peptide main-chain atoms and conserved class II residues obviously will not impart specificity of binding. As for class I, several of the peptide side chains appear to fit into pockets at the bottom of the peptide binding site. These contacts increase the binding affinity and provide a specific orientation of the peptide such that the upper face of the peptide can be recognized by T cells.The peptide side chains that point down into class II pockets are referred to as anchor residues. Although obvious in the crystal structure of the HLA-DR1 molecule complexed with a peptide from the influenza virus A hemagglutinin protein, such anchor residues had not been easily identified from the sequencing of peptides eluted from class II molecules because of their staggered ends. A more powerful approach for the identification of peptide motifs that bind specific class II molecules was based on binding of libraries of random peptide sequences and sequencing of those peptides recovered after binding to class II molecules (3). Polymorphic residues in the α and β chains of class II molecules define the specific pockets. In the case of the most prevalent class II molecule in humans, namely HLA-DR, only the β chain is polymorphic. The α chain does not contribute to the specificity of peptide binding, even though it provides important conserved contact residues.

An intriguing result from the crystal structure of class II molecules is that these heterodimeric molecules crystallized as a dimer of dimers, in which each $\alpha\beta$ heterodimer paired specifically with another. Contacts between class II molecules were at four interfaces. First, residues 49-55 of the β1 domain form homotypic contacts with a second molecule. Second, a homotypic interaction also occurs between residues 88 and 111 of the α2 domain. Finally, two identical interfaces occur in the membrane-proximal domains, between seven residues in the β2 domain and seven residues on the α2 domain (4). Although there has been much speculation on the significance of these dimers, experimental evidence for their existence at the cell surface of antigen-presenting cells or for their role in T-cell stimulation is still lacking.

Most class II–restricted T-cell responses are critically dependent on the binding of the CD4 coreceptor of the TCR to class II molecules. CD4 binding to class II molecules is of low affinity and may require multimerization at the cell surface to provide the necessary signal. An exposed loop, including residues 137-143 on the β2 domain, of class II molecules is critical for binding to the first Ig domain (D1) of CD4.

B. Primary Structure and Isotypes

Class II molecules consist of two transmembrane glycoproteins, the α and β chains, that are tightly but noncovalently associated. The gene exons for each chain reflect their domain organization (Fig. 1). The first extracellular domain, following a

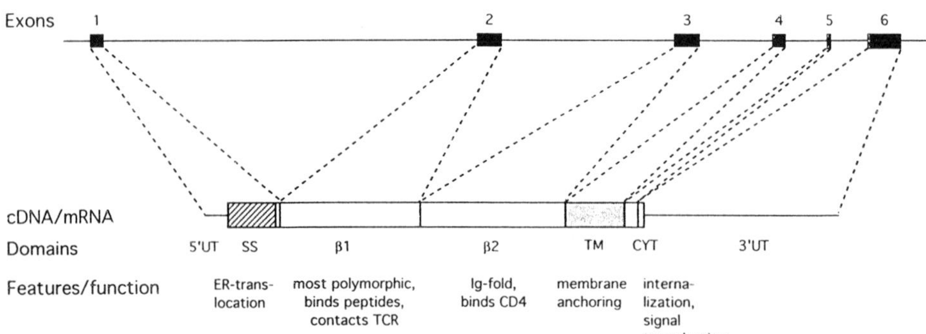

Figure 1 Domain organization of an MHC class II β chain. Top: Exon-intron organization of a class II β-chain gene. Middle: Primary structure of a class II β mRNA. The coding region is indicated by a box. The signal sequence is hatched and the transmembrane region is shaded. Bottom: Properties associated with the respective domains. Abbreviations: UT, untranslated region; SS, signal sequence; TM, transmembrane region; CYT, cytoplasmic tail; ER, endoplasmic reticulum; Ig, immunoglobulin.

signal sequence encoded in a separate exon, carries most of the allelic polymorphism. The second domain, less polymorphic, carries structural information for interaction with CD4. The next domain consists of the connecting peptide, which links the Ig-like domains with the plasma membrane, and a transmembrane region with unique features. In addition to the usual hydrophobic residues, these transmembrane regions contain several glycine residues involved in the α/β chain interaction (5). Thus, the membrane-spanning segments of class II α and β chains are not independent and contribute to the stability of heterodimers. Finally, the cytoplasmic tails are encoded by one or two exons, for the α and for some of the β chains, respectively. Despite their short length, these cytoplasmic tails carry important information for internalization from the cell surface (6) and for intracellular signaling (7).

Most animal species studied express multiple class II molecules encoded in nonallelic genes (isotypes). Mice carry two classical class II isotypes, the I-A and I-E molecules, each composed of polymorphic α and β chains. Curiously, many wild strains of mice lack expression of the I-E isotype, due to different mutations in the E_α and E_β genes. The reason for this high frequency of defective I-E alleles is not clear, particularly considering that some antigens stimulate T-cell responses that are uniquely I-E-restricted (8). The closest structural counterparts of I-A and I-E molecules in humans are the HLA-DQ and HLA-DR molecules, respectively. Strong sequence conservation between such pairs (e.g., I-E and HLA-DR) implies that these genes evolved from a common ancestor that preceded mammalian radiation. However, this structural conservation is not reflected at the functional level. First, whereas I-E molecules can be dispensable in many strains of mice, HLA-DR is the predominant class II–restricting element in human immune responses. Second, an additional isotype, called HLA-DP, for which there is no expressed counterpart in mice, is used in humans. Finally, most human chromosomes carry two expressed copies of HLA-DR β genes. The high degree of allelic polymorphism in these genes and the outbred nature of human populations are such that many individuals express up to eight different class II molecules: four isotypes (HLA-DP, HLA-DQ, and two HLA-DR molecules) with two alleles each. The reported pairings in *trans* between allelic forms of HLA-DQ and mixed isotypic pairing between DR α and DQ β chains provide an even greater potential for diversity within individuals. Such diversity is presumably useful in providing a wider range of potential immune responses. It is also possible that different isotypes have specialized functions. It is intriguing that very few HLA-DQ-restricted T cells have been described in human immune responses, even though HLA-DQ alleles have been often linked to increased disease susceptibilities. However, such allelic and isotypic diversity is not found in all species.

The cytoplasmic domains of class II molecules vary considerably between isotypes, even though sequence conservation exists between species (e.g., HLA-DR and I-E), suggesting that isotypes of class II may serve different but conserved functions.

III. GENETICS

A. Molecular Organization

Early genetic studies defined the HLA-D region—distinct from the HLA class I loci A, B, and C—as a locus controlling the proliferation of mixed lymphocyte cultures derived from HLA class I-matched donors. It took another 15 years to obtain a full molecular description of the genes in HLA-D. A combination of molecular cloning, DNA sequencing, and of mapping using pulse-field gel electrophoresis to resolve large DNA fragments resulted in a molecular map of the human MHC class II region, situated on the short arm of chromosome 6 at 6p21 (Fig. 2). In addition to the expected genes encoding the α and β chains of HLA-DP, -DQ, and -DR molecules, there are several inactive genes that are either pseudogenes (e.g., HLA-DPA2) or essentially nontranscribed genes (e.g., HLA-DQA2). The DR subregion is particularly complex and exists in different configurations on human chromosomes. In contrast to the DP and DQ subregions, there is only one α chain gene in

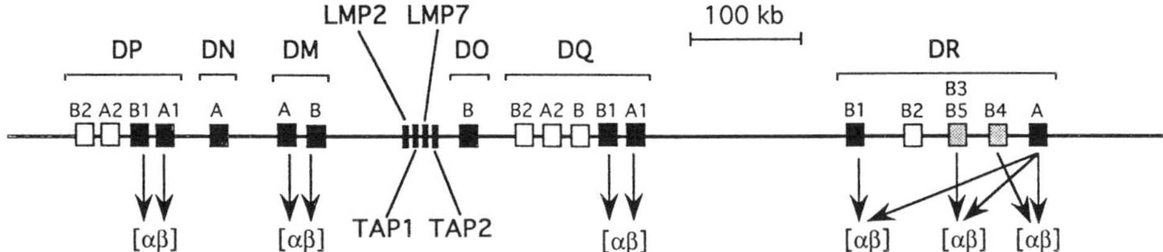

Figure 2 Molecular map of the human MHC class II region. The chromosome 6 centromere is to the left, class I genes and telomere are to the right. Genes, grouped within the subregions DM, DN, DO, DP, DQ, and DR and in the LMP-TAP cluster are represented by boxes. Distances are roughly to scale, but the size of genes is not. Following official HLA nomenclature, genes encoding α chains are designated A, those encoding β chains B. Filled boxes represent functional genes, open boxes represent nonfunctional genes, and shaded boxes represent genes that are either expressed or not, depending on the haplotype. Most haplotypes carry two expressed DRB genes: B1 and either B3, B4, or B5. The known $\alpha\beta$ pairs produced by expression of class II genes are indicated.

DR. Interestingly, the DR α is unique among class II α chains in that it does not display allelic polymorphism except for a conservative amino acid change in the transmembrane region. Most extended haplotypes include two expressed DR β genes and one or two pseudogenes. However, the DR1 and DR8 haplotypes express only one DR β chain. An additional and often confusing complication is that the most polymorphic DR β chain is encoded by the DRB1 gene except in the DR2 haplotypes, which can be subdivided into subtypes that differ mostly in the product of the DRB5 gene.

The control of class II gene expression is complex. Natural mutations that cause defects in class II expression, resulting in severe combined immunodeficiencies, have been very useful for the identification of important transcription factors (9). Shared promoter sequences among class II genes and the invariant chain gene ensure coordinate regulation of their expression. Besides constitutive expression in antigen-presenting cells, there is inducible expression of these genes in many different cell types after treatment with interferon-γ. A central transcription control element, CIITA, is required for both the inducible and constitutive expression of class II genes.

The mouse MHC class II region was called the H-2 *I* region, containing *Ir* (immune response) genes that control the strength of immune responses to various antigens. Recombinational analysis had divided the *I* region into I-A and I-E as well as other subregions such as *I-J* that turned out not to exist once the entire *I* region was isolated with molecular clones (10). The mouse class II molecules, also called Ia (*I*-region–associated) antigens, are encoded by α and β genes in the *I* region. Interestingly, a recombination hotspot falls right within the I-Eβ gene and defines the genetic boundary between the I-A and I-E subregions. The overall mouse class II gene organization mirrors that in man with some differences. The mouse counterparts of the HLA-DP, -DQ, and -DR subregions in man have the same orientation: centromeric-telomeric. There are fewer pseudogenes and expressed class II genes in mouse. The Aβ_3 is a pseudogene related to HLA-DP. The I-A molecules are encoded by a single pair of transcribed genes for the α and β chains. A pair of transcribed genes for the α and β chains of I-E are also present, but with the addition of a transcribed gene called Eβ_2, whose function has remained unknown. Many mouse strains, including wild mice, do not express functional I-E molecules yet thrive in their natural environment. This fact, along with the replacement of the HLA-DP ancestor by a pseudogene, clearly shows that during evolution different class II isotypes have been favored to predominate in their usage.

B. The MHC Class II Region Contains Nonclassical Class II Genes and Other Genes Related to MHC Function

One of the most fascinating rewards in the molecular analysis of the MHC class II region was the discovery of several other genes that are either nonclassical class II or structurally unrelated genes. Most of them appear to be involved in some aspect of MHC function.

The first nonclassical class II genes found were DNA and DOB. Although separated by about 200 kb, and despite a different regulation of expression, this new pair of α and β chains suggested that they may represent a new class II heterodimer. Whereas expression of protein from these genes has not been demonstrated in humans, similar genes were found in mice and shown to encode a new heterodimeric class II molecule (11). The function of these molecules is still unknown, but their structural similarity with classical class II molecules suggests that they may be involved in the presentation of specialized antigens, possibly to specialized T cells. This situation may be analogous to that described for the presentation to T cells of special antigens by the nonclassical class I CD1 molecules (12). The greater conservation in expression of DOB than other class II genes, like HLA-DP, suggests that this molecule has some important function.

The DMA and DMB genes were later found in both human and mouse. The domain organization of these two molecules is the same as that of class II molecules, but the sequence similarity indicated that these genes were as distantly related to class II genes as they were to class I genes. The function of DM molecules was discovered later, with the surprising finding that DM genes encoded the long-sought important function for class II–restricted antigen presentation that had been defined and mapped in mutant cells (13).

Several other genes between the DP and the DQ subregions were identified by molecular cloning and their function defined by reverse genetics. Interestingly, they all turned out to be involved in some aspect of antigen presentation (14). However, unlike DM, these genes play important roles in the pathway of class I–restricted antigen presentation. Two of them each encode a subunit of a heterodimeric ATP-dependent transporter molecule called TAP (for transporter associated with antigen presentation). TAP is essential for the delivery of peptides from the cytosol to the lumen of the endoplasmic reticulum where they bind to MHC class I molecules. This transport requires ATP hydrolysis and is not particularly selective for peptide sequences except for lengths of about 7 to 20 residues. Two other genes, called LMP2 and LMP7, encode subunits of the proteasome, a multisubunit proteolytic complex that degrades ubiquitinated cytosolic proteins. These MHC-encoded subunits are alternate subunits that substitute for two of the constitutive subunits of the proteasome complex. Upregulation of the LMP2 and LMP7 gene expression by interferon-γ leads to a change in the subunit composition of the proteasome complex and a change of substrate specificity such that the carboxy-terminal ends of peptides become optimal for binding to class I molecules.

C. Allelic Polymorphism, HLA Class II Typing, and Disease Susceptibilities

The MHC system was discovered because of its extreme allelic polymorphism. No gene complex displays as much polymorphism as the MHC. Graft rejection and graft-versus-host disease (GVHD) are both caused by mismatches in MHC alleles between donor and recipient. Many theories have been proposed to explain the MHC polymorphism and what selective pressures operated on it during evolution. The mutation rate and the type of mutations in the coding regions of MHC genes suggest that a positive selection was driving the polymorphism, particularly in the first domain of the class II α and β molecules. The selective pressure for MHC polymorphism at the individual level can only be that heterozygosity provides an advantage. The extensive degree of allelic polymorphism may also provide some advantage to the species. Presumably, a greater number of alleles within a population provides a wider range of potential immune responses and protects the species from newly emerging pathogens. Interestingly, existing polymorphic alleles of class II molecules represent ancient alleles that have been maintained over long evolutionary time and inherited from precursor species.

Sequence comparisons between polymorphic alleles in humans and those in different species (in particular for the most polymorphic DRB1 gene) led to the *transspecies* hypothesis for the origin of existing alleles (15). This hypothesis proposes that ancestral alleles preexisted current species and that they have been maintained by selective pressure for a very long time. Analysis of the molecular clock in the polymorphic class II genes revealed that these genes did not mutate at a significantly greater rate than nonpolymorphic genes but that allelic polymorphism is ancient. Such molecular evolution studies have led to interesting conclusions about the origin of human populations and have posed a challenge to the prevailing view that all humans are descendants of an ancestral woman who lived in Africa about 200,000 years ago (based on sequence comparisons of maternally inherited mitochondrial DNA). The data for class II genes suggest rather that preexisting human populations were replaced by populations migrating from Africa (16).

Typing of HLA class II alleles was first achieved using serological reagents. Most of the HLA typing done today for clinical purposes is still based on serological reagents. Several alleles for HLA-DR and for HLA-DQ were described serologically. Only later, cellular typing using primed T cells revealed the existence of a third subset of human class II molecules called HLA-DP. Such cellular typing also led to the identification of distinct alleles within single serological specificities (e.g., DR4 represents several closely related alleles). Molecular typing, initially done by restriction fragment length polymorphism (RFLP) and later replaced by the polymerase chain reaction (PCR) amplification and oligonucleotide-specific hybridization, has refined serological typing of HLA-DR and HLA-DQ and cellular typing for HLA-DP. The 18 DR specificities identified with serological reagents have been expanded to 56 alleles distinguishable by sequence differences in the DR β chain. The 9 DQ specificities have been expanded into 13 DQ α and 17 DQ β sequences. Similarly, the 6 DP specificities can be divided into 4 DP α and 21 DP β sequences. These numbers are based on the 1990 World Health Organization (WHO) update on HLA typing (17), and they keep increasing. The usefulness of such refined molecular typing is that it can help to improve matching between donor and recipients of allografts.

Another clear advantage of molecular typing is that it led to a more accurate definition of the correlation between certain diseases associated with MHC class II and specific HLA class II alleles and isotypes (18,19). A great many diseases are more prevalent among individuals who carry particular HLA class II alleles. Most of these diseases have an autoimmune component. In contrast, only a few diseases have shown association with HLA class I alleles, HLA-B27 being the most frequently associated allele. Interpretation of such associations has been difficult because of the strong linkage disequilibrium between polymorphic HLA class II alleles. Linkage disequilibrium (in other words, the association of several closely linked alleles on haplotypes found in populations) precluded the attribution of a predisposition to a given locus because the phenotype (or disease) may be caused by another locus that remained linked to the first throughout the population. Even if selective pressure is applied to one locus, closely linked loci may have also been fixed in a population by "hitchhiking" with the one under selection. Molecular typing has clarified and refined some of these associations. A good example is provided by insulin-dependent diabetes mellitus (IDDM), which is associated primarily with the HLA-DR3 and -DR4 alleles. The finding that the association with HLA-DR4 was restricted to a subset of DR4 alleles, distinguishable only by sequence or by T-cell responses, suggested that the association may be due to the closely linked polymorphic HLA-DQ molecules.

HLA disease associations are not only positive, as "protective" alleles have also been described, such as HLA-DR2 for IDDM. Combination of alleles matter also, as DR3 and DR4 homozygous, as well as DR3,4 heterozygous individuals, are at even greater risk of diabetes relative to DR3,- and DR4,- individuals. A strong correlation was established between the presence of a given amino acid at position 57 of the DQ β chain and resistance to IDDM, whereas several other amino acids at that position are associated with an increased risk for IDDM. This amino acid residue influences both the nature of peptides that can bind to HLA-DQ and the interaction between the α and β chains. However, linkage with disease susceptibility is not simply determined by amino acids in class II molecules. It is certain that multiple unlinked genes outside of the MHC, at least seven in the case of IDDM, contribute to the disease etiology. In many cases of other autoimmune diseases, it is not known yet which class II molecule carries the predisposing amino acid sequence.

Despite intensive research into the role of specific class II alleles in establishing or influencing the progression of disease, little is known about the basis for these associations. In a few cases of autoimmune diseases, the self antigens that trigger the destructive immune response have been identified. For most, the autoantigen is still unknown. Disease can be caused by autoreactive T cells or antibodies. In some cases, transfer of antibodies from patients to experimental animals recapitulated the disease, thus implicating these antibodies in autoimmunity. Animal models of autoimmune diseases (e.g., experimental autoimmune encephalomyelitis, or EAE) imply that immunodominant peptides derived from an autoantigen (e.g., myelin basic protein, or MBP) bind to certain I-A alleles and provoke activation of autoreactive $CD4^+$ T cells. Such T cells can be transferred to nonimmunized animals and confer disease. Such models have been a rich source of experimental approaches to overcome activation of the autoreactive T cells, in particular by use of analog peptides that bind tightly but do not trigger T cells (20). Unfortunately, these encouraging results in animal models have not translated into similar successes in human diseases. The main challenges remain: What are the immunodominant peptides presented by class II molecules in autoimmunity? Which HLA class II allele or isotype is involved in this presentation? And, above all, how can such responses be turned off? Many promising approaches are currently under investigation, including the use of monoclonal antibodies to prevent the specific T-cell responses, of synthetic polymers that may block the class II/peptide interactions, tolerance induction by oral antigen, and addition or blocking of cytokines to reduce the autoreactivity of T cells or augment the protection mediated by inhibitory T cells (20). Our increased understanding of antigen presentation by class II molecules and of antigen-specific T-cell activation provides hope that useful therapeutic applications will emerge.

The presence of multiple genes within the MHC class II region suggested the possibility that some of the observed disease associations were due to polymorphism in those linked genes, as opposed to class II genes themselves. Polymorphism in the TAP genes has been proposed to be linked to diabetes (21). However, no convincing linkage between a disease and a non–class I or -class II gene in the MHC class II region has been reported to date.

IV. BIOSYNTHESIS AND ANTIGEN PROCESSING

A. Differences in Biosynthesis and Transport of Class I and Class II Molecules Control Their Functional Dichotomy

MHC class I and class II molecules serve essentially the same function: to present peptides to T cells. However, class I molecules have specialized in the presentation of internal antigens, whereas class II serve to present external antigens (1). There are fundamental biological reasons for this division. $CD8^+$ class I–restricted T cells kill target cells that display a foreign peptide. Therefore, it is important to ensure that only infected or transformed cells become targets of cytotoxic T cells. To achieve this, the immune system has developed a tightly controlled mechanism for the presentation of endogenous peptides by class I molecules. In contrast, $CD4^+$ T cells secrete important lymphokines that regulate both the humoral and cellular immune responses. These cells must sense the presence of foreign organisms, irrespective of whether host cells have been infected or not. A specialized set of antigen-presenting cells, mostly dendritic cells, macrophages, and B cells have developed the capacity to take up extracellular antigens and present them on class II molecules in order to trigger helper-T-cell responses. Despite the functional and structural similarities between class I and class II molecules, the important distinction in their antigen presentation properties is achieved immediately at the time and the site of their biosynthesis through interactions with other accessory molecules. Briefly, for class I, heavy chains and β_2-microglobulin do not assemble efficiently in the endoplasmic reticulum unless peptides of the right size and sequence are provided. Assembly of class I trimeric complexes requires multiple interactions with TAP molecules, and with several chaperone molecules in the endoplasmic reticulum such as BiP and calnexin. Once properly assembled, such class I–peptide complexes are transported directly to the cell surface.

Both chains of class II heterodimers are cotranslationally inserted into the endoplasmic reticulum membrane. Class II assembly does not stop with the heterodimer (22). $\alpha\beta$ chains immediately assemble onto trimers of the invariant chain (Ii). Ii is a type II transmembrane glycoprotein synthesized in large excess over the class II molecules. Ii serves three essential functions that prevent class II molecules from following the class I pathway of antigen presentation. First, Ii prevents peptide binding to $\alpha\beta$Ii complexes. Purified $\alpha\beta$Ii complexes do not bind peptides detectably and do not release peptides under dissociation conditions. Furthermore, soluble Ii at high concentrations can interfere with peptide binding to class II molecules. Thus, it appears that, once formed, $\alpha\beta$Ii complexes cannot bind peptides. Since the formation of such complexes occurs rapidly after α and β chain biosynthesis, most newly synthesized class II molecules will not bind peptides until Ii dissociation from $\alpha\beta$Ii complexes occurs in endocytic compartments. However, blocking is mutual in that peptides bound to $\alpha\beta$ heterodimers prevent association with Ii. Therefore, it is possible that some high-affinity peptides may successfully compete with Ii for binding to class II molecules in the endoplasmic reticulum. Second, Ii promotes assembly of class II $\alpha\beta$ heterodimers and their transport out of the ER. This role of Ii was appreciated more fully when mice deficient in Ii were generated in which surface expression of class II molecules was reduced by one order of magnitude relative to wild-type levels. In the absence of Ii, newly synthesized class II α and β chains form large aggregates in the endoplasmic reticulum. Third, Ii provides a targeting signal for the transport of class II molecules to endocytic compartments. In contrast to class I molecules that are transported directly to the cell surface, class II molecules reach acidic endosomal compartments prior to the dissociation of Ii, peptide loading, and transport to the cell surface. The cytoplasmic tail of Ii carries a di-leucine-based motif that is required for efficient transport to such endosomal compartments. The same motif also provides a powerful endocytosis signal for the internalization of cell surface class II-Ii complexes.

The removal of Ii from $\alpha\beta$Ii complexes occurs in discrete steps. An intermediate easily seen is an Ii fragment of about 10 kDa that has lost the carboxy-terminal domain. This short Ii fragment still provides the essential functions of Ii in terms of class II assembly, transport to endosomes, and blocking of peptide binding. The carboxy-terminal part of this 10-kDa fragment, up to residue 104 of Ii, is critical for blocking peptide binding. In fact, peptides ranging from residues 80 to 104 of Ii (also called CLIP, for class II–associated invariant chain peptide) are found associated with class II molecules upon further processing of Ii. A large body of evidence indicates that the CLIP region of Ii actually occupies the peptide-binding groove prior to Ii processing.

During transport from the ER to antigen processing compartments, class II molecules acquire complex carbohydrate modifications. Of the two N-linked glycosylation groups on the α chain of HLA-DR, only one is modified to a complex type. The single N-linked glycosylation group on the β chain is also modified into a complex high-mannose carbohydrate. The glycosylation of Ii is more complex. Ii contains two N-linked glycosylation groups and an O-linked carbohydrate. Ii becomes highly sialylated in the *trans*-Golgi compartment. In addition, a fraction of Ii becomes modified by addition of a sulfated proteoglycan. The reason for these complex modifications of Ii are unknown, although it has been suggested that Ii molecules residing transiently at the surface of APC may provide ligands to receptors on other cells.

Ii in both mouse and human comes in different isoforms. Through alternative splicing, a minor fraction of Ii acquires an additional exon in the extracellular domain. The real function of this alternative form of Ii, called p41, is unknown, although data with mouse p41 showed that it enhanced class II–restricted antigen presentation. In human but not in mouse, some Ii is translated from an alternative initiation codon resulting in a 16–amino acid extension of the cytoplasmic tail. This longer form of Ii is strongly retained in the ER except when fully assembled into $(Ii)_3(\alpha\beta)_3$ complexes. Although the precise function of this longer form of Ii (called p35) is unclear, it probably is required for proper HLA class II biosynthesis, because cells expressing only the short predominant form of Ii (called p33) develop abnormal endosomal compartments.

B. Antigen Processing and Presentation

Presentation of antigen by MHC class II molecules occurs after antigen has been taken up by antigen-presenting cells (APC) and processed intracellularly into peptides that can bind to class II molecules, and after class II–peptide complexes have returned to the cell surface. An effective immune surveillance will be achieved only if class II molecules can capture a wide range of peptides. Not only is it necessary for each class II allele to bind many different peptide sequences, but it would also be advantageous for class II molecules to bind peptides that have been generated in several subcellular sites. Since processing requirements for antigens with different chemical properties must vary, different repertoires of peptides are likely to be found among subcellular compartments in APC. Late endosomal structures where intracellular MHC class II molecules accumulate were first described in human B cells and termed MIIC (for MHC class II compartment). MIIC share features with lysosomes but represent unique compartments distinct from both endosomes and lysosomes. Newly synthesized class II molecules are transported to MIIC where they colocalize with HLA-DM molecules. Removal of CLIP and the loading of peptides most likely occurs in that compartment. The transition from CLIP-associated to peptide-loaded class II molecules has been assayed by following the stability of $\alpha\beta$ heterodimers in SDS detergent. For unknown but convenient reasons, class II molecules fall apart in SDS at ambient temperature unless they are associated with a stably bound peptide.

The existence of a specialized class II compartment implies specific transport pathways for the delivery of class II molecules to the compartment and for the transport of mature, peptide-loaded class II to the cell surface. A large fraction of the biosynthetic pool of class II molecules is transported directly from the *trans*-Golgi network to endosomes, whereas some of that pool reaches the cell surface before gaining access to endosomes by internalization. In either case, signals in the cytoplasmic tail of Ii are crucial for proper targeting of class II molecules. Steady-state studies by electron microscopic localization of intracellular class II molecules and pulse-chase studies of newly synthesized class II molecules clearly indicate that class II molecules accumulate in MIIC before their transport to the cell surface. How this final transport step to the surface is regulated is still unknown. In addition to a specialized targeting of class II molecules, there may also be specialized transport pathways to MIIC for proteins and peptides that are precursors to the antigenic peptides destined to bind to class II molecules.

The removal of CLIP from class II and the loading of peptides is catalyzed by HLA-DM, as demonstrated by in vitro assays with recombinant soluble molecules (13). This explains why cells deficient in DM have surface class II molecules that are occupied mostly by Ii-derived CLIP. It also implies that the selection of peptides presented by class II molecules will be based in part on the peptides' ability to gain access to compartments containing DM, such as the MIIC. However, the peptides that have been eluted from class II molecules, ranging from 12 to 25 amino acids in length, may not correspond in size to what was initially bound to class II. There is good evidence that unfolded proteins can bind to class II molecules. Processing and trimming of the peptides to their final size may follow the binding step. Once bound to class II, a peptide sequence is well protected from further proteolytic attack. This has interesting functional implications in that a dominant binding motif within a larger protein may preclude another weaker binding motif from being presented (23). There is functional evidence that such epitope selection occurs in some antigens.

Efficient delivery of foreign antigens to class II processing compartments requires active receptor-mediated uptake. Fluid-phase uptake of soluble antigen is an inefficient process and is unlikely to result in functional antigen presentation in vivo. Specialized APC have mechanisms for antigen capture. Dendritic cells use at least two types of receptors for antigen uptake: the mannose binding protein and another receptor (called DEC-205) with multiple lectinlike domains (24,25). Macrophages have powerful phagocytic properties that are triggered by the engagement of their Fc receptors. They are particularly good at processing large particulate or aggregated antigen. Finally, B cells internalize antigens through the membrane forms of Ig. Therefore, dendritic cells and macrophages are relatively nonspecific in the antigens they process, whereas B cells are highly specific. The specificity of antigen presentation by B cells serves to provide help from CD4$^+$ T cells mostly to antigen-specific B cells.

Antigens from different subcellular sources may reach class II processing compartments. Multiple processing pathways for class II–restricted antigen presentation are used, presumably to expand the range of peptides that can be used to mount immune responses (26). Some endogenous antigens can gain access to a class II processing compartment for presentation. Furthermore, some antigens can be presented by cells that lack Ii and HLA-DM. For some of those antigens, presentation is mediated by mature cell-surface class II molecules that internalize and recycle back to the cell surface (6). Peptides that have been eluted from class II molecules and sequenced confirm that the bulk of proteins that are sources of class II–restricted determinants are those expected to be in endosomes but also that some cytosolic proteins can provide peptides for class II-mediated presentation.

Understanding how endogenous self peptides can be presented by class II molecules is important because these peptides include minor histocompatibility antigens. Graft rejections in HLA-matched donor/recipient combinations can result from the presentation of such a self protein that differs between the two individuals.

V. FUNCTION

A. Peptide Presentation to CD4$^+$ T Cells

It is important to realize that engagement of a TCR by a class II/peptide complex can have very different outcomes depending on the developmental stage of the T cell and on the nature of costimulatory signals that the APC can provide. Early in T-cell development, CD4$^+$CD8$^+$ double-positive thymocytes with low TCR levels undergo sequentially a positive and a negative selection in the thymus. After maturation, CD4$^+$ and CD8$^+$ T cells receive proliferation and differentiation signals through their TCR that depend on costimulatory signals provided by CD28 binding to B7-1 and B7-2 molecules on APC. On the other hand, activation of effector functions, such as cytotoxicity, does not require a costimulatory signal.

T cells encounter class II molecules very early in their lifetime during differentiation in the thymus. Much of the T-cell repertoire is shaped during these early encounters. The current view (27) holds that class II molecules on epithelial cells in the cortical region of the thymus apply a positive selection for T cells that express a TCR with a low affinity for self class II. T cells are not positively selected for specific recognition of a given peptide because many different peptides can serve to positively select T cells. Although most of the experimental data have been derived with peptides on class I molecules selecting $CD8^+$ T cells, it is most likely also the case of class II–mediated positive selection. The essential role of class II molecules in the positive selection of T cells has been firmly established with class II–deficient mice, in which very few $CD4^+$ cells develop. At a later stage, class II molecules on bone marrow–derived dendritic cells in the thymic medulla negatively select T cells with receptors that display a high affinity for self class II. Interestingly, the same type of APC that can so powerfully stimulate T cells in the periphery cause them to be eliminated in the thymus. Clearly, the signal delivered by the TCR must be different at these different developmental stages. Tolerance induction in the T-cell population is extraordinarily sensitive, as very low doses of soluble antigen are sufficient to achieve tolerance (28). Class II molecules in the peripheral immune system are also involved in tolerance induction. This is achieved either by clonal anergy or by clonal deletion, the latter being achieved if the signal is strong. Anergy results when the costimulatory signal is missing. Nonprofessional APC induce tolerance because they lack ligands for CD28.

In most T-cell responses, whether positive or negative, the TCR-associated CD4 molecule plays an important role (29). Coengagement of CD4 with TCR dramatically enhances the T-cell response. CD4 binds to an exposed loop of the membrane-proximal $\beta 2$ domain of the class II β chain. Co-cross-linking of CD4 contributes to TCR-mediated signaling through the association of the src-family kinase lck with the cytoplasmic tail of CD4.

B cells require help in the form of lymphokines produced by helper T cells. They obtain help by presenting T-cell antigenic determinants on their class II molecules. As B cells process and present primarily antigens for which they have a specific Ig, it is essential that the epitope for antibody recognition be linked to that for T-cell recognition. B cells do not stimulate virgin T cells because they fail to provide the second signal. Nevertheless, B cells can receive help from mature T cells because the second signal is not needed to trigger T-helper (Th) functions.

The ligand density of APC influences the outcome of T-cell responses. At low densities, a Th2 response that provides help for B cells is favored. At high ligand densities, an inflammatory response is favored, mediated by Th1 cells that stimulate macrophages, NK cells, and cytotoxic T cells.

B. Peptide Specificity

Two types of specificities have to be distinguished: specificity of the peptide for the binding site in class II molecules and specificity of peptide recognition by T cells. Initially, the sequencing of individual peptides isolated from class II molecules yielded sufficient information for the prediction of some binding motifs for several class II molecules (30). As peptides bound to class II molecules extend outside of the binding site and have staggered ends, pool sequencing of peptides eluted from class II molecules does not produce data as clear as that for class I–eluted peptides. The main differences between the class I and class II modes of peptide binding are in the conserved contacts that involve mostly the ends of peptides bound to class I and the backbone of peptides bound to class II. However, the specificity of peptide binding is contributed largely by peptide side chains that point down into "pockets," very much in the way specificity is also achieved for binding to class I molecules.

A powerful tool to delineate the specificity in peptide binding to class II molecules is to screen random peptide libraries expressed by use of recombinant single-strand DNA phages. This approach was used very successfully to identify motifs for binding to different class II alleles (3). This information, together with the sequences of many peptides that had been eluted from class II molecules, has led to the definition of binding motifs for many different class II alleles (Table 1).

In vitro binding studies have revealed complex properties of the class II/peptide interaction with the existence of different conformations (31). Peptides bind very rapidly to soluble class II molecules, but this "fast on" binding results in complexes that dissociate rapidly. Stable peptide binding occurs only after a slow or pH-dependent reaction. Electrophoretic analysis of these complexes suggest that different folding conformations exist and that the formation of stable complexes requires a conformational change in class II molecules.

The CDR3 regions of the α and β chains of the TCR control most of the specificity for class II–bound peptides (32). The interaction between TCR and MHC-peptide complexes can be rather "fluid" in that the same class II/peptide combination can be recognized by different TCR sequences with different topologies. Peptide residues that most often confer TCR-specific recognition are those side chains that point up from the peptide binding site. Residues on the α helices of both the class II α and β chains also influence recognition by the TCR.

One of the most exciting and potentially useful developments in our understanding of MHC class II/peptide recognition by T cells is that modified peptide ligands can have dramatically different effects on the T cell response (33). In a fully immunogenic response, T cells are stimulated to produce effector functions (e.g., lymphokine production or cytotoxicity) and to proliferate. However, modified peptides can result in a partial activation of the T cells, resulting in effector functions but not growth. In other cases, modified peptides can even act as antagonists and block the T-cell responses or produce a state of anergy in the T cells even when presented by functional APC. Even a single amino acid substitution in a class II–bound peptide can change the T-cell response from a full activation to a state of long-lived tolerance. The different outcome in T cells responding to these related peptides is not simply due to different strengths of TCR-mediated signals, because qualitative differences were observed in the pattern of protein tyrosine phosphorylation upon engagement of the TCR by the different ligands.

C. Superantigens

Some antigens stimulate powerful T-cell responses without the need for processing. These antigens, called superantigens (34), constitute a family of molecules that can bind with high affinity to MHC class II molecules and stimulate entire families of T cells according to the Vβ or Vδ chain expressed in their TCR. Depending on the frequency of specific Vβ families, typically 5 to 25% of T cells are activated, sometimes with dire consequences for the host, as in food poisoning caused by the staphylococcal enterotoxins and toxic shock syndrome caused by the staphylococcal

Table 1 Peptide Binding Motifs for Human HLA-DR Molecules[a]

Allele	Relative Position 1	2	3	4	5	6	7	8	9
DRB1*0101	**Y,V**			**L,A**		**A,G**			L,A
	L,F			I,V		S,T			I,V
	I,A			M,N		P			N,F
	M,W			Q					Y
DRB1*0301	**L,I**			**D**		K,R			Y,L
	F,M					E,Q			F
	V					N			
DRB1*0401	**F,Y**			F,W		N,S	polar		polar
	W,I			I,L		T,Q	charged		aliphatic
	L,V			V,A		H,R	aliphatic		K
	M			D,E					
				no R,K					
DRB1*0402	**V,I**			Y,F		**N,Q**	R,K		polar
	L,M			W,I		**S,T**	H,N		aliphatic
				L,M		**K**	Q,P		**H**
				R,N					
				no D,E					
DRB1*0404	**V,I**			F,Y		N,T	polar		polar
	L,M			W,I		S,Q	charged		aliphatic
				L,V		R	aliphatic		K
				M,A					
				D,E					
				no R,K					
DRB1*0405	**F,Y**			V,I		N,S	polar		**D**,E
	W,V			L,M		T,Q	charged		Q
	I,L			D,E		K,D	aliphatic		
	M								
DRB1*1101	W,Y			M,L		R,K			
	F			V,I					
DRB1*1201	**I,L**		**L,M**			V,Y			**Y,F**
	F,Y		**N,V**			F,I			**M,I**
	V		**A**			N,A			**V**
DRB1*1501	L,V			F,Y			I,L		
	I			I			V,M		
							F		
DRB5*0101	**F,Y**			Q,V					**R,K**
	L,M			I,M					

[a]Anchor residues are shown (in the single-letter code) with the predominant amino acids in bold. Position 1 is defined as the peptide residue that binds into the first pocket in the class II peptide binding site. As class II–bound peptides can extend outside of the binding site, position 1 is rarely the first residue in the peptide. These data have been derived from a combination of degenerate peptide libraries that were tested for direct binding to HLA-DR molecules and of sequencing of peptides eluted from HLA-DR molecules that had been purified from human B cells. *Source*: Ref. 36.

toxic shock syndrome toxin 1 (TSST-1). Superantigens are mostly products of bacterial species, notably *Staphylococcus* and *Mycoplasma*. In addition, the murine mammary tumor retroviruses encode superantigens in an open reading frame at the 3' end of their genome. These retroviral superantigens act on T cells in a similar manner as the bacterial exoproteins, such as the staphylococcal enterotoxin A (SEA), SEB, SEE, and TSST-1.

The crystal structure of two superantigen–class II complexes (HLA-DR with SEB and TSST-1) has confirmed earlier conclusions that superantigens make external contacts with the $\alpha1$ domain of class II. Superantigens most likely contact a loop in the hypervariable region 4 of the TCR Vβ region, which lies outside the antigen combining site. Although superantigens do not occupy the peptide binding groove of class II molecules, they form very close contacts with the α helix of the $\alpha1$ domain and extend over the peptide itself, implying that the way a TCR contacts MHC class II in the presence of a superantigen must be different from the contacts made during antigen-specific recognition.

The biological reason for the existence of superantigens is still unclear. They must in some way provide an advantage to the pathogens that produce them. In the case of the mouse mammary tumor virus, a milk-transmitted retrovirus that encodes a superantigen, the strong immune response induced by the MMTV-encoded superantigen permits the survival of the virus through T-cell dependent clonal expansion of infected B cells (35). The possible involvement of superantigens in the pathogenesis of many diseases has been investigated (34). Potential viral superantigens have been reported for rabies virus and for HIV. A role for superantigens in autoimmunity has also been suggested. Disease models in mice revealed that autoreactive T cells, normally kept in check by tolerance mechanisms, can become activated nonspecifically (besides Vβ specificity) by superantigens and exacerbate autoimmune reactions (20).

Activation of the same cloned T cell by superantigen bound to a class II molecule and by an antigenic peptide bound to that class II molecule differ biochemically and in the final outcome of the T-cell response. The signals transmitted by the TCR result either in unresponsiveness or depletion in the case of superantigen or in T-cell responsiveness and the establishment of memory T cells in the case of antigenic peptide.

D. Signal Transduction

The intracellular part of MHC class II molecules has important functions, even though the extracellular domains and their ligands have attracted most of the attention. The α and β chains of class II molecules carry short cytoplasmic tails without any obvious sequence motifs for signal transduction. Nevertheless, signals are transmitted through class II molecules that can alter cellular responses as well as class II intracellular traffic. Natural cross-linking of class II molecules may occur when they are engaged by specific TCR or when superantigens bind. Cross-linking of class II molecules on B cells has several outcomes (7). First, it augments homotypic adhesion. As B and T cells share several surface adhesion molecules, this class II–mediated augmentation of adhesion may serve to increase the antigen-specific B–T-cell interactions. Second, it upregulates expression of the B7 costimulatory molecule. Finally, it induces B-cell differentiation and Ig production.

Superantigens, such as SEA and SEB, can stimulate B cells in the absence of T cells, even though the stimulation is much less pronounced than in the presence of T cells. This is presumably due to class II cross-linking mediated by the superantigen. How this cross-linking is achieved is not clear. It is possible that multimers can form, assuming a divalent binding of superantigen to class II. SEA apparently binds with high affinity to one site on HLA-DR and with a lower affinity to another. Superantigens are potent inducers of interleukin-1 (IL-1), tumor necrosis factor-alpha (TNFα), and nitric oxide in monocytes, mimicking the effect of cross-linking class II molecules.

Signals transduced by class II molecules are mediated by the accumulation of intracellular cAMP. Cross-linking of class II, or addition of exogenous cAMP, causes the recruitment of the protein kinase C (PKC) from the cytosol to a detergent-insoluble fraction. As with all antigen receptors, cross-linking of class II molecules results in the phosphorylation of tyrosine residues on several cytoplasmic proteins of the class II–expressing cells. Protein tyrosine kinases of the src family are activated in B cells and monocytes as a result of class II–mediated signaling. Activation of the protein tyrosine kinase begins a cascade of activation events leading to enhanced adhesion, proliferation, and differentiation. Signal transduction events initiated by MHC class II molecules also result in activation of transcription factors that control expression of cytokine genes in monocytes.

Mature HLA-DR molecules (molecules that are no longer associated with Ii) internalize and recycle back to the cell surface constitutively on B cells. The signal that controls this internalization is contributed jointly by the combination of the cytoplasmic tails of both class II α and β chains (6). The amino acid residues in those tails that provide the internalization signal have not been defined. Class II recycling through early endosomes may be an alternative antigen presentation pathway, used for antigens that are very rapidly degraded and processed after uptake into APC.

VI. CONCLUSIONS

MHC class II–restricted CD4$^+$ T cells contribute to GVHD. It is therefore essential to optimize the match between class II molecules of the donor and recipient to avoid potent class II alloreactivities. Serological typing for HLA class II does not guarantee a perfect match in the class II alleles, because the sequence diversity among class II molecules is greater than that detected by serological reagents. Molecular typing can be used to refine the distinctions between class II alleles and improve matching. Obviously, the greater the distinction between class II alleles, the less likely it becomes to find a matched donor. Nevertheless, such molecular approaches have been applied clinically and have resulted in improved tolerance of transplanted organs.

It is important to realize that even a perfect match between HLA class II alleles cannot avoid the possibility of GVHD mediated by the presentation of minor histocompatibility antigens. A low level of allelic polymorphism exists in most genes. It is therefore possible, albeit rare, that self peptides bound to class II molecules will differ slightly between individuals but sufficiently to trigger a class II–restricted T-cell response. Fortunately, great progress has been made in understanding how endogenous proteins are processed for presentation of peptides by class II molecules and very sensitive techniques have been developed to search and find individual peptides bound to class II molecules. These tools are now available to search for the source of minor histocompatibility antigens and for the specific class II molecule responsible for their presentation. An avenue with tremendous therapeutic and preventive potential is the manipulation of the nature of the class II-restricted T-cell responses according to the precise sequence of the peptide bound to class II molecules. Antagonist peptides that can bind to class II molecules as tightly as the antigenic peptide but cause T-cell unresponsiveness could be used to prevent unwanted alloresponses or responses to minor histocompatibility antigens. The problems faced in GVHD are very similar to those in autoimmunity. The intense efforts in these related fields may provide a common solution.

REFERENCES

1. Germain RN. MHC-dependent antigen processing and peptide presentation: providing ligands for T lymphocyte activation. Cell 1994; 76:287–299.
2. Stern LJ, Wiley DC. Antigenic peptide binding by class I and class II histocompatibility proteins. Structure 1994; 2:245–251.
3. Sinigaglia F, Hammer J. Defining rules for the peptide—MHC class II interaction. Curr Opin Immunol 1994; 6:52–56.
4. Brown JH, Jardetzky TS, Gorga JC, et al. Three-dimensional structure of the human class II histocompatibility antigen HLA-DR1. Nature 1993; 364:33–39.
5. Cosson P, Bonifacino JS. Role of transmembrane domain interactions in the assembly of class II MHC molecules. Science 1992; 258:659–662.
6. Pinet V, Vergelli M, Martin R, et al. Antigen presentation mediated by recycling of surface HLA-DR molecules. Nature 1995; 375:603–606.
7. Scholl PR, Geha RS. MHC class II signaling in B-cell activation. Immunol Today 1994; 15:418–422.
8. Jones PP, Begovich AB, Tacchini-Cottier FM, Vu TH. Evolution of class II genes: Role of selection in both the maintenance of polymorphism and the retention of non-expressed alleles. Immunol Res 1990; 9:200–211.
9. Mach B, Steimle V, Reith W. MHC class II-deficient combined immunodeficiency: A disease of gene regulation. Immunol Rev 1994; 138:207–221.
10. Steinmetz M, Minard K, Horvath S, et al. A molecular map of the immune response region from the major histocompatibility complex of the mouse. Nature 1982; 300:35–42.
11. Karlsson L, Surh CD, Sprent J, Peterson PA. An unusual class II molecule. Immunol Today 1992; 13:469–470.
12. Beckman EM, Porcelli SA, Morita CT, et al. Recognition of a lipid antigen by CD1-restricted alpha-beta$^+$ T cells. Nature 1994; 372:691–694.
13. Roche PA. HLA-DM: An in vivo facilitator of MHC class II peptide loading. Immunity 1995; 3:259–262.
14. Monaco JJ. Structure and function of genes in the MHC class II region. Curr Opin Immunol 1993; 5:17–20.
15. Klein J, Satta Y, O'Huigin C, Takahata N. The molecular descent of the major histocompatibility complex. Annu Rev Immunol 1993; 11:269–295.
16. Ayala FJ, Escalante A, O'Huigin C, Klein J. Molecular genetics of speciation and human origins. Proc Natl Acad Sci USA 1994; 91:6787–6794.
17. Bodmer JG, Marsh SGE, Albert ED, et al. Nomenclature for factors of the HLA system, 1990. Tissue Antigens 1991; 37:97–104.

18. Nepom GT, Erlich H. MHC class-II molecules and autoimmunity. Annu Rev Immunol 1991; 9:493–525.
19. Nepom GT. Class II antigens and disease susceptibility. Annu Rev Med 1995; 46:17–25.
20. Steinman L. Escape from "Horror Autotoxicus": Pathogenesis and treatment of autoimmune disease. Cell 1995; 80:7–10.
21. Faustman D. Mechanisms of autoimmunity in type 1 diabetes. J Clin Immunol 1993; 13:1–7.
22. Cresswell P. Assembly, transport, and function of MHC class II molecules. Annu Rev Immunol 1994; 12:259–293.
23. Sercarz EE, Lehmann PV, Ametani A, et al. Dominance and crypticity of T cell antigenic determinants. Annu Rev Immunol 1993; 11:729–766.
24. Jiang W, Swiggard WJ, Heufler C, et al. The receptor DEC-205 expressed by dendritic cells and thymic epithelial cells is involved in antigen processing. Nature 1995; 375:151–155.
25. Sallusto F, Cella M, Danieli C, Lanzavecchia A. Dendritic cells use macropinocytosis and the mannose receptor to concentrate macromolecules in the major histocompatibility complex class II compartment: Downregulation by cytokines and bacterial products. J Exp Med 1995; 182:389–400.
26. Long EO, Roche PA, Malnati MS, et al. Multiple pathways of antigen processing for MHC class II-restricted presentation. In: Humphreys RE, Pierce SK, eds. Antigen Processing and Presentation. San Diego, CA: Academic Press, 1994:67–79.
27. Von Boehmer H. Positive selection of lymphocytes. Cell 1994; 76:219–228.
28. Nossal GJV. Negative selection of lymphocytes. Cell 1994; 76:229–239.
29. Weiss A, Littman DR. Signal transduction by lymphocyte antigen receptors. Cell 1994; 76:263–274.
30. Chicz RM, Urban RG, Gorga JC, et al. Specificity and promiscuity among naturally processed peptides bound to HLA-DR alleles. J Exp Med 1993; 178:27–47.
31. Sadegh-Nasseri S, Stern LJ, Wiley DC, Germain RN. MHC class II function preserved by low-affinity peptide interactions preceding stable binding. Nature 1994; 370:647–650.
32. Davis MM, Chien Y. Topology and affinity of T-cell receptor mediated recognition of peptide-MHC complexes. Curr Opin Immunol 1993; 5:45–49.
33. Sloan-Lancaster J, Allen PM. Significance of T-cell stimulation by altered peptide ligands in T cell biology. Curr Opin Immunol 1995; 7:103–109.
34. Kotzin BL, Leung DY, Kappler J, Marrack P. Superantigens and their potential role in human disease. Adv Immunol 1993; 54:99–166.
35. Held W, Acha-Orbea H, MacDonald HR, Waanders GA. Superantigens and retroviral infection: Insights from mouse mammary tumor virus. Immunol Today 1994; 15:184–190.
36. Rammensee H-G, Friede T, Stevanovic S. MHC ligands and peptide motifs: First listing. Immunogenetics 1995; 41:178–228.

4

Biological Inhibitors of Lymphocyte Coreceptors for Antigen-Specific Immunosuppression

Jeffrey A. Ledbetter, Gary L. Schieven, and Peter S. Linsley

Bristol-Myers Squibb Pharmaceutical Research Institute
Seattle, Washington

I. INTRODUCTION

Graft-versus-host disease (GVHD) is caused by T-cell activation in response to allogeneic major histocompatibility complex (MHC) molecules following histoincompatible bone marrow transplantation (BMT) (1). Although GVHD can be prevented by removal of T cells from donor marrow (2), this increases the risk of failure of engraftment and relapse of leukemia (3,4). Therefore a primary goal in the treatment of GVHD disease is to achieve antigen-specific immunoregulation so that host-reactive T cells are tolerized or deleted without preventing T-cell responses to foreign antigens. Current therapies are not ideal because of nonspecific immunosuppression and toxicity. Recent advances in understanding the molecular basis of T-cell activation and differentiation have suggested new approaches to this problem.

Specificity of T-cell activation is determined by T-cell receptor (TCR) engagement with MHC-peptide complexes during antigen-presenting cell (APC): T-cell interaction, but it is now widely recognized that T cells require additional signals from adhesion receptors to respond. This concept, first proposed as the two-signal model of T-cell activation (5), has been expanded to incorporate multiple signals from adhesion receptors including CD2, CD28, CD4, and $\beta1$ and $\beta2$ integrins, which provide the T cell with a wider range of choices than previously imagined. Additional signals given by activated T cells to the APC, such as those through the CD40 receptor, are also required to support T-cell responses (6). Current approaches to modulation of T-cell responses by selective blockade of adhesion receptors have already shown promise in models of autoimmunity, transplantation, and GVHD. Here we review the function of adhesion receptors in the regulation of signal transduction in T cells and APC, and the new opportunities for immunoregulation by targeting of biological inhibitors to these interactions.

II. DUAL ROLE OF CD4, CD2, CD28, AND LFA-1(CD11a/CD18) AS ADHESION RECEPTORS AND SIGNALING CORECEPTORS FOR TCR/CD3 ACTIVATION

The binding of TCR to peptide/MHC is a primary determinant of T-cell activation, but the affinity of this interaction is low (7). Similarly, a restricted number of MHC molecules containing each immunogenic peptide limits the number of TCR molecules that can be bound. To solve these problems, T cells use molecules such as CD4/CD8, CD2, CD28/CTLA-4, and $\beta 1$ and $\beta 2$ integrins to mediate adhesion by binding to specific ligands on the APC. Following engagement, these molecules play a dual role by making critical contributions to the intracellular signals leading to activation responses. Although many questions remain, there has been rapid progress in understanding the molecular basis of the effects of adhesion molecules on intracellular signals. The key is the association of the cytoplasmic tails of these receptors with tyrosine kinases that phosphorylate CD3 ζ and ϵ chains to orchestrate the connection between the signalling motifs of the CD3 complex and activation of effector molecules that are recruited to the membrane by SH2 interactions. SH2 domains in signaling molecules such as ZAP70 and PLCγ1 bind phosphotyrosine in the context of specific amino acid sequences. Tyrosine phosphorylation can thus induce the assembly of specific signal complexes based on the identify of the sequences phosphorylated and the sequence specificity of the SH2 domains. After receptor cross-linking, multiple tyrosine kinases work together to activate downstream signaling cascades through phospholipase Cγ1 (PLCγ1), phosphatidylinositol-3 kinase (PI-3K), and microtubule associated protein kinase (MAP kinase) to control cytokine expression and proliferation responses.

A. Multiple Tyrosine Kinases Contribute During T-Cell Activation

The central role of tyrosine kinases in T-cell activation and differentiation has been demonstrated from gene overexpression and knockout experiments (8). Tyrosine kinases that have been identified in T cells physically linked to surface receptors, include members of the Src family (Lck and Fyn) and the Syk family (ZAP 70) (9). The activity of these kinases is regulated by the interaction of members of the two families in a process that requires the presence CD3 ζ or ϵ chains to form a scaffold for kinase binding (10–13). The tyrosine kinases of the Src family are thought to be activated first by cross-linking of their associated receptors (CD4, CD2, and CD8 for Lck, and CD3 for Fyn) followed by phosphorylation of membrane substrates including CD3 chains and the CD5 and CD6 molecules. This induces translocation of the ZAP70 kinase from the cytosol to the membrane by specific tandem SH2 binding to CD3 chains where ZAP70 can interact with Lck and Fyn (14–16). The CD5 and CD6 molecules may recruit additional enzymes to the membrane by specific SH2 interactions. ZAP70 probably plays a primary role in mediating early events in signal transduction such as phosphorylation and activation of PLCγ1, since patients with defective ZAP70 have a selective T-cell deficiency and are unresponsive to TCR signals in assays of calcium mobilization and IL2 production (17,18).

Cross-linking of CD3 alone can activate Fyn, but purified resting T cells do not proliferate unless high concentrations of anti-CD3 are immobilized on plastic to provide prolonged signals. Under conditions of antigen recognition where small numbers of CD3/TCR molecules are bound, T cells require help from activated Lck provided by other coreceptors. The contribution of CD4, CD8, and CD2-associated Lck to activation is dependent on physical approximation of coreceptors with the CD3/TCR complex during contact with APC.

A small fraction of CD4, CD8 and CD2 are constitutively associated with CD3/TCR (19–21). However, by binding directly to MHC class I and II outside the peptide binding site, CD8 and CD4 are actively redistributed into close contact with CD3/TCR during antigen recognition (22). In the case of CD2, the association of its major ligand, CD58 (LFA-3) with MHC molecules on APC (23) may be sufficient to stabilize interactions and functional synergy between CD2 and the CD3/TCR complex (24,25). Association of coreceptors with the TCR may also alter TCR avidity, as was recently shown for CD8-TCR interactions (26). It is not yet clear, however, how multiple coreceptors can make distinct contributions to overall activation signals through the same tyrosine kinase. One possibility is that coreceptors can direct intracellular kinase signals toward different substrates. Some evidence for this model (Fig. 1) has been presented from studies using monoclonal antibodies (mAbs) to crosslink CD3 with CD4 or CD2, in primary T cells followed by examination of tyrosine-phosphorylated substrates. Co-cross-linking of CD2 or CD4 has a synergistic effect, giving much more extensive cellular tyrosine phosphorylation than the crosslinking of each of these receptors alone, as illustrated in Fig. 2A. Crosslinking of CD4 with CD3 primarily directed signals toward membrane substrates such as the CD5 and CD6 molecules, whereas cross-linking of CD2 with CD3 primarily directed signals toward intracellular substrates such as PLCγ1 (27). These results suggest that CD4 and CD2 do not simply provide redundant functions during activation and that their association with the CD3/TCR complex is highly specific and asymmetrical.

B. Immunosuppression with mAbs to CD4 or CD2

In contrast to the augmentation of signals by CD4 or CD2 cross-linking with CD3/TCR, separate binding of mAbs or ligands to CD4 or CD2 has been associated with inhibition of T-cell activation, leading to early ideas of negative or inhibitory signals by these receptors (28–35). Other studies showed that under certain conditions of CD2 cross-linking with two antibodies, T-cell activation, IL2 production, and proliferation could be induced (36). CD4 mAbs were not found to be mitogenic alone or in combinations, and mitogenic effects of CD2 mAbs were dependent upon expression of CD3/TCR (37,38). Although the molecular basis of these effects is not yet fully clear, CD2 or CD4 cross-linking has been shown to activate Lck (39,40). Evidence has also been presented that ligands binding to CD4, including HIV-1 gp120, may trigger negative signals in T cells (41–43) to increase their sensitivity to apoptosis by mechanisms that include expression of the FAS receptor (44).

Studies in murine models have shown promise for the use of anti-CD4 mAbs for generating immunosuppression in autoimmunity (see Ref. 45 for review). CD4 mAbs at high doses were effective in preventing an immune response to the CD4

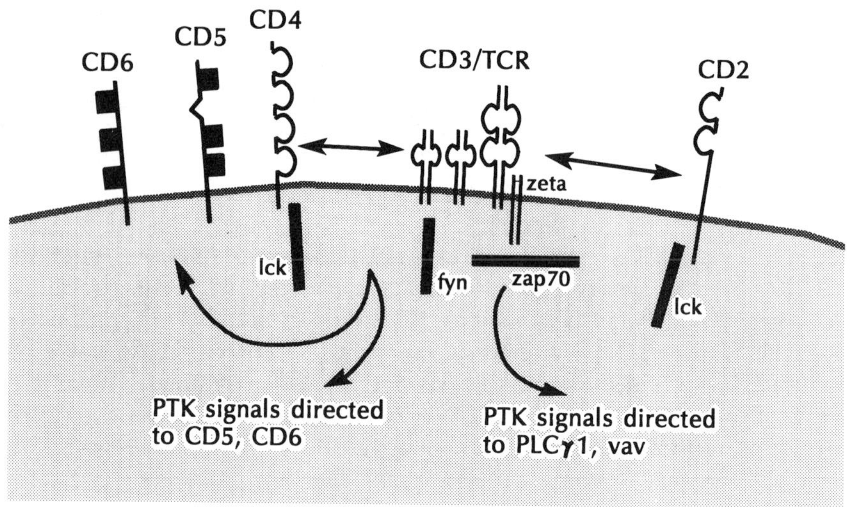

Figure 1 CD4 and CD2 coreceptors direct TCR-induced PTK signals. During T-cell interaction with APC, the APC ligands MHC class II and CD58 bind CD4 and CD2 to induce or strengthen their physical interaction with CD3/TCR. This allows efficient tyrosine phosphorylation of CD3 signaling motifs and subsequent activation of ZAP70. Although both CD4 and CD2 associate with the Src-family kinase Lck, they preferentially direct signals toward different intracellular substrates.

mAb itself (46) and prevented development of diabetes in NOD mice (47,48), arthritis in collagen type-II immunized animals (49), and lupus in NZBxNZW mice (45). However, these effects were associated with depletion of CD4 cells by mAb Fc-dependent effects. In later experiments, CD4 mAb $F(ab')_2$ fragments were found to be effective without depletion of CD4 cells and resulted in antigen-specific tolerance (50,51). Murine and chimeric anti-human CD4 mAbs have been tested in rheumatoid arthritis patients, but there was CD4 cell depletion in these studies (52–55). It will be critical in development of future CD4-directed therapies to prevent depletion of target cells by Fc-mediated clearance to avoid nonspecific immunosuppression.

Encouraging results with CD2 mAbs for induction of tolerance in vivo have also been presented (56–59). CD2 mAbs were found to inhibit generation of alloantigen specific CTL and prevented contact sensitivity in vivo. CD2 was downregulated after in vivo treatment but T cells were not depleted. CD2 mAb or $F(ab')_2$ fragments prevented normal receptor adhesion function and promoted the generation of a $CD4^+$ T-cell subset secreting IL4 and TGBβ (58). A soluble form of the CD2 ligand LFA-3 (CD58) expressed as an Ig-fusion protein (LFA-3Ig) had immunosuppressive activity but also caused T-cell depletion because of the Fc receptor–binding properties of the Ig tail (60).

How might CD4 or CD2-specific ligands generate negative signals? Cross-

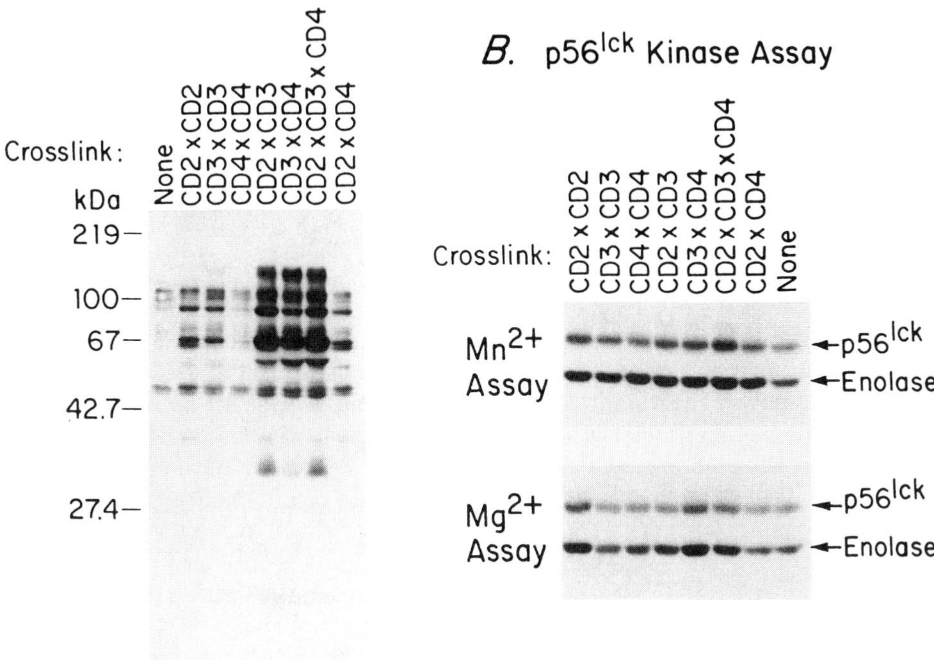

Figure 2 Differential activation of Lck after cross-linking CD4 separately or together with CD3 revealed by kinase assays in Mg^{2+} versus Mn^{2+}. CD3, CD2, and CD4 expressed on peripheral blood T cells were crosslinked separately or together using biotin-conjugated mAbs followed by avidin. A. Tyrosine phosphorylation of substrates in whole cell lysates was determined by a p-tyr blot. B. The autophosphorylation of Lck and its activity of towards enolase in the corresponding cell lysates was measured by immunoprecipitation with anti-Lck specific antisera followed by kinase assays in the presence of (γ-32p-ATP) plus either Mn^{2+} or Mg^{2+}. Phosphorylated Lck and enolase were separated by gel electrophoresis and detected by autoradiography. C. PhosphorImager analysis of the kinase activity towards enolase in the presence of Mn^{2+} or Mg^{2+}.

linking of CD4 alone can activate Lck (40), even though this does not result in optimal phosphorylation of cellular substrates (61). The data shown in Fig. 2 suggests that Lck is not fully activated by CD4 cross-linking, since increases in Lck activity could be detected in the presence of Mn^{2+} but not in the presence of Mg^{2+}. Even though Mn^{2+} is more effective in supporting activity by cellular tyrosine kinases (62,63), Mg^{2+} is the divalent action that must be used by Src-family kinases under physiological conditions, since virtually all cellular ATP is present as Mg-ATP. Cross-linking of CD4 with CD3 caused full activation of Lck, since increased kinase activity could be supported by either Mn^{2+} or Mg^{2+}. These data suggest that the CD4 interaction with CD3/TCR that results in activation of ZAP70 also alters the activation state of Lck itself. The detection of an altered activation state of Lck also suggests a possible explanation for the negative signals following CD4 cross-linking. After CD4 cross-linking, Lck dissociates from the CD4 receptor (40) and may then be unable to interact with ZAP 70 and CD3/TCR. Altered Lck activation was not observed after CD2 cross-linking (Fig. 2), so the functional coupling of CD4 versus CD2 to Lck seems to differ. This is also consistent with the differences between CD2 and CD4 in their potential for directly inducing mitogenic responses under special conditions. The inhibitory effects of CD2 mAbs or ligands may be partly due to effects on Lck directly and partly due to the prevention of critical regulatory signals from CD58 during T-cell/APC interactions.

C. The CD28 Receptor System

The CD28 and CTLA-4 receptors on T-cells and their ligands CD80 and CD86 on activated APC constitute another important adhesion/signaling system that is required for immune responses to antigen (64). Figure 3 summarizes this receptor system and shows the structural features of the soluble CTLA4-Ig immunoligand that is a specific inhibitor of CD80 and CD86 binding (65). CTLA4-Ig, composed of the extracellular domain of CTLA-4 and the CH2 and CH3 domain of IgG1 (human) or IgG2a (mouse), has already been used in vivo in models of autoimmunity, transplantation and GVHD to reveal the role of CD28 in T-cell activation and anergy.

Although mAbs to CD28 were shown to possess remarkable properties in stimulation of T cells in studies over the last 10 years, the importance of CD28 has been recognized only since the identification of natural ligands CD80 (66) and CD86 (67,68) and the demonstration of their ability to activate the CD28 receptor during T-cell binding to APC (69–71). Studies by Tan et al. showed that blockade of CD28 signals with CTLA4-Ig results in alloantigen-specific unresponsiveness in vitro (72),

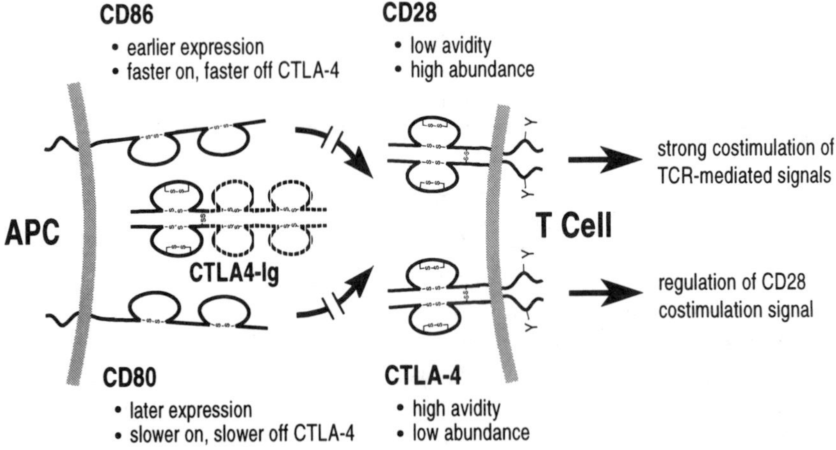

Figure 3 The CD28 receptor system. The CD80 and CD86 ligands for CD28 and CTLA-4 are expressed by activated APC and bind both receptors with equal overall avidities but with distinct kinetics. CD28, expressed on resting T cells, provides critical costimulatory signals, while CTLA-4, expressed on activated T cells, regulates the CD28 signals. The high avidity CTLA-4 receptor is a potent inhibitor of CD80 and CD86 binding when expressed in a soluble form with Ig CH2 and CH3 domains (CTLA4-Ig, shown with Ig tail in dashed line).

and Harding et al. used stimulatory anti-CD28 mAbs to prevent the development of anergy in murine T-cell clones (73). Evidence was presented that the role of CD28 in regulation of T-cell responsiveness is related to its effects on T-cell production of IL2. In other studies, transfection of CD80 into HLA-DR–positive 3T3 cells prevented development of clonal anergy to a tetanus toxoid antigen by human T-cell clones, whereas transfection of intracellular adhesion molecule-1 (ICAM-1) did not (74,75). These reports from in vitro studies have demonstrated the importance of the CD28 signal in T-cell activation or inactivation during recognition of antigen.

CD28-deficient mice have further clarified the role of CD28 in T-cell activation (76). Although T and B lymphocyte development was not affected, serum immunoglobulin levels were reduced to only 20% of normal. T cells were impaired in their ability to respond to mitogenic lectins, and antibody responses to T-dependent antigens were reduced (76). These results show that CD28 signals are required for T-cell helper function for B cells and agree with reports showing inhibition of T-dependent B-cell responses in vitro and in vivo by CTLA4-Ig (77,78).

The function of CTLA-4 is less well understood than that of CD28. Although CTLA-4 is a high-avidity receptor for CD80 and CD86, it is undetectable on resting T cells and is expressed in low amounts after T-cell activation. CTLA-4 is coexpressed with CD28 after activation and is upregulated by CD28 signaling (79–81). Since CD28 and CTLA-4 bind the same ligands, they are likely to be coclustered during T-cell/APC engagement. However, the effect of CTLA-4 ligation on CD28 signals has been reported to be either enhancement or inhibition of T-cell responses (79,82,83). A recent study showed that restimulation of primed T cells with antigen plus specific CTLA4 cross-linking caused apoptosis of antigen-specific T cells (84). Studies with lymphocytes from CD28-deficient mice showed that CTLA-4 cannot duplicate the function of CD28 (76,85), so CTLA-4 is likely to modulate CD28 adhesion and signaling properties. Further studies will be needed to clarify the natural role of CTLA-4 in T cells.

CD80 (formerly called B7 or B7-1) (86) was the first ligand identified for CD28 and CTLA-4 (65,66). Using expression cloning with CTLA4-Ig, a second ligand, CD86 (B70 or B7-2) (67,68,71) was identified that has a similar overall structure but only 25% sequence homology with CD80. Either CD80 or CD86 can trigger CD28 responses when immobilized or transfected into CHO or 3T3 cells (69,70), but they are inactive or even inhibitory when used in solution as Ig-fusion proteins. Similarly, either CD80 or CD86 can induce immune responses after expression in immunogenic tumors, resulting in tumor regression (87,88). These observations raise questions about the possibilities of different functions for these molecules. Evidence that CD80 and CD86 are not simply redundant molecules but serve distinct functions has come from findings that they show differences in expression patterns. CD86 is expressed on unactivated monocytes and dendritic cells, but CD80 is not (71,89,90). After activation, CD86 is upregulated before CD80 is expressed, and there are differences in regulation of expression by GM-CSF and γ interferon. CD80 and CD86 also show distinct kinetics of binding to CD28 and CTLA-4 (91), suggesting that they may be able to trigger different CD28 signals through different rates of CD28 clustering. This possibility is consistent with early studies with CD28 mAbs that showed different signals that are dependent on the degree of CD28 clustering (92).

D. CD28 Signal Transduction Pathways

Like the CD2 and CD4 coreceptors, the CD28 receptor generates signals that interact with and modify the signals from the TCR/CD3 complex. However, CD28 signals differ from these other receptors since CD28 can be efficiently triggered by a third-party CD80$^+$ cell or by cross-linking with mAbs without incorporating the TCR/CD3 complex (64). CD28 signals are also distinct from those generated by the TCR, since they are partially resistant to inhibition by cyclosporin A (93). CD28 therefore signals at least in part through a calcium-independent pathway. Interestingly, the calcium-independent arm of the CD28 signal is activated by bivalent binding of CD28 mAbs, whereas calcium-dependent signals require a higher order of cross-linking (92). Both the calcium-dependent and calcium-independent signals from CD28 are active in regulation of IL2 gene expression (94–98).

CD28 is similar to the other T-cell coreceptors since it depends on activation of tyrosine kinases for signal transduction (99,100). During stimulation, CD28 becomes phosphorylated on tyrosine residues and binds the 85-kDa subunit of PI-3K by an SH2 interaction (101–105). The tyrosine kinase Emt (also called Itk) binds CD28 and is activated by CD28 cross-linking (106). The multifunctional Src-family kinase Lck is also activated by CD28 cross-linking (101,107), and substrates that become phosphorylated on tyrosine include the vav protooncogene and PLCγ1 (99,108). Although activation of PLCγ1 can explain the calcium-dependent arm of the CD28 pathway, the molecular mechanisms for the calcium-independent arm are not yet clear. CD28 has been linked to activation of *N*-terminal c-Jun kinase JNK, a member of the MAP kinase family whose activation is required for IL-2 transcription (109). CD28 cross-linking with mAbs can also lead to downstream MAP kinase (ERK2) activation, but the CD80 ligand was not active in this study, suggesting that the strength of the CD28 signal can control which effector pathways are used (110). Figure 4 summarizes the properties of the CD28 signal transduction pathway.

E. Therapeutic Effects of CTLA4-Ig

CTLA4-Ig is a potent inhibitor of CD28 signals in vitro. CTLA4-Ig blocks CD80-dependent stimulation at low concentrations but requires about 100-fold higher concentrations to block CD86-dependent signals (91). CTLA4-Ig has been tested in animals in multiple studies and found to have several attractive features for an immunosuppressive drug, including a long serum half-life, low toxicity, and the induction of antigen-specific unresponsiveness.

The initial studies with human CTLA4-Ig (hCTLA4-Ig) in mice showed that it was effective in preventing antibody responses to T-dependent antigens sheep red blood cells (SRBC) or keyhole limpet hemocyanin (KLH) (78). Responses were prevented when hCTLA4-Ig was given up to 2 days after antigen administration, but this treatment was less effective if delayed further. Responses to a second challenge with antigen were blunted but not completely prevented (111). Splenic T cells from treated animals showed significantly reduced responses to antigen but normal responses to mitogens. The nonresponsive (tolerized) state could be enhanced by simultaneous treatment with hCTLA4-Ig plus a neutralizing anti-IL4 mAb to cause a long-lasting unresponsiveness to SRBC.

In transplantation models, rejection of cardiac allografts in rats was also delayed in treated animals but tolerance was not induced unless animals were pre-

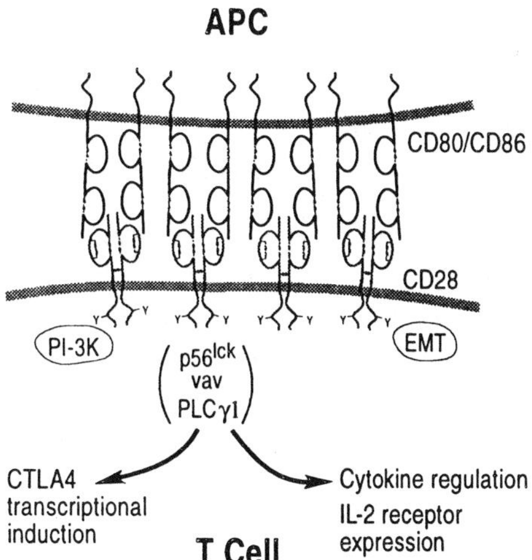

Figure 4 Signal transduction by the CD28 receptor. Cross-linking activates the CD28 signal through the associated EMT tyrosine kinase, inducing tyrosine phosphorylation of CD28 and binding of PI-3K by a specific SH2 interaction. The Lck kinase is also activated and PLCγ1 and vav are substrates, leading to CTLA-4 expression and augmentation of cytokine and cytokine receptor expression by transcriptional and posttranscriptional mechanisms.

treated with donor spleen cells plus hCTLA4-Ig prior to transplantation (112). In murine models of cardiac transplantation, hCTLA4-Ig alone was sufficient to cause transplantation tolerance, and similar results were obtained with pancreatic islet-cell xenografts (113–115). Thus CTLA4-Ig is able to induce transplantation tolerance. Later studies found that hCTLA4-Ig is less effective than murine CTLA4-Ig (mCTLA4-Ig) in blocking murine CD80 and CD86 ligands and that its effectiveness in mice is limited by immunogenicity of hCTLA4-Ig. Therefore these results are very encouraging for the use of CTLA4-Ig in transplantation.

CTLA4-Ig has been tested in several autoimmune disease models. In one study, mCTLA4-Ig was used to treat spontaneous lupus in NZB/NZW F1 (B/W) mice (116). Autoantibody production and proteinuria was blocked in treated mice, and life span was significantly prolonged. When treatment was delayed until a more advanced stage of illness, beneficial effects of CTLA4-Ig were still clear. These results provide the first evidence that CTLA4-Ig may be beneficial in chronic advanced autoimmune disease. CTLA4-Ig has also shown activity in other experimental autoimmune models where production of autoantibodies plays a role. For example, in autoimmune glomerulonephritis, treatment with hCTLA4-Ig blocked antibody production to glomerular basement membrane and reduced the severity of disease (117). Again, beneficial effects in this model were clear even when treatment was started after the beginning of disease. Autoantibody production in another model using hepatitis B eAg-expressing mice was presented by hCTLA4-Ig after triggering of disease by injection of a peptide containing a T-cell recognition site (118).

Indirect evidence for a role of the CD28 receptor system in other autoimmune diseases derives from the abnormal expression of CD80 and CD86 in diseased tissue.

In psoriasis and mycosis fungoides, CD80 and CD86 expression is highest on dermal dendritic cells in lesions (119), and these cells have enhanced ability to stimulate spontaneous T-cell proliferation. Aberrant CD80 expression was described in autoimmune thyroid disease (120), and it also accompanies T-cell infection with the retrovirus HTLV-1 in vitro (121). Chronically stimulated T-cell lines and CD4 T cells from HIV-1 infected donors also show CD80 and CD86 expression (122–124). These results suggest a more widespread involvement of the CD28 receptor in immune dysregulation during viral infection and disease.

In a lethal model of GVHD using transplantation of bone marrow cells across major and minor histocompatibility differences, acute symptoms were prevented in CTLA4-Ig treated mice, and survival was prolonged (125,126). Some hematological abnormalities were still found in treated mice, including pancytopenia and alterations in cellular composition of the spleen. CTLA4-Ig was not very effective in treatment of chronic GVHD. Taken together, the results suggest that CTLA4-Ig will be most useful for treatment in autoimmunity, where production of autoantibodies makes a major contribution to disease, but may be less effective than CD2 or CD18 ligands in blocking activity of cytotoxic T cells. The expression of CD80 on tumor cells has been identified as a critical determinant for induction of a cytotoxic $CD8^+$ T-cell response, but once activated, the cells were capable of killing tumor cells that did not express a CD28 ligand (127). Therefore treatment with CTLA4-Ig is likely to block priming of new cytotoxic T cells but not the activity of primed effector cells that have already responded to antigen.

F. The CD40 Receptor System

CD40 (formerly called Bp50) is a 50-kDa glycoprotein expressed by B cells, dendritic cells, activated endothelial cells, activated T cells, and some carcinomas and melanomas (128–132). CD40 is a member of the TNF receptor family (133), whose other members include CD27, 4-1BB, FAS, nerve growth factor receptor, and both the 55- and 75-kDa TNF receptors (134–138). A ligand for murine CD40 was isolated by expression cloning using a soluble CD40-Ig fusion protein and found to be a type II membrane protein closely related to TNF and expressed by activated T cells (139). Human CD40 ligand (CD40L or gp39) was rapidly identified and found to be defective in an X-linked immunodeficiency disease called hyper-IgM syndrome (140–144). These patients are unable to make IgG antibody responses to T-cell–dependent antigens and are susceptible to bacterial infections. Mice deficient in expression of gp39 have been generated and found to be unresponsive to T-dependent antigens and unable to generate germinal centers where B-cell maturation and differentiation take place (145). CD40 signals are therefore required for B-cell function and cannot be replaced by cytokines or by other adhesion receptors. In addition to activated T cells, mast cells and basophils also express gp39 and stimulate CD40 signals to enhance IgE synthesis (146).

CD40 activation occurs primarily during T-cell/B-cell interactions and is required for IgG antibody production. CD40 is also functionally active on macrophages, where it can stimulate production of cytokines, including IL-1 and TNF (128). CD40 can also transmit signals on activated epithelial cells (130) and causes upregulation of CD80 and CD86 on dendritic cells and B cells (147). CD40 therefore plays an important role in APC activation to promote efficient support for cognate

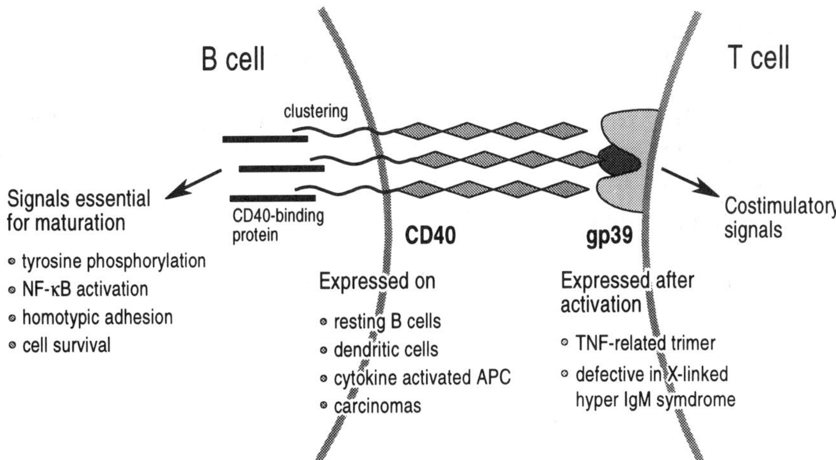

Figure 5 The CD40 receptor system. CD40 signals are required for B-cell maturation, since defects in binding of the CD40 ligand (gp39) cause immunodeficiency with failure of B-cell isotype switching and affinity maturation. A novel RING finger protein (CD40-binding protein) that binds the CD40 cytoplasmic tail has recently been isolated.

T-cell activation through CD28. The engagement of CD40 by gp39 expressed on activated T cells may also send direct signals to the T cell through the cytoplasmic tail of gp39 (148). Since CD28 signals in T cells also promote expression of gp39 (149), the CD40 and CD28 receptors form a circuit to promote each other's activation (150).

In agreement with the genetic data showing the critical nature of CD40 signals, inhibition of the CD40 receptor has already been found to prevent T-dependent Ab responses in vivo (151). A neutralizing mAb to murine gp39, MR1 (152), was an effective inhibitor of responses to antigen and prevented formation of germinal centers where B-cell maturation and selection occurs (153). MR1 seems to induce a state of antigen-specific tolerance but does not deplete antigen-primed T cells (154). MR1 has shown specific and nontoxic immunosuppressive activity in autoimmune disease models including collagen type II arthritis (155), spontaneous lupus (156), and both acute and chronic GVHD (157). An inhibitory mAb to human gp39 was also described, but data have so far been limited to in vitro experiments (158).

Soluble ligands that bind to CD40, including mAbs and gp39-CD8 fusion proteins, are potent agonists in vitro (129,142). Cross-linking of CD40 is required for full activation (159,160), and—under natural conditions—this is provided by the trimeric structure of gp39. Stimulatory mAbs to CD40 have now been recognized to be only partial agonists when compared to natural CD40 ligand (159). Fab fragments of CD40 mAb G28-5 were better inhibitors than the intact mAb, but it is not clear whether it will be possible to inhibit CD40 signals in vivo by ligands that bind to CD40 itself.

CD40 signals have been associated with maintenance of B-cell viability and responsiveness to later stimulation with IL-4 (161–163). CD40 cross-linking prevents activation-induced apoptosis after antigen-receptor triggering in normal B cells (164–168) and can either promote growth or directly induce apoptosis in malignant B cells (169,170). Early signals associated with CD40 activation include nuclear translocation of NF-κB (171,172) and induction of cellular tyrosine phosphorylation with activation of Src-family kinases (173–175). These two responses are probably related, since the nontoxic tyrosine kinase inhibitor herbimycin A blocked NF-κB activation after CD40 stimulation (172). A novel protein that associates with the CD40 cytoplasmic tail was recently identified by yeast two-hybrid cloning of its cDNA (176). This protein may be a transcriptional regulator because it contains a RING finger motif found in other DNA binding proteins. In addition, the CD40-binding protein shows substantial homology with the tumor necrosis factor–receptor-associated factors TRAF-1 and TRAF-2 (177). It is not yet known whether the CD40-binding protein is independent of the tyrosine kinase arm of the CD40 signal.

G. β2 Integrins as Targets for Immunosuppression

The integrins are a diverse family of cell surface heterodimers that mediate adhesion and signal transduction in multiple cell lineages (178,179). The β2 integrins are restricted to leukocytes and consist of CD11a/CD18 (LFA-1), CD11b/CD18 (complement receptor 3), and CD11c/CD18 (p150,95). Neutrophils depend on β2 integrins for their activation, since neutrophils from patients with leukocyte adhesion deficiency type 1 (LAD 1), caused by defective β2 integrins, are unable to make a respiratory burst in response to cytokines or to chemotactic peptides (180–183). Similarly, neutrophil activation in vitro requires adhesion mediated by β2 integrins (184,185). The β2 integrins are also involved in T-cell, B-cell, NK-cell, and macrophage function, since LAD 1 patients exhibit deficiencies in generation of cytotoxic T cells and show low T-cell responses to alloantigen in MLR (183). B-cell responses to T-cell-dependent antigens are low or absent in some patients (186), but lymphocyte responses such as delayed-type hypersensitivity are normal (187). The β1 integrins may provide overlapping signals that can compensate in the absence of β2 integrins to partially support T- and B-cell function, but neutrophils do not have backup support from other integrins. In vitro assays using mAbs to β2 integrins have also implicated these adhesion receptors in diverse leukocyte functions, including cytotoxicity by T cells and NK cells, production of IL-2 by activated T cells, and proliferation and differentiation by B cells (188–193). These functional responses are all inhibited by mAbs to β2 integrins and could be caused simply by prevention of adhesion. However, there is increasing evidence that β2 integrins are also providing transmembrane activation signals directly to responding leukocytes.

Immobilized CD18 or LFA-1 mAbs have been reported to enhance T-cell proliferation responses, and the LFA-1 adhesion ligands ICAM-1 and VCAM-1 also have costimulatory properties (194–198). Similarly, significant enhancement of the monocyte oxidative burst occurred after cross-linking of CD11b with mAbs (199) or by cross-linking with ICAM-1 (200). Cross-linking of either β1 or β2 integrins has been reported to induce tyrosine phosphorylation in fibroblasts or leukocytes (201-204), and some progress has been made in identification of integrin-associated kinases. The focal adhesion kinase (FAK) (205,206) is activated by β1 integrin engagement and is localized in focal adhesions, where it may phosphorylate cytoskeletal substrates such as paxillin and induce cytoskeletal reorganization (207). FAK kinase activation is regulated by β1 integrin aggregation and by receptor occupancy with extracellular matrix or Arg-Gly-Asp (RGD)-containing peptides (207).

CD18 or LFA-1 cross-linking has been found to induce calcium mobilization in T cells and neutrophils (208–210) and to synergize with CD3 cross-linking to increase tyrosine phosphorylation of PLCγ1 (211) without activation of FAK. The tyrosine kinases associated with β2 integrins and their mechanism of association are not yet clear, but a likely candidate is the protein closely related to FAK named fak-B, which has been recently identified in lymphocytes (212). Fak-B becomes associated with ZAP70 in activated T cells and is likely to play a role in TCR signaling pathways (212).

Evidence for the involvement of CD18 in signals leading to apoptosis has also been seen in responses of antigen-specific T-cell lines to bacterial superantigens. CD18 mAbs were found to prevent superantigen-induced apoptosis and were effective if added up to 3 hr after addition of superantigens (213). Apoptosis could also be prevented by herbimycin A or by cyclosporin A, consistent with CD18 signals through a tyrosine kinase pathway and PLCγ1 activation leading to calcium mobilization. The ICAM-1 and ICAM-2 ligands (214,215) expressed as Ig-fusion proteins have stimulatory properties for proliferation of resting T cells when coimmobilized with TCR mAbs and enhance the responsiveness to subsequent CD28 stimulation. However, with alloantigen-primed T cells, costimulation with ICAM-1 increased the frequency of apoptotic cells (216). An inhibitory effect of β1 integrin binding to extracellular matrix on apoptosis in mammary epithelial cells was also reported (217). Blocking mAbs to β1 integrins or destruction of extracellular matrix by protease activation induced apoptosis in these cells, suggesting a broad link between integrin signals and apoptosis.

Signals from multiple leukocyte receptors including CD40 induce homotypic adhesion through increased β2 integrin binding affinity (218). The contributions of late signals from β2 integrins to functional effects initiated from other receptors has not yet been fully explored. In the case of the CD40 receptor, however, induction of IgE synthesis and prevention of B-cell apoptosis by CD40 agonists were both dependent on β2 integrins, since they could be blocked by LFA-1 or CD18 mAbs (219,220). CD40 agonists also stimulate B-cell adhesion through β1 integrins (221); thus CD40 provides an example of a receptor-signaling cascade that depends on sequential activation through integrin adhesion receptors for biological responses.

Inhibitory mAbs to β2 integrins have been studied in vivo and found to be most effective in prevention of reperfusion injury by preventing neutrophils from binding and becoming activated during reperfusion (222–224). CD18 (common β chain) and CD11b mAbs have shown activity in preventing myocardial reperfusion injury or internal organ injury if administered at the time of reperfusion. The combination of an LFA-1 mAb plus an ICAM-1 mAb improved graft acceptance in heart allografts (225) and induced tolerance to an antigen given in the airways to sensitized mice (226). Thus inhibitors of β2 integrin function may be useful for immunosuppression and induction of tolerance during transplantation (227) and are very effective at preventing reperfusion injury by blocking neutrophil migration and activation. Toxicity was not seen in these studies. However, the utility in vivo of β2 integrin inhibitors for treatment of chronic autoimmune diseases may be limited by inhibitory effects on neutrophil activation and increased susceptibility to bacterial infections.

III. CLINICAL PROSPECTS FOR INHIBITORS OF COSTIMULATION

The costimulatory receptors on T cells and APC are attractive targets for development of biological inhibitors because of their potential for induction of tolerance. Each of the receptors discussed here signals by coupling to cytoplasmic tyrosine kinases that contribute to activation through complex interactions with other tyrosine kinases and phosphorylation of key substrates. The mAbs and soluble ligands that have shown promise for tolerance induction in vivo all seem to work by disrupting the delicate balance that is maintained between tyrosine kinases and phosphatases (228).

Each costimulatory receptor has a special role in signal transduction, even when it uses the same tyrosine kinase, as do CD4 and CD2 through associated Lck. The tolerance that develops following receptor binding and the mechanisms of action differ for each costimulatory receptor target. Ligands that bind CD2 and CD4 are both thought to give negative signals, probably by disrupting Lck interactions with the TCR. CD2 ligands cause tolerance through the emergence of an immunoregulatory T-cell subset secreting TFGβ and IL4 (58,229), while CD4 ligands may prime T cells to enter apoptosis when stimulated by antigen. These receptor-specific responses must be distinguished from immunosuppression by CD4 or CD2 ligands that can result from T-cell depletion by Fc-dependent mechanisms.

The CD28 and CD40 receptor systems are important new targets for immunomodulation that have emerged in the past several years. In both cases, effective inhibitors block receptor engagement during cell-cell adhesion. The CTLA4-Ig fusion protein prevents CD28 stimulation by binding with high avidity to the CD80 and CD86 ligands on activated APC. CTLA4-Ig induces T-cell anergy in vitro and in vivo by preventing the transmission of key signals through CD28. These signals involve the activation of tyrosine kinases, and T-cell unresponsiveness occurs because of disrupted signals. Because of the effectiveness of CTLA4-Ig in models of chronic autoimmune diseases, it is likely to be the next receptor inhibitor to be tested in clinical trials.

Inhibitors of the CD40 receptor have been made from neutralizing mAbs to gp39 expressed on activated T cells. In the mouse, the MR1 mAb promoted development of T-cell anergy in vivo without depleting antigen-primed T cells. Since the CD40 signal is associated with induction of CD80 and CD86 expression on APC, these results suggest that inhibitors of APC coreceptors such as CD40 can prevent signals that would otherwise be transmitted back to the antigen-specific T cell. MR1 was also capable of preventing T-cell responses in vivo and was effective in autoimmune mouse models and GVHD. In the human, soluble CD40-Ig fusion protein prevented CD40 responses in vitro, and blocking mAbs to human gp39 have also been effective. Clinical potential for CD40 inhibitors appears promising, but production of molecules for use in humans may take several years.

Antibodies to β2-integrins LFA-1, CD11b, or CD18 inhibit some lymphocyte effector functions such as T-cell cytotoxicity by preventing adhesion to target cells. Blocking activation signals is also likely to play a role in inhibitory properties of these mAbs. Although there has been encouraging results in T-cell tolerance induction when both LFA-1 and ICAM-1 are blocked by specific mAbs, the uses in vivo for treatment of chronic diseases may be limited by immunosuppression caused by blocking the widespread function of β2-integrins in diverse leukocyte responses.

Another approach to induction of antigen-specific tolerance uses soluble CD3 agonists to rapidly internalize the antigen receptor and provide transient polyclonal signals without full T-cell activation. The CD3 mAb OKT3 is based on this approach, but its activity is limited by toxicity provided by Fc receptor interactions with OKT3 that can induce inflammatory cytokine release (230). Tolerogenic peptides (231) derived from altered T-cell recognition sequences have recently been shown to induce partial activation signals to T-cell clones when compared with the native peptide (232,233). There are therefore multiple receptors and approaches that can alter T-cell/APC interactions to promote T-cell unresponsiveness through altered tyrosine kinase signals. Some of these approaches are likely to be complementary, but only a few studies have begun to identify desirable combinations (57,229). In addition, since requirements for induction of unresponsiveness differs among different subsets (234–236), it is likely that in some cases a tolerant state develops because of changes in the balance of subsets of antigen-specific T cells. The nature of the unresponsive state may therefore differ depending on the costimulatory receptor that is targeted, and future studies to address these questions will be needed.

REFERENCES

1. Clift RA, Storb R. Histoincompatible bone marrow transplants in humans. Annu Rev. Immunol 1987; 5:43–64.
2. Korngold R, Sprent J. Lethal graft-versus-host disease after bone marrow transplantation across minor histocompatibility barriers in mice: Prevention by removing mature T cells from marrow. J Exp Med 1987; 148:1687–1690.
3. Vallera DA, Blazar BR. T-cell depletion for graft-versus-host disease (GVHD) prophylaxis: A perspective on engraftment in mice and humans. Transplantation 1989; 47: 751–760.
4. Goldman JM, Gale RP, Horowitz MM. Bone marrow transplantation for chronic myelogenous leukemia in chronic phase: Increased risk to relapse associated with T cell depletion. Ann Intern Med 1988; 108:806–814.
5. Bretscher P, Cohn M. A theory of self-nonself discrimination. Science 1970; 169:1042–1049.
6. Hollenbaugh D, Ochs HD, Noelle RJ, et al. The role of CD40 and its ligand in the regulation of the immune response. Immunol Rev 1994; 138:23–37.
7. Matsui K, Boniface JJ, Reay PA, et al. Low affinity interaction of peptide-MHC complexes with T cell receptors. Science 1991; 254:1788–1791.
8. Perlmutter RM. In vivo dissection of lymphocyte signaling pathways. Clin Immunol Immunopathol 1993; 67:S44–S49.
9. Chan AC, Irving BA, Fraser JD, Weiss A. The zeta chain is associated with a tyrosine kinase and upon T-cell antigen receptor stimulation associates with ZAP-70, a 70-kDa tyrosine phosphoprotein. Proc Natl Acad Sci USA 1991; 88:9166–9170.
10. Weiss A. T cell antigen receptor signal transduction: A tale of tails and cytoplasmic protein-tyrosine kinases. Cell 1993; 73:209–212.
11. Wange RL, Kong AN, Samelson LE. A tyrosine-phosphorylated 70-kDa protein binds a photoaffinity analogue of ATP and associates with both the zeta chain and CD3 components of the activated T cell antigen receptor. J Biol Chem 1992; 267:11685–11688.
12. Bolen JB, Rowley RB, Spana C, Tsygankov AY. The Src family of tyrosine protein kinases in hemopoietic signal transduction. FASEB J 1992; 6:3403–3409.

13. Weiss A, Littman DR. Signal transduction by lymphocyte antigen receptors. Cell 1994; 76:263–274.
14. Iwashima M, Irving BA, van Oers NS, et al. Sequential interactions of the TCR with two distinct cytoplasmic tyrosine kinases. Science 1994; 263:1136–1139.
15. Timson Gauen LK, Zhu Y, Letourneur F, et al. Interactions of p59fyn and ZAP-70 with T-cell receptor activation motifs: defining the nature of a signaling motif. Mol Cell Biol 1994; 14:3729–3741.
16. Wange RL, Malek SN, Desiderio S, Samelson LE. Tandem SH2 domains of ZAP-70 bind to T cell antigen receptor zeta and CD3 epsilon from activated Jurkat T cells. J Biol Chem 1993; 268:19797–19801.
17. Arpaia E, Shahar M, Dadi H, et al. Defective T cell receptor signaling and $CD8^+$ thymic selection in humans lacking zap-70 kinase. Cell 1994: 76:947–958.
18. Chan AC, Kadlecek TA, Elder ME, et al. ZAP-70 deficiency in an autosomal recessive form of severe combined immunodeficiency. Science 1994; 264:1599–15601.
19. Saizawa K, Rojo J, Janeway CAJ. Evidence for a physical association of CD4 and the CD3: Alpha:beta T cell receptor. Nature 1987; 238:260–263.
20. Takada S, Engleman EG. Evidence for an association between CD8 molecules and the T cell receptor complex on cytotoxic T cells. J Immunol 1987; 139:3231–3235.
21. Brown MH, Cantrell DA, Brattsand G, et al. The CD2 antigen associates with the T-cell antigen receptor CD3 antigen complex on the surface of human T-lymphocytes. Nature 1989; 339:551–553.
22. Kupfer A, Singer SJ, Janeway CAJ, Swain SL. Coclustering of CD4 (L3T4) molecule with the T-cell receptor is induced by specific direct interaction of helper T cells and antigen-presenting cells. Proc Natl Acad Sci USA 1987; 84:5888–5892.
23. Bierer BE, Golan DE, Brown CS, et al. A monoclonal antibody to LFA-3, the CD2 ligand, specifically immobilizes major histocompatibility complex proteins. Eur J Immunol 1989; 19:661–665.
24. Bierer BE, Peterson A, Gorga JC, et al. Synergistic T cell activation via the physiological ligands for CD2 and T cell receptor. J Exp Med 1988; 168:1145–1156.
25. Kanner SB, Damle NK, Blake J, et al. CD2/LFA-3 ligation induces phospholipase-C gamma-1-tyrosine phosphorylation and regulates CD3 signaling. J Immunol 1992; 148:2023–2029.
26. Luescher IF, Vivier E, Layer A, et al. CD8 modulation of T-cell antigen receptor-ligand interactions on living cytotoxic T lymphocytes. Nature 1995; 373:353–356.
27. Wee S, Schieven GL, Kirihara JM, et al. Tyrosine phosphorylation of CD6 by stimulation of CD3: Augmentation by the CD4 and CD2 coreceptors. J Exp Med 1993; 177: 219–223.
28. Wilde DB, Marrack P, Kappler J, et al. Evidence implicating L3T4 in class II MHC antigen reactivity: monoclonal antibody GK1.5 (anti-L3T4a) blocks class II MHC antigen-specific proliferation, release of lymphokines, and binding by cloned murine helper T lymphocyte lines. J Immunol 1983; 131:2178–2183.
29. Wassmer PJ, Chan C, Lodgberg L, Shevach EM. Role of the L3T4-antigen in T cell activation: II. Inhibition of T cell activation by monoclonal anti-L3T4 antibodies in the absence of accessory cells. J Immunol 1985; 135:2237–2242.
30. Tite J, Sloan A, Janeway CA. The role of L3T4 in T cell activation: L3T4 may be both an Ia-binding protein and a receptor that transduces a negative signal. J Mol Cell Immunol 1986; 2:179–190.
31. Miller G, Hochman PS, Meier W, et al. Specific interaction of LFA-3 with CD2 can inhibit T cell responses. J Exp Med 1993; 178:211–222.
32. Martin PJ, Longton G, Ledbetter JA, et al. Functionally distinct epitopes of human Tp50. J Immunol 1983; 131:180–185.
33. Ohno H, Nakamura T, Yagita H, et al. Induction of negative signal through CD2 during antigen-specific T cell activation. J Immunol 1991; 147:2100–2106.

34. Lamb JR, Zanders ED, Sewell W, et al. Antigen-specific T cell unresponsiveness in cloned helper T cells mediated via the CD2 or CD3/Ti receptor patheways. Eur J Immunol 1987; 17:1641–1644.
35. Yokoyama A, Suzuki H, Kamitani T, et al. Characterization of inhibitory effect of an anti-murine CD2 monoclonal antibody on the proliferation of T cell clones. Immunol Lett 1991; 28:219–225.
36. Meuer SC, Hussey RE, Fabbi M, et al. An alternative pathway of T-cell activation: A functional role for the 50 kd T11 sheep erythrocyte receptor protein. Cell 1984; 36: 897–906.
37. Bockenstedt LK, Goldsmith MA, Dustin M, et al. The CD2 ligand LFA-3 activates T cells but depends on the expression and function of the antigen receptor. J Immunol 1988; 141:1904–1911.
38. Alcover A, Alberini C, Acuto O, et al. Interdependence of CD3-T1 and CD2 activation pathways in human T lymphocytes. EMBO J 1988; 7:1973–1977.
39. Danielian S, Fagard R, Alcover A, et al. The tyrosine kinase activity of p56lck is increased in human T cells activated via CD2. Eur J Immunol 1991; 21:1967–1970.
40. Veillette A, Bookman MA, Horak EM, et al. Signal transduction through the CD4 receptor involves the activation of the internal membrane tyrosine-protein kinase p56lck. Nature 1989; 338:257–259.
41. Banda NK, Bernier J, Kurahara DK, et al. Crosslinking CD4 by human immunodeficiency virus gp120 prime cells for activation-induced apoptosis. J Exp Med 1992; 176: 1099–1106.
42. Wang ZQ, Orlikowsky T, Dudhane A, et al. Deletion of T lymphocytes in human CD4 transgenic mice induced by HIV-gp120 and gp120-specific antibodies from AIDS patients. Eur J Immunol 1994; 24:1553–1557.
43. Terai C, Kombluth RS, Pauza CD, et al. Apoptosis as a mechanism of cell death in cultured T lymphoblasts acutely infected with HIV-1. J Clin Invest 1991; 87:1710–1715.
44. Wang Z-Q, Dudhane A, Orlikowsky T, et al. CD4 engagement induces Fas antigen-dependent apoptosis of T cells in vivo. Eur J Immunol 1994; 24:1549–1552.
45. Wofsy D. Treatment of murine lupus with anti-CD4 monoclonal antibodies. Immunol Ser 1993; 59:221–234.
46. Wofsy D, Mayes DC, Woodcock J, Seaman WE. Inhibition of humoral immunity in vivo by monoclonal antibody to L3T4: Studies with soluble antigens in intact mice. J Immunol 1985; 135:1698–1701.
47. Koike T, Itoh Y, Ishi T, et al. Preventive effect of monoclonal anti-L3T4 antibody on development of diabetes in NOD mice. Diabetes 1987; 36:539–541.
48. Shizuru JA, Taylor-Edwards C, Banks BA, et al. Immunotherapy of the nonobese diabetic mouse: treatment with an antibody to T-helper lymphocytes. Science 1988; 240:659–661.
49. Ranges GE, Sriram S, Cooper SM. Prevention of type II collagen-induced arthritis by in vivo treatment with anti-L3T4. J Exp Med 1985; 162:1105–1110.
50. Gutstein NL, Wofsy D. Administration of $F(ab')_2$ fragments of monoclonal antibody to L3T4 inhibits humoral immunity in mice without depleting $L3T4^+$ cells. J Immunol 1986; 137:3414–3419.
51. Carteron NL, Schimenti CL, Wofsy D. Treatment of murine lupus with $F(ab')_2$ fragments of monoclonal antibody to L3T4: Suppression of autoimmunity does not depend on T helper cell depletion. J Immunol 1989; 142:1470–1475.
52. Herzog CH, Walker CH, Muller W, et al. Anti-CD4 antibody treatment of patients with rheumatoid arthritis: I. Effect on clinical couse and circulating T cells. J Autoimmun 1989; 2:627–642.
53. Horneff G, Burmester GR, Emmrich F, Kalder JR. Treatment of rheumatoid arthritis with an anti-CD4 monoclonal antibody. Arthritis Rheum 1991; 34:129–140.

54. Reiter C, Kakavand B, Rieber EP, et al. Treatment of rheumatoid arthritis with monoclonal CD4 antibody M-T151: Clinical results and immunopharmacologic effects in an open study, including repeated administration. Arthritis Rheum 1991; 34:525–536.
55. Moreland LW, Bucy R, Pratt PW, et al. Treatment of refractory rheumatoid arthritis with a chimeric anti-CD4 monoclonal anti-body. Clin Res 1991; 39:309A.
56. Chavin KD, Lau HT, Bromberg JS. Prolongation of allograft and xenograft survival in mice by anti-CD2 monoclonal antibodies. Transplantation 1992; 54:286–291.
57. Chavin KD, Qin L, Woodard JE, et al. Anti-CD2 monoclonal antibodies synergize with FK506 but not with cyclosporine or rapamycin to induce tolerance. Transplantation 1994; 57:736–740.
58. Guckel B, Berek C, Lutz M, et al. Anti-CD2 antibodies induce T cell unresponsiveness in vivo. J Exp Med 1991; 174:957–967.
59. Chavin KD, Qin L, Lin J, et al. Anti-CD2 and anti-CD3 monoclonal antibodies synergize to prolong allograft survival with decreased side effects. Transplantation 1993; 55:901–908.
60. Majeau GR, Meier W, Jimmo B, et al. Mechanism of lymphocyte function-associated molecule 3-Ig fusion proteins inhibition of T cell responses. J Immunol 1994; 152: 2753–2767.
61. June CH, Ledbetter JA, Linsley PS, Thompson CB. Role of the CD28 receptor in T cell activation. Immunol Today 1990; 11:211–216.
62. Cooper JA, King CS. Dephosphorylation or antibody binding to the carboxy terminus stimulates pp60c src. Mol Cell Biol 1986; 6:4467–4477.
63. Schieven G, Martin GS. Nonenzymatic phosphorylation of tyrosine and serine by ATP is catalyzed by manganese but not magnesium. J Biol Chem 1988; 263:15590–15593.
64. Linsley PS, Ledbetter JA. The role of the CD28 receptor during T cell responses to antigen. Annu Rev Immunol 1993; 11:191–212.
65. Linsley PS, Brady W, Urnes M, et al. CTLA-4 is a second receptor for the B cell activation antigen B7. J Exp Med 1991; 174:561–569.
66. Linsley PS, Clark EA, Ledbetter JA. T cell antigen CD28 mediates adhesion with B cells by interacting with activation antigen B7/BB-1. Proc Natl Acad Sci USA 1990; 87:5031–5035.
67. Azuma M, Ito D, Yagita H, et al. B70 antigen is a second ligand for CTLA-4 and CD38. Nature 1993; 366:76–79.
68. Freeman GJ, Gribben JG, Boussiotis VA, et al. Cloning of B7-2: A CTLA-4 counter-receptor that costimulates human T cell proliferation (see comments). Science 1993; 262:909–911.
69. Linsley PS, Brady W, Grosmaire L, et al. Binding of the B cell activation antigen B7 to CD28 costimulates T cell proliferation and interleukin 2 mRNA accumulation. J Exp Med 1991; 173:721–730.
70. Freeman GJ, Borriello F, Hodes RJ, et al. Murine B7-2, an alternative CTLA4 counter-receptor that costimulates T cell proliferation and interleukin 2 production. J Exp Med 1993; 178:2185–2192.
71. Caux CB, Van Bervhet C, Massacrier MA, et al. B70/B7-2 is identical to CD86 and is the major functional ligand for CD28 expressed on hyman dendritic cells. J Exp Med 1994; 180:1841–1847.
72. Tan P, Anasetti C, Hansen JA, et al. Induction of alloantigen-specific hyporesponsiveness in human T lymphocytes by blocking interaction of CD28 with its natural ligand B7/BB1. J Exp Med 1993; 177:165–173.
73. Harding FA, McArthur JG, Gross JA, et al. CD28-mediated signaling co-stimulates murine T cells and prevents induction of anergy in T-cell clones. Nature 1992; 356: 607–609.

74. Gimmi CD, Freeman GJ, Gribben JG, et al. Human T-cell clonal anergy is induced by antigen presentation in the absence of B7 costimulation. Proc Natl Acad Sci USA 1993; 90:6586–6590.
75. Boussiotis VA, Freeman GJ, Gray G, et al. B7 but not intercellular adhesion molecule-1 costimulation prevents the induction of human alloantigen-specific tolerance. J Exp Med 1993; 178:1753–1763.
76. Shahinian A, Pfeffer K, Lee KP, et al. Differential T cell costimulatory requirements in CD28-deficient mice. Science 1993; 261:609–612.
77. Damle NK, Linsley PS, Ledbetter JA. Direct helper T cell-induced B-cell differentiation involves T-cell antigen CD28 and B-cell activation antigen B7. Eur J Immunol 1991; 21:1277–1282.
78. Linsley PS, Wallace PM, Johnson J, et al. Immunosuppression in vivo by a soluble form of the CTLA-4 T cell activation molecule. Science 1992; 257:792–795.
79. Linsley PS, Greene JL, Tan P, et al. Coexpression and functional cooperation of CTLA-4 and CD28 on activated T lymphocytes. J Exp Med 1992; 176:1595–1604.
80. Freeman GJ, Lombard DB, Gimmi CD, et al. CTLA-4 and CD28 mRNA are coexpressed in most T cells after activation: Expression of CTLA-4 and CD28 mRNA does not correlate with the pattern of lymphokine production. J Immunol 1992; 149:3795–3801.
81. Lindsten T, Lee KP, Harris ES, et al. Characterization of CTLA-4 structure and expression on human T cells. J Immunol 1993; 151:3489–3499.
82. Damle NK, Klussman K, Leytze G, et al. Costimulation of T lymphocytes with integrin ligands intercellular adhesion molecule-1 or vascular cell adhesion molecule-1 induces functional expression of CTLA-4, a second receptor for B7. J Immunol 1994; 152: 2686–2697.
83. Walunas TL, Lenschow DJ, Bakker CY, et al. CTLA-4 can function as a negative regulator of T cell activation. Immunity 1994; 1:405–413.
84. Gribben JG, Freeman GJ, Boussiotis VA, et al. CTLA4 mediated antigen-specific apoptosis of human T cells. Proc Natl Acad Sci USA 1995; 92:811–815.
85. Green JM, Noel PJ, Sperling AI, et al. Absence of B7-dependent responses in CD28-deficient mice. Immunity 1994; 1:501–508.
86. Freeman GJ, Freedman AS, Segil JM, et al. B7, a new member of the Ig superfamily with unique expression on activated and neoplastic B-cells. J Immunol 1989; 143:2714–2722.
87. Ramarathinam L, Castle M, Wu Y, Liu Y. T cell costimulation by B7/BB1 induces CD8 T cell-dependent tumor rejection: an important role of B7/BB1 in the induction, recruitment, and effector function of antitumor T cells. J Exp Med 1994; 179:1205–1214.
88. Chen L, McGowan P, Ashe S, et al. Tumor immunogenicity determines the effect of B7 costimulation on T cell-mediated tumor immunity. J Exp Med 1994; 179:523–532.
89. Hathcock KS, Laszlo G, Pucillo C, et al. Comparative analysis of B7-1 and B7-2 costimulatory ligands: Expression and function. J Exp Med 1994; 180:631–640.
90. Larsen CP, Ritchie SC, Hendrix R, et al. Regulation of immunostimulatory function and costimulatory molecule (B7-1 and B7-2) expression on murine dendritic cells. J Immunol 1994; 152:5208–5219.
91. Linsley PS, Greene JL, Brady W, et al. Human B7-1 (CD80) and B7-2 (CD86) bind with similar avidities but distinct kinetics to CD28 and CTLA-4-receptors. Immunity 1994; 1:793–801.
92. Ledbetter JA, Imboden J, Schieven GL, et al. CD28 ligation in T-cell activation: Evidence for two signal transduction pathways. Blood 1990; 75:1531–1539.
93. June CH, Ledbetter JA, Gillespie MM, et al. T-cell proliferation involving the CD28 pathway is associated with cyclosporine-resistant interleukin 2 gene expression. Mol Cell Biol 1987; 7:4472–4481.

94. Linsley PS, Ledbetter JA. Immunoligands: CTLA4-Ig and the CD28 T cell costimulatory pathway. In press.
95. Fraser JD, Irving BA, Crabtree GR, Weiss A. Regulationi of interleukin-2 gene enhancer activity by the T cell accessory molecule CD28. Science 1991; 251:313–316.
96. Fraser JD, Weiss A. Regulation of T-cell lymphokine gene transcription by the accessory molecule CD28. Mol Cell Biol 1992; 12:4357–4363.
97. Verweij CL, Geerts M, Aarden LA. Activation of interleukin-2 gene transcription via the T-cell surface molecule CD28 is mediated through an NF-kB-like response element. J Biol Chem 1991; 266:14179–14182.
98. Lindsten T, June CH, Ledbetter JA, et al. Regulation of lymphokine messenger RNA stability by a surface-mediated T-cell activation pathway. Science 1989; 244:339–343.
99. Lu Y, Granelli-Piperno A, Bjorndahl JM, et al. CD28-induced T cell activation: Evidence for a protein-tyrosine kinase signal transduction pathway. J Immunol 1992; 149:24–29.
100. Vandenberghe P, Freeman GJ, Nadler LM, et al. Antibody and B7/BB1-mediated ligation of the CD28 receptor induces tyrosine phosphorylation in human T cells. J Exp Med 1992; 175:951–960.
101. Hutchcroft JE, Bierer BE. Activation-dependent phosphorylation of the T-lymphocyte surface receptor CD28 and associated proteins. Proc Natl Acad Sci USA 1994; 91: 3260–3264.
102. Pages F, Ragueneau M, Rottapel R, et al. Binding of phosphatidylinositol-3-OH kinase to CD28 is required for T-cell signalling. Nature 1994; 369:327–329.
103. Prasad KV, Cai YC, Raab M, et al. T-cell antigen CD28 interacts with the lipid kinase phosphatidylinositol 3-kinase by a cytoplasmic Tyr(P)-Met-Xaa-Met motif. Proc Natl Acad Sci USA 1994; 91:2834–2838.
104. Stein PH, Fraser JD, Weiss A. The cytoplasmic domain of CD28 is both necessary and sufficient for costimulation of interleukin-2 secretion and association with phosphatidylinositol 3′-kinase. Mol Cell Biol 1994; 14:3392–3402.
105. Truitt KE, Hicks CM, Imboden JB. Stimulation of CD28 triggers an association between CD28 and phosphatidylinositol 3-kinase in Jurkat T cells. J Exp Med 1994; 179:1071–1076.
106. August A, Gibson S, Kawakamis Y, et al. CD28 is associated with and induces the immediate tyrosine phosphorylation and activation of the tec family kinase itk/tskemt in the jurkat leukemic T-cell line. Proc Natl Acad Sci USA 1994; 91:9347–9351.
107. August A, Dupont B. Activation of src family kinase lck following CD28 crosslinking in the Jurkat leukemic cell line. Biochem Biophys Res Commun 1994; 199:1466–1473.
108. Ledbetter JA, Linsley PS. CD28 receptor crosslinking induces tyrosine phosphorylation of PLCy-1. Adv Exp Med Biol 1992; 323:23–27.
109. Su B, Jacinto E, Hibi M, et al. JNK is involved in signal integration during costimulation of T lymphocytes. Cell 1994; 77:727–736.
110. Nunes JA, Collette Y, Truneh A, et al. The role of p21ras in CD28 signal transduction: Triggering of CD28 with antibodies, but not the ligand B7-1, activates p21ras. J Exp Med 1995; 180:1067–1076.
111. Wallace PM, Rodgers JN, Leytze GM, et al. Induction and reversal of long-lived specific unresponsiveness to a T-dependent antigen following treatment with soluble CTLA-4. Submitted for publication.
112. Lin H, Bolling SF, Linsley PS, et al. Long-term acceptance of major histocompatibility complex mismatched cardiac allografts induced by CTLA4Ig plus donor-specific transfusion. J Exp Med 1993; 178:1801–1806.
113. Pearson TC, Alexander DZ, Winn KJ, et al. Transplantation tolerance induced by CTLA4-Ig. Transplantation 1994; 57:1701–1706.
114. Turka LA, Linsley PS, Lin H, et al. T-cell activation by the CD28 ligand B7 is required for cardiac allograft rejection in vivo. Proc Natl Acad Sci USA 1992; 89:11102–11105.

115. Lenschow DJ, Zeng Y, Thistlethwaite JR, et al. Long-term survival of xenogeneic pancreatic islet grafts induced by CTLA4lg (see comments). Science 1992; 257:789-792.
116. Finck BK, Linsley PS, Wofsy D. Treatment of murine lupus with CTLA4lg. Science 1994; 265:1225-1227.
117. Nishikawa K, Linsley PS, Collins AB, et al. Effect of CTLA-4 chimeric protein on rat autoimmune anti-glomerular basement membrane glomerulonephritis. Eur J Immunol 1994; 24:1249-1254.
118. Milich DR, Linsley PS, Hughes JL, Jones JE. Soluble CTLA-4 can suppress autoantibody production and elicit long term unresponsiveness in a novel transgenic model. J Immunol 1994; 153:429-435.
119. Nestle FO, Turka LA, Nickoloff BJ. Characterization of dermal dendritic cells in psoriasis: Autostimulation of T lymphocytes and induction of the Th1 type cytokines. J Clin Invest 1994; 94:202-209.
120. Tandon N, Metcalfe RA, Barnett D, Weetman AP. Expression of the costimulatory molecule B7/BB1 in autoimmune thyroid disease. Q J Med 1994; 87:231-236.
121. Valle AP, Garrone JY, Bonnefoy J-Y, et al. mAb 104, a new monoclonal antibody, recognizes the B7 antigen that is expressed on activated B cells and HTLV-1-transformer cells. Immunology 1990; 69:531-535.
122. Haffar OK, Smithgall MD, Bradshaw J, et al. Costimulation of T-cell activation and virus production by B7 antigen on activated CD4$^+$ T cells from human immunodeficiency virus type 1-infected donors. Proc Natl Acad Sci USA 1993; 90:11094-11098.
123. Sansom DM, Hall ND. B7/BB1, the ligand for CD28, is expressed on repeatedly activated human T cells in vitro. Eur J Immunol 1993; 23:295-298.
124. Azuma M, Yssel H, Phillips JH, et al. Functional expression of B7/BB1 on activated T lymphocytes. J Exp Med 1993; 177:845-850.
125. Blazar BR, Taylor PA, Linsley PS, Vallera DA. In vivo blockade of CD28/CTLA4: B7/BB1 interaction with CTLA4-Ig. Blood 1994; 83:3815-3825.
126. Wallace PM, Johnson JS, MacMaster JF, et al. CTLA4-Ig treatment ameliorates the lethality of murine graft-versus-host disease across major histocompatibility complex barriers. Transplantation 1994; 58:602-610.
127. de Boer M, Kasran A, Kwekkeboom J, et al. Ligation of B7 with CD28/CTLA-4 on T cells results in CD40 ligand expression, interleukin-4 secretion and efficient help for antibody production by B cells. Eur J Immunol 1993; 23:3120-3125.
128. Alderson MR, Armitage RJ, Tough TW, et al. CD40 expression by human monocytes: Regulation by cytokines and activation of monocytes by the ligand CD40. J Exp Med 1993; 178:669-674.
129. Clark EA, Ledbetter JA. Activation of human B cells mediated through two distinct cell surface differentiation antigen, Bp35 and Bp50. Proc Natl Acad Sci USA 1986; 83: 4494-4498.
130. Galy AH, Spits H. CD40 is functionally expressed on human thymic epithelial cells. J Immunol 1992; 149:775-782.
131. Paulie S, Ehlin-Hendricksson B, Mellstedt H, et al. A p50 surface antigen restricted to human urinary bladder carcinomans and B lymphocytes. Cancer Immunol Immunother 1985; 20:23-28.
132. Ledbetter JA, Clark EA, Norris NA, et al. Expression of a functional B cell receptor Bp50 on carcinomas. Leukocyte Typing III 1987; 432-435.
133. Stamenkovic I, Clark EA, Seed B. A B-lymphocyte activation molecule related to the nerve growth factor receptor and induced by cytokines in carcinomas. EMBO J 1989; 8:1403-1410.
134. Camerini D, Walz G, Loenen WA, et al. The T cell activation antigen CD27 is a member of the nerve growth factor/tumor necrosis factor receptor gene family. J Immunol 1991; 147:3165-3169.

135. Durkop H, Latza U, Hummel M, et al. Molecular cloning and expression of a new member of the nerve growth factor receptor family that is characteristic for Hodgkin's disease. Cell 1992; 68:421–427.
136. Kwon BS, Weissman SM. cDNA sequences of two inducible T-cell genes. Proc Natl Acad Sci USA 1989; 86:1963–1967.
137. Heller RA, Song K, Onasch MA, et al. Complementary DNa cloning of a receptor for tumor necrosis factor and demonstration for a shed form of the receptor. Proc Natl Acad Sci USA 1990; 87:6151–6155.
138. Loetscher H, Pan Y-CE, Lahm HW, et al. Molecular cloning and expression of the human 55 kd tumor necrosis factor receptor. Cell 1990; 61:351–359.
139. Armitage RJ, Strockbine L, Sato TA, et al. Molecular and biological characterization of a murine ligand for CD40. Nature 1992; 357:80–82.
140. Aruffo A, Farrington M, Hollenbaugh D, et al. The CD40 ligand, gp39, is defective in activated T cells from patients with X-linked hyper-IgM syndrome. Cell 1993; 72:291–300.
141. DiSanto JP, Bonnefoy JY, Gauchat JF, et al. CD40 ligand mutations in X-linked immunodeficiency with hyper-IgM. Nature 1993; 361:541–543.
142. Hollenbaugh D, Grosmaire LS, Kullas CD, et al. The human T cell antigen gp39, a member of the TNF gene family, is a ligand for the CD40 receptor: expression of a soluble form of gp39 with B cell co-stimulatory activity. EMBO J 1992; 11:4313–4321.
143. Spriggs MK, Armitage RJ, Strockbine L, et al. Recombinant human CD40 ligand stimulates B cell proliferation and immunoglobulin E secretion. J Exp Med 1992; 176: 1543–1550.
144. Allen RC, Armitage RJ, Conley ME, et al. CD40 Ligand gene defects responsible for X-linked hyper-IgM syndrome. Science 1993; 259:990–993.
145. Xu J, Foy TM, Laman JD, et al. Mice deficient for the CD40 ligand. Immunity 1994; 1:423–431.
146. Gauchat J-F, Henchoz S, Mazzel G, et al. Induction of human IgE synthesis in B cells by mast cells and basophils. Nature 1993; 365:340–343.
147. Ranheim EA, Kipps TJ. Activated T-cells induce expression of B7/BB1 on normal or leukemic B cells through a CD40 dependent signal. J Exp Med 1993; 177:925–935.
148. Armitage RJ, Tough TW, Macduff BM, et al. CD40 ligand is a T cell growth factor. Eur J Immunol 1993; 23:2326–2331.
149. Klaus SJ, Pinchuk LM, Ochs HD, et al. Costimulation through CD28 enhances T cell-dependent B cell activation via CD40-CD40L interaction. Journal of Immunology 1994; 152:5643–5652.
150. Clark EA, Ledbetter JA. How B and T cells talk to each other. Nature 1994; 367:425–429.
151. VandenEertwegh JM, Noelle RJ, Roy M, et al. In vivo CD40-gp39 interactions are essential for thymus-dependent humoral immunity: I. In vivo expression of CD40 ligand, cytokines, and antibody production delineates sites of cognate T-B cell interactions. J Exp Med 1993; 178:1555–1565.
152. Noelle RJ, Roy M, Shepherd DM, et al. A 39-KDa protein on activated helper T cells binds CD40 and transduces the signal for cognate activation of B cells. Proc Natl Acad Sci USA 1992; 89:6550–6554.
153. Foy TM, Shepherd DM, Durie FH, et al. gp39-CD40 Interactions are essential for germinal center formation and the development of B cell memory. J Exp Med 1994; 180:157–163.
154. Foy TM, Shepherd DM, Durie FH, et al. In vivo CD40-gp39 interactions are essential for thymus-dependent humoral immunity: II. Prolonged suppression of the humoral immune response by an antibody to the ligand for CD40, gp39. J Exp Med 1993; 178: 1567–1575.

155. Durie FH, Fava RA, Foy TM, et al. Prevention of collagen-induced arthritis with an antibody to gp39, the ligand for CD40. Science 1993; 261:1328–1330.
156. Mohan C, Shi Y, Laman JD, Datta SK. Interaction between CD40 and its ligand gp39 in the development of murine lupus nephritis. J Immunol 1995; 154:1471–1480.
157. Durie FH, Aruffo A, Ledbetter J, et al. Antibody to the ligand of CD40, gp39, blocks the occurrence of the acute and chronic forms of graft-vs-host disease. J Clin Invest 1994; 94:1333–1338.
158. Lederman S, Yellin MJ, Krichevsky A, et al. Identification of a novel surface protein on activated $CD4^+$ T cells that induces contact dependent B cell differentiation (Help). J Exp Med 1992; 175:1091–1101.
159. Ledbetter JA, Grosmaire LS, Hollenbaush D, et al. Agonistic and antagonistic properties of CD40 mAb G28-5 are dependent on binding valency. Circ Shock 1994; 44:67–72.
160. Paulie S, Rosen A, Ehlin-Henriksson B, et al. The Human B lymphocyte and carcinoma antigen, CDw40, is a phosphoprotein involved in growth signal transduction. J Immunol 1989; 142:590–595.
161. Gordon J, Millsum MJ, Guy GR, Ledbetter JA. Synergistic interaction between interleukin 4 and anti-B-50 (CD40) revealed in a novel B cell restimulation assay. Eur J Immunol 1987; 17:1535–1538.
162. Gordon J, Millsum MJ, Guy GR, Ledbetter JA. Resting B lymphocytes can be triggered directly through the CD40 (Bp50) antigen: A comparison with IL-4 mediated signaling. J Immunol 1988; 140:1425–1430.
163. Banchereau J, dePaoli J, Valle A, et al. Long-term human B cell lines dependent on interleukin-4 and antibody to CD40. Science 1991; 251:70.
164. Parry SL, Hasbold J, Holman M, Klaus GGB. Hypercross-linking surface IgD receptors on mature B cells induces apoptosis that is reversed by costimulation with IL-4 and anti-CD40. J Immunol 1994; 152:2821–2829.
165. Knox KA, Gordon J. Protein tyrosine phosphorylation is mandatory for CD40-mediated rescue of germinal center B cells from apoptosis. Eur J Immunol 1993; 23: 2578–2584.
166. Tsubata T, Wu J, Honjo T. B-cell apoptosis induced by antigen receptor crosslinking is blocked by a T-cell signal through CD40. Nature 1993; 364:645–648.
167. Valentine MA, Licciardi KA. Rescue from anti-IgM-induced programmed cell death by the B cell surface proteins CD20 and CD40. Eur J Immunol 1992; 22:3141–3148.
168. Holder MJ, Wang H, Milner AE, et al. Suppression of apoptosis in normal and neoplastic human B lymphocytes by CD40 ligand is independent of Bc1-2 induction. Eur J Immunol 1993; 23:2368–2371.
169. Ledbetter JA, Shu G, Gallahger M, Clark EA. Augmentation of normal and malignant B cell proliferation by monoclonal antibody to the B cell-specific antigen BP50 (CDW40). J Immunol 1987; 138:788–794.
170. Funakoshi S, Longo DL, Beckwith M, et al. Inhibition of human B-cell lymphoma growth by CD40 stimulation. Blood 1994; 83:2787–2794.
171. Lalmanach-Girard A-C, Chiles TC, Parker DC, Rothstein TL. T cell-dependent induction of NF-kB in B cells. J Exp Med 1993; 177:1215–1219.
172. Berberich I, Shu GL, Clark EA. Crosslinking CD40 on B cells rapidly activates NF-kB. J Immunol 1994; 153:4357–4366.
173. Uckun FM, Schieve GL, Dibirdik I, et al. Stimulation of protein tyrosine phosphorylation, phosphoinositide turnover, and multiple previously unidentified serine/threonine-specific protein kinases by the Pan-B-cell receptor CD40/Bp50 at discrete developmental stages of human B-cell ontogeny. J Biol Chem 1991; 266:17478–17485.
174. Faris M, Gaskin F, Parsons JT, Fu SM. CD40 signaling pathway: Anti-CD40 mAb induces rapid dephosphorylation and phosphorylation of tyrosine-phosphorylated pro-

teins including protein tyrosine kinsase Lyn, Fyn and Syk and the appearance of a 28-kD phosphorylated protein. J Exp Med 1994; 179:1923–1931.

175. Ren CL, Morio T, Fu SF, Geha RS. Signal transduction via CD40 involves activation of lyn kinase and phosphatidylinositol-3-kinase, and phosphorylation of phospholipase Cgamma2. J Exp Med 1994; 179:673–680.
176. Hu HM, O'Rourke K, Boguski MS, Dixit VM. A novel RING finger protein interacts with the cytoplasmic domain of CD40. J Biol Chem 1994; 269:30069–30072.
177. Rothe M, Wong SC, Henzel WJ, Goeddel DV. A novel family of putative signal transducers associated with cytoplasmic domain of the 75 kDa tumor necrosis factor receptors. Cell 1994; 78:681–692.
178. Patarroyo M, Makgoba MW. Leucocyte adhesion to cells: Molecular basis, physiological relevance, and abnormalities (editorial rev). Scand J Immunol 1989; 30:129–164.
179. Hynes RO. Integrins: Versatility, modulation, and signaling in cell adhesion. Cell 1992; 69:11–25.
180. Kishimoto TK, Hollander N, Roberts TM, et al. Heterogeneous mutations in the beta subunit common to the LFA-1, Mac-1, and p150,95 glycoproteins cause leukocyte adhesion deficiency. Cell 1987; 50:193–202.
181. Krensky AM, Mentzer SJ, Clayberger C, et al. Heritable lymphocyte function-associated antigen-1 deficiency: Abnormalities of cytotoxicity and proliferation associated with abnormal expression of LFA-1. J Immunol 1985; 135:3102–3108.
182. Bowen TJ, Ochs HD, Altman LC, et al. Severe recurrent bacterial infections associated with defective adherence and chemotaxis in two patients with neutrophils deficient in a cell-associated glycoprotein. J Pediatr 1982; 101:932–940.
183. Beatty PG, Ochs HD, Harlan JM, et al. Absence of monoclonal-antibody-defined protein complex in boy with abnormal leukocyte function. Lancet 1984; 1:535–537.
184. Nathan C, Srimal S, Farber C, et al. Cytokine-induced respiratory burst of human neutrophils: Dependence on extracellular matrix proteins and CD11/CD18 integrins. J Cell Biol 1989; 109:1341–1349.
185. Shappell SB, Toman C, Anderson DC, et al. Mac-1 (CD11b/CD18) mediates adherence-dependent hydrogen peroxide production by human and canine neutrophils. J Immunol 1990; 144:2702–2711.
186. Fischer A, Seger R, Durandy A, et al. Deficiency of the adhesive protein complex lymphocytic function antigen 1, complement receptor type 3, glycoprotein pl50,95 in a girl with recurrent bacterial infections: Effects on phagocytic cells and lymphocyte functions. J Clin Invest 1985; 76:2385–2392.
187. Anderson DC, Springer TA. Leukocyte adhesion deficiency: An inherited defect in the Mac-1, LFA-1, and pl50, 95 glycoproteins. Annu Rev Med 1987; 38:175–194.
188. Beatty PG, Ledbetter JA, Martin PJ, et al. Definition of a common leukocyte cell-surface antigen (Lp95-150) associated with diverse cell-mediated immune functions. J Immunol 1983; 131:2913–2918.
189. Howard DR, Eaves AC, Takei F. Lymphocyte function-associated antigen (LFA-1) is involved in B cell activation. J Immunol 1986; 136:4013–4018.
190. Lindqvist C, Patarroyo M, Betty PG, Wigzell H. A monoclonal antibody inhibiting leukocyte adhesion blocks induction of IL-2 production but not IL-2 receptor expression. Immunology 1987; 60:579–584.
191. Krensky AM, Robbins E, Springer TA, Burakoff SJ. LFA-1, LFA-2 and LFA-3 antigens are involved in CTL-target conjugation. J Immunol 1984; 132:2180–2182.
192. Krensky AM, Sanchez-Madrid F, Robbins E, et al. The functional significance, distribution, and structure of LFA-1, LFA-2, and LFA-3: cell surface antigens associated with CTL-target interaction. J Immunol 1983; 131:611–616.
193. Moy VT, Brian AA. Signaling by lymphocyte function-associated antigen 1 (LFA-1)

in B cells: Enhanced antigen presentation after stimulation through LFA-1. J Exp Med 1992; 175:1–7.
194. Wacholtz MC, Patel SS, Lipsky PE. Leukocyte function-associated antigen 1 is an activation molecule for human T cells. J Exp Med 1989; 170:431–448.
195. van Seventer G, Shimizu Y, Horgan KJ, Shaw S. The LFA-1 ligand ICAM-1 provides an important co-stimulatory signal for T cell receptor-mediated activation of resting T cells. J Immunol 1990; 144:4579–4586.
196. van Seventer GA, Newman W, Shimizu Y, et al. Analysis of T cell stimulation by superantigen plus major histocompatibility complex class II molecules or by CD3 monoclonal antibody: Costimulation by purified adhesion ligands VCAM-1, ICAM-1, but not ELAM-1. J Exp Med 1991; 174:901–913.
197. Kuhlman P, Moy VT, Lollo BA, Brian AA. The accessory function of murine intercellular adhesion molecule-1 in T lymphocyte activation: Contributions of adhesion and co-activation. J Immunol 1991; 146:1773–1782.
198. Damle NK, Klussman K, Aruffo A. Intercellular adhesion molecule-2, a second counter-receptor for CD11a/CD18 (leukocyte function-associated antigen-1), provides a costimulatory signal for T-cell receptor-initiated activation of human T cells. J Immunol 1992; 148:665–671.
199. Fan S-T, Edgington TS. Integrin regulation of leukocyte inflammatory function—CD11b/CD18 enhancement of the tumor necrosis factor-alpha responses of monocytes. J Immunol 1993; 150:2872–2980.
200. Rothlein R, Kishimoto TK, Mainolfi E. Cross-linking of ICAM-1 induces co-signaling of an oxidative burst from mononuclear leukocytes. J Immunol 1994; 152:2488–2495.
201. Nojima Y, Rothstein DM, Sugita K, et al. Ligation of VLA-4 on T cells stimulates tyrosine phosphorylation of a 105-kD protein. J Exp Med 1992; 175:1045–1053.
202. Wang SC-T, Kanner SB, Ledbetter JA, et al. Evidence for LFA-1/ICAM-1 dependent stimulation of protein tyrosine phosphorylation in human B-lymphoid cell lines during homotypic adhesion. J Leukoc Biol; In press.
203. Guan JL, Trevithick JE, Hynes RO. Fibronectin/integrin interaction induces tyrosine phosphorylation of a 120-kDa protein. Cell Regul 1991; 2:951–964.
204. Kornberg LJ, Earp HS, Turner CE, et al. Signal transduction by integrins: Increased protein tyrosine phosphorylation caused by clustering of beta 1 integrins. Proc Natl Acad Sci USA 1991; 88:8392–8396.
205. Schaller MD, Borgman CA, Cobb BS, et al. pp125FAK a structurally distinctive protein-tyrosine kinase associated with focal adhesions. Proc Natl Acad Sci USA 1992; 89:5192–5196.
206. Hanks SK, Calalb MB, Harper MC, Patel SK. Focal adhesion protein-tyrosine kinase phosphorylated in response to cell attachment to fibronectin. Proc Natl Acad Sci USA 1992; 89:8487–8491.
207. Miyamoto S, Akiyama SK, Yamada KM. Synergistic roles for receptor occupancy and aggregation in integrin transmembrane function. Science 1995; 267:883–897.
208. van Seventer GA, Bonvini E, Yamada H, et al. Costimulation of T cell receptor/CD3-mediated activation of resting human $CD4^+$ T cells by leukocyte function-associated antigen-1 ligand intercellular cell adhesion molecule-1 invo prolonged inositol phospholipid hyudrolysis and sustained inc of intracellular Ca^{2+} levels. J Immunol 1992; 149:3872–3880.
209. Pardi R, Bender JR, Dettori C, et al. Heterogeneous distribution and transmembrane signaling properties of lymphocyte function-associated antigen (LFA-1) in human lymphocyte subsets. J Immunol 1989; 143:3157–3166.
210. Richter J, Ng-Sikorski J, Olsson I, Andersson T. Tumor necrosis factor-induced degranulation in adherent human neutrophils is dependent on CD11b/CD18-integrin-

triggered oscillations of cytosolic free Ca^{2+}. Proc Natl Acad Sci USA 1990; 87:9472–9476.

211. Kanner SB, Grosmaire LS, Ledbetter JA, Damle NK. Beta $_2$-integrin LFA-1 signaling through phospholipase C-gamma1 activation. Proc Natl Acad Sci USA 1993; 90:7099–7103.
212. Kanner SB, Aruffo A, Chan PY. Lymphocyte antigen receptor activation of a focal adhesion kinase-related tyrosine kinase substrate. Proc Natl Acad Sci USA 1994; 91: 10484–10487.
213. Damle NK, Leytze G, Klussman K, Ledbetter JA. Activation with superantigens induces programmed death in antigen-primed $CD4^+$ class II^+ major histocompatibility complex T lymphocytes via a CD11a/CD18-dependent mechanism. Eur J Immunol 1993; 23:1513–1522.
214. Marlin SD, Springer TA. Pruified intercellular adhesion molecule-1 (ICAM-1) is a ligand for lymphocyte function-associated antigen 1 (LFA-1). Cell 1987; 51:813–819.
215. Staunton DE, Dustin ML, Springer TA. Functional cloning of ICAM-2, a cell adhesion ligand for LFA homologous to ICAM-1. Nature 1989; 339:61–64.
216. Damle NK, Klussman K, Leytze G, et al. Costimulation with integrin ligands intercellular adhesion molecule-1 or vascular cell adhesion molecule-1 augments activation-induced death of antigen-specific $CD4^+$ T lymphocytes. J Immunol 1993; 151:2368–2379.
217. Boudreau N, Sympson CJ, Werb Z, Bissell MJ. Suppression of ICE and apoptosis in mammary epithelial cells by extracellular matrix. Science 1995; 267:891–893.
218. Barrett TB, Shu G, Clark EA. CD40 signaling activates CD11a/CD18 (LFA-1)-mediated adhesion in B-cells. J Immunol 1991; 146:1722–1729.
219. Bjorck P, Paulie S. Inhibition of LFA-1-dependent human B-cell aggregation induced by CD40 antibodies and interleukin-4 leads to decreased IgE synthesis. Immunology 1993; 78:218–225.
220. Sumimoto S-I, Heike T, Kanazashi S-I, et al. Involvement of LFA-1/intracellular adhesion molecule-1-dependent cell adhesion in CD40-mediated inhibition of human B lymphoma cell death induced by surface IgM crosslinking. J Immunol 1994; 153: 2488–2496.
221. Flores-Romo L, Estoppey D, Bacon KB. Anti-CD40 antibody stimulates the VLA-4 dependent adhesion of normal and LFA-1 deficient B cells to endothelium. Immunology 1993; 79:445–451.
222. Arfors KE, Lundberg C, Lindbon L, et al. A monoclonal antibody to the membrane glycoprotein complex CD18 inhibits polymorphonuclear leukocyte accumulation and plasma leakage in vivo. Blood 1987; 69:338–340.
223. Vedder NB, Winn RK, Rice CL, et al. A monoclonal antibody to the adherence-promoting leukocyte glycoprotein, CD18, reduces organ injury and improves survival from hemorrhagic shock and resuscitation in rabbits. J Clin Invest 1989; 81:939–944.
224. Simpson PJ, Todd RF III, Fantone JC, et al. Reduction of experimental canine myocardial reperfusion injury by a monoclonal antibody (anti-M01, anti-CD11b) that inhibits leukocyte adhesion. J Clin Invest 1988; 81:624–629.
225. Isobe M, Yagita H, Okumura K, Ihara A. Specific acceptance of cardiac allograft after treatment with antibodies to ICAM-1 and LFA-1. Science 1992; 25:1125–1127.
226. Nakao A, Nakajima H, Tomioka H, et al. Induction of T cell tolerance by pretreatment with anti-ICAM-1 and anti-lymphocyte function-associated antigen-1 antibodies prevents antigen-induced eosinophil recruitment into the mouse airways. J Immunol 1994; 153:5819–5825.
227. Gotoh M, Fukuzaki T, Monden M, et al. A potential immunosuppressive effect of anti-lymphocyte function-associated antigen-1 monoclonal antibody on islet transplantation. Transplantation 1994; 57:123–126.

228. Hunter T. Protein kinases and phosphatases: The yin and yang of protein phosphorylation and signaling. Cell 1995; 80:225–236.
229. Chavin KD, Qin L, Lin J, et al. Combination anti-CD2 and anti-CD3 monoclonal antibodies induce tolerance while altering IL-2, IL-4, TNF and TGFBeta production. Ann Surg 1993; 218:492–501.
230. Hirsch R, Bluestone JA, Bare CV, Gress RE. Advantages of F(ab′)2 fragments of anti-CD3 monoclonal antibody as compared to whole antibody as immunosuppressive agents in mice. Transplant Proc 1991; 23:270–271.
231. Tisch R, McDevitt HO. Antigen-specific immunotherapy: Is it a real possibility to combat T-cell-mediated autoimmunity? Proc Natl Acad Sci USA 1994; 91:437–438.
232. Madrenas J, Wange RL, Wang JL, et al. Zeta Phosphorylation without ZAP-70 activation induced by TCR antagonists or partial agonists. Science 1995; 267:515–518.
233. Sloan-Lancaster J, Shaw AS, Rothbard JB, Allen PM. Partial T cell signaling: Altered phospho-zeta and lack of ZAP70 recruitment in APL-induced T cell anergy. Cell 1994; 79:913–922.
234. Williams ME, Lichtman AH, Abbas AK. Anti-CD3 antibody induces unresponsiveness to IL-2 in Th2 clones but not in Th2 clones. J Immunol 1990; 144:1208–1214.
235. Gilbert KM, Hoang KD, Weigle WO. Th1 and Th2 clones differ in their response to a tolerogenic signal. J Immunol 1990; 144:2063–2071.
236. Corry DB, Reiner SL, Linsley PS, Locksley RM. Differential effects of blockade of CD28-B7 on the development of Th1 or Th2 effector cells in experimental leishmaniasis. J Immunol 1994; 153:4142–4148.

5

Immunosuppression and Immunophilin Ligands: Cyclosporin A, FK506, and Rapamycin

Amy Crum Vander Woude and Barbara E. Bierer
Dana-Farber Cancer Institute
Boston, Massachusetts

I. OVERVIEW

Advances in cellular and molecular immunology have heralded the application of novel modalities in clinical and experimental transplantation. The successful outcome of bone marrow and solid organ transplantation has been greatly enhanced in the last thirty years not only by improvements in surgical techniques and by progressive understanding of HLA histocompatibility and typing, but also by the development of effective immunosuppressive agents. Activation of both T and B lymphocytes is essential for the generation of an antigen-specific immune response, and the inappropriate or undesired activation of these cells can lead to autoimmunity, or, in the setting of allograft transplantation, graft rejection or graft-versus-host disease (GVHD). T-lymphocyte function is central to the maintenance and regulation of the immune response; T cells not only mediate cytotoxicity and immune suppression but, through the production and secretion of cytokines, T cells also control the proliferation of B cells as well as their differentiation to antibody-secreting cells. Therefore, regulation of the T-cell arm of the immune response is essential for the maintenance of immune homeostasis and for the prevention of graft rejection and GVHD.

Many immunosuppressive regimens use combinations of immunosuppressive drugs. Ideally, these agents are nonoverlapping for toxicity and have complementary mechanisms of action. Understanding the mechanism(s) of action of these agents involves an appreciation of the normal pathways of T-cell activation and proliferation and thereby of the site of actions of specific inhibitors. Resting, G_0 peripheral T cells express on their cell surface a heterodimeric antigen-specific T-cell receptor (TcR) complexed to an array of at least five nonpolymorphic polypeptides termed CD3. The TcR-CD3 complex recognizes processed peptide antigen presented in the groove of molecules of the major histocompatibility complex

(MHC), which, in the human, is defined by products of the histocompatibility locus (HLA) located on chromosome 6. Upon recognition of a specific antigen/MHC complex in concert with an appropriate costimulatory signal, the TcR-CD3 complex transduces activating signals from the surface to the cytoplasm of the cell. The earliest biochemical signals that can be delineated following TcR-CD3 ligation involve the generation of protein tyrosine kinase activity and of phosphatidylinositol hydrolysis. These pathways are interdependent, but both ultimately result in the induction of gene transcription involving immediate early, early, and late activation genes, which results, finally, in proliferation of T cells and differentiation towards effector function. Costimulation can be provided by a number of T-cell coreceptor molecules, including but not limited to CD4 or CD8, CD28, CD2, and CD40L. In the absence of costimulation, engagement of the TcR-CD3 complex alone can lead to a T-cell hypo- or unresponsiveness and the development of T-cell anergy.

Immunosuppressive agents can be categorized by their site of action in T-cell activation pathways (Fig. 1). It should be noted that many obvious complexities and details are sacrificed in this attempt to simplify the complex and arcane field. Although the precise mechanism of action is poorly understood, 15-deoxyspergulatin, MW496.9 (1), a derivative of spergualin isolated from *Bacillus laterosporus*, is thought to inhibit antigenic processing and MHC presentation of antigen. It has been shown to associate and interact with a member of the heat-shock protein (hsp) 70 family (2), and this may relate to its mechanism of immunosuppression. It has been tested and found useful in preclinical models of allograft transplantation and has been shown to control a single patient with cyclosporin A (CsA)–and steroid-resistant GVHD (3).

Upon TcR-CD3 engagement of antigen successfully presented by antigen-presenting cells (APC), the APC is stimulated to produce a number of cytokines, which, in turn, propagate the immune response. Cytokine inhibitors such as interleukin-1 (IL-1) receptor antagonist (IL-1ra), recombinant soluble tumor necrosis factor-alpha (TNF-α) receptor, or neutralizing monoclonal antibodies (mAbs) directed against TNF-α, directly antagonize cytokine by binding to the receptor and competing for ligand binding. A number of these agents have been shown to be useful in the prevention or treatment of acute GVHD in humans (4,5) or in preclinical models (6), and their function may relate to cytokine dysregulation as an important pathophysiological concomitant of this disease (7–9). A myriad of cytokine antagonists are now available, and it is interesting to note that many cytokine receptors have a naturally occurring form that acts in vitro and possibly in vivo as an antagonist. Cytokine inhibitors may modulate the clinical manifestations of rejection or GVHD and ameliorate the tissue destruction associated with preparative conditioning and with GVHD; whether they reduce underlying T-cell alloreactivity remains to be shown.

T-cell activation and costimulation may be inhibited by a number of inhibitors of signal transduction or by agents that interact or interfere with the cell surface receptors important for stimulation. Leflunomide (previously termed HWA 486) has been shown to inhibit the tyrosyl phosphorylation of a number of proteins, including those residues catalyzed by the src-related tyrosine kinases p561ck and p59fyn and the autophosphorylation of the epidermal growth factor (EGF) receptor (for review, see Ref. 10). T-cell surface receptor antagonists, including OKT3, a

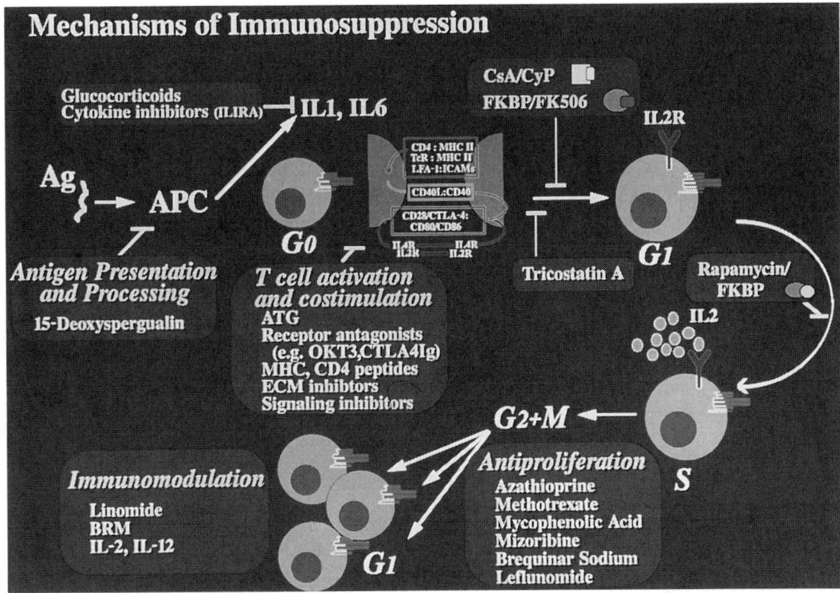

Figure 1 Overview of site of action of immunosuppressive agents. In the presence of costimulatory signals, T lymphocytes are stimulated upon engagement of the TcR-CD3 complex by peptide antigen embedded in the groove of MHC molecules. Antigen processing and MHC presentation appear to be inhibited by 15-deoxyspergualin, a derivative of spergualin. In addition, early TcR-CD3 engagement can be inhibited by agents that block either the TcR-CD3 itself (e.g., OKT3 mAb) or MHC molecules (e.g., MHC-derived peptides), costimulatory molecules (e.g., CD4-derived peptides, CTLA4Ig), secondary cytokines (e.g., IL-lra, TNF-α inhibitors), or extracellular matrix proteins (ECM) involved in early T-cell signaling. T-cell signaling recruits complex biochemical signaling machinery, resulting in nuclear gene transcription. The induction of mRNA for cytokines (e.g., IL-2) is inhibited by the immunosuppressive agents cyclosporin A (CsA) and FK506 (tacrolimus) when complexed to their intracellular receptors. IL-2 binding to the IL-2 receptor induces a number of further biochemical changes that are, in aggregate, inhibited by rapamycin, a structural homolog of FK506. T cells are thereby stimulated to undergo proliferation, which can be inhibited by a number of antimetabolites including both purine and pyrimidine inhibitors. Immune responses can also be modulated by a number of biological response modifiers (BRM) such as cytokines (e.g., IL-2, IL-12) or other agents (e.g., linomide).

monoclonal antibody (mAb) directed against the CD3ϵ chain of the TcR-CD3 complex, and CTLA4Ig, a recombinant protein which inhibits ligand binding to CD28 (and its closely associated family member CTLA4) are examples of agents that have been approved for clinical use or are in phase II clinical trials. Peptides directed against the T-cell coreceptor CD4 or against the nonpolymorphic determinants of the MHC molecule itself are in development. These and other agents are directed toward the interruption of appropriate T cell : APC interactions, thereby inhibiting activating signals to the cell.

A number of inhibitors of transcriptional activation of early genes have been developed and are now approved for clinical use. Because of their specificity of action, both cyclosporin A (CsA, Sandimmune) and FK506 (tacrolimus, Prograf) have been widely used in solid organ and bone marrow transplantation and are the focus of this chapter. Discovered by Borel in 1976, CsA was purified from the fungus *Tolypocladium inflatum* based on its ability to inhibit a mixed lymphocyte reaction (MLR) (11). CsA, a cyclic undecapeptide of MW 1203 (Fig. 2), was recently shown to be synthesized by a single enzyme, CsA synthetase. It was shown to be profoundly immunosuppressive and to lack myelotoxicity or other severe side effects (12). In animal studies, CsA was shown to be useful in models of transplantation and in autoimmunity (reviewed in Refs. 12 and 13). FK506 (Fig. 2) was isolated from soil samples containing *Streptomyces tsukubaensis* in 1987 by Fujisawa Pharmaceutical Co. (14,15). It too was purified to homogeneity based on its ability to inhibit an MLR and was shown to be a member of the macrolide antibiotic family. When the structure of FK506 was determined, it was shown to be homologous to another macrocyclic compound, rapamycin (Fig. 2). Rapamycin was isolated from *Streptomyces hygroscopicus*, found in Rapa Nui in 1975 by Wyeth-Ayerst Pharmaceuticals, and had been demonstrated to have antifungal, antitumor, and antiproliferative activity (16,17). It was later found to have immunosuppressive activity as well and specifically to inhibit later phases of T-cell activation such as those required for growth factor-dependent proliferation (18,19). Rapamycin is being studied in clinical trials at this time.

CsA and FK506 both share the ability to inhibit T-cell activation–dependent induction of early gene transcription, specifically the genes encoding cytokines such as IL-2. Early signal transduction events, including tyrosine kinase activation and phosphatidylinositol hydrolysis, are not perturbed by CsA or FK506. It is now appreciated that both CsA and FK506 diffuse freely into the cell and bind to specific intracellular receptors termed immunophilins (discussed in detail below). CsA binds to a family of receptors termed cyclophilins, initially purified by Handschumacher and coworkers as a CsA-binding protein (20). FK506 and its structural homolog rapamycin bind to a family of proteins termed FKBPs (FK506 binding proteins). A significant advance in understanding occurred when it was shown that an isoform of cyclophilin was identical to a yeast enzyme shown to function as a *cis-trans* peptidyl prolyl isomerase (PPIase or rotamase), able to catalyze the refolding of proteins in vitro (21). FKBPs were also shown to be rotamase enzymes (22,23). CsA inhibited the rotamase activity of cyclophilins, while FK506 and rapamycin inhibited the rotamase activity of FKBPs. However, inhibition of rotamase activity did not explain immunosuppressive activity. It was subsequently shown that the binding of drug to receptor resulted in the formation of an active moiety able to bind to and inhibit specific molecular targets within the cell. CsA-cyclophilin and FK506-FKBP complexes targeted the serine/threonine phosphatase calcineurin, while rapamycin-FKBP targeted a protein termed TOR (target of rapamycin) (reviewed below). Thus calcineurin, inhibited by CsA and FK506, is required for transcriptional activation of cytokine genes, while TOR, inhibited by rapamycin, is required for growth factor–dependent proliferation, although the details of signaling remain to be determined. Rapamycin inhibits T cells at the late G_1/S interface.

The antimetabolites act to inhibit cellular proliferation (Fig. 3) by depleting the cell of essential metabolic intermediates required for DNA synthesis. Both purine (Fig. 4) and pyrimidine inhibitors have been extensively explored. While lymphocytes depend on salvage pathways more than other cells, the clinical usefulness of

(a) Cyclosporin A (CsA)

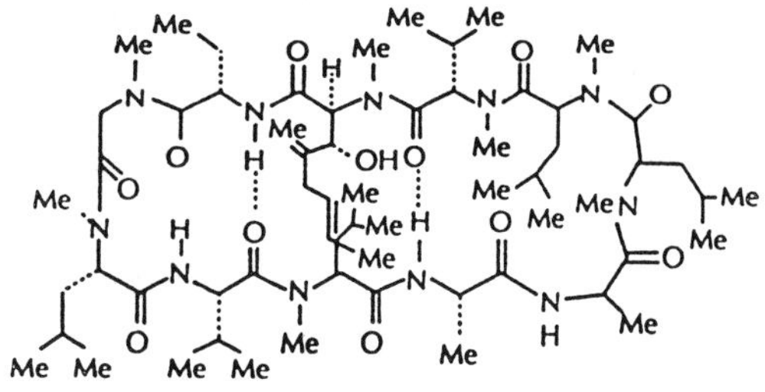

(b) FK506

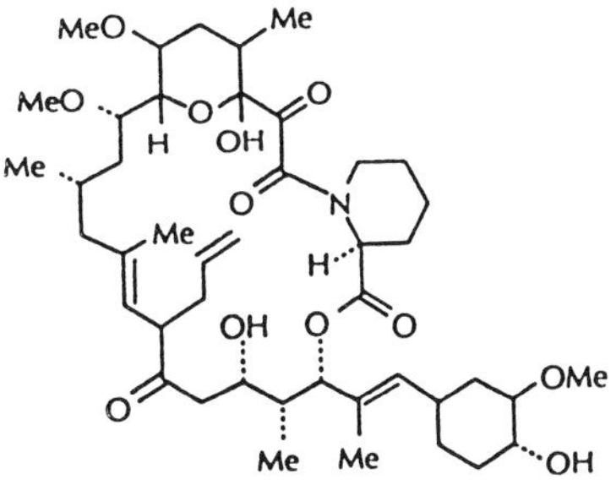

(c) Rapamycin

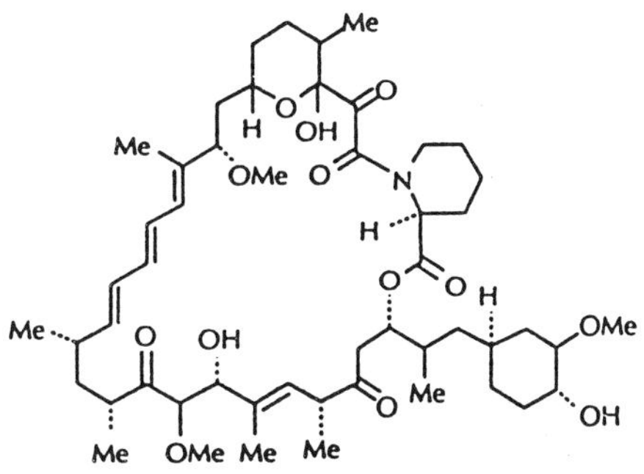

Figure 2 Chemical structure of three immunosuppressant drugs: (a) Cyclosporin A (CsA, Sandimmune), a cyclic undecapeptide of M_r 1203 Da; (b) FK506 (tacrolimus, Prograf), a macrolide antibiotic of M_r 822 Da; and (c) rapamycin, another macrolide antibiotic, with M_r 914 Da. ME = methyl group.

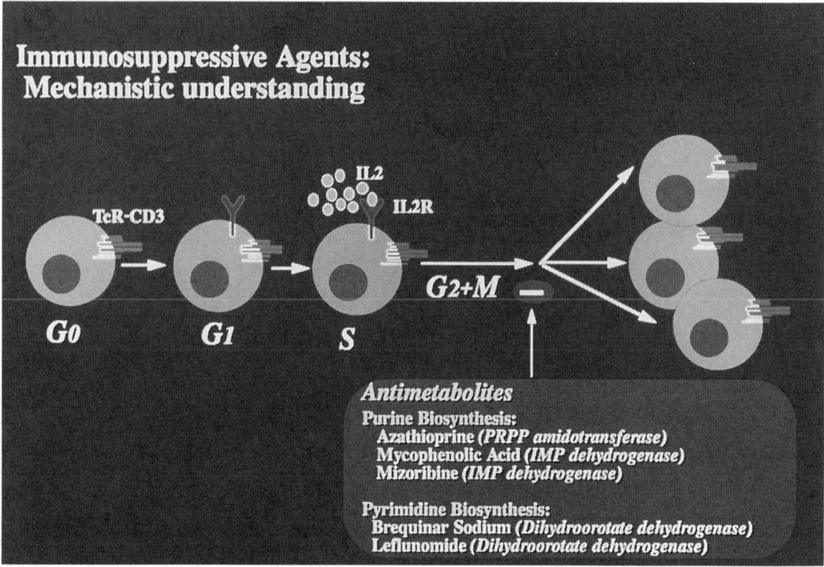

Figure 3 Inhibition of cellular proliferation by antimetabolites. Purine biosynthesis is inhibited by azathioprine, which inhibits PRPP amidotransferase, and by mycophenolic acid and mizoribine, which both target IMP dehydrogenase, as delineated in greater detail in Fig. 4. Pyrimidine biosynthesis is affected by brequinar sodium and leflunomide, which both appear to target dihydroorotate dehydrogenase. Other compounds are currently in development.

these drugs is limited by their lack of specificity. Nevertheless, in combination with other agents, antimetabolite drugs have a place in the armamentarium of immunosuppressive drugs.

It should be appreciated that the majority of agents mentioned above are primarily involved in lymphocyte inhibition. A growing body of evidence suggests that post-transplant immunomodulation may also be important. A variety of biological response modifiers may limit the toxicity of prolonged immunosuppression and help to improve graft function following transplantation. Indeed, many of these agents are thought to promote T-cell reactivity against the tumor and may thereby improve the event-free survival of this patient population.

This chapter reviews our current understanding of the molecular mechanisms of action of CsA, FK506, and rapamycin. A brief description of the clinical applications of CsA and FK506, both approved for use in transplantation, will follow.

II. IMMUNOPHILINS ARE THE INTRACELLULAR RECEPTORS FOR CsA, FK506, AND RAPAMYCIN

For their immunosuppressive effects to be recognized, CsA, FK506, and rapamycin must traverse the cellular membrane and bind to their respective intracellular receptors. These receptors, generically termed immunophilins, are highly abundant proteins, accounting for as much as 0.1 to 0.4% of total cellular protein (24–26). The immunophilins are divided into two distinct families based on amino acid homology

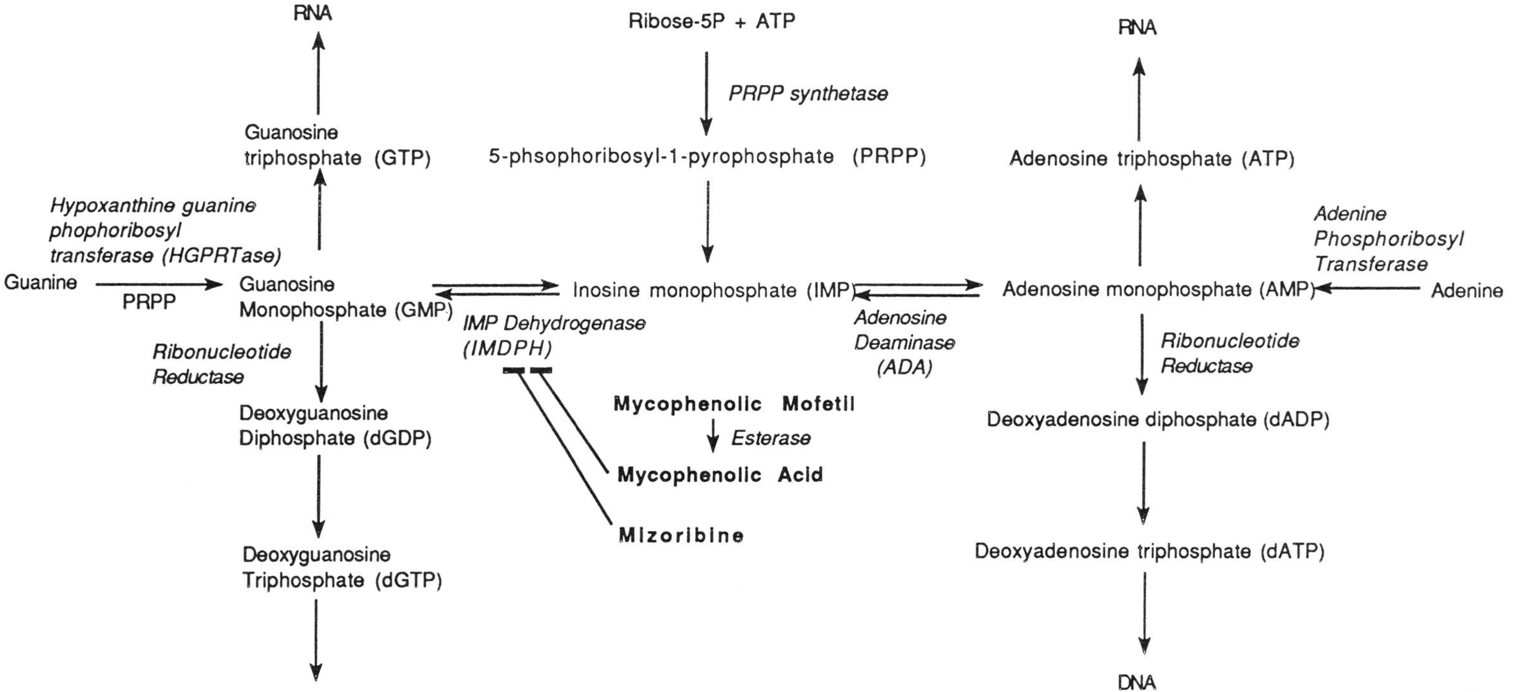

Figure 4 Pathways of purine biosynthesis and site of action of several antimetabolite agents. Synthesis of the purine nucleotides adenylic acid (AMP), inosinic acid (IMP), and guanylic acid (GMP) occurs via one of two pathways: either directly from the purine bases guanine, hypoxanthine, and adenine or de novo from nonpurine precursors such as ribose 5-phosphate. IMP is a common intermediate in both routes of synthesis. The conversion of IMP to GMP by IMP dehydrogenase (IMPDH) is inhibited by mycophenolic mofetil, mycophenolic acid, and mizoribine. By depleting the cell of essential metabolic intermediates required for DNA synthesis, these agents inhibit cellular proliferation.

and binding specificity for drug. CsA binds to members of the cyclophilin (CyP) family, while FK506 and rapamycin bind to the FK506-binding protein (FKBP) family of immunophilins. The two receptor types are phylogenetically unrelated and are not cross-reactive: CsA cannot bind to members of the FKBP family and neither FK506 nor rapamycin can bind to cyclophilins. Within each immunophilin family, the amino acid sequences are evolutionarily well conserved, suggesting that immunophilins mediate an essential cellular process. Although the precise nature of their endogenous function is unknown, it has been suggested that immunophilins may be involved in the regulation of protein folding and trafficking within the cell (24,27).

All immunophilins possess rotamase activity capable of catalyzing the *cis-trans* interconversion of peptidyl-prolyl bonds (21–23,25,26,28–30). Binding of immunosuppressant to immunophilin results in inhibition of rotamase activity. It was therefore initially postulated that inhibition of enzymatic activity was responsible for the observed immunosuppressive properties of these agents (31). It is now known that the immunosuppressive agent alone functions only as a prodrug. Binding of drug to its appropriate immunophilin results in formation of an active drug-immunophilin complex which is capable of inhibiting specific signal transduction pathways (19,30,32). Despite the structural similarity between rapamycin and FK506 and their shared intracellular receptors, the molecular targets of these drug-immunophilin complexes are distinct. The molecular target of both CsA/CyP and FK506/FKBP complexes is the serine-threonine phosphatase calcineurin; rapamycin/FKBP complexes target members of the TOR (target of rapamycin) family of intracellular proteins.

A. Cyclophilins

A number of cyclophilin isoforms have been described. CyPA is by far the most abundant isoform in mammalian cells and has been shown to be localized mainly to the cytoplasm (25,33). This isoform was initially purified in 1984 from bovine spleen on the basis of its high affinity for CsA. Five years later, it was noted to be identical to a previously described enzyme known as peptidyl-prolyl *cis-trans* isomerase (PPIase or rotamase) (21). Like all immunophilins, CyPA possesses rotamase activity which is inhibited by binding of CsA (K_i = 6 nM) (21).

CyPB is a 21-kDa protein containing a 25–amino acid sequence directing its localization to the endoplasmic reticulum (ER) and to a lesser degree to the Golgi apparatus and plasma membrane (34–36). Expression of CyPB mRNA is slightly less than that of CyPA mRNA in most cells; the isomerase activity of CyPB has been shown to be approximately one-third that of CyPA (34,37). The affinity for substrate also differs between the two isoforms: while CyPB binds CsA with less affinity (K_i = 9 nM) (38) than does CyPA, once bound, the inhibition of calcineurin phosphatase activity by CyPB is greater (39). Studies of s-cyclophilin, the avian homolog of CyPB, have confirmed its localization in the ER and have further demonstrated sequestration of s-cyclophilin within calciosomes in the ER lumen (36). CyPB itself has been shown to be associated with an ER protein termed CAML, which is thought to regulate calcium release into the cytoplasm (40). Overexpression of the CAML protein in Jurkat T cells resulted in enhancement of lymphokine gene transcription via a calcineurin-dependent mechanism (40).

Like CyPB, CyPC is also localized to the ER (38,41). However, its tissue distribution is more restricted than either CyPA or CyPB, being expressed primarily in the kidney and to a lesser degree in the spleen (38,41). This observation has led to speculation that this particular isoform may mediate the nephrotoxic effects often observed with administration of CsA in the clinical setting. In the unbound state, CyPC interacts with a 77-kDa protein with homology to the scavenger receptor (41,42). This association is disrupted in the presence of CsA (41). CyPD contains a signal sequence that is thought to direct localization in the mitochondria, but little else is known about its function (25,37). The protein appears to be expressed ubiquitously, but at much lower levels than CyPA (37). CyP40 is slightly larger than cyclophilins A through D. Its aminoterminal domain contains a region with homology to other cyclophilins (43,44). Interestingly, its carboxy terminus is 31% identical to FKBP52 (formerly hsp59) (43). Both CyP40 and FKBP52 have been shown to be components of the inactive steroid receptor complex, although their roles in this complex have not been defined. Other molecules with significant homology to the cyclophilin family have been described, including the 150-kDa molecule NK-TR, which is a component of a putative tumor recognition complex on the surface of natural killer cells (45,46). The amino acid sequence of NK-TR contains a cyclophilin-like domain near the aminoterminus, but rotamase activity of this protein has not yet been documented. Tissue distribution of NK-TR is highly restricted, being expressed mainly on NK cells and in lesser amounts on other hematopoietic cells (45,46).

B. FK506 Binding Proteins

Like the cyclophilins, a number of FKBP isoforms have been characterized which differ in their subcellular localization and affinity for drug (26). All proteins that contain an FK506 binding site and rotamase active site are capable of binding both FK506 and rapamycin, although the affinities for the two agents often differ. The predominant FKBP isoform in mammalian cells is the 12-kDa FKBP12, which is found mainly in the cytoplasm. The human gene for FKBP12 predicts a 108–amino acid protein with 57% homology to its yeast counterpart (47,48). In the absence of drug, FKBP12 has been shown to associate with the ryanodine receptor in the sarcoplasmic reticulum (SR) of skeletal muscle (49,50). It has been suggested that FKBP12 may assist in the folding of this large protein; alternatively, it may regulate calcium flux based on its location in the SR and the known function of ryanodine as a calcium release channel (see below).

A homologous protein to FKBP12, FKBP12.6 has been identified but its role in vivo is still unknown. Although the molecular weight of FKBP12.6 is slightly greater than that of FKBP12, this isoform actually migrates more slowly than FKBP12 by SDS-PAGE (51). Only 16 amino acids differ between the two isoforms, including the replacement of a well-conserved tryptophan residue in the drug binding site with a phenylalanine (51). Functionally, the two isomers are similar in terms of rotamase activity and affinity for drug.

Like cyclophilins B and C, FKBP13 is found mainly in the endoplasmic reticulum (52–54). Its aminoterminus contains a 21–amino acid signal sequence responsible for localization in the ER and a putative carboxyterminal ER retention sequence. Many of its amino acid residues, including those composing the drug binding and rotamase active sites, are identical to those of FKBP12 (52–54). Overall, the two isoforms share 47% amino acid sequence homology. Binding studies have shown that human FKBP13 (K_d = 55 nM) binds FK506 with lower affinity than does FKBP12 (K_d = 0.4 nM) (38). FKBP25 is nuclear in location and demonstrates 44% sequence homology to FKBP12 in its carboxy terminal domain (55–57).

Like FKBP13, the sequence of FKBP25 also contains unique regions not found in other immunophilins, including a 101-amino acid amino terminal alpha helical domain of unknown function. Although the affinity of FKBP25 for FK506 (K_i = 160 nM) is significantly less than that of FKBP12, FKBP25 uniquely demonstrates higher affinity for rapamycin (K_i = 0.2 nM) than for FK506; the structural basis for this wide discrepancy in drug binding remains to be shown (58). Rotamase activity of FKBP25 is estimated to be approximately two times that of FKBP12 (55), perhaps suggesting that the two isoforms have different preferred substrate specificities in vivo. In vitro, FKBP25 has been shown to form a nuclear complex with casein kinase II and nucleolin (59). Although nucleolin appears to be involved in production of ribosomes, the function of the complex containing FKBP25 is presently unknown.

FKBP51 is a newly identified immunophilin that is also an enzymatically active rotamase (60,61). Like other immunophilins, FK506 and rapamycin both inhibit its rotamase activity, and FK506 when complexed with FKBP51 (60,61) can inhibit calcineurin phosphatase activity (60). Expression of FKBP51 was initially thought to be restricted to T cells (60), but it is now clear that FK51 is expressed in a wide variety of tissues (61).

A fifth immunophilin, FKBP52 (hsp59), is a component of the inactive steroid receptor complex, which also contains the glucocorticoid receptor, heat-shock protein (hsp) 90, and hsp70 (62–65). Binding of FK506 to FKBP52 has no effect on assembly of the cytosolic complex. FKBP52 has also been shown to associate with hsp90 in the absence of the other complex members. The amino acid sequence of FKBP52 contains three regions with homology to FKBP12. The amino terminal domain contains a rotamase active site similar to other described immunophilins (62). The second region of FKBP12 homology lacks rotamase activity but has been shown to bind ATP and GTP in vitro (66). The third region also lacks rotamase activity but binds calmodulin in vitro and appears to be involved in the association of FKBP52 with hsp90 (67,68).

C. The Endogenous Cellular Function of Immunophilins

The cellular abundance, broad tissue distribution, and evolutionary conservation of immunophilins suggests that their function is essential for cell survival. However, this hypothesis has not been supported by experimental data in lower eukaryotes. In yeast, disruption of the gene for either CyPA or FKBP12 resulted in resistance to drug but had no effect on cellular viability. This may, of course, be explained if other cyclophilin or FKBP analogs in yeast subserve a conserved function. In all, four cyclophilin genes and three FKBP genes have been identified in *Saccharomyces cerevisiae*. Yeast strains lacking two cyclophilin genes (CPR1, CPR2, and CPR3) are viable, as are yeast strains lacking two FKBP genes (FPR1, FPR2). Thus it appears that either cyclophilin and FKBP genes are nonessential for viability or that other homologous proteins subserve overlapping functions (69–72). Similar studies have not been performed in mammalian systems, and it is therefore not known what effect, if any, genetic disruption of immunophilins would have on mammalian cells.

Immunophilins may be critical for cell survival under specific conditions, including conditions that may not have been tested in initial experiments. The response to heat shock is one example of such a cellular stress. Heat shock promotes expression of the yeast cyclophilin genes CPR1 and CPR2; disruption of either gene confers sensitivity to heat shock. These proteins may be involved in refolding proteins whose structure is perturbed by thermal conditions. Indeed, FKBP52 was first identified as a heat-shock protein, complexed with hsp70 and hsp90 in the steroid receptor complex. In vitro, CyPA has been shown to refold carbonic anhydrase (73), and FKBP12 has been shown to increase refolding of ribonuclease T1 (74). The ER-associated FKBP13 homolog (FPR2) is induced by conditions that increase the burden of unfolded or misfolded proteins. It is also interesting that CyP40 and FKBP52 are both components of the inactive steroid receptor complex (43,44,63). Cyclophilins have been shown to protect cells from the destructive effects of heat shock (75). Perhaps under conditions of cellular stress, such as those eliciting function of heat-shock proteins, immunophilin function becomes critical to ensure cellular integrity.

The cellular function of immunophilins may not rest entirely in refolding proteins or protein transport (see Refs. 27, 76, and 77). Complexes of immunophilins have been increasingly recognized. In the absence of FK506, FKBP12 has been shown to be associated with the ryanodine receptor of skeletal muscle (49,50,78) and with the 1,4,5-triphosphate receptor (IP_3R) (79). FK506 regulates calcium (Ca^{+2}) release by dissociating FKBP12 from the receptors, altering Ca^{+2} flux (50,79). Regulation by FKBP12 is not due to its isomerase activity (80) but, at least in the case of the IP_3R, to association of calcineurin and regulation of the phosphorylate state of the receptor (79). Calcineurin appears to affect the activity of voltage-gated Ca^{+2} channels and thereby may regulate neuronal transmitter release, as has recently been shown for the regulation of glutamate release from isolated synaptosomes (81). These findings may have direct relevance to the neurotoxicity observed with CsA and FK506 administration. In addition, the cytoplasmic domain of TGFβ interacts with FKBP12, although the functional significance of this observation is not clear (82). CyPC binds to a 77-kDa protein with homology to the scavenger receptor (83). Finally, CyPA and CyPB bind to HIV gag protein and modify infectivity (84,85). The molecular mechanisms of immunophilin regulation require further investigation.

D. The Biologically Relevant Immunophilins for Immunosuppressive Effect

Although all immunophilins have been shown to bind drug, it is likely that specific isoforms mediate the majority of immunosuppressive effects induced by CsA, FK506, and rapamycin. In mammalian cells, it appears that either CyPA or CyPB can mediate the effects of CsA (38). Overexpression of either isoform in Jurkat T cells resulted in enhanced CsA sensitivity. CsA/CyPC complexes have also been shown to inhibit calcineurin activity in vitro, but this has not been substantiated in vivo, perhaps secondary to sequestration of CyPC in the ER lumen (38,86). Although CyPB is also localized mainly to the ER, its orientation may be such that it is still able to interact with calcineurin. The relevant intracellular receptor for FK506 appears to be FKBP12 (38,87,88). Similar to the experiments described above, overexpression of FKBP12 in Jurkat T cells resulted in increased sensitivity to FK506. In contrast, overexpression of FKBP13 or FKBP25 had no effect on drug sensitivity (38). Note that FKBP12.6, FKBP51, and FKBP52 were not examined in this system. In yeast, FKBP12 also appears to be responsible for expression of the biological effects of rapamycin. Deletion of the gene encoding *RBP1* (*FPR1*), the homolog of mammalian FKBP12, conferred rapamycin resistance (70,71,89). Overexpression of human FKBP12 restored sensitivity to rapamycin (70,71,89). This not only indicates that FKBP12 is able to mediate the effects of rapamycin in yeast but also demonstrates the high degree of homology conserved among members of the immunophilin family. Finally, the observed effects of rapamycin were reversed in the presence of excess concentrations of FK506, indicating that the two drugs competed for binding to their immunophilin receptors within the cell (18,70,71,89–91).

Primary murine bone marrow mast cells (BMMC) provided a system in which to further study the role of FKBP immunophilins in mediating the immunosuppressive effects of FK506 and rapamycin in mammalian cells. Lymphokine gene transcription and calcineurin activity in BMMC were noted to be sensitive to CsA but not to FK506. The cells were subsequently found to express very low levels of FKBP12 and FKBP25 but normal levels of FKBP13 and FKBP52. Overexpression of FKBP12, but not of FKBP25, or of vector alone in a murine mast cell line restored FK506 sensitivity (87,88). BMMC were also relatively resistant to treatment with rapamycin; overexpression of FKBP12 restored rapamycin sensitivity (87,88). Interestingly, despite the higher affinity of FKBP25 for rapamycin than for FK506 in vitro, overexpression of this isoform had no effect on rapamycin sensitivity (87,88). Thus, FKBP12 may be a biologically relevant immunophilin for the actions of both FK506 and rapamycin.

III. GAIN-OF-FUNCTION MODEL FOR DRUG-IMMUNOPHILIN COMPLEXES

Several observations challenged the hypothesis that inhibition of immunophilin rotamase activity was responsible for the observed immunosuppressive properties of CsA, FK506, and rapamycin. First, immunophilins are abundant intracellularly and the concentration of drug required to fully saturate all respective receptors would be much greater than the nanomolar concentrations capable of inhibiting T-cell activation (22,30). In addition, despite potent inhibition of FKBP rotamase activity by both FK506 and rapamycin, their observed biological actions differed (18,19). Furthermore, the two drugs were shown to inhibit the biological actions of each other, suggesting that FK506 and rapamycin competed for binding to FKBPs (19,92,93). Finally, analogs of FK506 (32,94) and CsA (31,86) were developed that lacked immunosuppressive properties, but still bound to and inhibited the rotamase action of immunophilins. These observations indicated that inhibition of rotamase activity alone was insufficient to explain the observed biological properties of CsA, FK506, and rapamycin. It was subsequently proposed that the action of these agents was dependent on binding of drug to immunophilin, resulting in the formation of an active drug-immunophilin complex capable of inhibiting specific steps in T-cell signal transduction pathways (19,30,32). This gain-of-function model suggested that both drug and immunophilin were inactive in unbound form, but together formed a complex capable of binding to a molecular target within the cell. Based on their identical biological activities, CsA/CyP and FK506/FKBP complexes were predicted to share the same intracellular target; the molecular target of rapamycin/FKBP complexes was anticipated to be distinct.

IV. CALCINEURIN IS THE TARGET OF CsA/CyP AND FK506/FKBP COMPLEXES

In the presence of costimulatory signals, activation of T cells can be achieved by ligation of the surface T-cell receptor (TcR)-CD3 complex. A rapid rise in intracellular calcium concentration results and is followed by the initiation of transcriptional activation (95). Following binding of various cytokines to their respective membrane receptors, a second wave of stimulation is initiated, ultimately resulting in T-cell activation and proliferation. In T cells, IL-2 is the primary growth factor responsible for stimulation of proliferation.

Both CsA and FK506 have been shown to inhibit calcium-dependent signaling pathways in T cells (28,96–98). Initial studies investigating their mechanism(s) of action therefore focused on cellular events that were known to be calcium-sensitive. Neither drug was found to have any effect on tyrosine phosphorylation, inositol triphosphate release, protein kinase C activation, or cellular calcium flux. Yet IL-2 production was consistently decreased in the presence of these drugs, suggesting that a critical intermediate in T-cell signaling was affected.

In 1991, it was found that CsA/CyPA, CsA/CyPC, and FK506/FKBP12 complexes bound three polypeptides isolated from extracts of calf brain and thymus (41,86). Two of these peptides were identified as the A and B subunits of the cellular phosphatase calcineurin; the third was shown to be calmodulin, a cofactor required for calcineurin activity. Binding of these specific drug-immunophilin complexes inhibited the phosphatase activity of calcineurin in vitro, while drugs alone, immunophilins alone, or the complex of rapamycin/FKBP12 had no effect (86). Subsequent studies indicated that complexes of CsA/CyPB, FK506/FKBP12.6, and FK506/FKBP51 were also able to inhibit calcineurin activity; those of FK506/FKBP13, FK506/FKBP25, and FK506/FKBP52 were not (38,51,61,99,100). Inhibition of calcineurin phosphatase activity correlated with inhibition of IL-2 production (91) and affected other immune functions such as activation-dependent induction of apoptosis (90) and degranulation of CTL (101), basophils and mast cells (87,88,102–108). Furthermore, inhibition was specific for calcineurin, as the activity of other cellular phosphatases was unaffected in the presence of nanomolar concentrations of either CsA or FK506 in vivo (91,109). Similarly, in vivo treatment of cells with rapamycin at nanomolar concentrations failed to inhibit calcineurin activity, but did reverse the inhibition mediated by FK506 (86). Based on these observations, it was hypothesized that calcineurin was the molecular target of both CsA and FK506 and that it served as a critical link between the rapid rise in calcium observed following ligation of cell surface receptors and the ultimate production of lymphokines such as IL-2 (see Fig. 5).

Calcineurin (Cn), also known as serine/threonine phosphatase 2B (or PP2B), is a heterodimeric protein that is dependent on binding of calcium and calmodulin for enzymatic activity (110,111). The enzyme is composed of two subunits, termed

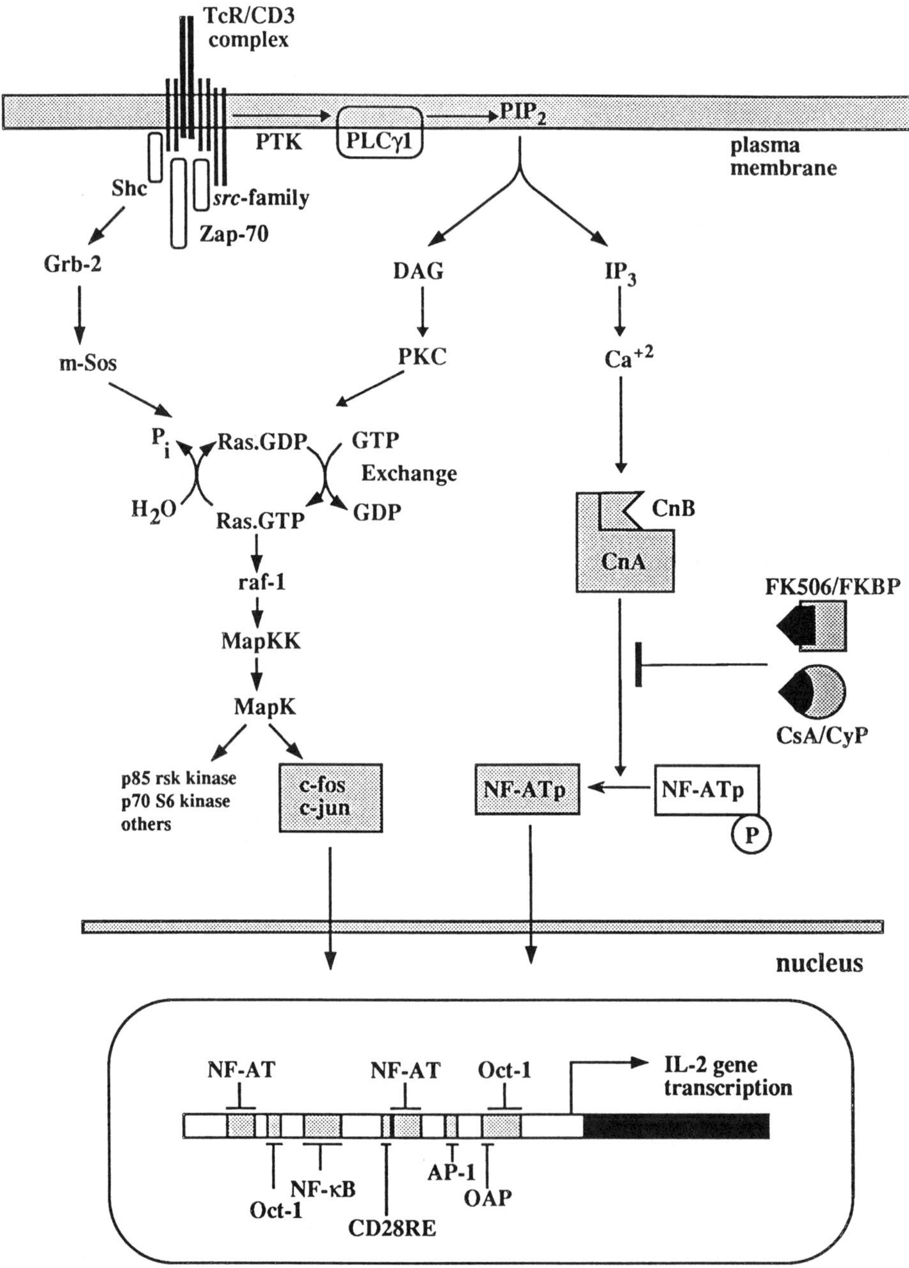

Figure 5 Simplified schematic of T-cell signaling events following ligation of the TcR-CD3 complex on the cell surface. Binding of ligand to the TcR-CD3 complex in the presence of an appropriate costimulatory signal induces protein tyrosine kinase (PTK) activity, which in turn results in activation of phospholipase Cγl (PLCγl). PLCγl stimulates activity of protein kinase C (PKC) as well as an increase in intracellular calcium levels. In its activated state, PKC activates the mitogen-activated (MAP) kinase cascade, ultimately leading to induction of AP-1 family members such as *fos* and *jun* in the nucleus. Other transcription factors, such as NFATp, have been shown to be regulated by the serine/threonine phosphatase calcineurin.

calcineurin A (CnA) and calcineurin B (CnB), which are noncovalently but stably associated (112). The 59-kDa calcineurin A is the larger of the two units and is composed of an amino terminal catalytic domain, a B-subunit binding domain, a calmodulin (CaM)-binding domain, and a carboxy terminal autoinhibitory domain (113). The smaller 19-kDa subunit B is referred to as the regulatory subunit and contains four EF-hand sequence motifs, each of which binds a single calcium ion (114). CnB is constitutively associated with CnA and is required for phosphatase activity of calcineurin. Likewise, calmodulin must bind to CnA in the presence of Ca^{2+} for calcineurin to be enzymatically active. Enhancement of enzymatic activity has been shown to occur following limited proteolysis of calcineurin to remove only the carboxy terminal portion of CnA, which contains the CaM binding site and a putative autoinhibitory domain (110,115). Similarly, a 25-amino acid peptide derived from this region has been synthesized and appears to inhibit calcineurin activity in vitro (116). While data suggest that this inhibition may occur via either a competitive (117) or noncompetitive (116,118) mechanism, our current understanding is that the autoinhibitory domain acts as a competitive inhibitor of Cn activity by binding at the active site (Sagoo, manuscript submitted). This model is supported by the recent crystallographic structure of calcineurin (119).

Three isoforms of CnA have been cloned (CnA α, β, and γ, or PP2Bα 1, 2, and 3) (113,120,121). All are similar in structure and share 75 to 80% amino acid sequence homology. Multiple alternatively spliced forms of each isoform have been identified, and a 30-bp alternatively spliced exon is present between the CaM-binding and autoinhibitory domains in all three genes (121–123). While the expression of CnAγ is testis-specific (120), the other two isoforms are found in all tissues. Like the CnA isoforms, one of the two cloned CnB isoforms is widely expressed while the other is found only in the testis (114,124,125).

V. ROLE OF CALCINEURIN IN T-CELL ACTIVATION

The apparent selectivity of FK506 and CsA for calcium-sensitive signal transduction pathways is consistent with the knowledge that calcineurin is the cellular target of these agents. Treatment of Jurkat T cells with either CsA or FK506, but not with rapamycin, resulted in inhibition of calcineurin activity (91). Furthermore, inhibition of calcineurin activity following stimulation via the TcR-CD3 complex in the presence of either CsA or FK506 correlated with inhibition of lymphokine production (91). Drug concentrations resulting in a 50% decrease in calcineurin activity induced a similar decrease in IL-2 production, resulting in a shift in the dose-response curve (91).

On a molecular level, overexpression of one or both chains of calcineurin in Jurkat T cells resulted in decreased sensitivity to CsA and FK506 (126–128). In the

---

This enzyme is activated by increasing intracellular calcium levels generated by activation of PLCγl. In concert with other known transcription factors, NFATp and AP-1 family members have been shown to participate in regulation of IL-2 gene transcription. Cyclosporin A and FK506, once bound to their respective intracellular receptors, both act by inhibiting calcineurin, thereby disrupting a critical pathway in T-cell signaling. (From Ref. 225.)

presence of protein kinase C activators such as phorbol myristate acetate (PMA), IL-2 transcription in the transfected cells could be achieved with lower concentrations of calcium ionophore (128,129). This observation suggested not only that calcineurin was a critical intermediate in T cell signaling, but that levels of the phosphatase were limiting in the pathway. Transfection of a mutant CaM-independent form of calcineurin (termed ΔCaM-AI) resulted in the ability to partially induce IL-2 promoter activity using PMA alone (117,127). Transient transfection of the ΔCaM-AI construct also indicated that calcineurin not only affected production of IL-2, but also regulated activation of IL-4, granulocyte-macrophage colony stimulating factor (GM-CSF), and TNF-α gene transcription as well (130–132). Furthermore, calcineurin and $p21^{ras}$ have been shown to act cooperatively to induce IL-2 production (126).

Complementary studies used synthetic analogs of CsA and FK506 to confirm that inhibition of calcineurin activity correlated with immunosuppressive efficacy (86,94,109,133). Agents possessing immunosuppressive capability effectively inhibited calcineurin activity; those lacking immunosuppressive qualities but still able to bind to immunophilins had no effect on calcineurin activity. Several analogs of CsA were highly immunosuppressive yet bound inefficiently to cyclophilins. However, those drug-immunophilin complexes that were able to form demonstrated an exceptionally high affinity for calcineurin, explaining their ability to induce immune suppression. These studies confirmed that binding of drug to its immunophilin receptor was required for expression of immunosuppressive properties and that the target of these drug-immunophilin complexes was indeed calcineurin.

VI. IDENTIFIED TARGETS OF CALCINEURIN

Activation of T cells by ligation of the TcR-CD3 complex induces transcription of a large number of genes that have been classified according to the time frame in which they are expressed (134). Immediate early (IE) genes are expressed within minutes of activation and encode proteins such as c-fos, NF AT, and c-myc, which function to regulate expression of other genes. Expression of early (E) genes such as *lck*, IL-2 (and other lymphokines), and the alpha chain of the IL-2 receptor, occurs between 2 to 6 hr following activation. Late (L) gene expression does not begin until 2 to 14 days following antigen presentation. Genes in this category encode cell surface markers such as the transferrin receptor and TNF-β. In activated T cells, mRNA levels of IE and L genes were unaffected by treatment with either CsA or FK506 (135,136). However, accumulation of IL-2, IL-3, IL-4, IFN-γ, TNF-α, GM-CSF, and c-myc mRNA was completely inhibited in the presence of either drug (135,136). This inhibition was secondary to decreased gene transcription rather than enhanced degradation of mRNA as determined by nuclear runoff experiments (135,136).

These observations and the knowledge that CsA and FK506 inhibited calcineurin activity stimulated interest in determining the downstream substrates of calcineurin. Specifically, it was hypothesized that calcineurin might affect nuclear proteins involved in regulation of lymphokine gene transcription. One candidate substrate was NFAT (nuclear factor of activated T cells), a family of related transcription factors known to be involved in regulation of a number of lymphokine genes, including IL-2, IL-3, IL-4, GM-CSF, and TNF-α (137). Following T-cell activation, NFAT (NFAT1) is translocated from the cytoplasm to the nucleus, where it forms a multimeric complex with members of the AP-1 family (i.e., *fos* and *jun*), which in turn binds to a specific site(s) on the IL-2 promoter (138–141). Dephosphorylation of $NFAT_p$ has been shown to be mediated by calcineurin and is required for translocation of NFAT to the nucleus (139,142). Translocation of $NF\text{-}AT_p$ is inhibited by CsA or FK506, consistent with the hypothesis that calcineurin activity is required for translocation of $NFAT_p$ from the cytoplasm to the nucleus (138,142–144).

A physical interaction between calcineurin and $NFAT_p$ has recently been shown (145). Purified bovine calcineurin bound to calmodulin-sepharose beads was able to precipitate $NFAT_p$ from lysates of T lymphocytes. Of note, both the phosphorylated and dephosphorylated forms (from resting and activated T cells, respectively) of $NFAT_p$ were able to bind to calcineurin, demonstrating that binding of substrate to calcineurin occurs at a site distinct from the catalytic site and that an interaction with the active site is not a requirement for binding. The complex of FK506-FKBP12 was able to inhibit $NFAT_p$ binding to calcineurin. The recent x-ray crystallographic structures of calcineurin/FK506/FKBP12 (119) and calcineurin/calmodulin/FK506/FKBP12 (146) demonstrating that FK506/FKBP12 binds to calcineurin at a site 10 Å away from the phosphatase active site is consistent with this data.

The role of other NFAT family members in IL-2 gene induction and their regulation by CsA or FK506 is less well defined. None of the NFAT family members are expressed exclusively in the immune system (147). While $NFAT_p$ is highly expressed in resting T cells, $NFAT_c$ (also termed NFAT2) is induced by T-cell activation (148). CsA or FK506 treatment of T cells inhibits the accumulation of $NFAT_c$ mRNA (149). NFAT4 (NFATα), of which multiple splice variants are known (147), is highly expressed in the thymus (147,150); regulation by inhibitors of calcineurin activity has not been shown. A fourth family member, NFAT3, is present in low amounts in spleen and thymus, absent in peripheral blood lymphoaytes (PBL), and is expressed abundantly outside the immune system (147). The ability to bind DNA and to associate with AP-1 elements is similar among all NFAT family members (147). It is clear that multiple NFAT binding sites are present in the IL-2 and other cytokine promoters; the occupancy of these NFAT sites by individual family members and their regulation by signal transduction machinery and by drug remain to be determined.

Other transcription factors are also sensitive to FK506 and CsA. NFκB and rel belong to a family of transcription factors that is distantly related to $NFAT_p$. In the cytoplasm, NFκB and rel are sequestered in an inactive state by the binding of a third family of proteins termed IκBs (see Refs. 151 to 153). Phosphorylation of IκB members results in release of NFκB and rel, permitting translocation to the nucleus following T-cell activation (154,155). It has been suggested that calcineurin may function as an upstream regulator of IκB activity, thereby permitting translocation of NFκB and stimulation of lymphokine gene transcription. The activity of Oct-1/OAP, another transcription factor that binds to the IL-2 promoter, has similarly been shown to be sensitive to treatment with either CsA or FK506 (156).

Substrates other than transcription factors have also been identified as targets of calcineurin. Nitric oxide synthase, whose function in lymphocytes is not presently known, has been shown to serve as a substrate of calcineurin in vitro (157). Furthermore, cAMP-dependent PKA and one isoform of phosphodiesterase appear to be substrates for calcineurin in vitro (158). Dephosphorylation of PKA or phosphodiesterase appears to decrease PKA activity and may serve to oppose calcineurin in T-cell activation pathways (159). An adenylyl cyclase has been shown to contain an FKBP12-like domain and to be regulated by calcineurin (160). Similarly, apoptosis in immature T cells, such as thymocytes or T-cell hybridomas, following ligation of the TcR-CD3 complex was inhibited in the presence of CsA or FK506, and such inhibition correlated with inhibition of calcineurin activity (90,161). These observations suggest that calcineurin is involved in cellular processes other than signal transduction in T cells. Nor are the effects of calcineurin confined solely to T cells, as cellular processes in other hematopoietic lineages have been shown to be sensitive to calcineurin inhibition as well. Degranulation of mast cells and basophils in some systems, as well as serine esterase release from cytotoxic T lymphocytes (CTL), was inhibited in the presence of CsA and FK506 (101–107). Both of these processes are independent of new protein synthesis and, in the case of mast cells and basophils, can be induced within 5 minutes of stimulation. Activation of B lymphocytes by either anti-immunoglobulin antibodies or by PMA plus calcium ionophore was also inhibited by treatment with CsA or FK506 (162–165). Calcium-dependent neutrophil chemokinesis on vitronectin has been shown to be sensitive to inhibition by FK506 (166). The immunophilin proteins cyclophilin A (167) and FKBP12 (168) have been shown to promote neutrophil chemotaxis, a function inhibitable by CsA and FK506, respectively. Thus, calcineurin not only appears to be a critical intermediate in T-cell signaling pathways, but is involved in other cellular processes as well. Furthermore, its activity is not limited solely to T cells, but is found in other hematopoietic lineages as well.

VII. THE BIOLOGICAL EFFECTS OF RAPAMYCIN

Rapamycin is structurally similar to FK506 and binds to the same family of immunophilins, the FKBPs. Like CsA and FK506, binding of rapamycin to its intracellular receptor appears to be required for expression of its immunosuppressive effects. However, the target of rapamycin is not calcineurin, nor does rapamycin affect transcription of lymphokine genes (18,19,32). Rather, it acts later in the cell cycle to interrupt growth factor mediated signaling pathways (see Fig. 6). Furthermore, whereas the antiproliferative effect of CsA and FK506 is confined primarily to hematopoietic cells, rapamycin inhibits proliferation of a number of cell lines, including some of nonhematopoietic origin (17,18,24,28).

Response to stimulation with a number of growth factors and other mitogenic stimuli is inhibited in the presence of rapamycin. Initial efforts to define the mechanism of action of this agent therefore focused on early signaling events following growth-factor stimulation. Ligation of many growth-factor receptors results in rapid tyrosine phosphorylation of multiple cellular substrates via protein tyrosine kinases (PTK) and the subsequent activation of mitogen-activated kinase (MAP) cascades. These events were not affected by treatment with rapamycin (169–172). Phosphorylation of the 40S subunit of the S6 ribosome occurs later in growth-factor signaling and is thought to promote more efficient synthesis of proteins involved in cell cycle regulation. The S6 kinases, which catalyze 40S phosphorylation, have been divided into two distinct families which differ in amino acid sequence and substrate specificity. Members of the p85 S6 kinase family were not sensitive to treatment with rapamycin (169–173). In contrast, enzymatic activity of p70 S6 kinase family

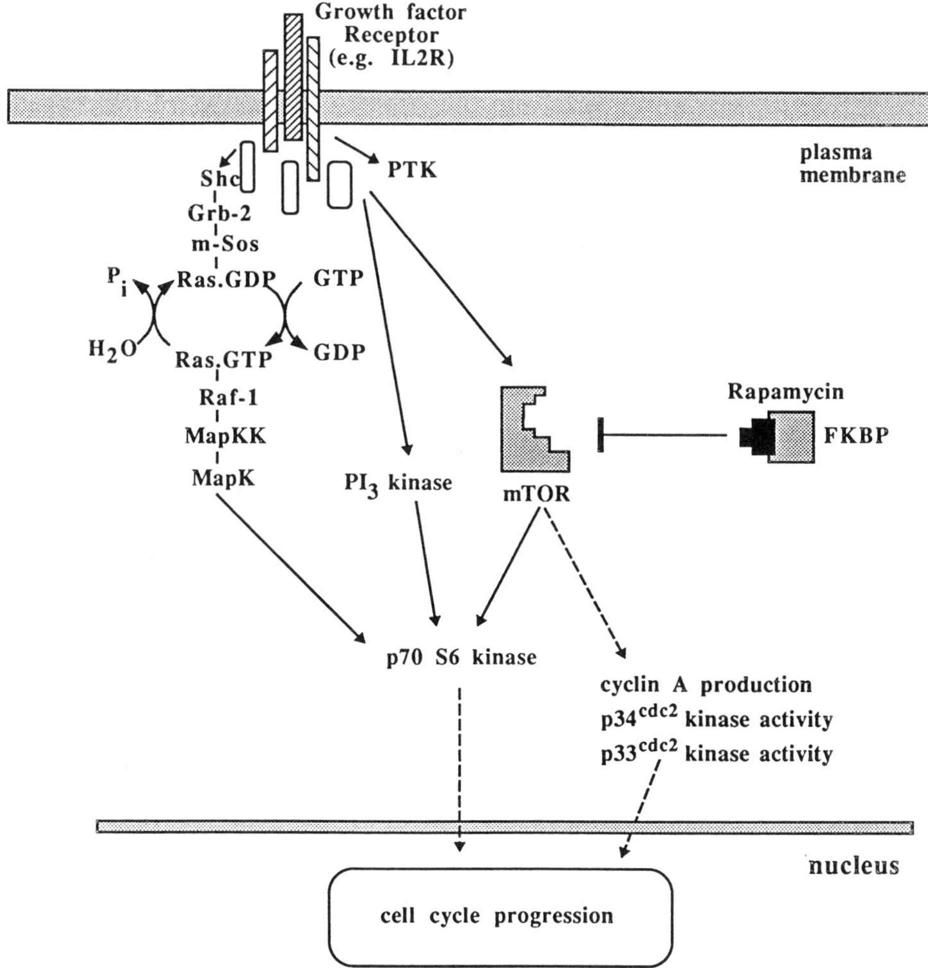

Figure 6 Rapamycin inhibits cell cycle progression in late G1 phase by interacting with the mammalian TOR (mTOR) protein. Binding of growth factor or mitogen to its respective receptor initiates early biochemical events such as protein tyrosine kinase (PTK) activity and activation of phosphatidylinositol (PI) kinase activity. Downstream effects include activation of p70 S6 kinase as well as effects on various cyclins and their associated cyclin-dependent kinases (cdk). Rapamycin/FKBP complexes induce rapid inactivation of p70 S6 kinase as well as inhibition of cyclin A production, association of cyclin A with $p34^{cdc2}$, and decreased $p34^{cdc2}$ and $p33^{cdk2}$ activity. In vitro, rapamycin/FKBP12 complexes have been shown to bind to the TOR family of intracellular proteins. The relationship of this interaction to the observations noted above has not yet been determined. (From Ref. 225.)

members was inhibited in the presence of rapamycin (169–173). Inhibition did not appear to result from direct interaction of drug with p70 S6 kinase, as rapamycin had no effect in a cell-free system (170,172).

Because rapamycin inhibited proliferation in a number of cell lines, it was hypothesized that the drug might affect proteins involved in regulation of cell cycle progression. Indeed, rapamycin has been shown to induce cell cycle arrest specifically in late G1 phase (78,174–176). Studies therefore focused on the effect of rapamycin on regulatory proteins known to be critical during this portion of the cell cycle. The eukaryotic cell cycle appears to be controlled by a series of regulatory cascades involving the cyclins and associated cyclin-dependent kinases (cdk) (177,178). Progression from one phase to the next is characterized by cyclical changes in both the concentration and/or activity of various regulatory proteins as well as their association with other regulatory proteins. For instance, activity of $p34^{cdc2}$ has been shown to increase abruptly prior to entry into S-phase (175); furthermore, this burst in activity correlated with formation of $p34^{cdc2}$/cyclin A complexes (175). In some cell systems, treatment with rapamycin inhibited the normally observed late rise in $p34^{cdc2}$ activity without affecting protein levels; inhibition was reversed in the presence of excess concentrations of FK506 (175). Other studies have demonstrated decreased expression of cyclin A and in nonhematopoietic cells, cyclin E, in the presence of rapamycin during G1 phase (176). Activity of $p33^{cdk2}$ has also been shown to be inhibited by rapamycin in a human osteosarcoma cell line (174). Thus, rapamycin may influence multiple proteins involved in regulation of the cell cycle, but the precise mechanism by which this occurs remains unclear.

Although the above observations informed our understanding of cellular events affected by rapamycin, they did not identify the direct molecular target of rapamycin/FKBP complexes. In fact, the cellular target of rapamycin/FKBP complexes in mammalian cells was not identified until 1994 (179,180). However, earlier studies in yeast systems provided some clues regarding the mechanism of action of rapamycin in higher eukaryotes. Two gene loci, termed TOR1 (DRR1) and TOR2 (DRR2), were identified in *S. cerevisiae* which, when mutated, conferred rapamycin resistance (89,181). Interestingly, however, the phenotypes of the two mutations differed. Genomic disruption of the TOR1 gene resulted only in a subtle growth defect (10 to 15% longer generation time than wild-type) (182). In contrast, mutation of the TOR2 gene was lethal, although it did not cause a cell cycle–specific arrest (183). Disruption of both TOR1 and TOR2 resulted in cell cycle arrest in G1-phase (182,183). Because disruption of TOR1 was nonlethal and resulted only in mild inhibition of growth, it is likely that the cellular function of this gene product was not essential for cell viability. Furthermore, that neither TOR1 or TOR2 disruption alone induced G1 arrest suggested that the function of the two proteins may at least partially overlap, enabling the remaining protein to compensate for loss of the other. TOR1 and TOR2 are highly homologous, sharing 67% identity overall (181,183). Similarity increases to 77% in the carboxy terminal domain, which contains a region with homology to the lipid kinase domain of phosphatidylinositol (PI) kinases (181,183). Although the intracellular function of PI kinases is unknown, it has been suggested that these proteins function as second messengers within the cell. A number of PI kinases also have serine/threonine kinase activity (184). A similar role has therefore been proposed for the TOR proteins. Data to support this hypothesis have been controversial.

A number of independent groups have now identified a mammalian protein with homology to the yeast TOR proteins that appears to bind selectively to the rapamycin/FKBP12 complex in vitro (179,180). The protein, referred to as mammalian (m)TOR (also termed RAFT1, FRAP, or RAPT1) is a 2549 amino acid protein that bears significant homology to TOR1 and TOR2 (39 and 43%, respectively) (179,180). Like TOR1 and TOR2, the carboxy terminal domain of mTOR contains a putative PI kinase domain, suggesting a role in intracellular signaling for this protein. Immunoprecipitated mTOR from rat brain has been shown to have phosphatidylinositol 4-kinase activity (185). However, the complex of rapamycin-FKBP12 was unable to inhibit PI4 kinase activity. Whether the predominant enzymatic activity of mTOR is a lipid kinase or serine/threonine kinase remains to be shown. In addition, over twenty consensus sites for phosphorylation by protein kinase C (PKC) have also been identified. Furthermore, a 133 amino acid region which is sufficient for binding to the rapamycin/FKBP12 complex has been isolated; Ser-2035 appears to be a crucial residue within this domain (186) and has been shown to correlate with those mutations of TOR1 and TOR2 that conferred rapamycin resistance in yeast (187). The rapamycin-sensitive protein mTOR has been shown to be an upstream regulator of p70 S6 kinase activity in vivo (186). Other regions of mTOR show no apparent homology to other known proteins. Thus, although mTOR is in many respects similar to the yeast proteins TOR1 and TOR2, it also carries within it unique sequences whose function are at present unknown.

IX. CLINICAL APPLICATIONS OF IMMUNOSUPPRESSIVE THERAPY

CsA and, more recently, FK506 have been critical for the improved outcome of both solid organ and bone marrow transplantation that has been observed over the last two decades. Prior to the introduction of CsA to the clinical arena approximately fifteen years ago, glucocorticosteroids and azathioprine were the main agents available to physicians for the prevention and treatment of allograft rejection. While these agents were highly effective, they induced significant morbidity with both long- and short-term administration. Furthermore, once steroid therapy had been initiated, it was often difficult to taper the dose without reinducing rejection. Although equally efficacious in preventing and treating graft rejection, CsA also has a spectrum of undesirable side effects that often accompany its administration. The drug can be both nephrotoxic and neurotoxic, findings consistent with the ubiquitous expression of calcineurin. Other side effects that limit its usefulness for prolonged therapy include hirsutism, hyperglycemia, and hypertension. Furthermore, maintenance of an immunosuppressed state for an extended period of time increases the risk of infectious complications, some of which may be life-threatening. Nevertheless, availability of CsA allowed physicians to use combination immunosuppressive therapy, thereby permitting administration of lower doses of steroids for shorter periods of time.

Because they share a common intracellular target, the toxicity profiles of CsA and FK506 are very similar. Common side effects encountered with administration of either agent include nephrotoxicity, neurotoxicity (insomnia, tremor, headache), gastrointestinal disturbances, hyperglycemia, hyperkalemia, and glucose intolerance (188). While hypertension is more commonly seen with CsA, headache and other neurologic side effects are more often associated with administration of FK506. Hirsutism and gingival hypertrophy are unique to CsA. In contrast, hair loss has been reported as a side effect of FK506. Both medications have parenteral and oral formulations and both are metabolized by the liver. Drugs that inhibit activity of cytochrome P450, such as ketoconazole and erythromycin, may cause an increase in drug levels and associated toxicity (see Table 1). The incidence of posttransplant lymphoproliferative disorders occurring during treatment with either drug appears to be similar at approximately 1.5% (189). Of note, young children treated with FK506 following liver transplantation were reported to have a higher incidence of Epstein-Barr virus (EBV) infection and of EBV-associated lymphoproliferative disorder (190). Whether this was related to the increased immunosuppression of patients on FK506 is unclear (191).

Although initially isolated in 1984, FK506 was not approved by the U.S. Food and Drug Administration (FDA) for use in orthotopic liver transplantation until 1994 (192,193). Early trials investigating the efficacy of FK506 often administered the drug to patients who had failed conventional therapies for rejection. The first

Table 1 Comparison of Toxicities Between CsA and FK506[a]

	U.S. study (%)		European study (%)	
	FK506 (n = 250)	CsA (n = 250)	FK506 (n = 262)	CsA (n = 261)
Nervous system				
Headache	64	60	31	20
Tremor	56	46	44	30
Insomnia	64	68	29	21
Paresthesia	40	30	29	21
Gastrointestinal				
Diarrhea	72	47	32	23
Nausea	46	37	30	22
Constipation	24	27	19	20
LFT abnormalities	36	30	5	2
Anorexia	34	24	6	4
Vomiting	27	15	12	9
Hypertension	47	56	31	35
Urogenital				
Kidney function	40	27	33	18
Oliguria	18	15	16	8
Metabolic				
Hyperkalemia	45	26	10	7
Hypokalemia	29	34	11	14
Hyperglycemia	47	38	29	16
Hypomagnesemia	48	45	15	8
Hematologic				
Anemia	47	38	4	1
Leukocytosis	32	26	8	7
Thrombocytopenia	24	20	10	14
Pain	63	57	19	14
Rash	24	19	8	3

[a]Percentages taken from two recently published large randomized trials (192,193) investigating the use of CsA versus FK506 following orthotopic liver transplantation.

phase II trial to be reported compared the combination of FK506 and prednisone to a historical control group receiving a CsA-based regimen for prevention of hepatic allograft rejection (194). Patients receiving FK506 were more often rejection-free at 1 month following transplantation and experienced fewer episodes of steroid-refractory rejection. Although a significant decrease in renal function was noted in a small percentage of patients receiving FK506, this generally correlated with suboptimal hepatic function, which complicated dosing and often led to toxic levels of drug. Patients receiving FK506 had fewer infectious complications overall, probably secondary to the much lower doses of corticosteroids required to control or prevent rejection. Hypertension was more common in those receiving CsA, with only 22% of those receiving FK506 requiring antihypertensive medication. Overall survival at 1 year was slightly better in the FK506 group, suggesting that this agent might be useful in the prevention of hepatic allograft rejection. Two prospective randomized trials comparing prophylaxis with FK506 to traditional CsA-based regimens have now been published (192,193). More than 500 patients were enrolled in both trials and similar conclusions were drawn from the two studies. In the United States, the U.S. Multicenter FK506 Liver Study Group randomized patients undergoing ABO-matched orthotopic liver transplantation to receive either a CsA-based regimen or FK506 and corticosteroids as prophylaxis for graft rejection (192). Patients were monitored for clinical evidence of graft rejection. In addition, liver biopsies were performed if there was clinical suspicion of rejection as well as routinely on days 7, 28, and 360 following transplantation. Initial episodes of rejection in adults were managed with high-dose methylprednisolone followed by 200 mg of prednisone, which was subsequently tapered over an undefined period. If this measure failed to control the rejection, the monoclonal antibody OKT3 was administered. Patients with rejection refractory to all the above treatments were managed at the discretion of the treating physician.

At the time of initial publication, the 1-year overall survival of 88% was equivalent in the two arms. FK506 prophylaxis was associated with an 82% rate of graft survival at 1 year versus 79% in those receiving CsA-based regimens. Importantly, at least two different dose schedules of FK506 were administered during the course of the study. Furthermore, while the incidence of neurotoxicity and renal insufficiency was higher in those receiving FK506, the data was not stratified for the dose of drug administered (see Table 2). Finally, those randomized to receive CsA-based prophylaxis received a myriad of regimens based on the current standard at participating institutions. Of the twelve centers, 10 administered CsA (1 mg/kg intravenously every 12 hr) and azathioprine (2 mg/kg intravenously each day) preoperatively followed by steroid therapy which was started during the procedure. The remaining institutions employed different CsA dosing schedules, usually in combination with either azathioprine, corticosteroids, or both. A single institution administered antilymphocyte globulin for 5 days with concomitant administration of steroids and CsA. These differences in treatment complicate interpretation of the reported data, although it is encouraging that similar results were reported in a second randomized trial.

The European FK506 Multicenter Liver Study Group simultaneously conducted a similar trial comparing the use of FK506 versus CsA for prevention of graft rejection in liver transplant recipients (193). As in the U.S. trial, dosing of FK506 was adjusted during the course of the study and CsA-based regimens, although

Table 2 Drugs that alter FK506 and CsA concentrations[a]

Increase levels	Decrease levels
Calcium channel blockers	Anticonvulsants
Diltiazem	Carbamazepine
Nicardipine	Phenobarbital
Verapamil	Phenytoin
Antifungal agents	Antibiotics
Clotrimazole	Rifabutin
Fluconazole	Rifampin
Itraconazole	
Ketoconazole	
Other drugs	
Bromocriptine	
Cimetidine	
Clarithromycin	
Cyclosporine	
Danazol	
Erythromycin	
Methylprednisolone	
Metoclopramide	

[a]Certain drugs, including several commonly used in the treatment of posttransplantation complications, may either increase or decrease effective serum concentrations of CsA and/or FK506 by interfering with clearance of these immunosuppressive agents. Possible interactions must be watched for closely to avoid either increased toxicity or decreased efficacy of CsA or FK506.

similar to those described above, were not standardized. One-year overall survival rates were similar between the two arms, with 77% of those receiving CsA-based regimens and 82% of those receiving FK506 alive at 1 year. Those receiving CsA for prophylaxis had higher rates of both acute and chronic graft rejection. Furthermore, of those with documented rejection episodes, a greater proportion of patients receiving CsA were considered refractory to treatment. In contrast, episodes of rejection in those receiving FK506 were controlled with lower doses of corticosteroids and, as a result, FK506-treated patients demonstrated a lower incidence of infectious complications. Although FK506 appeared to have equal if not greater efficacy than traditional CsA-based regimens, the side effects associated with drug administration, such as neurotoxicity and renal insufficiency, were somewhat more common in those receiving FK506 (Table 2). Thus, the results of both trials suggest that while CsA- and FK506-based regimens were equivalent in terms of graft survival and overall survival, the incidence of both acute rejection refractory to treatment with corticosteroids and of chronic rejection were lower in those patients receiving FK506. Unfortunately, greater toxicity was associated with administration of FK506, making it difficult to support use of one regimen over the other. Of note however, the results and toxicities of both higher and more moderate doses of FK506 were pooled; whether lower doses of FK506—which have been shown to be equally efficacious and are now recommended—would be associated with decreased toxicity in comparison to CsA has not as yet been determined. It is interesting to note that the 1-year inpatient cost of liver transplantation is lower in patients treated with FK506 as compared to CsA secondary to different rates and severity of graft rejection (191). Analyses of resource utilization such as this will become increasingly important as health care delivery systems are more closely scrutinized in the future.

Numerous phase II trials have also investigated the role of FK506 in prevention of allograft rejection in renal, cardiac, lung, pancreatic, small bowel transplantation and in allogeneic bone marrow transplantation. These were for the most part small, nonrandomized trials in which results were compared to historical controls (195–202). As with the results obtained in liver transplantation, it appears that FK506 is as effective as CsA in preventing rejection in recipients of renal allografts. Although a prospective randomized trial has not yet been published, the experience at single institutions indicates that FK506 provides equal prophylaxis of graft rejection while allowing rapid tapering of corticosteroids (196). Infectious complications are therefore less common, as is the need for pharmacological management of hypertension. A single randomized trial investigated whether addition of azathioprine to the combination of FK506 and prednisone following renal transplantation was of benefit (195). At a mean follow-up of 5.5 months, preliminary results indicated no difference between the two treatment arms. However, further follow-up will be required to determine whether the incidence of chronic graft rejection and long-term side effects are similar in the two treatment groups. Limited experience demonstrating FK506 rescue of steroid-resistant and CsA-resistant renal transplant recipients has been published (203,204). These reports confirm the utility of conversion from CsA to FK506 in liver allograft recipients (205,206) and show that, despite targeting the same molecular species in the cell, FK506 and CsA may have different clinical spectra in specific circumstances. Use of FK506 in lung transplantation has also been investigated (197). Infection is the major cause of morbidity and mortality in these patients during the early posttransplant period. In one small study, patients receiving a FK506-based regimen for prophylaxis experienced fewer episodes of rejection in the 6 months following transplantation than did those receiving CsA-based therapy. However, the incidence of serious infection was similar in the two groups, emphasizing the need for development of more effective and specific immunosuppressive regimens. Finally, a number of small studies have shown FK506 to be effective in the prevention and treatment of graft rejection in both adult and pediatric cardiac allograft recipients (198,207,208). As with transplantation of other solid organs, patients receiving FK506 required significantly lower doses of corticosteroids and developed fewer infections than those who received CsA. Importantly, the incidence of hypertension and hyperlipidemia, both of which can adversely affect cardiac function, was also lower in patients receiving FK506 as compared to historical controls. Furthermore, those who did require pharmacological management of their blood pressure were all controlled with single-agent therapy.

Many other studies investigating the role of FK506 in solid-organ transplantation have now been published. It is clear that FK506 demonstrates equal if not greater efficacy than traditional CsA-based regimens for both the prevention and treatment of allograft rejection. In addition, there appear to be several advantages to administering FK506 rather than CsA for maintenance of immunosuppression. The ability to quickly taper corticosteroid therapy has reduced the incidence of infectious complications in this patient population. Furthermore, the commonly observed side effects of hirsutism and gingival hyperplasia associated with CsA administration do not occur with FK506. These improvements in therapy may translate to improved quality of life for patients following transplantation. One single-institution study evaluated posttransplant quality of life following cardiac transplantation as perceived by the patient (209), a study which confirmed the results of an evaluation of patients converted from CsA to FK506 following orthotopic liver transplantation (210). Patients receiving FK506-based therapy reported better quality of life at 7 months posttransplant than did those receiving CsA. Furthermore, at no time during the study was quality of life ever rated inferiorly in the FK506 group. Although the exact reason for these findings was not apparent from the information obtained, it was suspected that improved physical appearance (i.e., decreased cushingoid features and hirsutism) may have contributed to the enhanced sense of well-being. It was also suggested that FK506 may have an as yet uncharacterized effect on mood. In any case, these and other factors appear to contribute to the acceptance of FK506 as a first-line therapy following allograft transplantation.

The ability to administer lower doses of corticosteroids with FK506 therapy has important implications for the pediatric population (207,211). In addition to the complications seen in adults, long-term administration of corticosteroids in children impairs growth of long bones and results in growth retardation and short stature. Use of FK506 may lessen these side effects by permitting rapid taper and lower overall doses of corticosteroids in the posttransplant period. In addition, children appear to be less susceptible to the nephrotoxic effects of FK506, making administration of the medication easier and safer than in adults (207). Other areas of active investigation include determination of the most effective postoperative dosing of FK506 (intravenous bolus versus continuous infusion) and the design of other immunosuppressive regimens, both of which aim to decrease the incidence of nephrotoxicity associated with administration of FK506.

Bone marrow transplantation is unique in that graft rejection is much less common than the converse situation, in which the graft recognizes alloantigens on recipient cells. This condition, termed graft-versus-host disease (GVHD), is a commonly encountered complication of bone marrow transplantation (for review, see Ref. 8). Although GVHD can at times be life-threatening or even fatal, a small degree of GVHD may be desirable in leukemic patients, as it may coincide with a graft-versus-leukemia effect. CsA has traditionally been used in both the treatment and prevention of GVHD. However, several nonrandomized studies involving small numbers of patients have now been published indicating that FK506 is also effective in this setting and has an acceptable level of associated toxicity (202,212,213). Phase III randomized trials are now being conducted to determine the role of FK506 in the treatment and prophylaxis of GVHD in allogenic matched related and matched unrelated bone marrow transplant recipients.

Although options for management of graft rejection have increased significantly since the first solid-organ and bone marrow transplantations were performed, use of immunosuppressive agents is still associated with significant morbidity. It is not surprising that CsA and FK506 have similar toxicity profiles since they share a common molecular target. As a result, it is unlikely that the two agents would be synergistic if administered together. In fact, since both CsA and FK506 are metabolized through the cytochrome p450 enzyme mixed function oxidase, FK506 can enhance CsA toxicity (214–217). Because rapamycin affects a different signaling pathway than CsA and FK506, it may be effective in treating rejection episodes that have failed to respond to treatment with either of the former. Furthermore, combination therapy with rapamycin and either CsA or FK506 may enhance efficacy while maintaining a permissible incidence of side effects. However, little is presently known regarding the toxicity of rapamycin in humans and clinical trials have only recently been initiated. Rapamycin may also be effective in treating disorders unrelated to transplantation as, unlike CsA and FK506, the effects of rapamycin are not limited solely to hematopoietic cells. For instance, rapamycin has been shown to inhibit the proliferation of vascular smooth muscle cells following balloon catheter injury, suggesting that it may have a role in the prevention of restenosis following angioplasty (218–221). Rapamycin may also be effective in the treatment of autoimmune disorders (222,223). Studies in animal models have shown that rapamycin prevents or retards progression of a number of autoimmune diseases. Onset of diabetes in the nonobese diabetic (NOD) mouse was inhibited by rapamycin (222). Similarly, disease progression in the MRL/lpr mouse, a model of systemic lupus erythematosus, was also inhibited by rapamycin (222). MRL/lpr mice develop progressive lymphadenopathy with associated autoimmune disorders and immunosuppression at an early age. This process is thought to be mediated by the activation and proliferation of T cells and is inhibitable by rapamycin but not CsA. Rapamycin was also effective in retarding progression of disease in a mouse model of rheumatoid arthritis (222). Clinical trials investigating the use of rapamycin in the treatment of human autoimmune disease have not yet been published.

The introduction of CsA to clinical transplantation in the early 1980s revolutionized the approach to solid-organ and bone marrow transplantation. Since that time, advances in surgical techniques and in the preservation of cadaveric organs have contributed to the improved outcome observed in solid-organ transplantation. Similarly, improvements in supportive care, such as more effective antibiotics and improved manipulation of blood products, have decreased the morbidity associated with bone marrow transplantation. Unfortunately, significant barriers still exist to the effective prevention and management of both graft rejection and, in the case of bone marrow transplantation, GVHD. CsA and FK506 have improved our ability to treat these conditions, and newer drugs are always being developed. However, their side effects are often prohibitive, leaving physicians with few alternative options for maintenance of adequate immunosuppression in transplant recipients. As new agents become available, combination therapy using non-crossreactive drugs may alleviate some of the associated toxicity while enhancing immunosuppressive efficacy. Other areas of research have focused on the state of tolerance induced in transplant recipients. It has been reported that some liver allograft recipients are able to eventually discontinue immunosuppressive therapy without rejection of their graft (224). Indeed, karyotypic analysis of cadaveric livers transplanted from donors of the opposite sex revealed that while the hepatocytes and endothelium of major blood vessels within the allograft were of donor origin, the entire macrophage system had been replaced with recipient cells. This state of tolerance is thought to result from a situation in which donor and recipient cells coexist, permitting existence of the graft despite differing MHC antigens on recipient and donor cells. In animal models, simultaneous transplantation of a solid organ and bone marrow from the same donor is being investigated as a mechanism to induce tolerance in recipients. If successfully developed, this may abrogate the need for aggressive immunosuppressive therapy, thereby lessening the associated toxicity often encountered in the clinical setting at present.

X. SUMMARY

Study of the mechanisms of action of CsA, FK506, and rapamycin has furthered our understanding of T-cell signaling pathways. In order to exert their immunosuppressive effects, all three agents must bind to immunophilin receptors within the cell. Although not structurally similar, CsA and FK506 share a common molecular target, the serine/threonine phosphatase calcineurin. Inhibition of calcineurin activity has been shown to correlate with decreased production of IL-2 and inhibition of T-cell proliferation. Rapamycin also inhibits T-cell proliferation yet has no effect on lymphokine production. Although FK506 and rapamycin are structurally similar and bind to the same family of intracellular receptors, rapamycin acts later in the cell cycle to inhibit growth factor–mediated signaling pathways. Members of the TOR family of intracellular proteins appear to be the molecular target of rapamycin. Although initially identified and characterized in yeast, a mammalian homolog of the yeast TOR proteins has now been identified and is referred to as mammalian (m) TOR. All three TOR proteins contain regions with homology to the lipid kinase domain of phosphatidylinositol (PI) kinases, suggesting a possible role in intracellular signaling.

These agents have not only contributed to our scientific understanding of the mechanisms by which T cells function, but have also improved the outcome of both solid organ and bone marrow transplantation dramatically. With continued basic science investigation it is hoped that newer agents with greater efficacy and/or less toxicity will be developed. Furthermore, clinical trials currently in progress will hopefully improve our ability to prevent and treat graft rejection (and in the case of bone marrow transplantation, GVHD), ultimately resulting in improved outcome for transplant recipients.

REFERENCES

1. Amemiya H. 15-Deoxyspergualin. In: Kupiec-Weglinski JW, ed. New Immunosuppressive Modalities in Organ Transplantation. Austin, TX: Landes, 1994:75–91.
2. Nadler SG, Tepper MA, Schacter B, Mazzucco CE. Interaction of the immunosuppressant deoxyspergualin with a member of the Hsp70 family of heat shock proteins. Science 1992; 258:484–486.
3. Kasai M, Higa T, Naohara T, et al. 15-deoxyspergualin controls cyclosporin- and steroid-resistant intestinal acute graft-versus-host disease after allogeneic bone marrow transplantation. Bone Marrow Transplant 1994; 14:315–317.
4. McCarthy PL, Abhyankar S, Neben S, et al. Inhibition of interleukin-1 by an interleukin-1 receptor antagonist prevents graft-versus-host disease. Blood 1991; 78:1915–1918.
5. Holler E, Kolb HJ, Mittermuller J, et al. Modulation of acute graft-versus-host disease after allogeneic bone marrow transplantation by tumor necrosis factor α (TNFα)

release in the course of pretransplant conditioning: Role of conditioning regimens and prophylactic application of a monoclonal antibody neutralizing human TNFα (MAK 195F). Blood 1995; 86:890–899.
6. Vallera DA, Taylor PA, Vannice JL, et al. Interleukin-1 or tumor necrosis factor-α antagonists do not inhibit graft-versus-host disease induced across the major histocompatibility barrier in mice. Transplantation 1995; 60:1371–1374.
7. Antin JH, Ferrara JLM. Cytokine dysregulation and acute graft-versus-host disease. Blood 1992; 80:2964–2968.
8. Ferrara JLM, Deeg HJ. Graft-versus-host disease. N Engl J Med 1991; 324:667–674.
9. Remberger M, Ringden O, Markling L. TNFα levels are increased during bone marrow transplantation conditioning in patients who develop acute GVHD. Bone Marrow Transplant 1995; 15:99–104.
10. Williams JW, McChesney LP, Sankary HN, et al. Leflunomide. In: Kupiec-Weglinski JW, ed. New Immunosuppressive Modalities in Organ Transplantation. Austin, TX: Landes, 1994:65–73.
11. Borel JF, Feurer C, Gubler HU, Stähelin H. Biological effects of cyclosporin A: A new antilymphocytic agent. Agents Actions 1976; 6:468–475.
12. Borel JF. Pharmacology of cyclosporine (Sandimmune): IV. Pharmacological properties in vivo. Pharmacol Rev 1989; 41:260–272.
13. Shevach EM. The effects of cyclosporin A on the immune system. Annu Rev Immunol 1985; 397–423.
14. Kino T, Hatanaka H, Miyata S, et al. FK-506, a novel immunosuppressant isolated from a Streptomyces II: Immunosuppressive effect of FK-506 in vitro. J Antibiot 1987; 40:1256–1265.
15. Kino T, Hatanaka H, Hashimoto M, et al. FK-506, a novel immunosuppressant isolated from a Streptomyces I: Fermentation, isolation, and physico-chemical and biological characteristics. J Antiobiot 1987; 40:1249–1255.
16. Vézina C, Kudelski A, Sehgal SN. Rapamycin (AY-22,989), a new antifungal antibiotic: I. Taxonomy of the producing streptomycete and isolation of the active principle. J Antibiot 1975; 28:721–726.
17. Sehgal SN, Baker H, Vezina C. Rapamycin (AY-22,989), a new antifungal antibiotic: II. Fermentation, isolation and characterization. J Antibiot 1975; 28:727–732.
18. Dumont FJ, Staruch MJ, Koprak SK, et al. Distinct mechanisms of suppression of murine T cell activation by the related macrolides FK-506 and rapamycin. J Immunol 1990; 144:251–258.
19. Bierer BE, Mattila PS, Standaert RF, et al. Two distinct signal transmission pathways in T lymphocytes are inhibited by complexes formed between an immunophilin and either FK506 or rapamycin. Proc Natl Acad Sci USA 1990; 87:9231–9235.
20. Handschumacher RE, Harding MW, Rice J, et al. Cyclophilin: A specific cytosolic binding protein for cyclosporin A. Science 1984; 226:544–547.
21. Fischer G, Wittman-Liebold B, Lang K, et al. Cyclophilin and peptidyl-prolyl cis-trans isomerase are probably identical proteins. Nature (Lond) 1989; 337:476–478.
22. Siekierka JJ, Hung SHY, Poe M, et al. A cytosolic binding protein for the immunosuppressant FK506 has peptidyl-prolyl isomerase activity but is distinct from cyclophilin. Nature (Lond) 1989; 341:755–757.
23. Harding MW, Galat A, Uehling DE, Schreiber SL. A receptor for the immunosuppressant FK 506 is a cis-trans peptidyl-prolyl isomerase. Nature (Lond) 1989; 341:758–760.
24. Fruman DA, Burakoff SJ, Bierer BE. Immunophilins in protein folding and immunosuppression. FASEB J 1994; 8:391–400.
25. Walsh CT, Zydowsky LD, McKeon FD. Cyclosporin A, the cyclophilin class of peptidylprolyl isomerases, and blockade of T cell signal transduction. J Biol Chem 1992; 267:13115–13118.

26. Rosen MK, Schreiber SL. Natural products as probes of cellular function: Studies of immunophilins. Angewandte Chemie 1992; 31:384–400.
27. Gething M-J, Sambrook J. Protein folding in the cell. Nature (Lond) 1992; 355:33–45.
28. Sigal NH, Dumont FJ. Cyclosporin A, FK-506, and rapamycin: Pharmacological probes of lymphocyte signal transduction. Annu Rev Immunol 1992; 10:519–560.
29. Bierer BE. Advances in therapeutic immunosuppression: Biology, molecular actions, and clinical implications. Curr Opin Hematol 1993; 149–159.
30. Schreiber SL. Chemistry and biology of the immunophilins and their immunosuppressive ligands. Science 1991; 251:283–287.
31. Sigal NH, Dumont F, Durette P, et al. Is cyclophilin involved in the immunosuppressive and nephrotoxic mechanism of action of cyclosporin A? J Exp Med 1991; 172: 619–628.
32. Bierer BE, Somers PK, Wandless TJ, et al. Probing immunosuppressant action with a nonnatural immunophilin ligand. Science 1990; 250:556–558.
33. Haendler B, Hofer-Warbinek R, Hofer E. Complementary DNA for human T-cell cyclophilin. EMBO J 1987; 6:947–950.
34. Price ER, Zydowsky LD, Jin M, et al. Human cyclophilin B: A second cyclophilin gene encodes a peptidyl-prolyl isomerase with a signal sequence. Proc Natl Acad Sci USA 1991; 88:1903–1907.
35. Hasel KW, Glass JR, Godbout M, Sutcliffe JG. An endoplasmic reticulum-specific cyclophilin. Mol Cell Biol 1991; 11:3483–3491.
36. Arber S, Krause K-H, Caroni P. s-Cyclophilin is retained intracellularly via a unique COOH-terminal sequence and colocalizes with the calcium storage protein calreticulin. J Cell Biol 1992; 116:113–125.
37. Bergsma DJ, Eder C, Gross M, et al. The cyclophilin multigene family of peptidyl-prolyl isomerases. J Biol Chem 1991; 266:23204–23214.
38. Bram RJ, Hung DT, Martin PK, et al. Identification of the immunophilins capable of mediating inhibition of signal transduction by cyclosporin A and FK506: Roles of calcineurin and cellular location. Mol Cell Biol 1993; 13:4760–4769.
39. Etzkorn FA, Chang Z, Stolz LA, Walsh CT. Cyclophilin residues which affect noncompetitive inhibition of calcineurin's protein phosphatase activity by the cyclophilin/cyclosporin A complex. Biochemistry 1994; 33:2380–2388.
40. Bram RJ, Crabtree GR. Calcium signalling in T cells stimulated by a cyclophilin B-binding protein. Nature (Lond) 1994; 371:355–358.
41. Friedman J, Weissman I. Two cytoplasmic candidates for immunophilin action are revealed by affinity for a new cyclophilin: One in the presence and one the absence of CsA. Cell 1991; 66:799–806.
42. Friedman J, Trahey M, Weissman I. Cloning and characterization of cyclophilin C-associated protein: A candidate natural cellular ligand for cyclophilin C. Proc Natl Acad Sci USA 1993; 90:6815–6819.
43. Kieffer LJ, Seng TW, Li W, et al. Cyclophilin-40, a protein with homology to the p59 component of the steroid receptor complex. J Biol Chem 1993; 268:12303–12310.
44. Kieffer LJ, Thalhammer T, Handschumacher RE. Isolation and characterization of a 40-kDa cyclophilin-related protein. J Biol Chem 1992; 267:5503–5507.
45. Cacalano NA, Chen B-X, Cleveland WL, Erlanger BF. Evidence for a functional receptor for cyclosporin A on the surface of lymphocytes. Proc Natl Acad Sci USA 1992; 89:4353–4357.
46. Anderson SK, Gallinger S, Roder J, et al. A cyclophilin-related protein involved in the function of natural killer cells. Proc Natl Acad Sci USA 1993; 90:542–546.
47. Standaert RF, Galat A, Verdine GL, Schreiber SL. Molecular cloning and overexpression of the human FK506-binding protein FKBP. Nature (Lond) 1990; 346:671–674.

48. Maki N, Sekiguchi F, Nishimaki J, et al. Complementary DNA encoding the human T-cell FK506-binding protein, a peptidylprolyl cis-trans isomerase distinct from cyclophilin. Proc Natl Acad Sci USA 1990; 87:5440–5443.
49. Timerman AP, Ogunbumni E, Freund E, et al. The calcium-release channel of sarcoplasmic reticulum is modulated by FK-506-binding protein. J Biol Chem 1993; 268: 22992–22999.
50. Brillantes A-MB, Ondrias K, Scott et al. Stabilization of calcium release channel (ryanodine receptor) function by FK506-binding protein. Cell 1994; 77:513–523.
51. Sewell TJ, Lam E, Martin MM, et al. Inhibition of calcineurin by a novel FK-506-binding protein. J Biol Chem 1994; 269:21094–21102.
52. Jin Y-J, Albers MW, Lane WS, et al. Molecular cloning of a membrane-associated human FK506- and rapamycin-binding protein, FKBP-13. Proc Natl Acad Sci USA 1991; 88:6677–6681.
53. Nigam SK, Jin YJ, Jin MJ, et al. Localization of the FK506 binding protein, FKBP 13, to the lumen of the endomplasmic reticulum. Biochem J 1993; 294:511–515.
54. Nielsen JB, Foor F, Sierkerka JJ, et al. Yeast FKBP-13 is a membrane-associated FK506-binding protein encoded by the nonessential gene FKB2. Proc Natl Acad Sci USA 1992; 89:7471–7475.
55. Jin Y-J, Burakoff SJ, Bierer BE. Molecular cloning of a 25-kDa high affinity rapamycin binding protein, FKBP25. J Biol Chem 1992; 267:10942–10945.
56. Hung DT, Schreiber SL. cDNA cloning of a human 25 kDa FK506 and rapamycin binding protein. BBRC 1992; 184:733–738.
57. Wiederrecht G, Martin MM, Sigal NH, Siekierka JJ. Isolation of a human cDNA encoding a 25 kDa FK-506 and rapamycin binding protein. BBRC 1992; 185:298–303.
58. Galat A, Lane WS, Standaert RF, Schreiber SL. A rapamycin-selective 25-kDa immunophilin. Biochemistry 1992; 31:2427–2434.
59. Jin YJ, Burakoff SJ. The 25-kDa FK506-binding protein is localized in the nucleus and associates with casein kinase II and nucleolin. Proc Natl Acad Sci USA 1993; 90: 7769–7773.
60. Baughman G, Wiederrecht GJ, Campbell NF, et al. FKBP51, a novel T-cell-specific immunophilin capable of calcineurin inhibition. Mol Cell Biol 1995; 15:4395–4402.
61. Yeh W-C, Li T-K, Bierer BE, McKnight SL. Identification and characterization of an immunophilin expressed during the clonal expansion phase of adipocyte differentiation. Proc Natl Acad Sci USA 1995; 92:11081–11085.
62. Callebaut I, Renoir J-M, Lebeau M-C, et al. An immunophilin that binds M_r 90,000 heat shock protein: Main structural features of a mammalian p59 protein. Proc Natl Acad Sci USA 1992; 89:6270–6274.
63. Lebeau M-C, Massol N, Herrick J, et al. p59, an hsp 90-binding protein: Cloning and sequencing of its cDNA and preparation of a peptide-directed polyclonal antibody. J Biol Chem 1992; 267:4281–4284.
64. Renoir J-M, Radanyi C, Faber LE, Baulieu E-E. The non-DNA-binding heterooligomeric form of mammalian steroid hormone receptors contains a hsp90-bound 59-kilodalton protein. J Biol Chem 1990; 265:10740–10745.
65. Sanchez ER, Faber LE, Hemzel WJ, Pratt WB. The 56-59-kilodalton protein identified in untransformed steroid receptor complexes is a unique protein that exists in cytosol in a complex with both the 70- and 90-kilodalton heat shock proteins. Biochemistry 1990; 29:5145–5152.
66. Le Bihan S, Renoir J-M, Radanyi C, et al. The mammalian heat shock protein binding immunophilin (p59/HBI) is an ATP and GTP binding protein. BBRC 1993; 195:600–607.
67. Massol N, Lebeau MC, Renoir JM, et al. Rabbit FKBP59-heat shock protein binding immunophilin (HBI) is a calmodulin binding protein. BBRC 1992; 187:1330–1333.

68. Peattie DA, Harding MW, Fleming MA, et al. Expression and characterization of human FKBP52, an immunophilin that associates with the 90 kDa heat shock protein and is a component of steroid receptor complexes. Proc Natl Acad Sci USA 1992; 89: 10974–10978.
69. Brizuela L, Chrebet G, Bostian KA, Parent SA. Antifungal properties of the immunosuppressant FK-506: Identification of an FK-506-responsive yeast gene distinct from FKB1. Mol Cell Biol 1991; 11:4616–4626.
70. Heitman J, Movva NR, Hiestand PC, Hall MN. FK506-binding protein proline rotamase is a target for the immunosuppressive agent FK 506 in Saccharomyces cerevisiae. Proc Natl Acad Sci USA 1991; 88:1948–1952.
71. Koltin Y, Faucette L, Bergsma DJ, et al. Rapamycin sensitivity in Saccharomyces cerevisiae is mediated by a peptidyl-prolyl cis-trans isomerase related to human FK506-binding protein. Mol Cell Biol 1991; 11:1718–1723.
72. Tropschug M, Barthelmess IB, Neupert W. Sensitivity to cyclosporin A is mediated by cyclophilin in Neurospora crassa and Saccharomyces cerevisiae. Nature (Lond) 1989; 342:953–955.
73. Freskgard P-O, Bergenham N, Jonsson B-H, et al. Isomerase and chaperone activity of prolyl isomerase in the folding of carbonic anhydrase. Science 1992; 258:466–468.
74. Schonbrunner ER, Schmid FX. Peptidyl-prolyl cis-trans isomerase improves the efficiency of protein disulfide isomerase as a catalyst of protein folding. Proc Natl Acad Sci USA 1992; 89:4510–4513.
75. Sykes K, Gething M-J, Sambrook J. Proline isomerases function during heat shock. Proc Natl Acad Sci USA 1993; 90:5853–5857.
76. Fischer G, Schmid FX. The mechanism of protein folding: Implications of in vitro refolding models for de novo protein folding and translocation in the cell. Biochemistry 1990; 29:2205–2212.
77. Schmid FX. Prolyl isomerase: Enzymatic catalysis of slow protein-folding reactions. Annu Rev Biophys Biomol Struct 1993; 22:123–143.
78. Jayaraman T, Brillantes A-M, Timerman AP, et al. FK506 binding protein associated with the calcium release channel (ryanodine receptor). J Biol Chem 1992; 267:9474–9477.
79. Cameron AM, Steiner JP, Roskams AJ, et al. Calcineurin associated with the inositol 1,4,5-triphosphate receptor-FKBP12 complex modulates Ca^{2+} flux. Cell 1995; 83:463–472.
80. Timerman AP, Wiederrecht G, Marcy A, Fleischer S. Characterization of an exchange reaction between soluble FKBP12 and the FKBP-ryanodine receptor complex. J Biol Chem 1995; 270:2451–2459.
81. Sihra TS, Nairn AC, Kloppenburg P, et al. A role for calcineurin (protein phosphatase-2B) in the regulation of glutamate release. BBRC 1995; 212:609–616.
82. Wang T, Donahoe PK, Zervos AS. Specific interaction of type I receptors of the TGF-β family with the immunophilin FKBP12. Science 1994; 265:674–676.
83. Freedman RB. A protein with many functions? Nature (Lond) 1989; 337:407–408.
84. Thali MB, Kondo E, Rosenwirth B, et al. Functional association of cyclophilin A with HIV-1 virions. Nature (Lond) 1994; 372:363–365.
85. Franke EK, Yuan HEH, Luban J. Specific incorporation of cyclophilin A into HIV-1 virions. Nature (Lond) 1994; 372:359–362.
86. Liu J, Farmer JDJ, Lane WS, et al. Calcineurin is a common target of cyclophilin-cyclosporin A and FKBP-FK506 complexes. Cell 1991; 66:807–815.
87. Fruman DA, Bierer BE, Benes JE, et al. The complex of FK506-binding protein 12 and FK506 inhibits both IgE activation-induced cytokine transcripts and calcineurin phosphatase activity in mouse mast cells. J Immunol 1995; 154:1846–1851.
88. Fruman DA, Wood MA, Gjertson CK, et al. FK506 binding protein 12 mediates

sensitivity to both FK506 and rapamycin in murine mast cells. Eur J Immunol 1995; 25:563–571.

89. Heitman J, Movva NR, Hall MN. Targets for cell cycle arrest by the immunosuppressant rapamycin in yeast. Science 1991; 253:905–909.
90. Fruman DA, Mather PE, Burakoff SJ, Bierer BE. Correlation of calcineurin phosphatase activity and programmed cell death in T cell hybridomas. Eur J Immunol 1992; 22:2513–2517.
91. Fruman DA, Klee CB, Bierer BE, Burakoff SJ. Calcineurin phosphatase activity in T lymphocytes is inhibited by FK 506 and cyclosporin A. Proc Natl Acad Sci USA 1992; 89:3686–3690.
92. Dumont FJ, Melino MR, Staruch MJ, et al. The immunosuppressive macrolides FK-506 and rapamycin act as reciprocal antagonists in murine T cells. J Immunol 1990; 144:1418–1424.
93. Bierer BE, Schreiber SL, Burakoff SJ. The effect of the immunosuppressant FK-506 on alternate pathways of T cell activation. Eur J Immunol 1991; 21:439–445.
94. Dumont FJ, Staruch MJ, Koprak SL, et al. The immunosuppressive and toxic effects of FK-506 are mechanistically related: Pharmacology of a novel antagonist of FK-506 and rapamycin. J Exp Med 1992; 176:751–760.
95. Weiss A, Littman DR. Signal transduction by lymphocyte antigen receptors. Cell 1994; 76:263–274.
96. Bierer BE, Jin YJ, Fruman DA, et al. FK506 and rapamycin: Molecular probes of T-lymphocyte activation. Transplant Proc 1991; 23:2850–2855.
97. Schreiber SL, Crabtree GR. The mechanism of action of cyclosporin A and FK506. Immunol Today 1992; 13:136–142.
98. Fruman DA, Burakoff SJ, Bierer BE. Molecular actions of cyclosporin A, FK506, and rapamycin. In: Thomson WA, Starzl TE, eds. Immunosuppressive Drugs: Developments in Anti-Rejection Therapy. London: Edward Arnold, 1994:15–35.
99. Swanson SK-H, Born T, Zydowsky LD, et al. Cyclosporin-mediated inhibition of bovine calcineurin by cyclophilins A and B. Proc Natl Acad Sci USA 1992; 89:3741–3745.
100. Wiederrecht G, Hung S, Chan HK, et al. Characterization of high molecular weight FK-506 binding activities reveals a novel FK-506-binding protein as well as a protein complex. J Biol Chem 1992; 267:21753–21760.
101. Dutz JP, Fruman DA, Burakoff SJ, Bierer BE. A role for calcineurin in degranulation of murine cytotoxic T lymphocytes. J Immunol 1993; 150:2591–2598.
102. Lancki DW, Kaper BP, Fitch FW. The requirements for triggering of lysis of cytolytic T lymphocyte clones: II. Cyclosporin A inhibits TCR-mediated exocytosis but only selectively inhibits TCR-mediated lytic activity by cloned CTL. J Immunol 1989; 142: 416–424.
103. Trenn G, Taffs R, Hohman R, et al. Biochemical characterization of the inhibitory effect of CsA on cytolytic T lymphocyte effector functions. J Immunol 1989; 142: 3796–3802.
104. Cirillo R, Triggiana M, Siri L, et al. Cyclosporin A rapidly inhibits mediator release from human basophils presumably by interacting with cyclophilin. J Immunol 1990; 144:3891–3897.
105. de Paulis A, Cirillo R, Ciccarelli A, et al. Antiinflammatory effect of FK506 on human basophils. Transplant Proc 1991; 23:2905–2906.
106. de Paulis A, Cirillo R, Ciccarelli A, et al. FK-506, a potent novel inhibitor of the release of proinflammatory mediators from human $Fc\epsilon RI^+$ cells. J Immunol 1991; 146:2374–2381.
107. Hultsch T, Albers MW, Schreiber SL, Hohman RJ. Immunophilin ligands demonstrate common features of signal transduction leading to exocytosis or transcription. Proc Natl Acad Sci USA 1991; 88:6229–6233.

108. Kaye RE, Fruman DA, Bierer BE, et al. Effects of cyclosporin A and FK506 on Fc_ϵ receptor type I-initiated increases in cytokine mRNA in mouse bone marrow-derived progenitor mast cells: Resistance to FK506 is associated with a deficiency in FK506-binding protein FKBP12. Proc Natl Acad Sci USA 1992; 89:8542–8546.
109. Liu J, Albers MW, Wandless TJ, et al. Inhibition of T cell signalling by immunophilin-ligand complexes correlates with loss of calcineurin phosphatase activity. Biochemistry 1992; 31:3896–3901.
110. Merat DL, Hu ZY, Carter TE, Cheung WY. Bovine brain calmodulin-dependent protein phosphatase: Regulation of subunit A activity by calmodulin and subunit B. J Biol Chem 1985; 260:11053–11059.
111. Stemmer PM, Klee CB. Dual calcium ion regulation of calcineurin by calmodulin and calcineurin B. Biochem 1994; 33:6859–6866.
112. Stemmer P, Klee CB. Serine/threonine phosphatases in the nervous system. Curr Opin Neurobiol 1991; 1:53–64.
113. Guerini D, Klee CB. Cloning of human calcineurin A: Evidence for two isozymes and identification of a polyproline structural domain. Proc Natl Acad Sci USA 1989; 86: 9183–9187.
114. Guerini D, Krinks MH, Sikela JM, et al. Isolation and sequence of a cDNA clone for human calcineurin B, the Ca2+-binding subunit of the Ca2+/calmodulin-stimulated protein phosphatase. DNA 1989; 8:675–682.
115. Manalan AS, Klee CB. Activation of calcineurin by limited proteolysis. Proc Natl Acad Sci USA 1983; 90:4291–4295.
116. Hashimoto Y, Perrino BA, Soderling TR. Identification of an autoinhibitory domain in calcineurin. J Biol Chem 1990; 265:1924–1927.
117. Parsons JN, Wiederrecht GJ, Salowe S, et al. Regulation of calcineurin phosphatase activity and interaction with the FK-506/FK-506 binding protein complex. J Biol Chem 1994; 269:19610–19616.
118. Perrino BA, Ng LY, Soderling TR. Calcium regulation of calcineurin phosphatase activity by its B subunit and calmodulin: Role of the autoinhibitory domain. J Biol Chem 1995; 270:340–346.
119. Kissinger CT, Parge HE, Knighton DR, et al. Crystal structures of human calcineurin and the human FKBP12-FK506-calcineurin complex. Nature (Lond) 1995; 378:641–644.
120. Muramatsu T, Giri PR, Higuchi S, Kincaid RL. Molecular cloning of a calmodulin-dependent phosphatase from murine testes: Identification of a developmentally expressed nonneural isoenzyme. Proc Natl Acad Sci USA 1992; 89:529–533.
121. Kincaid RL, Giri PR, Higuchi S, et al. Cloning and characterization of molecular isoforms of the catalytic subunit of calcineurin using nonisotopic methods. J Biol Chem 1990; 265:11312–11319.
122. McPartlin AE, Barker HM, Cohen PTW. Identification of a third alternatively spliced cDNA encoding the catalytic subunit of protein phosphatase 2Bβ. Biochim Biophys Acta 1991; 1088:308–310.
123. Muramatsu T, Kincaid RL. Molecular cloning and chromosomal mapping of the human gene for the testis-specific catalytic subunit of calmodulin-dependent protein phosphatase (calcineurin A). BBRC 1992; 188:265–271.
124. Mukai H, Chang C-D, Tanaka H, et al. cDNA cloning of a novel testis-specific calcineurin B-like protein. BBRC 1991; 179:1325–1330.
125. Ueki K, Muramatsu T, Kincaid RL. Structure and expression of two isoforms of the murine calmodulin-dependent protein phosphatase regulatory subunit (calcineurin B). BBRC 1992; 187:537–543.
126. Woodrow M, Clipstone NA, Cantrell D. $p21^{ras}$ and calcineurin synergize to regulate the nuclear factor of activated T cells. J Exp Med 1993; 178:1517–1522.

127. O'Keefe SJ, Tamura J, Kincaid RL, et al. FK-506- and CsA-sensitive activation of the interleukin-2 promoter by calcineurin. Nature (Lond) 1992; 357:692–694.
128. Clipstone NA, Crabtree GR. Identification of calcineurin as a key signalling enzyme in T-lymphocyte activation. Nature (Lond) 1992; 357:695–697.
129. Fruman DA, Pai S-Y, Burakoff SJ, Bierer BE. Characterization of a mutant calcineurin Aα gene expressed by EL4 lymphoma cells. Mol Cell Biol 1995; 15:3857–3863.
130. Kubo M, Kincaid RL, Webb DR, Ransom JT. The Ca^{2+}/calmodulin-activated, phosphoprotein phosphatase calcineurin is sufficient for positive transcriptional activation of the mouse IL-4 gene. Int Immunol 1994; 6:179–188.
131. Tsuboi A, Masuda ES, Naito Y, et al. Calcineurin potentiates activation of the granulocyte-macrophage colony-stimulating factor gene in T cells: Involvement of the conserved lymphokine element 0. Mol Biol Cell 1994; 5:119–128.
132. Goldfeld AE, Tsai E, Kincaid RL, et al. Calcineurin mediates human tumor necrosis factor α gene induction in stimulated T and B cells. J Exp Med 1994; 180:763–768.
133. Nelson PA, Akselband Y, Kawamura A, et al. Immunosuppressive activity of $[MeBm_2t]^1$-D-Diaminobutyryl-8-, and D-Diaminopropyl-8-cyclosporin analogues correlates with inhibition of calcineurin phosphatase activity. J Immunol 1993; 150:2139–2147.
134. Crabtree G. Contingent genetic regulatory events in T lymphocyte activation. Science 1989; 243:355–361.
135. Kronke M, Leonard WJ, Depper JM, et al. Cyclosporin A inhibits T-cell growth factor gene expression at the level of mRNA transcription. Proc Natl Acad Sci USA 1984; 81:5214–5218.
136. Tocci MJ, Matkovich DA, Collier KA, et al. The immunosuppressant FK506 selectively inhibits expression of early T cell activation genes. J Immunol 1989; 143:718–726.
137. Rao A. NFATp: A transcription factor required for the co-ordinate induction of several cytokine genes. Immunol Today 1994; 15:274–281.
138. Flanagan WM, Corthesy B, Bram RJ, Crabtree GR. Nuclear association of a T-cell transcription factor blocked by FK-506 and cyclosporin A. Nature (Lond) 1991; 352:803–807.
139. Jain J, McCaffrey PG, Valge-Arthur VE, Rao A. Nuclear factor of activated T cells contains Fos and Jun. Nature (Lond) 1992; 356:801–804.
140. Northrop JP, Ullman KS, Crabtree GR. Characterization of the nuclear and cytoplasmic components of the lymphoid specific nuclear factor of activated T cells (NF-AT). J Biol Chem 1993; 268:2917.
141. Boise LH, Petryniak B, Mao X, et al. The NFAT-1 DNA binding complex in activated T cells containing Fra-1 and JunB. Mol Cell Biol 1993; 13:1911.
142. McCaffrey PG, Perrino BA, Soderling TR, Rao A. NF-AT_p, a T lymphocyte DNA-binding protein that is a target for calcineurin and immunosuppressive drugs. J Biol Chem 1993; 268:3747–3752.
143. Jain J, McCaffrey PG, Miner Z, et al. The T-cell transcription factor NFATp is a substrate for calcineurin and interacts with Fos and Jun. Nature (Lond) 1993; 365:352–355.
144. Shaw KT-Y, Ho AM, Raghavan A, et al. Immunosuppressive drugs prevent a rapid dephosphorylation of transcription factor NFAT1 in stimulated immune cells. Proc Natl Acad Sci USA 1995; 92:11205–11209.
145. Wesselborg S, Fruman DA, Sagoo JK, et al. Identification of a physical interaction between calcineurin and nuclear factor of activated T cells (NFATp). J Biol Chem 1996; 271:1274–1277.
146. Griffith JP, Kim JL, E. KE, et al. X-ray structure of calcineurin inhibited by the immunophilin-immunosuppressant FKBP12-FK506 complex. Cell 1995; 82:507–522.

147. Hoey T, Sun Y-L, Williamson K, Xu S. Isolation of two new members of the NF-AT gene family and functional characterization of the NF-AT proteins. Immunity 1995; 2: 461–472.
148. Jain J, Burgeon E, Badalian TM, et al. A similar DNA-binding motif in NFAT family proteins and the Rel homology region. J Biol Chem 1995; 270:4138–4145.
149. Jain J, Loh C, Rao A. Transcriptional regulation of the IL-2 gene. Curr Opin Immunol 1995; 7:333–342.
150. Masuda ES, Naito Y, Tokumitsu H, et al. NFATx: A novel member of the NFAT family that is predominantly expressed in the thymus. Mol Cell Biol 1995; 15:2697–2706.
151. Baeuerle PA, Henkel T. Function and activation of NF-κB in the immune system. Annu Rev Immunol 1994; 12:141–179.
152. Beg AA, Baldwin AS. The IκB proteins: multifunctional regulators of Rel/NF-κB transcription factors. Genes Dev 1993; 7:2064–2070.
153. Gilmore T, Morin P. The IκB proteins: Members of a multifunctional family. Trends Genet 1993; 9:427–433.
154. Venkataraman L, Burakoff SJ, Sen R. FK506 inhibits antigen receptor-mediated induction of c-rel in B and T lymphoid cells. J Exp Med 1995; 181:1091–1099.
155. Frantz B, Nordby EC, Bren G, et al. Calcineurin acts in synergy with PMA to inactivate IκB/MAD3, an inhibitor of NF-κB. EMBO J 1994; 13:861–870.
156. Ullman KS, Flanagan M, Edwards CA, Crabtree GR. Activation of early gene expression in T lymphocytes by Oct-1 and an inducible protein, OAP[40]. Science 1991; 254: 558–562.
157. Dawson TM, Steiner JP, Dawson VL, et al. Immunosuppressant FK506 enhances phosphorylation of nitric oxide synthase and protects against glutamate neurotoxicity. Proc Natl Acad Sci USA 1993; 90:9808–9812.
158. Cohen P, Cohen PTW. Protein phosphatases come of age. J Biol Chem 1989; 264: 21435–21438.
159. Paliogianni F, Kincaid RL, Boumpas DT. Prostaglandin E_2 and other cyclin AMP elevating agents inhibit interleukin-2 gene transcription by counteracting calcineurin-dependent pathways. J Exp Med 1993; 178:1813–1817.
160. Paterson JM, Smith SM, Harmar AJ, Antoni FA. Control of a novel adenylyl cyclase by calcineurin. BBRC 1995; 214:1000–1008.
161. Holländer GA, Fruman DA, Bierer BE, Burakoff SJ. Calcineurin inhibition in vivo disrupts T cell development and repertoire selection. Transplantation 1994; 58:1037–1043.
162. Walliser P, Benzie CR, Kay JE. Inhibition of murine B-lymphocyte proliferation by the novel immunosuppressive drug FK-506. Immunology 1989; 68:434–435.
163. Wicker S, Boltz RCJ, Matt V, et al. Suppression of B cell activation by cyclosporin A, FK506 and rapamycin. Eur J Immunol 1990; 20:2277–2283.
164. Muraguchi A, Butler JL, Kehrl JH, et al. Selective suppression of an early step in human B cell activation by cyclosporin A. J Exp Med 1983; 158:690–702.
165. Klaus GGB: Cyclosporine-sensitive and cyclosporine-insensitive modes of B cell stimulation. Transplantation 1988; 46:11S–14S.
166. Hendey B, Klee CB, Maxfield FR. Inhibition of neutrophil chemokinesis on vitronectin by inhibitors of calcineurin. Science 1992; 258:296–299.
167. Xu Q, Leiva MC, Fischkoff SA, et al. Leukocyte chemotactic activity of cyclophilin. J Biol Chem 1992; 267:11968–11971.
168. Leiva MC, Lyttle CR. Leukocyte chemotactic activity of FKBP and inhibition by FK506. BBRC 1992; 186:1178–1183.
169. Calvo V, Crews CM, Vik TA, Bierer BE. Interleukin 2 stimulation of p70 kinase activity is inhibited by the immunosuppressive rapamycin. Proc Natl Acad Sci USA 1992; 89:7571–7575.

170. Price DJ, Grove JR, Calvo V, et al. Rapamycin-induced inhibition of the 70 kilodalton S6 protein kinase. Science 1992; 257:973–976.
171. Kuo CJ, Chung J, Fiorentino DF, et al. Rapamycin selectively inhibits interleukin-2 activation of p70 S6 kinase. Nature (Lond) 1992; 358:70–73.
172. Chung J, Kuo CJ, Crabtree GR, Blenis J. Rapamycin-FKBP specifically blocks growth-dependent activation of and signaling by the 70 kd S6 protein kinases. Cell 1992; 69:1227–1236.
173. Terada N, Franklin RA, Lucas JL, et al. Failure of rapamycin to block proliferation once resting cells have entered the cell cycle despite inactivation of p70 S6 kinase. J Biol Chem 1993; 268:12062–12068.
174. Albers MW, Williams RT, Brown EJ, et al. FKBP-rapamycin inhibits a cyclin-dependent kinase activity and a cyclin D1-cdk association in early G1 of an osteosarcoma cell line. J Biol Chem 1993; 266:22825–22829.
175. Morice WG, Brunn GJ, Wiederrecht G, et al. Rapamycin-induced inhibition of $p34^{cdc2}$ kinase activation is associated with G_1/S-phase growth arrest in T lymphocytes. J Biol Chem 1993; 268:3734–3738.
176. Morice WG, Wiederrecht G, Brunn GJ, et al. Rapamycin inhibition of interleukin-2-dependent $p33^{cdk2}$ and $p34^{cdc2}$ kinase activation in T lymphocytes. J Biol Chem 1993; 268:22737–22745.
177. Norbury C, Nurse P. Animal cell cycles and their control. Annu Rev Biochem 1992; 61:441–470.
178. Sherr CJ. Mammalian G_1 cyclins. Cell 1993; 73:1059–1065.
179. Brown EJ, Albers MW, Shin TB, et al. A mammalian protein targeted by G1-arresting rapamycin-receptor complex. Nature (Lond) 1994; 369:756–758.
180. Sabatini DM, Erdjument-Bromage H, Liu M, et al. RAFT1: A mammalian protein that binds to FKBP12 in a rapamycin-dependent fashion and is homologous to yeast TORs. Cell 1994; 78:35–43.
181. Cafferkey R, Young PR, McLaughlin MM, et al. Dominant missense mutations in a novel yeast protein related to mammalian phosphatidylinositol 3-kinase and VPS34 abrogate rapamycin cytotoxicity. Mol Cell Biol 1993; 13:6012–6023.
182. Helliwell SB, Wagner P, Kunz J, et al. TOR1 and TOR2 are structurally and functionally similar but not identical phosphatidylinositol kinase homologues in yeast. Mol Biol Cell 1994; 5:105–118.
183. Kunz J, Henriquez R, Schneider U, et al. Target of rapamycin in yeast, TOR2, is an essential phosphatidylinositol kinase homolog required for G1 progression. Cell 1993; 73:585–596.
184. Hunter T. When is a lipid kinase not a lipid kinase? When it is a protein kinase. Cell 1995; 83:1–4.
185. Sabatini DM, Pierchala BA, Barrow RK, et al. The rapamycin and FKBP12 target (RAFT) displays phosphatidylinositol 4-kinase activity. J Biol Chem 1995; 270:20875–20878.
186. Brown EJ, Beal PA, Keith CT, et al. Control of p70 S6 kinase by kinase activity of FRAP in vivo. Nature (Lond) 1995; 377:441–446.
187. Chiu MI, Katz H, Berlin V. RAPT1, A mammalian homologue of yeast TOR, interacts directly with the FKBP12/rapamycin complex. Proc Natl Acad Sci USA 1994. In press.
188. Tacrolimus (FK506) for organ transplants. Med Lett 1994; 36:82–83.
189. Reyes J, Tzakis A, Green M. Posttransplant lymphoproliferative disorders occurring under primary FK506 immunosuppression. Transplant Proc 1991; 23:3044–3046.
190. Cox KL, Lawrence-Miyasaki LS, Garcia-Kennedy R, et al. An increased incidence of Epstein-Barr virus infection and lymphoproliferative disorder in young children on FK506 after liver transplantation. Transplantation 1995; 59:524–529.
191. Lake JR, Gorman KJ, Esquivel CO, et al. The impact of immunosuppressive regimens

on the cost of liver transplantation—Results from the U.S. FK506 multicenter trial. Transplantation 1995; 60:1089–1095.

192. The U.S. Multicenter FK506 Liver Study Group. A comparison of tacrolimus (FK506) and cyclosporine for immunosuppression in liver transplantation. N Engl J Med 1994; 331:1110–1115.
193. European FK506 Multicenter Liver Study Group. Randomised trial comparing tacrolimus (FK506) and cyclosporin in prevention of liver allograft rejection. Lancet 1994; 344:423–428.
194. Todo S, Fung JJ, Tzakis A, et al. One hundred ten consecutive primary orthotopic liver transplants under FK506 in adults. Transplant Proc 1991; 23:1397–1402.
195. Shapiro R, Jordan ML, Scantlebury V, et al. Randomized trial of FK506/prednisone vs FK506/azothioprine/prednisone after renal transplantation: Preliminary report. Transplant Proc 1993; 25:669–672.
196. Shapiro R, Jordan M, Scantlebury V, et al. FK506 in clinical kidney transplantation. Transplant Proc 1991; 23:3065–3067.
197. Griffith BP, Bando K, Hardesty RL, et al. A prospective randomized trial of FK506 versus cyclosporine after human pulmonary transplantation. Transplantation 1994; 57:848–851.
198. Armitage JM, Kormos RL, Morita S. Clinical trial of FK506 immunosuppression in adult cardiac transplantation. Ann Thorac Surg 1992; 54:205–211.
199. Todo S, Tzakis A, Reyes J. Intestinal transplantation in humans under FK506. Transplant Proc 1993; 25:1202–1203.
200. Ricordi C, Tzakis AG, Carroll PB. Human islet isolation and allotransplantation in 22 consecutive cases. Transplantation 1992; 53:407–414.
201. Nauhaus P, Blumhardt G, Bechstein WF, et al. Comparison of FK506- and cyclosporine-based immunosuppression in primary orthotopic liver transplantation: A single center experience. Transplantation 1995; 59:31–40.
202. Fay JW, Wingard JR, Antin JH, et al. FK506 (Tacrolimus) monotherapy for prevention of graft-versus-host disease after histocompatible sibling allogeneic bone marrow transplantation. Blood 1996; 87:3514–3515.
203. Jordan ML, Shapiro R, Jensen CW, et al. FK506 conversion of renal allografts failing cyclosporine immunosuppression. Transplant Proc 1991; 23:3078–3081.
204. Mathew A, Talbot D, Minford EJ, et al. Reversal of steroid-resistant rejection in renal allograft recipients using FK506. Transplantation 1995; 60:1182–1184.
205. Fung JJ, Todo S, Tsakis A, et al. Current status of FK-506 in liver transplantation. Transplant Proc 1991; 23:1902–1905.
206. Demetris AJ, Fung JJ, Todo S, et al. Conversion of liver allograft recipients from cyclosporine to FK506 immunosuppressive therapy: A clinical pathologic study of 96 patients. Transplantation 1992; 53:1056–1062.
207. Armitage JM, Kormos RL, Fung J, Starzl TE. The clinical trials of FK506 and primary and rescue immunosuppression in adult cardiac transplantation. Transplant Proc 1991; 23:3054–3057.
208. Armitage JM, Kormos TL, Fung JJ, et al. Preliminary experience with FK506 in thoracic transplantation. Transplantation 1991; 52:164–170.
209. Dew MA, Harris RC, Simmons RG, et al. Quality-of-life advantages of FK506 versus conventional immunosuppressive drug therapy in cardiac transplantation. Transplant Proc 1991; 23:3061–3064.
210. Felser I, Wagner S, Depee J, et al. Changes in quality of life following conversion from CyA to FK506 in orthotopic liver transplant patients. Transplant Proc 1991; 23: 3032–3034.
211. Jensen CWB, Scantlebury V, Fung J, et al. Pediatric renal transplantation under FK506 immunosuppression. Transplant Proc 1991; 23:3075–3077.
212. Fay JW, Collins RH, Pineiro A. FK506 to prevent graft-versus-host disease (GVHD)

after allogeneic marrow transplantation (AMT) using unrelated marrow donors (UMD)—A Phase II study. Blood 1993; 82:420a.

213. Fay JW, Weisdorf DJ, Wingard JR. FK506 monotherapy for prevention of graft versus host disease after histocompatible sibling marrow transplantation. Blood 1992; 80:135a.
214. Burke MD, Omar G, Thompson AW, Whiting RH. Inhibition of the metabolism of cyclosporine by human liver microsomes by FK506. Transplantation 1990; 50:901–902.
215. Shah IA, Whiting PH, Omar G, et al. Effects of FK506 on human hepatic microsomal cytochrome P-450-dependent drug metabolism in vitro. Transplant Proc 1991; 23:2783–2785.
216. Moochhala SM, Lee EJD, Earnest L, et al. Inhibition of drug metabolism in rat and human liver microsomes by FK506 and cyclosporine. Transplant Proc 1991; 23:2786–2788.
217. Shiraga T, Matsuda H, Nagase K, et al. Metabolism of FK506, a potent immunosuppressant agent, by cytochrome P450 3A enzymes in rat, dog and human liver microsomes. Biochem Pharmacol 1994; 47:727–735.
218. Askelband Y, Harding MW, Nelson PA. Rapamycin inhibits spontaneous and fibroblast growth factor beta-stimulated proliferation. Transplant Proc 1991; 23:2833–2836.
219. Gregory CR, Morris RE, Pratt R, et al. The use of new antiproliferative immunosuppressants is a novel and highly effective strategy for the prevention of vascular occlusive disease. J Heart Lung Transplant 1992; 11:197.
220. Gregory CR, Huie P, Billingham MB, Morris RE. Rapamycin inhibits arterial intimal thickening caused by both alloimmune and mechanical injury: Its effect on cellular, growth factor, and cytokine response in injured vessels. Transplantation 1993; 55:1409–1418.
221. Gregory CR, Pratt RE, Huie P, et al. Effects of treatment with cyclosporine, FK506, rapamycin, mycophenolic acid, or deoxyspergualin on vascular smooth muscle proliferation in vitro and in vivo. Transplant Proc 1993; 25:770–771.
222. Carlson RP, Baeder WL, Caccese RG, et al. Effects of orally administered rapamycin in animal models of arthritis and other autoimmune diseases. Ann NY Acad Sci 1993; 685:86–113.
223. Carlson RP, Hartman DA, Tomchek LA, et al. Rapamycin, a potential disease-modifying antiarthritic drug. J Pharmacol Exp Ther 1993; 266:1125–1138.
224. Starzl TE, Demetris AJ, Trucco M. Cell migration, chimerism and graft acceptance. Lancet 1993; 339:1579–1582.
225. Bierer BE. Cyclosporin, FK506, and rapamycin: Binding to immunophilins and biological action. In: Samelson L, ed. Lymphocyte Signal Transduction; Chemical Immunology. Basel: Karger, 1994; 50:128–155.

6

Leukocyte Adhesion, Trafficking, and Migration

Takashi Kei Kishimoto, Bruce Walcheck, and Robert Rothlein
Boehringer Ingelheim Pharmaceuticals, Inc.
Ridgefield, Connecticut

I. INTRODUCTION

The trafficking of leukocytes is a central feature of host defense. Leukocytes require ready access to tissue sites of injury or infection. The mechanisms of leukocyte trafficking require that a circulating leukocyte be able to attach to the vascular endothelium at the appropriate time. It is clear that the inappropriate recruitment of leukocytes can lead to massive destruction of healthy tissue. The cell adhesion molecules that help to mediate this highly regulated response have been the focus of intense research. Adhesion molecules also play an important role as accessory molecules in antigen presentation and in mediating effector-cell functions, such as CTL–target cell interactions and myeloid-cell–mediated phagocytosis. Furthermore adhesion molecules are not just static binding molecules but can have cosignaling properties. As the field expands, the amount of data to be assimilated becomes almost overwhelming. Each year new adhesion molecules are discovered and characterized. Molecular analysis has yielded rich insights into the structure-function relationships, receptor-ligand relationships, cell signaling activity, and regulation of expression and function. Two themes have emerged that help to clarify how the numerous adhesion molecules are orchestrated to provide a dynamic mechanism for cell trafficking and how this information can be used to develop novel therapeutics: (a) a multistep model of leukocyte–endothelial cell interaction that unifies much of the experimental data and defines sequential roles for specific adhesion molecules and (b) development of animal models of disease and inflammation to test the potential efficacy of anti-adhesion agents. This review is not intended as an exhaustive review of the literature but rather focuses on leukocyte trafficking in the context of the multistep model and the potential therapeutic applications of anti–adhesion molecule therapy for the treatment of immunological and inflammatory diseases, with particular emphasis on organ transplantation.

II. A PARADIGM FOR LEUKOCYTE–ENDOTHELIAL CELL INTERACTIONS

A. Initial Interactions of Circulating Leukocytes with Endothelial Cells

In order for leukocytes to adhere to vascular endothelium in vivo, they must overcome several physical barriers: first, the circulating leukocytes must be in a quiescent, nonadhesive state but be capable of becoming adherent almost instantly; second, the circulating leukocytes must be able to distinguish inflamed endothelium from noninflamed endothelium; and third, leukocytes must be able to resist the tremendous shear forces generated by the flow of blood. One of the earliest observable events is the phenomenon of leukocyte rolling (1). Researchers using intravital microscopy techniques have known for decades that some leukocytes can roll along the surface of vascular endothelium at a velocity of about two orders of magnitude slower than the cells in the main flow of the blood. This rolling behavior is thought to be an early inflammatory response to tissue damage caused by the surgical manipulation needed to prepare an animal for intravital microscopy. Neutrophil rolling is minimal or absent in those studies that require little or no surgical preparation. Furthermore, leukocyte rolling precedes firm adhesion at sites of inflammation (2,3). It has become apparent that the selectin family of adhesion molecules plays a major role in mediating rolling of neutrophils, monocytes, and some subsets of lymphocytes (reviewed in Refs. 4–7). More recently, there has been evidence that the VLA-4 integrin, binding to its endothelial ligand VCAM-1, can also mediate the rolling of eosinophils and some subsets of lymphocytes.

1. Selectins

The selectins are a family of three closely related molecules, L-selectin, E-selectin, and P-selectin (reviewed in Refs. 4–7). All three selectins share a common structural motif: an *N*-terminal C-type lectin domain, an epidermal growth factor–like domain, a variable number of short consensus repeats (2 repeats in L-selectin, 6 in E-selectin, and alternatively spliced forms with 8 or 9 SCRs in P-selectin), a transmembrane domain, and a cytoplasmic domain (8–15). The lectin domain is largely responsible for the Ca^{2+}-dependent carbohydrate-binding properties of the selectins. Extensive mutagenesis of the selectins and crystal structure of the E-selectin lectin domain reveals a probable binding pocket for sialylated, fucosylated lactosamines (see below) (16,17). Selectins exhibit distinct tissue distribution and modes of regulation. L-selectin expression is restricted to leukocytes: about 60% of circulating lymphocytes, including virtually all naive lymphocytes, and essentially all monocytes and neutrophils constitutively express L-selectin on their surfaces (18). However L-selectin can be rapidly downmodulated upon cell activation or receptor cross-linking (19–22). L-selectin is cleaved at a membrane-proximal site resulting in release of the extracellular domain of L-selectin and loss of L-selectin adhesive function. L-selectin mediates homing of naive lymphocytes to peripheral lymph nodes (23–25) and is involved in the more general recruitment of myeloid and lymphoid cells to sites of inflammation (18,21). E-selectin expression is restricted to cytokine-stimulated endothelium (26). E-selectin is synthesized de novo, resulting in maximal expression 3 to 4 hr following stimulation (26). Expression of E-selectin is downmodulated primarily by internalization over the course of 12 to 24 hr in vitro.

The pattern of expression is consistent with a major role in acute inflammation in vivo (27), although it is apparent that E-selectin can be found at some sites of chronic inflammation, such as skin (28) or synovium (29). Neutrophils and monocytes bind E-selectin (26), as do a subset of skin-homing T cells (28,30) and γ-δ T cells (31). P-selectin expression is restricted to activated platelets and endothelial cells. Unlike E-selectin, the primary mechanism of P-selectin upregulation is through mobilization of intracellular granules containing P-selectin (32–34). Stimulation of platelets or endothelium with thrombin or histamine will result in immediate upregulation of P-selectin. The cytoplasmic domain of P-selectin contains sequences that direct P-selectin localization to Weibel-Palade bodies of endothelium or to the alpha granules of platelets (35). Once on the cell surface, P-selectin is rapidly cleared by internalization (36). However P-selectin has also been implicated in some chronic inflammatory diseases. Like E-selectin, P-selectin supports the adhesion of neutrophils, monocytes, and a subset of lymphocytes (37–41). However, it appears that E- and P-selectin may bind to distinct subpopulations of lymphocytes (42). Gene-targeted knockouts for all three selectins have been reported (43–45). Mice deficient in L-selectin expression exhibit abnormal peripheral lymph node development, consistent with a critical role for L-selectin in homing, and show depressed acute inflammatory responses (45). Similarly P-selectin knockout animals exhibit deficient inflammatory reactions at the early time points, but the inflammatory infiltrate was relatively normal at 4 to 6 hr, consistent with a role for P-selectin at the earliest stages of inflammation (43). Interestingly, E-selectin knockouts were relatively normal in their inflammatory responses. However, addition of an anti-P-selectin MAb profoundly depressed neutrophil recruitment compared to that of anti-P-selectin–treated wild-type animals (44). These results suggest a degree of functional redundancy among the selectins.

2. Selectin Ligands

The lectin domain of the selectins serves as the major ligand-binding domain. Although major advances have led to an understanding of the carbohydrate determinants involved in selectin binding, the precise nature of selectin ligands has remained controversial. This ambiguity reflects the subtle complexities of carbohydrate recognition—carbohydrates can be joined via different linkages and exist as branched structures—and the fact that carbohydrate epitopes can be displayed on a wide range of carrier proteins and lipids. Early evidence indicated that the sialyl Lewis X, a sialylated, fucosylated lactosamine, is the ligand for E-selectin. Sialyl Lewis X is appropriately expressed on myeloid cells and a subset of lymphocytes (46–49). Similarly, sialyl Lewis A, which differs from SLeX only in the linkage between *N*-acetylglucosamine with galactose and fucose, has been implicated in E-selectin binding (50,51). Sulfated Lewis X can also bind selectins (52–54). Complicating this scheme is the observation that P-selectin and L-selectin can also bind SLeX, SLeA, and sulfated Lewis X, yet the binding characteristics of the selectins are distinct (51,54–58).

It has become apparent that while carbohydrates are an essential component of selectin ligands, the specific carrier protein contributes significantly to selectin specificity and binding affinity. A putative ligand for L-selectin was identified by Butcher and colleagues on high endothelial venules with the MECA-79 MAb (59,60). In a parallel line of investigation, Rosen, Lasky and colleagues utilized a soluble L-selectin-Ig chimera to identify, purify, and clone a highly glycosylated mucin, termed GlyCAM-1 (61,62). GlyCAM-1 is an unusual protein that contains a C-terminal amphipathic helix and lacks a conventional transmembrane domain (62). Sialic acid, fucose, and sulfation are critical components of the GlyCAM-1 ligand (63). A second mucin, CD34, was identified as a putative ligand for L-selectin (64). CD34 is widely expressed on endothelium and hematopoietic stem cells. Its regulation as an L-selectin ligand is unknown but may involve selective glycosylation at sites of inflammation. Using a similar strategy, McEver and colleagues identified a ligand for P-selectin on neutrophils (65). Cloning of this molecule, termed PSGL-1, revealed a mucin expressed as a homodimer, which requires appropriate decoration with sialic acid and fucose to serve as a functional ligand for P-selectin (66). Evidence for high-affinity ligands for E-selectin also exists. A 250-kDa molecule has been purified from bovine $\gamma\delta$ T cells on an E-selectin affinity matrix (31). Unlike the 240-kDa dimeric form of PSGL, the $\gamma\delta$ T-cell ligand remains a monomer upon reduction. Similarly a 160-kDa E-selectin ligand has been identified on mouse neutrophils (67). Finally, there is indirect functional evidence that L-selectin and E-selectin may operate in the same adhesion pathway. Whether they act as specific receptor-ligand pairs is unresolved, although clearly L-selectin is not a high-affinity ligand that can be purified on E-selectin affinity columns.

3. VLA-4

VLA-4 is a member of the integrin family of adhesion molecules (68). Integrins are involved in many fundamental processes in development, wound healing, hemostasis, and immunity (69). All integrins have a similar basic structure, comprising an α subunit, containing multiple divalent cation binding domains, noncovalently associated with a cysteine-rich β subunit. Historically, integrin subfamilies were defined by the β subunit, which could associate with different α subunits. One subfamily involved in leukocyte trafficking is the CD18 or $\beta 2$ integrins (see below). The VLA-4 integrin is composed of the $\alpha 4$ and $\beta 1$ subunits ($\alpha 4\beta 1$ heterodimer). The $\beta 1$ subfamily is the largest integrin subfamily (68,69) and includes the classic fibronectin receptor ($\alpha 5\beta 1$). The $\alpha 4$ subunit is unusual in that it is capable of pairing with two different β subunits, $\beta 1$ and $\beta 7$ (70). Of the other known integrin α subunits, only the αv subunit is known to pair with multiple β subunits. $\alpha 4\beta 1$ is expressed on lymphocytes, monocytes, and eosinophils but not on neutrophils; it mediates both cell-matrix and cell-cell interactions. $\alpha 4\beta 1$ binds fibronectin, but interestingly at a site distinct from the RGD recognition sequence bound by the classical $\alpha 5\beta 1$ fibronectin receptor (71). Lymphocyte–endothelial cell interactions are also mediated in part by $\alpha 4\beta 1$ binding to endothelial cell VCAM-1 (72), a molecule that is structurally related to the ICAMs (see below). In addition, $\alpha 4\beta 1$ can mediate LFA-1–independent lymphocyte aggregation by binding an undefined ligand on lymphocyte surfaces. $\alpha 4\beta 7$ was first defined in the mouse as LPAM-2, a molecule involved in lymphocyte trafficking to the Peyer's patches (70,73). The human homologue of $\beta 7$ was identified and shown to be a leukocyte-specific antigen. $\alpha 4\beta 7$ mediates lymphocyte binding to HEV of Peyer's patches by recognizing the MAdCAM-1 adhesion protein (74–76).

4. VCAM-1

VCAM-1 was first identified functionally as an endothelial cell adhesion molecule for lymphocytes (77–79). Like E-selectin, VCAM-1 expression is induced by stimulation of endothelial cells with proinflammatory cytokines, such as IL-1 and TNF (78,79). Interestingly γ-interferon induces expression of VCAM-1 but not E-selectin. VCAM-1 is a member of the immunoglobulin supergene family (77). There are two main alternatively spliced forms with six and seven Ig-like domains. VCAM-1 has two distinct binding sites for VLA-4, one located in domain 1 and the other in domain 3 (80). VCAM-1 expression is generally restricted to endothelial cells, although it is expressed in other tissues during development.

5. Molecular Basis of Neutrophil Rolling

An early indication that L-selectin may mediate the initial binding events between circulating neutrophils and inflamed endothelium was based upon the observation that L-selectin and the Mac-1 integrin are inversely regulated upon neutrophil exposure to chemotactic agents (19,21). These results indicate that L-selectin and Mac-1 mediate distinct adhesion events, and that L-selectin-dependent adhesion involves unstimulated neutrophils and precedes Mac-1-dependent adhesion. Experimental evidence to support this model came from two lines of investigation: (a) An in vitro flow chamber was constructed to simulate shear stress found in venules, and neutrophils were allowed to interact with cytokine-stimulated endothelium under conditions of flow. Neutrophil rolling and binding under these conditions were not affected by antibodies directed against the CD18 integrins (81) but were inhibited by anti-L-selectin MAb (82). (b) Intravital microscopy allowed investigators to observe neutrophil rolling events in vivo on exteriorized venules. Both polyclonal and monoclonal antibodies directed against L-selectin and an L-selectin–Ig chimera effectively inhibited neutrophil rolling (83,84). Inhibition of neutrophil rolling prevented downstream events, including neutrophil extravasation (2,3). L-selectin gene knockout mice exhibit a deficient neutrophil rolling response (45). L-selectin also contributes to the rolling responses of monocytes (85). Moreover, transfection of L-selectin–negative cells with L-selectin gene confers the ability to roll on endothelial cells in vivo (86,87) and on purified MAdCAM-1 in vitro (88). Interestingly, leukocyte rolling requires an intact L-selectin cytoplasmic domain, suggesting that interactions with cytoskeleton or other cytosolic proteins are critical to maintain function (89). The subcellular distribution of L-selectin has been localized to the tips of microvilli projections (90,91). This unusual distribution is thought to be important in presenting L-selectin in an optimal manner to mediate neutrophil rolling.

These observations were further extended to demonstrate that E-selectin and P-selectin also support neutrophil rolling (92–94). Purified molecules incorporated in artificial planar membranes or selectin transfectants were shown to directly support leukocyte rolling in vitro under flow conditions. Interestingly neutrophil rolling on E-selectin transfectants has been shown to be partially blocked by anti-L-selectin MAb in a variety of different models (94–96). Anti-P selectin MAb has also been shown to inhibit rolling in vivo by intravital microscopy. Indeed much of the spontaneous rolling of neutrophils observed in exteriorized venules can be attributed to a P-selectin–dependent rolling event (97). The P-selectin–dependent component can be increased by perfusing the venules with histamine (98,99). P-selectin–knockout animals exhibit deficient rolling behavior at early time points, which is consistent with a role for P-selectin in mediating very early inflammatory events (43). Anti-E-selectin MAb inhibits neutrophil rolling on IL-1-treated rabbit mesentery venules

(100). In addition to rolling on cytokine-activated endothelial cells, neutrophils have also been shown to roll on adherent platelets, where rolling is P-selectin–dependent (101), and on adherent neutrophils, where rolling is strictly dependent upon L-selectin (102). These other neutrophil rolling interactions may play an important role in recruiting additional leukocytes to inflammatory sites. More recently subsets of T cells have been shown to roll on P- and E-selectin (42). Interestingly, distinct subsets and ligands appear to be involved.

Recently there has been evidence that the VLA-4 integrin can also mediate rolling interactions of eosinophils (103) and some T lymphocytes (104). This type of interaction is unlikely to be significant for neutrophil rolling, since neutrophils are devoid of VLA-4 expression. Since eosinophils and many T cells also express L-selectin, it is unclear which molecules are more important for rolling or if they mediate rolling under different inflammatory conditions. VLA-4 is likely to have multiple roles in mediating rolling as well as tethering and perhaps transendothelial migration. In addition, VLA-4 contributes to adhesion to matrix (fibronectin) and in lymphocyte-lymphocyte adhesion.

B. Triggering of Leukocytes by Chemoattractants

Once leukocytes begin to localize to the vascular endothelium at a site of inflammation, they require a second signal that instructs the leukocytes to enter the tissue and triggers a transition from a quiescent circulating leukocyte to a primed, surface-mobile leukocyte. This signal is provided by chemoattractants which serve to both attract and activate leukocytes. Recently a large class of chemoattractants, termed chemokines, has been characterized (105). Many chemokines are specific for subclasses of leukocytes, which adds another level of selectivity to the recruitment of leukocytes. Acute inflammatory infiltrates are typically dominated by neutrophils, while more chronic inflamed sites may involve monocytes, eosinophils, or subsets of lymphocytes. It is clear that many of these cell types express L-selectin or ligands for P- and E-selectin; thus initial binding via selectins is not sufficient to account for the specificity of leukocyte recruitment. Chemokines and other chemoattractants may provide the crucial "go or no-go" signal to enter inflamed tissue. In this scenario, selectin-mediated rolling of leukocytes on endothelium would be readily reversible unless there is an appropriate chemokine signal. Bovine $\gamma\delta$ T cells express high levels of L-selectin and have been shown to bind to peripheral lymph node HEV; however, they are unable to enter the lymph node (220). One possibility is that these cells lack the appropriate chemokine receptor to receive the secondary signal to enter the tissue. Neutrophil chemokines trigger what is likely to be an irreversible commitment of the neutrophil to migrate into the inflamed tissue.

1. Chemokines

Chemokines are low-molecular-weight cytokines that serve to attract and activate leukocytes (reviewed in Ref. 105). Amino acid homology among chemokines varies considerably; however, all chemokines have four conserved cysteine residues. Moreover the chemokines can be broadly divided into two major families based upon the positioning of the first pair of cysteines: in the C-X-C family, the first two cysteine residues are separated by a single amino acid; in the C-C family, the first pair of cysteines are adjacent. These structural subfamilies also target different classes of leukocytes and map to different chromosomes (C-X-C to chromosome 4 and C-C chemokines to chromosome 17).

The C-X-C chemokines primarily target neutrophils. The best studied C-X-C chemokine is IL-8 (106), whose structure has been revealed by NMR spectroscopy and x-ray crystallography (107). Other members of this family include GROα, GROβ, GROγ, NAP-2, ENA-78, PF4, IP-10, and GCP-2. The *N*-terminal segment preceding the first cysteine is critical for activity towards neutrophils. All C-X-C chemokines acting on neutrophils have a short *N*-terminal segment that includes a Glu-Leu-Arg (ELR) motif adjacent to the first cysteine. Removal or mutagenesis of this ELR motif abrogates activity (108,109). The C-X-C chemokines can be produced by a wide variety of cells, including monocytes, lymphocytes, neutrophils, endothelial cells, epithelial cells, fibroblasts, and others in response to proinflammatory cytokines.

The C-C chemokines primarily target mononuclear leukocytes. The C-C chemokines include MCP-1, HC14, MCP-3, MIP-1α, MIP-1β, and RANTES. The C-C chemokines are structurally similar to the C-X-C chemokines; however, they lack a common *N*-terminal motif, such as the ELR motif of the C-X-C chemokines. C-C chemokines can also be produced by a wide variety of cell types in response to proinflammatory cytokines.

2. Other Chemoattractants

It is important to note that chemokines are not the only molecules that attract and activate leukocytes. Classic neutrophil chemoattractants include such diverse and unrelated products as the C5a fragment of complement, platelet activating factor (PAF), leukotriene LTB4, and the fMet-Leu-Phe peptide. All of these molecules exhibit potent chemoattractant and cell-activating activities and can often be found in the same sites that chemokines are produced.

3. Chemokine and Chemoattractant Receptors

The receptors for both the chemokines and many classical chemoattractants share a number of structural similarities. These receptors belong to a family of molecules termed "serpentine" receptors, so named because they are single-chain molecules that span the membrane seven times (105,110). The serpentine receptors are coupled to intracellular trimeric G-proteins. Other G-coupled serpentine receptors are involved in signal transduction for neurotransmission, vision, olfaction, and hormone action. Serpentine receptors for fMLP (111), C5a (112), PAF (113), IL-8 (114,115), and MIP-1a/RANTES (116) have been identified. Thus despite the great structural dissimilarities between fMLP, C5a, PAF, and the chemokines, these chemoattractants mediate their biological effects by binding to the same class of receptors. However the overall sequence homology among serpentine receptors is quite low. One exception is two different types of IL-8 receptors: IL8-RA and IL8-RB (114,115). These receptors are highly homologous (77% identity), yet IL8-RA shows high specifity for IL-8 while IL8-RB is more promiscuous in that it binds all C-X-C chemokines that have the ELR motif (117,118).

Binding of chemoattractants to their respective serpentine receptors transduces a signal via heterotrimeric G proteins. Chemoattractant binding induces phosphoinositide-specific phospholipase C (PI-PLC) and calcium mobilization. The G-coupled serpentine receptors can be inactivated by pertussis toxin, indicating involvement of Gi-type G proteins.

4. Biological Consequences of Chemokine Activity

Chemokines can elicit a broad range of responses from leukocytes, dependent largely upon their local concentration. At nanomolar concentrations, chemokines are chemotactic for those leukocytes expressing the appropriate serpentine receptors. Chemokines also modulate adhesion molecule expression and function. Neutrophil chemoattractants induce rapid proteolysis of L-selectin (19) and mobilization of intracellular stores of Mac-1 to the surface (119,120), resulting in rapid downregulation of L-selectin and upregulation of Mac-1. This inverse regulation of L-selectin and Mac-1 is one of the hallmarks of this transition from selectin-dependent initial binding to Mac-1-dependent transendothelial migration. IL-8 has also been shown to have antiadhesive effects at concentrations which are independent of its affect on L-selectin expression (121,122). At high concentrations, chemoattractants induce exocytosis of primary and secondary granules and provide potent costimulatory signals for neutrophil oxidative burst (123).

The chemotactic activity of chemokines can be easily measured in vitro. Neutrophil chemoattractants—such as fMLP, C5a, LTB4, PAF, and IL-8—are all well characterized. Cytokine-stimulated endothelial cells can produce several chemoattractants, including IL-8 and PAF. Neutrophil transendothelial migration across cytokine-stimulated endothelium can be blocked by an antiserum against IL-8, suggesting that in 3- to 4-hr-stimulated endothelial cell cultures IL-8 is the major neutrophil chemoattractant (124). The C-C chemokines show strong chemoattractant activity towards monocytes. The identification of chemokines which are active toward lymphocytes has been more difficult, but it is one of the fastest-emerging areas in this field. RANTES was among the first chemokines shown to be chemotactic for memory T cells but not for neutrophils (125). More recent evidence suggests that MIP-1α, MIP-1β (126,127), and MCP-1 (128) can also act as T-cell chemoattractants.

The triggering of a transition in neutrophil adhesiveness has also been demonstrated in vitro. Under static conditions, the adhesion of resting neutrophils to cytokine-stimulated endothelium is partially selectin-dependent and partially CD18/ICAM-1 dependent. However, neutrophils stimulated with chemotactic agents adhere to endothelial cells in a strictly CD18/ICAM-1–dependent manner. Similarly, under conditions of flow, neutrophils roll and do not stop on an artificial planar membrane containing P-selectin and ICAM-1 (93). If fMLP is infused into the chamber, the rolling velocity decreases dramatically and neutrophils eventually stop and spread on the lipid bilayer. Interestingly if only P-selectin is present in the bilayer, neutrophils do not become arrested even with the infusion of fMLP. Thus, even in this artificial system, all three components—selectins, chemoattractants, and CD18/ICAM-1—are required for the transition from a rolling interaction to firm adhesion. Triggering of VLA-4–mediated adhesion can be triggered in lymphoid cell lines by transfection of an fMLP receptor and exposure of the transfectants to fMLP (129). The triggering event is rapid and inhibited by pertussis toxin.

Bargatze et al. (130) provided an elegant demonstration for the in vivo requirement of a G-coupled receptor-mediated signaling event in this transition from rolling interactions to transendothelial migration. Intravital microscopy showed that treatment of mice with pertussis toxin disrupted the rolling interactions of lymphocytes with high endothelial venules of lymphoid organs. The requirement for a

G-coupled receptor could be bypassed with the infusion of phorbol ester, which allowed lymphocytes to become firmly adherent to venules.

Although chemokines are primarily used experimentally as soluble factors, this may not be the most physiologically relevant form. Soluble chemokines would quickly be carried downstream by blood flow. It would be more efficient if chemokines were physically associated with the endothelial cell surface, as this would limit diffusion and ensure specific localization of leukocytes. IL-8 can be immunolocalized to both endothelial cell surfaces and the underlying collagen bed (124). It has been proposed that proteoglycans can serve as carriers for chemokines and immobilize chemokines at the appropriate site (127,131,132). Shaw and colleagues demonstrated that heparin and other proteogylcans can immobilize MIP-1b and promote T-cell adhesion to VCAM-1 (133). Rot and coworkers similarly showed that IL-8 immobilized onto heparin enhances the chemotactic response (132). Zimmerman and colleagues have proposed a similar model for PAF (40,134). Endothelial cells produce a membrane-associated PAF that is synthesized rapidly upon stimulation with histamine or thrombin. PAF and P-selectin become coexpressed on the surfaces of endothelial cells and may act cooperatively, with P-selectin acting as a tether to slow the circulating neutrophil and PAF providing the secondary signal to trigger firm adhesion and transendothelial migration.

C. Transendothelial Migration

Once a leukocyte receives the appropriate chemotactic signal, it must be able to migrate across the vascular endothelial barrier. Classic studies indicate that leukocytes first crawl on the surface of the endothelial monolayer and then migrate between endothelial junctions and proceed through the basement membrane (reviewed in Ref. 135). Many molecules have been implicated in leukocyte transendothelial migration, including the CD18 integrins, $\alpha 4$ integrins, ICAM-1, VCAM-1, and PECAM-1. The CD18 integrins play a key role as evidenced by the identification of patients that are genetically deficient in CD18 integrin expression (136). Neutrophils from patients with this disease, termed leukocyte adhesion deficiency (LAD), are capable of rolling on endothelial cells but are unable to transmigrate across the endothelial monolayer (82,137,138).

1. CD18 Integrins

The CD18 integrins—LFA-1, Mac-1, and p150,95—have distinct α subunits which share a common $\beta 2$ (or CD18) subunit (139–143). The α subunits of LFA-1, Mac-1, and p150,95 are unusual in that they have a large 200–amino acid insertion (I) domain, which is homologous to the A domain of von Willebrand factor, the complement factors C2 and B, and cartilage matrix protein. Most other integrin α subunits lack this inserted domain. MAb mapping studies have indicated that most function-blocking MAbs bind to the I domain (144). Recently the I domain has been expressed as a separate entity and shown to have some of the divalent cation-binding (145) and functional properties of the intact molecule. These results indicate that, for the CD18 integrins, the I domain is a major component of the ligand-binding structure.

While integrins in general are expressed on diverse cell types, the CD18 integrins are restricted in expression to leukocytes. LFA-1 is constitutively expressed on the cell surfaces of most leukocytes. Mac-1 and p150,95 are primarily expressed by myeloid cells but can be induced on subsets of NK cells and activated lymphocytes. Mac-1 is stored in intracellular vesicles in unstimulated neutrophils and monocytes (119). Upon activation with chemotactic agents, the vesicles are mobilized and recruited to the cell surface, resulting in rapid upregulation of Mac-1 surface expression. In addition to quantitative upregulation of Mac-1 expression, both Mac-1 and LFA-1 function are qualitatively regulated (146–148). On quiescent cells, LFA-1 and Mac-1 are expressed in an inactive conformation. Upon stimulation, LFA-1 and Mac-1 assume an active conformation, which is readily detected by binding activity and by MAbs that recognizes activation-specific epitopes (149–151).

Both LFA-1 and Mac-1 are capable of recognizing multiple ligands. The intercellular adhesion molecules (ICAMs) have been defined functionally as LFA-1 ligands. The three known ICAM molecules are all members of the immunoglobulin supergene family (see below). Mac-1 also binds ICAM-1 but shows more promiscuous binding activity in binding to such diverse molecules as the iC3b fragment of complement, fibrinogen, factor X, and an undefined ligand on neutrophils (152–154).

While the contributions of LFA-1 and Mac-1 to leukocyte trafficking are emphasized in this review, it is important to note that these integrins play at least a contributing role in leukocyte effector function and immune cell regulation. Cytolytic T-cell–target cell binding (155), myeloid cell phagocytosis (156), and antigen presentation all involve integrins as accessory molecules. In addition, ligation through integrins has been shown to provide costimulatory signals for T-cell activation (157) and for neutrophil oxidative burst (123).

2. ICAM-1

ICAM-1 was the first of three ICAMs identified as specific ligands for LFA-1 (158). Both ICAM-1 and ICAM-3 have a five Ig-like domain structure, while ICAM-2 has only two Ig-like domains (159–164). LFA-1 binds to contact sites within the first two Ig domains of ICAM-1 (165). Mac-1 has also been shown to bind ICAM-1, but at a distinct site localized to domain 3 (166). There is no definitive evidence that Mac-1 can also bind ICAM-2 or ICAM-3. ICAM-1 is expressed at low levels on unstimulated endothelium and mononuclear leukocytes; however, many cell types can be induced to express ICAM-1 upon stimulation with proinflammatory cytokines, such as IL-1 and TNF, and the levels of ICAM-1 expressed on stimulated endothelial cells and lymphocytes is markedly elevated (158,167). In contrast, ICAM-2 is constitutively expressed on endothelial cells (168) and ICAM-3 is expressed on leukocytes, including neutrophils (169). Only ICAM-1 has been clearly implicated in mediating leukocyte trafficking to sites of inflammation. In addition, ICAM-1 has been shown to be involved in antigen presentation and CTL–target cell interactions. Recently cross-linking of ICAM-1 has been shown to transduce a costimulatory signal to monocytes (170).

3. PECAM-1

PECAM-1 (CD31) is also a member of the immunoglobulin supergene family with six Ig-like domains (171). PECAM-1 is widely expressed by cells in the vascular compartment, including platelets, neutrophils, monocytes, subsets of T lymphocytes, and vascular endothelial cells. Unlike ICAMs and VCAM-1, PECAM-1 can participate in homophilic interactions. There is also evidence that PECAM-1 can bind to a distinct but yet unidentified receptor (172). PECAM-1 on endothelial cells is localized between endothelial cell junctions (173). Endothelial cells cultured in the presence of anti-PECAM-1 MAb do not form normal cell-to-cell contacts. MAb against PECAM-1 blocks neutrophil recruitment in vivo in a murine model of peritonitis (174).

4. Molecular Basis of Transendothelial Migration

The first indication that the CD18 integrins are involved in leukocyte transendothelial migration came from the study of LAD patients who are genetically deficient in their expression of CD18 integrins. These patients suffer from severe and recurrent bacterial infections of soft tissues. Leukocytes from these patients exhibit a wide spectrum of defects in adhesion-related functions; however, clinically the primary impairment is in the ability of leukocytes to migrate out of the vascular compartment (136). Blood levels of leukocytes are markedly elevated, but infected lesions are virtually devoid of a leukocyte infiltrate. Normal neutrophils transfused into these patients are capable of responding to an inflammatory insult. In vitro study of these CD18-deficient neutrophils revealed some deficiency in their ability to adhere to cytokine-stimulated endothelium under static conditions (137,138). Yet these leukocytes bound as well as normal leukocytes to stimulated endothelium under conditions of flow (82). However, CD18-deficient leukocytes show an almost complete defect in their ability to transmigrate through a monolayer of cytokine-stimulated endothelium (137,138).

MAbs directed against the CD18 complex also effectively inhibited leukocyte transendothelial migration in vitro (137,138). The use of antibodies directed against the individual CD18 integrins, LFA-1 and Mac-1, indicated that both integrins contribute to neutrophil transendothelial migration, although antibodies against LFA-1 were more effective than anti-Mac-1 MAbs in blocking migration (138). The process of how integrins promote directed migration is not clear. However, in the case of Mac-1, elegant studies by Smith and colleagues suggest that neutrophils exposed to small stepwise increases of a chemotactic factor, mimicking a chemotactic gradient, respond by stepwise recruitment of Mac-1 from intracellular pools to the leading edge (175). As the neutrophil migrates in response to small increases in chemoattractant levels, the cell surface Mac-1 continues down the surface of the leukocyte until it reaches the trailing uropod, and a new wave of Mac-1 is recruited to the leading edge. Migration continues only as long as there are continuous stepwise increases in chemoattractant levels.

A major ligand for CD18-dependent transmigration appears to be ICAM-1 (137,138). Anti-ICAM-1 also blocks neutrophil transendothelial migration, although not to the same extent as an anti-CD18 MAb. The inhibitory effect of anti-ICAM-1 MAb was additive with that of anti-Mac-1 MAb but not with anti-LFA-1 MAb. These results suggest that LFA-1 mediates transmigration primarily through its interaction with ICAM-1 on endothelial cells, while Mac-1, which can also bind ICAM-1, may use other ligands as well. T-lymphocyte transendothelial migration has been extensively studied by Oppenheimer-Marks and colleagues. $CD8^+$ T cells show a greater transendothelial migratory capacity than $CD4^+$ cells. Migrating cells of both subsets are enriched for CD29 bright cells, although $CD8^+$ cells are predominately $CD45RA^+$ while $CD4^+$ cells are predominately $CD45RO^+$ (176). Although T cells bind to both ICAM-1 and VCAM-1 on stimulated endothelium, antibody-blocking experiments indicate that the LFA-1-ICAM-1 interaction is the primary mechanism for transendothelial migration. Consistent with this model, T-cell clones from CD18-deficient LAD patients are able to bind to endothelium via VLA-4/VCAM-1 interactions but are deficient in their ability to transmigrate (177). However, Chuluyan and Issekutz have found that monocytes from LAD patients can undergo transendothelial migration in a VLA-4–dependent manner (178). Thus VLA-4 may have multiple roles in both mediating leukocyte rolling and participating in transendothelial migration of some cell types. Interestingly Oppenheimer-Marks demonstrated that ICAM-1 and VCAM-1 have distinct subcellular distributions which might account for the differences in their involvement in T-cell transendothelial migration (179). ICAM-1 is expressed on both the apical and basal surfaces of endothelial cells as well as at endothelial junctions, while VCAM-1 is restricted to the apical surface. Thus ICAM-1 is appropriately expressed to allow migration to the basal side of the endothelium.

Recent evidence suggests that antibodies directed against PECAM-1 can block transendothelial migration of monocytes. PECAM-1 is also appropriately expressed at vascular endothelial cell junctions. Pretreatment of either the monocytes or the endothelial monolayer is sufficient to block transendothelial migration (180). From electron microscopy studies, it appears that anti-PECAM-1–treated monocytes are stuck on the apical surface above endothelial cell junctions (180). However PECAM-1 has also been implicated in providing a secondary chemokinelike signal which triggers integrin-mediated adhesion (191). Thus it is not entirely clear whether PECAM-1 is directly involved in transendothelial migration or if it mediates its effects by transducing a signal to the leukocyte.

III. THERAPEUTIC POTENTIAL OF ANTI–ADHESION MOLECULE ANTAGONISTS

The therapeutic potential of anti–adhesion molecule antagonists was first realized with the identification and characterization of the LAD patients. The lesson learned from this experiment of nature was that the CD18 integrins are in the critical pathway for neutrophil recruitment to sites of inflammation. Fischer and colleagues treated several severely deficient LAD patients by bone marrow transplantation and observed that engraftment and survival was significantly better than expected (182). These observations suggested that antagonists of CD18 may be therapeutically useful for attenuating a broad spectrum of inflammatory and immunological diseases, including graft rejection. More recently, patients deficient in fucose-containing carbohydrates, including components of selectin ligands, have been identified (183). Like the CD18-deficient patients, these patients suffer from recurrent infections. However, their primary immunological defect appears to affect selectin-dependent functions (183–185). Gene-targeted knockout animals have also provided experimental systems to assess the contributions of various adhesion molecules (43–45,186). The multistep model for leukocyte-endothelial interactions has important therapeutic implications: the model predicts that selectin-dependent leukocyte rolling, chemokine-triggering, and CD18 integrin/ICAM-1-dependent transendothelial migration are sequential steps, not parallel events. Thus blockade at any one of these steps should inhibit the ultimate recruitment of leukocytes into inflammatory sites. This concept has been tested in vivo with anti–adhesion molecule MAbs in a variety of clinically relevant animal models of ischemia-reperfusion injury of the heart, gut, lungs, nerve tissue, and models of immunological and inflammatory disease, such as asthma and autoimmune disease (187). Indeed, mouse MAbs directed against LFA-1 and ICAM-1 are being tested clinically for a variety of indications. Presently the in vivo efficacy of chemokine or chemokine-receptor antagonists is not as well documented; however, this is a rapidly growing and promising area of research. This review focuses on the use of anti–adhesion molecule therapy in animal models of transplantation and preliminary indications of the first clinical trials.

A. Animal Models of Transplantation

Proof of the principle that anti–adhesion molecule therapy may be beneficial in graft survival has been studied in a variety of models, although primarily involving rodent species and the use of anti-integrin or anti-ICAM MAbs. Although selectin antagonists have been shown to be useful in many ischemia-reperfusion injury models, there is little experimental data for organ transplantation. Similarly the use of chemokine- or chemokine-receptor antagonists have not been extensively tested in animal models of transplantation. However this is an active area of research, and this situation is likely to change rapidly.

Early damage to transplanted cardiac tissue as a result of neutrophil-mediated reperfusion injury can be attenuated by MAbs against either CD18 or ICAM-1 (188). Treatment of rats with anti-ICAM-1 as the sole immunosuppressant for 10 days after cardiac transplantation prolonged allograft survival from a mean of 10 days to 18 days (189). Similarly, an anti-LFA-1 MAb prolonged cardiac allograft survival in mice, and anti-CD18 MAb reduced both cellular and vascular rejection of cardiac grafts in a rabbit model (190,191). Interestingly VCAM-1 expression is selectively induced in rejecting cardiac tissue. However initial studies indicated that anti-VCAM-1 MAb treatment prolonged graft survival by only a few days and had no significant effect on leukocyte infiltration or subsequent rejection (192). More recent studies from the same group indicate that increased doses of MAb and prolonged MAb therapy resulted in a significant improvement in cardiac graft survival (193). MAb against either LFA-1 or VLA-4 inhibit graft vasculitis in cardiac allografts (194,195); however anti-CD18 but not anti VLA-4 blocked cellular rejection as well (195). Antisense DNA directed against the ICAM-1 mRNA message prolonged cardiac allograft survival and reduced graft damage in mice (196). This study indicates that targeting adhesion molecules at the transcriptional level may also be therapeutically useful in vivo. Rejection of islet cells can be prevented by treatment of the recipient with anti-LFA-1 MAb (197,198) or pretreatment of the islet cells with anti-ICAM-1 MAb (199). Antibodies to both LFA-1 (200,201) and ICAM-1 (201) have been shown to improve engraftment and survival of allogeneic bone marrow transplants and reduce the severity of graft-versus-host disease in mice. Anti-ICAM-1 has also been shown to prevent early graft rejection of transplanted small bowel in rats (202) and prolong heterotopic corneal allograft survival in mice (203,204). Hepatic allograft survival in rats was prolonged from a mean of 11 days to a mean of 24 days with anti-LFA-1 and anti-ICAM-1 MAb therapy (205). In a mouse skin allograft model, anti-LFA-1 MAb but not anti-ICAM-1 MAb was found to significantly prolong graft survival from a mean of 24 days to a mean of 75 to 80 days (206).

Isobe et al. made an intriguing observation that a combination of anti-ICAM-1 and anti-LFA-1 MAb together, but not separately, induced specific acceptance of cardiac allografts in mice (207). A 6-day course of therapy prolonged allograft survival from a mean of 8 days to well over 70 days when the study was ended. Interestingly, after 65 days the transplanted mice accepted skin grafts from the donor strain but not from a third-party strain, suggesting that specific tolerance had been induced. Treatment with a combination of anti-VCAM-1 and anti-VLA-4 MAbs also promoted much longer survival of cardiac graft tissue than either MAb alone; however, only one animal out of four showed long term acceptance of a skin graft from the same donor strain (208). Similarly an ICAM-1 antisense used in conjunction with anti-LFA-1 MAb allowed indefinite survival of transplanted cardiac grafts in mice and induced donor-specific tolerance to other grafted tissue (196). Subsequent reports from other groups suggest that anti-LFA-1 MAb can promote long-term thyroid- (209) and skin-graft survival (206). In the thyroid allograft model a single dose of anti-LFA-1 MAb prevented graft rejection for over 70 days in all transplanted mice and promoted graft survival beyond 470 days in 50% of the recipients. However, long-term graft survival does not necessarily mean that specific tolerance was achieved. Zeng et al. (199) observed that pretreatment of islet cells with anti-ICAM-1 promoted long-term graft survival (40% survival beyond 100 days) but did not induce systemic tolerance. One hypothesis is that anti-LFA-1 MAb may block crucial secondary signals to T lymphocytes and possibly induce a state of anergy. However these results from rodent models of transplantation must be interpreted with caution, since it is apparently easier to induce tolerance in rodents than in humans, and it is unknown how well these results will carry over to the clinic.

In a more clinically relevant model, Cosimi et al. tested the efficacy of an anti-ICAM-1 MAb in a nonhuman primate model of renal allograft rejection (210). The anti-ICAM-1 was given as the sole form of immunosuppressive therapy over a course of 12 days and was shown to prolong graft survival from a mean of 10 days in controls to a mean of over 22 days. In addition, when monkeys were treated with anti-ICAM-1 MAb as the sole form of induction therapy, the initial postoperative deterioration in kidney function manifest by a rise in serum creatinine was mitigated. Another series of experiments showed that anti-ICAM-1 treatment could also reverse ongoing acute rejection episodes. In this study, cyclosporine A was administered initially as the sole form of immunosuppressive therapy, and the dose of CyA was gradually reduced until an acute rejection episode occurred, as determined by a rise in serum creatinine. Anti-ICAM-1 was then administered and was found to reverse the serum creatinine levels back to baseline and prolong allograft survival. These results indicate anti-ICAM-1 is acting at the level of blocking leukocyte effector function or immune regulation, in addition to its effects on cell trafficking. In another nonhuman primate model, anti-ICAM-1 was again used as the sole form of immunosuppressive therapy and shown to prolong survival of heterotopic cardiac allografts from a mean of 9 days to 23 to 27 days (211).

B. Clinical Trials with Anti-Adhesion Molecule Antibodies

Organ transplantation elicits two distinct responses from the host: an acute inflammatory reaction and a chronic immunological reaction. The immunological response to foreign MHC is well characterized, and general T-cell immunosuppressants, such as cyclosporine and FK506, have radically improved the long-term outlook for many types of organ transplantation. However, organ transplant can be thought of as an unusual case of ischemia-reperfusion injury. In this case ischemia begins with the removal of the organ from the donor, and the organ becomes reperfused upon implantation into the recipient. With the increased success of long-term graft survival due to general immunosuppressive therapy, it is becoming more apparent that the acute inflammatory component may play a substantial role in early graft failure and possibly exacerbate the chronic immunological component. The surgical trauma compounds the acute inflammatory component. Not surprisingly, vascular adhesion molecules, such as ICAM-1 and VCAM-1, have been shown to be upregulated on transplanted organs undergoing rejection, and levels of circulating, soluble adhesion molecules in serum have been shown to be elevated in patients undergoing graft rejection. Presently MAb directed against the LFA-1 integrin and its ligand, ICAM-1, are in clinical trials as an add-on therapy to general immunosuppressives. Since LFA-1–ICAM-1 interactions are involved in antigen-presentation and CTL effector function as well as in leukocyte trafficking, it is likely that anti-LFA-1 and anti-ICAM-1 may have an impact on the inflammatory component as well as the immunological component. The use of antilymphocyte or antithymocyte serum for induction therapy may work in part because of its reactivity with LFA-1 and ICAM-1.

1. The 25/3 Anti-LFA-1 MAb

The first clinical trial involving the use of anti-LFA-1 MAb for transplantation of bone marrow into HLA nonidentical recipients actually preceded most of the work with animal models of transplantation (212). The impetus to proceed with these studies was based upon the observation of Fischer et al. (182) that CD18-deficient LAD patients given a lifesaving bone marrow transplant showed a much higher success of engraftment than (5 of 5 successful engraftment) compared to that of other recipients treated for other congenital immunodeficiency diseases (about 25% successful engraftment). These results suggested that LFA-1 may play an important role in rejection of HLA-incompatible graft rejection. The 25/3 anti-LFA-1 MAb was chosen for an open-label, uncontrolled study of HLA-nonidentical bone marrow transplantation to children with congenital immunodeficiencies. The MAb was given at the time of transplant as an add-on therapy to more conventional ablative and immunosuppressive therapy (212). The anti-LFA-1 MAb was well tolerated and all 7 patients showed early engraftment, compared to only 1 in 7 in historical controls. The study was expanded to 46 children with malignant osteopetrosis, Fanconi's anemia, or inherited immunodeficiency disorders, such as Wiskott-Aldrich syndrome and functional T-cell immunodeficiency (213). Bone marrow from HLA-nonidentical related donors was depleted of T lymphocytes prior to transplantation. Anti-LFA-1 MAb was administered from day −3 to day 6 of transplantation, along with conventional immunosuppressive therapy. Of the total number of patients, 72% showed successful engraftment, compared to only 26% success in historical controls.

In another trial, the same MAb was administered to 10 patients undergoing steroid-resistant graft-versus-host disease (214). After a 5-day course of therapy, 2 patients showed a complete response to therapy while a third had a partial reduction in the overall severity of graft-versus-host disease. Five other patients had a response in at least one of the involved organs (usually skin). However 7 of the 8 responding patients relapsed upon cessation of MAb therapy.

The 25/3 anti-LFA-1 MAb was also used in clinical trials for cadaveric kidney transplantation. The MAb was initially tested for its ability to reverse acute rejection episodes (215). The MAb was administered as an add-on therapy at the onset of rejection. Although the course of treatment was intended for 10 days, only 1 of 7 patients received the full treatment because of the poor prognosis. In contrast, a separate open-label trial showed efficacy for the use of anti-LFA-1 MAb given at the time of transplantation as an add-on to azathioprine and steroid therapy (216). "Low-risk" patients were enrolled and transplanted with cadaveric kidneys with less than a 48-hr cold ischemia time. The 10-day course of MAb administration was well tolerated and was sufficient to give blood levels of MAbs to saturate sites on LFA-1–bearing cells. There were no acute rejection episodes in the first month, although 6 patients had rejection episodes within 1 to 3 months. Of 15 transplanted kidneys, 14 remained functional during a 12- to 19-month follow-up, with 1 kidney lost due to technical complications. These studies showed that anti-LFA-1 therapy may be more effective when given prophylactically at the time of transplantation, where it would have maximal effect on preventing the neutrophil-mediated tissue damage.

2. The R6.5 Anti-ICAM-1 MAb (Enlimomab)

The anti-ICAM-1 MAb, R6.5 (BIRR1; enlimomab), has also been evaluated in clinical trials for kidney transplant, liver transplant, rheumatoid arthritis, stroke, and burn. This review will focus on the use of anti-ICAM-1 in transplantation. The anti-ICAM-1 was first tested in a phase I-IIa open-label study of cadaveric renal allografts into patients that were considered "high risk" for posttransplant complications, such as delayed graft function or acute rejection (217,218). Anti-ICAM-1 was given prophylactically over a course of 6 to 14 days in addition to conventional therapy with cyclosporine A, azathioprine, and steroids. In vitro studies with the R6.5 MAb inidicated that 10 μg/mL was a critical concentration to achieve maximal function-blocking activity; thus 10 μg/mL was set as the target blood trough level for a therapeutic dose. Early dosing regimens (150 to 300 mg over 13 to 14 days) indicated that only 1 of 7 patients reached the pharmokinetic target for blood levels of anti-ICAM-1 MAb.

The dosing regimen was initially based upon the experience with R6.5 MAb in the nonhuman primate model of renal transplantation. However it is possible that sick humans express significantly more ICAM-1, an inflammatory cell surface marker, than healthy monkeys and therefore require more anti-ICAM-1 to saturate all sites. Alternatively humans are known to have a basal level of 100 to 200 ng/mL of a soluble form of ICAM-1 in serum (219), which is elevated in inflammatory conditions and may act as a sink for anti-ICAM-1 MAb. A circulating form of ICAM-1 has not been detected in monkey serum, although this has not been exhaustively examined.

Subsequent patients who were enrolled in the study were given a higher total dose of MAb over a shorter course of therapy (300 to 560 mg over 6 days). Ten of eleven of these patients achieved target blood trough levels of at least 10 μg/mL of anti-ICAM-1 MAb. Although this was not intended to be a controlled study, efficacy comparisons can be made between the 11 patients who achieved target blood levels of MAb (therapeutic dose) and the 7 patients who did not achieve target blood levels (subtherapeutic dose). All seven patients who received a subtherapeutic dose had at least one acute rejection episode within the first 3 months after transplant. In marked contrast, only 3 of 11 patients who achieved a therapeutic dose had a rejection episode in the first 3 months. Similarly 6 of the 7 patients given the subtherapeutic dose had delayed graft function compared with 6 of 11 for the patients that achieved a therapeutic dose. The MAb was well tolerated in both groups and in all dosing regimens. These results were very promising, particularly given the "high-risk" population enrolled. However it is important to note that this was an open-label phase I-IIa trial. The efficacy of the anti-ICAM-1 MAb is currently being evaluated in a ongoing phase IIb and a separate phase III placebo-controlled, double-blinded renal transplant trial.

Preliminary indications of a phase I study to evaluate safety and dosing in a liver transplant model are now available. Anti-ICAM-1 was administered prophylactically as an add-on to conventional immunosuppressive therapy with cyclosporine A, azathioprine, and steroids. Liver transplant patients needed even more MAb than renal transplant patients to achieve the target blood trough level of 10 μg/mL. The highest dosing regimen was 880 mg of MAb over a 6-day course. Even at the highest dosing regimen, the safety profile remained good.

IV. SUMMARY

The recognition that different classes of adhesion molecules and chemoattractants work cooperatively but sequentially has provided a useful framework to understand how leukocytes traffic to sites of inflammation. Basic research discoveries are now being exploited to develop novel therapeutic drugs for the treatment of inflammatory and immunological diseases, including organ transplantation. Early clinical trials with anti-LFA-1 and with anti-ICAM-1 are promising, and the results of the first placebo-controlled, double-blinded clinical trials are eagerly awaited. Animal models of transplantation will be extended to test selectin antagonists and chemokine or chemokine-receptor antagonists. The main limitation of the current mouse MAb therapy is its inherent immunogenicity in humans. Second-generation therapies will include modified antibodies with reduced immunogenicity, such as CDR-grafted antibodies, or alternative strategies, such as antisense inhibitors, to modulate adhesion molecule expression. The ultimate goal is to identify small molecule inhibitors of adhesion molecules that are safe, orally available, and effective in vivo. Such a drug has tremendous potential for treating a wide spectrum of inflammatory and immunological diseases.

REFERENCES

1. Atherton A, Born GVR. Quantitative investigations of the adhesiveness of circulating polymorphonuclear leukocytes to blood vessel walls. J Physiol 1972; 222:447–474.
2. von Andrian UH, Hansell P, Chambers JD, et al. L-selectin function is required for β_2-integrin-mediated neutrophil adhesion at physiological shear rates in vivo. Am J Physiol Heart Circ Physiol 1992; 263:H1034–H1044.
3. Lindbom L, Xie X, Raud J, Hedqvist P. Chemoattractant-induced firm adhesion of leukocytes to vascular endothelium in vivo is critically dependent on initial leukocyte rolling. Acta Physiol Scand 1992; 146:415–421.

4. Lasky LA. Selectins: Interpreters of cell-specific carbohydrate information during inflammation. Science 1992; 258:964–969.
5. Kishimoto TK, Rothlein R. Integrins, ICAMs, and selectins: Role and regulation of adhesion molecules in neutrophil recruitment to inflammatory sites. In: Advances in Pharmacology. Vol. 25. New York, Academic Press, 1994:117–169.
6. McEver RP. Selectins. Curr Opin Immunol 1994; 6:75–84.
7. Bevilacqua MP, Nelson RM. Selectins. J Clin Invest 1993; 91:379–387.
8. Johnston GI, Cook RG, McEver RP. Cloning of GMP-140, a granule membrane protein of platelets and endothelium: Sequence similarity to proteins involved in cell adhesion and inflammation. Cell 1989; 56:1033–1044.
9. Bevilacqua MP, Stengelin S, Gimbrone MA, Seed B. Endothelial leukocyte adhesion molecule 1: An inducible receptor for neutrophils related to complement regulatory proteins and lectins. Science 1989; 243:1160–1165.
10. Lasky LA, Singer MS, Yednock TA, et al. Cloning of a lymphocyte homing receptor reveals a lectin domain. Cell 1989; 56:1045–1055.
11. Siegelman MH, Van de Rijn M, Weissman IL. Mouse lymph node homing receptor cDNA clone encodes a glycoprotein revealing tandem interaction domains. Science 1989; 243:1165–1172.
12. Siegelman MH, Weissman IL. Human homologue of mouse lymph node homing receptor: Evolutionary conservation at tandem cell interaction domains. Proc Natl Acad Sci USA 1989; 86:5562–5566.
13. Tedder TF, Isaacs CM, Ernst TJ, et al. Isolation and chromosomal localization of cDNAs encoding a novel human lymphocyte cell surface molecule, LAM-1. J Exp Med 1989; 170:123–133.
14. Camerini D, James SP, Stamenkovic I, Seed B. Leu-8/TQI is the human equivalent of the Mel-14 lymph node homing receptor. Nature 1989; 342:78–80.
15. Bowen BR, Nguyen T, Lasky LA. Characterization of a human homologue of the murine peripheral lymph node homing receptor. J Cell Biol 1989; 109:421–427.
16. Erbe DV, Wolitzky BA, Presta LG, et al. Identification of an E-selectin region critical for carbohydrate recognition and cell adhesion. J Cell Biol 1992; 119:215–227.
17. Graves BJ, Crowther RL, Chandran C, et al. Insight into E-selectin/ligand interaction from the crystal structure and mutagenesis of the lec/EGF domains. Nature 1994; 367: 532–538.
18. Lewinsohn DM, Bargatze RF, Butcher EC. Leukocyte-endothelial cell recognition: Evidence of a common molecular mechanism shared by neutrophils, lymphocytes, and other leukocytes. J Immunol 1987; 138:4313–4321.
19. Kishimoto TK, Jutila MA, Berg EL, Butcher EC. Neutrophil Mac-1 and MEL-14 adhesion proteins inversely regulated by chemotactic factors. Science 1989; 245:1238–1241.
20. Kahn J, Ingraham RH, Shirley F, et al. Membrane proximal cleavage of L-selectin: Identification of the cleavage site and a 6-kD transmembrane peptide fragment of L-selectin. J Cell Biol 1994; 125:461–470.
21. Jutila MA, Rott L, Berg EL, Butcher EC. Function and regulation of the neutrophil MEL-14 antigen in vivo: Comparison with LFA-1 and Mac-1. J Immunol 1989; 143: 3318–3324.
22. Palecanda A, Walcheck B, Bishop DK, Jutila MA. Rapid activation-independent shedding of leukocyte L-selectin induced by cross-linking of the surface antigen. Eur J Immunol 1992; 22:1279–1286.
23. Gallatin WM, Weissman IL, Butcher EC. A cell-surface molecule involved in organ-specific homing of lymphocytes. Nature 1983; 304:30–34.
24. Butcher EC. The regulation of lymphocyte traffic. Curr Topics Microbiol Immunol 1986; 128:85–122.

25. Yednock TA, Rosen SD. Lymphocyte homing. Adv Immunol 1989; 44:313–378.
26. Bevilacqua MP, Pober JS, Mendrick DL, et al. Identification of an inducible endothelial-leukocyte adhesion molecule, E-LAM 1. Proc Natl Acad Sci USA 1987; 84:9238–9242.
27. Cotran RS, Gimbrone MA, Bevilacqua MP, et al. Induction and detection of a human endothelial activation antigen in vivo. J Exp Med 1986; 164:661–666.
28. Picker LJ, Kishimoto TK, Smith CW, et al. ELAM-1 is an adhesion molecule for skin-homing T cells. Nature 1991; 349:796–799.
29. Koch AE, Burrows JC, Haines GK, et al. Immunolocalization of endothelial and leukocyte adhesion molecules in human rheumatoid and osteoarthritic synovial tissues. Lab Invest 1991; 64:313–320.
30. Shimizu Y, Shaw S, Graber N, et al. Activation-independent binding of human memory T cells to adhesion molecule ELAM-1. Nature 1991; 349:799–802.
31. Walcheck B, Watts G, Jutila MA. Bovine gamma/delta T cells bind E-selectin via a novel glycoprotein receptor: First characterization of a lymphocyte/E-selectin interaction in an animal model. J Exp Med 1993; 178:853–863.
32. Stenberg PE, McEver RP, Shuman MA, et al. A platelet alpha granule membrane protein (GMP-140) is expressed on the plasma membrane after activation. J Cell Biol 1985; 101:880–886.
33. McEver RP, Beckstead JH, Moore KL, et al. GMP-140, a platelet alpha-granule membrane protein, is also synthesized by vascular endothelial cells and is localized in Weibel-Palade bodies. J Clin Invest 1989; 84:92–99.
34. Bonfanti R, Furie BC, Furie B, Wagner DD. PADGEM (GMP140) is a component of Weibel-Palade bodies of human endothelial cells. Blood 1989; 73:1109–1112.
35. Disdier M, Morrissey JH, Fugate RD, et al. Cytoplasmic domain of P-selectin (CD62) contains the signal for sorting into the regulated secretory pathway. Mol Biol Cell 1992; 3:309–321.
36. Green SA, Setiadi H, McEver RP, Kelly RB. The cytoplasmic domain of P-selectin contains a sorting determinant that mediates rapid degradation in lysosomes. J Cell Biol 1994; 124:435–448.
37. Larsen E, Celi A, Gilbert GE, et al. PADGEM protein: A receptor that mediates the interaction of activated platelets with neutrophils and monocytes. Cell 1989; 59:305–312.
38. Geng J-G, Bevilacqua MP, Moore KL, et al. Rapid neutrophil adhesion to activated endothelium mediated by GMP-140. Nature 1990; 343:757–760.
39. Patel KD, Zimmerman GA, Prescott SM, et al. Oxygen radicals induce human endothelial cells to express GMP-140 and bind neutrophils. J Cell Biol 1991; 112:749–759.
40. Lorant DE, Patel KD, McIntyre TM, et al. Coexpression of GMP-140 and PAF by endothelium stimulated by histamine or thrombin: A juxtacrine system for adhesion and activation of neutrophils. J Cell Biol 1991; 115:223–234.
41. Moore KL, Thompson LF. P-Selectin (CD62) binds to subpopulations of human memory T lymphocytes and natural killer cells. Biochem Biophys Res Commun 1992; 186:173–181.
42. Alon R, Rossiter H, Wang X, et al. Distinct cell surface ligands mediate T lymphocyte attachment and rolling on P and E selectin under physiological flow. J Cell Biol 1994; 127:1485–1495.
43. Mayadas TN, Johnson RC, Rayburn H, et al. Leukocyte rolling and extravasation are severely compromised in P selectin–deficient mice. Cell 1993; 74:541–554.
44. Labow MA, Norton CR, Rumberger JM, et al. Characterization of E-selectin-deficient mice: Demonstration of overlapping function of the endothelial selectins. Immunity 1994; 1:709–720.
45. Arbones ML, Ord DC, Ley K, et al. Lymphocyte homing and leukocyte rolling and migration are impaired in L-selectin–deficient mice. Immunity 1994; 1:247–260.

46. Phillips ML, Nudelman E, Gaeta FCA, et al. ELAM-1 mediates cell adhesion by recognition of a carbohydrate ligand, sialyl-Le^{x}. Science 1990; 250:1130–1132.
47. Walz G, Aruffo A, Kolanus W, et al. Recognition by ELAM-1 of the sialyl-Lex determinant on myeloid and tumor cells. Science 1990; 250:1132–1134.
48. Lowe JB, Stoolman LM, Nair RP, et al. ELAM-1-dependent cell adhesion to vascular endothelium determined by a transfected human fucosyltransferase cDNA. Cell 1990; 63:475–484.
49. Goelz SE, Hession C, Goff D, et al. ELFT: A gene that directs the expression of an ELAM-1 ligand. Cell 1990; 63:1349–1356.
50. Berg EL, Robinson MK, Mansson O, et al. A carbohydrate domain common to both sialyl Le^{a} and sialyl Le^{X} is recognized by the endothelial cell leukocyte adhesion molecule ELAM-1. J Biol Chem 1991; 266:14869–14872.
51. Tyrrell D, James P, Rao N, et al. Structural requirements for the carbohydrate ligand of E- selectin. Proc Natl Acad Sci USA 1991; 88:10372–10376.
52. Yuen C-T, Bezouska K, O'Brien J, et al. Sulfated blood group Lewis^{a}: A superior oligosaccharide ligand for human E-selectin. J Biol Chem 1994; 269:1595–1598.
53. Yuen C-T, Lawson AM, Chai W, et al. Novel sulfated ligands for the cell adhesion molecule E- selectin revealed by the neoglycolipid technology among O-linked oligosaccharides on an ovarian cystadenoma glycoprotein. Biochemistry 1992; 31:9126–9131.
54. Green PJ, Tamatani T, Watanabe T, et al. High affinity binding of the leukocyte adhesion molecule L-selectin to 3′-sulphated-Le^{a} and -Le^{x} oligosaccharides and the predominance of sulphate in this interaction demonstrated by binding studies with a series of lipid-linked oligosaccharides. Biochem Biophys Res Commun 1992; 188:244–251.
55. Polley MJ, Phillips ML, Wayner E, et al. CD62 and endothelial cell-leukocyte adhesion molecule 1 (ELAM-1) recognize the same carbohydrate ligand, sialyl-Lewis x. Proc Natl Acad Sci USA 1991; 88:6224–6228.
56. Larsen GR, Sako D, Ahern TJ, et al. P-selectin and E-selectin: Distinct but overlapping leukocyte ligand specificities. J Biol Chem 1992; 267:11104–11110.
57. Berg EL, Magnani J, Warnock RA, et al. Comparison of L-selectin and E-selectin ligand specificities: The L-selectin can bind the E-selectin ligands sialyl Le^{x} and sialyl Le^{a}. Biochem Biophys Res Commun 1992; 184:1048–1055.
58. Foxall C, Watson SR, Dowbenko D, et al. The three members of the selectin receptor family recognize a common carbohydrate epitope, the sialyl Lewis^{x} oligosaccharide. J Cell Biol 1992; 117:895–902.
59. Streeter PR, Rouse BT, Butcher EC. Immunohistologic and functional characterization of a vascular addressin involved in lymphocyte homing into peripheral lymph nodes. J Cell Biol 1988; 107:1853–1862.
60. Berg EL, Robinson MK, Warnock RA, Butcher EC. The human peripheral lymph node vascular addressin is a ligand for LECAM-1, the peripheral lymph node homing receptor. J Cell Biol 1991; 114:343–349.
61. Imai Y, Singer MS, Fennie C, et al. Identification of a carbohydrate-based endothelial ligand for a lymphocyte homing receptor. J Cell Biol 1991; 113:1213–1221.
62. Lasky LA, Singer MS, Dowbenko D, et al. An endothelial ligand for L-selectin is a novel mucin-like molecule. Cell 1992; 69:927–938.
63. Imai Y, Lasky LA, Rosen SD. Sulphation requirement for GlyCAM-1, an endothelial ligand for L-selectin. Nature 1993; 361:555–557.
64. Baumhueter S, Singer MS, Henzel W, et al. Binding of L-selectin to the vascular sialomucin CD34. Science 1993; 262:436–438.
65. Moore KL, Stults NL, Diaz S, et al. Identification of a specific glycoprotein ligand for P-selectin (CD62) on myeloid cells. J Cell Biol 1992; 118:445–456.

66. Sako D, Chang X-J, Barone KM, et al. Expression cloning of a functional glycoprotein ligand for P-selectin. Cell 1993; 75:1179–1186.
67. Levinovitz A, Måhlhoff J, Isenmann S, Vestweber D. Identification of a glycoprotein ligand for E-selectin on mouse myeloid cells. J Cell Biol 1993; 121:449–459.
68. Hemler ME. VLA proteins in the integrin family: Structures, functions, and their role on leukocytes. Annu Rev Immunol 1990; 8:365–400.
69. Hynes RO. Integrins: Versatility, modulation, and signaling in cell adhesion. Cell 1992; 69:11–25.
70. Holzmann B, Weissman IL. Peyer's patch–specific lymphocyte homing receptors consist of a VLA-4-like alpha chain associated with either of two integrin beta chains, one of which is novel. EMBO J 1989; 8:1735–1741.
71. Wayner EA, Garcia-Pardo A, Humphries MJ, et al. Identification and characterization of the T lymphocyte adhesion receptor for an alternative cell attachment domain (CS-1) in plasma fibronectin. J Cell Biol 1989; 109:1321–1330.
72. Elices MJ, Osborn L, Takada Y, et al. VCAM-1 on activated endothelium interacts with the leukocyte integrin VLA-4 at a site distinct from the VLA-4/fibronectin binding site. Cell 1990; 60:577–584.
73. Holzmann B, McIntyre BW, Weissman IL. Identification of a murine Peyer's patch-specific lymphocyte homing receptor as an integrin molecule with an alpha chain homologous to human VLA-4 alpha. Cell 1989; 56:37–46.
74. Berlin C, Berg EL, Briskin MJ, et al. Alpha 4 beta 7 integrin mediates lymphocyte binding to the mucosal addressin MAdCAM-1. Cell 1993; 74:185–195.
75. Andrew DP, Berlin C, Honda S, et al. Distinct but overlapping epitopes are involved in $\alpha_4\beta_7$-mediated adhesion to vascular cell adhesion molecule-1, mucosal addressin-1, fibronectin, and lymphocyte aggregation. J Immunol 1994; 153:3847–3861.
76. Briskin MJ, McEvoy LM, Butcher EC. MAdCAM-1 has homology to immunoglobulin and mucin-like adhesion receptors and to IgA1. Nature 1993; 363:461–464.
77. Osborn L, Hession C, Tizard R, et al. Direct expression cloning of vascular cell adhesion molecule 1, a cytokine-induced endothelial protein that binds to lymphocytes. Cell 1989; 59:1203–1211.
78. Schwartz BR, Wayner EA, Carlos TM, et al. Identification of surface proteins mediating adherence of CD11/CD18-deficient lymphoblastoid cells to cultured human endothelium. J Clin Invest 1990; 85:2019–2022.
79. Rice GE, Munro JM, Bevilacqua MP. Inducible cell adhesion molecule 110 (INCAM-110) is an endothelial receptor for lymphocytes. A CD11/CD18-independent adhesion mechanism. J Exp Med 1990; 171:1369–1374.
80. Vonderheide RH, Springer TA. Lymphocyte adhesion through very late antigen 4: Evidence for a novel binding site in the alternatively spliced domain of vascular cell adhesion molecule 1 and an additional α4 integrin counter-receptor on stimulated endothelium. J Exp Med 1992; 175:1433–1442.
81. Lawrence MB, Smith CW, Eskin SG, McIntire LV. Effect of venous shear stress on CD18-mediated neutrophil adhesion to cultured endothelium. Blood 1990; 75:227–237.
82. Smith CW, Kishimoto TK, Abbassi O, et al. Chemotactic factors regulate lectin adhesion molecule-1 (LECAM-1)-dependent neutrophil adhesion to cytokine-stimulated endothelial cells in vitro. J Clin Invest 1991; 87:609–618.
83. Ley K, Gaehtgens P, Fennie C, et al. Lectin-like cell adhesion molecule 1 mediates leukocyte rolling in mesenteric venules in vivo. Blood 1991; 77:2553–2555.
84. von Andrian UH, Chambers JD, McEvoy LM, et al. Two-step model of leukocyte-endothelial cell interaction in inflammation: Distinct roles for LECAM-1 and the leukocyte β_2 integrins in vivo. Proc Natl Acad Sci USA 1991; 88:7538–7542.
85. Luscinskas FW, Kansas GS, Ding H, et al. Monocyte rolling, arrest and spreading on

IL-4-activated vascular endothelium under flow is mediated via sequential action of L-selectin, β_1-integrins, and β_2-integrins. J Cell Biol 1994; 125:1417–1427.
86. Von Andrian UH, Chambers JD, Berg EL, et al. L-selectin mediates neutrophil rolling in inflamed venules through sialyl Lewis^X-dependent and -independent recognition pathways. Blood 1993; 82:182–191.
87. Ley K, Tedder TF, Kansas GS. L-selectin can mediate leukocyte rolling in untreated mesenteric venules in vivo independent of E- or P-selectin. Blood 1993; 82:1632–1638.
88. Berg EL, McEvoy LM, Berlin C, et al. L-selectin mediated lymphocyte rolling on MAdCAM-1. Nature 1993; 366:695–698.
89. Kansas GS, Ley K, Munro JM, Tedder TF. Regulation of leukocyte rolling and adhesion to high endothelial venules through the cytoplasmic domain of L-selectin. J Exp Med 1993; 177:833–838.
90. Picker LJ, Warnock RA, Burns AR, et al. The neutrophil selectin LECAM-1 presents carbohydrate ligands to the vascular selectins ELAM-1 and GMP-140. Cell 1991; 66: 921–933.
91. Erlandsen SL, Hasslen SR, Nelson RD. Detection and spatial distribution of the β_2 integrin (Mac-1) and L-selectin (LECAM-1) adherence receptors on human neutrophils by high-resolution field emission SEM. J Histochem Cytochem 1993; 41:327–333.
92. Lawrence MB, Springer TA. Neutrophils roll on E-selectin. J Immunol 1993; 151: 6338–6346.
93. Lawrence MB, Springer TA. Leukocytes roll on a selectin at physiologic flow rates: Distinction from and prerequisite for adhesion through integrins. Cell 1991; 65:1–20.
94. Abbassi O, Kishimoto TK, McIntire LV, et al. E-selectin supports neutrophil rolling in vitro under conditions of flow. J Clin Invest 1993; 92:2719–2730.
95. Bargatze RF, Kurk S, Watts G, et al. In vivo and in vitro functional examination of a conserved epitope of L- and E-selectin crucial for leukocyte-endothelial cell interactions. J Immunol 1994; 152:5814–5825.
96. Lawrence MB, Bainton DF, Springer TA. Neutrophil tethering to and rolling on E-selectin are separable by requirement for L-selectin. Immunity 1994; 1:137–145.
97. Dore M, Korthuis RJ, Granger DN, et al. P-selectin mediates spontaneous leukocyte rolling in vivo. Blood 1993; 82:1308–1316.
98. Ley K. Histamine can induce leukocyte rolling in rat mesenteric venules. Am J Physiol Heart Circ Physiol 1994; 267:H1017–H1023.
99. Kubes P, Kanwar S. Histamine induces leukocyte rolling in post-capillary venules: A P-selectin–mediated event. J Immunol 1994; 152:3570–3577.
100. Olofsson AM, Arfors K-E, Ramezani L, et al. E-selectin mediates leukocyte rolling in interleukin-1-treated rabbit mesentery venules. Blood 1994; 84:2749–2758.
101. Buttrum SM, Hatton R, Nash GB. Selectin-mediated rolling of neutrophils on immobilized platelets. Blood 1993; 82:1165–1174.
102. Bargatze RF, Kurk S, Butcher EC, Jutila MA. Neutrophils roll on adherent neutrophils bound to cytokine-induced endothelial cells via L-selectin on the rolling cells. J Exp Med 1994; 180:1785–1792.
103. Sriramarao P, Von Andrian UH, Butcher EC, et al. L-selectin and very late antigen-4 integrin promote eosinophil rolling at physiological shear rates in vivo. J Immunol 1994; 153:4238–4246.
104. Jones DA, McIntire LV, Smith CW, Picker LJ. A two-step adhesion cascade for T cell/endothelial cell interactions under flow conditions. J Clin Invest 1994; 94:2443–2450.
105. Baggiolini M, Dewald B, Moser B. Interleukin-8 and related chemotactic cytokines—CXC and CC chemokines. Adv Immunol 1994; 55:97–179.
106. Robinson EA, Yoshimura T, Leonard EJ, et al. Complete amino acid sequence of a

human monocyte chemoattractant, a putative mediator of cellular immune reaction. Proc Natl Acad Sci USA 1989; 86:1850–1854.
107. Baldwin ET, Weber IT, St Charles R, et al. Crystal structure of interleukin 8: Symbiosis of NMR and crystallography. Proc Natl Acad Sci USA 1991; 88:502–506.
108. Clark-Lewis I, Schumacher C, Bagglioni M, Moser B. Structure-activity relationships of interleukin-8 determined using chemically synthesized analogs: Critical role of NH2-terminal residues and evidence for uncoupling of neutrophil chemotaxis, exocytosis, and receptor binding activities. J Biol Chem 1991; 266:23128–23134.
109. Hebert CA, Vitangcol RV, Baker JB. Scanning mutagenesis of interleukin-8 identifies a cluster of residues required for receptor binding. J Biol Chem 1991; 266:18989–18994.
110. Murphy PM. The molecular biology of leukocyte chemoattractant receptors. Annu Rev Immunol 1994; 12:593–633.
111. Boulay F, Tardif M, Brouchon L, Vignais P. Synthesis and use of a novel N-formyl peptide derivative to isolate a human N-formyl peptide receptor DNA. Biochem Biophys Res Commun 1990; 168:1103–1109.
112. Gerard NP, Gerard C. The chemotactic receptor for human C5a anaphylatoxin. Nature 1991; 349:614–617.
113. Honda Z, Nakamura M, Miki I, et al. Cloning by functional expression of platelet-activating factor receptor from guinea pig lung. Nature 1991; 349:342–346.
114. Holmes WE, Lee J, Kuang W-J, et al. Structure and functional expression of a human interleukin-8 receptor. Science 1991; 253:1278–1280.
115. Murphy PM, Tiffany HL. Cloning of complementary cDNA encoding a functional human interleukin-8 receptor. Science 1991; 253:1280–1283.
116. Neote K, DiGregorio D, Mak JY, et al. Molecular cloning, functional expression, and signaling characteristics of a C-C chemokine receptor. Cell 1993; 72:415–425.
117. Lee J, Horuk R, Rice GC, et al. Characterization of two high affinity human interleukin-8 receptors. J Biol Chem 1992; 267:16283–16287.
118. LaRosa GJ, Thomas KM, Kaufman ME, et al. Amino terminus of the interleukin-8 receptor is a major determinant of receptor subtype specificity. J Biol Chem 1992; 267: 25402–25406.
119. Todd RF III, Arnaout MA, Rosin RE, et al. Subcellular localization of the large subunit of Mo1 (Mo1 alpha; formerly gp 110), a surface glycoprotein associated with neutrophil adhesion. J Clin Invest 1984; 74:1280–1290.
120. Borregaard N, Miller LJ, Springer TA. Chemoattractant-regulated fusion of a novel, mobilizable intracellular compartment with the plasma membrane in human neutrophils. Science 1987; 237:1204–1206.
121. Ley K, Baker JB, Cybulsky MI, et al. Intravenous interleukin-8 inhibits granulocyte emigration from rabbit mesenteric venules without altering L-selectin expression or leukocyte rolling. J Immunol 1993; 151:6347–6357.
122. Gimbrone MA, Obin MS, Brock AF, et al. Endothelial interleukin-8: A novel inhibitor of leukocyte-endothelial interactions. Science 1989; 246:1601–1603.
123. Shappell SB, Toman C, Anderson DC, et al. Mac-1 (CD11b/CD18) mediates adherence-dependent hydrogen peroxide production by human and canine neutrophils. J Immunol 1990; 144:2702–2711.
124. Huber AR, Kunkel SL, Todd RF, Weiss SJ. Regulation of transendothelial neutrophil migration by endogenous Il-8. Science 1991; 254:99–102.
125. Schall TJ, Bacon K, Toy KJ, Goeddel DV. Selective attraction of monocytes and T lymphocytes of the memory phenotype by cytokine RANTES. Nature 1990; 347:669–671.
126. Taub DD, Conlon K, Lloyd AR, et al. Preferential migration of activated $CD4^+$ and $CD8^+$ T cells in response to MIP-1alpha and MIP-1beta. Science 1993; 260:355–358.

127. Tanaka Y, Adams DH, Hubscher S, et al. T-cell adhesion induced by proteoglycan-immobilized cytokine MIP-1α. Nature 1993; 361:79–82.
128. Carr MW, Roth SJ, Luther E, et al. Monocyte chemoattractant protein 1 acts as a T-lymphocyte chemoattractant. Proc Natl Acad Sci USA 1994; 91:3652–3656.
129. Honda S, Campbell JJ, Andrew DP, et al. Ligand-induced adhesion to activated endothelium and to vascular cell adhesion molecule-1 in lymphocytes transfected with the N-formyl peptide receptor. J Immunol 1994; 152:4026–4035.
130. Bargatze RF, Butcher EC. Rapid G protein-regulated activation event involved in lymphocyte binding to high endothelial venules. J Exp Med 1993; 178:367–372.
131. Rot A. Neutrophil attractant/activation protein-1 (interleukin-8) induces in vitro neutrophil migration by haptotactic mechanism. Eur J Immunol 1993; 23:303–306.
132. Webb LM, Ehrengruber MU, Clark-Lewis I, et al. Binding to heparin sulfate or heparin enhances neutrophil responses to interleukin 8. Proc Natl Acad Sci USA 1993; 90:7158–7162.
133. Holter W, Majdic O, Liszka K, et al. Kinetics of activation antigen expression by in vitro-stimulated human T lymphocytes. Cellular Immunol 1985; 90:322–330.
134. Lorant DE, Topham MK, Whatley RE, et al. Inflammatory roles of P-selectin. J Clin Invest 1993; 92:559–570.
135. Smith CW. Transendothelial migration. In: Harlan JM, Liu DY, eds. Adhesion: Its Role in Inflammatory Disease. New York: Freeman, 1992:83–116.
136. Anderson DC, Springer TA. Leukocyte adhesion deficiency: An inherited defect in the Mac-1, LFA-1, and p150,95 glycoproteins. Annu Rev Med 1987; 38:175–194.
137. Smith CW, Rothlein R, Hughes BJ, et al. Recognition of an endothelial determinant for CD18-dependent neutrophil adherence and transendothelial migration. J Clin Invest 1988; 82:1746–1756.
138. Smith CW, Marlin SD, Rothlein R, et al. Cooperative interactions of LFA-1 and Mac-1 with intercellular adhesion molecule-1 in facilitating adherence and transendothelial migration of human neutrophils in vitro. J Clin Invest 1989; 83:2008–2017.
139. Larson RS, Corbi AL, Berman L, Springer TA. Primary structure of the LFA-1 alpha subunit: An integrin with an embedded domain defining a protein superfamily. J Cell Biol 1989; 108:703–712.
140. Corbi AL, Kishimoto TK, Miller LJ, Springer TA. The human leukocyte adhesion glycoprotein Mac-1 (Complement receptor type 3, CD11b) alpha subunit: Cloning, primary structure, and relation to the integrins, von Willebrand factor and factor B. J Biol Chem 1988; 263:12403–12411.
141. Corbi AL, Miller LJ, O'Connor K, et al. cDNA cloning and complete primary structure of the alpha subunit of a leukocyte adhesion glycoprotein, p150,95. EMBO J 1987; 6:4023–4028.
142. Arnaout MA, Remold-O'Donnell E, Pierce MW, et al. Molecular cloning of the alpha subunit of human and guinea pig leukocyte adhesion glycoprotein Mo1: Chromosomal localization and homology to the alpha subunits of integrins. Proc Natl Acad Sci USA 1988; 85:2776–2780.
143. Kishimoto TK, O'Connor K, Lee A, et al. Cloning of the beta subunit of the leukocyte adhesion proteins: Homology to an extracellular matrix receptor defines a novel supergene family. Cell 1987; 48:681–690.
144. Diamond MS, Garcia-Aguilar J, Bickford JK, et al. The I domain is a major recognition site on the leukocyte integrin Mac-1 (CD11b/CD18) for four distinct adhesion ligands. J Cell Biol 1993; 120:1031–1043.
145. Michishita M, Videm V, Arnaout MA. A novel divalent cation-binding site in the A domain of the β2 integrin CR3 (CD11b/CD18) is essential for ligand binding. Cell 1993; 72:857–867.
146. Buyon JP, Abramson SB, Philips MR, et al. Dissociation between increased surface

expression of Gp165/95 and homotypic neutrophil aggregation. J Immunol 1988; 140: 3156–3160.
147. Dustin ML, Springer TA. T cell receptor cross-linking transiently stimulates adhesiveness through LFA-1. Nature 1989; 341:619–624.
148. Van Kooyk Y, Van de Wiel-van Kemenade P, Weder P, et al. Enhancement of LFA-1-mediated cell adhesion by triggering through CD2 or CD3 on T lymphocytes. Nature 1989; 342:811–813.
149. Dransfield I, Hogg N. Regulated expression of Mg^{2+} binding epitope on leukocyte integrin α subunits. EMBO J 1989; 8:3759–3765.
150. Keizer GD, Visser W, Vliem M, Figdor CG. A monoclonal antibody (NKI-L16) directed against a unique epitope on the alpha-chain of human leukocyte function-associated antigen 1 homotypic cell-cell interactions. J Immunol 1988; 140:1393–1400.
151. Robinson MK, Andrew D, Rosen H, et al. Antibody against the Leu-CAM β-chain (CD18) promotes both LFA-1 and CR3-dependent adhesion events. J Immunol 1992; 148:1080–1085.
152. Altieri DC, Agbanyo FR, Plescia J, et al. A unique recognition site mediates the interaction of fibrinogen with the leukocyte integrin Mac-1 (CD11b/CD18). J Biol Chem 1990; 265:12119–12122.
153. Altieri DC, Edgington TS. The saturable high affinity association of factor X to ADP-stimulated monocytes defines a novel function of the Mac-1 receptor. J Biol Chem 1988; 263:7007–7015.
154. Beller DI, Springer TA, Schreiber RD. Anti-Mac-1 selectively inhibits the mouse and human type three complement receptor. J Exp Med 1982; 156:1000–1009.
155. Krensky AM, Sanchez-Madrid F, Robbins E, et al. The functional significance, distribution, and structure of LFA-1, LFA-2, and LFA-3: Cell surface antigens associated with CTL-target interactions. J Immunol 1983; 131:611–616.
156. Rothlein R, Springer TA. Complement receptor type three-dependent degradation of opsonized erythrocytes by mouse macrophages. J Immunol 1985; 135:2668–2672.
157. Van Seventer GA, Shimizu Y, Horgan KJ, Shaw S. The LFA-1 ligand ICAM-1 provides an important costimulatory signal for T cell receptor-mediated activation of resting T cells. J Immunol 1990; 144:4579–4586.
158. Rothlein R, Dustin ML, Marlin SD, Springer TA. A human intercellular adhesion molecule (ICAM-1) distinct from LFA-1. J Immunol 1986; 137:1270–1274.
159. Simmons D, Makgoba MW, Seed B. ICAM, an adhesion ligand of LFA-1, is homologous to the neural cell adhesion molecule NCAM. Nature 1988; 331:624–627.
160. Staunton DE, Marlin SD, Stratowa C, et al. Primary structure of intercellular adhesion molecule 1 (ICAM-1) demonstrates interaction between members of the immunoglobulin and integrin supergene families. Cell 1988; 52:925–933.
161. Vazeux R, Hoffman PA, Tomita JK, et al. Cloning and characterization of a new intercellular adhesion molecule ICAM-R. Nature 1992; 360:485–488.
162. De Fougerolles AR, Klickstein LB, Springer TA. Cloning and expression of intercellular adhesion molecule 3 reveals strong homology to other immunoglobulin family counter-receptors for lymphocyte function-associated antigen 1. J Exp Med 1993; 177: 1187–1192.
163. Fawcett J, Holness CL, Needham LA, et al. Molecular cloning of ICAM-3, a third ligand for LFA-1, constitutively expressed on resting leukocytes. Nature 1992; 360: 481–484.
164. Staunton DE, Dustin ML, Springer TA. Functional cloning of ICAM-2, a cell adhesion ligand for LFA-1 homologous to ICAM-1. Nature 1989; 339:61–64.
165. Staunton DE, Dustin ML, Erickson HP, Springer TA. The LFA-1 and rhinovirus binding sites of ICAM-1 and arrangement of its Ig-like domains. Cell 1990; 61:243–254.
166. Diamond MS, Staunton DE, Marlin SD, Springer TA. Binding of the integrin Mac-1

(CD11b/CD18) to the third immunoglobulin-like domain of ICAM-1 (CD54) and its regulation by glycosylation. Cell 1991; 65:961–971.
167. Dustin ML, Rothlein R, Bhan AK, et al. Induction by IL-1 and interferon, tissue distribution, biochemistry, and function of a natural adherence molecule (ICAM-1). J Immunol 1986; 137:245–254.
168. De Fougerolles AR, Stacker SA, Schwarting R, Springer TA. Characterization of ICAM-2 and evidence for a third counter-receptor for LFA-1. J Exp Med 1991; 174: 253–267.
169. De Fougerolles AR, Springer TA. Intercellular adhesion molecule 3, a third adhesion counter-receptor for lymphocyte function-associated molecule 1 on resting lymphocytes. J Exp Med 1992; 175:185–190.
170. Rothlein R, Kishimoto TK, Mainolfi E. Cross-linking of ICAM-1 induces co-signalling of an oxidative burst from mononuclear leukocytes. J Immunol 1994; 152:2488–2495.
171. Newman PJ, Berndt MC, Gorski J, et al. PECAM-1 (CD31) cloning and relation to adhesion molecules of the immunoglobulin gene superfamily. Science 1990; 247:1219–1222.
172. Muller WA, Berman ME, Newman PJ, et al. A heterophilic adhesion mechanism for platelet/endothelial cell adhesion molecule 1 (CD31). J Exp Med 1992; 175:1401–1404.
173. Albelda SM, Oliver PD, Romer LH, Buck CA. EndoCAM: A novel endothelial cell-cell adhesion molecule. J Cell Biol 1990; 110:1227–1237.
174. Vaporciyan AA, DeLisser HM, Yan H-C, et al. Involvement of platelet-endothelial cell adhesion molecule-1 in neutrophil recruitment in vivo. Science 1993; 262:1580–1582.
175. Hughes BJ, Hollers JC, Crockett-Torabi E, Smith CW. Recruitment of CD11b/CD18 to the neutrophil surface and adherence-dependent cell locomotion. J Clin Invest 1992; 90:1687–1696.
176. Pietschmann P, Cush JJ, Lipsky PE, Oppenheimer-Marks N. Identification of subsets of human T cells capable of enhanced transendothelial migration. J Immunol 1992; 149:1170–1178.
177. Kavanaugh AF, Lightfoot E, Lipsky PE, Oppenheimer-Marks N. Role of CD11/CD18 in adhesion and transendothelial migration of T cells: Analysis utilizing CD18-deficient T cell clones. J Immunol 1991; 146:4149–4156.
178. Chuluyan HE, Issekutz AC. VLA-4 integrin can mediate CD11/CD18-independent transendothelial migration of human monocytes. J Clin Invest 1993; 92:2768–2777.
179. Oppenheimer-Marks N, Davis LS, Bogue DT, et al. Differential utilization of ICAM-1 and VCAM-1 during the adhesion and transendothelial migration of human T lymphocytes. J Immunol 1991; 147:2913–2921.
180. Muller WA, Weigl SA, Deng X, Phillips DM. PECAM-1 is required for transendothelial migration of leukocytes. J Exp Med 1993; 178:449–460.
181. Tanaka Y, Albelda SM, Horgan KJ, et al. CD31 expressed on distinctive T cell subsets is a preferential amplifier of $\beta 1$ integrin-mediated adhesion. J Exp Med 1992; 176:245–253.
182. Le Deist F, Blanche S, Keable H, et al. Successful HLA nonidentical bone marrow transplantation in three patients with the leukocyte adhesion deficiency. Blood 1989; 74:512–516.
183. Etzioni A, Frydman M, Pollack S, et al. Brief report: Recurrent severe infections caused by a novel leukocyte adhesion deficiency. N Engl J Med 1992; 327:1789–1792.
184. Von Andrian UH, Berger EM, Ramezani L, et al. In vivo behavior of neutrophils from two patients with distinct inherited leukocyte adhesion deficiency syndromes. J Clin Invest 1993; 91:2893–2897.
185. Price TH, Ochs HD, Gershoni-Baruch R, et al. In vivo neutrophil and lymphocyte function studies in a patient with leukocyte adhesion deficiency type II. Blood 1994; 84:1635–1639.

186. Sligh JE Jr, Ballantyne CM, Rich SS, et al. Inflammatory and immune responses are impaired in mice deficient in intercellular adhesion molecule 1. Proc Natl Acad Sci USA 1993; 90:8529–8533.
187. Harlan JM, Winn RK, Vedder NB, et al. In vivo models of leukocyte adherence to endothelium. In: Harlan JM, Liu DY, eds. Adhesion: Its Role in Inflammatory Disease. New York: Freeman, 1992:117–150.
188. Byrne JG, Smith WJ, Murphy MP, et al. Complete prevention of myocardial stunning, contracture, low-reflow, and edema after heart transplantation by blocking neutrophil adhesion molecules during reperfusion. J Thorac Cardiovasc Surg 1992; 104:1589–1596.
189. Kobayashi H, Miyano T, Yamataka A, et al. Prolongation of rat cardiac allograft survival by a monoclonal antibody: Anti-rat intercellular adhesion molecule-1. Cardiovasc Surg 1993; 1:577–582.
190. Nakakura EK, McCabe SM, Zheng B, et al. Potent and effective prolongation by anti-LFA-1 monoclonal antibody monotherapy of non-primarily vascularized heart allograft survival in mice without T cell depletion. Transplantation 1993; 55:412–417.
191. Nakakura EK, McCabe SM, Zheng B, et al. A non-lymphocyte-depleting monoclonal antibody to the adhesion molecule LFA-1 (CD11a) prevents sensitization to alloantigens and effectively prolongs the survival of heart allografts. Transplant Proc 1993; 25:809–812.
192. Orosz CG, Van Buskirk A, Sedmak DD, et al. Role of the endothelial adhesion molecule VCAM in murine cardiac allograft rejection. Immunol Lett 1992; 32:7–12.
193. Orosz CG, Ohye RG, Pelletier RP, et al. Treatment with anti-vascular cell adhesion molecule 1 monoclonal antibody induces long-term murine cardiac allograft acceptance. Transplantation 1993; 56:453–460.
194. Paul LC, Davidoff A, Benediktsson H, Issekutz TB. The efficacy of LFA-1 and VLA-4 antibody treatment in rat vascularized cardiac allograft rejection. Transplantation 1993; 55:1196–1199.
195. Sadahiro M, McDonald TO, Allen MD. Reduction in cellular and vascular rejection by blocking leukocyte adhesion molecule receptors. Am J Pathol 1993; 142:675–683.
196. Stepkowski SM, Tu Y, Condon TP, Bennett CF. Blocking of heart allograft rejection by intercellular adhesion molecule-1 antisense oligonucleotides alone or in combination with other immunosuppressive modalities. J Immunol 1994; 153:5336–5336.
197. Gotoh M, Fukuzaki T, Monden M, et al. A potential immunosuppressive effect of anti-lymphocyte function-associated antigen-1 monoclonal antibody on islet transplantation. Transplantation 1994; 57:123–126.
198. Gotoh M, Fukuzaki T, Dono K, et al. Induction of unresponsiveness to islet allograft by anti-LFA-1 monoclonal antibody treatment. Transplant Proc 1993; 25:973–974.
199. Zeng Y, Gage A, Montag A, Rothlein R, et al. Inhibition of transplant rejection by pretreatment of xenogeneic pancreatic islet cells with anti-ICAM-1 antibodies. Transplantation 1994; 58:681–689.
200. Van Dijken PJ, Ghayur T, Mauch P, et al. Evidence that anti-LFA-1 in vivo improves engraftment and survival after allogeneic bone marrow transplantation. Transplantation 1990; 49:882–886.
201. Harning R, Pelletier J, Lubbe K, Takei F, Merluzzi VJ. Reduction in the severity of graft-versus-host disease and increased survival in allogeneic mice by treatment with monoclonal antibodies to cell adhesion antigens LFA-1α and MALA-2. Transplantation 1991; 52:842–845.
202. Yamataka T, Kobayashi H, Yagita H, et al. The effect of anti-ICAM-1 monoclonal antibody treatment on the transplantation of the small bowel in rats. J Pediatr Surg 1993; 28:1451–1457.
203. Guymer RH, Mandel TE. Monoclonal antibody to ICAM-1 prolongs murine heterotopic corneal allograft survival. Austr NZ J Ophthalmol 1991; 19:141–144.

204. He Y, Mellon J, Apte R, Niederkorn JY. Effect of LFA-1 and ICAM-1 antibody treatment on murine corneal allograft survival. Invest Ophthalmol Vis Sci 1994; 35: 3218–3225.
205. Harihara Y, Sakamoto H, Sanjo K, Otsubo O, et al. Prolongation of hepatic allograft survival with antibodies to ICAM-1 and LFA-1. Transplant Proc 1994; 26:2258–2258.
206. Van Kooyk Y, De Vries-van der Zwan A, De Waal LP, Figdor CG. Efficiency of antibodies directed against adhesion molecules to prolong skin graft survival in mice. Transplant Proc 1994; 26:401–403.
207. Isobe M, Ihara A. Tolerance induction against cardiac allograft by anti-ICAM-1 and anti-LFA-1 treatment: T cells respond to in vitro allostimulation. Transplant Proc 1993; 25:1079–1080.
208. Isobe M, Suzuki J, Yagita H, et al. Immunosuppression to cardiac allografts and soluble antigens by anti-vascular cellular adhesion molecule-1 and anti-very late antigen-4 monoclonal antibodies. J Immunol 1994; 153:5810–5818.
209. Talento A, Nguyen M, Blake T, et al. A single administration of LFA-1 antibody confers prolonged allograft survival. Transplantation 1993; 55:418–422.
210. Cosimi AB, Conti D, Delmonico FL, et al. In vivo effects of monoclonal antibody to ICAM-1 (CD54) in nonhuman primates with renal allografts. J Immunol 1990; 144: 4604–4612.
211. Flavin T, Rothlein R, Faanes R, et al. Monoclonal antibody against intercellular adhesion molecule (ICAM)-1 prolongs cardiac allograft survival in cynomologus monkeys. Transplant Proc 1990; 23:533–534.
212. Fischer A, Blanche S, Veber F, et al. Prevention of graft failure by an anti-HLFA-1 monoclonal antibody in HLA-mismatched bone-marrow transplantation. Lancet 1986; 2:1058–1061.
213. Fischer A, Friedrich W, Fasth A, et al. Reduction of graft failure by a monoclonal antibody (anti-LFA-1 CD11a) after HLA nonidentical bone marrow transplantation in children with immunodeficiencies, osteopetrosis, and Fanconi's anemia: A European group for immunodeficiency/European group for bone marrow transplantation report. Blood 1991; 77:249–256.
214. Stoppa A-M, Maraninchi D, Blaise D, et al. Anti-LFA1 monoclonal antibody (25.3) for treatment of steroid-resistant grade III-IV acute graft-versus-host disease. Transplant Int 1991; 4:3–7.
215. Le Mauff B, Hourmant M, Rougier J-P, et al. Effect of anti-LFA1 (CD11a) monoclonal antibodies in acute rejection in human kidney transplantation. Transplantation 1991; 52:291–296.
216. Hourmant M, Le Mauff B, Le Meur Y, et al. Administration of an anti-CD11a monoclonal antibody in recipients of kidney transplantation: A pilot study. Transplantation 1994; 58:377–380.
217. Cosimi AB, Rothlein R, Auchincloss H Jr, et al. Phase I clinical trial of anti-ICAM-1 (CD54) monoclonal antibody immunosuppression in renal allograft recipients. In: Lipsky PE, Rothlein R, Kishimoto TK, et al, eds. Structure, Function, and Regulation of Molecules Involved in Leukocyte Adhesion. New York: Springer-Verlag, 1992:373–387.
218. Haug CE, Colvin RB, Delmonico FL, et al. A phase I trial of immunosuppression with anti-ICAM-1 (CD54) mAb in renal allograft recipients. Transplantation 1993; 55:766–773.
219. Rothlein R, Mainolfi EA, Czajkowski M, Marlin SD. A form of circulating ICAM-1 in human serum. J Immunol 1991; 147:3788–3793.
220. Walcheck B, Jutila MA. Bovine gamma delta T cells express high levels of functional peripheral lymph node homing receptor (L-selectin). International Immunol 1994; 6: 81–91.

7

Cytokine Networks

Andrew H. Lichtman
Brigham and Women's Hospital and Harvard Medical School
Boston, Massachusetts

Werner Krenger
Dana-Farber Cancer Institute and Harvard Medical School
Boston, Massachusetts

James L. M. Ferrara
Dana-Farber Cancer Institute, Children's Hospital, and Harvard Medical School
Boston, Massachusetts

I. INTRODUCTION

The goal of this chapter is to review the basic biological properties of the major cytokines and to provide a basic understanding of the complexity of cellular and molecular interactions during the immune response to foreign molecules. The first part of this chapter describes cytokines that are predominantly produced by T cells and that act primarily on T cells, while the second part discusses the inflammatory cytokines predominantly produced by mononuclear phagocytes. The discussion of hematopoietic cytokines, including interleukin (IL)-3, IL-7, and colony stimulating factors (CSFs) are beyond the scope of this chapter; excellent reviews concerning the function of these cytokines have been published elsewhere (1–6). Advances of our understanding of the cytokine networks are likely to provide us with the ability to modulate cytokine responses in multiple immune responses, including those involved in the transplantation of organs.

II. T-CELL–DERIVED CYTOKINES

In this first section, we discuss cytokines that are produced by T lymphocytes and/or influence T-lymphocyte differentiation and function. The functions of $CD4^+$ effector T cells include the regulation of both cell-mediated and humoral immune responses. These functions are mediated in large part by a variety of cytokines produced by antigen-activated $CD4^+$ T lymphocytes. Populations of helper T cells are often differentiated into two polar subsets: T helper 1 $CD4^+$ cells producing IL-2 and interferon (IFN)-γ and T-helper 2 $CD4^+$ cells producing IL-4, IL-5, and IL-10 (7,8). More recently, it has been demonstrated that $CD8^+$ T cells can polarize in a similar way into two subsets with different cytokine production profiles (9,10). In this chapter, we therefore refer to these two subsets as "type 1" and "type 2." Due to secretion of distinct combinations of cytokines with distinct effector functions, the differential activation of type 1 versus type 2 T cells will determine the character of an ensuing immune response.

The following discussion includes a description of the biochemical and functional characteristics of the T-cell–derived cytokines and their receptors (Table 1), followed by a description of the roles of subsets of helper T cells that secrete different sets of these cytokines.

A. Interleukin-2 and Interleukin-15

IL-2 is a 14- to 17-kDa glycoprotein that functions as the major autocrine growth factor for T lymphocytes (11–15). IL-2 is produced by both $CD4^+$ and, in lesser quantities, by $CD8^+$ cells. New IL-2 synthesis occurs in response to T-cell-receptor (TCR) binding of peptide-MHC antigen and is a consequence of upregulated IL-2 gene transcription. The regulation of IL-2 gene transcription has served as a paradigm for the study of activation of other cytokine genes in T cells as well as other cell types. The promoter of the IL-2 gene has been extensively mapped and includes binding sites for several constitutive and inducible transcription factors, including Oct-1, AP-1, NFκB, NFAT, and NFIL2A (16). The activation of two of the factors, NFAT and NFIL2A, is dependent on TCR-induced calcium signals and is inhibitable by the immunosuppressive drugs cyclosporine and FK506 (17). The coordinate activation of all of these factors is probably necessary for in vivo transcription of the IL-2 gene. In addition to signals generated after engagement of the TCR, maximal IL-2 production requires signals generated by the binding of costimulatory molecules to T-cell surface receptors. The best-defined costimulators are B7-1 and B7-2, expressed on professional antigen-presenting cells such as activated B cells, macrophages, and dendritic cells (18). The B7 molecules bind to CD28 and CTLA-4 on T cells. Costimulation of IL-2 production may involve both enhanced transcription and mRNA molecule stability. Antigen stimulation in the absence of costimulators results in little or no IL-2 production and may lead to a state of T-cell functional unresponsiveness, or anergy. The anergic phenotype is characterized by a long-term block in the T cell's ability to produce IL-2 upon subsequent exposure to antigen, even with costimulators present. This form of anergy has been implicated as a mechanism of peripheral tolerance to antigens (19,20).

IL-2 binds to a high-affinity, multimeric IL-2 receptor (IL-2R), which is a member of the type 1 cytokine receptor family (21,22). The members of this family, which also include receptors for IL-3, IL-4, IL-5, IL-6 and IL-7, all share certain structural features in their extracellular domains, including a five–amino acid motif, tryptophan-serine-X-tryptophan-serine (WSXWS). All cytokines which bind to these type 1 receptors share a particular tertiary structure which includes four α helices. The high-affinity IL-2 receptor is composed of a complex of α, β, and γ chains (15,23,24). The γ chain is essential for signal transduction and is also a subunit of the receptors for IL-4, IL-7, IL-9, and IL-15. IL-2R$\beta\gamma$ has a lower affinity for IL-2 than the IL-2$\alpha\beta\gamma$ receptor, but it can transduce growth signals through the γ chain. Antigen-induced signals upregulate IL-2Rα expression and therefore lead to the formation of high-affinity receptors. As with other cytokines, most of our understanding of IL-2 function derives from in vitro studies. In T lymphocytes, IL-2 binding to its receptor stimulates mitosis, but the signaling pathways are poorly understood. Tyrosine kinases, including p56 lck and Jak family

Table 1 Cytokines—Sources, Targets, and Principal Biological Effects

Cytokine	Cell sources	Targets	Effects	References
IL-1α,β	Activated mononuclear phagocytes, many other cell types (e.g., epithelium, endothelium)	Mononuclear phagocytes, (primarily IL-1β), vascular endothelium, T and B cells, NK cells, hepatocytes, hypothalamus	Costimulators of T and B cells. Upregulate cytokine gene expression, adhesion molecules. Activate neutrophils (via IL-8), endothelium, complement, stem cells. Inducers of neuropeptides, fever, hypotension, acute phase response proteins and cachexia. Central to inflammatory response.	107–151, 153, 154, 159–163, 165–181, 192–202, 218, 226, 228, 241, 246, 247, 257, 270–274, 278, 295
IL-1ra	Activated mononuclear phagocytes, keratinocytes	Shares receptor with IL- 1α and IL-1β	Specific inhibitor of the action of IL-1, upregulated by type 2 cytokines and immunoglobulins. Important mediator of anti-inflammatory effects.	182–191, 257, 270
IL-2	Activated T cells ($CD4^+$ and $CD8^+$)	T and B cells, mononuclear phagocytes, NK cells	T-cell growth factor, stimulates growth and cytocidal function of NK cells, enhances IFN-γ production by T and NK cells and susceptibility of T cells to activation-induced death.	7–9, 11–17, 19–29, 96–101, 140, 270, 271, 277, 285, 294
IL-4	Activated type 2 T cells, mast cells, basophils, $NK1.1^+CD4^+$ T cells, eosinophils, thymocytes	T and B cells, mononuclear phagocytes	T-cell growth factor and inducer of IgE synthesis by B cells. Inhibits macrophage inflammatory function, upregulates MHC II on APC, promotes type 2 T-cell differentiation, induces vascular cell adhesion molecules.	7–9, 13, 32–42, 48, 96–102, 236, 274, 275, 278, 292, 294
IL-5	Activated type 2 T cells, mast cells	B cells, eosinophils	Promoter of eosinophil growth and differentiation, enhances IgA production by B cells.	46–51
IL-6	Activated mononuclear phagocytes, endothelial cells, activated T cells, fibroblasts	T and B cells, hepatocytes	Terminal differentiation factor for B cells, stimulates antibody production, costimulates T cells and thymocytes, promotes acute phase response proteins. Growth factor for malignant plasma cells, hematopoietic stem cells, cofactor for growth of hemopoietic stem cells.	220, 228, 248–260

(continued)

Table 1 Continued

Cytokine	Cell sources	Targets	Effects	References
IL-8	Mononuclear phagocytes, platelets, endothelial cells, fibroblasts, T cells	Neutrophils, T cells, fibroblasts	Activator of neutrophils, eosinophils, basophils, lymphocytes. Promoter of hemoattraction. Inducer of adherence and extravasation.	164, 261–263
IL-9	Activated type 2 T cells	Bone marrow precursors, mast cells, T cells	Promoter of erythropoiesis, growth factor for activated T cells, induces growth and activation of mast cells.	52–54
IL-10	Activated type 2 T cells, mononuclear phagocytes, B cells, thymocytes, keratinocytes	T cells, mononuclear phagocytes, langerhans cells, NK cells, mast cells	Inhibitor of macrophage inflammatory functions, including cytokine production and cytotoxic effector activities. Inhibits MHC II and B7 expression and type 1 T cell differentiation, inhibits T-cell activation and B7 expression on APC, enhances antibody production.	7–9, 55–67, 96–101
IL-12	Mononuclear phagocytes, B cells, other accessory cells	T cells, NK cells	Activator of NK cells, promotes type 1 T-cell differentiation. Strong inducer of IFN-γ production. Important initiator of cell-mediated immunity.	7–9, 68–80, 96–101, 103, 106
IL-13	Activated type 2 T cells, mast cells, EBV cell lines	Mononuclear phagocytes, B cells	Similar effects to IL-4 but no effect on T cells.	43–45
IL-15	Mononuclear phagocytes, smooth muscle cells, placenta, epithelial cells	T cells, NK cells	Similar effects to IL-2 on T-cell growth. Activates NK cytotoxicity via IL-2 receptor.	30, 31
IFN-γ	Activated type 1 T cells, type 0 T cells, NK cells, $CD8^+$ T cells	Mononuclear phagocytes, T and B cells, granulocytes and many other cell types	Promotes B-cell isotype switching and type 1 T-cell differentiation. Activates endothelium, macrophages and neutrophils. Upregulates MHC class I and II and adhesion molecules. Central role in cell-mediated immunity.	7–9, 13, 41, 77, 78, 81–88, 96–102, 105, 120, 160, 204, 236, 267, 288

TGF-β	Activated T cells, activated mononuclear phagocytes	T cells, mononuclear phagocytes, neutrophils	Inhibitor of T-cell activation. Stimulates IgA production by B cells, inhibits macrophage and neutrophil activation.	89–93
TNF-α	Activated mononuclear phagocytes, type 0, 1 and 2 T cells, eosinophils, NK-cells, polymorph. leukocytes; multiple other cell types	Neutrophils, endothelial cells, lymphocytes, lung, liver, muscle, fat tissue, hypothalamus, tumor cells	Stimulator of mononuclear phagocytes. Costimulator of T cells and B cells; upregulates MHC on APCs, potentiates CTL-mediated lysis, enhances NK activity. Activates vascular endothelium (cell adhesion molecules) and inflammatory leukocytes (neutrophils, eosinophils), Growth factor for fibroblasts and endothelial cells. hemopoietic tissues. Induces necrosis, apoptosis, fever, acute phase response proteins (liver), coagulation system. Suppresses bone marrow stem cell division. At high concentrations: induces cachexia, reduces tissue perfusion, depresses blood glucose concentrations, relaxes vascular smooth muscle tone.	94, 95, 120, 151, 175, 177, 193, 203–247, 267, 270, 277, 279–295
TNF-β	Activated type 1 T cells	Binds to same receptors as TNF- α	Similar to TNF-α, but action is local and paracrine rather than systemic.	94, 95

kinases, associate with the $\beta\gamma$ chains of the IL-2 receptor and become phosphorylated. IL-2 also stimulates the growth and cytocidal functions of natural killer cells, but only at high concentrations, since NK cells only express the $\beta\gamma$ form of the receptor. Other activities of IL-2 observed in vivo include enhancing interferon-γ (IFN-γ) production by T lymphocytes and NK cells and promoting growth and antibody production by B lymphocytes. Another potentially important role for IL-2 is to render T lymphocytes susceptible to activation-induced apoptotic death as a normal regulatory mechanism for the downregulation of immune responses and maintenance of self tolerance (25,26).

In vivo, IL-2 acts in an autocrine and paracrine manner. IL-2 knockout mice have normal numbers and subset distribution of T cells, suggesting that this cytokine is not required for thymic development. Furthermore, these mice are capable of mounting specific immune responses suggesting that other T-cell growth factors can substitute for IL-2 (27). The major pathology in these mice is the development of systemic autoimmune disease, anemia, and an inflammatory bowel disease similar to ulcerative colitis. The autoimmune disease in this setting is consistent with a role for IL-2 in promoting peripheral deletion of self-reactive T cells. An IL-2Rγ chain-deficient mouse line has also been developed; this mouse shows a profound block in T- and B-cell development (28). Since the IL-2Rγ chain is also a signaling subunit of several other cytokine receptors, including interleukin-4 and interleukin-7, the lymphocyte developmental defects observed in the γ-chain–deficient mice probably reflect the requirement of one or more of these latter cytokines in early lymphocyte maturation. Consistent with this is the finding that mutations in the IL-2Rγ chain gene are a cause of human X-linked severe combined immunodeficiency disease (29).

Interleukin 15 (IL-15) is a recently identified cytokine which shares many of the biological properties of IL-2 including growth factor activity for T cells (30,31). Although it does not share sequence homology with IL-2, it has a similar predicted tertiary structure and it requires the IL-2Rβ and γ chains for binding and signal transduction. IL-15 is produced by several cell types, including monocytes, epithelial cells, smooth muscle and placenta, but not T lymphocytes. The role of IL-15 in immune responses is presently unknown.

B. Interleukin-4 and Interleukin-13

IL-4 is a 20-kDa protein produced by activated T cells that has important biological effects on T and B lymphocytes, macrophages, and endothelium (13,32,33). The major IL-4-producing cell is the antigen-activated type 2 $CD4^+$ T lymphocyte, but type 2 $CD8^+$ T cells, mast cells, eosinophils, basophils, and double-negative thymocytes can also produce the cytokine. In addition, a population of cells expressing CD4 and the natural killer (NK) cell marker NK1.1 produce abundant IL-4 and may be an important source of the cytokine early in immune responses. T-cell production of IL-4 is largely regulated by T-cell-receptor–mediated enhancement of IL-4 gene transcription, and involves cyclosporin A–sensitive NFAT activation. Similar to IL-2, IL-4 has a four-α-helix structure. The IL-4 receptor includes at least two polypeptide chains, one WSXWS-containing member of the type 1 cytokine receptor family and a second chain identical to the γ chain of the IL-2R (34). Signaling by this receptor involves receptor-associated tyrosine kinases Jak1 and

Jak3, and tyrosine phosphorylation of a DNA binding protein IL-4 Stat (or Stat6), which, after dimerization, translocates into the nucleus and induces gene transcription (35).

IL-4 has several effects on B lymphocytes. It is the major identified factor that promotes heavy-chain isotype switching to the ϵ chain, and it is required for IgE synthesis. Therefore, IL-4 likely has a fundamental role in allergic diseases. In addition, IL-4 increases B-cell class II MHC expression and enhances B-cell proliferation responses to certain stimuli in vitro. The physiologic relevance of these effects in vivo is not known. IL-4 has two significant and related effects on T lymphocytes. First, it is the autocrine growth factor for type 2 $CD4^+$ T cells. Second, IL-4 is required for the differentiation of naive T cells into IL-4 producing type 2 T cells. Therefore, if IL-4 is present at the time of primary antigen exposure in an immune response, the responding T cells will tend to differentiate into type 2 T cells (13,36–38). It is not clear what the initial source of IL-4 is in such circumstances; candidates include mast cells, T cells bearing the $\gamma\delta$ form of antigen receptor, and $CD4^+$-$NK1.1^+$ cells (39). IL-4 has important downregulatory effects on macrophage function, effects which are also shared by IL-10 (see below). These effects include inhibition of lipopolysaccharide or IFN-γ activation responses. Thus, IL-4 blocks activation of monocyte/macrophage transcription and expression of proinflammatory cytokines, chemokines, and hematopoietic growth factors, including IL-1, IL-6, IL-12, IL-8, macrophage inflammatory protein (MIP)-1α, tumor necrosis factor (TNF)-α, granulocyte-macrophage colony-stimulating factor (GM-CSF), and granulocyte colony-stimulating factor (G-CSF). IL-4 also inhibits IFN-γ stimulated production of nitric oxide and prostaglandins by macrophages (40). Furthermore, IL-4 antagonizes the actions of the inflammatory cytokine IL-1 by inducing secretion of a specific receptor antagonist (IL-1ra) (41). Thus, IL-4 exerts a general suppressive effects on inflammatory processes by negatively influencing or preventing the actions of IL-1 and also of type 1 cytokines, and these effects are important for regulating cell mediated immune responses. IL-4 also stimulates endothelial cells to express vascular cell adhesion molecule-1 (VCAM-1) and monocyte chemotactic protein-1 (MCP-1). IL-4 gene knockout mice do not produce IgE. T cells from these mice also do not produce other type 2 cytokines, such as interleukin-5, indicating that IL-4 may be essential for differentiation into type 2 T cells in vivo (42).

IL-13 is a recently characterized cytokine produced by activated T cells which has many of the same biological effects as IL-4 (43–45). The amino acid sequences of IL-4 and IL-13 are about 30% homologous, and the tertiary structure of IL-13 is predicted to include four α-helices arranged in a similar way to IL-4. It is likely that IL-13 utilizes a distinct receptor which shares the same signaling subunit as the IL-4 receptor. Similar to IL-4, IL-13 has down-regulatory effects on monocytes/macrophages including inhibition of proinflammatory cytokine production and suppression of macrophage cytotoxic functions and it also promotes the switch to IgE in B cells. In contrast to IL-4, IL-13 does not affect T-cell growth or differentiation.

C. Interleukin-5

IL-5 is a 40-kDa protein composed of two identical polypeptide chains, produced by activated type 2 $CD4^+$ and $CD8^+$ T cells and by activated mast cells (46–51). The cytokine contains a four α-helix conformation and the α-chain of the two subunit IL-5 receptor belongs to the type 1 cytokine receptor family. The β chain of the IL-5 receptor is a signal-transducing chain which is identical to the one used by receptors for IL-3 and GM-CSF. IL-5 has its most important effects on eosinophils. It promotes eosinophil growth and differentiation in the bone marrow, enhances eosinophil chemotaxis in response to other cytokines and it activates parasite-killing mechanisms in mature eosinophils. In addition, IL-5 acts together with IL-2 and IL-4 to promote B-cell growth and differentiation, and it enhances IgM and IgA production by mature B cells.

D. Interleukin-9

IL-9 is a pleiotropic cytokine that may have important roles in hematopoiesis and mature T-cell growth (52,53). Human IL-9 is variably glycosylated, with a molecular weight ranging from 20 to 30 kDa. To date, the only significant source of IL-9 identified is the activated CD4$^+$ T cell, usually with the type 2 cytokine pattern. A high-affinity IL-9 receptor complex has been characterized and includes a subunit with an extracellular hematopoietin receptor family WSXWS motif as well as the common γ subunit present in the IL-2, IL-4, IL-7 and IL-15 receptors (54). The major functions of IL-9, as defined by in vitro assays, include the support of early erythroid differentiation from bone marrow precursors, growth of activated T lymphocytes, and the growth and activation of mast cells.

E. Interleukin-10

IL-10 was originally called "cytokine synthesis inhibiting factor" (CSIF), and it is an important regulatory cytokine that functions to downregulate immune responses (55–58). It is an 18-kDa member of the four α-helix family of cytokines. IL-10 is secreted mainly by type 2 CD4$^+$ T cells, but macrophages, fetal thymocytes, keratinocytes, and both CD5$^+$ and CD5$^-$ murine peritoneal B cells can also produce this cytokine (56). Both CD4$^+$ and CD8$^+$ T cells secrete IL-10, although the level of production is higher in CD4$^+$ cells. In contrast to murine IL-10, which is produced exclusively by type 2 CD4$^+$ T cells, human IL-10 can be produced by type 0, type 1, and type 2 T-cell clones (59). Activated monocytes secrete large amounts of IL-10, but maximal synthesis occurs with slower kinetics than for IL-1 and TNF-α. IL-10 mediates its effects via interaction with a specific receptor (IL-10R) which is now well characterized and this receptor is expressed on the surface of T and B cells, thymocytes, mast cells, macrophages, and hematopoietic cells (60). The human IL-10R exhibits 70% sequence homology with the murine IL-10R cDNA.

The major effects of IL-10 are to inhibit macrophage inflammatory responses. IL-10 blocks macrophage production of several cytokines, including TNF-α, IL-1, chemokines, and IL-12 (61–63). Moreover, IL-10 inhibits the induction of nitric oxide synthase and the production of nitric oxide; it thus decreases the cytotoxic effector activities of macrophages (61). These effects on macrophages are also induced by IL-4, and often IL-10 and IL-4 are expressed coordinately by type 2 T cells. In addition, IL-10 inhibits class II MHC, B7-1, and B7-2 expression by macrophages and Langerhans cells, and thereby downregulates antigen-presenting functions of these cells (64). These combined effects indicate that IL-10 controls immune responses in which macrophage activation is the major effector mechanism. For example, in models of lipopolysaccharide-induced sepsis, the administration of

IL-10 is very effective in preventing lethality and downregulates the circulating levels of tumor necrosis factor-α (65,66). IL-10–deficient mice have abundant macrophage infiltrates in many tissues and they develop an inflammatory bowel disease similar to that observed in IL-2–deficient mice (67).

F. Interleukin-12

IL-12 plays important roles in regulating T-cell and NK cell–mediated responses (68–73). IL-12 is a heterodimeric molecule composed of a 35-kDa polypeptide chain (p35) and a 40-kDa chain (p40). The p35 chain has a four-α-helix structure shared by IL-2, IL-4, IL-5 and IL-10. The p40 chain is highly homologous to the extracellular portion of the ligand-binding chain of the IL-6 receptor. Although several cell types, including T lymphocytes, produce the p35 chain, synthesis of a fully functional IL-12 molecule composed of both p35 and p40 chains is restricted to monocytes and B lymphocytes. The receptor for IL-12 is expressed on T cells and NK cells but not on monocytes (74), and it is not well characterized at present. Recent work indicates that it is linked to a signal transduction pathway involving members of the Jak and STAT family of molecules, in particular Jak2, Stat3, and Stat4 (75). Jak-STAT pathways are also involved in signal transduction by several other cytokine receptors including IL-4, IL-6 and IFN-γ receptors. IL-12 is a potent NK-cell activator and it enhances the growth, cytolytic activity, and IFN-γ production by these cells. All these effects are increased synergistically by IL-2. IL-12 is also a potent inducer of the differentiation of naive T cells toward an IFN-γ–producing type 1 phenotype, and therefore, IL-12 is important for the development of macrophage-dependent T-cell–mediated immune responses to intracellular microbes (36,76–78). Due to the powerful effects of IL-12 in the induction of cell-mediated immunity, it is likely that a natural IL-12 antagonist may exist. One such antagonist could be p40 itself, which binds to the IL-12 receptor but does not trigger biological activity (79). p40 may act as an endogenous regulator of IL-12 activity because it is produced in large excess over IL-12 both in vitro and in vivo after lipopolysaccharide stimulation of mononuclear phagocytes (80).

G. Interferon-γ

IFN-γ plays a central role in cell mediated immune responses (13,81–85). It is a 20- to 25-kDa glycoprotein produced by activated type 1 $CD4^+$ and $CD8^+$ T cells and NK cells. The regulation of IFN-γ expression is incompletely understood, but T cell receptor signals as well as those provided by IL-2 and IL-12 enhance transcription of the IFN-γ gene. IFN-γ binds to a unique widely distributed cell surface receptor, which includes an IFN-γ binding subunit and at least one additional signaling subunit. Cytokine binding to the receptor initiates the formation of a multicomponent receptor-kinase complex, which includes Jak-1 and Jak-2 kinases and leads to the tyrosine phosphorylation and nuclear translocation of the Stat1 transcription factor (86). After dimerization, Stat1 (now called STF-IFN-γ) binds to IFN-γ activation sites in the promoters of various genes and mediates induction of the gene encoding interferon response factor-1 (IRF-1) (87). IFN-γ is critical for the effector phase of cell-mediated immune responses because of various effects on cells of both the specific and natural immune systems. Prominent among these effects is the activation of macrophages and other phagocytes for the killing of intracellular microbes and, along with signals provided by other cytokines, activation of macrophage killing of tumor cells. IFN-γ also activates neutrophils, enhances NK-cell cytolytic capabilities, and promotes the differentiation of cytotoxic T cells (CTL). IFN-γ stimulates both class I and class II MHC molecule expression on many cell types and thereby enhances the cognitive and amplification phases of T-cell-mediated immune responses. T-cell extravasation into tissues is also enhanced by IFN-γ effects on endothelial morphology and adhesion molecule expression. IFN-γ directly affects B cells, promoting differentiation and inhibiting IL-4 stimulation of IgE switching. IFN-γ promotes B-cell switching to IgG subtypes, which are most efficient at fixing complement, and IFN-γ is also implicated in promoting the differentiation of naive T cells toward IFN-γ secretion, as is IL-12. IFN-γ–deficient mice show a decreased resistance to intracellular microbial infections such as *Leishmania major* and *Mycobacterium tuberculosis* (88).

H. Transforming Growth Factor-β

Transforming growth factor-β (TGF-β) is a member of a family of cytokine/growth factor polypeptides which have pleiotropic growth stimulatory and inhibitory effects on various cell types (89–91). This family includes five forms of TGF-β (1 through 5), inhibins, and activins (92). The major T-cell-derived member of this family is a 25-kDa glycoprotein homodimer, TGF-β1. The actions of TGF-β are mediated by a complex and incompletely characterized family of receptors which are widely distributed. TGF-β1 exerts largely inhibitory influences on cells of the specific and natural immune systems. This includes the inhibition of T-cell proliferative responses to antigens, the blockade of CTL development, the inhibition of the respiratory burst in macrophages, and the suppression of inflammatory cytokine stimulation of neutrophils. In addition, TGF-β1 has distinct stimulatory activities including stimulation of fibroblast growth and matrix synthesis, and stimulation of IgA secretion by B lymphocytes. TGF-β1–deficient mice suffer from a lethal inflammatory disease characterized by diffuse tissue infiltration by neutrophils (93).

I. Tumor Necrosis Factor-β (Lymphotoxin)

Tumor necrosis factor-β (TNF-β) is a T-cell-derived cytokine that shares many properties with TNF-α described later in this chapter (94,95). TNF-β is a 20- to 25-kDa cytokine whose primary amino acid structure is 30% homologous to TNF-α. Unlike TNF-α, TNF-β is expressed as a secretory protein with a leader sequence and does not require proteolytic processing for release from the cell. Both type 1 $CD4^+$ T cells and $CD8^+$ T cells produce TNF-β, but mononuclear phagocytes (the primary source of TNF-α) do not. TNF-β binds to the same receptors as TNF-α and therefore stimulates the same biological responses. Generally, the amount of TNF-β released by T cells is much less than the levels of TNF-α released by activated mononuclear phagocytes; therefore the biological effects of TNF-β are usually paracrine rather than systemic. Such local effects include cytolysis, neutrophil activation, and endothelial activation, and these responses to TNF-β can be enhanced by the simultaneous presence of IFN-γ. Systemic effects of TNF-β may occur when massive polyclonal T-cell stimulation ensues, such as in the setting of toxic shock syndrome caused by bacterial superantigen stimulation of large numbers of $CD4^+$ T lymphocytes.

J. T-Cell Subsets

Subsets of helper T lymphocytes were first identified among long-term mouse $CD4^+$ T-cell clones (7,96,97). Th1 clones produce IL-2, IFN-γ, and TNF-β and utilize IL-2 as their autocrine growth factor. Th2 clones produce IL-4, IL-5, IL-10, and IL-13 and utilize IL-4 as their autocrine growth factor (Fig. 1). As mentioned earlier in this chapter, $CD8^+$ T cells can also polarize into two subsets with different cytokine production profiles, similar to the Th1 and Th2 subsets of $CD4^+$ T cells (9,10,46); we therefore refer to these two subsets as "type 1" and "type 2." A third phenotype, "type 0" cells, are usually defined as producers of IL-2, IL-4, and IFN-γ and possibly other cytokines. Type 0 $CD4^+$ T cells have been proposed to be precursors of type 1 and type 2 $CD4^+$ clones (98); however, it is not clear at present whether T cells pass through a type 0 stage of unrestricted cytokine expression before polarization into type 1 or type 2 subsets (99). Subsequent to the description of mouse type 1 or type 2 $CD4^+$ clones, human counterparts were described, although the frequency of rigidly defined type 1 or type 2 clones isolated from bulk human lymphocyte populations is considerably lower than for mouse lymphocytes (100,101).

A type 1 response is critically important for the eradication of intracellular infectious organisms, presumably because of the macrophage-activating properties of IFN-γ. In contrast, a type 2 response appears to be important for humoral and cellular defenses against certain types of extracellular infections, such as helminths. This is largely because of the dependence of IgE production on IL-4 and eosinophil growth and differentiation on IL-5. Perhaps a more generally significant role of type 2 responses is the inhibition of macrophage function by IL-4 and IL-10, with the consequent downregulation of the inflammatory effector phase of type 1 responses and suppression of type 1 responses by type 2 cells may be a potential basic mechanism for the maintenance of peripheral tolerance to antigens and/or self antigens. An imbalance in Th subset responses to particular antigens may lead to

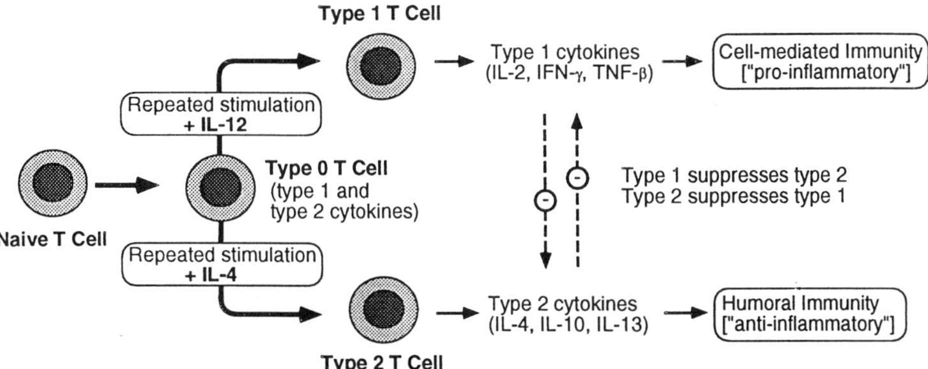

Figure 1 Differentiation and function of T-cell subsets. Naive T cells can differentiate in the presence of IL-4 or IL-12 into two polarized subsets, distinguished by their cytokine profiles. Type 1 $CD4^+$ or $CD8^+$ T cells preferentially produce IL-2 and IFN-γ, whereas type 2 cells produce IL-4, as described in the text. It should be noted that it has to be still established whether passage through a type 0 stage is a prerequisite step for T cells before acquisition of a more restricted cytokine profile.

pathological situations. For example, there is evidence that certain infections are poorly controlled when type 2 T cells predominate (102), and organ-specific immunity may be generally associated with type 1–dominated responses (80). Thus, it is clear that selective cytokine production by type 1 and 2 cells is a fundamental determinant of the quality and quantity of immune responses to different antigens. Imbalances in the ratio of type 1 to type 2 cells have been evoked in the immunopathogenesis of various autoimmune, infectious, and immunodeficiency diseases.

$CD4^+$ T helper cells, the major cytokine-producing effector cells, differentiate from naive precursors. Naive T cells, identified by phenotypic markers (e.g., in the mouse $CD44^{lo}$, L-selectin^{hi}, $CD45RB^{hi}$) or by absence of previous antigen exposure (e.g., T cells from an unimmunized, TCR -transgenic mouse) produce small amounts of IL-2 and no detectable IFN-γ or IL-4 when they are stimulated for the first time in vitro. Naive T-cell populations can be driven to differentiate into type 1–or type 2–like populations in vitro by providing TCR stimulation (either antigen or anti-TCR/CD3 antibodies) plus exogenously added cytokines. TCR transgenic mice have provided a reliable way to study this differentiation process because they are sources of uniform populations of naive $CD4^+$ T cells that can be stimulated in vitro by physiological antigen presentation. The results of several reported experiments of this kind indicate that IL-4 is required to drive differentiation of naive cells into type 2–like $CD4^+$ T cells, which produce IL-4, but not IL-2 or IFN-γ (76,78). It is also clear that IL-2, which is produced by the naive T cell, is required for initiating the IL-4–dependent type 2 differentiation response. The effect of IL-4 in subset differentiation appears to be directly on T cells, since it can be observed in experiments using anti-CD3 in the absence of antigen-presenting cells. Although it has remained difficult for investigators to rule out the possibility that IL-4 promotes the outgrowth of cells precommitted to the type 2 cytokine phenotype in these experiments, the rapid change in the population phenotype and the lack of detectable IL-4 expression in the starting population argue for a phenotypic change of uncommitted precursor cells. The molecular mechanism by which IL-4 promotes IL-4 expression and inhibits IL-2 and IFN-γ expression remains to be elucidated.

Differentiation toward the type 1 cytokine phenotype requires the absence of IL-4 and the presence of IL-12 and perhaps IFN-γ (76,78). There is evidence that IL-12 may act directly on T cells in the absence of IFN-γ (103); new studies also suggest that IL-12 enhancement of IFN-γ production by accessory cells contributes to the development of IFN-γ–producing type 1 T cells (76). Thus, it appears that the combination of TCR and IL-12–induced signals in naive T cells leads to a block in the ability of the progeny T cells to transcribe the IL-4 gene and to enhanced ability to transcribe IL-2 and IFN-γ genes. It is clear that IL-4 has a dominant effect over IL-12, causing differentiation to type 2 T cells even when both cytokines are present. Again, the mechanism by which transcriptional regulation of IL-4, IFN-γ, and IL-2 are altered during type 1 differentiation are unknown. In addition to exogenous cytokines, other factors may play a role in subset differentiation, including the type of antigen-presenting cell, different costimulatory molecules, and exogenous hormones. Some recent evidence suggests that costimulation provided by B7-2 molecules preferentially enhances in vitro and in vivo differentiation of type 2 $CD4^+$ T cells (104).

Type 1 and type 2 T cells can only be distinguished according their cytokine profile, a cumbersome process involving the generation of T-cell lines or clones. At present, molecular distinctions between these two differentiated T-cell subsets remain poorly defined. However, recent reports established differences in signal transduction pathways between murine type 1 and type 2 $CD4^+$ cells. Type 1 but not type 2 clones lack the accessory factor-1 (AF-1; also referred to as IFN-γRβ-chain) and thus can not induce the transcription factor STF-IFN-γ after binding of IFN-γ to its receptor (105). Moreover, type 2 cells have a signaling defect after ligand binding to the IL-12 receptor and can not phosphorylate Jak2, Jak3 and Jak4 (106).

Recently, the argument has been raised that individual T cells display a remarkable diversity in their cytokine secretion patterns, collectively forming a continuous spectrum in which type 1 and type 2 T cells merely represent two of the possible extreme phenotypes (99). The significance of type 1 and type 2 clones may derive from their reflection of physiological immune responses, in which the predominant effector cytokines being produced by T cells are either IL-2 and IFN-γ or IL-4 and IL-10, respectively.

III. MONONUCLEAR CELL-DERIVED CYTOKINES

The cytokines described above are either derived from T cells or act on T cells and are mainly produced during specific (acquired) immunity. By contrast, the proinflammatory cytokines IL-1 and TNF-α are in large part secreted during processes of natural (innate) immunity to infectious microbes or other foreign macromolecules. In addition, IL-1 and TNF-α are also produced by activated mononuclear cells during processes of acquired immunity, thereby enhancing natural immunity. Although IL-1 and TNF-α are often called monokines, the cellular source of these cytokines is not always a distinguishing characteristic because many cell types other than mononuclear cells can also produce them. A hallmark of these cytokines is their synergistic, pleiotropic and sometimes redundant effects on target cells. In addition to their role as mediators of an effector phase, monokines can also act as co-stimulators of lymphocyte activation. This part of the chapter reviews the current knowledge about production and function of these cytokines in vitro and in vivo (Table 1).

A. Interleukin-1

IL-1 is a polypeptide cytokine with two 17-kDa isoforms, IL-1α and IL-1β. IL-1 was originally described in the 1940s as "endogenous pyrogen" and later as a lymphocyte activating factor. It is an important cytokine in inflammatory and defense responses and has pleiotropic effects on a variety of tissues. The IL-1 genes are transcriptionally silent in unstimulated peripheral blood mononuclear cells (PBMC), fibroblasts, vascular smooth muscle cells and vascular endothelial cells. However, these genes can be rapidly induced by a variety of agents as described below. In contrast, IL-1 is constitutively expressed in several cell types, including epithelial cells, large granular lymphocytes, Kupffer cells, and some transformed cell lines. Neutrophil granulocytes, fibroblasts, synovial lining cells, dermal dendritic cells, T and B cells, keratinocytes, microglia and astrocytes, also have been shown to possess the ability to synthesize IL-1 protein or at least transcribe IL-1 mRNA (reviewed in Refs. 107–109).

1. Production of IL-1

The genomic organization of IL-1, its protein structure, and the control of transcription, translation, secretion, and processing have been elucidated to a considerable extent. The most powerful inducer of transcription of the IL-1 gene (and other inflammatory cytokines), is endotoxin/lipopolysaccharide (LPS), a product of the cell wall from gram-negative bacteria (110). Two cDNAs coding for IL-1α or IL-1β have been cloned from activated human and murine mononuclear phagocytes (109,111,112). The 17-kDa polypeptides are products from distinct genes with nearly identical genomic organization, and the two forms of IL-1 appear to be under separate transcriptional control (113), but both mature proteins are initially synthesized as a pro-IL-1 precursor protein with a MW of approximately 33 kDa (114). The inactive IL-1β precursor is processed by the IL-1β converting enzyme (ICE) to its proinflammatory 17-kDa form, while pre-IL-1α is not a substrate for ICE (115,116). Structural analysis revealed that IL-1β consists of 12 β strands held together by hydrogen bonds and its overall folding is similar to that of the soybean trypsin inhibitor (117). In the absence of LPS but in the presence of other cytokines (e.g., IFN-γ), IL-1 mRNA expression can occur without synthesis of IL-1 protein; cells containing untranslated IL-1 mRNA are considered to be "primed" (118). The transcription of IL-1 is rapid and occurs within 15 min in macrophage cell lines and human PBMC, with peak accumulation at 8 hr, followed by a rapid decrease (119). In primed cells, small amounts of LPS or other stimuli (TNF-α, IFN-γ, or IL-1 itself) can trigger rapid translation of preformed mRNA, resulting in higher IL-1 and TNF-α protein synthesis than in unprimed cells (81,120).

Numerous observations suggest that the majority of cell types can produce both isoforms of IL-1, although various cell types contain markedly different steady-state levels of their mRNAs; the synthesis of IL-1β mRNA is usually more than an order of magnitude greater than that of IL-1α mRNA in human PBMC, and it is the more common IL-1 isoform found in the circulation (121). On the other hand, production of IL-1 by some T-cell clones or Epstein-Barr virus (EBV)-transformed B cells is restricted to either IL-1α or IL-1β. (122,123). Differential production of the two isoforms has also been found in mononuclear cells from rheumatoid arthritis joints and in human keratinocytes, where IL-1α is the predominant mRNA species (124).

2. IL-1 Receptors

Both IL-1α and IL-1β polypeptides bind in a competitive manner to the same IL-1 receptors (IL-1R) and therefore share various biological activities when present at picomolar levels. The IL-1 receptor exists in two isoforms, p80 (type 1) and p68 (type 2), which are encoded by two separate genes (125). The IL-1Rs have extracellular Ig-like domains and therefore they are members of the Ig-gene superfamily. The type 1 IL-1R appears to be present on all cell types that respond to IL-1. The expression of this receptor does not appear to be regulated tightly and surprisingly, is the sole known signal transducing receptor for IL-1 (126–128). While both the 31-kDa and processed 17-kDa forms of IL-1α bind to the type 1 IL-1R, only the 17-kDa form of IL-1β can bind and transduce a signal. A variety of intracellular signaling pathways have been implicated in the IL-1 response, including arachidonic acid, protein kinase C, cyclic AMP, ceramide, and a cascade of novel protein kinases that results in the phosphorylation of heat shock protein 27. Presently, the evidence is inconclusive as to the relative importance and interrelationships of many of these pathways (129–132).

The type 2 IL-1R (p68) is widely distributed throughout tissues and its expression is tightly regulated. This receptor can be shed efficiently from the cellular surface and p68 may thus act as a "decoy" target for IL-1 and play a significant role in the downregulation of IL-1 responses. In addition, the binding of IL-1 to its receptor downregulates its expression in a negative feedback mechanism (133).

3. Stimuli for IL-1 Production

As mentioned above, the most important known stimulus for IL-1 production is endotoxin/LPS (110), with about five molecules per monocyte being sufficient to stimulate mRNA transcription. In addition, other potent stimulators include polypeptide exotoxins from gram-positive bacteria (staphylococci, streptococci), live viruses, synthetic adjuvants from bacterial cell walls, complement, thrombin, bile salts, androgen metabolites, phorbol esters, calcium ionophores, UV light, and, importantly, cytokines (134). In addition, a recent study suggests that cells undergoing apoptosis, or "programmed cell death," acquire the capacity to produce IL-1 more efficiently (135). Under normal physiological conditions, IL-1 mRNA expression is not significant except in some cell types in the epidermis or in neuroendocrine tissues (136,137). It is unclear whether increased mRNA expression in normal tissues is accompanied by the translation into protein; thus the role of IL-1 in homeostasis remains to be clarified (138).

4. Biological Functions of IL-1

The effects of IL-1 on different tissues are pleiotropic, with further potential differences between local and systemic effects. At low levels, the predominant effects of IL-1 in the local microenvironment are primarily immunoregulatory. First, IL-1 is a costimulator of T-cell proliferation and B-cell activation (growth and Ig production). Assays with suboptimal concentrations of antigen suggest that IL-1 amplifies T-cell activation and induces IL-2, IL-2R, IL-3, IL-4, and IL-5 gene expression, particularly in conjunction with antigens, mitogens, calcium ionophores, or stimulators of protein kinase C (108,139–141). Whether IL-1 is absolutely essential for the generation of a T-cell–dependent immune response to a foreign antigen is still an open question. Only type 2 $CD4^+$ T cells have receptors for IL-1 ($>$20,000 receptors per cell), whereas type 1 cells express much less IL-1R, comparable to leukocytes (100 to 200 per cell). Thus, IL-1 may function as a more effective costimulator for certain subsets of T cells compared to others. A second group of target cells for the costimulation of IL-1 is hematopoietic stem cells. Here, IL-1 acts in synergy with others CSFs (IL-3, IL-6, GM-CSF, CSF-1) (142). IL-1α seems to stimulate the growth and differentiation of purified progenitors cells both directly and indirectly (143), and it can further promote hematopoiesis by inducing production of GM-CSF, G-CSF, and macrophage CSF (M-GSF) (134,144,145). Injection of IL-1β protects mice from cytopenia caused by cytotoxic agents and total-body irradiation, possibly via protection of early hematopoietic progenitor cells (146–148). Incubation of bone marrow ex vivo with IL-1 can dramatically expand the number of hematopoietic progenitor cells, although IL-1 can inhibit formation of B-cell colonies in mice (149,150). Importantly, a requirement for IL-1α (and TNF-α) in fetal thymocyte commitment and differentiation has recently been demonstrated, where it appears to be necessary for the induction of IL-2 receptor (CD25) expression (151).

A second important biologic function of IL-1 appears to be the regulation of apoptosis. Overexpression of IL-1–converting enzyme (ICE), a member of a subfamily of cysteine proteases originally described as the cell death gene ced-3 in *Caenorhabditis elegans* (152), induced apoptosis in transfected cell lines. Knockout mice carrying a disrupted enzyme (ICE$^{-/-}$) are resistant to apoptosis induced by an antibody to Fas (153,154). The Fas antigen (CD95) is a cell surface protein that has high homology to the TNF-α receptor, and its ligation mediates apoptosis in activated T cells (155,156). Recent studies indicate that both TNF-α and IL-1 stimulate cells via the intracellular messenger ceramide (157), and ceramide has been implicated as a endogenous regulator of apoptosis (158). The specifics of the involvement of the IL-1 pathway in Fas-mediated apoptosis awaits further investigation.

The third important activity of IL-1 may be its principal function: the mediation of host defenses against invading organisms. The elimination of foreign proteins is achieved in part through the activation of mononuclear cells and the ensuing combined action of proinflammatory cytokines. A vigorous host defense is therefore invariably associated with inflammatory processes that lead to nonspecific destruction of self tissues and to disturbances of normal host functions. Most studies of the role of IL-1 in inflammation use bacterial products or cytokines to stimulate mononuclear phagocytes. The major cellular targets of IL-1 during these responses are mononuclear phagocytes, endothelial cells, and NK-cells. Important proinflammatory activities of low concentrations of IL-1 are the induction and upregulation of adhesion molecules, including selectins, intercellular adhesion molecule-1 (ICAM-1) and VCAM-1, the priming and activation of neutrophil leukocytes and endothelial cells, the promotion of vascular permeability, the induction of complement proteins, and the induction of additional inflammatory cytokines such as TNF-α, IL-6, IL-8 and IL-1 itself (159–161). Increased numbers of neutrophils are often a hallmark of infectious and inflammatory diseases; IL-1 administration causes elevations of circulating neutrophils in humans and animals and their peak elevation occurs 3 to 4 hr after injection (162,163), but high doses of IL-1 result in granulocytopenia due to increased endothelial cell adherence by marginated neutrophils. IL-1 also upregulates the production of IL-8, called neutrophil-activating protein-1 (164). IL-8 belongs to a family of neutrophil and monocyte chemotactic cytokines that are important contributors to local inflammation (see below).

Acute inflammation is often accompanied by a systemic response. When IL-1 is produced in large amounts, it is instrumental in mediating an acute-phase response that includes fever, hypotension, and the production of large amounts of hepatic proteins as well as metabolic alterations in muscle and fat (cachexia). The systemic effects of IL-1 are similar to those of TNF-α; however, IL-1 alone does not produce direct tissue injury and only the combination of high levels of circulating IL-1 and TNF-α is lethal in experimental animals (134). IL-1 is an endogenous pyrogen in the central nervous system (CNS) (165). However, this cytokine does not cross the blood-brain barrier (unlike other molecules the same size), and it is therefore likely that IL-1 acts on special endothelial cells of the periventricular organs in areas where the barrier is interrupted (166). A major systemic vascular effect of high IL-1 levels is hypotension, probably related to the induction of cyclooxygenase products, platelet activating factor, and/or nitric oxide (167). TNF-α potentiates this hypotensive effect of IL-1, whereas cyclooxygenase inhibitors can prevent it (168). IL-1 also depresses myocardial function and induced generalized vascular leaks. In multiple inflammatory conditions such as bacterial infections, rheumatoid arthritis, or inflammatory bowel disease, IL-1 increases production of normal hepatic proteins about 100- to 1000-fold (108). One such protein, serum amyloid A, contributes to the development of secondary amyloidosis. In addition, IL-1 induces hepatocytes to produce fatty acids, complement, fibrinogen, and various clotting factors. Some of these actions occur probably via IL-6 (108). Finally, the catabolic effects of high concentrations of IL-1 include the induction of tachyphylaxis, anorexia, and hypoglycemia (169–171). In general, the systemic effects induced by IL-1 resemble those induced by TNF-α, and both cytokines contribute to the observed syndromes in inflammation and infection.

Thus far, the critical role for IL-1 in disease has been revealed via the specific blockade of this cytokine; despite extensive studies, however, the physiological importance of IL-1 in vivo has not been fully elucidated. However, IL-1β-deficient mice have recently been generated (172), which should make it possible to study the role of IL-1 more in detail. IL-1β-deficient mice were unable to mount a normal acute-phase inflammatory response to turpentine, which normally causes formation of local abscesses and tissue injury. In contrast, when mice were infected with pathogens, the development of systemic inflammation in IL-1 knockout mice was indistinguishable from that in IL-1 wild-type mice (172).

5. Experimental Models to Study IL-1 Dysregulation

The induction of proinflammatory cytokines appears to be a central element in the development of gram-negative septic shock syndrome, which is a major focus of critical patient care (173). Experimental endotoxemia has proven a useful model for the pleiotropic systemic effects of IL-1. Infusion of LPS from *E. coli* into healthy human subjects induces fever, cytokinemia, and several hematological and endocrinological changes characteristic of the native infection (reviewed in Ref. 174). Elevated levels of IL-1β have also been found in plasma of patients with infections (175), and similar effects have been observed in animal models of septic shock (168). Intravenous infusion of IL-1α or IL-1β causes many of the same physiological effects as bacterial sepsis (septic shock), including fever, increased neutrophils and hepatic acute phase proteins, hypotension, and cachexia. Even at low doses, the injection of exogenous IL-1 as an adjuvant chemotherapy for malignancy has caused fever, hypotension, anorexia, sleepiness, neuropeptide release, myalgias, and gastrointestinal disturbances in bone marrow transplantation patients (162,163). The range of potentially therapeutic levels appears to be quite narrow, with dose-limiting toxicity observed at approximately 300 ng/kg. Further evidence that the pathophysiology of sepsis is mediated through IL-1 is that tissue expression of the IL-1 gene is dramatically increased after LPS infusion. Plasma levels of IL-1β peak after 1 to 2 hr (176,177), and the highest cytokine levels are found in the spleen, lung, and liver; IL-1 mRNA levels in these organs correlate with the degree of hypotension (176,178).

6. IL-1 Antagonism

Glucocorticoids (dexamethasone) belong to the best-known inhibitors of IL-1 production (179–181). In addition, several naturally occurring IL-1 antagonists have been found, including lipoprotein, lipids, and α-2 macroglobulin. These molecules are not specific IL-1 antagonists, however, because they inhibit other inflammatory cytokines as well. Specific inhibitors have been identified and can be detected in serum, plasma, or urine from patients with leukemia or other disease states or in the supernatant from monocyte/macrophage cell lines (182,183). The best studied specific IL-1 inhibitor is the IL-1 receptor antagonist (IL-1ra). IL-1ra was originally named "IL-1 inhibitor"; it was isolated from human mononuclear phagocytes and its cDNA has been sequenced (184–186). IL-1ra is a 17-kDa polypeptide (glycosylated form is 25 kDa) and has a 26% homology to IL-1β and 19% to IL-1α. These homologies, together with a conserved intron-exon organization in all three proteins, strongly suggest that IL-1ra is a third member of the IL-1 gene family. IL-1ra, which contains a leader sequence and a signal peptide, is secreted by cells through a classic pathway and acts as a pure antagonist with no known agonist activity (187).

The IL-1 system is one of the most tightly regulated cytokine systems known. Both purified and recombinant soluble IL-1ra compete with the binding of IL-1 to its surface receptor with approximately the same affinity as either IL-1α or IL-1β. Despite its high affinity for the receptor, IL-1ra does not undergo receptor-mediated endocytosis; consequently IL-1ra blocks signal transduction from the receptor to the nucleus. IL-1ra blocks IL-1 activity in vitro and in vivo, including thymocyte proliferation, endothelial and neutrophil adhesion, and cytokine synthesis (188). To inhibit 50% of these IL-1–induced responses in vitro, a 100-fold excess of IL-1ra is required (189). In addition to the secreted form of IL-1ra, an intracellular form of this antagonist (icIL-1ra) was discovered in keratinocytes and other epithelial cells; this molecule is now recognized as an alternatively spliced product of the IL-1ra gene (190), but its function is not yet completely understood. As mentioned earlier, the expression of IL-1ra is upregulated by type 1 T-cell cytokines and downregulated by type 2 cytokines (41). Furthermore, it has recently been shown that immunoglobulins (Ig) can induce the production of IL-1ra (191) and thus the therapeutic effects of a regimen of intravenous immunoglobulin (IV-Ig) in several immune-mediated disorders may be explained by the direct downregulatory effect of Ig on the action of inflammatory cytokines.

5. Other Biological Properties of IL-1

In addition to the biological effects mentioned above, IL-1 influences a host of mechanisms both in health and disease. IL-1 has a profound effect on fibroblast proliferation, synovial cells, bone, and collagen and therefore plays a role in fibrosis and arthritis (192–194). IL-1 also increases the expression of genes for complement, several enzymes and protooncogenes and it induces synthesis of protaglandins, platelet activating factor, and blood clotting factors in endothelial cells (134). Finally, IL-1 induces several neuropeptides, including corticotropin releasing factor, adenocorticotrope hormone, vasopressin, and somatostatin (108). In contrast, the production of thyreotropine releasing hormone (TRH) is downregulated by IL-1.

In health, serum levels of IL-1β do not usually exceed 60 pg/mL (195). However, excess IL-1 is produced in various disease states and may lead either to a beneficial or detrimental net effect. For example, PBMC from patients with rheumatoid arthritis produce more IL-1 than do cells from normal individuals. Increases in IL-1 or IL-1R production has also been reported during allograft rejection, several types of cancer, human immunodeficiency virus (HIV) infection, hepatitis B, insulin-dependent diabetes mellitus, strenuous exercise, smoking, bacterial infection, psoriasis, hepatitis, burns, high-dose IL-2 therapy, GVHD, and meningitis (108,196,197–202). In contrast, IL-1 production is diminished in systemic lupus erythematosus, scleroderma, atopic dermatitis, lung cancer, and severe trauma (174). It is important to note that some of these studies report correlations between IL-1 levels and clinical symptoms. The causal relationship of IL-1 and related molecules to the pathogenesis of any individual disease remains hypothetical at present and needs further investigation. Systemic IL-1 levels may not always correlate with the severity of disease, due to compartmentalization of IL-1 that produces regional effects despite undetectable serum levels. In addition, the synergy of IL-1 with other inflammatory cytokines, particularly TNF-α, is important in inducing acute and chronic inflammatory changes in the diseases mentioned above.

B. Tumor Necrosis Factor-α

TNF-α and TNF-β are two closely related polypeptide cytokines encoded by separate genes but share similar functions with respect to inflammation and antitumor activity both in vitro and in vivo. Unlike TNF-β, which is produced primarily by T cells, the major source of TNF-α is the activated mononuclear phagocyte; however, a wide range of cell types can also secrete this protein after appropriate activation, including NK cells, mast cells, polymorphonuclear leukocytes, eosinophils, astrocytes, Langerhans cells, and Kupffer cells (203–206). In addition, both type 1 and type 2 T cells can produce TNF-α (99). Like IL-1, TNF-α mediates processes of natural immunity, including infection and host inflammatory reactions that protect against pathogens. The multiple overlapping activities with IL-1 and the pleiotropic and synergistic functions are important features of this cytokine (Table 1). However, TNF-α is characterized by additional functions that are not shared with IL-1: TNF-α is directly cytotoxic in vitro and in vivo and induces necrosis of tumors. In addition, TNF-α in high concentrations is pivotal in triggering the lethal effects of endotoxin shock, cachexia and other systemic manifestations of disease.

1. Production of TNF-α

TNF-α was discovered originally in sera of mice injected with LPS and BCG (bacille Calmette-Guérin) (207). This substance induced hemorrhagic necrosis of transplanted tumors in mice. TNF-α was then also implicated as a mediator of the severe wasting syndrome observed in terminal cancer patients, from which it derived its name, *cachectin* (206,208–210). Protein purification and sequencing led to the cloning of human and murine TNF-α in the 1980s. The gene for human TNF-α encodes a 26-kDa nonglycosylated transmembrane protein. After stimulation of cells with LPS, this molecule is proteolytically cleaved into a 17-kDa polypeptide with 157 amino acids. Subsequently, polypeptide chains associate noncovalently to form a trimer with three identical subunits, which represents the predominant biologically active form. Sequence data indicate that 79% of amino acids are conserved between human and murine cDNA. A leader peptide is normally removed cotranslationally to yield the 17-kDa secreted form, but evidence suggests that TNF-α may also exist as a 26-kDa membrane-associated protein with cytotoxic activity (211). As is the case for IL-1, the major stimulus for TNF-α production from mononuclear phagocytes is LPS (110). However, additional stimuli induce its transcription and secretion. These stimuli include viruses (HIV, influenza virus), mycobacteria, fungi, parasites, products of complement activation, antigen-antibody complexes, and cytokines (206). Once translated, the TNF-α protein is relatively unstable; its serum half-life after bolus injection is only about 6 to 20 min (212). As is the case for IL-1, mononuclear cells primed by IFN-γ produce large amounts of TNF-α rapidly after triggering with LPS (120).

2. TNF-α Receptors

Two distinct receptors for TNF-α have been identified: type I (TNF-R55) and type II (TNF-R75) (213,214). While the type I receptor seems to be more ubiquitous, the type II receptor is predominantly expressed on hematopoietic cells. Both TNF-α and TNF-β interact with the same membrane receptors, but the 75-kDa receptor possesses greater affinity for TNF-α than the 55-kDa receptor. The extracellular domains of the two receptors share 28% homology. The receptor-ligand interaction is unusually weak when compared with other cytokines (approximately 10^{-9} M), but TNF-α is often synthesized in large quantities and thus can easily saturate its receptor. In addition, maximal responses can be triggered when as little as 10% of the cell membrane receptors are occupied. Target cells include neutrophils, endothelial cells, lymphocytes, fibroblasts, and cells in tissues of liver, muscle, fat, intestines, lung, and hematopoietic organs; most of these tissues express both receptor types (206,215). Notable exceptions are erythrocytes and unstimulated T cells.

Soluble forms of the TNF-α receptor (sTNF-αR) can be released from the cell surface by proteolytic cleavage and are detected in serum and urine in pathological situations (216). DNA sequencing revealed that the proteins represent the extracellular portions of p55 and p75 (217). The release of sTNF-αR results in the downregulation of cell surface receptors and therefore enables target cells to decrease their responsiveness to TNF-α. However, assessments of the biological relevance of circulating sTNF-αR are complicated by the wide range of levels reported with different assays.

3. Principal Biological Actions of TNF-α

Several different experimental approaches have been employed to explore the extraordinarily diverse biological effects of TNF-α. It should be noted that, unlike most other cytokines, TNF-α possesses considerable species-specific differences regarding its in vivo activities (218). In particular, the administration of murine but not human TNF-α caused lethality when injected in mice. In contrast, the cytotoxic activities of TNF-α from both species were similar (219). Human TNF-α appears to interact with murine p55 but not with p75 and, based on this observation, it has been suggested that binding to both receptor chains is necessary to induce lethality and antitumor function (220).

The first biological property ascribed to TNF-α was its antineoplastic activity; the precise mechanism of this direct cytotoxic effect of TNF-α on tumor cells is still under investigation. Necrosis by TNF-α is probably mediated by direct tumor cell lysis, a process not well understood but believed to involve the binding of this cytokine to the TNF-αR on the surface of target cells. This receptor-ligand interaction results in the induction of several intracellular enzymes, including protein kinase C and phospholipases and also of free radicals. TNF-α seems to exert its necrotizing effect by causing a local Schwartzman-like reaction around tumor blood vessels. A Schwartzman reaction can be local or systemic and it is an exaggerated form of a host response to microbes. Tissue injury during a localized Schwartzman reaction is due to the effect of TNF-α on neutrophil activation and on blood vessels, causing intravascular coagulation.

It has been demonstrated that TNF-α induces cell death not only by necrosis but also by apoptosis (221). Apoptotic or "programmed" cell death is distinguished from necrosis by a different physical appearance of target-cell membranes and by the induction of DNA fragmentation. The induction of apoptotic mechanisms seems to be a common pathway in the superfamily of TNF-α receptors because, as noted above, the Fas antigen is also a member of this TNF-α receptor superfamily and the interaction of Fas ligand with Fas results in apoptosis (155). TNF-α does not seem to bind directly to Fas (222) and thus Fas and TNF-αR possess different ligands. Both these receptor-ligand interactions may induce similar downstream second-messenger mechanisms, however, which lead to DNA fragmentation. The activation of intracellular proteases is possibly a common step after induction of apoptosis after receptor binding, and the molecular mechanisms of TNF-α–induced cytotoxicity may also be target cell–specific (223).

In addition to its antitumor activity, TNF-α causes an extremely wide variety of biological effects. As is the case for IL-1, the actions of TNF-α vary as a function of the quantity of cytokine produced (Table 1). Low amounts of TNF-α (e.g., approximately 10^{-9} M) act locally to induce surface adhesion molecules on vascular endothelial cells. TNF-α activates inflammatory leukocytes—including neutrophils, eosinophils, and mononuclear phagocytes—to produce further proinflammatory cytokines such as IL-1, IL-6, IL-8 and TNF-α itself. TNF-α also acts as a costimulator for T- and B-cell activation. A comparison between TNF-α and IL-1β shows that both cytokines can augment mitogen-induced T-cell proliferation; however, TNF-α is less effective than IL-1 in promoting IL-2 production and ongoing T-cell growth (224). TNF-α can induce the synthesis of several CSFs from vascular endothelial cells and from fibroblasts, stimulate fibroblast proliferation, and also promote the migration of inflammatory cells into the intercellular matrix. Finally, TNF-α suppresses bone marrow stem-cell division, and it promotes CTL-mediated lysis and expression of MCH molecules.

When TNF-α is produced at high levels, it can act as an endocrine hormone and exert the full spectrum of its biological activities. Systemic effects after acute exposure to TNF-α include the generation of fever, shock, tissue injury, and the production of hepatic acute-phase serum proteins; the same effects observed in septic shock syndrome and endotoxemia (173,212,225,226). The proinflammatory actions of TNF-α have been implicated in the protective mechanisms during the early phases of infection, neoplastic transformation, injury, and wound healing (reviewed in Ref. 206). Data from TNF-R55 knockout mice reveal that TNF-α plays a decisive role in some of these protection mechanisms and it cannot be substituted by other cytokines or by TNF-R75 (227). After chronic exposure, TNF-α induces metabolic alterations in muscle and fat tissues, leading to cachexia characterized by anorexia, weight loss, and dehydration. Furthermore, extremely high concentrations (exceeding 10^{-7} M) of the protein lead to severe metabolic disturbances, which include the reduction of tissue perfusion, relaxation of vascular smooth muscle tone, activation of coagulation, promotion of intravascular thrombosis, and depression of blood glucose concentrations. Finally, chronic administration may lead to lymphopenia and immunodeficiency due to its suppressive effects on stem-cell division. All these responses are mediated either by TNF-α directly or indirectly via upregulation of additional inflammatory cytokines. Despite its short half-life, TNF-α is a pivotal molecule in these mechanisms because it triggers a cascade of cytokines that persist for hours after serum TNF-α has been cleared: following injection of LPS, a temporal relationship in the production of TNF-α, IL-1, and IL-6 is observed, whereby TNF-α is always produced earlier than IL-1. Injection of TNF-α itself leads to two successive waves of cytokines; first IL-1 and then IL-6. In the presence of antibody to TNF-α, LPS-induced plasma levels of IL-1 and IL-6 are inhibited, underscoring the importance of TNF-α in this systemic process (228,229).

4. TNF-α in Disease

TNF-α has been implicated in the pathophysiology of a number of human diseases. First, as mentioned above, it is involved in the sequelae of septic shock syndrome, where it induces hypotension, vascular leakage, necrosis, activating the clotting cascade and also stimulating the release of secondary inflammatory mediators (173,177,230). Second, TNF-α has strong antitumor effects due to its cytotoxic and antiproliferative potential in certain cancers—e.g., astrocytoma, ovarian cancer, lung cancer and melanoma (reviewed in Ref. 231). Thus, phase I and II trials of TNF-α administration in cancer patients have been conducted to determine the antitumor efficiency of this cytokine. At present, data from systemic TNF-α administration have been disappointing, whereas local administration of this cytokine seems more promising. Further complicating efforts to treat cancer with TNF-α is the observation that not all tumors appear to be amenable to treatment, due to their resistance to the actions of TNF-α (232). Third, TNF-α appears to be a key mediator of the effector phase of GVHD and allograft rejection after bone marrow transplantation (BMT) (233–236), and it has been implicated in venoocclusive disease. Fourth, TNF-α promotes rheumatoid arthritis by inducing activation of tissue inflammation, and it has also been associated with joint destruction (237). Fifth, in diabetes, TNF-α mediates the destruction of β-islet cells and resistance to insulin (238). Sixth, besides its induction during cachexia related to acquired human immunodeficiency syndrome (AIDS), TNF-α can stimulate viral proliferation that may injure the CNS; importantly, anti-TNF-α drugs can inhibit HIV-1 replication (239). In addition, TNF-α may play a role in diseases as diverse as meningitis, trauma, adult respiratory distress syndrome, malaria, and multiple sclerosis (94,206,240,241).

The magnitude of any individual responses is usually dependent on the amount of TNF-α present. However, exact correlations between TNF-α levels and the severity of disease are not always possible. For example, local compartmentalization of TNF-α secretion may produce regional effects that do not correlate with serum levels. Interpretation of serum levels may also be hampered by a lack of consensus regarding the normal range of TNF-α levels during homeostasis. Naturally occurring binding proteins are also critical to the biological effects of TNF-α, and they can both neutralize and prolong TNF-α bioactivity. TNF-α production may be discontinuous during a protracted illness, and cytokines induced by TNF-α may produce additional or synergistic effects with low and undetectable levels of TNF-α. Such synergy of TNF-α with other proinflammatory cytokines appears to be important in acute GVHD, which is described in detail in a later chapter.

Finally, an interesting and important phenomenon regarding the reduced potential of mononuclear phagocytes to secrete TNF-α has been termed "adaptation" (or "endotoxin tolerance" or "desensitization") (242). Adaptation has been demonstrated in both animals and in human cancer patients who become tolerant to endotoxin after low-dose injections of LPS (243,244). In vitro studies using murine macrophages have confirmed these data; secretion of TNF-α is completely inhibited in response to a high-dose LPS stimulus if cells had been pretreated with low doses of LPS (245). Recent studies suggest that cytokine production may be differentially affected during endotoxin tolerance: TNF-α and IL-6 production is downregulated, whereas IL-1β is only marginally affected or even upregulated (246,247). Such refractoriness to stimulation with LPS is reversible with administration of IFN-γ or PMA (245). Macrophage activation by LPS is therefore complex, and the intensified study of mechanisms that regulate inflammatory cytokine production will be relevant to improved therapeutic strategies for toxic shock syndrome and inflammatory responses.

C. Interleukin-6 and Interleukin-8

IL-6 was originally named BSF-2 (B-cell stimulatory factor 2) and purified from supernatants of murine T-cell lines, fibroblasts, and human peripheral PBMC (248–251). Both human and murine IL-6 have been cloned (252,253). They differ considerable in their NH2-terminus and the molecular weights of the proteins range between 21 to 28 kDa (human) and 22 to 29 kDa (mouse), depending on cell source and preparation. IL-6 is produced by a wide variety of cells, including activated T cells, endothelial cells, mononuclear phagocytes, fibroblasts, mast cells, and tumor-cell lines. Accessory cells may be the major source of IL-6, but T cells can be a significant source of IL-6 in vivo and murine helper T-cell lines also often produce enormous amounts of IL-6 (254,255). IL-6 is not produced constitutively by normal cells, but it is readily induced after stimulation with LPS, IL-1, or TNF-α or after viral infections (256). Blockade of the action of TNF-α or IL-1 with specific antibodies results in the failure to produce IL-6 during host inflammatory responses (228,257). The principal biological functions are similar to those of IL-1 and TNF-α (Table 1). IL-6 is an endogenous pyrogen and an inducer of hepatic acute-phase proteins. Since IL-1 and TNF-α both induce IL-6 production, levels of IL-6 often correlate with the amount of fever and severity of disease in patients with infections. In fact, correlations of the severity of the disease with IL-6 is sometimes better than with IL-1 or TNF-α. However, IL-6 alone does not cause shock in experimental animals. It is important to note that several aspects formerly ascribed to IL-1 are indeed the result of a combined action of IL-1 and IL-6 (see below). Another important biological property of IL-6 is its function as a late differentiation factor of B cells (reviewed in Ref. 258); it can also act in a synergistic manner with IL-1 to promote antibody production from plasma cells and stimulates growth of malignant plasma cells (259,260). In addition to these actions, IL-6 acts on T cells to enhance their responsiveness to IL-2 and is therefore required mainly in the initial stages of T-cell activation. Finally, IL-6 can also act as a growth factor together with other cytokines (GM-CSF, G-CSF) for early bone marrow hemopoietic progenitor cells.

IL-8 is a member of a large family of structurally related 8- to 10-kDa proinflammatory polypeptides called chemokines (reviewed in Refs. 261 and 262). This family is divided into two subfamilies (CXC and CC), based on the position of cystein residues in the amino acid sequences. IL-8, together with melanoma growth-stimulating activity and platelet factor 4, belongs to the CXC family, while molecules like RANTES, monocyte chemotactic protein-1, or macrophage inflammatory protein-1 are members of the CC family. Cellular sources of chemokines are TNF-α-, IL-1, or LPS-activated mononuclear phagocytes, antigen-activated T cells, endothelial cells, fibroblasts, epithelial cells, and platelets. Target cells can express two forms of the IL-8 receptor (IL-8RA or IL-8RB) (263): the IL-8RA gene is expressed on CD4$^+$ T cells, monocytes, melanoma cells, fibroblasts, neutrophils, and myeloid precursor cells, whereas IL-8RB expression is more restricted and confined primarily to myeloid cells. It is now believed that IL-8 is a principal secondary mediator of inflammation induced by IL-1 or TNF-α via its activation and attraction of neutrophils and to a lesser extent eosinophils, basophils, and lymphocytes. IL-8 triggers transendothelial migration, degranulation, shape change, and the respiratory burst in neutrophils, which are its major targets. This induced production of peroxide, superoxide radicals, and the release of enzymes leads to efficient killing of pathogens.

TNF-α, IL-1, and IL-6 appear to share biological activities to a remarkable extent. Thus, synergy, pleiotropy, and redundancy are common properties of these cytokines. In inflammatory responses, these three cytokines activate the same targets which include neutrophils, fibroblasts, and of endothelial cells to increase vascular permeability and cellular adhesion (IL-6 does not mediate the latter). TNF-α shares several lymphocyte activating functions with IL-1 and IL-6. In higher concentrations, the combined action of these cytokines results in fever and the formation of hepatic acute-phase proteins. The observed redundancy seems to be due to the induction of a common DNA-binding protein, NF-IL-6, after specific receptor-ligand interactions of each of the three cytokines. During the generation of fever, for example, this common pathway could lead to prostaglandin E_2 synthesis in the hypothalamus (226).

IV. CYTOKINE NETWORKS

The immune response to foreign proteins involves the activation of T lymphocytes after cognate interaction with accessory mononuclear cells. Macrophages therefore have important immunoregulatory roles: first, they can present many extracellular molecules to T and B cells in conjunction with class I or class II MHC antigens. Second, macrophages express surface receptors for cytokines and, following cytokine binding and internalization, macrophages acquire novel properties and become activated. Third, activated macrophages produce and release an array of soluble mediators, including proteases, complement proteins, and cytokines, thus further promoting T-cell activation and the immune response to foreign antigens (reviewed in Ref. 264).

Important intercellular communications, including those between antigen presenting cells and T cells, occur via cytokines. These cytokines form an intricate network of regulatory molecules with complex reciprocal and occasional asymmetrical interactions among various cell types during an immune response. These interactions include the regulation of macrophage activation by T cells and the effects of monokines on lymphocyte function, effectively forming either positive or negative feedback loops. Furthermore, T-cell cytokines and monokines can act together in a synergistic manner on a variety of target cells. A schematic and simplified representation of these interactions is shown in Fig. 2. It should be noted that the attributes

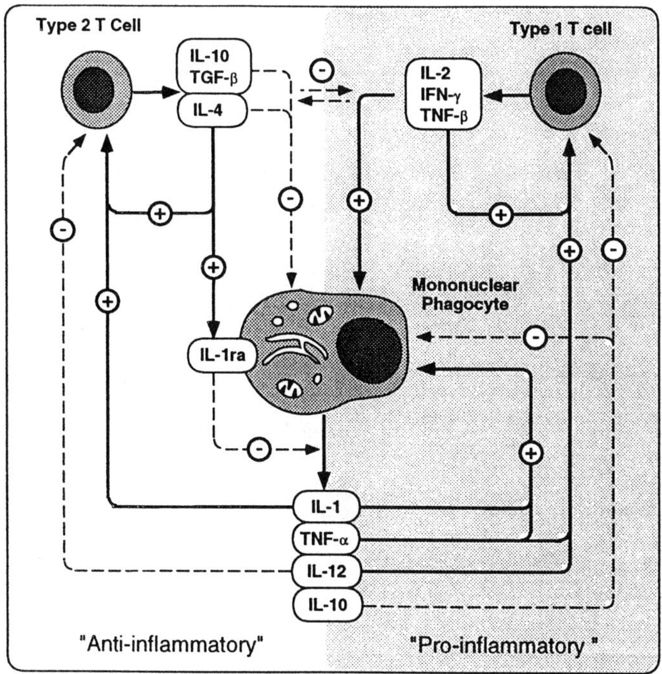

Figure 2 Schematic representation of the most important interactions of T-cell cytokines and mononuclear phagocyte-derived cytokines. Activation of type 1 T cells preferentially induces proinflammatory effects, whereas activation of type 2 T cells generally leads to anti-inflammatory effects. Positive feedback mechanisms are symbolized by →, whereas inhibitory influences are shown as --→. As described in the text, the attributes "proinflammatory" and "antiinflammatory" are generalizations that are not universally applicable.

"proinflammatory" and "anti-inflammatory" in this figure are generalizations that are not universally applicable. For example, diseases such as lupus erythematosus are associated with type 2 cytokine responses and high Ig production, but they can be understood as a form of chronic inflammation. However, with regard to acute inflammation, the terms used in Fig. 2 are reasonably accurate.

A. Modulation of Mononuclear Cells by T-Cell Cytokines

There is an abundant literature concerning interaction of T cells and mononuclear cells via cytokines during induction and progression of humoral or cell-mediated immune responses. As stated earlier, type 1 (IL-2, IFN-γ) and type 2 (IL-4, IL-10) cytokines have reciprocal effects on the activation and function of macrophages. Activation of effector function of mononuclear cells is stimulated by type 1 T cells, and IFN-γ is a central mediator. In particular, this cytokine upregulates the expression of class II MHC molecules on macrophages (265) and increases their cytocidal function upon stimulation with LPS (266). Many of the biological effects of TNF-α are induced and augmented by IFN-γ (81) because IFN-γ acts to prime mononuclear cells to secrete TNF-α and to upregulate TNF-α receptors in response to LPS (120,267). In nonseptic conditions, however, the mechanisms for macrophage activation seem to be either via cognate interactions of T cells with macrophages or via production of TNF-α by type 1 CD4$^+$ T cells (268). Thus, IFN-γ may act as a regulator that locally enhances the action of TNF-α without producing the high concentrations of TNF-α associated with systemic toxicity. Similarly, IL-2 directly stimulates TNF-α production in vitro by purified murine macrophages, but macrophages respond to IL-2 generally less well than monocytes both in vitro and in vivo (269). In addition, IL-2 induces not only the production of IL-1α and β, but also the production of IL-1ra by human PBMCs in vitro (270,271). Such opposite effects suggest the presence of a cytokine network that may attenuate the effects of IL-1 after its induction by IL-2.

Type 2 T cells exert a negative influence on macrophage activation and effector function. This effect is due not only to the lack of IFN-γ secretion by these cells but also to direct suppressive effects exerted by the type 2 cytokines IL-4 and IL-10. Both cytokines inhibit the induction of TNF-α production and antagonize LPS-induced responses in vivo (55,65,66,268,269,272). IL-4 also antagonizes the actions of TNF-α and IL-1 by regulating gene expression (273) and by increasing IL-1ra secretion (41,274). Thus, type 2 cytokines generally exert suppressive effects on inflammatory processes by negatively influencing or preventing the actions of TNF-α and IL-1 and also of type 1 cytokines. It has to be stressed, however, that IL-4 does not rigidly exert only anti-inflammatory effects because under certain circumstances, overproduction of this cytokine can promote inflammation. For example, the injection of type 2 CD4$^+$ T cells can mediate IL-4 local delayed-type hypersensitivity reactions as measured in a foot pad swelling assay (275).

B. Modulation of Lymphocyte Function by Monokines

Monokines also exert regulatory effects on T cells to form a feedback loop in the interactions between T cells and mononuclear cells (Fig. 2). Some important interactions between macrophages and T cells involve IL-1. As mentioned earlier in this chapter, IL-1 functions together with polyclonal activators to enhance the proliferation of CD4$^+$ T cells and the growth and differentiation of B cells. IL-1 induces receptors for IL-2, which would then allow T cells to respond to activation signals provided by IL-2. IL-1 and TNF-α, in turn, can also stimulate IL-2 production (276,277); IL-1 is one of the few known soluble costimulators for T-cell proliferation, but as most murine T-cell clones that express the IL-1R are producers of IL-4 but not of IL-2, IL-1 may function as a costimulator for only some T-cell subsets. The concept that IL-4 has proinflammatory effects is also supported by the finding that IL-4 induces cellular adhesion molecules on endothelial cells (278).

The effects of TNF-α on T-cell activation are more ambiguous. For example, TNF-α enhances thymocyte proliferation (151,279); it is comitogenic with anti-CD3 mAb-, phorbol ester- and CD2-induced human T-cell proliferation (280,281), and it acts as an autocrine growth factor for T cells in dendritic cell-mediated T-cell activation (282). Antigen-specific and mitogen-induced T-cell responses are enhanced by TNF-α (283), and this cytokine can also induce lymphocyte-activated killer (LAK) cells in PBMC in synergy with IL-2 (284,285). Furthermore, TNF-α has been reported to influence the human allogeneic mixed lymphocyte reaction (MLR) (286). TNF-α also acts as autocrine growth factor for B cells (287). In studies using human vascular endothelium, the adhesion of endothelial cells for lymphocytes and for polymorphonuclear neutrophils is increased both by TNF-α or IL-1 (159,288). Finally, TNF-α acts alone or in synergy with IFN-γ to upregulate expression of MHC molecules. Ia expression on murine macrophages as well as MHC II expression on human endothelial cells were significantly increased when cell cultures were incubated in the presence of TNF-α (289,290). Thus, a positive feedback mechanism in T-cell activation is mediated by IL-1 and TNF-α via their influence on the homing of and antigen-presentation to lymphocytes.

In contrast to these reported positive effects of TNF-α on T-cell function, this cytokine also exerts negative effects on T-cell activation. Despite the fact that the presence of TNF-α during an MLR upregulates the capacity of dendritic APCs to stimulate alloreactive T cells, the capacity to present soluble antigens is diminished (291), and thus high concentrations of TNF-α may cause generalized immunosuppression by inducing the loss of APC function. Furthermore, TNF-α can completely abrogate the response of an IL-4–dependent murine cell line to exogenous IL-4 (292). Chronic exposure to TNF-α alters the function of activated T cells because prolonged treatment in vitro with TNF-α impairs production of IL-2, IL-10, IFN-γ, TNF-α, and TNF-β following stimulation through the TCR/CD3 complex (293). In one report, TNF-α has been shown to suppress IL-2–stimulated cytotoxic activity of human T-cell clones (294). In addition to this inhibition of cytokine secretion, TNF-α as well as IL-1 can also downregulate immune responses by inhibiting the induction of MHC molecules on antigen-presenting cells. In this case, T-cell activation is prevented by TNF-α and IL-1 via downregulation of the IFN-γ–induced expression of Ia antigens on endothelial cells (295).

REFERENCES

1. Lindemann A, Mertelsmann R. Interleukin-3: Structure and function. Cancer Invest 1993; 11:609.
2. Yang YC, Clark SC. Interleukin-3: Molecular biology and biologic activities. Hematol Oncol Clin North America 1989; 3:441.
3. Sunderland MC, Roodman GD. Interleukin-3: Its biology and potential uses in pediatric hematology/oncology. Am J Pediatr Hematol Oncol 1991; 13:414.
4. Ihle JN. Interleukin-3 and hematopoiesis. Chem Immunol 1992; 51:65.
5. Rapoport AP, Abboud CN, DiPersio JF. Granulocyte-macrophage colony-stimulating factor (GM-CSF) and granulocyte colony-stimulating factor (G-CSF): receptor biology, signal transduction, and neutrophil activation. Blood Rev 1992; 6:43.
6. Kastelein RA, Shanafelt AB. GM-CSF receptor: Interactions and activation. Oncogene 1993; 8:231.
7. Mosmann TR, Cherwinski H, Bond MW, et al. Two types of murine helper T cell clone: I. Definition according to profiles of lymphokine activities and secreted proteins. J Immunol 1986; 136:2348.
8. Mosmann TR, Coffman RL. Heterogeneity of cytokine secretion patterns and functions of helper T cells. Adv Immunol 1989; 46:111.
9. Croft M, Carter L, Swain SL, Dutton RW. Generation of antigen-specific CD8 effector populations: Reciprocal action of interleukin (IL)-4 and IL-12 in promoting type 2 versus type 1 cytokine profiles. J Exp Med 1994; 180:1715.
10. Seder RA, Boulay JL, Finkelman FD, et al. CD8 T cells can be primed in vitro to produce IL-4. Immunology 1992; 148:1652.

11. Ciardelli T, Smith KA. Interleukin 2: Prototype for a new generation of immunoactive pharmaceuticals. TIPS 1989; 10:239.
12. Smith KA. Interleukin-2. Curr Opin Immunol 1992; 4:271.
13. Paul WE, Seder RA. Lymphocyte responses and cytokines. Cell 1994; 76:241–251.
14. Janssen RA, Mulder NH, The TH, De Leij L. The immunobiological effects of interleukin-2 in vivo. Cancer Immunol Immunother 1994; 39:207.
15. Waldmann TA. The IL-2/IL-2 receptor system: A target for rational immune intervention. Immunol Today 1993; 14:264.
16. Crabtree GR. Contingent genetic regulatory events in T lymphocyte activation. Science 1989; 243:355.
17. Schreiber SL, Crabtree GR. The mechanism of action of cyclosporin A and FK506. Immunol Today 1992; 13:136.
18. June CH, Bluestone JA, Nadler LM, Thompson CB. The B7 and CD28 receptor families. Immunol Today 1994; 15:321.
19. Harding FA, McArthur JG, Gross JA, et al. CD28-mediated signalling co-stimulates murine T cells and prevents induction of anergy in T-cell clones. Nature 1992; 356:607.
20. Schwartz RH. A cell culture model for T lymphocyte clonal anergy. Science 1990; 248: 1349.
21. Miyajima A, Kitamura T, Harada N, et al. Cytokine receptors and signal transduction. Annu Rev Immunol 1992; 10:295.
22. Taga T, Kishimoto T. Cytokine receptors and signal transduction. FASEB J 1992; 6: 3387.
23. Smith KA. The interleukin 2 receptor. Adv Immunol 1988; 42:165.
24. Waldmann TA. The IL-2/IL-2 receptor system: a target for rational immune intervention. Immunol Today 1993; 14:264.
25. Lenardo MJ. Interleukin-2 programs mouse alpha beta T lymphocytes. Nature 1991; 353:858.
26. Critchfield JM, Racke MK, Zuniga-Pflucker JC, et al. T cell deletion in high antigen dose therapy of autoimmune encephalomyelitis. Science 1994; 263:1139.
27. Kundig TM, Schorle H, Bachmann MF, et al. Immune responses in interleukin-2-deficient mice. Science 1993; 262:1059.
28. Cao X, Shores EW, Hu-Li J, et al. Defective lymphoid development in mice lacking expression of the common cytokine receptor γ chain. Immunity 1995; 2:223.
29. Leonard WJ, Noguchi M, Russell SM, McBride OW. The molecular basis of X-linked severe combined immunodeficiency: The role of the interleukin-2 receptor gamma chain as a common gamma chain, gamma c. Immunol Rev 1994; 138:61.
30. Carson WE, Giri JG, Lindemann MJ, et al. Interleukin (IL)-15 is a novel cytokine that activates human natural killer cells via components of the IL-2 receptor. J Exp Med 1994; 180:1395.
31. Grabstein KH, Eisenman J, Shanebeck K, et al. Cloning of a T cell growth factor that interacts with the beta chain of the interleukin-2 receptor. Science 1994; 264:965.
32. Boulay JL, Paul WE. The interleukin-4 family of lymphokines. Curr Opin Immunol 1992; 4:294.
33. Banchereau J, Briere F, Galizzi JP, et al. Human interleukin 4. J Lipid Med Cell Signal 1994; 9:43.
34. Keegan AD, Pierce JH. The interleukin-4 receptor: signal transduction by a hematopoietin receptor. J Leuk Biol 1994; 55:272.
35. Hou J, Schinder U, Henzel WJ, et al. An interleukin-4-induced transcription factor: IL-4 Stat. Science 1994; 265:1701.
36. Seder RA, Paul WE. Acquisition of lymphokine-producing phenotype by $CD4^+$ T cells. Annu Rev Immunol 1994; 12:635.
37. Swain SL, Weinberg AD, English M, Huston G. IL-4 directs the development of Th2-like helper effectors. J Immunol 1990; 145:3796.

38. Swain SL. IL4 dictates T-cell differentiation. Res Immunol 1993; 144:616.
39. Yoshimoto T, Paul WE. CD4^{pos}, NK1.1^{pos} T cells promptly produce interleukin 4 in response to in vivo challenge with anti-CD3. J Exp Med 1994; 179:1285.
40. Sands WA, Bulut V, Severn A, et al. Inhibition of nitric oxide synthesis by interleukin-4 may involve inhibiting the activation of protein kinase C epsilon. Eur J Immunol 1994; 24:2345.
41. Sone S, Orino E, Mizuno K, et al. Production of IL-1 and its receptor antagonist is regulated differently by IFN-gamma and IL-4 in human monocytes and alveolar macrophages. Eur Resp J 1994; 7:657.
42. Kopf M, Le Gros G, Bachmann M, et al. Disruption of the murine IL-4 gene blocks Th2 cytokine responses. Nature 1993; 362:245.
43. Minty A, Chalon P, Derocq JM, et al. Interleukin-13 is a new human lymphokine regulating inflammatory and immune respones. Nature 1993; 362:248.
44. Zurawski G, DeVries JE. Interleukin 13, an interleukin 4-like cytokine that acts on monocytes and B cells, but not on T cells. Immunol Today 1994; 15:19.
45. Zurawski SM, Vega F Jr., Huyghe B, Zurawski G. Receptors for interleukin-13 and interleukin-4 are complex and share a novel component that functions in signal transduction. EMBO J. 1993; 12:2663.
46. Carter LL, Dutton RW. Relative perforin- and fas-mediated lysis in T1 and T2 CD8 effector populations. J Immunol 1995; 155:1028.
47. Takatsu K, Tominaga A, Harada N, et al. T cell-replacing factor (TRF)/interleukin 5 (IL-5): Molecular and functional properties. Immunol Rev 1988; 102:107.
48. Lee HJ, Matsuda I, Naito Y, et al. Signals and nuclear factors that regulate the expression of interleukin-4 and interleukin-5 genes in helper T cells. J Allergy Clin Immunol 1994; 94:594.
49. Koike M, Takatsu K. IL-5 and its receptor: Which role do they play in the immune response? Int Arch Allergy Immunol 1994; 104:1.
50. Miyajima A, Mui AL, Ogorochi T, Sakamaki K. Receptors for granulocyte-macrophage colony-stimulating factor, interleukin-3, and interleukin-5. Blood 1993; 82:1960.
51. Mita S, Harada N, Naomi S, et al. Receptors for T cell-replacing factor/interleukin 5. Specificity, quantitation, and its implication. J Exp Med 1988; 168:863.
52. Chang MS, Engel G, Benedict C, et al. Isolation and characterization of the human interleukin-9 receptor gene. Blood 1994; 83:3199.
53. Yang YC. Human interleukin-9: A new cytokine in hematopoiesis. Leuk Lymph 1992; 8:441.
54. Renauld JC, Druez C, Kermouni A, et al. Expression cloning of the murine and human interleukin 9 receptor cDNAs. Proc Natl Acad Sci USA 1992; 89:5690.
55. Moore KW, O'Garra AO, De Waal Malefyt R, et al. Interleukin-10. Annu Rev Immunol 1993; 11:165.
56. Howard M, O'Garra A, Ishida H, et al. Biological properties of interleukin 10. J Clin Immunol 1992; 12:239.
57. Mosmann TR, Moore KW. The role of IL-10 in crossregulation of TH1 and TH2 responses. Immunol Today 1991; 12:A49.
58. Rennick D, Berg D, Holland G. Interleukin 10: An overview. Prog Growth Factor Res 1992; 4:207.
59. Yssel H, DeWaal Malefyt R, Roncarolo MG, et al. Il-10 produced by subsets of human CD4$^+$ T cell clones and peripheral blood T cells. J Immunol 1992; 149:2378.
60. Liu Y, Wei SH, Ho AS, et al. Expression cloning and characterization of a human IL-10 receptor. J Immunol 1994; 152:1821.
61. Bogdan C, Vodovotz Y, Nathan C. Macrophage deactivation by interleukin 10. J Exp Med 1991; 174:1549.
62. De Waal Malefyt R, Abrams J, Bennett B, et al. Interleukin 10 (IL-10) inhibits cyto-

kine synthesis by human monocytes: An autoregulatory role of IL-10 produced by monocytes. J Exp Med 1991; 174:1209.
63. Bogdan C, Nathan C. Modulation of macrophage function by transforming growth factor beta, interleukin-4, and interleukin-10. Ann NY Acad Sci 1993; 23:713.
64. DeWaal-Malefyt R, Haanen J, Spits H, et al. Interleukin-10 (IL-10) and viral IL-10 strongly reduce antigen-specific human T cell proliferation by diminishing the antigen-presenting capacity of monocytes via down-regulation of class II major histocompatibility complex expression. J Exp Med 1991; 174:915.
65. Howard M, Muchamuel T, Andrade S, Menon S. Interleukin-10 protects mice from lethal endotoxemia. J Exp Med 1993; 177:1205.
66. Gerard C, Bruyns C, Marchant A, et al. Interleukin 10 reduces the release of tumor necrosis factor and prevents lethality in experimental endotoxemia. J Exp Med 1993; 177:547.
67. Kuhn R, Lohler J, Rennick D, et al. Interleukin-10-deficient mice develop chronic enterocolitis. Cell 1993; 75:263.
68. Kobayashi M, Fitz L, Ryan M, et al. Identification and purification of natural killer cell stimulatory factor (NKSF), a cytokine with multiple biologic effects on human lymphocytes. J Exp Med 1989; 170:827.
69. Trinchieri G. Interleukin-12: A cytokine produced by antigen-presenting cells with immunoregulatory functions in the generation of T-helper cells type 1 and cytotoxic lymphocytes. Blood 1994; 84:4008.
70. Wolf SF, Sieburth D, Sypek J. Interleukin 12: A key modulator of immune function. Stem Cells 1994; 12:154.
71. Brunda MJ. Interleukin-12: J Leuk Biol 1994; 55:280.
72. Chehimi J, Trinchieri G. Interleukin-12: A bridge between innate resistance and adaptive immunity with a role in infection and acquired immunodeficiency. J Clin Immunol 1994; 14:149.
73. Scott P. IL-12: initiation cytokine for cell-mediated immunity. Science 1993; 260:496.
74. Desai BB, Quinn PM, Wolitzky AG, et al. IL-12 receptor: II. Distribution and regulation of receptor expression. J Immunol 1992; 148:3125.
75. Jacobson NG, Szabo SJ, Weber-Nordt RM, et al. Interleukin 12 signalling in Th1 cells involves tyrosine phosphorylation of Stat3 and Stat4. J Exp Med 1995; 181:1755.
76. Hsieh CS, Macatonia SE, Tripp CS, et al. Development of TH1 $CD4^+$ T cells through IL-12 produced by Listeria-induced macrophages. Science 1993; 260:547.
77. Manetti R, Gerosa F, Guidizi MG, et al. Interleukin 12 induces stable priming for interferon gamma (IFN-gamma) production during differentiation of human T helper (Th) cells and transient IFN-gamma production in established Th2 cell clones. J Exp Med 1994; 179:11273.
78. Seder RA, Gazzinelli R, Sher A, Paul WE. Interleukin 12 acts directly on $CD4^+$ T cells to enhance priming for interferon gamma production and diminishes interleukin 4 inhibition of such priming. Proc Natl Acad Sci USA 1993; 90:10188.
79. Mattner F, Fischer S, Guckes S, et al. The interleukin-12 subunit p40 specifically inhibits effects of the interleukin-12 heterodimer. Eur J Immunol 1993; 23:2202.
80. Trembleau S, Germann T, Gately MK, Adorini L. The role of IL-12 in the induction of organ-specific autoimmune diseases. Immunol Today 1995; 16:383.
81. DeMaeyer E, DeMaeyer-Guignard J. Interferon-γ. Curr Opin Immunol 1992; 4:321.
82. Farrar MA, Schreiber RD. The molecular cell biology of interferon-gamma and its receptor. Annu Rev Immunol 1993; 11:571.
83. Halloran PF. Interferon-gamma, prototype of the proinflammatory cytokines—Importance in activation, suppression, and maintenance of the immune response. Transplant Proc 1993; 25:10.
84. Ijzermans JN, Marquet RL. Interferon-gamma: A review. Immunobiology 1989; 179:456.

85. Vilcek J. Recent progress in the elucidation of interferon alpha/beta and interferon gamma actions. Semin Hematol 1993; 30:9.
86. Darnell JE Jr., Kerr IM, Stark GR. Jak-STAT pathways and transcriptional activation in response to IFNs and other extracellular signaling proteins. Science 1994; 264:1415.
87. Pine R, Canova A, Schindler C. Tyrosine phosphorylated p91 binds to a single element in the ISGF2/IRF-1 promoter to mediate induction by IFN alpha and IFN gamma, and is likely to autoregulate the p91 gene. EMBO J 1994; 13:158.
88. Dalton KD, Pitts-Meek S, Keshav S, et al. Multiple defects of immune cell function in mice with disrupted interferon gamma genes. Science 1993; 259:1739.
89. Attisano L, Wrana JL, Lopez-Casillas F, Massague J. TGF-beta receptors and actions. Biochim Biophys Acta 1994; 1222:71.
90. Ruscetti F, Varesio L, Ochoa A, Ortaldo J. Pleiotropic effects of transforming growth factor-beta on cells of the immune system. Ann NY Acad Sci 1993; 23:488.
91. Wahl SM. Transforming growth factor beta: the good, the bad, and the ugly. J Exp Med 1994; 180:1587.
92. Kingsley DM. The TGF-beta superfamily: New members, new receptors, and new genetic tests of function in different organisms. Genes Dev 1994; 8:133.
93. Shull MM, Ormsby I, Kier AB, et al. Targeted disruption of the mouse transforming growth factor-beta 1 gene results in multifocal inflammatory disease. Nature 1992: 359:693.
94. Ruddle NH. Tumor necrosis factor (TNF-alpha) and lymphotoxin (TNF-beta). Curr Opin Immunol 1992; 4:327.
95. Aggarwal BB. Comparative analysis of the structure and function of TNF-alpha and TNF-beta. Immunol Ser 1992; 56:61.
96. Mosmann TR. T lymphocyte subsets, cytokines, and effector functions. Ann NY Acad Sci 1992; 664:89.
97. Mosmann TR, Coffman RL. TH1 and TH2 cells: Different patterns of lymphokine secretion lead to different functional properties. Annu Rev Immunol 1989; 7:145.
98. Roecken M, Saurat JH, Hauser C. A common precursor for $CD4^+$ T cells producing IL-2 or IL-4. J Immunol 1992; 148:1031.
99. Kelso A. Th1 and Th2 subsets: paradigms lost? Immunol Today 1995; 16:374.
100. Romagnani S. Lymphokine production by human T cells in disease states. Annu Rev Immunol 1994; 12:227.
101. Romagnani S. Human TH1 and TH2 subsets: Doubt no more. Immunol Today 1991; 12:256.
102. Heinzel FP, Sadick MD, Holaday BJ, et al. Reciprocal expression of interferon-γ or interleukin-4 during the resolution or progression of murine leishmaniasis. J Exp Med 1989; 169:59.
103. Trinchieri G. Interleukin-12 and its role in the generation of TH1 cells. Immunol Today 1993; 14:335–338.
104. Kuchroo VK, Das MP, Brown JA, et al. B7-1 and B7-2 costimulatory molecules activate differentially the Th1/Th2 developmental pathways: Application to autoimmune disease therapy. Cell 1995; 80:707.
105. Pernis A, Gupta S, Gollob KJ, et al. Lack of interferon γ receptor β chain and the prevention of interferon γ signaling in Th1 cells. Science 1995; 269:245.
106. Szabo SJ, Jacobson NG, Dighe AS, et al. Developmental commitment to the Th2 lineage by extinction of IL-12 signaling. Immunity 1995; 2:665.
107. DiGiovine FS, Duff GW. Interleukin 1: The first interleukin. Immunol Today 1990; 11:13.
108. Dinarello CA. Interleukin-1 and interleukin-1 antagonism. Blood 1991; 77:1627.
109. Fenton MJ. Review: Transcriptional and post-transcriptional regulation of interleukin-1 gene expression. Int J Immunopharm 1992; 14:401.

110. Rietschel ET, Brade H. Bacterial endotoxins. Sci Am 1992; 267:54.
111. Auron PEW, Rosenwasser AC, Mucci LJ, et al. Nucleotide sequence of human monocyte IL-1 precursor cDNA. Proc Natl Acad Sci USA 1984; 81:7907.
112. Lomedico PTG, Hellmann R, Dukovich CP, et al. Cloning and expression of murine interleukin-1 cDNA in Escherichia coli. Nature 1984; 312:458.
113. Turner M, Chantry D, Buchan G, et al. Regulation of expression of human IL-1 alpha and IL-1 beta genes. J Immunol 1989; 143:3556.
114. Bensi GR, Palla G, Carinci E, et al. Human interleukin-1 beta gene. Gene 1987; 52:95.
115. Thornberry NA, Bull HG, Calaycay JR, et al. A novel heterodimeric cysteine protease is required for interleukin-1-beta processing in monocytes. Nature 1992; 356:768.
116. Black RA, Kronheim SR, Sleath PR. Activation of interleukin-1 beta by a co-induced protease. FEBS Lett 1989; 247:386.
117. Preistle JP, Schar HP, Grutter MG. Crystallographic refinement of interleukin 1 beta at 2.0 A resolution. Proc Natl Acad Sci USA 1989; 86:9667.
118. Schindler R, Clark BR, Dinarello CA. Dissociation between interleukin-1β mRNA and protein synthesis in human peripheral blood mononuclear cells. J Biol Chem 1990; 265:10232.
119. Fenton MJC, Collins BD, Webb KL, et al. Transcriptional regulation of the human prointerleukin-1 beta gene. J Immunol 1987; 138:3972.
120. Gifford GE, Lohmann-Matthes ML. Gamma interferon priming of mouse and human macrophages for induction of tumor necrosis factor production by bacterial lipopolysaccharide. J Natl Cancer Inst 1987; 78:121.
121. March CJ, Mosley B, Larsen D, et al. Cloning sequence and expression of two distinct human interleukin 1 complementary DNAs. Nature 1985; 315:641.
122. Acres RB, Larsen A, Conlon PJ. IL-1 expression in a clone of human T cells. J Immunol 1987; 138:2132.
123. Acres RB, Larsen A, Gillis S, Conlon PJ. Production of IL-1α and IL-1β by clones of EBV transformed human B cells. Mol Immunol 1987; 24:479.
124. Kupper TS, Ballard DW, Chua AO, et al. Human keratinocytes contain mRNA indistinguishable from monocyte interleukin 1α and β mRNA: Keratinocyte epidermal cell-derived thymocyte activating factor is identical to interleukin 1. J Exp Med 1986; 164:2095.
125. Savage N, Puren AJ, Orencole SF, et al. Studies on IL-1 receptors on D10S T-helper cells: Demonstration of two molecularly and antigenically distinct IL-1 binding proteins. Cytokine 1989; 1:23.
126. Sims J, Gayle M, Slack J, et al. Interleukin 1 signaling occurs exclusively via the type 1 receptor. Proc Natl Acad Sci USA 1990; 90:6155.
127. Colotta F, Re F, Muzio M, et al. Interleukin-1 type II receptor: a decoy target for IL-1 that is regulated by IL-4. Science 1993; 261:472.
128. Ye K, Dinarello C. Identification of the promoter region of human interleukin 1 type I receptor gene. Proc Natl Acad Sci USA 1993; 90:2295.
129. Freshney NW, Rawlinson Lea. Interleukin-1 activates a novel protein kinase cascade that results in the phosphorylation of hsp27. Cell 1994; 78:1039.
130. Chang J, Gilman SC, Lewis AJ. Interleukin 1 activates phospholipase A2 in rabbit chondrocytes: a possible signal for IL-1 action. J Immunol 1986; 136:1283.
131. Shirakawa F, Yamashita U, Chedid M, Mizel SB. Cyclin AMP-an intracellular second messenger for interleukin 1. Proc Natl Acad Sci USA 1988; 85:8201.
132. Mathias S, Younes A, Kan CC, et al. Activation of the sphingomyelin signaling pathway in intact EL-4 cells and in a cell-free system by IL-1 beta. Science 1993; 259:519.
133. Ye K, Koch KC, Clark BD, Dinarello CA. Interleukin-1β downregulates gene and surface expression of interleukin-1 receptor type I by destabilizing its mRNA whereas interleukin-2 increases its expression. Immunology 1992; 75:427.

134. Dinarello CA. Interleukin-1. Adv Pharmacol. 1994; 25:21.
135. Hogquist KA, Nett MA, Unanue ER, Chaplin DD. Interleukin-1 is processed and released during apoptosis. Proc Natl Acad Sci USA 1991; 88:8485.
136. Breder CD, Dinarello CA, Saper CB. Interleukin-1 immunoreactive innervation of the human hypothalamus. Science 1988; 240:321.
137. Hauser C, Saurat JH, Schmitt A, et al. Interleukin-1 is present in normal epidermis. J Immunol 1986; 136:3317.
138. Takaca L, Kovacs EJ, Smith MR, et al. Detection of IL-1 beta and IL-1 alpha gene expression by in situ hybridization. J Immunol 1988; 141:3081.
139. Simic MM, Stosic GS. The dual role of interleukin 1 in lectin-induced proliferation of T cells. Folia Biol 1985; 31:410.
140. Rothenberg EV, Diamond RA, Pepper KA, Yang JA. IL-2 gene inducibility in T cells before T cell receptor expression: Changes in signaling pathways and gene expression requirements during intrathymic maturation. J Immunol 1990; 144:1614.
141. Orencole SF, Dinarello CA. Characterization of a subclone (D10S) of the D10.G4 helper T-cell line which proliferates to attomolar concentrations of interleukin 1 in the absence of mitogens. Cytokine 1989; 1:14.
142. Crown J, Jakubowski A, Gabrilove J. Interleukin-1: biological effects in human hematopoiesis. Leuk Lymph 1993; 9:433.
143. Hestdal K, Ruscetti FW, Chizzonite R, et al. Interleukin-1 (IL-1) directly and indirectly promotes hematopoietic cell growth through type I IL-1 receptor. Blood 1994; 84:125.
144. Zsebo KM, Yuschenkoff VN, Schiffer S, et al. Vascular endothelial cells and granulopoiesis: Interleukin-1 stimulates release of G-CSF and GM-CSF. Blood 1988; 71:99.
145. Bagby GC. Interleukin-1 and hematopoiesis. Blood Rev 1989; 3:152.
146. Fibbe WE, van der Meer J, Falkenburg J, et al. A single low dose of human recombinant interleukin-1 accelerates the recovery of neutrophils in mice with cyclophosphamide-induced neutropenia. Exp Hematol 1989; 17:805.
147. Oppenheim JJ, Neta R, Tiberghien P, et al. Interleukin-1 enhances survival of lethally irradiated mice treated with allogeneic bone marrow cells. Blood 1989; 74:2257.
148. Tiberghien P, Laithier V, Mabed M, et al. Interleukin-1 administration before lethal irradiation and allogeneic bone marrow transplantation: Early transient increase of peripheral granulocytes and successful engraftment with accelerated leukocyte, erythrocyte, and platelet recovery. Blood 1993; 81:1933.
149. Hirayama F, Clark SC, Ogawa M. Negative regulation of early B lymphopoiesis by interleukin-3 and interleukin-1 alpha. Proc Natl Acad Sci USA 1994; 91:469.
150. Muench MO, Firbo MT, Moore MAS. Bone marrow transplantation with interleukin-1 plus kit ligand ex vivo expanded bone marrow accelerates hematopoietic reconstitution in mice without the loss of stem cell lineage and proliferative potential. Blood 1993; 81:2463.
151. Zuniga-Pflucker C, Jiang D, Lenardo MJ. Requirement for TNF-α and IL-1α in fetal thymocyte commitment and differentiation. Science 1995; 268:1906.
152. Yuan J, Shaham S, Ledoux S, et al. The C. elegans cell death gene ced-3 encodes a protein similar to mammalian interleukin-1 beta converting enzyme. Cell 1993; 75:641.
153. Kuida K, Lippke JA, Ku G, et al. Altered cytokine export and apoptosis in mice deficient in interleukin-1β converting enzyme. Science 1995; 267:2000.
154. Miura M, Zhu H, Rotello R, et al. Induction of apoptosis in fibroblasts by IL-1 beta converting enzyme, a mammalian homolog of the C. elegans cell death gene ced-3. Cell 1993; 75:653.
155. Itoh N, Yonehara S, Ishii A, et al. The polypeptide encoded by the cDNA for human cell surface antigen Fas can mediate apoptosis. Cell 1991; 66:233.
156. Ju ST, Panka DJ, Cui H, et al. Fas (CD95)/FasL interactions required for programmed cell death after T-cell activation. Nature 1995; 373:444.

157. Wright SD, Kolesnick RN. Does endotoxin stimulate cells by mimicking ceramide? Immunol Today 1995; 16:297.
158. Pushkareva M, Obeid LM, Hannun YA. Ceramide: An endogenous regulator of apoptosis and growth suppression. Immunol Today 1995; 16:294.
159. Cavender DE, Haskard DO, Joseph B, Ziff M. Interleukin-1 increases the binding of human B and T lymphocytes to endothelial cell monolayers. J Immunol 1986; 136:203.
160. Dustin ML, Rothlein R, Bhan AK, et al. Induction by IL-1 and interferon-gamma: Tissue distribution, biochemistry, and function of a natural adherence molecule (ICAM-1). J Immunol 1986; 137:245.
161. Groves RW, Ross E, Barker JN, et al. Effect of in vivo interleukin-1 on adhesion molecule expression in normal human skin. J Invest Dermatol 1992; 98:384.
162. Smith J, Urba W, Steis R, et al. Interleukin-alpha: Results of a phase I toxicity and immunomodulatory trial. Am Soc Clin Oncol 1990; 9:717.
163. Tewari A, Buhles WC, Starnes HF. Preliminary report: Effects of interleukin-1 on platelet counts. Lancet 1990; 336:712.
164. Baggiolini MW, Walz A, Kunkel SL. Neutrophil-activating peptide-1/interleukin-8, a novel cytokine that activates neutrophils. J Clin Invest 1989; 84:1045.
165. Kluger MJ. Fever: role of pyrogens and cryogens. Physiol Rev 1991; 71:93.
166. Coceani F, Lees J, Dinarello CA. Occurrence of interleukin-1 in cerebrospinal fluid of the conscious cat. Brain Res 1988; 446:245.
167. Beasley D, Schwartz JH, Brenner BM. Interleukin-1 induces prolonged L-arginine dependent cyclic guanosine monophosphate and nitrite production in rat vascular smooth muscle cells. J Clin Invest 1991; 87:602.
168. Okusawa S, Gelfand JA, Ikejima T, et al. Interleukin 1 induces a shock-like state in rabbits: Synergism with tumor necrosis factor and the effect of cyclooxygenase inhibition. J Clin Invest 1988; 81:1162.
169. Mrosovsky N, Molony LA, Conn CA, Kluger MJ. Anorexic effects of interleukin-1 in the rat. Am J Physiol 1989; 257:R1315.
170. Wogensen LD, Mandrup PT, Markholst H, et al. Interleukin-1 potentiates glucose stimulated insulin release in the isolated perfused pancreas. Acta Endocrinol 1988; 117:302.
171. Bird TA, Davies T, Baldwin SA, Saklatvala J. Interleukin-1 stimulates hexose transport in fibroblasts by increasing the expression of glucose transporters. J Biol Chem 1990; 265:13578.
172. Zheng H, Fletcher D, Kozak W, et al. Resistance to fever induction and impaired acute phase response in interleukin-1β-deficient mice. Immunity 1995; 3:9.
173. Parillo JE, Parker MM, Natanson C, et al. Septic shock in humans: Advances in the understanding of pathogenesis, cardiovascular dysfunction and therapy. Ann Intern Med 1990; 113:227.
174. Dinarello CA, Wolff SM. The role of interleukin-1 in disease. N Engl J Med 1993; 328:106.
175. Cannon JGF, Gelfand JS, Tompkins JA, et al. Circulating interleukin-1β and tumor necrosis factor-α after burn injury in humans. Crit Care Med 1992; 20:1414.
176. Wakabayashi G, Gelfand JA, Burke JF, et al. A specific receptor antagonist for interleukin-1 prevents Escherichia coli-induced shock. FASEB J 1991; 5:338.
177. Cannon JGT, Gelfand RG, Michie JA, et al. Circulating interleukin-1 and tumor necrosis factor in septic shock and experimental endotoxin fever. J Infect Dis 1990; 161:79.
178. Clark BD, Bedrosian I, Schindler R, et al. Detection of interleukin-1α and 1β in rabbit tissues during endotoxemia using sensitive radioimmunoassays. J Appl Physiol 1991; 71:2412.
179. Rordorf-Adam C, Lazdins J, Woods-Cook K, et al. An assay for the detection of

interleukin-1 synthesis inhibitors: Effects of antirheumatic drugs. Drugs Exp Clin Res 1989; 15:355.

180. Bochner BS, Rutledge BK, Schleimer RP. Interleukin 1 production by human lung tissue: II. Inhibition by anti-inflammatory steroids. J Immunol 1987; 139:2303.
181. Davidson J, Milton AS, Rotondo D. A study of the pyrogenic actions of interleukin-1 alpha and interleukin-1 beta: Interactions with a steriodal and a non-steroidal anti-inflammatory agent. Br J Pharm 1990; 100:542.
182. Seckinger P, Dayer JM. Interleukin-1 inhibitors. Ann Inst Pasteur Immunol 1987; 138:461.
183. Isono N, Kumagai K. Production of interleukin-1 inhibitors by the murine macrophage cell line P388D which produces interleukin-1. Microbiol Immunol 1989; 33:43.
184. Eisenberg SP, Evans RJ, Arend WP, et al. Primary structure and functional expression from complementary DNA of a human interleukin-1 receptor antagonist. Nature 1990; 343:341.
185. Seckinger P, Lowenthal JW, Williamson K, et al. An urine inhibitor of interleukin-1 activity that blocks ligand binding. J Immunol 1987; 138:1546.
186. Arend WP, Joslin FG, Thompson RC, Hannum CH. An IL-1 inhibitor from human monocytes: Production and characterization of biologic properties. J Immunol 1989; 143:1851.
187. Arend WP. Interleukin-1 receptor antagonist. Adv Immunol 1993; 54:167.
188. Granowitz EV, Clark BD, Mancilla J, Dinarello CA. Interleukin-1 receptor antagonist competitively inhibits the binding of interleukin-1 to the type II interleukin-1 receptor. J Biol Chem 1991; 266:14147.
189. Arend WP, Welgus HG, Thompson RC, Eisenberg SP. Biological properties of recombinant human monocyte-derived interleukin-1 receptor antagonist. J Clin Invest 1990; 85:1694.
190. Haskill S, Martin G, Van Le L, et al. cDNA cloning of an intracellular form of the human interleukin-1 receptor antagonist associated with epithelium. Proc Natl Acad Sci USA 1990; 88:3681.
191. Aukrust P, Froland S, Liabakk NB, et al. Release of cytokines, soluble cytokine receptors, and interleukin-1 receptor antagonist after intravenous immunoglobulin administration in vivo. Blood 1994; 84:2136.
192. Feige U, Karbowski A, Rordorf-Adam C, Pataki A. Arthritis induced by continuous infusion of hr-interleukin-1α into the rabbit knee-joint. Int J Tissue React 1989; 11:225.
193. Kohase M, May LT, Tamm I, et al. A cytokine network in human diploid fibroblasts: Interactions of β-interferons, tumor necrosis factor, platelet-derived growth factor and interleukin-1. Mol Cell Biol 1987; 7:273.
194. Zucali JR, Dinarello CA, Oblon DJ, et al. Interleukin-1 stimulates fibroblasts to produce granulocyte-macrophage colony-stimulating activity and prostaglandin E2. J Clin Invest 1986; 77:1857.
195. Cannon JG, van der Meer, Kwiatkowski D, et al. Interleukin-1 beta in human plasma: Optimization of blood collection, plasma extraction, and radioimmunoassay methods. Lymph Res 1988; 7:457.
196. Abhyankar S, Gilliland DG, Ferrara JLM. Interleukin 1 is a critical effector molecule during cytokine dysregulation in graft-versus-host disease to minor histocompatibility antigens. Transplantation 1993; 53:1518.
197. Rambaldi A, Torcia M, Bettoni S, et al. Modulation of cell proliferation and cytokine production in acute myeloblastic leukemia by interleukin-1 receptor antagonist and lack of its expression by leukemic cells. Blood 1990; 76:114.
198. Ristow HJ. A major factor contributing to epidermal proliferation in inflammatory skin diseases appears to be interleukin 1 or a related protein. Proc Natl Acad Sci USA 1987; 84:1940.

199. Cooper KD, Hammerberg C, Baadsgaard O, et al. IL-1 activity is reduced in psoriatic skin: Decreased IL-1 alpha and increased nonfunctional IL-1 beta. J Immunol 1990; 144:4593.
200. Groves RW, Sherman L, Dower SK, Kupper TS. Detection of interleukin-1 receptors in human epidermis: Induction of the type-2 receptor after organ culture and psoriasis. Am J Pathol 1994; 145:1048.
201. Tron VA, Rosenthal D, Sauder DN. Epidermal interleukin-1 is increased in cutaneous T cell lymphoma. J Invest Dermatol 1988; 90:378.
202. Oberyszyn TM, Sabourin CL, Bijur GN, et al. Interleukin-1 alpha gene expression and localization of interleukin-1 alpha protein during tumor promotion. Carcinogenesis 1993; 7:238.
203. Cuturi MC, Murphy M, Costa-Giomi MP, et al. Independent regulation of tumor necrosis factor and lymphotoxin production by human peripheral blood lymphocytes. J Exp Med 1987; 165:1581.
204. Beutler B, Tkacenko V, Milsark I, et al. Effect of γ-interferon on cachectin expression by mononuclear phagocytes: Reversal of the LPS^d (endotoxin resistance) phenotype. J Exp Med 1986; 164:1791.
205. Young JDE, Liu CC, Butler G, et al. Identification, purification and characterization of a mast cell-associated cytolytic factor related to tumor necrosis factor. Proc Natl Acad Sci USA 1987; 84:9175.
206. Tracey KJ, Cerami A. Tumor necrosis factor: Pleiotropic cytokine and therapeutic target. Annu Rev Med 1994; 45:491.
207. Carswell EA, Old LJ, Kassel RL, et al. An endotoxin-induced serum factor that causes necrosis of tumors. Proc Natl Acad Sci USA 1975; 72:3666.
208. Mannel DN, Moore RN, Mergenhagen SE. Macrophages as a source of tumoricidal activity (tumor necrotizing factor). Infect Immun 1980; 30:523.
209. Beutler B, Mahoney J, Le Trang NP, Cerami A. Purification of cachectin, a lipoprotein lipase-suppressing hormone by endotoxin-induced RAW 264.7 cells. J Exp Med 1985; 161:984.
210. Nissen-Meyer J, Hammerstrom J. Physicochemical characterization of cytostatic factors released from human monocytes. Infect Immun 1982; 38:67.
211. Perez C, Albert I, DeFay K, et al. A nonsecretable cell surface mutant of tumor necrosis factor (TNF) kills by cell-to-cell contact. Cell 1990; 63:251.
212. Tracey KJ, Beutler B, Lowry SF, et al. Shock and tissue injury induced by recombinant human cachectin. Science 1986; 234:470.
213. Lewis M, Tartaglia LA, Lee A, et al. Cloning and expression of cDNAs for two distinct tumor necrosis factor receptors demonstrate on receptor is species-specific. Proc Natl Acad Sci USA 1991; 88:2830.
214. Armitage RJ. Tumor necrosis factor receptor superfamily members and their ligands. Curr Opin Immunol 1994; 6:407.
215. Smith C, Davis T, Anderson D, et al. A receptor for tumor necrosis factor defines an unusual family of cellular and viral proteins. Science 1990; 248:1019.
216. Van Zee KJ, Kohno T, Fischer E, et al. Tumor necrosis factor soluble receptors circulate during experimental and clinical inflammation and can protect against excessive tumor necrosis factor-α in vitro and in vivo. Proc Natl Acad Sci USA 1992; 89: 4845.
217. Nophar Y, Kemper O, Brakebusch C, et al. Soluble forms of tumor necrosis factor receptors (TNF-Rs): The cDNA for the type I TNF-R, cloned using amino acid sequence data of its soluble form, encodes both the cell surface and a soluble form of the receptor. EMBO J 1990; 9:3269.
218. Everaerdt B, Brouckaert P, Fiers W. Recombinant IL-1 receptor antagonist protects against TNF-induced lethality in mice. J Immunol 1994; 152:5041.

219. Brouckaert P, Libert C, Everaerdt B, Fiers W. Selective species specifity of tumor necrosis factor for toxicity in the mouse. Lymph Cytokine Res 1992; 11:193.
220. Brouckaert P, Libert C, Everaerdt B, et al. Tumor necrosis factor, its receptors and the connection with interleukin 1 and interleukin 6. Immunobiology 1993; 187:317.
221. Laster SM, Wood JG, Gooding LR. Tumor necrosis factor can induce both apoptotic and necrotic forms of cell lysis. J Immunol 1988; 141:2629.
222. Brunner T, Mogli RJ, LaFace D, et al. Cell-autonomous Fas (CD95)/Fas-ligand interaction mediates activation-induced apoptosis in T-cell hybridomas. Nature 1995; 373:441.
223. Doherty P. Cell-mediated cytotoxicity. Cell 1993; 75:607.
224. Hackett RJ, Davis LS, Lipsky PE. Comparative effects of tumor necrosis factor-alpha and IL-1 beta on mitogen-induced T cell activation. J Immunol 1988; 140:2639.
225. Long NC, Otterness I, Kunkel S, et al. Roles of interleukin 1β and tumor necrosis factor in lipopolysaccharide fever in rats. Am J Physiol 1990; 259:724.
226. Dinarello CA, Cannon JG, Wolff SM, et al. Fever, tumor necrosis factor and interleukin-1. J Exp Med 1986; 162:2163.
227. Pfeffer K, Matsuyama T, Kundig TM, et al. Mice deficient for the 55kD tumor necrosis factor receptor are resistant to endotoxin shock, yet succumb to L. monocytogenes infection. Cell 1993; 73:457.
228. Fong YM, Tracey KJ, Moldawer LL, et al. Antibodies to cachectin/TNF reduce interleukin-1β and interleukin-6 appearance during lethal bacteremia. J Exp Med 1989; 170:1627.
229. Abbas AK, Lichtman AH, Pober JS. Cytokines. In: Cellular and Molecular Immunology. Philadelphia: Saunders 1991:225.
230. Tracey KJ. Tumor necrosis factor (cachectin) in the biology of septic shock syndrome. Circ Shock 1991; 35:123.
231. Hieber U, Heim ME. Tumor necrosis factor for the treatment of malignancies. Oncology 1994; 51:142.
232. Giaccone G, Kadoyama C, Maneckjee R, et al. Effects of tumor necrosis factor, alone or in combination with topoisomerase-II-targeted drugs, on human lung cancer cell lines. Int J Cancer 1990; 46:326.
233. Piguet PF. Tumor necrosis factor and graft-versus-host disease. In: Burakoff SJ, Deeg HJ, Ferrara JLM, Atkinson K, eds. Graft-vs.-Host Disease. New York: Marcel Dekker, 1990:258.
234. Holler E, Kolb HJ, Hintermeier-Knabe R, et al. The role of tumor necrosis factor alpha in acute graft-versus-host disease and complications following allogeneic bone marrow transplantation. Transplant Proc 1993; 25:1234.
235. Nestel FP, Price KS, Seemayer TA, Lapp WS. Macrophage priming and lipopolysaccharide-triggered release of tumor necrosis factor alpha during graft-versus-host disease. J Exp Med 1992; 175:405.
236. Krenger W, Snyder KM, Byon CH, et al. Polarized type 2 alloreactive $CD4^+$ and $CD8^+$ donor T cells fail to induce experimental acute graft-versus-host disease. J Immunol 1995; 155:585.
237. Kollias G. Tumor necrosis factor: a specific trigger in arthritis. Res Immunol 1993; 144:342.
238. Argiles JM, Lopez-Soriano J, Lopez-Soriano FJ. Cytokines and diabetes: the final step? Involvement of TNF-alpha in both type I and II diabetes mellitus. Horm Meth Res 1994; 26:447.
239. Fazely F, Dezube BJ, Allen-Ryan J, et al. Pentoxifylline (Trental) decreases the replication of the human immunodeficiency virus type I in human peripheral blood mononuclear cells and in cultured T cells. Blood 1991; 77:1653.
240. Grau GE, Piguet PF, Lambert PH. Immunopathology of malaria: Role of cytokine production and adhesion molecules. Mem Inst Oswaldo Cruz. 1992; 87(suppl 5):95.

241. Lopez-Cortes LF, Cruz-Ruiz M, Gomez-Mateos J, et al. Measurement of levels of tumor necrosis factor-alpha and interleukin-1 beta in the CSF of patients with meningitis of different etiologies: Utility in the differential diagnosis. Clin Infect Dis 1993; 16:534.
242. Kosland DE, Goldbeter A, Stock JB. Amplification and adaptation in regulatory and sensory systems. Science 1982; 217:220.
243. Freudenberg MA, Galanos C. Induction of tolerance to lipopolysaccharide (LPS)-D-galactosamine lethality by pretreatment with LPS is mediated by macrophages. Infect Immun 1988; 56:1352.
244. Mackensen A, Galanos C, Engelhardt R. Modulating activity of interferon-γ on endotoxin-induced cytokine production in cancer patients. Blood 1991; 78:3254.
245. Mengozzi M, Ghezzi P. Cytokine downregulation in endotoxin tolerance. Eur Cytokine Netw 1993; 4:89.
246. Erroi A, Fantuzzi G, Mengozzi M, et al. Differential regulation of cytokine production in lipopolysaccharide tolerance in mice. Infect Immun 1993; 61:4356.
247. Knopf HP, Otto F, Engelhardt R, et al. Discordant adaptation of human peritoneal macrophages to stimulation by lipopolysaccharide and the synthetic lipid A analogue SDZ MRL 953. J Immunol 1994; 153:287.
248. Hirano T, Taga T, Nakano N, et al. Purification to homogeneity and characterization of human B-cell differentiation factor (BCDF or BSF_p-2). Proc Natl Acad Sci USA 1985; 82:5490.
249. Van Damme J, Opdenakker G, Simpson RJ, et al. Identification of the human 26-kD protein, interferon beta 2 (IFN-beta 2), as a B cell hybridoma/plasmacytoma growth factor induced by interleukin 1 and tumor necrosis factor. J Exp Med 1987; 165:914.
250. Jones TH. Interleukin-6 and endocrine cytokine. Clin Endocrinol 1994; 40:703.
251. Borden EC, Chin P. Interleukin-6: A cytokine with potential diagnostic and therapeutic roles. J Lab Clin Med 1994; 123:824.
252. Hirano T, Yasukawa K, Harada H, et al. Complementary DNA for a novel human interleukin (BSF-2) that induces B lymphocytes to produce immunoglobulin. Nature 1986; 324:73.
253. Yasukawa K, Hirano T, Watanabe Y, et al. Structure and expression of human B cell stimulatory factor-2 (BSF-2/IL-6) gene. EMBO J 1987; 6:2939.
254. Van Snick J, Cayphas S, Vink A, et al. Purification and NH2-terminal amino acid sequence of a T-cell-derived lymphokine with growth factor activity for B-cell hybridomas. Proc Natl Acad Sci USA 1986; 83:9679.
255. Hirano T, Matsuda T, Turner M, et al. Excessive production of interleukin 6/B cell stimulatory factor-2 in rheumatoid arthritis. Eur J Immunol 1988; 18:1797.
256. Shalaby MR, Waage A, Espevik T. Cytokine regulation of interleukin 6 production by human endothelial cells. Cell Immunol 1989; 121:372.
257. Gershenwald JE, Fong YM, Fahey TJ, et al. Interleukin-1 receptor blockade attenuates the host inflammatory response. Proc Natl Acad Sci USA 1990; 87:4966.
258. Van Snick J. Interleukin-6: an overview. Annu Rev Immunol 1990; 8:253.
259. Kawano M, Hirano T, Matsuda T, et al. Autocrine generation and requirement of BSF-2/IL-6 for human multiple myelomas. Nature 1988; 332:83.
260. Kishimoto T, Hirano T. Molecular regulation of B lymphocyte response. Annu Rev Immunol 1988; 6:485.
261. Baggiolini M, Dewald B, Moser B. Interleukin-8 and related chemotactic cytokines-CXC and CC chemokines. Adv Immunol 1994; 55:97.
262. Oppenheim JJ, Zachariae COC, Mukaida N, Matsushima K. Properties of the novel proinflammatory supergene "intercrine" cytokine family. Annu Rev Immunol 1991; 9: 617.
263. Horuk R. The interleukin-8-receptor family: From chemokines to malaria. Immunol Today 1994; 15:169.

264. Unanue ER, Allen PM. The basis for the immunoregulatory role of macrophages and other accessory cells. Science 1987; 236:551.
265. Steeg PS, Moore RN, Oppenheim JJ. Regulation of murine macrophage Ia-antigen expression by products of activated spleen cells. J Exp Med 1980; 152:1734.
266. Meltzer MS. Macrophage activation for tumor cytotoxicity: Characterization of priming and trigger signals during lymphokine activation. J Immunol 1981; 127:179.
267. Ruggiero V, Tavernier J, Fiers W, Baglioni C. Induction of the synthesis of tumor necrosis factor receptors by interferon-γ. J Immunol 1986; 136:2445.
268. Stout RD. Macrophage activation by T cells: cognate and non-cognate signals. Curr Opin Immunol 1993; 5:398.
269. McBride WH, Economou JS, Nayersina R, et al. Influences of interleukins 2 and 4 on tumor necrosis factor production by murine mononuclear phagocytes. Cancer Res 1990; 50:2949.
270. Tilg H, Shapiro L, Vannier E, et al. Induction of circulating antagonists to IL-1 and TNF by IL-2 administration and their effects on IL-2-induced cytokine production in vitro. J Immunol 1994; 152:3189.
271. Numerof RP, Aronson FR, Mier JW. Interleukin 2 stimulates the production of IL-1-alpha and IL-1-beta by human peripheral blood mononuclear cells. J Immunol 1988; 141:4250.
272. Sher A, Gazzinelli RT, Oswald IP, et al. Role of T cell-derived cytokines in the downregulation of immune responses in parasitic and retroviral infection. Immunol Rev 1992; 127:183.
273. Essner R, Rhoades K, McBride WH, et al. IL-4 downregulates IL-1 and TNF gene expression in human monocytes. J Immunol 1989; 142:3857.
274. Wong HL, Costa GL, Lotze MT, Wahl SM. Interleukin (IL) 4 differentially regulates monocyte IL-1 family gene expression and synthesis in vitro and in vivo. J Exp Med 1993; 177:775.
275. Mueller KM, Jaunin F, Masouye I, et al. Th2 cells mediate IL-4-dependent local tissue inflammation. J Immunol 1993; 150:5576.
276. Larsson EL, Iscove NN, Coutinho A. Two distinct factors are required for induction of T-cell growth. Nature 1980; 283:664.
277. Lowenthal JW, Ballard DW, Bogerd H, et al. Tumor necrosis factor-alpha activation of the IL-2 receptor-alpha gene involves the induction of kappa B-specific DNA binding proteins. J Immunol 1989; 142:3121.
278. Masinovsky B, Urdal D, Gallatin WM. IL-4 acts synergistically with IL-1β to promote lymphocyte adhesion to microvascular endothelium by induction of vascular cell adhesion molecule-1. J Immunol 1990; 145:2886.
279. Ranges GE, Zlotnik A, Espevik T, et al. Tumor necrosis factor α/cachectin is a growth factor for thymocytes. J Exp Med 1988; 167:1472.
280. Munoz-Fernandez MA, Pimental-Muinos FX, Alonso MA, et al. Synergy of tumor necrosis factor with proteinase C activators on T cell activation. Eur J Immunol 1990; 20:605.
281. Santis AG, Campanero MR, Alonso JL, et al. Regulation of tumor necrosis factor (TNF)-α synthesis and TNF receptor expression in T lymphocytes through the CD2 activation pathway. Eur J Immunol 1992; 22:3155.
282. McKenzie JL, Calder VL, Starling GC, Hart DNJ. Role for tumor necrosis factor-alpha in dendritic cell-mediated primary mixed leukocyte reactions. Bone Marrow Transplant 1995; 15:163.
283. Yokota S, Geppert TD, Lipsky PE. Enhancement of antigen- and mitogen-induced human T lymphocyte proliferation by tumor necrosis factor-α. J Immunol 1988; 140: 531.
284. Robinet E, Branellec D, Termijtelen AM, et al. Evidence for tumor necrosis factor-α

involvement in the optimal induction of class I allospecific cytotoxic T cells. J Immunol 1990; 144:4555.

285. Chouaib S, Bertoglio J, Blay JY, et al. Generation of lymphokine-activated killer cells: Synergy between tumor necrosis factor and interleukin-2. Proc Natl Acad Sci USA 1988; 85:6875.
286. Shalaby MR, Espevik T, Rice GC, et al. The involvement of tumor necrosis factor-α and -β in the mixed lymphocyte reaction. J Immunol 1988; 141:499.
287. Boussiotis VA, Nadler LM, Strominger JL, Goldfeld AE. Tumor necrosis factor alpha is an autocrine growth factor for normal human B cells. Proc Natl Acad Sci USA 1994; 91:7007.
288. Thornhill MH, Wellicome SM, Mahiouz DL, et al. Tumor necrosis factor combines with IL-4 or IFN-γ to selectively enhance endothelial cell adhesiveness for T cells. J Immunol 1991; 146:592.
289. Leeuwenberg JF, Van Damme J, Maeger T, et al. Effects of tumor necrosis factor on the interferon-gamma-induced major histocompatibility complex class II antigen expression by human endothelial cells. Eur J Immunol 1988; 18:1469.
290. Chang RJ, Lee SH. Effects of interferon-gamma and tumor necrosis factor-alpha on the expression of an Ia antigen on a murine macrophage cell line. J Immunol 1986; 137:2853.
291. Sallusto F, Lanzavecchia A. Efficient presentation of soluble antigen by cultured dendritic cells is maintained by granulocyte/macrophage colony-stimulating factor plus interleukin 4 and is downregulated by tumor necrosis factor α. J Exp Med 1994; 179:1109.
292. Ramsdell F, Picha KS, Seaman MS, Kennedy MK. TNF abrogates the response of the CT.4S cell line to IL-4. J Immunol Meth 1994; 167:299.
293. Cope AP, Londei M, Chu NR, et al. Chronic exposure to tumor necrosis factor (TNF) in vitro impairs the activation of T cells through the T cell receptor/CD3 complex: Reversal in vivo by anti-TNF-α antibodies in patients with rheumatoid arthritis. J Clin Invest 1994; 94:749.
294. Pawelec G. Modulation of IL-2 and IL-4 induced cytotoxicities in human T helper lymphocyte clones by tumor necrosis factor-α. J Immunol 1991; 146:572.
295. Tanaka M, McCarron RM. The inhibitory effect of tumor necrosis factor and interleukin-1 on Ia induction by interferon-γ on endothelial cells from murine central nervous system microvessels. J Neuroimmunol 1990; 27:209.

8

Mechanisms of T-Cell–Mediated Cytotoxicity in Vivo and in Vitro

Michail V. Sitkovsky
National Institute of Allergy and Infectious Diseases
National Institutes of Health
Bethesda, Maryland

Pierre A. Henkart
National Cancer Institute
National Institutes of Health
Bethesda, Maryland

I. INTRODUCTION

T-lymphocyte–mediated cytotoxicity has attracted the interest of both basic researchers interested in the mechanisms of immunological recognition and effector functions as well as applied and clinically oriented scientists interested in diverse pathological processes and in the application of cytotoxic T lymphocytes (CTL) to prevent or to treat disease.

Several detailed reviews and books have recently been published (1,2), so this chapter is limited to an overview of the general features of CTL and concentrates on the latest important advances in understanding the mechanisms of the lethal hit delivery by CTL and the mechanisms of target cell death.

CTL are defined as thymus-derived cytotoxic cells with surface markers characteristic to T cells and with the ability to recognize and kill target cells in a MHC class I–or II–restricted manner in a relatively short time. The cell surface markers most commonly used include Thy-1, CD2, CD4, CD8, and TCR$\alpha\beta$ or $\gamma\delta$. All of these T-cell surface proteins are well defined with commercially available monoclonal antibodies.

II. CD8$^+$ AND CD4$^+$ CTL

The CD8 and CD4 surface antigens on T lymphocytes have been useful markers for distinguishing two subsets of T cells. These molecules serve as coreceptors that bind to respective MHC class I and II molecules bearing peptide antigen on antigen-presenting cells. The long-standing generalization that the CD8$^+$ subset contains cells that are precursors of CTL is still useful, but there are also many examples of highly potent CD4$^+$ CTL. Cloned lines of such mouse CD4$^+$ CTL have been found to display either the Th1 or Th2 cytokine pattern, although these two types may utilize different cytotoxicity pathways, as discussed below.

Similarities and differences between CD4$^+$ and CD8$^+$ CTL were the subject of several recent studies in which it was shown that the normal T-cell response against viral proteins (e.g., HIV gp120 and gp160) could be mediated not only by CD8$^+$ CTL, but also by CD4$^+$ CTL. The lysis by some CD4$^+$ CTL is characterized by similar time course, morphological changes in target cells, and DNA degradation in target cells such as those described for CD8$^+$ CTL; but in several instances, CD4$^+$ CTL kill more slowly and less specifically than do CD8$^+$ CTL. In contrast to CD8$^+$ CTL, some CD4$^+$ CTL are able to kill bystander, non-antigen-bearing cells by a mechanism that is presently unclear (3,4).

The cytotoxic properties of CD8$^+$ and CD4$^+$ CTL may have profound implications for immune regulation, since the cytotoxic process may have a role in shaping the population of antigen-presenting B cells and macrophages. An interesting new dimension to regulation of CD8$^+$ T cell responses was revealed by the recent demonstration that IL-4 could switch CD8$^+$ CTL to noncytolytic CD8$^-$CD4$^-$ cells that make IL-4, IL-5, and IL-10 and help to activate resting B cells but lose the ability to produce γ-interferon. This observation suggests the basis for a strategy to prevent transplant rejection by lymphokines (5).

The most detailed information about the molecular mechanisms of CTL–target cell interactions presented in this chapter was provided by studies of CD8$^+$ CTL.

III. RECOGNITION BY CTL AND THEIR RETARGETING

The sparing of "innocent bystanders" (i.e., cells without recognizable antigen) is an important property of CTL. Evidence of the ability of lymphocytes to specifically recognize other cells in cognate interactions was first provided in studies where cytotoxic cells were shown to specifically adhere to macrophage monolayers syngeneic to immunized cells (6). Thus, studies of CTL were among the first to reveal the unique recognition specificity of the cellular immune response (6–8). Understanding of these cellular phenomena led to cloning of antigen-recognizing molecules on T cells. It is now recognized that the unique specificity of recognition by CTL is the function of their surface antigen receptors (TCR), whose recognition repertoire is formed as a result of rearrangements of germline genes (9).

CTL could also be classified on the basis of differences in their mechanism of recognition as $\gamma\delta$ TCR$^+$ CTL (in contrast to $\alpha\beta$ CTL) that recognize target cells in an MHC-unrestricted manner (10). Attempts were made to identify specific features of TCR that determine the recognition of MHC class I or II peptide complexes. Indeed, the use of monoclonal antibodies to different epitopes of V regions established preferential use of some Vβ regions by CD8$^+$ or CD4$^+$ T cells. It is believed that antigen recognition repertoires for T cells are more restricted than those for B cells. It was also suggested that the size of the TCR repertoire of CTL specific for peptides homologous to self antigens could be significantly reduced by the natural tolerance to self peptides presented by MHC class I molecules (11).

Studies of TCR repertoires of CTL are of practical importance, since they may allow specific intervention in attempts to enhance or inhibit CTL response, as illustrated by the attempts to develop CTL vaccines to tumors (12) and viruses (13).

The ability of CTL to be triggered by cross-linking of the TCR suggested that it would be possible to use CTL for lysis of target cells even if they do not express the specific recognizable antigen. Indeed, inclusion of the anti-TCR IgG class monoclonal antibodies in the mixture of CTL and FcR expressing target cells resulted in their lysis due to TCR cross-linking and CTL–target cell bridging by anti-TCR monoclonal antibody (14); development of bispecific antibodies (anti-TCR and anti–target cell surface antigen) followed (15). Such bispecific antibodies achieved both CTL–target cell binding and CTL triggering, offering the possibility to redirect CTL-mediated lysis to a variety of tumor or virus-infected cells as long as monoclonal antibodies to the specific antigen and TCR are available. Intensive studies are now under way to develop different bispecific antibodies using biochemical techniques and genetic engineering (15), with the hope of using them in clinical situations where their specificity and differences in surface antigen densities between targeted tumor or virus-infected cells and normal cells will permit selective lysis by CTL.

IV. GENERATION OF CTL

The individual cellular and molecular events involved in the process of differentiation of precursor CTL (pCTL) into CTL are not well understood, but it is believed that cell-cell interactions involving recognition by pCTL TCR of MHC class I–or II-presented antigenic peptides is the required first signal (16).

Recent development of MHC class I-deficient mice with a disrupted β2-microglobulin gene confirmed the important role of MHC class I in CD8 CTL generation and demonstrated the striking sensitivity of pCTL to the presentation of antigen: even trace amounts of incorrectly folded MHC class I heavy chains were sufficient for the generation of $CD8^+$ CTL in such mice (17). Thus, CTL TCR engagement with antigenic peptides triggers a complex cascade of intracellular biochemical events leading to—among other changes—enhanced expression of high-affinity growth factor (IL-2) receptor and IL-2 mediated proliferation.

It was also shown that the most efficient proliferation takes place after the engagement of the CD28 molecule on pCTL with the complementary surface receptor on the opposing antigen-presenting cell surface, which have been identified as B7 molecules (18,19). As the result of these two signals, pCTL became enlarged, proliferated, developed exocytic granules with lytic molecules, and further differentiated into mature CTL and—later—into memory CTL.

Memory CTL are activated to deliver the lethal hit via TcR engagement of target cell antigen; this does not require costimulation or additional growth factors or cell division. In contrast to the cytotoxic effector CTL, a CD28-B7 interaction is necessary for generation of class I MHC–specific CTL. These studies suggest a promising strategy to enhance development of antitumor CTL by transfecting tumor cells with B7 antigen in vitro (20).

The development of CTL (their proliferation and differentiation) is regulated by several different lymphokines. Among the lymphokines shown to have such properties are IL-2, IL-4, IL-5, IL-6, IL-7, and IL-12 (21), but the precise contribution of individual lymphokines and the degree of redundancy of their action are still under study. Such studies are facilitated by the increased availability of lymphokine gene knockout mice.

VI. DISTINCT STAGES AND REGULATION OF CTL–TARGET CELL INTERACTIONS: CELL-CELL CONTACTS LEADING TO THE LETHAL HIT DELIVERY TO TARGET CELLS

CTL–target cell interactions require close cell-cell contacts, since prevention of such contacts in vitro inhibits killing, while their enhancement (e.g., by microcentrifugation) facilitates killing (1). It is believed that CTL on the surrounding cells—being in close contact (nonspecific adhesion, nonspecific "conjugates")—are able to "screen" the opposite surface for the expression of foreign antigens. By definition, not all such contacts are lethal to target cells, since innocent bystander cells are spared by CTL; but this "nonspecific" adhesion step should be considered crucial, since it allows for the recognition of antigen by TCR (1,2,22). Engagement of the antigen receptor results in specific conjugate formation, where events leading to the CTL activation and lethal hit delivery to the target cell take place. Enumeration of these conjugates by microscopy or the cell sorter is an important assay in studies of the mechanisms of CTL functions (23). The ability to form conjugates is not the unique property of CTL, since T-helper cells form conjugates, reflecting again the similarities between CTL and T-helper cells in interactions with antigen-presenting cells (24).

With the development of monoclonal antibodies to different surface antigens, it was demonstrated that the integrin superfamily of cell adhesion molecules—which are functionally dependent on the presence of divalent cations—is important in CTL–target cell conjugate formation. The interaction of LFA-1 (on the CTL surface) with molecules of ICAM-1 (on the target cell surface) is generally the major source of such antigen-independent adhesion, while additional contributions are provided by CD8 (on the CTL) interacting with MHC class I-peptide complex (on the target) and by CD-2 (on the CTL) interacting with LFA-3 (on the target) (25,26). Future studies will doubtless reveal additional adhesion molecules involved in CTL–target cell interactions, as was recently shown for CD43 interactions with ICAM-1 and ICAM-2 and for the importance of CD28 interaction with B7 (18) in CTL activation.

Recognition that LFA-1 was the major contributor in conjugate formation by T cells explained the Mg^{2+} dependence of CTL-target cell conjugate formation. Indeed, LFA-1—in contrast to some other integrins—requires Mg^{2+} but not Ca^{2+}. Studies of the contributions of these "accessory" molecules may offer novel approaches to modulation of CTL activity: by blocking conjugate formation, one can effectively block the CTL attack on target cells.

Evidence that CTL conjugate formation is regulated by a TCR-triggered phosphorylation event was provided by the observation that PMA alone can bypass the requirement in TCR engagement in increasing the adhesiveness of CTL to target cells (22). The detailed studies directly demonstrated that the ability of LFA-1, VLA, and CD8 antigens to bind their respective ligands can indeed be regulated through the changes in extracellular domains (27) and due to the engagement of TCR. LFA-1 phosphorylation correlated with a TCR-triggered transient increase in adhesiveness (28), while the CD8 antigen studies represent an interesting example of how TCR initiates the cascade of transmembrane signaling events culminating in changes in the ability of the surface receptor to participate in cell-cell contacts and feedback activation of the TCR complex (29,30). Thus, the rapid changes in avidity of integrins for their ligands are explained by TCR-triggered activation (phosphorylation) of, e.g., LFA-1 and increase in its avidity for its complementary ligand, ICAM-1. The mechanism of this avidity increase is unknown.

The biological efficiency of CTL could be explained by their ability to kill multiple targets, which assumes that CTL have mechanisms for engagement and disengagement with target cell and for triggering and interrupting the lethal hit delivery. Early and late events in transmembrane signaling following activation of CTL after TCR engagement are similar to those of other T cells. They include both the tyrosine kinase pathway and the protein kinase C–mediated pathway (31). Thus, TCR engagement is believed to involve tyrosine protein kinase–mediated activation of CD8, which in turn binds target cell MHC class I and provides enhanced phosphorylation of CD3 chains through CD8-associated p56*lck*, which, in turn, further enhances TCR signaling (32).

While calcineurin has been implicated in the regulation of TCR-triggered lymphokine production, it was also shown to be involved in regulation of protein synthesis–independent processes of lethal hit delivery and granule exocytosis (31,33). Interestingly, protein kinase A (PKA)—long known to be a negative regulator of such processes in the effector functions of CTL—was recently found to play a dual role: while protein kinase A inhibits lethal hit delivery and granule exocytosis, it is required in the synthesis of γ-interferon by activated CTL (31). It appears that this kinase is a downregulating enzyme in cytoplasmic processes which do not require a protein synthesis (e.g. granule exocytosis and lethal hit delivery), while its free catalytic subunit C-α is important in the production of γ-interferon by CTL and of IL-2 by T-helper cells.

VI. LETHAL HIT DELIVERY AND PATHWAYS OF TARGET CELL DAMAGE BY CTL

Understanding CTL-mediated cytotoxicity requires knowledge of the molecular mechanisms involved in target cell lysis. Different degrees of target cell impairment are described in the literature (cytostasis, loss of reproductive potential, cytocidal effects, and—the extreme form—physical breakdown of the cell membrane and dissolution of cellular structures, or cytolysis).

It has recently become clear that CTL, as studied in vitro, utilize two independent pathways in damaging target cells after recognition by the TCR. These two pathways—granule exocytosis and Fas—are illustrated in Fig. 1 and discussed below. While CD8$^+$ CTL utilize both these pathways, Th1 type CD4$^+$ clones seem to use only the Fas pathway while Th2 type CD4$^+$ clones utilize only granule exocytosis. Other CTL-mediated cytotoxicity pathways have also been described, but these kill targets more slowly and typically involve the soluble cytokines TNF and lymphotoxin. The latter effectors can undoubtedly be important to various biological processes in vivo.

A. Apoptosis versus Necrosis

In discussing the various CTL effector pathways, it is useful to consider the background literature on apoptotic versus necrotic cell death, as these terms have become ingrained in the literature. The term "apoptosis" was originally coined to describe a

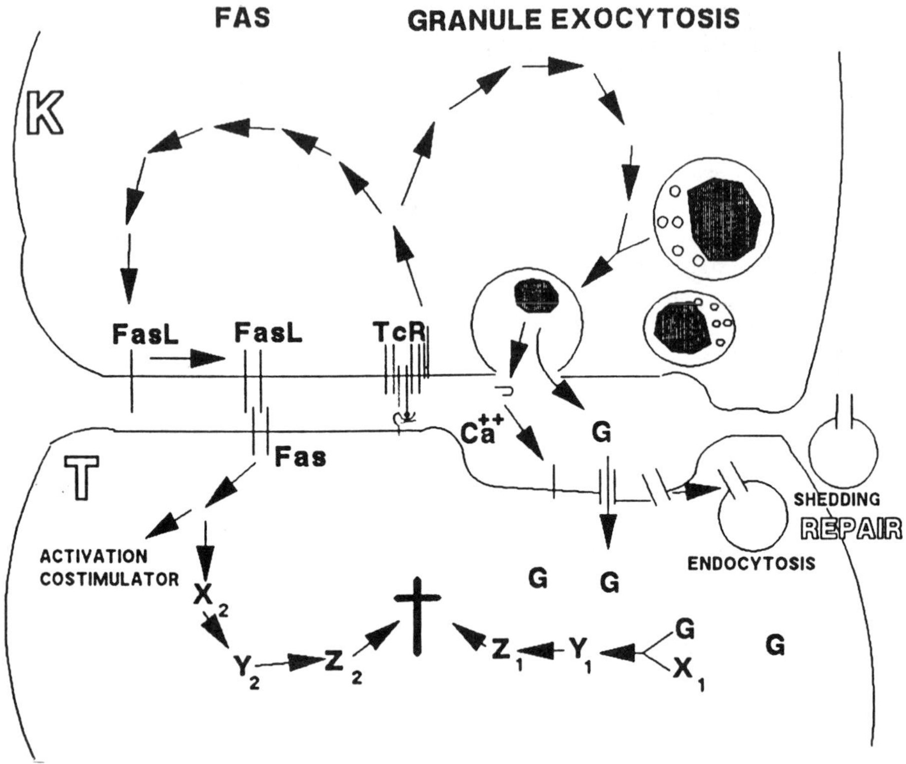

Figure 1 CTL-mediated cytotoxicity via the granule exocytosis pathway and the Fas pathway. Both cytotoxicity pathways are initiated by antigen recognition via the TcR. Receptor signaling is probably initially shared by both pathways. The right side shows the granule exocytosis pathway, in which the granule mediators, stored in an electrostatic complex within the granules, are released into the intercellular volume created by binding of the killer cell (K) to its target (T). Extracellular ionic conditions dissolve the matrix, and calcium induces conformational changes in cytolysin/perforin, rendering it amphipathic, so that it inserts into the target membrane, where it forms a pore. Granzymes (G) gain access to the target cytoplasm through the pore and trigger a death response in the target cell by a molecular pathway still not defined (X_1, Y_1, Z_1). The Fas pathway, shown on the left, is triggered by a TcR-induced expression of the Fas ligand on the surface of the killer cell. This ligand engages Fas on the target cell, leading to death by an undefined pathway (X_2, Y_2, Z_2), which may be different from the death pathway triggered by granzymes.

syndrome of morphological characteristics of cell death that was developmental or part of a physiological process (34).

The most prominent characteristics involve the nucleus. They include a redistribution of nuclear DNA around the nuclear membrane, often described as chromatin clumping. With time, the nuclei themselves fragment into smaller bodies. This nuclear damage seen morphologically is roughly correlated with biochemical measurements of DNA fragmentation. A characteristic ladder pattern with 200-bp spacing results from digestion of intact chromatin by nucleases, but this pattern is observed after larger fragments are initially generated during apoptosis.

The cytoplasm of apoptotic cells is characterized by overall shrinkage, swelling of the endoplasmic reticulum, and membrane blebbing. In some cases, the cells themselves can be seen to fragment. Typically, both the nuclear and cytoplasmic damage occurs prior to the disruption of the plasma membrane, which allows the release of chromium 51 or entry of dyes such as propidium iodide or trypan blue. Cells dying apoptotically are typically phagocytosed by nearby tissue macrophages without the inflammation characteristic of bacterial phagocytosis (35,36).

The described apoptotic nuclear changes are easily detectable, and the expanding list of conditions that induce them includes the withdrawal of growth factors and transmembrane signaling through specific ligand-receptor interactions, which could be mimicked by monoclonal antibodies to these receptors. In combination with cell division, such programmed cell death regulates the finely tuned balance between different subpopulations of cells in thymus, bone marrow, and peripheral lymphoid tissues.

The characteristic apoptotic death pattern has been contrasted with that seen when cells are injured by external stimuli such as complement, osmotic stress, or other types of membrane damage. The morphology of necrotic death is characterized by overall cell and mitochondrial swelling, while the nuclear morphology remains unchanged.

Target cells killed by CTL generally—but not always—have apoptotic features, including fragmented DNA (37). This apoptotic feature of cell death can originate from either of the two major death pathways utilized by CTL, as described below.

B. The Granule Exocytosis Pathway

Classically, lymphocytes have been regarded as nongranulated cells; compared to granulocytes and mast cells, the most granulated lymphocytes are only modestly endowed with granules. Cloned CTL grown in IL-2 show characteristic granules when examined by electron microscopy. These contain a number of components, which are listed in Table 1. These molecules are arranged in the membrane-bound cytoplasmic granule in two distinct regions: an insoluble matrix comprising the negatively charged proteoglycan complexed with the positively charged granzymes and cytolysin/perforin. These "core" complexes give a granular gray stain in the electron microscope. The rest of the volume within the granule contains soluble lysosomal enzymes along with membrane vesicles that have presumably arisen from compound endocytosis, similar to multivesicular bodies.

Upon degranulation, the core complexes dissolve in the altered extracellular pH and ionic conditions, releasing effector molecules that will damage the target cell (38). The status of granules in CTL found in vivo has been controversial, because both the number of granules and the expression of granule proteins are considerably

Table 1 Components of CTL Secretory Granules

Cytolysin/perforin
Granzymes A–H
Calreticulin
Lysosomal enzymes
Chondroitan sulfate-containing proteoglycan

less than in CTL grown in vitro. Some laboratories have reported cytolysin/perforin and granzyme protein and mRNA expression in such CTL (39), and subsequent perforin knockout results argue compellingly that the granule exocytosis pathway dominates cytotoxicity with target cells lacking Fas (see below).

Because degranulation in cytotoxic lymphocytes can be measured conveniently by monitoring granzyme A release into the supernatant using the sensitive BLT-esterase assay (57), a number of studies detailing signaling pathways in the effector cell have been carried out, as outlined above. It is probably fair to say that CTL degranulation occurs by molecular signaling similar to that found in other cells using the "regulated" pathway of protein secretion (40). The polarized stimulus provided by the target cell surface gives rise to a polarized degranulation, so that the granule contents are largely or completely deposited into the synapse-like junctional space between the killer cell and its bound target (41), as shown in Fig. 1.

C. Granule Effector Molecules

The known components of cytotoxic lymphocyte secretory granules are shown in Table 1. Of these, cytolysin/perforin has received the most attention as an effector of target cell damage. This 70-kDa protein, expressed only in cytotoxic lymphocytes (both T cells and large granular lymphocytes), shows sequence homology with proteins of the complement membrane attack complex. It is a major protein band on gels of purified granules and is a highly potent Ca^{2+}-dependent lytic agent due to its ability to form pores in lipid bilayers. The mechanism of this pore formation appears to be due to a Ca^{2+}-induced change in the conformation of this protein. In Ca^{2+}-free granule extracts of moderate ionic strength, the protein is soluble, but after secretion into the Ca^{2+}-containing extracellular medium it becomes amphipathic so that it spontaneously and rapidly inserts into lipid bilayers. There, the protein monomers aggregate and form functional aqueous pores that appear to be heterogeneous. The maximal aggregation state gives rise to structures, visualized by negative-stain electron microscopy, that are rather similar to those formed by the membrane attack complex of complement, but larger. Functional studies on proteins released from resealed red cell ghosts show that proteins of up to one-half million molecular weight can go through these pores (42–44).

CTL-secreted cytolysin/perforin is capable of delivering lethal damage to target cells, as shown by the properties of RBL mast-cell transfectants secreting it onto the membranes of target cells. Such artificial killer cells are very potent at killing red cell targets but only marginal in mediating lysis of tumor targets. This reflects the properties of cytolysis when cytolysin/perforin is added to the medium and also reflects the ability of nucleated cells to repair membrane damage (45,46).

Construction of knockout mice lacking functional cytolysin/perforin has allowed its functional role in lymphocyte cytotoxicity to be assessed both in vivo and in vitro (47). It is notable that $CD8^+$ T cells develop normally in such mice and also become activated normally in response to alloantigen or virus both in vivo and in vitro; however, these routes of activation in these mice produce CTL that are profoundly defective compared to wild-type mice in their ability to kill target cells lacking expression of the Fas antigen (47,48).

Such CTL retain the ability to upregulate the Fas ligand and allow a clear means of defining the Fas pathway as outlined below. These knockout mice are also markedly deficient in their ability to clear several types of viral infections, as predicted from previous studies that had implicated CTL in this process.

D. Granzymes

Another class of cytotoxic effector molecules in granules has been identified more recently. Granzymes are a subfamily of serine proteases defined by sequence homology and are found in granules of lymphocytes, mast cells, and the azurophilic granules of neutrophils (49). In cytotoxic lymphocytes, granzymes A and B are the principal granzymes expressed in vivo; these two proteases have distinct proteolytic specificities, cleaving proteins with complex sequence requirements dominated by positively charged amino acids (granzyme A) and aspartic acid (granzyme B) (49). Other granzymes in addition to these appear to be expressed in natural killer (NK) cells, while yet others appear in T lymphocytes activated and maintained in vitro.

The evidence is now quite convincing that granzymes play a major role in causing target cell damage. These proteases are not normally cytotoxic when added exogenously to cells; however, if the target membrane is permeabilized by detergent or pore-forming agents such as cytolysin/perforin, granzymes trigger an apoptotic death response in cells. This has been shown both by addition of purified components to cells and by their delivery via the transfected RBL mast cells (50–52). The enhanced cytotoxicity due to granzymes is associated with an apoptotic killing process, as it is accompanied by nuclear morphology changes and DNA fragmentation, but the granzyme-associated apoptotic death pathway accounts for most of the lysis seen with tumor target cells. Granzymes have no effect on the ability of RBL transfectants to kill red blood cells, which appears to involve only cytolysin/perforin.

There is other evidence confirming the role for granzymes in target cell damage. When the gene for granzyme B was inactivated in mice, generally normal immune responses were observed, but CTL showed slower rates of target cell killing and DNA breakdown (53). Another approach consisted of loading the granzyme inhibitor aprotinin into the target cell cytoplasm, which caused them to be resistant to both lysis and DNA damage by CTL and granzyme-expressing RBL transfectants (54). Since aprotinin fails to block when added exogenously, these experiments suggest that granzymes act in the target cell.

The mechanism by which granzymes lethally damage the target cell is still unclear. It has been shown that introduction of a granzyme B analog into the cytoplasm leads to activation of the protein kinase cdc2 (55), which normally becomes activated during the cell cycle after complexing with cyclin B at the beginning of mitosis. Cdc2 kinase phosphorylates a number of protein substrates, including the nuclear matrix protein lamin B, which leads to the breakdown of the nucleus and controls a number of nuclear events associated with mitosis. Since there are similarities between these nuclear events and those classically associated with apoptosis, it was hypothesized that granzyme-mediated activation of cdc2 kinase led to apopotic damage. In support of this, an inhibitor of this kinase blocked granzyme-mediated apoptotic nuclear damage.

Subsequent experiments make it clear that granzymes do not need target nuclei in order to mediate their cytotoxic effects after injection into cells. In these experiments, enucleated target cells behaved very differently from red cells and were equivalent to intact target cells with respect to the enhancement of cytotoxicity seen when RBL cells expressing granzymes were compared to those expressing only cytolysin/perforin. Thus, for the apoptotic granzyme-mediated death pathway, the nuclear damage is an epiphenomenon with respect to cell death as assessed by membrane integrity.

Another somewhat different potential granule effector molecule, termed TIA-1, has been described. Like granzymes, this molecule is granule-associated and has the ability to cause DNA fragmentation in permeabilized target cells; however TIA-1 lacks sequence homology to proteases and has not been demonstrated to have protease activity. The long isoform of TIA-1 has an RNA binding motif, but the functional significance of this is unclear (56). Definitive evidence for a physiological role for this interesting molecule is presently lacking.

E. The Fas Pathway of Target Cell Killing

The granule exocytosis model of cytotoxicity could not account for several observations of cell-mediated cytotoxicity. For example, some target cells could be killed by CTL in the presence of MgEGTA at very low [Ca^{2+}], when no granule exocytosis or polymerization of perforin could have taken place. In contrast to predictions of the granule exocytosis model, significant target cell lysis was observed, suggesting the existence of another pathway of $CD8^+$ CTL cytotoxicity that is not perforin-based and is Ca^{2+} independent (57,58).

The second major pathway of CTL-mediated cytotoxicity is termed the Fas pathway because it utilizes Fas antigen (also known as APO-1 or CD95) on the target cell. This molecule was identified as a unique cell surface antigen that triggers apoptotic cell death in the absence of complement when cross-linked by antibody (59). It is expressed at low levels on resting lymphocytes but upregulated upon their activation; it is found at moderate levels on various tumor cells. It is also expressed on nonlymphoid cells, especially in the liver.

The involvement of Fas in a CTL lytic pathway was recognized when it was shown that calcium-independent lysis occurred only when target cells expressed Fas (60). The strongest evidence for the role of Fas-mediated cytotoxicity was provided by recent studies with perforin knockout mice. The calcium-independent lysis is accounted for by the ability of CTL to cross-link target Fas antigen (48,61). While some monoclonal antibodies directed at this membrane protein are not cytotoxic and can costimulate proliferation when added to suboptimal levels of anti-CD3 monoclonal antibody (62), other IgM anti-Fas monoclonal antibodies are capable of triggering apoptotic cell death that, in some cells, is detectable within hours; however, there are examples of tumor cells that bind cytotoxic anti-Fas monoclonal antibodies but fail to die, most likely due to the absence of biochemical pathways coupling the Fas receptor to intracellular processes.

Fas is a transmembrane 45-kDa protein that is a member of the TNF-R/NGF-R family (63). It shows homology with the cysteine-rich extracellular domains of both TNF receptor chains, and its intracellular domain has a region of homology with the 55-kDa TNF-R1. Transfection studies of deleted constructs of both these receptors show this region is necessary for death signaling, leading to speculation that there is a common death pathway. However, other experimental approaches argue against this appealing idea, which remains controversial. As is the case for the granzyme-triggered death pathway, cell death triggered by Fas does not require a nucleus (64).

Cytotoxicity triggered by anti-Fas is independent of Ca^{2+} in the medium and does not require RNA or protein synthesis, thus distinguishing it from a number of other apoptotic death systems. It seems most likely that regulation of the Fas death pathway in vivo is mediated by the activation-dependent expression of Fas on target cells and Fas ligand on the surface of CTL.

The involvement of Fas in a second pathway of lymphocyte-mediated cytotoxicity has received further strong support from studies with cytotoxic hybridomas and identification of the Fas ligand as a cell surface molecule expressed in an activation-dependent manner (65). Fas ligand is described as a 31-kDa type II membrane protein, a member of the TNF family, which is expressed on activated T cells. Transfection of this molecule conferred a potent cytotoxic activity on COS cells when tested with Fas^+ targets, and purified Fas ligand had potent cytotoxic ability on such targets.

Several groups (66,67) have now provided strong evidence that the Fas pathway accounts for the cytotoxic activity of cloned $CD4^+$ Th1 cells, which were suggested not to use the granule exocytosis pathway of cytotoxicity (68). Activated T cells express a Fas ligand (FasL), which is capable of binding Fas and cross-linking it to trigger cytotoxicity. As perhaps expected, this multivalent cross-linking triggers a more rapid and profound death response in many Fas-bearing cells. Fas-mediated CTL cytotoxicity is generally calcium-dependent because calcium is required for TcR-triggered upregulation of Fas ligand. The signaling involved in this process appears to involve protein kinases and calcineurin, and thus it is likely that TcR engagement results in early signaling shared by both the granule exocytosis and Fas pathways (69).

Natural mutations in the mouse Fas and FasL genes, termed *lpr* and *gld*, respectively, have been studied for their autoimmune phenotype characterized by development of greatly enlarged lymphoid organs with age (70). When young, these mice have rather normal immune systems including CTL, and thus it is clear that the Fas pathway does not dominate in vivo CTL effector mechanisms. Interestingly, in both *lpr* and *gld* mice, activated mature T cells fail to die upon in vitro secondary TCR cross-linking, as do those of normal mice. It thus appears that the Fas pathway provides a means of downregulating T-cell numbers after they expand during an immune response and that failure of this pathway results in an accumulation of such T cells. Experiments in which CTL from the perforin knockout mice were used with *lpr* targets in various combinations make it clear that the Fas and granule exocytosis pathways together account for virtually all CTL activity as measured in short-term in vitro assays (48,61,71).

While Fas-induced cell death is typically accompanied by apoptotic nuclear changes, these are not necessary for cell death, as seen by experiments in which both anti-Fas antibodies and CTL-bearing Fas ligand induce death in enucleated fibroblasts (64).

F. The Cytotoxic Lymphokines TNF and Lymphotoxin (LT)

Soluble mediators of CTL cytotoxicity have been sought for many years, and LT was first described in the 1960s (72). When TNF and LT were cloned and sequenced, molecular studies revealed that these cytokines have membrane-associated forms as well as secreted forms. Soluble TNF comprises a homotrimer of a 17-kDa protein chain, and LT is a homologous trimer of 25-kDa chains. The membrane form of TNF is a longer 26-kDa chain, while the membrane form of LT consists of a complex of one LT chain and two LTβ chains (33 kDa), which have membrane domains. All forms are expressed by T cells and NK cells. The cytotoxicity of these cytokines depends on their binding to one of the two TNF-R expressed on a variety of transformed cells; however, these receptor-ligand interactions can lead to activation, no response, or apoptotic cell death, depending on the cells. Little is known about the molecular pathway leading to cell death induced by these TNF receptors.

VII. CONCLUDING REMARKS

With molecular approaches dominating the studies of cytotoxic lymphocyte mechanisms and gene knockout mice being increasingly available for studies, the definition of distinct cytotoxicity pathways and assessment of their relevance in vitro and in vivo are expected to proceed with great speed. The intracellular events leading to CTL activation and to cell death in both pathways remain to be precisely described. Thus, progress in the understanding of CTL generation and mechanisms of their recognition is now complemented by a better understanding of the mechanisms of lethal hit delivery. This all bodes well for the development of novel diagnostic tools and therapeutic approaches in pathologies that involve CTL.

ACKNOWLEDGMENTS

The authors wish to thank Brenda Marshall and Shirley Starnes for help in preparation of this manuscript.

REFERENCES

1. Martz E. Overview of CTL-target adhesion and other critical events in the cytotoxic mechanism. In: Sitkovsky M, Henkart P, eds. Cytotoxic Cells: Generation, Recognition, Effector Functions, Methods. New York: Birkhauser/Springer-Verlag, 1993.
2. Berke G. The functions and mechanisms of action of cytolytic lymphocytes. In: Paul WE, ed. Fundamental Immunology. New York: Raven Press, 1993.
3. Liu AY, Miskovsky EP, Stanhope PE, Siliciano RF. Production of transmembrane and secreted forms of tumor necrosis factor (TNF)-α by HIV-1-specific CD4$^+$ cytolytic T lymphocyte clones. J Immunol 1992; 148:3789–3798.
4. Ozdemirli M, el-Khatib M, Bastiani L, et al. The cytotoxic process of CD4 Th1 clones. J Immunol 1992; 149:1889.
5. Erard F, Wild MT, Garcia-Sanz JA, Le Gros G. Switch of CD8 T cells to noncytolytic CD8-CD4-cells that make TTH2 cytokines and help B cells. Science 1993; 260:1802–1805.
6. Brondz BD. Complex specificity of immune lymphocytes in allogeneic cell cultures. Fiolia Biol (Praha) 1968; 14:115–131.
7. Berke G, Sullivan KA, Amos DB. Tumor immunity in vitro: Destruction of a mouse ascites tumor through a cycling pathway. Science 1972; 177:433–434.
8. Golstein P, Svedmyr EAJ, Wigzell H. Cells mediating specific in vitro Cytotoxicity: I. Detections of receptor-bearing lymphocytes. J Exp Med 1971; 134:1385–1402.
9. Kranz DM, Tjoa B, β T-cell receptor repertoires among cytotoxic and helper T lympho-

cytes. In: Sitkovsky MV, Henkart PA, eds. Cytotoxic Cells: Recognition, Effector Function, Generation, and Methods. Boston/Basel/Berlin: Birkhauser, 1993.
10. Allison JP, Havran WL. The immunobiology T cells with invariant $\gamma\delta$ antigen receptors. Annu Rev Immunol 1991; 9:679–705.
11. Casanova JL, Cerottini JC, Matthes M, et al. H-2-restricted cytolytic T lymphocytes specific for HLA display T-cell receptors of limited diversity. J Exp Med 1992; 176:439–447.
12. Melief CJ, Kast WM. Lessons from T cell responses to virus induced tumours for cancer eradication in general. Cancer Surv 1992; 13:81–99.
13. Atlan H, Gersten MJ, Salk PL, Salk J. Can AIDS be prevented by T-cell vaccination? Immunol Today 1993; 14:200–202.
14. Ertl HC, Greene MI, Noseworthy JH, et al. Identification of idiotypic receptors on retrovirus-specific cytotoxic T cells. Proc Natl Acad Sci USA 1982; 79:7479–7483.
15. Segal DM, Jost CR, George AJT. Targeted cellular cytotoxicity. In: Sitkovsky MV, Henkart PA, eds. Cytotoxic Cells: Recognition, Effector Functions, Generation, and Methods. Boston-Basel-Berlin: Birkhauser, 1993.
16. Rammensee HG, Falk K, Rotzschke P. Peptides naturally presented by MHC class I molecules. Annu Rev Immunol 1993; 11:213–244.
17. Apasov S, Sitkovsky M. Highly lytic $CD8^+$, alpha beta T-cell receptor cytotoxic T cells with major histocompatibility (MHC) class I antigen-directed cytotoxicity in beta 2-microglobulin, MHC class I-deficient mice. Proc Natl Acad Sci USA 1993; 90:2837–2841.
18. Azuma M, Cayabyab M, Buck D, et al. CD28 interaction with B7 costimulates primary allogeneic proliferative responses and cytotoxicity mediated by small, resting T lymphocytes. J Exp Med 1992; 175:353–360.
19. Schwartz RH. Costimulation of T lymphocytes: The role of CD28, CTLA-4, and B7/BB1 in interleukin-2 production and immunotherapy. Cell 1992; 71:1065–1068.
20. Harding FA, Allison JP. CD28-B7 interactions allow the induction of $CD8^+$ cytotoxic T lymphocytes in the absence of exogenous help. J Exp Med 1993; 177:1791–1796.
21. Palladino G. Generation of effector cytotoxic T cells from cytotoxic T cell precursors: Role of soluble factors. J Neurol Sci 1993; 115(suppl):S24–S28.
22. Berrebi G, Takayama H, Sitkovsky MV. Antigen-receptor requirement for conjugate formation and lethal hit triggering by cytotoxic T lymphocytes can be bypassed by protein kinase C activators and Ca^{++} ionophores. Proc Natl Acad Sci USA 1987; 84:1364–1368.
23. Berke G. Enumeration of lymphocyte-target cell conjugates by cytofluorometry. Eur J Immunol 1985; 15:337–340.
24. Kupfer A, Singer SJ. Cell biology of cytotoxic and helper T-cell functions. Annu Rev Immunol 1989; 7:309–338.
25. Springer TA, Dustin ML, Kishimoto TK, Marlin SD. The lymphocyte function-associated LFA-1, CD2, and LFA-3 molecules: Cell adhesion receptors of the immune system. In: Paul WE, Carison FC, Metzger H, eds. Annual Review of Immunology. Palo Alto, CA: Annual Review, 1987.
26. Bierer BE, Burakoff SJ. T-lymphocyte activation: The biology and function of CD2 and CD4. Immunol Rev 1989; 111:267–294.
27. van Kooyk Y, Weder P, Hogervorst F, et al. Activation of LFA-1 through a Ca2(+)-dependent epitope stimulates lymphocyte adhesion. J Cell Biol 1991; 112:345.
28. Dustin ML, Springer TA. T-cell receptor cross-linking transiently stimulates adhesiveness through LFA-1. Nature 1989; 341:619–624.
29. O'Rourke AM, Mescher MF. T cell receptor-mediated signaling occurs in the absence of inositol phosphate production. J Biol Chem 1988; 263:18594–18597.
30. O'Rourke AM, Rogers J, Mescher MF. CD8 binding to class I is activated via the T cell receptor and results in signalling for response. Nature 1990; 346:187–189.

31. Sugiyama H, Apasov S, Trenn G, Sitkovsky M. Identification of protein kinases and protein phosphatases involved in CTL effector functions. "ON" and "OFF" signalling and immunopharmacological implications. In: Sitkovsky M, Henkart P. eds. Cytotoxic Cells. Boston-Basel-Berlin: Birkhauser, 1993; 331–339.
32. O'Rourke AM, Mesher MF. The role of $CD8^-$ class I interactions in CTL function. In: Sitkovsky MV, Henkart PA, eds. Cytotoxic Cells: Recognition, Effector Function, Generation, and Methods. Boston-Basel-Berlin: Birkhauser, 1993.
33. Dutz JP, Fruman DA, Burakoff SJ, Bierer BE. A role for calcineurin in degranulation of murine cytotoxic T lymphocytes. J Immunol 1993; 159:2591–2598.
34. Kerr JFR, Wyllie AH, Currie AR. Apoptosis: a basic biological phenomenon with wide-ranging implications in tissue kinetics. Br J Cancer 1972; 26:239–257.
35. Wyllie AH, Kerr JFR, Currie AR. Cell death: The significance of apoptosis. Int Rev Cytol 1980; 68:251–306.
36. Duvall ML, Wyllie AH. Death and the cell. Immunol Today 1986; 7:115–119.
37. Russell JH. Internal disintegration model of cytotoxic lymphocyte-induced target damage. Immunol Rev 1983; 72:97–118.
38. Peters PJ, Borst J, Oorschot V, et al. Cytotoxic T lymphocyte granules are secretory lysosomes, containing both perforin and granzymes. J Exp Med 1991; 173:1099–1109.
39. Nagler-Anderson C, Lichtenheld M, Eisen HN, Podack ER. Perforin mRNA in primary peritoneal exudate cytotoxic T lymphocytes. J Immunol 1989; 143:3440–3443.
40. Kelly RB. Pathways of protein secretion in eukaryotes. Science 1985; 230:25–32.
41. Podack ER, Kupper A. T-cell effector functions: Mechanisms for delivery of cytotoxicity and help. Annu Rev Cell Biol 1991; 7:479–504.
42. Henkart PA. Mechanism of lymphocyte-mediated cytotoxicity. Annu Rev Immunol 1985; 3:31–58.
43. Young JDE, Cohn ZA, Podack ER. The ninth component of complement and the pore-forming protein (perforin) from cytotoxic T cells: Structural, immunological and functional similarities. Science 1986; 233:184–190.
44. Yagita H, Nakata M, Kawasaki A, et al. Role of perforin in lymphocyte-mediated cytolysis. Adv Immunol 1992; 51:215–242.
45. Shiver JW, Henkart PA. A noncytotoxic mast cell tumor line exhibits potent IgE-dependent cytotoxicity after transfection with the cytolysin/perforin gene. Cell 1991; 64:1174–1181.
46. Henkart PA, Hayes MP, Shiver JW. The granule exocytosis model for lymphocyte cytotoxicity and its relevance to target cell DNA breakdown. In: Sitkovsky MV, Henkart PA, eds. Cytotoxic Cells: Recognition, Effector Function, Generation, and Methods. Boston: Birkhauser, 1992; 153–165.
47. Kagi D, Ledermann B, Burki K, et al. Cytotoxicity mediated by T cells and natural killer cells is greatly impaired in perforin-deficient mice. Nature 1994; 369:31–37.
48. Kojima H, Shinohara N, Hanaoka S, et al. Two distinct pathways of specific killing revealed by perforin mutant cytotoxic T lymphocytes. Immunity 1994; 1:357–364.
49. Jenne DE, Masson D, Zimmer M, et al. Isolation and complete structure of the lymphocyte serine protease granzyme G, a novel member of the granzyme multigene family in murine cytolytic T lymphocytes: Evolutionary origin of lymphocyte proteases. Biochemistry 1989; 28:7953–7961.
50. Shi L, Kam CM, Powers JC, et al. Purification of three cytotoxic lymphocyte granule serine proteases that induce apoptosis through distinct substrate and target cell interactions. J Exp Med 1992; 176:1521–1529.
51. Henkart PA, Williams MS, Nakajima H. Degranulating cytotoxic lymphocytes inflict multiple damage pathways on target cells: A cytolysin/perforin-mediated membrane damage pathway and a granzyme-mediated internal disintegration pathway. Curr Top Microbiol Immunol 1995; 198:75–93.

52. Nakajima H, Park H, Henkart PA. Synergistic role of granzymes A and B in mediating target cell death by RBL mast cell tumors also expressing cytolysin/perforin. J Exp Med 1995; 181:1037–1046.
53. Heusel JW, Wesselschmidt RL, Shresta S, et al. Cytotoxic lymphocytes require granzyme B for the rapid induction of DNA fragmentation and apoptosis in allogeneic target cells. Cell 1994; 76:977–987.
54. Nakajima H, Henkart PA. Cytotoxic lymphocyte granzymes trigger a target cell internal disintegration pathway leading to cytolysis and DNA breakdown. J Immunol 1994; 152: 1057–1063.
55. Shi L, Nishioka WK, Th'ng J, et al. Premature p34cdc2 activation required for apoptosis. Science 1994; 263:1143–1145.
56. Kawakami A, Tian Q, Duan X, et al. Identification and functional characterization of a TIA-1-related nucleoysin. Proc Natl Acad Sci USA 1992; 89:8681–8685.
57. Trenn G, Takayama H, Sitkovsky MV. Exocytosis of cytolytic granules may not be required for target cell lysis by cytotoxic T-lymphocytes. Nature 1987; 330:72–74.
58. Ostergaard HL, Kane KP, Mescher MF, Clark WR. Cytotoxic T lymphocyte-mediated lysis without release of serine esterase. Nature 1987; 330:71–72.
59. Yonehara S, Ishii A, Yonehara M. A cell-killing monoclonal antibody (anti-Fas) to a cell surface antigen co-downregulated with the receptor of tumor necrosis factor. J Exp Med 1989; 169:1747–1756.
60. Rouvier E, Luicani M-F, Golstein P. Fas involvement in Ca^{2+} independent T cell mediated cytotoxicity. J Exp Med 1993; 177:195–200.
61. Kagi D, Vignaux F, Ledermann B, et al. Fas and perforin pathways as major mechanisms of T cell-mediated cytotoxicity. Science 1994; 265:528–530.
62. Alderson MR, Armitage RJ, Maraskovsky E, et al. Fas transduces activation signals in normal human T lymphocytes. J Exp Med 1993; 178:2231–2235.
63. Clement M-V, Stamenkvic I. Fas and tumor necrosis factor receptor-mediated cell death: Similarities and distinctions. J Exp Med 1994; 180:557–567.
64. Schulze-Osthoff K, Walczak H, Drîge W, Krammer PH. Cell nucleus and DNA fragmentation are not required for apoptosis. J Cell Biol 1994; 127:15–20.
65. Suda T, Nagata S. Purification and characterization of the Fas-ligand that induces apoptosis. J Exp Med 1994; 179:873–879.
66. Stadler T, Hahn S, Erb P. Fas antigen is the major target molecule for $CD4^+$ T cell-mediated cytotoxicity. J Immunol 1994; 152:1127–1133.
67. Ju ST, Cui H, Pank DJ, et al. Participation of target Fas protein in apoptosis pathway induced by $CD4^+$ Th1 and $CD8^+$ cytotoxic T cells. Proc Natl Acad Sci USA 1994; 91: 4185–4189.
68. Lancki DW, Hsieh CS, Fitch FW. Mechanisms of lysis by cytotoxic T lymphocyte clones: Lytic activity and gene expression in cloned antigen-specific $CD4^+$ and $CD8^+$ T lymphocytes. J Immunol 1991; 146:3242–3249.
69. Anel A, Buferne M, Boyer C, et al. TCR-induced Fas ligand expression in CTL clones is blocked by protein tyrosine kinase inhibitors and cyclosporin A. Eur J Immunol 1994; 24:2469–2476.
70. Cohen PL, Eisenberg RA. Lpr and gld: Single gene models of systemic autoimmunity and lymphoproliferative disease. Annu Rev Immunol 1991; 9:243–269.
71. Lowin B, Hahne M, Mattmann C, Tschopp J. Cytolytic T-cell cytotoxicity is mediated through perforin and Fas lytic pathways. Nature 1994; 370:650–652.
72. Paul NL, Ruddle NH. Lymphotoxin. Annu Rev Immunol 1988; 6:407–438.

9

Natural Killer Cells

Giorgio Trinchieri
Wistar Institute
Philadelphia, Pennsylvania

I. DEFINITION OF NATURAL KILLER (NK) CELLS

NK cells were originally identified in the peripheral blood and other lymphoid organs of humans and experimental animals as cells capable of lysing in vitro, in the absence of previous deliberate or known sensitization, a variety of cell types including tumor-derived cell lines, virus-infected cells, and, in some instances, normal cells (1,2). NK cells are currently defined as cytotoxic cells with the predominant morphology of large granular lymphocytes (LGL) that do not express on their surface the CD3 antigen complex or any of the known T-cell receptor chains (TCR α, β, γ, δ) but that do express on the majority of the cells the CD16 (FcγRIIIA) and CD56 (N-CAM) antigens in humans, the NK1.1 antigen in the mouse, and the NKR-PI antigen in the rat and that mediate cytolytic reactions even in the absence of MHC class I or class II antigen expression on the target cells. The cytotoxicity mediated by NK cells is clearly distinct from that mediated by cytotoxic T lymphocytes (CTL), which recognize specific antigenic peptides in association with major histocompatibility complex (MHC) class I or class II molecules. Cytotoxicity mediated by NK cells is often defined as non-MHC-requiring, to distinguish it from the MHC-restricted one mediated by CTL. Certain T lymphocytes that expressed either an $\alpha\beta$ or a $\gamma\delta$ TCR may exhibit, particularly upon activation, a TCR-independent cytolytic activity resembling that of NK cells. These T lymphocytes are appropriately described as displaying NK-like cytotoxicity or non-MHC-requiring cytotoxicity.

II. MORPHOLOGY OF NK CELLS

Human peripheral blood cells with LGL morphology (i.e., with a high cytoplasm-to-nucleus ratio, indented nucleus, and azurophilic granules) were first described in 1911 by Pappenheim and Ferrata (3) and termed monocytoid or leukocytoid lymphocytes. Although a morphology of LGL has been attributed to all NK cells (4), it is now evident that a significant proportion of NK cells is similar in size to other lymphocyte subsets and may also be agranular (5). It is not known whether these different morphological forms of NK cells represent a heterogeneous population of mature NK cells or are representative of differentiation or activation status. In transmission electron microscopy (6), human LGL appear as medium- to large-sized lymphocytes, with round or indented nuclei, condensed chromatin, and usually prominent nucleoli. The cytoplasm is abundant and contains a variety of organelles. Membrane-bound granules (primary lysosomes), characteristic of these cells, range in diameter from 50 to 800 nm, with a circular to elongated profile, and contain an electron-dense core (internum) surrounded by a layer of lesser opacity (externum). In addition to lysosomal enzymes, the granules contain phospholipids, proteoglycans, and proteins important for cytotoxic lymphocytes function, such as serine esterases (granzymes) and pore-forming proteins (perforins) (7,8). The cytoplasm of LGL also contains other structures, probably representing differentiation or activation forms of the granules, including smooth vesicles, coated vesicles, myelinlike figures and multivesicular bodies, and the typical parallel tubular arrays (PTA), formed by tubules packed in wall-to-wall contact and often associated with granule membranes (9).

III. ORIGIN AND TISSUE DISTRIBUTION OF NK CELLS

NK cells originate in the bone marrow and most are short-lived, with a life span calculated to be from a few days to a few weeks (10,11). The increased number of NK cells and altered anatomical distribution in response to infection or other stimuli is primarily due to increased production in the bone marrow and possibly in part to proliferation of mature peripheral NK cells (12). Although relatively little is known of the characteristics of NK progenitor cells, the possible existence of a developmental relationship between NK and T cells is suggested by the similar functions mediated by the two cell types and by the sharing of surface markers, such as CD2, CD7, and CD8. Approximately 80% of NK cells express CD2 antigens, which are able to trigger the cytotoxic activity of these cells (13,14). CD8 is expressed on one-third of NK cells, at consistently lower density than on T cells (15); only the CD8 α chain is present on NK cells, unlike T cells, which express CD8 as a dimer of α and β chains (16). There is no evidence that in NK cells CD8 is involved in recognition of target cells MHC class I as in class I restricted cytotoxic T cells.

While NK cells do not rearrange any of the TCR genes and develop normally in mice with altered gene recombination mechanisms, such as SCID mice or mice deficient for the recombinase-associated gene RAG-2 (17), they do accumulate nonfunctional transcripts of the constant regions of the TCR β and δ genes. The transcripts of the TCR β- and δ-chain genes in NK cells are heterogeneous and correspond to a J region correctly spliced to the C region, preceded by a variable length of the genomic sequence upstream of the J region (18,19); thus, there is no evidence of even partial rearrangement of the two genes in NK cells, whereas in T$\gamma\delta$ cells, nonfunctional TCRβ mRNAs of similar size as those in NK cells (1kb) often reflect a nonfunctional D-J-C rearrangement (19). The high transcriptional activity of TCR β and δ genes in immature and mature NK cells is likely due to the shared expression between NK and T cells of lymphoid-specific transcription factors such as hGATA-3, involved in the regulation of TCR genes, in the absence of the expression of genes associated with rearrangement such as RAG-1 (19). NK cells also express on the surface the ζ chain of the TCR-associated CD3 complex associated with the FcγRIIIA (CD16) receptor (2,17). A further relationship between T and NK cells is suggested by the observations that human activated NK cells express cytoplasmic CD3 ε proteins and fetal liver NK cells express cytoplasmic CD3ε, δ, and γ proteins, and that the fetal murine thymus, in which most of the cells express the CD16 antigen, contains cell types able to generate T cells in the thymic environment and NK cells in an extrathymic environment (17,20).

Several lines of evidence suggests that NK cells originate and, at least in part, differentiate in the bone marrow. Treatment of mice with the bone-seeking isotope strontium 89 depresses splenic NK activity but leaves CTL generation and macrophage-mediated cytotoxicity intact (21–23). Bone marrow reconstitution of radiation chimeras between high- and low-NK reactive mouse strains resulted in restoration of levels of NK activity corresponding to that of the bone marrow donor strain and independent of host environment (24,25). NK-cell differentiation is also impaired in congenital or estradiol-induced osteopetrotic mice, confirming the necessary role of bone marrow microenvironment (26,27). Differentiation of cytotoxic lymphoid cells with NK characteristics ($CD3^-$, $CD56^+$) was obtained from bone marrow $CD34^+$ cells cultured in the presence of interleukin-2 (IL-2) (28–30); although only a small proportion of the NK-like cells generated in these cultures expressed CD2, it was demonstrated that interaction of the NK precursor cells with cultured bone marrow stromal cells induces the expression of CD2 on the maturing cells, analogously to the thymic effect on CD2 expression in immature T lymphocytes (29). Bone marrow $CD34^+$ NK precursor cells include a presumably more primitive $CD7^-$ subset and a more mature and committed $CD7^+$ subset (29).

The development of NK cells does not require the thymic microenvironment, as shown by the normal or augmented development of NK cells in athymic nude mice and rats (31,32) and in patients with DiGeorge's syndrome (33). Also, both differentiated NK cells (34) and NK cell precursors able to differentiate in vitro to NK cells (35) are present during human fetal development before the appearance of the thymic anlage. However, culture of $CD3^-$ human thymocytes with IL-2 induces the generation of $CD56^+$ $CD3^-$ cytotoxic cells (36–38). Triple negative ($CD3^-$, $CD4^-$, $CD8^-$) thymocytes expressing the CD7 antigens were shown to give origin to T$\gamma\delta$, T$\alpha\beta$, as well as $CD3^-$ $CD16^+$ NK-like clones (39). Within the triple negative (TN) thymocytes (representing 5 to 10% of total thymocytes), a small subset of $CD56^+$ $CD5^-$ cells (3 to 15% of TN thymocytes) was committed to develop into NK cells, whereas $CD56^-$ $CD5^+$ TN cells (75 to 96% of TN thymocytes) appear to represent the major T-cell-committed population in the thymus (40). Within the rare $CD56^-$ $CD5^-$ (1 to 10% of TN cells) are included possibly distinct precursor cells for T and NK lineage as well as pluripotent hematopoietic precursor cells (35,40). These results are consistent with the hypothesis that NK cells are related to the T-cell lineage and may share a common T/NK cell-committed progenitor. This hypothesis is also supported by the finding that early fetal murine TN thymocytes express FcγRII/III (CD16/CD32) and generate in vivo or in vitro NK cells when removed from the thymic environment (20). Thus, a common progenitor may give rise to T and NK lineage in a microenvironment-dependent manner.

Mature NK cells are mostly present in peripheral blood, where they represent approximately 15% of lymphocytes, with large individual variation, and in the spleen, but they are rare or absent in other lymphoid organs (2,41). NK cells do not normally recirculate through the thoracic duct. In the bone marrow, where they originate, they represent less than 1% of the cells, indicating that a pool of preformed NK cells is not sequestered in the bone marrow. Small numbers of NK cells can be identified in the liver (pit cells), lung, and intestinal mucosa (42,43). Upon activation—e.g., in response to interferon or to viral or bacterial infections—NK cells may accumulate in some organs in which they are normally rare, particularly in the liver and bone marrow (12). Cells with characteristics of activated NK cell (decidual granulocytes) represent the predominant hematopoietic cell type present in the human early pregnancy decidua (44): the physiological significance of the recruitment of these cells in the decidua is not clear but might have a role in facilitating embryonic implantation, in allowing placenta and embryo growth, or in the modulation of the maternal immune response against embryo antigens.

Data from irradiated patients and experimental animals suggest that mature NK cells are relatively short-lived and radiation-resistant (10,11,45–48). In mice, sublethal total body irradiation induces a decrease in NK activity beginning on day 14 after irradiation: the activity is fully restored after 8 weeks (49). These data suggest that murine mature NK cells are relatively radioresistant renewable cells with a life span up to 2 weeks and that their direct progenitors are radiosensitive. Leukemogenic split-dose irradiation determines a more persistent depression of NK activity (48,50). Similarly, in most irradiated patients, depression of NK activity is observed, with subsequent recovery after 3 to 4 months (45). The lack of recovery in some patients could be attributed either to the irradiation or immunosuppressive protocol used or to the effect of the underlying malignant disease that prompted irradiation. Experiments using the cell cycle-specific cytotoxic agent hydroxyurea indicated a much shorter half-life (on average, 1 day) of NK cells than suggested by the irradiation experiments (11). These contrasting results may be explained by the observations obtained with experiments of 3H-thymidine pulse-chase in vivo, which indicated that migration of labeled NK cells from bone marrow to spleen requires at least 2 days; some of the NK cells in the spleen survive up to 2 months, but in a resting state with reduced NK cytotoxic activity (51); these long-lived NK cells might have been underestimated in the experimental protocol measuring residual cytotoxic activity.

IV. NK CELL-MEDIATED CYTOTOXICITY

Cytotoxicity mediated by NK cells depends on binding to the target cells, followed by activation of the lytic mechanism, which usually involves secretion of the granules including molecules with lytic ability such as the pore-forming proteins (8). Lysis of the target cells is due both to the alteration of membrane permeability and to the degradation of target cell DNA (8). A number of surface molecules have been identified on NK cells which, when stimulated, activate the cytotoxic mechanism (52). The best-characterized of these molecules is the low-affinity receptor of the Fc fragment of IgG (FcγRIIIA or CD16) expressed on virtually all mature human NK cells (41,53). CD16 is associated with dimers of the ζ chain of CD3/TCR or of the γ chain of FcϵRI, and mediates signal transduction with similar mechanisms as those observed via the TCR/CD3 complex (54). Through CD16, NK cells recognize

IgG antibody-coated target cells and mediate antibody-dependent cytotoxicity (ADCC). However, CD16 does not appear to be involved in the induction of cytotoxicity in the absence of antibodies (2). Other molecules, including receptors able to activate the cytotoxic mechanism and adhesion molecules facilitating the effector/target cell contact, are probably involved in target cell recognition and triggering of the cytotoxic mechanisms, as CD16 is not required, in the absence of antibodies, for NK cell cytotoxicity (52).

Although resting peripheral blood NK cells are cytotoxic, their activity can be greatly enhanced both in vivo and in vitro by exposure to cytokines such as IFN-α/β, IL-2, and natural killer cell stimulatory factor (NKSF/IL-12) for a few hours (55–57). Resting NK cells express intermediate-affinity IL-2 receptors and IL-2 induces the progression of most NK cells into the cell cycle (58). IL-2–induced proliferation of NK cells can also be observed in vivo in patients treated with IL-2; in particular, prolonged infusion of low- dose recombinant IL-2 for as long as 3 months induced a maintained selective expansion of $CD3^-$ $CD56^+$ NK cells, which may become the most abundant lymphocyte subset in peripheral blood (59).

Although the activity of NK cells has been considered nonspecific and, unlike $CD8^+$ cytotoxic T lymphocytes (CTL), does not require the expression of major histocompatibility complex (MHC) antigens on target cells, evidence suggesting specificity in NK cell recognition has been accumulating for many years. Kiessling and collaborators (60) demonstrated that NK cells were the effector cells responsible for the rejection of parental bone marrow grafts in irradiated F1 mice (hematopoietic hybrid resistance), indicating a genetic specificity in NK cell action. The major locus responsible for this resistance, Hh-1, was mapped to the H-2DL region, and studies with H- $2D^d$ transgenic mice strongly suggested that the product of the class I allele D^d is a major determinant governing the genetic specificity of NK cells (61). In rats, NK cells rapidly eliminate in vivo allogeneic lymphocytes as well as bone marrow cells (allogeneic lymphocyte cytotoxicity, ALC), and alloreactive NK cells were also generated in vitro (62). The genetic elements controlling this alloreactivity are in a class I region (RT1-C) of the rat MHC, but, unlike murine hybrid resistance, in which the suspecitiblity to rejection was always inherited as a recessive trait (and resistance as a dominant one), susceptibility to both rejection and lysis by rat alloreactive NK cells was found to segregate dominantly, although rarely, in some strain combinations (62).

In several experimental systems, the susceptibility of target cells to NK cell-mediated lysis is inversely proportional to their expression of class I MHC antigens (63). One of the hypotheses to explain the ability of NK cells to recognize class I low target cells is the "missing self hypothesis," which postulates that one function of NK cells is to recognize and eliminate cells that do not express MHC class I molecules (63). This hypothesis needs to be modified, however, to accommodate findings suggesting that NK cells may be affected not only by the presence or absence of class I molecules but also by the nature of MHC-bound peptide fitting, either because, similarly to T cells, they might directly sense the combination of peptide and MHC or because they recognize changes in molecular conformations of the MHC molecules induced by the peptide binding (64). The peptide-binding class I $\alpha1/\alpha2$ domains have been shown to be necessary for NK cell recognition, and single amino acid substitutions in the peptide-binding groove of the class I molecules alter the ability of the molecules to protect target cells from NK cells (64). It has also been suggested that alteration of endogenous peptides by external peptide loading or by virus infection abrogates class I–mediated resistance of target cells and makes them susceptible to NK cell cytotoxicity (65).

Two hypotheses have been proposed to explain the mechanism of class I recognition by NK cells: (a) the effector inhibition hypothesis postulating that the presence of class I (or particular conformations of class I) on the target cells delivers a negative signal to the NK cells, which prevents the activation of cytotoxicity, or (b) the target interference hypothesis postulating that class I antigens or their peptides sterically mask recognition of an NK target structure on the target cells (63). Although many of the experimental data can be explained on the basis of either hypothesis or through intermediate interpretations, several recent lines of evidence, discussed below, appear to favor the effector inhibition hypothesis.

The first receptor identified on murine NK cells that is probably involved in recognition of class I MHC is the Ly-49 antigen. Ly-49 is expressed in 15 to 20% of NK cells in C57BL/6 mice (66). Both the Ly-49$^+$ and Ly-49$^-$ subsets of NK cells have similar cytotoxic activity against NK-sensitive cell lines, but the Ly- 49$^+$ subset, unlike the Ly-49$^-$ one, is unable to lyse target cells expressing H-2D^d or H-2D^k (66). The following observations suggest that interaction of Ly-49 with class I MHC D^d or D^k delivers a negative signal to the NK cells: (a) anti-Ly-49 or anti–class I α1/GKa2 domain antibodies restore lysis of H-2D^d or D^k target cells by Ly- 49$^+$ NK cells (66); (b) Ly-49$^+$ cells bind to purified D^d or D^k molecules, and this binding is prevented by anti-Ly-49 antibodies (67); and (c) the Ly-49$^+$ NK cells binding to a H-2D^d or D^k target cell are globally inactivated and cannot mediate ADCC against the same target cells (66). Ly-49 is a homodimeric type II integral membrane protein with carboxyl-terminal extracellular domains homologous to members of the C-type lectin superfamily. In addition to the Ly-49 gene, there are several genes highly homologous to Ly-49 (68), which may encode receptors recognizing class I antigens, possibly with a different specificity, and account for the class I–mediated protection of target cells against the majority of NK cells which are Ly-49$^-$ (68). The Ly-49 multigene family is encoded by a cluster of genes, the NK gene complex, which are in the distal portion of mouse chromosome 6, associated with the genes encoding the NK1.1, NKR-P1, and CD69 antigens. These are all disulfide-linked dimers of type II integral membrane proteins with type C lectin homology (68). The human CD69 antigen is encoded by a gene in the chromosome 12p13 near the NKG2 gene cluster, encoding other still uncharacterized type II integral membrane molecules preferentially expressed in NK cells (68). Although these lectinlike molecules have a specificity for carbohydrates, they might also bind to polypeptide or conformational sequences, as shown by the fact that CD23, one of the members of this family, binds to IgE independently of carbohydrates, whereas it binds to the carbohydrate structure of CD21 (69). However, the hypothesis of a role for carbohydrate recognition activity has recently been supported by the data of Bezouska et al. (70), indicating that oligosaccharides that bind to NKR-P1 with high affinity are able to inhibit binding of NKR-P1 protein to target cells, to prevent target cell killing, to activate signal transduction in NK cells, and, when incorporated in NK-resistant target cells, to make them sensitive to NK cell–mediated cytotoxicity. It is noteworthy that many members of this receptor family (e.g., NK1-1, NKR-P1, and CD69) are triggering molecules on NK cells, inducing cytotoxicity and cytokine production (68). Although the ligands for NK1.1, NKR-P1, and CD69 are not known, it cannot be excluded that they also recognize class I MHC and that interaction of different NK receptors with class I or of the same receptor with different conformations of class I might deliver either blocking or triggering signals. The data from alloreactive rat NK cells (62), indicating that in certain strain combinations the susceptibility to lysis by NK cells cosegregates with MHC class I in a dominant way, indeed suggest the possibility that at least in some instances NK cell cytotoxicity may be activated by direct recognition of class I MHC.

In the last few years, several molecules on human NK cells most likely responsible for class I recognition on target cells and presumably able to deliver a negative signal preventing cytotoxicity have been described (71). These NK-cell receptors include (a) the family of p58 receptors, recognized by antibodies GL183 and EB6, recognizing on HLA- C molecules an allelism in positions 77 and 80 (Asn-77-Lys-80 or Ser-77-Asn-80) (72,73), and (b) the NKB1 70-kDa glycoprotein and the type II C lectinlike transmembrane protein Kp43 (CD94), which appear to recognize on HLA-B molecules the supertypic specificity Bw4 and Bw6, respectively (74,75). These receptors on human NK cells appear to deliver a negative signal to NK cells which, in most cases, globally inhibit their ability to mediate cytotoxicity, even if activated through a different receptor, including ADCC mediated through CD16. These results are compatible with a model in which lysis of NK cells must be triggered by any one of a set of distinct target cell ligands, but where all of these signals can be overruled by class I–mediated inhibition (76). It is remarkable that the C-type lectinlike receptors, such as Ly-49, Kp43, and NKR-P1, on NK cells might be involved in delivering both activatory and inactivatory signals; also, recognition of class I MHC and delivery of a negative signal appear to be mediated on NK cells not only by the C-type lectinlike receptors such as Ly-49 and Kp43 but also by structurally unrelated molecules such as p58 and NKB1 receptors.

V. PRODUCTION OF CYTOKINES FROM NK CELLS

Many of the physiological functions of NK cells are mediated at least in part by their ability to secrete cytokines. NK cells are powerful producers of IFN-γ and granulocyte-macrophage colony-stimulating factors (GM-CSF), and they have also been shown to be able to produce tumor necrosis factor-α (TNF-α), macrophage-CSF (M-CSF), IL-3, IL-8, and other cytokines (2,56,77,78). Cytokines such as IL-2, IL-12, TNF-α, and IL-1; triggering of surface receptors, such as CD16 interaction with immune complexes; and the interaction of still undefined surface receptors with ligands on NK-sensitive target cells are among the stimuli that, acting individually or often in synergistic combination, induce NK cells to produce cytokines (2,79,80).

VI. NK CELLS AS EFFECTOR CELLS OF INNATE RESISTANCE AGAINST INFECTIOUS AGENTS AND TUMORS

Because of their ability to respond to external stimuli without previous sensitization, NK cells are able to respond rapidly, although nonspecifically, to the presence of infectious microorganisms or in some cases neoplastic cells. Together with phagocytic cells (monocyte/macrophages and neutrophils), NK cells are effectors of the innate or natural resistance, which represents the first line of defense against infection.

The ability of NK cells to participate in the resistance against infection by certain viruses is well documented in experimental animals (81) and is strongly suggested by the recurrent viral infections in the few patients described to have a selective deficiency of NK cells (82). In vitro NK cells selectively lyse virus-infected cells, with a mechanism that is at least in part dependent on the production of IFN-α, a potent stimulator of NK cell activity (83,84). In vivo virus-infection and IFN production are usually accompanied by a rapid activation of and increase in the number of NK cells, both systemic and localized, in the infected area (12). The NK response of virus infection usually peaks at 3 days postinfection and is followed by an antigen-specific T-helper and CTL response, which peaks 7 to 9 days postinfection (12). The early NK response induces a significant reduction in the titer of certain viruses, e.g., during infection with murine cytomegalovirus (81). Other viruses, such as lymphocyte choriomeningitis virus (LCMV), are resistant to the antiviral effects of NK cells; the IFN production and NK- cell activation induced by these viruses can even have pathogenic effects (81).

Although the role of NK cells in the natural resistance against bacteria and parasites has not been analyzed in depth, the ability of NK cells to be directly cytotoxic for bacteria and certain parasites has been described (85). The ability of NK cells to produce cytokines with potent activatory effects on phagocytic cells has led to the postulate of a role for this cell type in inflammation during infection (2,77). This hypothesis was strengthened by the observation that resting NK cells respond with production of IFN- γ and other cytokines to stimulation with IL-2, immune complexes, cellular interaction, and other stimuli with a faster kinetics than observed with antigenic stimulation of circulating T lymphocytes (56,77,79).

The original in vivo observation that NK cells, by producing IFN-γ and other cytokines, may have a central role in the antigen- and T-cell–independent activation of macrophage in infection was obtained in studies in athymic nude mice (86) and in mice with the SCID mutation (87) infected with the facultative intracellular bacterium *Listeria monocytogenes*. The SCID mice, although lacking B and T cells, achieve a partial control of *Listeria* growth and develop macrophages with increased expression of MHC class II and tumoricidal activity. This macrophage activation in SCID mice is blocked by treatment of the animals with either neutralizing anti-IFN-γ antibodies or anti-aGM1 before infection, to deplete NK cells: these results suggest that NK cells produce IFN-γ and thus activate phagocytic cells upon infection of the animals with *Listeria* (87). Very similar findings of phagocytic cell activation mediated by NK cell–produced IFN-γ has also been demonstrated in mice infected with *Toxoplasma gondii*, demonstrating that NK cells also play a central role in the innate resistance against this intracellular parasite (88). TNF produced by infected phagocytic cells was shown to be required for production of IFN-γ from NK cells (87–89). However, TNF by itself is not a sufficient stimulus for IFN-γ production, and it was clear that other humoral or cellular interactions were required for inducing NK cells to produce IFN-γ efficiently. A recently discovered cytokine, NK stimulatory factor or interleukin-12 (IL-12), is able to induce IFN-γ production by NK and T cells, alone or in synergy with TNF, IL-2, and other inducers; it probably represents the missing link between infected phagocytic cells and IFN-γ–producing NK cells.

IL-12 is an heterodimeric cytokine formed by two covalently linked glycosylated chains of 35 and 40 kDa. IL-12 was originally purified from the supernatant fluids of EBV- transformed human B lymphoblastoid cell lines (57). However, in addition to B cells, phagocytic cells—i.e., monocytes, macrophages, and neutrophils—have been identified as the major physiological producers of IL-12 (90). Phagocytic cells produce IL-12 in response to bacteria, bacterial products such as LPS, and intracellular parasites. The cell types on which IL-12 exert biological activity are T and NK cells. The major direct biological function of IL-12 on these cell types are the induction of cytokine production, primarily IFN-γ, the enhancement of a generation of cytotoxic cells, and a mitogenic effect on antigen-activated lymphocytes (57).

In part through its ability to induce IFN-γ production, IL-12, produced in response to infections, represents an important functional link between the effector cells of innate resistance, phagocytic cells, and NK cells and the effector cells of adaptive resistance, T and B lymphocytes. The ability of IL-12 to induce IFN-γ production from circulating NK cells and at least a proportion of T cells determines a rapid, antigen-independent production of IFN-γ during infections (57,90). IFN-γ acts as a potent enhancer of phagocytic and bactericidal activity of phagocytic cells, participating early in infection to activate some of the inflammatory mechanisms that represent the first innate resistance against infection. This antigen-independent activation of phagocytic cells, which involves, in addition to IL-12, other monocyte-derived cytokines such as TNF and IL-1, has been shown to be important in experimental animals for the resistance against infection by microorganisms such as *L. monocytogenes* and *T. gondii* (91,92).

The observation that NK cells lyse in vitro transformed or tumor-derived cell lines has been used to support the theory that, in immune surveillance, NK cells rather than T cells can recognize and lyse newly arising malignant tumor cells (93). In experimental animals, the in vivo activity of NK cells against tumors was investigated by evaluating their effect on long-term growth of tumors, metastasis formation, and short-term elimination of radiolabeled tumor cells (2). Although these experiments have clearly shown that NK cells can destroy tumor cells in vivo, the evidence for an effective role of NK cells in resistance to spontaneously arising neoplastic cells is much less compelling. In human cancer patients, NK-cell cytotoxic activity is often decreased and several studies have suggested that NK-cell activity in the patients tends to correlate with increased survival times and longer intervals before metastasis is observed (94,95). However, the hypothesis of a role for NK cells in immune surveillance is not yet supported by statistical evidence indicating a correlation between low tumor incidence and high NK cell cytotoxic activity (96). Because of their potential antileukemia cytotoxic activity, donor-derived NK cells may have an important role in the graft-versus-leukemia (GVL) reaction in bone marrow transplantation (97,98).

VII. REGULATION OF ADAPTIVE IMMUNITY BY NK CELLS

Like other effector cells of natural resistance, NK cells, by interacting with infectious agents and antigens early during the immune response, have either stimulatory or inhibitory effects on the function of B and T cells as well as on antigen-presenting cells (2). Evidence for an enhancing effect of NK cells on B-cell response has been shown both in vitro and in vivo by studies demonstrating that NK cells, in the absence of T cells, support antigen-specific B-cell responses, in part by producing IFN-γ (99,100).

IL-12 has a major effect in the antigen-specific adaptive immune response by facilitating the generation of a T-helper type 1 (Th-1) response and suppressing a Th-2 response (101). The presence of IL-12 during antigen stimulation in vitro using human peripheral blood lymphocytes (102), or both in vivo (103) and in vitro in experimental animals, induces generation of Th-1 cells producing IFN-γ and IL-2 and inhibits the generation of Th-2 cells producing IL-4. The physiological importance of this facilitating effect of IL-12 on Th-1 cell generation is shown by the ability of IL-12 to cure infection by *Leishmania major* in susceptible BALB/c mice by inducing a Th-1 type immune response when administered at the early times of infection (104,105). When admixed with soluble *Leishmania* antigen, IL-12 also acts as a potent adjuvant in a vaccination model by inducing a Th-1 memory response which protects BALB/c from subsequent infection with virulent *L. major* (103). A major role for NK cells in the early IFN-γ production and in the generation of Th-1 cells in response to *L. major* infection in resistant mouse strain, e.g., C3H, has been suggested by the finding that depletion of NK cells by anti-aGM1 induces decreased IFN-γ levels and promotes IL-4 production in both lymph nodes and spleen of these infected mice, resulting in enhanced disease as measured by parasite number and lesion development (106). In several experimental systems, it has been shown that the enhancing effect of IL- 12 on Th-1 responses is dependent on production of IFN-γ and on the presence of NK cells, possibly needed for the early production of IFN-γ. In particular, depletion of NK cells in vitro prevented the ability of IL-12 to induce Th-1 cell generation in cultures of peripheral blood lymphocytes from atopic patients stimulated with allergens (102) and in vivo prevented the ability of IL-12 to act as a potent Th-1 inducing adjuvant in the vaccination of BALB/c mice with *L. major* soluble antigen (103).

The importance of phagocytic cells and NK cells in determining the characteristics of the Th response during antigenic stimulation indicated that the mechanisms of innate resistance have a determining influence on the subsequent antigen-specific immune response: IL-12 appears to have a key role in mediating the interaction between phagocytic cells, NK cells, and T lymphocytes in these processes (101,107).

VIII. MODULATION OF HEMATOPOIESIS BY NK CELLS

The first suggestion of a role of NK cells in hematopoiesis came from the studies of Cudkowicz and collaborators (60,108–110) on the phenomenon of hybrid resistance to parental bone marrow transplantation. Parental hematopoietic tumors or bone marrow grafts do not survive in lethally irradiated F1 mice, even if these animals accept grafts of skin or any other type of parental tissue. The characteristics of the effector cells mediating hybrid resistance suggested their identity with NK cells (60). On the basis of these observations, Cudkowicz and Hochman (110) in 1979 originally postulated the hypothesis that NK cells might "engage in regulated reactions against self to ensure homeostasis." The hybrid resistance phenomenon has been, however, difficult to reproduce in vitro. In one study (111), purified murine NK cells from F1 animals have been shown to suppress parental CFU-GM colony formation somewhat more efficiently than syngeneic colony formation, but this complex experimental system was not amenable to a detailed genetic study. Fresh or activated NK cells from athymic rats lyse and inhibited colony formation by allogeneic hematopoietic progenitor cells but stimulated syngeneic hematopoiesis (112).

When purified preparations of polyclonal human NK cells are added to bone marrow cells or enriched preparations of peripheral blood hematopoietic progenitor cells, a significant although often incomplete inhibition of hematopoietic colony formation is observed (113,114). Even when highly enriched preparations of hematopoietic progenitor cells were used as target cells, NK-cell–mediated cytolysis of the progenitor cells could not be demonstrated (114). Rather, during incubation of NK cells with hematopoietic progenitor cell preparations, production of low levels of TNF was observed and neutralizing antibodies against TNF were shown to prevent the suppressive effect of NK cells on hematopoietic colony formation (115). These studies indicated that polyclonal NK-cell preparations in vitro inhibit hematopoietic colony formation by secreting TNF and, in some conditions, IFN-γ, a cytokine that synergizes with TNF in inhibiting colony formation (115–117). This nonspecific suppressive effect of NK cells was observed using NK cells either autologous or allogeneic to the hematopoietic progenitor cells: thus, this in vitro model of NK cells suppression of hematopoiesis did not reproduce the genetic specificity observed in the murine hybrid resistance phenomenon (113,114).

Although there is no evidence for a hybrid resistance phenomenon in humans, recent reports documenting the ability of mixed lymphocyte culture (MLC)-derived $CD3^-$, $CD16^+$ clones to specifically lyse PHA-induced blasts generated from the stimulating donor and a proportion of allogeneic donors but not those generated from autologous donors (118) point to the existence of a strikingly similar system. So far, at least five distinct NK allospecificities have been identified (119,120). The specificity of the alloreactive NK cells has been investigated in many recent studies; as discussed above, a variety of receptor molecules have been identified on NK cells that recognize specific class I HLA antigens and which, upon triggering deliver a negative signal preventing the activation of the cytotoxic mechanism (71). Human alloreactive NK clones are able to recognize allogeneic hematopoietic progenitor cells and significantly and often completely suppress colony formation by purified peripheral blood hematopoietic progenitor cells from susceptible donors (121). The alloreactive NK clones produced cytokines with a suppressive effect on in vitro hematopoiesis, such as IFN-γ and TNF-α, when exposed to hematopoietic cells from susceptible but not from resistant donors. However, the mechanism by which alloreactive NK cells inhibit colony formation is more consistent with a direct cytotoxic effect than with the production of inhibitory cytokines because antibodies (anti-IFN-γ, TNF-α, and lymphotoxin), which completely blocked the inhibition by polyclonal NK cells, had only a minimal effect on the inhibition by the alloreactive clones. Thus, alloreactive NK cells are likely the human counterpart of the cells mediating murine hybrid resistance, and these cells might play clinically important roles in rejection or in GVL reactions following allogeneic bone marrow transplantation (121).

NK cells, constitutively or upon activation, not only produce lymphokines with mostly inhibitory effects on hematopoiesis, such as TNF and IFN-γ, but also some with mostly positive effects, such as GM-CSF, M-CSF, and IL-3 (77,78). In vivo depletion of NK cells by treatment of mice with anti-NK cell antibodies demonstrated a differential effect of NK cells on various lineages. NK-cell depletion in normal mice increases phagocytopoiesis and decreases erythropoiesis and megakaryocytopoiesis (122,123). Consistent with these results, in mice receiving myelosuppressive irradiation, depletion of NK cells results in faster recovery of phagocytopoiesis and slower recovery of megakaryocytopoiesis and erythropoiesis (124).

Clinical evidence for a role of NK cells in the regulation of human hematopoiesis is provided by the demonstration that NK cells are the effector cells mediating suppression of hematopoiesis in some cases of acquired aplastic anemia, in both acute and chronic monoclonal NK lymphocytosis, and possibly in other clinical conditions (125). In vitro studies have shown that NK cells have a prevalent inhibitory effect on colony formation from hematopoietic progenitor cells (113,115). However, NK cells enhance formation of megakaryocytic colonies and, in some experimental conditions, of erythroid and granulocyte-macrophage colonies (78,126). The effect of NK cells is mostly mediated by secretion of humoral factors and may require the participation of accessory cells (115).

Although NK cell depletion in irradiated animals before both syngeneic and allogeneic bone marrow transplantation has been shown to enhance survival and hematopoietic recovery (127), in mice, donor-type activated NK cells promote both syngeneic and allogeneic bone marrow engraftment and B-cell development (128–130); these experimental findings suggest that NK cells may replace T cells in favoring engraftment when T-cell–depleted bone marrow is used in clinical transplantation.

After bone marrow transplantation, NK cells are the first lymphocyte population to reconstitute the patient (131,132). The engraftment of donor NK cells is observed also in SCID infants who have not been conditioned by cytoreductive treatment before transplantation, even when significant NK-cell function is present before transplantation (133). The pretransplant irradiation therapy in conditioned patients does not immediately abrogate NK activity, but the ability of their cells to maintain cytotoxic activity against NK-sensitive target cells or to generate activity against tumor cells during the culture in the presence of IL-2 is completely suppressed, suggesting a complete block in the proliferative ability of both NK cells and their more mature precursor cells (134). After transplantation, NK cells and LGL appear, both in humans (134) and in experimental animals (135), already at 1 week, and their number and activity increase to a peak at 30 to 50 days, slightly declining thereafter to normal or slightly subnormal levels (132,135). The appearance of NK cells precedes that of any other lymphocyte type and, at 20 to 30 days, NK cells may represent 50 to 90% of all peripheral lymphocytes (136). The appearance of cytotoxic NK cells parallels that of IL-2–inducible cytotoxic cells (134). The cytotoxic NK cells in the recipient are in an activated state, as suggested by their blastlike appearance and their ability to lyse efficiently not only the NK-sensitive K562 cells but also NK-resistant Daudi cells, tumor cells, and fresh leukemia cells (134,137). Acute graft-versus-host disease (GVHD) has been associated with an accelerated and elevated recovery of NK cytotoxic activity (138,139). These findings—together with a significant increase in the number of $CD16^+$ $CD3^-$ NK lymphocytes in the skin and patients with acute GVHD (140) and the ability of human activated NK cells to induce acute GVHD when transplanted into SCID mice (141)—suggest the possibility that NK cells and the cytokines released by NK cells, such as IFN-γ and TNF-α, may play a central role in the pathogenesis of clinical acute GVHD (141).

Because activated NK cells from patients with acute GVHD have been shown to have cytotoxic activity against leukemia cells, it is possible that one of the mechanisms by which GVHD augments the GVL effect involves the secondary activation of NK cells by cytokine released during the GVHD process (138,139).

IX. PATHOLOGICAL ALTERATIONS IN NK-CELL NUMBER AND FUNCTIONS

The NK cell function and in some cases the number of NK cells are often decreased in pathological conditions, e.g., the already mentioned depression observed in cancer patients and the severely depressed cytotoxic and cytokine production functions observed in patients with acquired immunodeficiency syndrome (AIDS) (94,142). The reduced activity or number of NK cells in patients may be secondary to altered hematological functions and cytokine production, but it may also contribute to the pathology of the disease, e.g., decreasing the innate resistance against tumor growth and metastasis in cancer patients or against opportunistic infections in AIDS patients. A complete congenital absence of NK cells is extremely rare and has been described only in a minute number of patients; it is characterized by a pathology of recurrent severe viral infections (82). A specific NK hyporesponsiveness is observed in patients with Chediak-Higashi syndrome (143), a rare autosomal recessive disease associated with cellular dysfunction, including fusion of cytoplasmic granules and defective degranulation of neutrophil lysosomes. NK cells in these patients are normal in number but present a single large granule in the cytoplasm and have a severely reduced ability to mediate cytotoxicity (143).

Malignant acute expansion of NK cells is quite rare and acute lymphocytic leukemia with phenotypic and genotypic characteristics of NK cells, including ability to mediate cytotoxicity, was described in a small group of children and adult patients (144). More commonly observed is a chronic monoclonal proliferative disorder of large granular lymphocytes with a clinical course that is often relatively benign (145). Most patients have lymphocytic infiltration of the bone marrow, and severe neutropenia and anemia are often observed. Associated diseases, most commonly rheumatoid arthritis, hepatitis, or cancer, are present in up to half of the patients (145). Although cells from all these patients are characterized by a morphology of LGL, in approximately two-thirds of the cases they represent a monoclonal expansion of $CD8^+$ T cells; in only less than one-third do they have the typical phenotype and genotype of $CD3^-$ $CD56^+$ and, in some patients, $CD16^+$ NK cells (145).

REFERENCES

1. Takasugi M, Mickey MR, Terasaki PI. Reactivity of lymphocytes from normal persons on cultured tumor cells. Cancer Res 1973; 33:2898–2902.
2. Trinchieri G. Biology of natural killer cells. Adv Immunol 1989; 47:187–376.
3. Pappenheim A, Ferrata A. Uber die verschiedenen lymphoiden Zellformen des normalen und pathologischen Blutes. Folia Haemat 1911; 10:78.
4. Timonen T, Ortaldo JR, Herberman RB. Characteristics of human large granular lymphocytes and relationship to natural killer and K cells. J Exp Med 1981; 153:569–582.
5. Ortaldo JR, Winkler-Pickett R, Kopp W, et al. Relationship of large and small $CD3^-$

CD56^{+} lymphocytes mediating NK-associated activties. J Leuk Biol 1992; 52:287–295.
6. Grossi CE, Cadoni A, Zicca A, et al. Large granular lymphocytes in human peripheral blood:ultrastructural and cytochemical characterization of granules. Blood 1982; 59: 277–283.
7. Caulfield JP, Hein A, Schmidt RE, et al. Ultrastructural evidence that the granules of human natural killer cell clones store membrane in a nonbilayer phase. Am J Pathol 1987; 127:305–316.
8. Young JD, Cohn ZA. Cellular and humoral mechanisms of cytotoxicity: Structural and functional analogies. Adv Immunol 1987; 41:269.
9. Payne CM, Glasser L. Evaluation of surface markers on normal human lymphocytes containing parallel tubular arrays: A quantitative ultrastructural study. Blood 1981; 57:567–573.
10. Hochman PS, Cudkowicz G, Dausset J. Decline of natural killer cell activity in sublethally irradiated mice. J Natl Cancer Inst 1978; 61:265–268.
11. Miller SC. Production and renewal of murine killer cells in the spleen and bone marrow. J Immunol 1982; 129:2282–2286.
12. Biron CA, Turgiss LR, Welsh RM. Increase in NK cell number and turnover rate during acute viral infection. J Immunol 1983; 131:1539–1545.
13. Schmidt RE, MacDermott RP, Bartley G, et al. Specific release of proteoglycans from human natural killer cells during target lysis. Nature 1985; 318:289–291.
14. Schmidt RE, Michon JM, Woronicz J, et al. Enhancement of natural killer function through activation of the T11 E rosette receptor. J Clin Invest 1987; 79:305–308.
15. Perussia B, Fanning V, Trinchieri G. A human NK and K cell subset shares with cytotoxic T cell expression of the antigen recognized by antibody OKT8. J Immunol 1983; 131:223–231.
16. Baume DM, Caligiuri MA, Manley TJ, et al. Differential expression of CD8α and CD8β associated with MHC-restricted and non-MHC-restricted cytolytic effector cells. Cell Immunol 1990; 131:352–359.
17. Lanier LL, Spits H, Phillips JH. The developmental relationship between NK cells and T cells. Immunol Today 1992; 13:392–395.
18. Fagioli M, Care A, Ciccone E, et al. Molecular heterogeneity of the 1.0-kb T beta transcript in natural killer and gamma/delta lymphocytes. Eur J Immunol 1991; 21: 1529–1534.
19. Biassoni R, Verdiani S, Cambiaggi A, et al. Human CD3^{-} CD16^{+} natural killer cells express the hGATA-3 T cell transcription factor and an unrearranged 2.3-kb TcR δ transcript. Eur J Immunol 1993; 23:1083–1087.
20. Rodewald HR, Moingeon P, Lucich JL, et al. A population of early fetal thymocytes expressing Fc gamma RII/III contains precursors of T lymphocytes and natural killer cells. Cell 1992; 69:139–150.
21. Haller O, Wigzell H. Suppression of natural killer cell activity with radioactive strontium: Effector cells are marrow dependent. J Immunol 1977; 118:1503–1506.
22. Kumar V, Ben-Ezra J, Bennett M, et al. Natural killer cells in mice treated with 89 strontium: Normal target-binding cell numbers but inability to kill even after interferon adminstration. J Immunol 1979; 123:1832–1838.
23. Levy EM, Kumar V, Bennett M. Natural killer activity and suppressor cells in irradiated mice repopulated with a mixture of cells from normal and 89Sr-treated mice. J Immunol 1981; 127:1428–1432.
24. Haller O, Kiessling R, Orn A, et al. Generation of natural killer cells: An autonomous function of the bone marrow. J Exp Med 1977; 145:1411–1416.
25. Roder JC. The beige mutation in the mouse: I. A stem cells predetermined impairment in natural killer cell function. J Immunol 1979; 123:2168–2173.
26. Hackett J, Tutt M, Lipscomb M, et al. Origin and differentiation of natural killer

cells: II. Functional and morphologic studies of purified NK1.1+ cells. J Immunol 1986; 136:3124–3131.
27. Seaman WE, Gindhart TD, Greenspan JS, et al. Natural killer cells, bone, and the bone marrow: Studies in estrogen-treated mice and in congenitally osteopetrotic (mi/mi). J Immunol 1979; 122:2541–2547.
28. Miller JS, Verfaillie C, McGlave P. The generation of human natural killer cells from CD34+/DR-primitive progenitors in long-term bone marrow culture. Blood 1992; 80: 2182–2187.
29. Miller JS, Alley KA, McGlave P. Differentiation of natural killer (NK) cells from human primitive marrow progenitors in a stroma-based long-term culture system: Identification of a $CD34^{+}7^{+}$ NK progenitor. Blood 1994; 83:2594–2601.
30. Lotzova E, Savary CA, Champlin RE. Genesis of human oncolytic natural killer cells from primitive $CD34^{+}$ $CD33^{-}$ bone marrow progenitors. J Immunol 1993; 150:5263–5269.
31. Herberman RB, Nunn MF, Lavrin DH. Natural cytotoxic reactivity of mouse lymphoid cells against syngeneic and allogeneic tumors: II. Characterization of effector cells. Int J Cancer 1975; 16:230.
32. Lotzova E, Savary CA, Gray KN, et al. Natural killer cell profile of two random-bred strains of athymic rats. Exp Hematol 1984; 12:633–640.
33. Sirianni MC, Businco L, Seminara R, et al. Severe combined immunodeficiencies, primary T-cell defects and DiGeorge syndrome in human: characterization by monoclonal antibodies and natural killer cell activity. Clin Immunol Immunopathol 1983; 28:361–370.
34. Phillips JH, Hori T, Nagler A, et al. Ontogeny of human natural killer (NK) cells: Fetal NK cells mediate cytolytic function and express cytoplasmic CD3 epsilon, delta proteins. J Exp Med 1992; 175:1055–1066.
35. Poggi A, Sargiacomo M, Biassoni R, et al. Extrathymic differentiation of T lymphocytes and natural killer cells from human embryonic liver precursors. Proc Natl Acad Sci USA 1993; 90:4465–4469.
36. Torten M, Sidell N, Golub SH. Interleukin 2 and stimulator lymphoblastoid cells induce human thymocytes to bind and kill K562 targets. J Exp Med 1982; 156:1545–1550.
37. Toribio ML, De Landazuri MO, Lopez-Betet M. Induction of natural killer-like cytotoxicity in cultured human thymocytes. Eur J Immunol 1983; 13:964–969.
38. Michon JM, Caligiuri MA, Hazanow SM, et al. Induction of natural killer effectors from human thymus with recombinant IL-2. J Immunol 1988; 140:3660–3667.
39. Denning SM, Jones DM, Ware RE, et al. Analysis of clones derived from human $CD7^{+}CD4^{-}CD8^{-}CD3^{-}$ thymocytes. Int Immunol 1991; 3:1015–1024.
40. Sanchez MJ, Spits H, Lanier LL, et al. Human natural killer cell committed thymocytes and their relation to the T cell lineage. J Exp Med 1993; 178:1857–1866.
41. Perussia B, Starr S, Abraham S, et al. Human natural killer cells anlayzed by B73.1, a monoclonal antibody blocking Fc receptor functions: I. Characterization of the lymphocyte subset reactive with B73.1. J Immunol 1983; 130:2133–2141.
42. Bouwens L, Wisse E. Pit cells in the liver. Liver 1992; 12:3–9.
43. Weissler JC, Nicod LP, Lipscomb MF, et al. Natural killer cell function in human lung is compartmentalized. Am Rev Respir Dis 1987; 135:941–949.
44. Starkey PM, Sargent IL, Redmann CWG. Cell populations in human early pregnancy decidua: Characterization and isolation of large granular lymphocytes by flow cytometry. Immunology 1988; 65:129–134.
45. Blomgren H, Baral E, Edsmyr F, et al. Natural killer activity in peripheral lymphocyte population following local radiation therapy. Acta Radiol Oncol Radiat Phys Biol 1980; 19:139–143.

46. Brovall C, Schacter B. Radiation sensitivity of human natural killer cell activity: Control by x-linked genes. J Immunol 1981; 126:2236–2239.
47. Dean DM, Pross HF, Kennedy JC. Spontaneous human lymphocyte-mediated cytoxicity against tumor target cells: III. Stimulating and inhibitory effects of ionizing radiaiton. Int J Radiat Oncol Biol Phys 1978; 4:633–641.
48. Gorelik E, Herbermann RB. Depression of natural antitumor resistance of C57BL/6 mice by leukemogenic doses of radiation and restoration of resistance by transfer of bone marrow or spleen cells from normal, but not beige, syngeneic mice. J Natl Cancer Inst 1982; 69:89–93.
49. Socinski MA, Ershler WB, Tosato G, et al. Pure red blood cell aplasia with chronic Epstein-Barr virus infection: Evidence for T-cell mediated suppression of erythroid colony-forming units. J Lab Clin Med 1984; 104:995–1006.
50. Parkinson DR, Brightman RP, Waksal SD. Altered natural killer cell biology in C57BL/6 mice after leukemogenic split-dose irradiation. J Immunol 1981; 126:1460–1464.
51. Pollack SB, Rosse C. The primary role of murine bone marrow in the production of natural killer cells: A cytokinetic study. J Immunol 1987; 139:2149–2156.
52. Yokoyama WM. Recognition structures on natural killer cells. Cur Opinion Immunol 1993; 5:67–73.
53. Ravetch JV, Perussia B. Alternative membrance forms of FcγRIII(CD16) on human NK cells and neutrophils: Cell-type specific expression of two genes which differ in single nucleotide substitutions. J Exp Med 1989; 170:481–497.
54. Pignata C, Prasad KVS, Robertson MJ, et al. FcγRIIIA-mediated signaling involves src-family lck in human natural killer cells. J Immunol 1993; 151:6794–6800.
55. Trinchieri G, Santoli D. Antiviral activity induced by culturing lymphocytes with tumor-derived or virus-transformed cells: Enhancement of human natural killer cell activity by interferon and antagonistic inhibition of susceptibility of target cells to lysis. J Exp Med 1978; 147:1314–1333.
56. Trinchieri G, Matsumoto-Kobayashi M, Clark SC, et al. Response of resting human peripherial blood natural killer cells to interleukin-2. J Exp Med 1984; 160:1147–1169.
57. Kobayashi M, Fitz L, Ryan M, et al. Identification and purification of natural killer cell stimulatory factor (NKSF), a cytokine with multiple biologic effects on human lymphocytes. J Exp Med 1980; 170:827–846.
58. London L, Perussia B, Trinchieri G. Induction of proliferation in vitro of resting human natural killer cells: IL-2 induces into cell cycle most peripheral blood NK cells, but only a minor subset of low density T cells. J Immunol 1986; 137:3845–3854.
59. Caligiuri MA, Murray C, Robertson MJ, et al. Selective modulation of human natural killer cells in vivo after prolonged infusion of low dose recombinant interleukin 2. J Clin Invest 1993; 91:123–132.
60. Kiessling R, Hochman PS, Haller O, et al. Evidence for a similar or common mechanism for natural killer cell activity and resistance to hemopoietic grafts. Eur J Immunol 1977; 7:655–663.
61. Yu YY, Kumar V, Bennett M. Murine natural killer cells and marrow graft rejection. Ann Rev Immunol 1992; 10:189–213.
62. Rolstad B, Wonigeit K, Vaage JT. Alloreactive rat natural killer (NK) cells in vivo and in vitro: The role of the major histocompatibility complex (MHC). In: Rolstad B, ed. Natural Immunity to Normal Hematopoietic Cells. Boca Raton, FL: CRC Press, 1994: 99–149.
63. Ljunggren HG, Karre K. Experimental strategies and interpretations in the analysis of changes in MHC gene expression during tumour progression: Opposing influences of T cell and natural killer mediated resistance? J Immunogenet 1986; 13:141.
64. Storkus WJ, Salter RD, Alexander J, et al. Class I-induced resistance to natural

killing: Identification of nonpermissive residues in HLA-A2. Proc Natl Acad Sci USA 1991; 88:5989–5992.
65. Kaufman DS, Schoon RA, Leibson PJ. Role for major histocompatibility complex class I in regulating natural killer cell-mediated killing of virus-infected cells. Proc Natl Acad Sci USA 1992; 89:8337–8341.
66. Karlhofer FM, Ribaudo RK, Yokoyama WM. MHC class I alloantigen specificity of Ly-49$^+$ IL-2-activated natural killer cells. Nature 1992; 358:66–70.
67. Kane KP. Ly-49 mediates IL 4 lymphoma adhesion to isolated class I major histocompatibility complex molecules. J Exp Med 1994; 179:1011–1015.
68. Yokoyama WM, Seaman WE. The Ly-49 and NKR-P1 gene families encoding lectin-like receptors on natural killer cells: The NK gene complex. Annu Rev Immunol 1993; 11:613–635.
69. Aubry J-P, Pochon S, Graber P, et al. CD21 is a ligand for CD23 and regulates IgE production. Natura 1992; 358:505–507.
70. Bezouska K, Yuen C, O'Brien J, et al. Oligosaccharide ligands for NKR-P1 protein activate NK cells and cytotoxicity. Nature 1994; 372:150–157.
71. Trinchieri G. Recognition of class I major histocompatibility complex antigens by natural killer cells. J Exp Med 1994; 180:417–421.
72. Moretta L, Ciccone E, Mingari MC, et al. Human natural killer cells: Origin, clonality, specificity, and receptors. Adv Immunol 1994; 55:341–380.
73. Colonna M, Borsellino G, Falco M, et al. HLA-C is the inhibitory ligand that determines dominant resistance to lysis by NK1- and NK2-specific natural killer cells. Proc Natl Acad Sci USA 1993; 90:12000–12004.
74. Moretta A, Vitale M, Sivori S, et al. Human natural killer cell receptors for HLA-class I molecules: Evidence that the Kp43 (CD94) molecule functions as receptor for HLA-B alleles. J Exp Med 1994; 180:545–555.
75. Litwin V, Gumperz J, Parham P, et al. NKB1: A natural killer cell receptor involved in the recognition of polymorphic HLA-B molecules. J Exp Med 1994; 180:537–543.
76. Correa I, Corral L, Raulet DH. Muliple natural killer cell-activating signals are inhibited by major histocompatibility complex class I expression in target cells. Eur J Immunol 1994; 24:1323–1331.
77. Cuturi MC, Anegón I, Sherman F, et al. Production of hemtopoietic colony- stimulating factors by human natural killer cells. J Exp Med 1989; 169:569–583.
78. Murphy WJ, Keller JR, Harrison CL, et al. Interleukin-2-activated natural killer cells can support hematopoiesis in vitro and promote marrow engraftment in vivo. Blood 1992; 80:670–677.
79. Anegón I, Cuturi MC, Trinchieri G, et al. Interaction of Fcγ receptor (CD16) with ligands induces transcription of IL-2 receptor (CD25) and lymphokine genes and expression of their products in human natural killer cells. J Exp Med 1988; 167:452–472.
80. Chan SH, Perussia B, Gupta JW, et al. Induction of IFN-γ production by NK cell stimulatory factor (NKSF): Characterization of the responder cells and synergy with other inducers. J Exp Med 1991; 173:869–879.
81. Welsh RM. Regulation of virus infections by natural killer cells: A review. Natl Immun Cell Growth Regul 1986; 5:169–199.
82. Biron CA, Byron KS, Sullivan JL. Severe herpesvirus infections in an adolescent without natural killer cells. N Engl J Med 1989; 320:1731–1735.
83. Santoli D, Trinchieri G, Koproswki H. Cell-mediated cytotoxicity in humans against virus-infected target cells: II. Interferon induction and activation of natural killer cells. J Immunol 1978; 121:532–538.
84. Bandyopadhyay S, Perussia B, Trinchieri G, et al. Requirement for HLA-DR positive accessory cells in natural killing of cytomegalovirus-infected fibroblasts. J Exp Med 1986; 164:180–195.

85. Garcia-Penarrubia P, Koster FT, Kelley RO, et al. Antibacterial activity of human natural killer cells. J Exp Med 1989; 169:99–114.
86. Newborg MS, North RJ. On the mechanism of T cell independent anti-Listeria resistance in nude mice. J Immunol 1980; 124:571–577.
87. Bancroft GJ, Sheehan KCF, Schreiber RD, et al. Tumor necrosis factor is involved in the T cell-independent pathway of macrophage activation in scid mice. J Immunol 1989; 143:127–130.
88. Sher A, Oswald J, Hieny S, et al. Toxoplasma gondii induces a T-independent IFN-γ response in NK cells which requires both adherent accessory cells and TNF- α. J Immunol 1993; 150:3982–3998.
89. D'Andrea A, Aste-Amezaga M, Valiante NM, et al. Interleukin-10 inhibits human lymphocyte IFN-γ production by suppressing natural killer cell stimulatory factor/interleukin-12 synthesis in accessory cells. J Exp Med 1993; 178:1041–1048.
90. D'Andrea A, Rengaraju M, Valiante NM, et al. Production of natural killer cell stimulatory factor (NKSF/IL-12) by peripheral blood mononuclear cells. J Exp Med 1992; 176:1387–1398.
91. Tripp CS, Wolf SF, Unanue ER. Interleukin 12 and tumor necrosis factor alpha are costimulators of interferon gamma production by natural killer cells in severe combined immunodeficiency mice with listeriosis, and interleukin 10 is a physiologic antagonist. Proc Natl Acad Sci USA 1993; 90:3725–3729.
92. Gazzinelli RT, Hieny S, Wynn TA, et al. Interleukin-12 is required for the T- lymphocyte independent induction of interferon-γ by an intracellular parasite and induces resistance in T-deficient hosts. Proc Natl Acad Sci USA 1993; 90:6115–6119.
93. Bloom BR. Natural killers to rescue immune surveillance? Nature 1982; 300:214–215.
94. Pross HF. Natural killer cell activity in human malignant disease. In: Lotzova E, Herberman RB, eds. Natural Immunity, Cancer and Biological Response Modification. Basel, Switzerland: Karger, 1986:196–205.
95. Schantz SP, Brown BW, Lira E, et al. Evidence for the role of natural immunity in the control of metastatic spread of head and neck cancer. Cancer Immunol Immunother 1987; 25:141–148.
96. Pross HF, Sterns E, MacGillis DRR. Natural killer activity in women at "high risk" for breast cancer, with and without benign breast syndrome. Int J Cancer 1984; 34:303.
97. Hauch M, Gazzolo MV, Small T, et al. Anti-leukemia potential of interleukin-2 activated natural killer cells after bone marrow transplantation for chronic myelogenous leukemia. Blood 1990; 75:2250–2262.
98. Drobyski WR, Piaskowski V, Ash RC, et al. Preservation of lymphokine- activated killer activity following T cell depletion of human bone marrow. Transplantation 1990; 50:625–632.
99. Mond JJ, Brunswick M. A role for IFN-gamma and NK cells in immune response to T cell-regulated antigens types 1 and 2. Immunol Rev 1987; 99:105–118.
100. Yuan D, Wilder J, Dang T, et al. Activation of B lymphocytes by NK cells. Int Immunol 1992; 4:1373–1380.
101. Trinchieri G. Interleukin-12 and its role in the generation of T_H1 cells. Immunol Today 1993; 14:335–338.
102. Manetti R, Parronchi P, Giudizi MG, et al. Natural killer cell stimulatory factor (NKSF/IL-12) induces Th1-type specific immune responses and inhibits the development of IL-4 producing Th cells. J Exp Med 1993; 177:1199–1204.
103. Afonso LCC, Scharton TM, Vieira LQ, et al. The adjuvant effect of interleukin- 12 in a vaccine against Leishmania major. Science 1994; 263:235–237.
104. Heinzel FP, Schoenhaut DS, Rerko RM, et al. Recombinant interleukin 12 cures mice infected with Leishmania major. J Exp Med 1993; 177:1505–1509.
105. Sypek JP, Chung CL, Mayor SEH, et al. Resolution of cutaneus leishmaniasis: Inter-

leukin-12 initiates a protective T helper type 1 immune response. J Exp Med 1993; 177: 1797–1802.
106. Scharton TM, Scott P. Natural killer cells are a source of interferon gamma that drives differentiation of CD4+ T cell subsets and induces early resistane to Leishmania major of mice. J Exp Med 1993; 178:567–577.
107. Romagnani S. Induction of T_H1 and T_H2 responses: A key role for the "natural" immune response? Immunol Today 1992; 13:379–381.
108. Cudkowicz G, Stimpfling JH. Deficient growth of C57B1 mouse marrow cells transplanted in F1 hybrid mice: Association with the histocompatibiltiy-2 locus. Immunology 1964; 7:291–306.
109. Cudkowicz G, Bennet M. Peculiar immunobiology of bone marrow allografts: I. Graft rejection by irradiated responder mice. J Exp Med 1971; 134:83–102.
110. Cudkowicz G, Hochman PS. Do natural killer cells engage in regulated reaction against self to ensure homeostasis? Immunol Rev 1979; 44:13–41.
111. Bordignon C, Daley JP, Nakamura I. Hematopoietic histoincompatibility reactions by NK cells in vitro: Model for genetic resistance to marrow grafts. Science 1985; 230: 1398–1401.
112. Rolstad B, Benestad HB. Spontaneous alloreactivity of natural killer (NK) and lymphokine-activated killer (LAK) cells from athymic rats against normal haemic cells: NK cells stimulate syngeneic but inhibit allogeneic haemopoiesis. Immunology 1991; 74:86–93.
113. Hansson M, Beran M, Andersson B, et al. Inhibition of in vitro granulopoiesis by autologous and allogeneic human NK cells. J Immunol 1982; 129:126–132.
114. Degliantoni G, Perussia B, Mangoni L, et al. Inhibition of bone marrow colony formation by human natural killer cells and by natural killer cell-derived colony-inhibiting activity. J Exp Med 1985; 161:1152–1168.
115. Degliantoni G, Murphy M, Kobayashi M, et al. Natural killer (NK) cell-derived hematopoietic colony-inhibiting activity and NK cytotoxic factor: Relationship with tumor necrosis factor and synergism with immune interferon. J Exp Med 1985; 162:1512–1530.
116. Murphy M, Loudon R, Kobayashi M, et al. Gamma interferon and lymphotoxin, released by activated T cells, synergize to inhibit granulocyte-monocyte colony formation. J Exp Med 1986; 164:263–279.
117. Murphy M, Perussia B, Trinchieri G. Effects of recombinant tumor necrosis factor, lymphotoxin and immune interferon on proliferation and differentiation of enriched hematopoietic precursor cells. Exp Hematol 1988; 16:131–138.
118. Ciccone E, Viale O, Pende D, et al. Specific lysis of allogeneic cells after activation of $CD3^-$ lymphocytes in mixed lymphocyte culture. J Exp Med 1988; 168:2403–2408.
119. Moretta A, Bottino C, Pende D, et al. Identification of four subsets of human $CD3^-$ $CD16^+$ natural killer (NK) cells by the expression of clonally distributed functional surface molecules: Correlation between subset assignment of NK clones and ability to mediate specific alloantigen recognition. J Exp Med 1990; 172:1589–1598.
120. Ciccone E, Pende D, Viale O, et al. Evidence of a natural killer (NK) repertoire for (allo)antigen recognition: Definition of five distinct NK-determined allospecificities in humans. J Exp Med 1992; 175:709–718.
121. Nunès J, Klasen S, Ragueneau M, et al. CD28 mAbs with distinct binding properties differ in their ability to induce T cell activation: Analysis of early and late activation events. Int Immunol 1992; 5:311–315.
122. Hansson M, Petersson M, Koo GC, et al. In vivo function of natural killer cells as regulators of myeloid precursor cells in the spleen. Eur J Immunol 1988; 18:485–488.
123. Pantel K, Nakeff A. Differential effect of natural killer cells on modulating CFU- Meg and BFU-E proliferation in situ. Exp Hematol 1989; 17:1017–1021.

124. Pantel K, Boertman J, Nakeff A. Inhibition of hematopoietic recovery from radiation-induced myelosuppression by natural killer cells. Radiat Res 1990; 122:168–171.
125. Trinchieri G. Natural killer cells inhæmatopoiesis. In: Lewis CE, McGee J O'D, eds. The Natural Immune System: Natural Killer Cells, vol. 1. Oxford, England: Oxford University Press, 1992:41–65.
126. Gewirtz AM, Xu WY, Mangan KF. Role of natural killer cells, in comparison with T lymphocytes and monocytes, in the regulation of normal human megakaryocytopoiesis in vitro. J Immunol 1987; 139:2915–2924.
127. Tiberghien P, Longo DL, Wine JW, et al. Anti-asialo GM1 antiserum treatment of lethally irradiated recipients before bone marrow transplantation: Evidence that recipient natural killer depletion enhances survival, engraftment, and hematopoietic recovery. Blood 1990; 76:1419–1430.
128. Murphy WJ, Keller JR, Harrison CL, et al. Interleukin-2-activated natural killer cells can support hematopoiesis in vitro and promote marrow engraftment in vivo. Blood 1992; 80:670–677.
129. Murphy WJ, Bennet M, Kumar V, et al. Donor-type activated natural killer cells promote marrow engraftment and B cell development during allogeneic bone marrow transplantation. J Immunol 1992; 148:2953–2960.
130. Siefer Ak, Longo DL, Harrison CL, et al. Activated natural killer cells and inteleukin-2 promote granulocytic and megakaryocytic reconstitution after syngeneic bone marrow transplantation in mice. Blood 1993: 82:2577–2584.
131. Rooney CM, Wimperis JZ, Brenner MK, et al. Natural killer cell activity following T-cell depleted allogeneic bone marrow transplantation. Br J Haematol 1986; 62:413–420.
132. Lum LG. The kinetics of immune reconstitution after human marrow transplantation. Blood 1987; 69:369–380.
133. Gaines AD, Schiff SE, Buckley RH. Donor type natural killer cells after haploidentical T cell-depleted bone marrow stem cell transplantation in a patient with adenosine deaminase-deficient severe combined immunodeficiency. Clin Immunol Immunopathol 1991; 60:299–304.
134. Keever CA, Welte K, Small T, et al. Interleukin 2-activated killer cells in patients following transplants of soybean lectin-separated and E rosette-depleted bone marrow. Blood 1987; 70:1893–1903.
135. Hokland M, Jacobsen N, Ellegaard J, et al. Natural killer function following allogeneic bone marrow transplantation: Very early reemergence but strong dependence of cytomegalovirus infection. Transplantation 1988; 45:1080–1084.
136. Ault KA, Antin JH, Ginsburg D, et al. Phenotype of recovering lymphoid cell populations after marrow transplantation. J Exp Med 1985; 161:1483–1502.
137. Hercend T, Takvorian T, Nowill A, et al. Characterization of natural killer cells with antileukemia activity following allogeneic bone marrow transplantation. Blood 1986; 67:722–728.
138. Dokhelar MC, Wiels J, Lipinski M, et al. Natural killer cell activity in human bone marrow recipients: Early reappearance of peripheral natural killer activity in graft-versus-host disease. Transplantation 1981; 31:61–65.
139. Keever CA, Klein J, Leong N, et al. Effect of GVHD on the recovery of NK cell activity and LAK precursors following BMT. Bone Marrow Transplant 1993; 12:289–295.
140. Rhoades JL, Cibull ML, Thompson JS, et al. Role of natural killer cells in the pathogenesis of human acute graft-versus-host disease. Transplantation 1993; 56:113–120.
141. Xun C, Brown SA, Jennings CD, et al. Acute grafte-versus-host-like disease induced by transplantation of human activated natural killer cells into SCID mice. Transplantation 1993; 56:409–417.

142. Chehimi J, Starr S, Frank I, et al. Natural killer cell stimulatory factor (NKSF) increases the cytotoxic activity of NK cells from both healthy donors and HIV-infected patients. J Exp Med 1992; 175:789–796.
143. Haliotis T, Roder J, Klein M, et al. Chediak-Higashi gene in humans: I. Impairment of natural-killer function. J Exp Med 1908; 151:1039–1048.
144. Robertson MJ, Ritz J. Biology and clinical relevance of human natural killer cells. Blood 1990; 76:2421–2438.
145. Reynolds CW, Foon KA. Tγ-lymphoproliferative disorders in man and experimental animals: A review of the clinical, cellular and functional characteristics. Blood 1984; 64:1146–1158.

10

The Immune System: Effector and Target of Graft-Versus-Host Disease

Frances T. Hakim and Crystal L. Mackall
National Cancer Institute
National Institutes of Health
Bethesda, Maryland

I. INTRODUCTION

A. Overview

Over the past two decades allogeneic bone marrow transplantation (BMT) has become a widely accepted treatment for malignancies and lymphohematopoietic failure syndromes. Despite advances in histocompatibility matching and immunosuppressive drugs, however, graft-versus-host disease (GVHD) has continued to a be a common and often lethal complication of marrow transplantation. The interaction of donor cells and host target tissues in GVHD has proven to be a complex conundrum, involving multiple target organs and shifting patterns of cytokines and effector cells. Acute GVHD (AGVHD) not only results in an immediate multiorgan inflammatory syndrome affecting the skin, liver, and digestive tract but also produces a long-term immune deficiency and an increased frequency of chronic GVHD (CGVHD). Initial attempts to prevent GVHD by T depletion have also resulted in increased failure of engraftment and increased leukemic relapse (1,2), with little overall improvement in long-term survival. The general objective of current studies of GVHD, therefore, is to gain a deeper understanding of the T-cell populations, cytokine networks, and cellular interactions of GVHD. These insights may then provide the next generation of treatments that prevent both the inflammation and immune dysfunction of GVHD while retaining its antileukemic efficacy.

Reviewing the pathophysiology of the immune system in GVHD differs in one major regard from analysis of other organ systems: the immune system is both the effector and the major target of GVHD. Hence this chapter focuses first upon the initial steps in acute GVHD: the activation of donor T cells, the expansion of anithost effector populations, and the elaboration of inflammatory cytokines. Second, the factors contributing to the prolonged immune deficiency associated with GVHD are examined: anergy, suppression, and reduced lymphopoiesis. Finally, the immune mechanisms contributing to the long-term functional alterations of chronic GVHD are examined: cytokine shifts and thymic dysfunction.

B. Animal Models of Graft-Versus-Host Disease

In order to review the effects of GVHD on the immune system, both clinical data and experimental models, the latter primarily in mice, are considered. Murine models provide the advantage of consistent inbred populations for comparison of different treatment groups. A broad range of donor/host strain combinations allow comparison of specific major histocompatibility complex (MHC) disparities on a variety of different genetic backgrounds. Specific deficiency mutations, use of antibody depletions in vivo and, most recently, transgenic and knockout strains have focused on specific effector populations and cytokines. Meanwhile, the broad array of recombinant cytokines and antagonists, molecular probes and cellular markers for flow cytometry have provided new insights into the cellular interactions of GVHD.

Two main models have been used to study acute GVHD (AGVHD); variants of these models used to rapidly induce the autoimmune symptoms of CGVHD are described in Section IV. In the first AGVHD model, mice are lethally irradiated (or, less frequently, treated with cyclophosphamide) and receive bone marrow and graded numbers of lymphocytes. Donor and host strain combinations can be chosen that differ at MHC class I or II loci or both, producing a rapidly lethal AGVHD. Alternatively, donor and host strains may be genetically identical at MHC (in mice termed H-2) loci, but of different backgrounds, hence incompatible for multiple minor antigens. As in humans, the latter differences are sufficient to produce a severe, often lethal disorder in many strain combinations, with many of the pathophysiologic characteristics of AGVHD occurring in HLA-identical, allogeneic BMT. GVHD in this model can be tracked by weight loss and mortality as well as by physical symptoms such as facial edema (squinty eyes), hunched posture, ruffled fur, and severe diarrhea. The pathological changes occurring in the skin, gut, and liver in this model correspond to those observed in humans. Many of the immunological characteristics are also comparable, including diminished lymphopoiesis and prolonged T and B cell dysfunction.

The second murine model that has been extensively utilized involves the injection of parental (P_1) splenic lymphocytes into unirradiated, immune competent ($P_1 \times P_2$)F1 adult hosts. This model will be referred to as parent-into-F1 ($P \rightarrow F1$) graft- versus-host reaction (GVHR), rather than GVHD, because the predominant effects are immunological, with minimal morbidity. (This chapter attempts to consistently refer to research done using this model as GVHR, even when the original authors often use the term "GVHD".) This model emphasizes the alloreaction of donor T cells to the "other" parental strain's antigens. The injected donor lymphocytes expand, develop into cytotoxic effectors, and attack the host lymphohematopoietic system, eliminating the host lymphocytes and stem cells (3). Because the initial splenic inoculum contains a high frequency of stem cells (10 to 20% as many as in bone marrow), these progenitor cells concurrently repopulate the host with donor-derived cells (4). Although the host animal receives no radiation or cytoreduction, within 3 to 4 weeks the lymphohematopoietic population becomes >85% donor-derived (3,4). As in irradiated models, there is a prolonged period of T- and B-cell dysfunction, lymphocytic infiltrates in multiple organs, and a markedly increased susceptibility to infection and CGVHD (4–10). Unlike irradiated models, however, AGVHR-associated immune deficiency typically develops only when donor and host differ at both class I and II MHC loci (4,11). Furthermore, despite the injection of as many as 10-fold more lymphocytes as in the irradiated model, mortality is very low. The clinical symptoms of GVHD (hunched posture, diarrhea, extensive weight loss) are rarely observed, and the histopathology of skin and gut is much less severe. Thus, the P $\rightarrow$ F1 GVHR model replicates and may even exaggerate the cellular immune responses of GVHD, yet it escapes the systemic inflammatory symptoms contributing to mortality in AGVHD. This discrepancy in pathology between AGVHR and AGVHD is one of several pieces of data contributing to current views of GVHD mechanisms.

II. AGVHD MECHANISMS: CELLS, CYTOKINES, AND INFLAMMATORY CYCLES

For many years the central paradigm of AGVHD has been that it is a cell-mediated immunological attack of donor T cells against the host. Whereas the T-cell alloresponse remains the core of AGVHD, recent research supports a complex interweaving of other cell populations and cytokines in the multiorgan pathophysiology of AGVHD. Ferrara and Lapp have recently contributed to models that incorporate three elements in the generation of AGVHD: donor T cells, donor (and host) macrophages and NK cells, and inflammatory stimulation from environmental pathogens or preparatory regimens. These three elements interact in a self- perpetuating cycle (Fig. 1). Cell damage from radiation and other components of common preparative regimens cause transient release of inflammatory cytokines, such as IL-1 and TNF-α, and increases the immunogenicity of host antigen presenting cells. Donor T cells responding to host alloantigens release IL-2 and, most important, IFN-γ, which activates macrophages and NK cells. Activated macrophages and NK cells can then be triggered by gut bacteria and by latent infections to release large quantities of inflammatory cytokines and active nitrogen intermediates, a "cytokine storm" (12,13), resulting in local tissue damage in the gut, liver, and skin. The critical aspects of AGVHD are therefore, first, that the donor T-cell population produces T-helper 1 (TH1) cytokines—IL-2 and IFN-γ—in response to host antigens. Second, the main effectors in AGVHD are not cytotoxic T cells but rather NK and proinflammatory macrophages. Finally, inflammatory cytokines released by these cells mediate tissue injury, weight loss, and mortality.

A. Activation of Host-Reactive Donor TH1 Cells Is Central to AGVHD

1. T-Cell Depletion Prevents GVHD

Donor T cells are indisputably necessary to induce GVHD. T-cell depletion from the donor inoculum has effectively prevented GVHD in clinical and murine studies. Recent studies have addressed effects of both marrow depletion or in vivo depletion of CD3, CD5, CD6, CD52, CD90 (Thy 1), TCR-$\alpha\beta$ expressing cells (1,14–16). (see also Chap. 23.)

Depletion studies have further determined that different T-cell subsets may be involved, depending upon the genetic disparity of donor and host. Depletion of

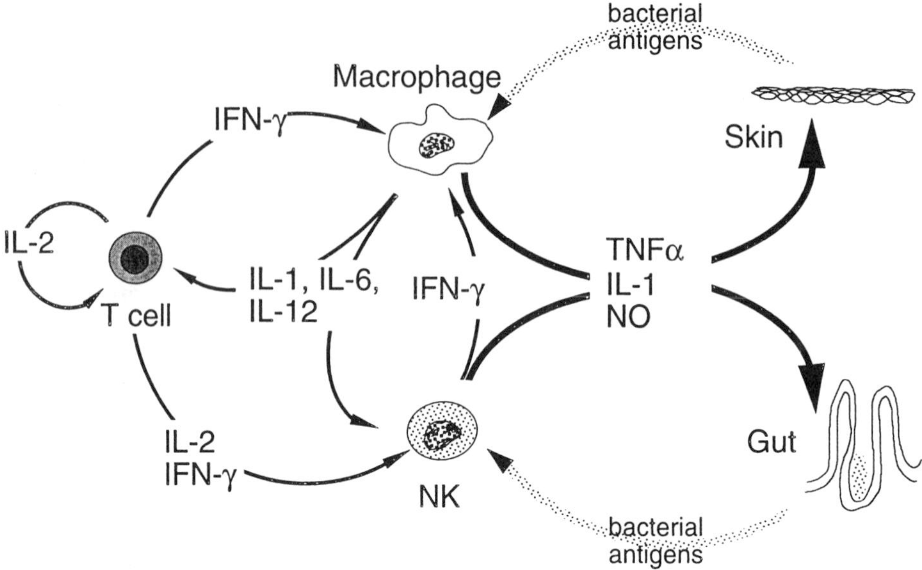

Figure 1 Diagram of the cells and cytokines involved in tissue damage in AGVHD. When donor T cells become activated by host alloantigens, they proliferate and secrete the cytokines IL-2 and IFN-γ, that, in turn, activate NK cells and macrophages. Host macrophages and other antigen-presenting cells secrete IL-1, IL-6, and IL-12, which increase donor T-cell and NK-cell activation and, particularly in the case of IL-12, enhance T-cell production of TH1 cytokines. NK cells and cytotoxic CD8 and CD4 T cells not only directly attack host cells, but also secrete elevated levels of IFN-γ. These elevated levels of IFN-γ result in the development of proinflammatory macrophages and activated NK cells. When these cells are triggered by bacterial or parasitic products, they secrete high titers of IL-1, TNF-α, and NO, resulting in tissue necrosis and systemic toxicity. Whereas the preparatory regimens prior to BMT stimulate the production of IL-1 and TNF-α in the skin and gut, this production is amplified manyfold during AGVHD due to the activation macrophages by IFN-γ and their triggering by local toxins.

$CD4^+$ but not of $CD8^+$ T cells delays or blocks the development of lethal AGVHD across a full MHC disparity (17,18). In donor/host strain combinations matched at class I and mismatched at class II antigens, CD4 T cells are similarly the dominant effectors (19,20); in those mismatched only at class I MHC antigens, in contrast, CD8 T cells are necessary and sufficient and CD4 depletion has little effect on mortality (21). CD8 cells are similarly required for the development of AGVHD in several MHC- matched, minor antigen–mismatched strain combinations (22). CD8 depletion prevents AGVHD; inclusion of CD4 as well as CD8 cells accelerates the development of lethal GVHD, but CD4 depletion alone alters AGVHD in only a few strains (22–24). Recent clinical trials similarly demonstrate a decrease in the frequency and severity of GVHD with CD8 depletion (25). In P → F1 GVHR in unirradiated hosts, in contrast, both CD4 and CD8 cells are necessary to induce an AGVHR; depletion of CD4 prevents the development of AGVHR (3,11,26), whereas depletion of CD8 prevents the development of antihost cytotoxic effectors and converts the reaction into an autoimmune CGVHR (see Section IV).

2. Host-Reactive Donor T Cells Expand Early in GVHD and GVHR

Donor T cells rapidly expand in number in early AGVHD. In patients who go on to develop AGVHD (as compared to those who do not) increased numbers of antihost T-helper precursors (THp) are seen in the first 30 days post-BMT. These persist throughout the clinical course of GVHD and resolve with its resolution. Phenotyping at week 2 after BMT has also shown increased numbers of $CD8^+$ cells in patients which go on to develop GVHD (27). Furthermore, $CD8^+CD3^+$ cells have been identified in lymphocytic infiltrates in the skin of patients undergoing acute GVHD (28,29). In murine marrow transplant models of GVHD, donor CD4 and, particularly, CD8 populations are found in much greater numbers in the host spleen in the first week after allogeneic as compared to syngeneic transplant. In nonlethal GVHR models, donor CD4 make up 15 to 25% of the total CD4 cells in the spleen within 2 days (Fig. 2). Donor CD4 and CD8 cells may comprise more than 50% of the total CD8 cells within 2 weeks (3).

This expansion is due to activation and proliferation of host- reactive donor T cells. Within the first hours of exposure to host alloantigens, donor T cells have become activated. This activation process requires two signals; one from the interaction of the TCR complex with antigen and the second from interaction of pairs of

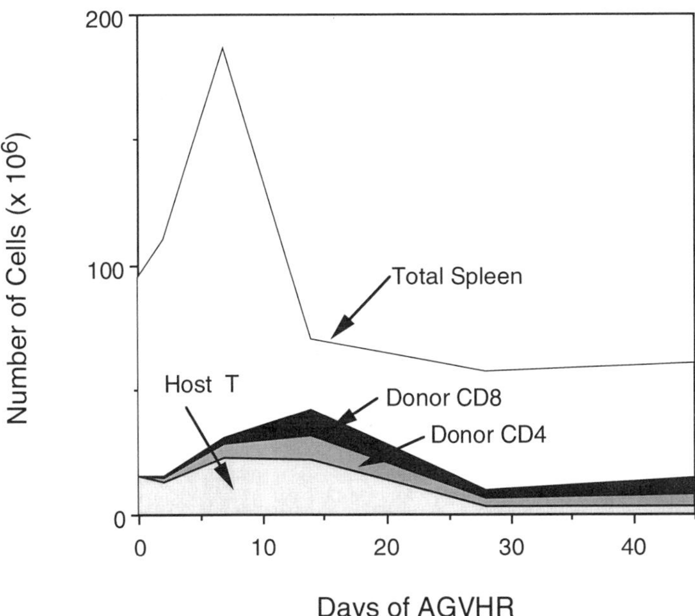

Figure 2 Alterations in donor and host CD4 and CD8 cells during AGVHR. Following injection of donor C57BL/6 (H-2 ^{b}) spleen cells into host B6D2F1 (H-2 $^{b/d}$) mice, donor CD4 (▩) and CD8 (■) cells rapidly increase in the host spleen. After 15 days of AGVHR, the donor CD4 and CD8 cells outnumber the host T-cell population (▢). During this period of cytotoxic attack, host populations and overall splenic cellularity (□) markedly decrease. By 28 to 45 days, not only have most host T cells have been eliminated but donor T cells are significantly reduced in number and remain low for many weeks.

costimulatory molecules located on T cells and antigen-presenting cells (APC) (30). Blockade of these constimulatory interactions reduces the development of GVHD (31–35). Alternatively, the depletion of activated T cells effectively blocks GVHD. Expression of IL-2R is upregulated early in T-cell activation. Depletion of IL-2R$^+$ cells in vivo by an antibody toxin conjugate has reduced GVHD severity in murine models (36); purging of host-reactive donor T cells by preculturing donor and host cells in the presence of anti-IL-2R- immunotoxin has similarly proven effective (37). Treatment with the murine anti-hIL-2R antibody has slightly reduced GVHD frequency in clinical trials (38).

Murine experiments have further identified the expanding T-cell populations as composed primarily of those cells specifically reactive to host antigens. Several of the MHC-matched, minor antigen–mismatched strain combinations used in murine GVHD studies are disparate at mls antigen loci. Mls antigens act as superantigens that stimulate the response of entire Vβ families of T-cell receptor β chains (TCR Vβ) (39). For example, T cells expressing TCR Vβ6 or Vβ8.1 are specifically stimulated by mls^a and Vβ3 cells are stimulated by mls^c. For the first few days after injection of donor lymphocytes into mls^{a+} irradiated hosts, those cells reactive with mls^a (T cells expressing V$\beta6^+$ and V$\beta8.1^+$) disappear from the thoracic duct drainage, the lymphocytic circulation, as they move into tissues and interact with host antigens. After 3 to 5 days the cells reemerge in the thoracic duct in greatly enhanced numbers (40). After 6 to 7 days, 75 to 90% of CD4 cells and more than 50% of the CD8 cells in the spleen express TCR Vβ families reactive to host mls antigens (Fig. 3) (41). Furthermore, these host-reactive cells play a crucial role in AGVHR. Depleting only those T cells expressing host-reactive TCR Vβ populations from the donor inoculum prevents the development of donor/host chimerism and GVHR-associated immune deficiency (42).

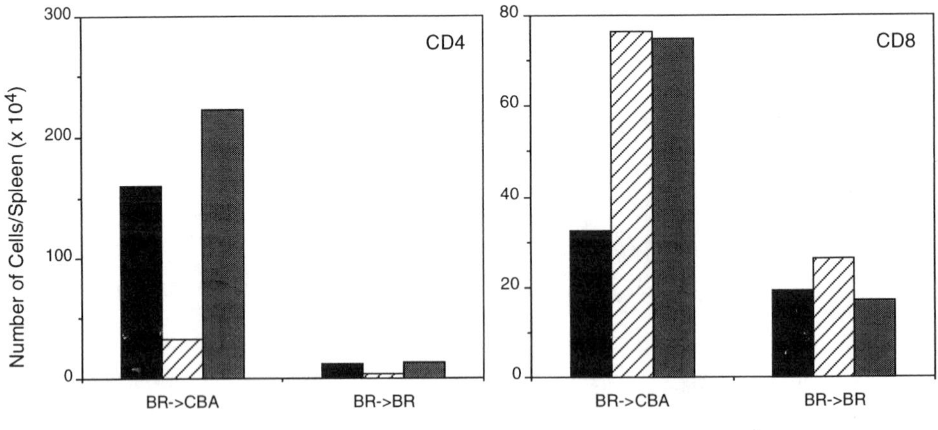

Figure 3 Expansion of host reactive T cells in AGVHD. At 1 week following injection of B10.BR (H-2^k) lymphocytes and bone marrow into irradiated CBA hosts (H-2^k), donor T cells expressing TCR Vβ populations reactive to host mls^{a,c} antigens expand far more than in BMT to syngeneic B10.BR hosts. Most of this expansion is specifically due to cells expressing Vβ3 (▩), Vβ6 (■) and Vβ8.1 (▨).

3. Activated Donor T Cells Produce TH1 Cytokines Crucial for GVHD

Donor T cells activated by host alloantigens elaborate cytokines, principally those associated with the development of the cellular immune response: IL-2 and IFN-γ. This pattern of cytokine production, recently termed the TH1 pattern (43) (see Chap. 17), enhances cell-mediated responses by stimulating cytotoxic T-cell differentiation, macrophase and NK activation, and increased immunogenicity of cells by upregulation of MHC antigens. Presumably these TH1 cytokines are produced by CD4 cells initially, because CD4 cells are the first T-cell subset to expand in the host and are the predominant donor cell at the time of early cytokine production (3). CD8 cells can also be major producers of the TH1 cytokines IL-2 and IFN-γ, particularly relevant in MHC-matched GVHD where CD8 cells are the main effectors. Within 2 days after induction of AGVHR, IL-2 is spontaneously produced and has been measured in unstimulated splenic cultures (44). The period of increased IL-2 production is a brief spike. Neither IL-2 mRNA nor the cytokine itself are detectable after the first week of GVHD (44,45). In contrast, IFN-γ mRNA and cytokine levels remain markedly elevated during the first 2 weeks of AGVHD or AGVHR in unstimulated splenic cells (46,47). Furthermore, these TH1 cells are the dominant population during AGVHD. Using an unusual combination of limiting dilution assay and PCR, Troutt observed that as many as 70% of the lymph node and spleen cells at 5 days of AGVHD produced IFN-γ mRNA when stimulated, compared to $<1\%$ of normal cells (48).

The TH1 cytokines appear to be crucial to the development of GVHD. Altering the cytokine production pattern of the donor cells from a TH1 pattern of IL-2 and IFN-γ production prevents the development of AGVHR and AGVHD (49–51) (see also Chap. 17). Blockade of IL-2 with anti-IL-2 monoclonal antibodies in B6 $\rightarrow$ B6D2F1 mice (an AGVHR model) aborts the development of antihost cytotoxic effectors and profound GVHR-associated immune deficiency (52). Treatment with soluble IFN-γ receptors reduces mortality, weight loss and the rise of serum amyloid protein, an acute-phase reactant that increases in GVHD (53). Exogenous IFN-γ treatment paradoxically also decreases lethal GVHD, but it may do so by decreasing endogenous production of this cytokine (54).

Thus host-reactive TH1 cells are the crucial element in the induction of GVHD. Days prior to the initial appearance of the clinical symptoms of GVHD, donor T cells become activated, secrete cytokines, proliferate, and differentiate into cytolytic effectors. Intervention by depleting T cells from the initial donor inoculum is the most effective means of blocking GVHD. Blockade of costimulatory interactions in activation, depletion of activated cells, or impedance of cytokine activity all substantially diminish the severity of GVHD.

B. Non-T Cells Are Key Effectors in AGVHD

1. NK Cells

Although T cells are central to initiating GVHD, non-T cells play a major role in both the tissue damage of GVHD and in the "cytokine storm," the cascade of inflammatory cytokines that produce systemic effects. One significant non-T population is NK cells. NK cells ($CD56^+$) are actually noted to decrease in the peripheral blood of patients destined to develop AGVHD (27,55). Data suggest, however, that

NK cells are infiltrating the tissues of developing AGVHD lesions. In murine GVHD, large granular lymphocytes (LGL) have been found in association with dead or dying epithelial cells in skin, liver, and colon, whereas CD8 T cells do not produce significant infiltrates in these organs (56). NK infiltrates have also been observed in GVHR associated with tissue damage in the thymus, liver, and pancreas (7,8). An increase in NK activity early in GVHR has been correlated with the development of histopathological lesions in lymphoid and nonlymphoid organs (7,8). When NK-deficient bg/bg mutant mice are used as the donors in GVHR, this early increase in NK activity does not occur and histopathological lesions fail to develop, although splenomegaly and immune dysfunction are still induced (57,58).

Depletion studies differ as to the importance of donor NK cells in determining the severity of GVHD. Depletion of endogenous NK cells from the donor inoculum did not block lethal GVHD in MHC- disparate mice (59), whereas depletion of poly IC-activated NK cells was effective (60,61), as was in vivo depletion during GVHD (62). This variance in results in different systems illustrates the diversity of NK subpopulations, which may be present endogenously or may be elicited by the stimulation of AGVHD.

NK cells are also important because of the cytokines they produce. Activated NK cells produce significant quantities of IFN-γ, which can contribute to the activation of proinflammatory macrophages (63,64). NK cells also produce mediators in common with macrophages that can contribute to the inflammatory response, including TNF-α, IL-1, and NO (65,66).

2. Macrophages

Donor and host macrophages increase in number during the first weeks of AGVHR, possibly in response to elevated production of IL-3 and granulocyte macrophage colony stimulating factor (GM-CSF) (3,5,46,67–69). During the donor repopulation of the lymphohematopoietic system in GVHR, granulocyte-macrophage colony forming units (GM-CFU) appear first in the spleen and later the bone marrow (4,5). Within a week after the rise in GM-CFU, Macl$^+$ cells become a major component of the spleen (3,5). Following allogeneic bone marrow transplantation (BMT), macrophages similarly are among the first populations differentiating from transplanted progenitor cells. Furthermore, macrophages are ubiquitous in affected tissues in GVHD.

Macrophages play a dual role in GVHD. Macrophages serve as APC to activate T cells against host alloantigens. As noted above, this is a crucial first step in the T-cell response. Macrophages activated by T- and NK-cell cytokines, in particular IFN-γ, play a further role as effector cells of GVHD. IFN-γ stimulation causes macrophages to differentiate into a proinflammatory state. When triggered by bacterial products such as endotoxin, these macrophages then secrete high titers of TNF-α, IL-1, IL-6 and NO (68,70) (Hakim and Gazzinelli, in preparation). These factors both increase APC stimulation of T cells and mediate the wasting and tissue damage of GVHD.

C. Inflammatory Cytokines Produce Systemic and Tissue-Specific Damage of GVHD

As noted above, despite involving the injection of 10-fold more donor lymphocytes, GVHR in unirradiated F1 hosts results in far less mortality and histopathological damage to skin, liver, or gut than does allogeneic BMT involving the same strain combinations. A major reason for this contrast may be the lack of a toxic preparative regimen in GVHR. Cytoreductive drugs or radiation immediately preceding injection of allogeneic donor cells result in high mortality, whereas delaying administration of donor T cells for 1 to 3 weeks after cytoxan or radiation significantly reduce lethality (71).

Preparatory regimens stimulate the production of inflammatory cytokines, including TNF-α, IL-1, and IL-6 in the skin, blood, and colon (45,72). The latter two, IL-1 and IL-6, act as cofactors (with antigen) in activating T cells. The differences in T-cell requirements and in reactivity to minor MHC loci in GVHD as opposed to GVHR may be linked to an increase in the immunogenicity of the host cells following lethal irradiation. Furthermore, expression of ICAM-1 is increased on epidermal and fibroblastlike cells within 3 to 4 days after BMT, resulting in an increase in the number of LFA-1$^+$ infiltrating lymphocytes (73). The binding of LFA-1 on T cells to ICAM-1 on APCs is a necessary costimulatory interaction in AGVHD (31). If both T-cell stimulatory cytokines and adhesion factors are increased by the preparatory regimens, then the activation of donor T cells would be enhanced.

Although the tissue damage of preparative regimens may trigger initial production of inflammatory cytokines, these rapidly disappear in the absence of AGVHD (72). Levels are sustained and increase manyfold during AGHVD because the IFN-γ-activated macrophages and NK cells of AGVHD are potent sources of these cytokines. Only low levels of TNF-α, IL-1, IL-6, and nitric oxide (NO) are observed in the serum and in unstimulated splenic supernatants during P → F1 GVHR (68,70,74). When triggered by low levels of LPS or parasite antigens, GVHR macrophages release 10- to 20-fold more of these factors, whereas normal host macrophages do not respond to these triggers (68,70,74) (Hakim and Gazzinelli, in preparation). Thus a synergy can occur between macrophage activation by IFN-γ from alloactivated T cells and macrophage triggering by bacterial and parasitic toxins.

At lower levels of stimulation, inflammatory cytokines may produce damage to those tissues with high concentrations of macrophage-lineage and NK cells and high exposure to pathogens. This circumstance is likeliest to occur in the skin, gut, and liver. All are organs that function as barriers to environmental pathogens. All are damaged by preparative regimens and all are major loci of tissue damage in GVHD. In AGVHD, mRNA for IL-1 and TNF-α increases dramatically in the skin and gut and remains elevated for weeks (45,72). Also consistent with this mechanism is evidence from the B6 → B6D2F1 AGVHR model. Injection of B6 donor spleen cells into B6D2F1 mice produces little mortality or skin pathology. When irradiated F1 skin was transplanted onto the unirradiated F1 host 1 week prior to induction of GVH *reaction* by injection of parental donor cells, only the patch of irradiated skin developed the characteristic lesions of GVH *disease*, including vacuolar degeneration of the epidermal-dermal junction and necrotic keratinocytes, accompanied by pronounce epidermal infiltrates (75). Thus the histopathology of GVHD depends upon both the radiation effects and the T-cell activation of GVHR.

This synergy can result in such high levels of inflammatory cytokines as to cause mortality due to septic shock (70). Early treatment with IL-1 in vivo accelerates GVHD mortality (76), whereas treatment with IL-1 receptor antagonist (IL-1ra) beginning at the time of transplant reduces mortality (77). Furthermore, treatment with IL-1ra beginning after 2 weeks of GVHD, that is, after the observed peak in IL-2 mRNA has passed, nonetheless reduces mortality (45). Similarly, treatment with soluble recombinant human TNF receptor (cross-reactive with one of the two

TNF receptors in mice) reduces GVHD mortality in allotransplanted SCID mice (72). Holler determined that a single injection of anti TNF-α prior to irradiation reduced GVHD mortality from 58 to 17% (78). This early increase in TNF-α has also been observed clinically and correlated with the frequency and severity of GVHD (79). Patients developing elevated levels of TNF-α during the conditioning regimen developed severe AGVHD with only 30% survival, those with increases in the first 90 days had 50% survival, whereas those with normal TNF- α for 90 days had 80% survival (78).

Thus AGVHD is composed to three main elements: the donor TH1 response to host alloantigens, the activation of proinflammatory macrophages and NK cells and the triggering of inflammatory factor release by environmental pathogens or their products.

III. GVHD-ASSOCIATED IMMUNE DEFICIENCY

One of the primary characteristics of GVHD is a profound and long-lasting immune deficiency. Clinically, this immune deficiency is an exacerbation of the predictable immune deficiency observed in all BMT recipients. The latter results from the ablation of host immunity via the preparative regimen followed by delayed reconstitution of immunity from donor marrow. Although many variables have been analyzed to determine what role they play in the immunodeficiency observed, only the time elapsed after BMT and the presence of GVHD have been shown to consistently affect the degree of immune recovery (80,81).

The etiology of GVHD-associated immune deficiency is complex and multifactorial. Clinical observations and data from murine models suggest that, at differing periods after onset of AGVHD, three main factors can contribute to immune deficiency: depletion and anergy of mature host-reactive lymphocytes, nonspecific suppression of lymphocyte function, and deficient lymphopoiesis of new B- and T-cell populations. Part of the complexity is due to the changing profile of lymphocytes during the period of deficiency. Initially after transplant, the main population of lymphocytes present consists of mature host-reactive donor lymphocytes. Immune functions are nonspecifically suppressed during this same period. Newly generated B and T lymphocytes appear, but more slowly than after BMT without AGVHD. Thus the predominant mechanism of immune deficiency may vary during the months of GVHD.

Although the mechanisms may vary, it is striking that the same three elements characterize the immune deficiency of AGVHD as were observed for the tissue damage and morbidity of this disorder. First, host-reactive donor T cells, in particular TH1 cells and the IFN-γ they produce, initiate AGVHD-associated immune deficiency. Second, the effectors are often non-T cells. Finally, cytokines mediate the effects which are therefore primarily MHC-nonspecific.

A. Host-Reactive TH1 Cells Are Deleted or Become Anergic

A paradox of AGVHD is that an immune-mediated disorder is associated with a rapid onset of profound immune deficiency. If donor populations are capable of rapidly responding to host antigens, why are they not capable of responding to in vitro stimulation? In murine models of GVHD, as noted above, the host- reactive cells in the donor T-cell complement expand disproportionately to become as much as 75 to 90% of the T cells present. These expanded populations may fail to respond to antigenic or allogeneic stimulation, because the T-cell repertoire is so sharply skewed toward host-responsive elements. Alternatively, further TCR stimulation may trigger programmed cell death in these host-activated cells. Recent research has demonstrated that activated T cells—including those activated by allogeneic cells—undergo apoptosis when stimulated by reagents cross-linking the T-cell receptor (82). Thus the polyclonal stimulation used in many in vitro assays may be triggering apoptosis rather than the response being assayed in the GVHD donor lymphocytes.

Indeed, evidence suggests that programmed cell death plays a major role in shifts in T-cell populations in vivo GVHD. After an initial expansion in response to host antigens, the donor T-cell population is rapidly reduced. Donor T cells expand severalfold more in allogeneic than in syngeneic BMT, but T-cell numbers in GVHD spleens subsequently decrease. Studies tracking T-cell populations by expression of specific TCR Vβ families suggest that this reduction is due to the development of anergy and clonal deletion of host-reactive cells. When BALB/c cells (H- 2^d; mls^c) are injected into DBA/2 hosts (H- 2^d; mls ^{a,c}), donor cells reactive against host mls^a antigens (TCR V$\beta6^+$) expand to become a 50 to 60% of the donor CD4 T cell repertoire at 1 week. The TCR V$\beta6^+$ population then rapidly decreases both in frequency and in total number until the hosts die at 4 weeks (Fig. 4). Similar experiments with other MHC matched, minor disparate combinations have demonstrated a similar expansion followed by clonal deletion and anergy to TCR Vβ specific stimulation, although the extent of deletion may vary depending on strain (83–86).

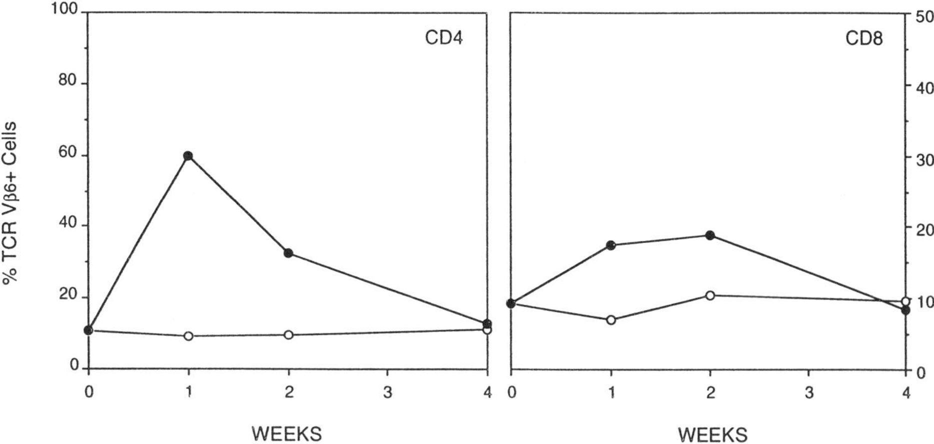

Figure 4 Expansion and deletion of host-reactive T cells in AGVHD .During the first week following injection of BALB/c (H-2^d) lymphocytes and bone marrow into irradiated DBA/2 hosts (H-2^d), the donor T cells expressing TCR Vβ6, that is, those reactive to host mls^a antigens, expanded to 60% of the CD4 T cell repertoire (●). Over subsequent weeks, these T cells diminished in frequency. In syngeneic BALB/c hosts (○), in contrast, the frequency of TCR Vβ6 expressing cells remained constant over time.

Similarly, in AGVHR, the donor T-cell population, both CD4 and CD8 cells, expands in the first weeks. But concurrent with the attack on host populations, the donor T-cell population is drastically reduced (3). In B6 → B6D2F1 GVHR there are fewer donor T cells present after 6 weeks than at 2 days (Fig. 2). The remaining donor T cells are anergic not merely to normal stimulation with mitogens (3) but even in response to PMA and calcium ionophore (87). At 3 to 6 months after induction of GVHR, the T-cell population is primarily derived from mature lymphocytes present in the donor inoculum (88) yet is unable to generate cytotoxic effectors against the host strain (88,89). This unresponsiveness is not due to lack of T-cell help, for it is not corrected by addition of IL-2 (88). Nor is it due to suppressor cells, for normal donor reactivity to host cells in vitro is not suppressed in cocultures (88,89). Furthermore, this tolerance is host-specific, for spleen cells at this point have recovered from AGVHR sufficiently to generate cytotoxic effectors against nonhost allogeneic targets (88,89). This host-specific tolerance is consistent with the development of anergy toward host antigens and/or the peripheral clonal deletion of host-reactive cells from the mature lymphocytes in the original donor inoculum.

B. T- and B-cell Function Is Suppressed

Thus many of the lymphocytes that expand during the initial period of activation and antihost attack in AGVHD may become deleted or anergic to further stimulation. Yet clonal deletion or anergy cannot in itself explain the general state of immune deficiency in GVHD. Indeed, in GVHR models, a rapid loss of host immune function occurs within the first 2 days, when the donor T cells are still a minority. Within 1 week, T and B cell responses in AGVHD and AGVHR are actively suppressed (4). The basic criteria of suppression are a reduction in the T- or B-cell responses of normal host, donor, or allogeneic populations when these are cocultured with AGVHR and AGVHD cells. Some of this suppression may be specific for the host; cytotoxic antihost effectors may reduce the population of host responder cells in these cocultures. Much of the suppression, however, is non-MHC specific.

Three main suppressor populations have been identified, all linked to the initial production of TH1 cytokines: $CD8^+$ T cells, macrophages and natural suppressor (NS) cells (Fig. 5). CD8 suppressor cells have been identified in both murine and clinical studies (90–92). Depletion of CD8 cells from AGVHR spleens reduces the suppression of normal cells in cocultures, whereas depletion of CD4 has little effect (91). In humans, suppression of B-cell function and T-cell proliferation in the setting of acute and chronic GVHD (93,94) has primarily been associated with $CD8^+$ T cells, although CD4 cells have been shown to exert nonspecific suppressor activity as well (95). A specific subpopulation of CD8 T cells, those expressing CD57, have been identified as having suppressor activity (92). This population expands in the post-BMT period, remaining elevated in the peripheral blood of patients with both acute and chronic GVHD for >3 years after BMT (96). These cells are not NK cells; they are negative for the CD16 antigen and do not lyse NK-sensitive targets (97). Recently, proinflammatory macrophages, isolated from the spleens or livers of mice undergoing AGVHD, have also been found to inhibit T- and B-cell responses to mitogens (98,99), particularly when stimulated with LPS

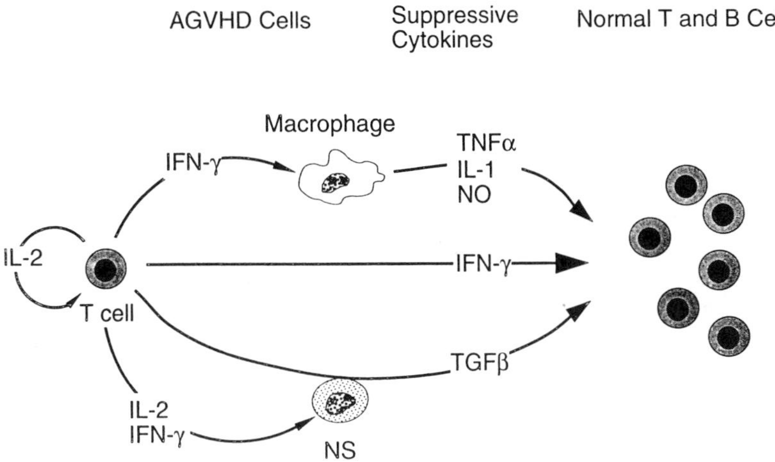

Figure 5 Diagram of immune suppression in AGVHD. The production of IL-2 and IFN-γ by host-reactive donor T cells, particularly CD8 cells, activates macrophages and NS cells. IFN-γ may reduce normal T- and B-cell proliferation directly or may indirectly stimulate production of suppressive factors by activated macrophages (including NO, TNF-α, and IL-1). TGF-β, produced in a latent form by T cells, may be converted into an active suppressor form by NS cells.

(98). The presence of these macrophages, however, is dependent upon CD8 cells; in the absence of CD8 cells, the suppressive macrophages do not appear (98). Finally, NS cells may contribute to suppression in GVHD. NS cells are null cells, lacking NK activity or expression of Thy 1, CD4, CD8, sIg, or macrophage markers (100). These cells appear in the first weeks after marrow transplant and have been demonstrated to inhibit both Con A- and LPS-stimulated proliferation in a non-MHC restricted manner (100–102). While not T cells, NS cells are stimulated by the IL-2 and IFN-γ produced by activated donor T cells in GVHD (103).

The inhibitory function of these suppressor cells is primarily mediated by release of factors rather that a direct attack on target cells. IFN-γ and TGF-β are the main T-cell cytokines that have been implicated. These factors are elevated either in vivo during the course of AGVHD or are produced in elevated levels in cultures of GVHD cells. As noted before, high levels of IFN-γ are present early in AGVHD (46,47); anti-IFN-γ reverses suppression of Con A-stimulated T-cell proliferation (104,105) and somewhat reduces the suppression of LPS stimulated B-cell proliferation (105). TGF-β which is also produced by T cells in AGVHD may affect B cell but not T cell function; anti TGF-β reversed suppression of LPS stimulated proliferation and anti Br-MRBC plaque forming cells (105). Huchet makes the point that neither IFN-γ in the levels produced by GVHD spleen cells, nor TGF-β in the latent form secreted, are able to suppress T- or B-cell function (105). They suggest that these factors either act upon NS cells or are converted by NS cells into a more active form. Thus the suppression could involve interaction of T and NS cells. Additional T-cell-derived factors may be involved; the suppressive factor produced by $CD8^+CD57^+$ cells is an as yet uncharacterized, low-molecular-weight, glycosylated factor distinct from TGF-β or IFN-γ (92,106).

Factors produced by proinflammatory macrophages also play a major role in suppression (Fig. 5). TNF-α, elevated in spleen, peripheral blood, and gut in AGVHD (45,70,72), enhances suppression of Con A–stimulated proliferating cells in cocultures (107). Anti-TNF-α reduces T-cell suppression, but addition of TNF-α to cocultures treated with anti-IFN does not reinstate the suppression (107), suggesting that other IFN- induced mediators are necessary. A possible candidate is NO, which, like TNF-α is a product of IFN-γ–activated macrophages and has been demonstrated to contribute to tissue damage in GVHD (66,74). Blockade of NO synthesis reduces the suppression of the Con A response in GVHD spleen (108). IL-1, another macrophage product elevated in GVHD, may also be involved, in that in vivo treatment with IL-1RA significantly increases the frequency of splenic T cells responsive to mitogens (77). Earlier work by Lapp has also implicated prostaglandins released by macrophages in immune suppression (109).

Thus the mechanisms of suppression of the immune response in GVHD follow a common path with the mechanisms of tissue damage. Suppression is dependent upon IFN-γ production by donor cells, primarily $CD8^+$ T cells, either directly, as suggested by Wall (104), or indirectly via IFN-γ induced development of NS cells and proinflammatory macrophages. The inflammatory cytokines released by these cells, including TNF- α and NO, then modulate the immune responsiveness of T and B cells.

C. Lymphopoiesis and Thymic Maturation Are Diminished and Delayed

The final element contributing to immune deficiency, and indeed the most important one in the prolonged immune deficiency of clinical GVHD, is the alteration in lymphopoiesis (Fig. 6). Whereas suppression is measurable for only the first few weeks in murine GVHR or GVHD (91), repopulation of the host with normal numbers of lymphocytes may require several months (3). Part of this deficit may be related to a decrease in progenitor cells. Both the number and the self-renewal capacity of the bone marrow stem cells is reduced in GVHD versus non-GVHD mice even several months after the transplant (110). Reductions in bone marrow progenitors have similarly been observed in GVHR (4,111,112). All of these studies are based, moreover, on assays of early erythroid and myeloid progenitors: splenic colony forming units (CFU-s) and granulocyte macrophage colony forming units (CFU-GM). Perhaps more significant than the quantitative reduction in progenitor cells is a skewing of lymphohematopoietic system away from the generation of NK, B, and T cells. Although bone marrow cellularity and peripheral blood counts of neutrophils and platelets were found to be little affected by GVHD (110), lymphocyte recovery was significantly delayed (86).

Clinical studies of BMT have consistently demonstrated the association of GVHD with delayed lymphocytic recovery. NK, B, and T cells are all affected. NK cells are the first of the lymphoid cells observed to reconstitute the peripheral blood of BMT recipients (55,113,114), appearing in high numbers as early as 10 to 20 days post-BMT without AGVHD. In the setting of GVHD, decreased numbers of NK^+ cells have been observed (27,55), although Keever (115) has reported increased killing of NK-sensitive targets, consistent with increased levels of the NK- activating cytokines IL-2 and IFN-γ noted previously.

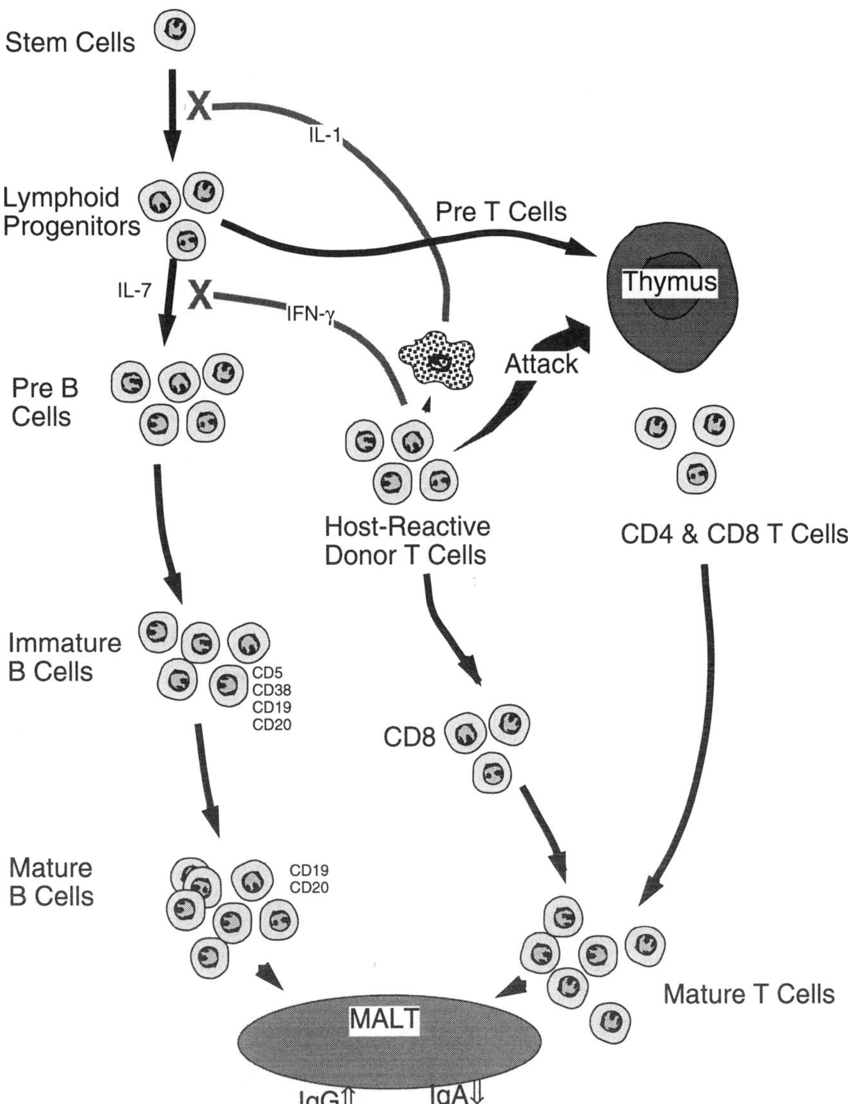

Figure 6 Diagram of impaired lymphopoiesis in GVHD. During AGVHD, host-reactive donor T cells and activated macrophages produce cytokines, which affect lymphopoiesis. IL-1 reduces production of lymphoid progenitors and IFN-γ interferes with the IL-7 stimulated production of pre-B cells in the bone marrow. Peripheral blood B cells are reduced, in particular $CD5^+$ B cells, in comparison to BMT without AGVHD. T-cell repopulation is affected both by a decrease in lymphoid progenitors and by thymic damage due to attack during early AGVHD. Repopulation of CD4 cells is dependent upon the thymus, but nonthymic pathways may contribute to CD8 levels. Antibody production in the MALT and antibody levels in plasma are altered toward increased IgG and reduced IgA.

The recovery of B-cell numbers generally begins approximately 1 month post-BMT and normalizes between 4 and 8 months (114,116). In the presence of GVHD, however, B-cell reconstitution is delayed until approximately 9 months post-BMT (116). Furthermore, B-cell maturation is abnormal. Non-GVHD reconstituting B cells initially resemble cord blood B cells ("recapitulation of ontogeny") (117) in having an elevated frequency of $CD5^+$ cells (116,118). There are fewer $CD5^+$ B cells in GVHD and no comparable CD5 overshoot period (118,119). Finally B-cell function remains impaired for a prolonged period even after quantitative reconstitution. This is evidenced by impaired T-cell-independent responses such as the production of isohemagluttinin titers and impaired B-cell responses to immunization with pneumococcal polysaccharide vaccine (80,120). T-cell-dependent B-cell responses are impaired as well. There is diminished IgG production to recall antigens such as tetanus and diphtheria, as well as essentially absent IgG production to neoantigens such as bacteriophage ØX174 and Keyhole limpet hemocyanin (80). In vitro evaluation of B cells confirms these deficits and provides evidence for a range of defects including impaired B-cell function, impaired T-cell help, and increased T-cell-mediated suppression (93,121).

Normal T-dependent isotype switching may also be affected in GVHD. Serum IgM and IgG levels have been reported to be increased in the setting of cGVHD (120,122). Further assessment of these immunoglobulins, however, has revealed the presence of monoclonal gammopathies or homogenous Ig components indicative of clonal dysregulatation (122,123). Mitus et al. have correlated the incidence of oligoclonal gammopathy with GVHD suggesting that the degree of clonal dysregulation is greater in the setting of GVHD (124). An IgA deficit is seen both in plasma levels and tissue levels in GVHD. IgA- and IgM-bearing plasma cells are deficient in the MALT (125) and there is decreased IgA secretion in saliva (126). The result of this B-cell deficiency, which is so apparent in patients with GVHD, is a prolonged susceptibility to infection with a particular susceptibility to infection with pneumococcus and other encapsulated organisms.

CD8 populations, in contrast, may be consistently elevated in BMT recipients with GVHD. $CD8^+$ T cell populations ($CD8^+CD3^+$) appear in substantial numbers from approximately 30d post-BMT (28,55,127–129). These cells progressively increase in number to supranormal levels and may remain elevated for several years after BMT (128). In the setting of GVHD, several investigators have reported increased numbers of $CD8^+$ T-cell numbers in the peripheral blood compared to BMT recipients who have not developed AGVHD (127,130), and some investigators note persistently high $CD8^+$ numbers in the setting of CGVHD (127,131) as well. As noted above, however, a significant subpopulation of $CD8^+$ T cells in recipients with GVHD express abnormal markers such as CD57 and CD11a (S6F1) for several years after BMT (92,96,97).

Although some investigators have noted a transient dominance of $CD4^+$ cells in the peripheral blood very early (15 to 25 days) after BMT (28,128), these cells rapidly diminish to very low levels after this time. The extent and duration of CD4 depletion has varied depending upon the study, but it appears to be present for at least 4 to 6 months post-BMT and up to years in some patients (28,128,129,132). Because of the overshoot in CD8 T-cell number discussed above, a severely depressed CD4/CD8 ratio exists for prolonged periods after BMT. In the setting of

GVHD, CD4 T-cell numbers remain depleted for an even greater time than in patients without GVHD (29,127,133).

In both murine GVHR and GVHD studies, a delay in B-cell repopulation has similarly been observed. In GVHR, host-derived mature B cells are eliminated from the spleen by 2 to 3 weeks (3), but new donor-derived B cells appear only after 6 to 8 weeks (3). The delay is due to a delay in B-cell generation. Pre-B cells in the bone marrow are eliminated by 16 days and do not reappear until after 40 days (6). In murine BMT models of GVHD, a similar 2-week delay was observed in the development of bone marrow pro-B and pre-B cells compared with non-GVHD (T-depleted) allogeneic controls (86). In B10.D2 → BALB/c GVHD, Garvy observed a reduction in IL-7 induced CFU from the marrow, consistent with the decrease in pro-B cells. Furthermore, this inhibition of IL-7 CFU could be linked to secretion of IFN-γ by host-reactive donor T cells in the marrow (86). IFN-γ could have suppressed generation of new B-lineage cells by a direct effect on proliferation. Alternatively, IFN-γ in the marrow could have stimulated macrophage activation and secretion of IL-1, similar to the postulated linkage of IFN-γ and inflammatory macrophage products in tissue damage and immune suppression. Although IL-1 has an overall stimulatory effect on hematopoiesis, it primarily enhances myelopoiesis while reducing the generation of B cells and pre-T cells from the bone marrow (134). Consistent with an IL-1–dependent suppression of lymphopoiesis, treatment with IL-1ra increased the number of thymocytes in GVHD mice (77).

Although alterations in lymphopoiesis may be sufficient to explain a delay in B-cell maturation or generation of pre-T cells, another contributing factor in the delay in T-cell recovery is thymic damage. Animal models have shown that the thymus plays a crucial role in $CD4^+$ T-cell regeneration even after syngeneic BMT (135). Studies of thymic changes after marrow transplantation have demonstrated profound thymic atrophy followed by a long-delayed recovery of epithelial and lymphoid elements (136,137). The thymus is a target organ of cytolytic attack early in AGVHR; donor NK and T cells invade the thymus (7,138,139). Thymic structure is destroyed. The cortex shrinks, the cortical-medullary demarcation disappears, and the characteristic clusters of pale epithelial cells and Hassall's bodies are lost (115). Recovery of normal structure requires as much as 6 months in severe GVHR models. First the thymic cortex regenerates, at about the same time that new pre-B cells appear in the bone marrow (6,115); this correlation is consistent with a common recovery of pre-B and pre-T-cell lymphopoiesis. Subsequently medullary thymocytes appear, and finally medullary epithelia and Hassall's bodies. Recovery of thymic structure occurs coincident with recovery of mitogen-stimulated T-cell proliferation and T-dependent B-cell responses to sRBC (115). Tracking of the appearance of T cells derived from bone marrow progenitors has demonstrated that all splenic CD4 cells at 2 months after induction of GVHR were derived from mature donor lymphocytes; only after 9 months were 75% of the CD4 cells derived from bone marrow progenitors (88). Thus the delayed recovery of T-dependent responses correlated with a delayed production of new T cells from progenitors.

The mechanism for the disparity in recovery rates of $CD4^+$ and $CD8^+$ T cells after BMT has not been clarified. Recently, however, we have shown that $CD4^+$ immune reconstitution after intensive chemotherapy is directly correlated with age, such that younger patients show improved $CD4^+$ T-cell regeneration compared to older patients (140). Further, this reconstitution correlates with the generation of CD45RA$^+$ T cells and with radiographic evidence of thymic enlargement, suggesting that active thymopoiesis is required for CD4$^+$ immune reconstitution. Thus successful CD4$^+$ T-cell immune reconstitution appears stringently thymic-dependent. In contrast, CD8$^+$ regeneration after intensive chemotherapy is less tightly correlated with age and thymic enlargement (Mackall, manuscript in preparation). After BMT as well, the relatively rapid reconstitution of CD8$^+$ T-cell populations occurs during a period of thymic dysfunction. This suggests that alternative, thymic-independent pathways may substantially contribute to reconstitution of CD8$^+$ T lymphocytes. As noted previously, many of the CD8 cells in the peripheral blood express abnormal markers. Furthermore, while CD8 cells recovered to normal numbers more rapidly than CD4 cells in murine GVHR, only 50% of the CD8 cells at 9 months were derived from pre-T populations (88). This disparity suggests that expansion of existing mature CD8 populations may play a significant role in early CD8 recovery.

As is it known that thymic function diminishes with age and may be severely affected by irradiation (141,142), decreased thymic function post-BMT may be the primary reason for the impaired CD4$^+$ T-cell reconstitution. Attempts to utilize thymic transplantation from unrelated donors matched for one HLA locus to improve immune reconstitution after BMT has been unsuccessful (143). Whether this reflects a technical problem with thymic transplantation (i.e., rejection, inadequate HLA matching, impaired pre-T-cell trafficking to subcutaneously implanted thymic tissue, etc.) or provides evidence that impaired thymic production is not playing a role in humans is not clear. In a murine model in which AGVHR was induced for 1 month, followed by lethal irradiation and transplantation of donor (or in some cases host) marrow and T cells, the T-cell deficiency was prolonged. When parental thymus grafts (which would not be attacked by GVHR effectors) were implanted 1 week before BMT, the T-cell populations recovered both function and normal numbers rapidly (144).

Thus multiple factors contribute to the prolonged immune deficiency in GVHD. The early expansion of host-reactive T cells is short-lived; through processes that probably include clonal deletion and anergy, the expanded donor T-cell population is diminished. The production of suppressor factors by CD8 cells, macrophages, and NS cells inhibits responses of the remaining T and B cells. Many of the same cells and factors may also function to reduce the development of T- and B-cell progenitors. Finally, the extensive damage to the thymus in AGVHD delays normal CD4 maturation until thymic structure is regenerated.

IV. CGVHD: LONG-TERM DYSFUNCTIONS

A. CGVHD Is a TH2-Mediated B-Cell Stimulatory Disorder

Although the immune deficits observed initially in AGVHD merge gradually into the long-lasting deficiencies of CGVHD, CGVHD is a disorder of immune dysregulation, not merely deficiency. CGVHD is characterized by autoantibody production and increased collagen deposition, resulting in clinical symptoms similar to those seen in patients with autoimmune disease, particularly scleroderma and Sjögren's disease. Whereas AGVHD is associated with hypogammaglobulinemia, serum IgM and IgG levels are elevated in CGVHD (122,145), associated with monoclonal gammopathies or homogenous Ig components indicative of clonal dysregulation (123,124). Even when the same organs are affected, the pathology may be distinct in AGVHD and CGVHD, with necrosis dominating in AGVHD and fibrosis characteristic of CGVHD. The skin lesions of AGVHD are characterized by necrosis of epithelial cells of the basal layer, with lymphoid infiltrates being minimal. In CGVHD, in contrast, there is a significant lymphocytic or lymphoplasmacytic infiltration and extensive dermal fibrosis.

As in AGVHD, animal models have provided useful insights into the pathophysiology of CGVHD. Two main categories of models have been studied: direct induction of P → F1 CGVHR and long-term development of CGVHR following AGVHR. In the first model, a P → F1 GVHR is induced using T-cell subsets or strain combinations that produce a chronic autoimmune GVHR, based on a cognate interaction between donor CD4 cells and host B cells (146,147). For example, injecting C57Bl/6 (B6) spleen cells into unirradiated (B6 × $B6^{bm12}$)F1 hosts, which differ only in I-A^b, results in a CGVHR with many of the pathological findings of the clinical syndrome (148,149). The basic paradigm of this model is the stimulation of donor CD4 cells by disparate class II antigen expressing host B cells (150,151); the B cells, in turn, respond to CD4 cytokines by proliferating and producing a variety of autoantibodies (149,152). B-cell numbers increase severalfold in spleen and lymph nodes and autoantibodies are measurable within 2 to 4 weeks (149). Hypergammaglobulinemia is common, with IgG1 and, particularly, IgE being elevated (151). Mortality increases only after several months and is due to autoimmune pathology, such as immune-complex-mediated glomerulonephritis and to an increased frequency of lymphoma (149,153). Few donor CD8 cells engraft; indeed, depletion studies have demonstrated that CD4 cells are sufficient to induce a CGVHR (11,90). Furthermore, full MHC disparate combinations, such as B6 → B6D2F1, can be converted from AGVHR into CGVHR by depletion of donor CD8 cells (26).

It is striking that the most commonly studied CGVHR strain combination, DBA/2 → B6D2F1, paradoxically involves a full MHC disparity. Such a strain combination might be expected to produce an acute suppressive GVHR. CD8 cells are reduced in frequency in DBA/2 mice, however, and have a ninefold lower frequency of anti-B6 pCTL than do comparable H-2^d strains (26). Thus this strain combination is comparable to the CD8-depleted model. Indeed, adding additional CD8 cells or total spleen cells converts this strain combination into an AGVHR, in which the host hematopoietic system is attacked and replaced by donor cells (154).

Also informative is a BMT model, extensively studied by Claman (155), which involves injection of B10.D2 bone marrow and lymphocytes into sublethally irradiated BALB/c hosts. The sublethal irradiation (optimally 600R) is crucial. Lethal irradiation results in AGVHD, sublethal irradiation in a rapid-onset CGVHD syndrome characterized by extensive sclerodermalike changes in the skin. As in the CGVHR models, the sublethal radiation may be necessary to retain extensive donor/host mixed chimerism and rapidly induce donor CD4 activation.

Research in the CGVHR models has demonstrated two key elements in the mechanism of CGVHD. The first is that the disease pathology in CGVHR is dependent upon the continued presence of host-reactive donor T cells that, unlike those in

AGVHD, fail to become tolerant of the host. Depletion of T cells in vivo with anti-Thy 1.2 antibodies even at 6 weeks after induction of cGVHR blocks further autoantibody production (156). This is consistent with clinical evidence correlating CGVHD with T-replete allogeneic grafts; T depletion reduces the incidence of CG-VHD as well as of AGVHD (1). Moreover, these donor T cells remain reactive to host antigens and do not become tolerized or anergic to host antigens even after several weeks. Ten weeks after induction of cGVHR in DBA/2 → B6D2F1 mice, donor-derived $CD4^+$ T cells reacted to host $I\text{-}A^b$ (but not $I\text{-}A^d$) alloantigens in vitro, providing helper factors for B-cell anti- sRBC plaque-forming cell assay (156). Class II antigen expression is elevated on cGVHR B cells even at 12 weeks, consistent with continued production of B-cell stimulatory cytokines (157). Finally, the disorder remains transferable to new hosts by transfer of T cells. At 7 to 9 weeks, DBA/2 → B6D2F1 cGVHR splenic T cells can induce autoantibody production in new secondary B6D2F1 hosts but not in DBA/2 (donor strain) hosts (156). This transfer is particularly remarkable in comparison with AGVHR, in which donor T cells become tolerant to the host and do not induce lethal AGVHD even on transfer into irradiated host strain recipients (10). Hence CGVHR is dependent upon a population of donor T cells that, unlike those in AGVHR, do not become deleted or tolerized to host antigens.

The second insight from CGVHR models is that the cytokine production patterns of AGVHR and CGVHR differ markedly. Whereas the predominant cytokines produced in AGVHR are T-helper 1 (TH1) cytokines; those in CGVHR are T-helper 2 (TH2). The skewing of the cytokine mRNA and protein production profile toward TH2 cytokines is evident within the first weeks of CGVHR. In the first 2 days after induction of CGVHR, a marked increase in IL-2 mRNA synthesis and cytokine content in supernatants has been observed in CGVHR mice, as in AGVHR models (44,158). Early IL-2 production is not inimicable with development of TH2 cells; indeed IL-2 is necessary for development of TH2 cells (159) and high levels of IL-2 stimulate TH2 activity in vivo (50). At day 2, however, an increase in IL-4 mRNA was also observed in unstimulated CGVHR splenocytes (158). By days 7, IL-2 mRNA had returned to normal levels while IL-4 and in particular IL-10 mRNA were elevated (158). Elevation of IL-4 and IL-10 mRNA, but not of IL2 or IFN-γ was also observed in unstimulated cultures after 2 to 3 weeks (47,157). Elevated Il-4 cytokine content in unstimulated CGVHR supernatants has also been demonstrated using a sensitive bioassay of induction of increased class II antigen in B cells; similarly, elevated expression of class II antigen on B cells has been observed from as early as 2 weeks to as late as 12 weeks after induction of CGVHR (157).

These TH2 cytokines are central to both the pathology and the immune dysfunctions of CGVHR. Anti IL-4 treatment in vivo not only blocks the elevation of IgG1 and IgE observed in CGVHR (160,161), it also reduces the onset of proteinuria and decreases the glomerulonephritis-associated mortality (160). Anti IL-10 in vitro reverses the suppression of production of TH1 cytokines IL- 2 and IFN-γ (157). Furthermore, in vivo treatment with IL-12, which stimulates TH1 cytokine production, converts the DBA/2 → B6D2F1 CGVHR into an acute suppressive GVHR (162).

The elevation of TH2 cytokines is consistent with many of the symptoms of CGVHD. Elevated IL-5 is associated with the increased eosinophilia observed clinically in CGVHD as well as in TH2 cytokine associated parasitic infections (163). IL-4 has been demonstrated to stimulate not only B-cell production of IgG1 and IgE, as noted, but also production of mast cells, which play a prominent role in the skin changes in Claman's scleroderma-like CGVHD model (164). Although clinical data on cytokine production in CGVHD are limited, the presence of these symptoms suggests a role for TH2 cytokines in the immune dysfunctions of this disorder.

B. Thymic Selection May Be Altered After AGVHD

Despite their utility, one shortcoming of the CGVHR models is their dependence upon extensive retention of host cells to directly stimulate donor CD4 cells. CGVHD develops long after AGVHD, when the host hematopoietic system has been thoroughly purged of host-originated cells. A second type of murine model provides evidence for the third element in CGVHR, the development of self reactivity in T cells maturing in a thymus damaged by AGVHD. Among long-term survivors of AGVHR, mice sometimes develop a secondary CGVHR, characterized by moderate lymphoid stimulation as well as perivascular and periductal lymphoid infiltrates in liver and salivary glands (10). Increased frequencies of autoimmune symptoms such as polychondritis, particularly in ear cartilage, and scleroderma-like changes in skin and an increased prevalence of lymphoma have also been observed (165,166). These mice have immune deficits in CD4 function quite similar to those observed in CGVHR mice. Although capable of generating a cytotoxic response to allogeneic stimulators, generation of cytotoxic effectors or of IL-2 in response to hapten-modified syngeneic cells is absent in both long-term AGVHR survivors and CGVHR mice (26,67). This same pattern of immune deficit has been observed in other autoimmune models, including the MRL lpr/lpr mice and the LP-BM5 virus induced murine AIDS model (167,168). Furthermore, the majority of these dysfunctional T cells have matured in the host after AGVHR. When AGVHR was induced in (B10 × B10.BR)F1 mice by injection of a mixture of B6 (Thy 1.2^+) lymph node and B6.PL (Thy 1.1^+) T- depleted bone marrow, the cells involved in the initial attack on the host were entirely Thy 1.2^+, that is, derived from the mature donor T-cell populations. After 9 months, however, more than 75% of the CD4 cells and 50% of the CD8 cells expressed Thy 1.1, indicating derivation from pre-T cells in the donor marrow (88). Thus the majority of the T cells during the period of immune dysfunction following AGVHR had matured in the host thymus.

Because the host thymus is extensively damaged in AGVHR, errors in thymic deletion of host-reactive T cells could contribute to autoreactivity. Desbarats has recently observed a failure of negative selection during thymic maturation, which correlated with a dramatic decrease in thymic medullary class II expression (169). In GVHD models involving irradiated hosts, Onoe (138) and recently Hollander (170) have also demonstrated a failure to clonally delete T-cell populations expressing TCR Vβ chains reactive with host mls antigens. Similar observations have also been made following cyclosporine treatment (171,172) or total lymphoid irradiation (173), both of which can result in development of autoimmune disorders (173,174). Thus autoreactive or, more accurately, host-reactive cells may mature following AGVHR.

It must be noted that existence of autoreactive cells in the thymus or even in the periphery in the early weeks of AGVHR does not establish a complete link between thymic dysfunction and the development of CGVHR. The thymic selection deficits have been observed in the first weeks after AGVHR (138,169), whereas significant peripheral repopulation from the recovered thymus (115) or development of CGVHR symptoms (10) does not occur for several months. The presence of host-reactive Vβ populations in skin or other organs involved in CGVHR has never been demonstrated. Furthermore, the duration of these shifts in T-cell repertoire has not been established. At 12 months after induction of B10 → (B10 × B10.BR)F1 AGVHR, we have failed to detect CD4 cells expressing host-reactive Vβ11 + TCR (88). This disparity in results could reflect strain differences in TCR affinity or in the severity of depletion of host populations, for thymic clonal deletion has been determined to be dependent on expression of antigens on host marrow-derived elements (175,176). Alternatively, the loss of Vβ11 + CD4 cells could reflect peripheral deletion (83) during the longer time course of this study. Finally, in order to explain the development of CGVHD, it is necessary to demonstrate not only the appearance of host-reactive cells but also the means for the development of a Th2-mediated immune dysfunction.

C. Differences in Host Tolerance of Th1 and Th2 Cells May Produce CGVHD

Thus we come to the final element in the development of CGVHD, the differences in the response of TH1 and TH2 cells to activation by host antigen. We would postulate the following scenario (Fig. 7). Two donor T-cell populations may be reactive to host antigens: the mature T cells in the original donor inoculum and newly matured host-reactive T cells that fail to be deleted during thymic maturation following AGVHR. These cells upon encountering host antigen in the periphery may then become activated. The evidence from AGVHD studies suggests that cells following a TH1 pattern will be clonally deleted or rendered anergic. TH2 cytokine directed responses, in contrast, do not appear to lead to deletion or anergy in CGVHR models, as described above. Indeed, TH2 clones have been found to be less subject to deletion following TCR cross-linking than are TH1 clones (177). Consistent with this hypothesis, Pals (10) has determined that long-term AGVHR cells, which could not induce an AGVHR against host-strain mice, were nonetheless able to stimulate antibody production in vitro by host-strain B cells. Injection of long-term GVHD cells into unirradiated F1 hosts produced popliteal lymph node enlargement and increased production of IgG plaque forming cells, evidence of expansion of host-reactive TH2 helper cells (10). We would therefore suggest that whether originating in the donor inoculum or maturing in the post-GVHR host thymus, host-reactive TH1 cells would be peripherally tolerized whereas host-reactive TH2 cells would be retained. Over time this disparity would result in a skewing of the population toward host-reactive TH2 cells. Such cells could then generate the autoimmune symptoms of CGVHR.

V. CONCLUSIONS

Research in recent years has substantiated the role of host- reactive donor T cells as the initiators of GVHD. More specifically, the pattern of cell populations and cytokines of AGVHD is that of the TH1 pathway of cell-mediated immunity. TH1

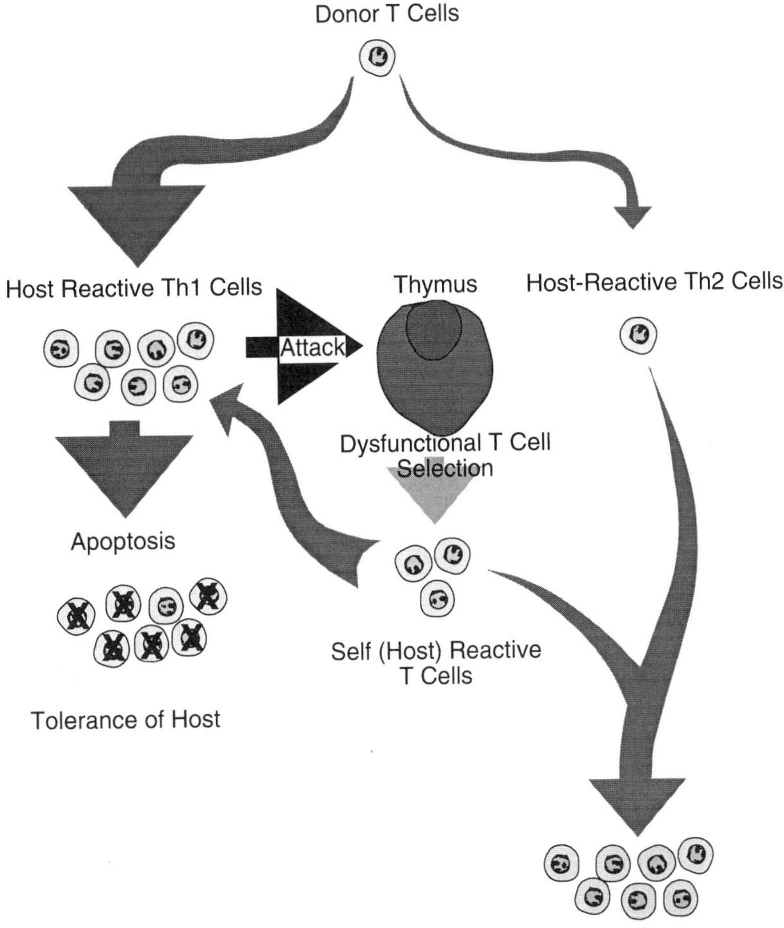

Figure 7 Diagram of proposed shift from AGVHD to CGVHD. Initially Th1 cytokine-producing T cells predominate in the expansion of host-reactive donor T cells, producing the inflammatory symptoms of AGVHD. These cells subsequently undergo clonal deletion by apoptosis or become anergic to host antigens, resulting in tolerance of host antigens. Host-reactive T cells producing the Th2 cytokines do not develop tolerance. New T cells emerging from the AGVHD-damaged thymus may contain self (host)-reactive cells. Those developing a Th1 cytokine pattern would undergo peripheral deletion, whereas those developing a Th2 cytokine pattern remain. Thus, over time, Th2 cytokine-producing cells would predominate in the host reactive population, giving rise to the symptoms of CGVHD.

cytokines produced early in GVHD stimulate the development of multiple effector cells: CD8 cytotoxic cells, NK cells, and proinflammatory macrophages. The cell-mediated attack these cells initiate and the inflammatory cytokines released are responsible for the multiorgan tissue damage of AGVHD. Furthermore, these cells and cytokines contribute to the suppression of immune function and the reduction in lymphopoiesis. Finally, thymic damage occurring during AGVHD may alter thymic regulation of host reactivity, establishing the conditions for the development of the prolonged immune deficiency and autoimmune pathology of CGVHD. CGVHD, by comparison, is mediated by host-reactive T cells producing cytokines of the TH2 pathway. These may arise out of the original donor inoculum or from self-reactive T cells maturing in a dysfunctional GVHD-damaged thymus or be due to a shift in TH1/TH2 cytokine patterns of host-stimulated cells in the periphery. Evidence suggests that while TH1 cells eventually become deleted or anergized peripherally, TH2 cells may continue to be reactive to host.

REFERENCES

1. Hale G, Waldmann H. CAMPATH-1 monoclonal antibodies in bone marrow transplantation. J Hematother 1994; 3:15–31.
2. Cobbold SP, Hale G, Clark MR, Waldmann H. Purging in auto- and allografts: Monoclonal antibodies which use human complement and other natural effector mechanisms. Prog Clin Biol Res 1990; 333:139–151.
3. Hakim FT, Sharrow SO, Payne S, Shearer GM. Repopulation of host lymphohematopoietic systems by donor cells during graft-vs-host reaction in unirradiated adult F1 mice injected with parental lymphocytes. J Immunol 1991; 146:2108–2115.
4. Hakim FT, Shearer GM. Immunologic and hematopoietic deficiencies of graft-vs.-host disease. In: Burakoff SJ, Deeg HJ, Ferrara J, Atkinson K, eds. Graft-vs.-Host Disease: Immunology, Pathophysiology, and Treatment. New York: Marcel Dekker, 1990:133–160.
5. Hakim FT, Pluznik DH, Shearer GM. Factors contributing to the decrease in concanavalin A-induced colony-stimulating factors in acute suppressive graft-versus-host disorder. Transplantation 1990; 49:781–787.
6. Xenocostas A, Lapp WS, Osmond DG. Suppression of B lymphocyte genesis in the bone marrow by systemic graft-versus- host reactions. Transplantation 1987; 43:549–555.
7. Ghayur T, Seemayer TA, Lapp WS. Association between the degree of thymic dysplasia and the kinetics of thymic NK cell activity during the graft-versus-host reaction. Clin Immunol Immunopathol 1988; 48:19–30.
8. Ghayur T, Seemayer TA, Lapp WS. Kinetics of natural killer cell cytotoxicity during the graft-versus-host reaction: Relationship between natural killer cell activity, T and B cell activity, and development of histopathological alterations. Transplantation 1987; 44:254–260.
9. Cray C, Levy RB. Virus-associated immune responses in mice undergoing GVHR exacerbated by concurrent MCMV infection. Transplantation 1990; 50:1027–1032.
10. Pals ST, Gleichmann H, Gleichmann E. Allosuppressor and allohelper T cells in acute and chronic graft-vs-host disease: V. F1 mice with secondary chronic GVHD contain F1-reactive allohelper but no allosuppressor T cells. J Exp Med 1984; 159:508–523.
11. Moser M, Sharrow SO, Shearer GM. Role of L3T4$^+$ and Lyt- 2$^+$ donor cells in graft-versus-host immune deficiency induced across a class I, class II, or whole H-2 difference. J Immunol 1988; 140:2600–2608.
12. Ferrara JL. Cytokine dysregulation as a mechanism of graft versus host disease. Curr Opin Immunol 1993; 5:794–799.
13. Antin JH, Verrara JL. Cytokine dysregulation and acute graft-versus-host disease. Blood 1992; 80:2964–2968.
14. Okunewick JP, Kociban DL, Machen LL, Buffo MJ. Comparison of the effects of CD3 and CD5 donor T cell depletion on graft-versus-leukemia in a murine model for

MHC-matched unrelated-donor transplantation. Bone Marrow Transplant 1994; 13: 11–17.

15. Soiffer RJ, Ritz J. Selective T cell depletion of donor allogeneic marrow with anti-CD6 monoclonal: rationale and results. Bone Marrow Transplant 1993; 12:S7–S10.
16. Blazar BR, Taylor PA. Snover DC, et al. Nonmitogenic anti-CD3F(ab′)2 fragments inhibit lethal murine graft-versus- host disease induced across the major histocompatibility barrier. J Immunol 1993; 150:265–277.
17. Sykes M, Harty MW, Szot GL, Pearson DA. Interleukin-2 inhibits graft-versus-host disease-promoting activity of $CD4^+$ cells while preserving CD4- and CD8-mediated graft-versus- leukemia effects. Blood 1994; 83:2560–2569.
18. Sprent J, Schaefer M, Gao EK, Korngold R. Role of T cell subsets in lethal graft-versus-host disease (GVHD) directed to class I versus class II H-2 differences: I. $L3T4^+$ cells can either augment or retard GVHD elicited by $Lyt\text{-}2^+$ cells in class I different hosts. J Exp Med 1988; 167:556–569.
19. Korngold R, Sprent, J. Surface markers of T cells causing lethal graft-vs-host disease to class I vs class II H-2 differences. J Immunol 1985; 135:3004–3010.
20. Sprent J, Surh CD, Agus D, et al. Profound atrophy of the bone marrow reflecting major histocompatibility complex class II-restricted destruction of stem cells by $CD4^+$ cells. J Exp Med 1994; 180:307–317.
21. Sprent J, Schaefer M, Lo D, Korngold R. Properties of purified T cell subsets: II. In vivo responses to class I vs class II H-2 differences. J Exp Med 1986; 163:998–1011.
22. Korngold R, Sprent J. Variable capacity of $L3T4^+$ T cells to cause lethal graft-versus-host disease across minor histocompatibility barriers in mice. J Exp Med 1987; 165: 1552–1564.
23. Hamilton BL. L3T4-positive T cells participate in the induction of graft-vs-host disease in response to minor histocompatibility antigens. J Immunol 1987; 139:2511–2515.
24. Truitt RL, Atasoylu AA. Contribution of $CD4^+$ and $CD8^+$ T cells to graft-versus-host disease and graft-versus-leukemia reactivity after transplantation of MHC-compatible bone marrow. Bone Marrow Transplant 1991; 8:51–58.
25. Nimer SD, Giorgi J, Gajewski JL, et al. Selective depletion of $CD8^+$ cells for prevention of graft-versus-host disease after bone marrow tranplanatation: A randomized controlled trial. Transplantation 1994; 57:82–87.
26. Via CS, Sharrow SO, Shearer GM. Role of cytotoxic T lymphocytes in the prevention of lupus-like disease occurring in a murine model of graft-vs-host disease. J Immunol 1987; 139:1840–1849.
27. Soiffer RJ, Gonin R, Murray C, et al. Prediction of graft-versus-host disease by phenotypic analysis of early immune reconstitution after CD6-depleted allogeneic bone marrow transplantation. Blood 1993; 82:2216–2223.
28. Favrot M, Janossy G, Tidman N, et al. T cell regeneration after allogeneic bone marrow transplantation. Clin Exp Immunol 1983; 54:59–72.
29. Atkinson K. Chronic graft-versus-host diesease. Bone Marrow Transplant 1990; 5:69–82.
30. Guinan EC, Gribben JG, Boussiotis VA, et al. Pivotal role of the B7:CD28 pathway in transplantation tolerance and tumor immunity. Blood 1994; 84:3261–3282.
31. Blazar BR, Carroll SF, Vallera DA. Prevention of murine graft-versus-host disease and bone marrow alloengraftment across the major histocompatibility barrier after donor graft preincubation with anti-LFA1 immunotoxin. Blood 1991; 78:3093–3102.
32. Harning R, Pelletier J, Lubbe K, et al. Reduction in the severity of graft-versus-host disease and increased survival in allogenic mice by treatment with monoclonal antibodies to cell adhesion antigens LFA-1 alpha and MALA-2. Transplantation 1991; 52: 842–845.

33. Durie FH, Aruffo A, Ledbetter J, et al. Antibody to the ligand of CD40, gp39, blocks the occurrence of the acute and chronic forms of graft-vs-host disease. J Clin Invest 1994; 94:1333–1338.
34. Blazar BR, Taylor PA, Linsley PS, Vallera DA. In vivo blockade of CD28/CTLA4: B7/BB1 interaction with CTLA4-Ig reduces lethal murine graft-versus-host disease across the major histocompatibility complex barrier in mice. Blood 1994; 15:3815–3825.
35. Wallace PM, Johnson JS, MacMaster JF, et al. CTLA4Ig treatment ameliorates the lethality of murine graft-versus-host disease across major histocompatibility complex barriers. Transplantation 1994; 58:602–610.
36. Ferrara JL, Marion A, McIntyre JF, et al. Amelioration of acute graft vs host disease due to minor histocompatibility antigens by in vivo adminstration of anti-interleukin 2 receptor antibody. J Immunol 1986; 137:1874–1877.
37. Cavazzana-Calvo M, Stephan JL, Sarnacki S, et al. Attenuation of graft-versus-host disease and graft rejection by ex vivo immunotoxin elimination of alloreactive T cells in an H-2 haplotype disparate mouse combination. Blood 1994; 83:288–298.
38. Anasetti C, Martin PJ, Storb R, et al. Prophylaxis of graft-versus-host disease by administration of the murine anti- IL-2 receptor antibody 2A3. Bone Marrow Transplant 1991; 7:375–381.
39. Herman A, Kappler JW, Marrack P, Pullen AM. Superantigens: Mechanism of T-cell stimulation and role in immune responses. Annu Rev Immunol 1991; 9:745–772.
40. Webb SR, Sprent J. Response of mature unprimed $CD8^+$ T cells to Mlsa determinants. J Exp Med 1990; 171:953–958.
41. MacDonald HR, Lees RK, Chvatchko Y. $CD8^+$ T cells respond clonally to Mls-1a-encoded determinants. J Exp Med 1990; 171:1381–1386.
42. Muluk SC, Hakim FT, Shearer GM. Regulation of graft- versus-host-reaction by Mls^a-reactive donor T cells. Eur J Immunol 1992; 22:1967–1973.
43. Powrie F, Coffman RL. Cytokine regulation of T-cell function: Potential for therapeutic intervention. Immunol Today 1993: 14:270–274.
44. Via CS. Kinetics of T cell activation in acute and chronic forms of murine graft-versus-host disease. J Immunol 1991; 146:2603–2609.
45. Abhyankar S, Gilliland DG, Ferrara JL. Interleukin-1 is a critical effector molecule during cytokine dysregulation in graft versus host disease to minor histocompatibility antigens. Transplantation 1993; 56:1518–1523.
46. Troutt AB, Kelso A. Lymphokine synthesis in vivo in an acute murine graft-versus-host reaction: mRNA and protein measurements in vivo and in vitro reveal marked differences between actual and potential lymphokine production levels. Int Immunol 1993; 5:399–407.
47. Allen RD, Staley T, Sidman CL. Differential cytokine expression in acute and chronic murine graft-versus-host-disease. Eur J Immunol 1993; 23:333–337.
48. Troutt AB, Kelso A. Enumeration of lymphokine mRNA- containing cells in vivo in a murine graft-versus-host reaction using the PCR. Proc Natl Acad Sci USA 1992; 89: 5276–5280.
49. Szebeni J, Wang MG, Pearson DA, et al. IL-2 inhibits early increases in serum gamma interferon levels associated with graft-versus-host-disease. Transplantation 1994; 58: 1385–1393.
50. Fowler DH, Kurasawa K, Husebekk A, et al. Cells of Th2 cytokine phenotype prevent LPS-induced lethality during murine graft-versus-host-reaction: Regulation of cytokines and $CD8^+$ lymphoid engraftment. J Immunol 1994; 152:1004–1013.
51. Fowler DH, Kurasawa K, Smith R, et al. Donor CD4- enriched cells of Th2 cytokine phenotype regulate graft-versus- host disease without impairing allogeneic engraftment in sublethally irradiated mice. Blood 1994; 84:3540–3549.

52. Via CS, Finkelman FD. Critical role of interleukin-2 in the development of acute graft-versus-host disease. Int immunol 1993; 5:565–572.
53. Ozmen L, Fountoulakis M, Gentz R, Garotta G. Immunomodulation with soluble IFN-γ receptor: preliminary study. Int Rev Exp Pathol 1993; 34:137–147.
54. Brok HP, Heidt PJ, van der Meide PH, et al. Interferon- γ prevents graft-versus-host disease after allogeneic bone marrow transplantation in mice. J Immunol 1993; 151: 6451–6459.
55. Smith BR, Rappeport JM, Burakoff SJ, Ault KA. Clinical correlates of unusual circulating lymphocytes appearing post marrow transplantation. In: Gale RP, Champlin R, eds. Progress in Bone Marrow Transplantation. New York: Liss, 1987:659–663.
56. Guillen FJ, Ferrara J, Hancock WW, et al. Acute cutaneous graft-versus-host disease to minor histocompatibility antigens in a murine model: Evidence that large granular lymphocytes are effector cells in the immune response. Lab Invest 1986; 55:35–42.
57. Ghayur T, Seemayer TA, Kongshavn PA, et al. Graft- versus-host reactions in the beige mouse: An investigation of the role of host and donor natural killer cells in the pathogenesis of graft-versus-host disease. Transplantation 1987; 44:261–267.
58. Knobloch C, Dennert G. Asialo-GM1-positive T killer cells are generated in F1 mice injected with parental spleen cells. J Immunol 1988; 140:744–749.
59. Blazar BR, Soderling CC, Koo GC, Vallera DA. Absence of a facilitory role for NK 1.1-positive donor cells in engraftment across a major histocompatibility barrier in mice. Transplantation 1988; 45:876–883.
60. MacDonald GC, Gartner JG. Prevention of acute lethal graft-versus-host disease in F1 hybrid mice by pretreatment of the graft with anti-NK-1.1 and complement. Transplantation 1992; 54:147–151.
61. MacDonald GC, Gartner JG. Prevention of acute lethal graft-versus-host disease in F1 hybrid mice by pretreatment of the graft with anti-NK-1.1 and complement. Transplantation 1992; 54:147–151.
62. Johnson BD, Truitt RL. A decrease in graft-vs.-host disease without loss of graft-vs.-leukemia reactivity after MHC- matched bone marrow transplantation by selective depletion of donor NK cells in vivo. Transplantation 1992; 54:104–112.
63. Denkers EY, Gazzinelli RT, Martin D, Sher A. Emergence of $NK1.1^{+}$ cells as effectors of IFN-gamma dependent immunity to Toxoplasma gondii in MHC class I-deficient mice. J Exp Med 1993; 178: 1465–1472.
64. Sher A, Oswald IP, Hieny S, Gazzinelli RT. Toxoplasma gondii induces a T-independent IFN-gamma response in natural killer cells that requires both adherent accessory cells and tumor necrosis factor-alpha. J Immunol 1993; 150:3982–3989.
65. Murphy WJ, Reynolds CW, Tiberghien P, Longo DL. Natural killer cells and bone marrow transplantation. J Natl Cancer Inst 1993; 85:1475–1482.
66. Garside P, Hutton AK, Severn A, et al. Nitric oxide mediates intestinal pathology in graft-vs-host disease. Eur J Immunol 1992; 22:2141–2145.
67. Hakim FT, Pluznik DH, Shearer GM. Alterations in T cell- derived colony-stimulating factors associated with GVH-induced immune deficiency. Transplantation 1990; 49: 773–781.
68. Smith SR, Terminelli C, Kenworthy-Bott L, Phillips DL. A study of cytokine production in acute graft-vs-host disease. Cell Immunol 1991; 134:336–348.
69. Crapper RM, Schrader JW. Evidence for the in vivo production and release into the serum of a T-cell lymphokine, persisting-cell stimulating factor (PSF), during graft-versus- host reactions. Immunology 1986; 57:553–558.
70. Nestel FP, Price KS, Seemayer TA, Lapp WS. Macrophage priming and lipopolysaccharide-triggered release of tumor necrosis factor alpha during graft-versus-host disease. J Exp Med 1992; 175:405–413.
71. Johnson BD, Drobyski WR, Truitt RL. Delayed infusion of normal donor cells after

MHC-matched bone marrow transplantation provides an antileukemia reaction without graft-versus-host disease. Bone Marrow Transplant 1993; 11:329–336.
72. Xun CQ, Thompson JS, Jennings CD, et al. Effect of total body irradiation, busulfan-cyclophosphamide, or cyclophosphamide conditioning on inflammatory cytokine release and development of acute and chronic graft-versus-host disease in H-2-incompatible transplanted SCID mice. Blood 1994; 83:2360–2367.
73. Schiltz PM, Giorno RC, Claman HN. Increased ICAM-1 expression in the early stages of murine chronic graft-versus- host disease. Clin Immunol Immunopathol 1994; 71: 136–141.
74. Hoffman RA, Langrehr JM, Simmons RL. The role of inducible nitric oxide synthetase during graft-versus-host disease. Transplant Proc 1992; 24:2856.
75. Desbarats J, Seemayer TA, Lapp WS. Irradiation of the skin and systemic graft-versus-host disease synergize to produce cutaneous lesions. Am J Pathol 1994; 144: 883–888.
76. Atkinson K, Matias C, Guiffre A, et al. In vivo administration of granulocyte colony-stimulating factor (G-CSF), granulocyte-macrophage CSF, inteleukin-1 (IL-1), and IL-4, alone and in combination, after allogeneic murine hematopoietic stem cell transplantation. Blood 1991; 77:1376–1382.
77. McCarthy PL Jr, Abhyankar S, Neben S, et al. Inhibition of interleukin-1 by interleukin-1 receptor antagonist prevents graft-versus-host disease. Blood 1991; 78:1915–1918.
78. Holler E, Kolb HJ, Hintermeier-Knabe R, et al. The role of TNFα in acute graft-versus-host disease and complications following allogeneic bone marrow transplantation. Transplant Proc 1993; 25:1234–1236.
79. Holler E, Kolb HJ, Möller A, et al. Increased serum levels of TNFα precede major complications of bone marrow transplantation. Blood 1990; 75:1011.
80. Witherspoon RP, Storb R, Ochs HD, et al. Recovery of antibody production in human allogeneic marrow graft recipients: Influence of time posttransplantation, the presence or absence of chronic graft-versus-host disease, and antithymocyte globulin treatment. Blood 1981; 58:360–368.
81. Storek J, Saxon A. Reconstitution of B cell immunity following bone marrow transplantation. Bone Marrow Transplant 1992; 9:395–408.
82. Kabelitz D, Pohl T, Pechhold K. Activation-induced cell death (apoptosis) of mature peripheral T lymphocytes. Immunol Today 1993; 14:338–339.
83. Webb S, Morris C, Sprent J. Extrathymic tolerance of mature T cells: Clonal elimination as a consequence of immunity. Cell 1990; 63:1249–1256.
84. Sprent J, Kosaka H, Gao EK, et al. Intrathymic and extrathymic tolerance in bone marrow chimeras. Immunol Rev 1993; 133:151–176.
85. Webb SR, Hutchinson J, Hayden K, Sprent J. Expansion/deletion of mature T cells exposed to endogenous superantigens in vivo. J Immunol 1994; 152:586–597.
86. Garvy BA, Elia JM, Hamilton BL, Riley RL. Suppression of B-cell development as a result of selective expansion of donor T cells during the minor H antigen graft-versus-host reaction. Blood 1993; 82:2758–2766.
87. Levy RB, Jones M, Cray C. Isolated peripheral T cells from GvHR recipients exhibit defective IL-2R expression, IL-2 production, and proliferation in response to activation stimuli. J Immunol 1990; 145:3998–4005.
88. Hakim FT, Payne S, Shearer GM. Recovery of T cell populations after acute graft-vs-host reaction. J Immunol 1994; 152:58–64.
89. Pals ST, Radaszkiewicz T, Gleichmann E. Allosuppressor- and allohelper-T cells in acute and chronic graft-vs-host disease: IV. Activation of donor allosuppressor cells in confined to acute GVHD. J Immunol 1984; 132:1669–1678.
90. Rolink AG, Gleichmann E. Allosuppressor- and allohelpher-T cells in acute and

chronic graft-vs.-host (GVH) disease: III. Different Lyt subsets of donor T cells induce different pathological syndromes. J Exp Med 1983; 158:546–558.
91. Hurtenbach U, Shearer GM. Analysis of murine T lymphocyte markers during the early phases of GvH-associated suppression of cytotoxic T lymphocyte responses. J Immunol 1983; 130:1561–1566.
92. Autran B, Leblond V, Sadat-Sowti B, et al. A soluble factor released by $CD8^+CD57^+$ lymphocytes from bone marrow transplanted patients inhibits cell-mediated cytolysis. Blood 1991; 77:2237–2241.
93. Lum LG, Seigneuret MC, Storb R, et al. In vitro regulation of immunoglobulin synthesis after marrow transplantation: I. T-cell and B-cell deficiencies in patients with and without chronic graft-versus-host disease. Blood 1981; 58:431–439.
94. Tsoi M, Storb R, Dobbs S, et al. Nonspecific suppressor cells in patients with chronic graft-vs-host disease after marrow grafting. J Immunol 1979; 123:1970–1976.
95. Lum LG, Orcutt-Thordarson N, Seigneuret MC, Storb R. The regulation of Ig synthesis after marrow transplantation: IV. T4 and T8 subset function in patients with chronic graft-versus-host disease. J Immunol 1982; 129:113–119.
96. Fukuda H, Nakamura H, Tominaga N, et al. Marked increase of $CD8^+S6F1^+$ and $CD8^+57^+$ cells in patients with graft-versus-host disease after allogeneic bone marrow transplantation. Bone Marrow Transplant 1994; 13:181–185.
97. Gorochov G, Debre P, Leblond V, et al. Oligoclonal expansion of $CD8^+CD57^+$ T cells with restricted T-cell receptor β chain variability after bone marrow transplantation. Blood 1994; 83:587–595.
98. Ikarashi Y, Kawai K, Watanabe H, et al. Immunosuppressive activity of macrophages in mice undergoing graft-versus-host reaction due to major histocompatibility complex class I plus II difference. Immunology 1993; 79:95–102.
99. Howell CD, Yoder TD, Vierling JM. Suppressor function of hepatic mononuclear inflammatory cells during murine chronic graft-vs-host disease: I. Macrophage-enriched cells mediate suppression in the liver. Cell Immunol 1991; 132:256–268.
100. Holda JH, Maier T, Claman HN. Murine graft-versus-host disease across minor barriers: Immunosuppressive aspects of natural suppressor cells. Immunol Rev 1985; 88: 87–105.
101. Holda JH, Maier T, Claman HN. Evidence that IFN-γ is responsible for natural suppressor activity in GVHD spleen and normal bone marrow. Transplantation 1988; 45:772–777.
102. Choi KL, Maier T, Holda JH, Claman HN. Suppression of cytotoxic T-cell generation by natural suppressor cells from mice with GVHD is partially reversed by indomethacin. Cell Immunol 1988; 112:271–278.
103. Holda JH, Maier T, Claman HN. Natural suppressor activity in graft-vs-host spleen and normal bone marrow is augmented by IL 2 and interferon-gamma. J Immunol 1986;137:3538–3543.
104. Wall DA, Hamberg SD, Reynolds DS, et al. Immunodeficiency in graft-versus-host disease: I. Mechanism of immune suppression. J Immunol 1988; 140:2970–2976.
105. Huchet R, Bruley-Rosset M, Mathiot C, et al. Involvement of IFN-gamma and transforming growth factor-beta in graft-vs-host reaction-associated immunosuppression. J Immunol 1993; 150:2517–2524.
106. Sadat-Sowti B, Debre P, Mollet L, et al. An inhibitor of cytotoxic functions produced by $CD8^+CD57^+$ T lymphocytes from patients suffering from AIDS and immunosuppressed bone marrow recipients. Eur J Immunol 1994; 24:2882–2888.
107. Wall DA, Sheehan KC. The role of tumor necrosis factor and interferon gamma in graft-versus-host disease and related immunodeficiency. Transplantation 1994; 57:273–279.
108. Hoffman RA, Langrehr JM, Wren SM, et al. Characterization of the immunosuppressive effects of nitric oxide in graft vs host disease. J Immunol 1993; 151:1508–1518.

109. Lapp WS, Mendes M, Kirchner H, Gemsa D. Prostaglandin synthesis by lymphoid tissue of mice experiencing a graft-versus- host reaction: relationship to immunosuppression. Cell Immunol 1980; 50:271–281.
110. van Dijken PJ, Wimperis J, Crawford JM, Ferrara JL. Effect of graft-versus-host disease on hematopoiesis after bone marrow transplantation in mice. Blood 1991; 78: 2773–2779.
111. Iwasaki T, Fujiwara H, Shearer GM. Loss of proliferative capacity and T cell immune development potential by bone marrow from mice undergoing a graft-vs-host reaction. J Immunol 1986; 137:3100–3108.
112. Seddik M, Seemayer TA, Lapp WS. The graft-versus-host reaction and immune function: IV. B cell functional defect associated with a depletion of splenic colony-forming units in marrow of graft-versus-host-reactive mice. Transplantation 1986; 41:242–247.
113. Franceschini F, Gale RP. Immune reconstitution following bone marrow transplantation in man. In: Gale RP, Champlin R, eds. Progress in Bone Marrow Transplantation, 4th ed. New York: 1987:607.
114. Ault KA, Antin JH, Ginsburg D, et al. Phenotype of recovering lymphoid cell populations after marrow transplantation. J Exp Med 1985; 161:1483–1502.
115. Ghayur T, Seemayer TA, Xenocostas A, Lapp WS. Complete sequential regeneration of graft-vs-host-induced severely dysplastic thymuses: Implications for the pathogenesis of chronic graft-vs-host disease. Am J Pathol 1988; 133:39–46.
116. Small TN, Keever CA, Weiner-Fedus S, et al. B cell differentiation following autologous, conventional or T cell depleted bone marrow transplantation: A recapitulation of normal B cell ontogeny. Blood 1990; 76:1647–1656.
117. Storek J, Ferrara S, Ku N, et al. B cell reconstitution after human bone marrow transplantation: recapitulation of ontogeny? Bone Marrow Transplant 1993; 12:387–398.
118. Storek J, Ferrara S, Ku N, et al. B cell reconstitution after human bone marrow transplantation: Recapitulation of ontogeny? Bone Marrow Transplant 1993; 12:387–398.
119. Antin JH, Ault KA, Rappeport JM, Smith BR. B lymphocyte reconstitution after human bone marrow transplantation: Leu-1 antigen defines a distinct populations of B lymphocytes. J Clin Invest 1987; 80:325–332.
120. Noel DR, Witherspoon RP, Storb R, et al. Does graft- versus-host disease influence the tempo of immunologic recovery after allogeneic human marrow transplantation? An observation of 56 long-term survivors. Blood 1978; 51:1087–1105.
121. Lum LG, Seigneuret MC, Orcutt-Thordarson N, et al. The regulation of immunoglobulin synthesis after HLA-identical bone marrow transplantation: VI. Differential rates of maturation of distinct functional groups within lymphoid subpopulations in patients after human marrow grafting. Blood 1985; 65:1422–1433.
122. Graze PR, Gale RP. Chronic graft versus host disease: A syndrome of disordered immunity. Am J Med 1994; 66:611–620.
123. Gerritsen EJA, van Tol MJD, Lankester AC, et al. Immunoglobulin levels of monoclonal gammopathies in childre after bone marrow transplantation. Blood 1993; 82: 3493–3502.
124. Mitus AJ, Stein R, Rappeport JM, et al. Monoclonal and oligoclonal gammopathy after bone marrow transplantation. Blood 1989; 74:2764–2788.
125. Beschorner WE, Yardley JH, Tutschka PJ, Santos GW. Deficiency of intestinal immunity with graft-vs.-host disease in humans. J Inf Dis 1981; 144:38–46.
126. Izutsu K, Sullivan KM, Schubert MM, et al. Disordered salivary immunoglobulin secretion and sodium transport in human chronic graft-versus-host disease. Transplantation 1983; 35:441–446.

127. Friedrich W, O'Rielly RJ, Koziner B, et al. T-lymphocyte reconstitution in recipients of bone marrow transplants with and without GVHD: Imbalances of T-cell subpopulations having unique regulatory and cognitive functions. Blood 1982; 59:696–701.
128. Atkinson K, Hansen JA, Storb R, et al. T-cell subpopulations identified by monoclonal antibodies after human marrow transplantation: I. Helper-inducer and cytotoxic- suppressor subsets. Blood 1982; 59:1292–1298.
129. Forman SJ, Nocker P, Gallagher M, et al. Pattern of T cell reconstitution following allogeneic bone marrow transplantation for acute hematological malignancy. Transplantation 1982; 34:967–998.
130. Witherspoon RP, Goehle S, Kretschmer M, Storb R. Regulation of immunoglobulin production after human marrow grafting: The role of helper and suppressor T cells in acute graft-versus-host disease. Transplantation 1986; 41:328–335.
131. Klingemann HG, Lum LG, Storb R. Phenotypical and functional studies on a subtype of suppressor cells ($CD8^+/CD11^+$) in patients after bone marrow transplantation. Transplantation 1987; 44:381–386.
132. Schneider LC, Antin JH, Weinstein H, et al. Lymphokine profile in bone marrow transplant recipients. Blood 1991; 78:3076–3080.
133. Witherspoon RP, Lum LG, Storb R. Immunologic reconstitution after human marrow grafting. Semin Hematol 1984; 21:2–10.
134. Morrissey P, Charrier K, Bressler L, Alpert A. The influence of IL-1 treatment on the reconstitution of the hemopoietic and immune systems after sublethal radiation. J Immunol 1988; 140:4202–4210.
135. Mackall CL, Granger L, Sheard MA, et al. T cell regeneration after bone marrow transplantation: Differntial CD45 isoform expression on thymic-derived versus thymic-independent progeny. Blood 1993; 82:2585–2594.
136. Beschorner WE, Hutchins GM, Elfenbein GJ, Santos GW. The thymus in patients with allogenic bone marrow transplants. Am J Pathol 1978; 92:173–186.
137. Muller-Hermelink HK, Sale GE, Borisch B, Storb R. Pathology of the thymus after allogeneic bone marrow transplantation in man: A histologic immunohistochemical study of 36 patients. Am J Pathol 1987; 129:242–256.
138. Fukushi N, Arase H, Wang B, et al. Thymus: A direct target tissue in graft-versus-host reaction after allogeneic bone marrow transplantation that results in abrogation of induction of self- tolerance. Proc Natl Acad Sci USA 1990; 87:6301–6305.
139. Cray C, Levy RB. Evidence that donor cells are present in the thymus of recipients undergoing a P----F1 graft-versus-host reaction exacerbated by concurrent murine cytomegalovirus infection. Transplantation 1992; 53:696–699.
140. Mackall CL, Fleisher TA, Brown MR, et al. Age, thymopoiesis, and $CD4^+$ T-lymphocyte regeneration after intensive chemotherapy (see comments). N Engl J Med 1995; 332:143–149.
141. Adkins B, Gandour D, Strober S, Weissman I. Total lymphoid irradiation leads to transient depletion of the mouse thymic medulla and persistent abnormalities among medullary stromal cells. J Immunol 1988; 140:3373–3379.
142. Bass H, Mosmann T, Strober S. Evidence for mouse Th1- and Th2-like helper T cells in vivo: Selective reduction of Th1-like cells after total lymphoid irradiation. J Exp Med 1989; 170:1495–1511.
143. Witherspoon RP, Sullivan KM, Lum LG, et al. Use of thymic grafts or thymic factors to augment immunologic recovery after bone marrow transplantation: Brief report with 2 to 12 years follow-up. Bone Marrow Transplant 1988; 3:425–435.
144. Fukuzawa M, Via CS, Shearer GM. Defective thymic education of L3T4+ T helper cell function in graft-vs-host mice. J Immunol 1988; 141:430–439.

145. Storek J, Saxon A. Reconstitution of B cell immunity following bone marrow transplantation. Bone Marrow Transplant 1992; 9:394–408.
146. Morris SC, Cheek RL, Cohen PL, Eisenberg RA. Autoantibodies in chronic graft versus host result from cognate T-B interactions. J Exp Med 1990; 171:503–517.
147. Morris SC, Cheek RL, Cohen PL, Eisenberg RA. Allotype- specific immunoregulation of autoantibody production by host B cells in chronic graft-versus-host disease. J Immunol 1990; 144:916–922.
148. Saitoh T, Fujiwara M, Asakura H. L3T4+ T cells induce hepatic lesions resembling primary biliary cirrhosis in mice with graft-versus-host reactions due to major histocompatibility complex class II disparity. Clin Immunol Immunopathol 1991; 59:449–461.
149. Gleichmann E, Pals ST, Rolink AG, et al. Graft-vs-host reactions: Clues to the etiopathology of a spectrum of immunological diseases. Immunol Today 1984; 5:324–32.
150. Via CS, Shearer GM. T-cell interactions in autoimmunity: Insights from a murine model of graft-versus-host disease. Immunol Today 1988; 9:207–213.
151. Goldman M, Druet P, Gleichmann E. TH2 cells in systemic autoimmunity: Insights from allogeneic diseases and chemically- induced autoimmunity. Immunol Today 1991; 12:223–227.
152. Kuppers RC, Suiter T, Gleichmann E, Rose NR. The induction of organ-specific antibodies during the graft-vs-host reaction. Eur J Immunol 1988; 18:161–166.
153. Rolink AG, Gleichmann H, Gleichmann E. Diseases caused by reactions of T lymphocytes to incompatible structures of the major histocompatibility complex: VII. Immune-complex glomerulonephritis. J Immunol 1983; 130:209–215.
154. Rozendaal L, Pals ST, Melief CJM, Gleichmann E. Protection from lethal graft-vs-host disease by donor stem cell repopulation. Eur J Immunol 1992: 22:575–579.
155. Claman HN, Jaffee BD, Huff JC, Clark RA. Chronic graft- versus-host disease as a model for scleroderma: II. Mast cell depletion with deposition of immunoglobulins in the skin and fibrosis. Cell Immunol 1985; 94: 73–84.
156. Rozendaal L, Pals ST, Gleichmann E, Melief CJ. Persistence of allospecific helper T cells is required for maintaining autoantibody formation in lupus-like graft-versus-host disease. Clin Exp Immunol 1990; 82:527–532.
157. De Wit D, van Mechelen M, Zanin C, et al. Preferential activation of Th2 cells in chronic graft-versus-host reaction. J Immunol 1993: 150:361–366.
158. Garlisi CG, Pennline KJ, Smith SR, et al. Cytokine gene expression in mice undergoing chronic graft-versus-host disease. Mol Immunol 1993; 30:669–677.
159. Ben-Sasson SZ, Le Gros G, Conrad DH, et al. IL-4 production by T cells from naive donors. IL-2 is required for IL- 4 production. J Immunol 1990; 145:1127–1136.
160. Umland SP, Razac S, Nahrebne DK, Seymour BW. Effects of in vivo administration of interferon-gamma, anti-IFN-gamma or anti- interleukin-4 monoclonal antibodies in chronic autoimmune graft- versus-host disease. Clin Immunol Immunopathol 1992; 63:66–73.
161. Doutrelepont JM, Moser M, Leo O, et al. Hyper IgE in stimulatory graft-versus-host disease: role of interleukin-4. Clin Exp Immunol 1991; 83:133–136.
162. Via CS, Rus V, Gately MK, Finkelman FD. IL-12 stimulates the development of acute graft-versus-host disease in mice that normally would develop chronic, autoimmune graft-versus-host disease. J Immunol 1994; 153;4040–4047.
163. Sher A, Coffman RL, Hieny S, Cheever AW. Ablation of eosinophil and IgE responses with anti-IL-5 or anti-IL-4 antibodies fails to affect immunity against Schistosoma mansoni in the mouse. J Immunol 1990; 145:3911–3916.
164. Levi-Schaffer F, Mekori YA, Segal V, Claman HN. Histamine release from mouse and rat mast cells cultured with supernatants from chronic murine graft-vs-host splenocytes. Cell Immunol 1990; 127:146–158.

165. Pals ST, Radaszkiewicz T, Roozendaal L, Gleichmann E. Chronic progressive polyarthiritis and other symptoms of collagen vascular disease induced by graft-vs-host reaction. J Immunol 1985; 134:1475–1482.
166. Pals ST, Zijstra M, Radaszkiewicz T, et al. Immunologic induction of malignant lymphoma: Graft-vs-host reaction-induced B cell lymphomas contain integrations of predominantly ecotropic murine leukemia proviruses. J Immunol 1986; 136:331–339.
167. Via CS, Shearer GM. Functional heterogeneity of L3T4$^+$ T cells in MRL-lrp/lrp mice. L3T4$^+$ T cells suppress major histocompatibility complex-self-restricted L3T4$^+$ T helper cell function in association with autoimmunity. J Exp Med 1988; 168:2165–2181.
168. Morse HC, Yetter RA, Via CS, et al. Functional and phenotypic alterations in T cell subsets during the course of MAIDS, a murine retrovirus-induced immunodeficiency syndrome. J Immunol 1989; 143:844–850.
169. Desbarats J, Lapp WS. Thymic selection and thymic major histocompatibility complex class II expression are abnormal in mice undergoing graft-versus-host reactions. J Exp Med 1993; 178:805–814.
170. Hollander GA, Widner B, Burakoff SJ. Loss of normal thymic repertoire selection and persistence of autoreactive T cells in graft vs host disease. J Immunol 1994; 152: 1609–1617.
171. Hollander GA, Fruman DA, Bierer BE, Burakoff SJ. Disruption of T cell development and repertoire selection by calcineurin inhibition in vivo. Transplantation 1994; 58: 1037–1043.
172. Cairns JS, Mainwaring MS, Cacchione RN, et al. Regulation of apoptosis in thymocytes. Thymus 1993; 21:177–193.
173. Sakaguchi N, Miyai K, Sakaguchi S. Ionizing radiation and autoimmunity: Induction of autoimmune disease in mice by high dose fractionated total lymphoid irradiation and its prevention by inoculating normal T cells. J Immunol 1994; 152:2586–2595.
174. Bucy RP, Xu XY, Li J, Huang G. Cyclosporin A-induced autoimmune disease in mice. J Immunol 1993; 151:1039–1050.
175. Roberts JL, Sharrow SO, Singer A. Clonal deletion and clonal anergy in the thymus induced by cellular elements with different radiation sensitivities. J Exp Med 1990; 171:935–940.
176. Gao EK, Lo D, Sprent J. Strong T cell tolerance in parent → F1 bone marrow chimeras prepared with supralethal irradiation. Evidence for clonal deletion and anergy. J Exp Med 1990; 171:1101–1121.
177. Ramsdell F, Seaman MS, Miller RE, et al. Differential ability of Th1 and Th2 T cells to express Fas ligand and to undergo activation-induced cell death. Int Immunol 1994; 6:1545–1553.

11

Cellular Pathology of Cutaneous Graft-Versus-Host Disease

Anita C. Gilliam
Case Western Reserve University
Cleveland, Ohio

George F. Murphy
University of Pennsylvania School of Medicine
Philadelphia, Pennsylvania

I. PATHOLOGY OF CUTANEOUS GVHD

A. General Considerations: The Enigma

The pathology of cutaneous graft-versus-host disease (GVHD) is subtle yet clinically devastating, experimentally reproducible yet etiologically mysterious, and target- cell-specific yet promiscuous regarding epidermal or dermal injury. The enigma of cutaneous GVHD is emphasized by its typical clinical features. Acute lesions occur after allogeneic bone marrow transplantation, and degree of histocompatibility disparity between donor and host correlates with severity. However, not all recipients of partially unmatched transplants develop clinical disease, and the characteristic exanthem may even occur in syngeneic (identical twin) transplants or independent of transplantation altogether. Acute GVHD generally is observed as a maculopapular rash that may be generalized (Fig. 1A). The onset may be as early as several weeks after marrow transplantation, and clinical confusion with viral and drug-related exanthems is common. Often there is palm and sole involvement, a valuable clue to GVHD as a cause. In addition, the rash may be punctate, corresponding to early involvement of hair follicles. Because cutaneous signs may precede visceral disease, the triad of skin rash, diarrhea, and abnormal liver function may not be present. In rare individuals, cutaneous involvement may be so severe as to cause epidermal sloughing in a manner similar to toxic epidermal neurolysis.

Chronic GVHD occurs at least several months after transplantation and may be either localized or generalized in distribution. The initial alterations are limited to the more superficial skin layers, with the formation of lichen planus–like papules or scaling erythematous plaques often first involving facial skin, palms, and soles. Gradual spread to other body sites generally occurs within 4 weeks and may be associated with diffuse erythema and induration, mottled hypo- and hyperpigmentation, and alopecia (Fig. 1B). Mucous membrane involvement results in excessive

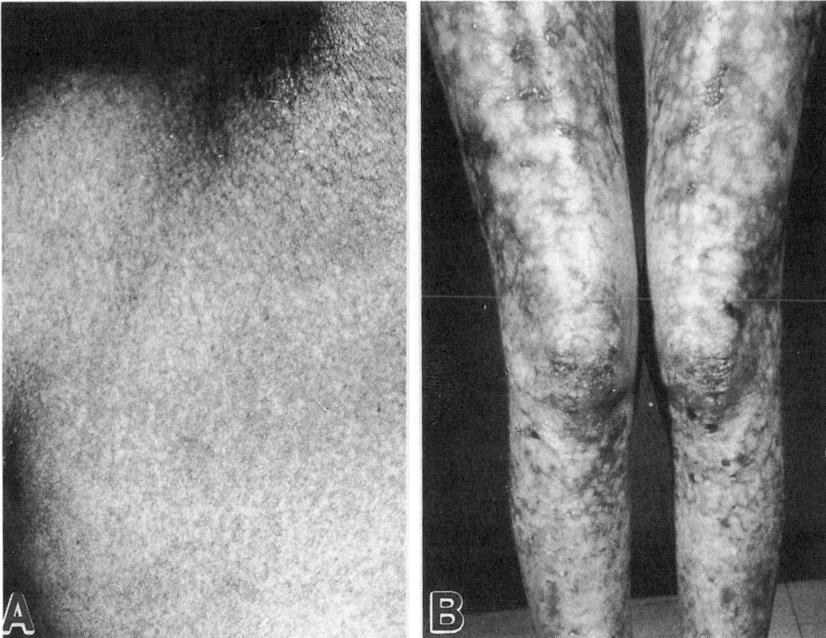

Figure 1 Clinical manifestations of epidermal (acute) and dermal (chronic) forms of GVHD. A. Mottled maculopapular erythema of acute GVHD. (Courtesy Yale Dermatology Residents' Slide Collection.) B. Chronically sclerotic skin of dermal GVHD covered by "poikilodermatous" epidermal layer showing atrophy, telangiectatic vessels, and mottled hypo- and hyperpigmentation.

dryness of the mouth, conjunctiva, trachea, and vagina to produce a siccalike syndrome. Ultimately, persistent alterations include brawny induration indistinguishable from skin lesions of progressive systemic sclerosis, epidermal thinning with prominent telangiectasia, and anomalous pigment distribution.

Not all patients who develop acute GVHD progress to chronic GVHD, and the latter may occur de novo, without antecedent acute disease. Therefore, it remains unclear whether acute and chronic GVHD are continua of the same disorder or independent but temporally related conditions. Perhaps either form of GVHD may sometimes be clinically covert, accounting for the overt predominance of one or the other in certain individuals. Chronic GVHD, on the other hand, may represent a distinctive autoimmune phenomenon set into motion by immunological imbalances resulting from acute cytotoxicity to the immune system, one cause of which might be acute GVHD. The clues to these and other mysteries remain locked in GVHD target tissues, which include skin, liver, gut, and lymphoid organs. As the most visible and accessible organ for clinical and experimental study, affected skin in GVHD is providing critical insights into the causes and potential cures to this enigmatic and important disease paradigm for cutaneous inflammation and fibrosis.

B. Acute GVHD

1. Endothelial Phase

The first histological alterations that occur in acute GVHD involve adhesion and transvascular diapedesis of lymphocytes through postcapillary venules situated within the uppermost dermis (superficial vascular plexus) (Fig. 2A). Such changes are often observed in biopsies 2 to 3 weeks after transplantation or in association with the first clinical signs and symptoms of cutaneous involvement. The molecular cascade responsible for these events is only beginning to be understood (see "Pathobiology," below). However, mast-cell degranulation about the affected venules appears to be related to activation of microvascular endothelial cells responsible for initial recruitment of effector cells. It is of interest, therefore, that pruritus, a common sign of mast-cell degranulation, may also accompany early clinical lesions of acute GVHD. The result of adhesive interaction between microvascular endothelial cells and effector cells is migration of the latter into the perivascular interstitium of the superficial (papillary) dermis. Remarkably few cells seem to be involved in this phase, and their migratory fate appears to be influenced by secondary induction of chemokines and adhesion molecules in target tissue, such as the overlying epidermal layer.

The diagnostic histology of the endothelial phase of acute GVHD is nonspecific, and serial biopsies are often required to establish a definitive diagnosis. Maculopapular viral exanthems are probably the most common cause of a superficial perivascular lymphocytic infiltrate, and this possibility must always be considered when the alternative possibility of acute GVHD is entertained. Although viral exanthems may be hemorrhagic and therefore associated with superficial perivascular extravasation of erythrocytes, altered coagulation status may also produce this finding. Drug eruptions must also be considered in the early endothelial phase of acute GVHD. Generally, drug eruptions will involve both superficial and deep dermal vessels, and the inflammatory infiltrate will include eosinophils as well as lymphocytes. However, in the setting of the immunosuppression that accompanies the posttransplant period, these characteristic features may be lacking. Cutaneous eruption of lymphocyte recovery, which is seen after chemotherapy and a period of marrow aplasia, shows an upper dermal, usually perivascular infiltrate with variable exocytosis of lymphocytes and spongiosis. Dyskeratotic keratinocytes are seen rarely. Thus, histological and clinical evolution over time is often the best diagnostic indicator of the presence of evolving acute GVHD.

2. Epidermotropic Phase

Lymphocytes that initially accumulate about superficial dermal venules migrate from the perivascular interstitium into the overlying epidermal layer (epidermotropism). Some of these cells may seem to align along the dermal-epidermal junction (Fig. 2B), while others are present at all levels of the epidermis (Fig. 2C). The finding of lymphocytes in the epidermis is diagnostically important in early acute GVHD, for it is the harbinger of target-cell injury. Unlike other forms of dermatitis showing lymphoid epidermotropism, such as various forms of eczematous dermatitis, acute GVHD fails to show intercellular edema (spongiosis) within the epidermal layer. Moreover, there generally is little or no vacuolization of the basal cell layer (Fig. 2D) associated with initial alignment of lymphocytes along the dermal-

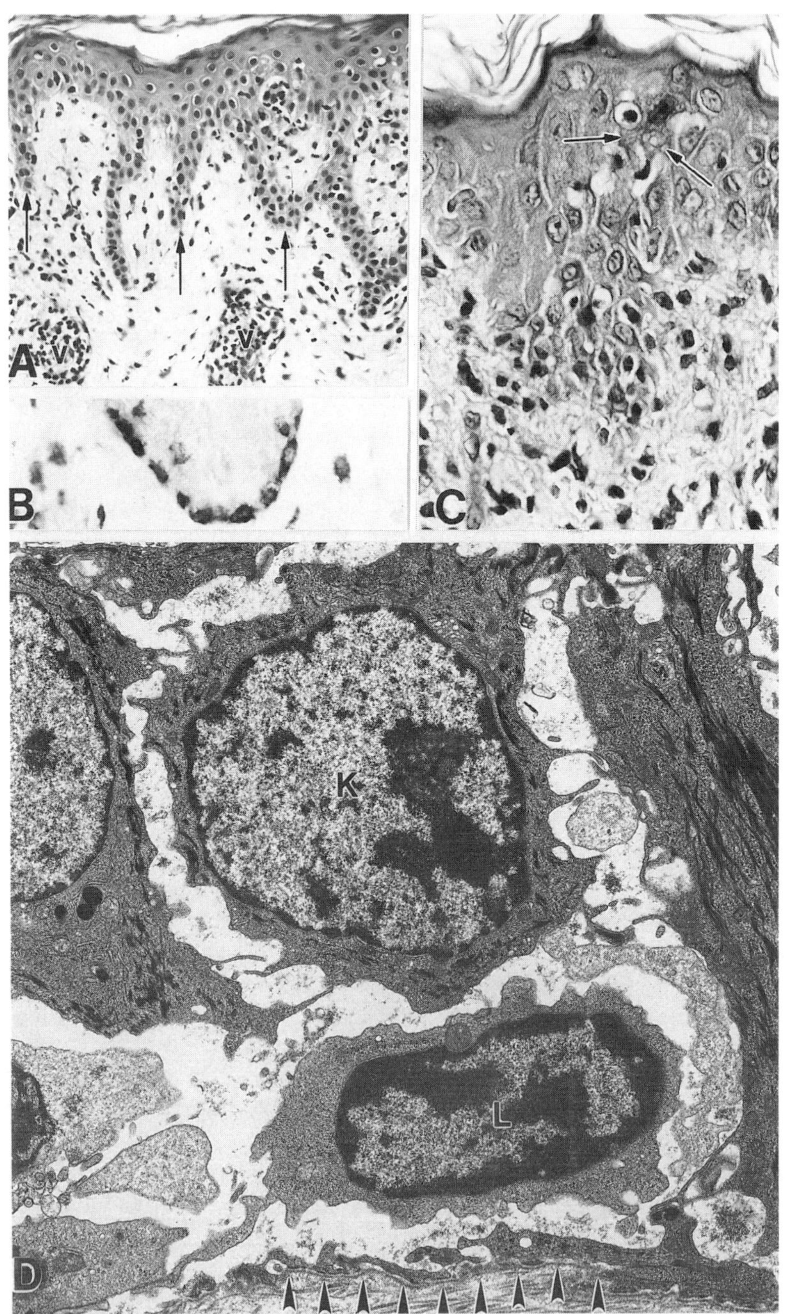

Figure 2 Acute GVHD: endothelial and epidermotropic phases. A. Early acute GVHD shows a sparse superficial perivascular (V) infiltrate of mononuclear cells and foci of migration of these cells into a relatively normal-appearing epidermal layer. Early migration may preferentially involve the rete ridges (arrows). B. The tip of an epidermal rete ridge stained immunohistochemically for the T-lymphocyte glycoprotein CD5. Note the alignment of T cells along the basal cell layer, a pattern often observed in early acute GVHD and believed to correlate with lymphocyte binding to the integral basement membrane protein, epiligrin (see text). C. Early epidermotropism of T cells about a centrally located keratinocyte (arrows).

epidermal interface, whereas early basal cell layer destruction is a relatively consistent finding in acute forms of interface dermatitis, such as erythema multiforme, where lymphocytes also tend to align along the dermal-epidermal junction.

In addition to lymphoid infiltration of the epidermis, migration into the upper third of the hair follicle (follicular infundibulum) is also commonly observed in acute GVHD (Fig. 3D). This phenomenon has been termed "cytotoxic folliculitis" and is a helpful indicator of early GVHD even in biopsies that fail to show significant lymphocytic infiltration of the interfollicular epidermis.

3. Target-Cell Phase

The most characteristic histologic finding in acute GVHD is the finding of "satellitosis," indicating target-cell injury within the epidermis or follicular epithelium (Fig. 3A and B). Satellitosis consists of multiple lymphocytes intimately surrounding a keratinocyte that shows signs of eosinophilic degeneration and necrosis. Such keratinocytes usually contain condensed, hyperchromatic, and sometimes fragmented nuclei. The cytoplasm is dark red due to increased eosin uptake (acidophilia). Although keratinocytes so affected have been referred to as "dyskeratotic," this term fails to describe whether these cells are actually undergoing necrosis or apoptosis (see below). In general, the degree of epidermal injury seems out of proportion to the sparse numbers of lymphocytes present within the superficial dermal and epidermal layers. Indeed, in rare instances, epidermal necrosis in the setting of a sparse lymphoid infiltrate may be so extensive as to produce extensive and life-threatening blisters and sloughing. It is important to realize that a small number of degenerating keratinocytes independent of lymphocytic apposition may be the sequelae of the pretransplant conditioning regimen alone. Accordingly, care should be taken to attribute epidermal necrosis to acute GVHD only when such changes are associated with clear-cut clustering of epidermotropic lymphocytes. With disease progression, basal-cell-layer vacuolization may accompany satellitosis, and the former may be so pronounced in some patients as to result in diffuse epidermal sloughing in a manner akin to toxic epidermal necrolysis.

Ultrastructural analysis of the target-cell phase of acute GVHD permits demonstration of putative effector mononuclear cells with characteristics of lymphocytes in direct apposition to degenerating and necrotic target keratinocytes (Fig. 3C). Interestingly, these target epidermal cells appear to lose intercellular desmosomal attachments at an early stage in this degenerative process (Yoo YH, in preparation). Occasionally lymphocytes forming satellite aggregates within the epidermis contain membrane-bound, lysosomelike cytoplasmic granules, consistent with those of cytotoxic lymphocytes. Similar alterations may be observed in the follicular infundibulum (Fig. 3D); in experimental disease, target-cell injury at this site appears to preferentially involve the "bulge" region near the insertion site of the arrector pili muscle.

Most of the changes described above (endothelial, epidermotropic, and target-cell phases) occur within the first month after transplantation, and the interval

---

Such cells are likely candidates for the degeneration and necrosis that characterizes target cell injury (see Fig. 3). D. Transmission electron micrograph of acute GVHD. Note the epidermotropic lymphocyte (L) directly above the dermal-epidermal junction (arrowheads). The adjacent keratinocyte (K) at this juncture appears viable.

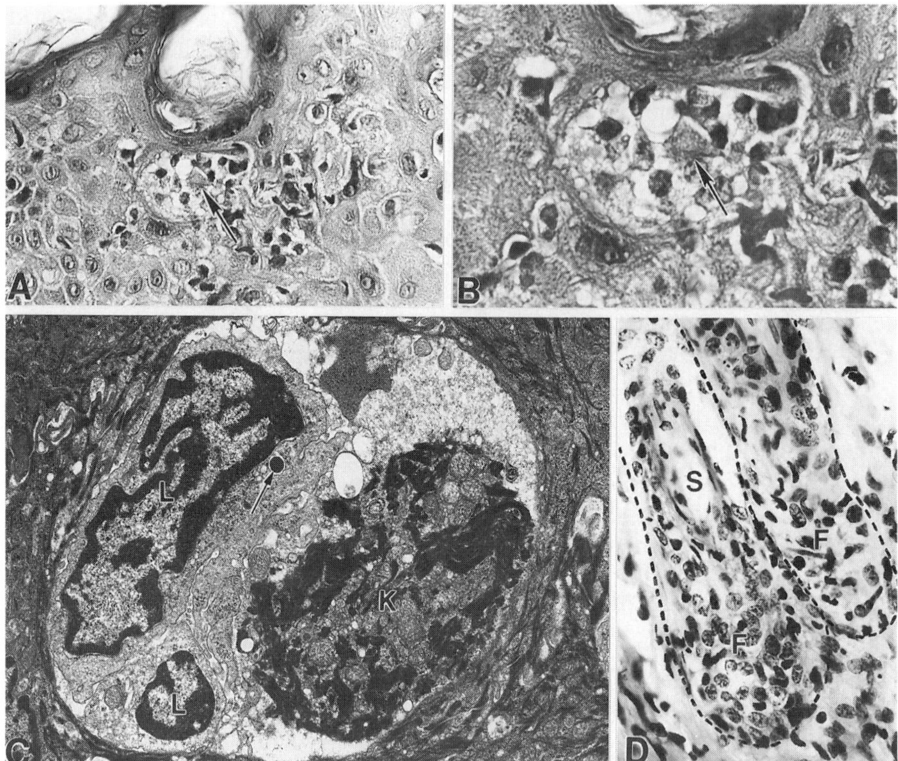

Figure 3 Acute GVHD: target cell phase. A and B. Epidermotropic lymphocytes characteristically surround keratinocytes (arrows) showing nuclear fragmentation and eosinophilic cytoplasmic degeneration and necrosis ("satellitosis"). C. Ultrastructural analysis of target keratinocyte (K) discloses cell shrinkage, membrane blebs, cytoplasmic condensation, and aggregation of tonofilaments consistent with cell death; note that the adjacent putative effector lymphocytes (L) appear viable and contain occasional membrane-bound organelles (arrow) consistent with cytotoxic granules. D. Experimental murine GVHD showing pronounced infiltration of follicular (F) epithelium by lymphocytes. Satellitosis at these sites often involves the bulge region where epithelial stem cells are believed to reside. S = hair shaft.

separating initial inflammatory infiltration from target-cell injury may be as short as 7 to 10 days. Therefore, if an initial biopsy proves nondiagnostic in an individual suspected of developing acute GVHD, a repeat biopsy in 1 to 2 weeks often reveals characteristic findings. The rapid evolution of the epidermal injury in acute GVHD is underscored by the stratum corneum pattern, which generally retains a normal "basket-weave" architecture. This is not the case in more chronic dermatoses, where perturbations in the underlying epidermis are translated into an abnormal scale pattern that may be appreciated both clinically and histologically.

C. Chronic GVHD

1. Epidermal Alterations

The epidermal manifestations of chronic GVHD are far less subtle than those observed in acute disease. Common to both is the finding of satellitosis, with epidermotropic lymphocytes surrounding degenerating and necrotic keratinocytes. The inflammatory infiltrate in chronic GVHD is not sparse and angiocentric, however. Rather, it may fill the papillary dermis in a bandlike manner (Fig. 4A). Moreover, it is associated with transformation of degenerating basal cells into cells with flattened, polyhedral contours ("squamitization" of the basal-cell layer). The papillary dermis may contain melanin-laden histiocytes, sequelae of basal-cell-layer injury

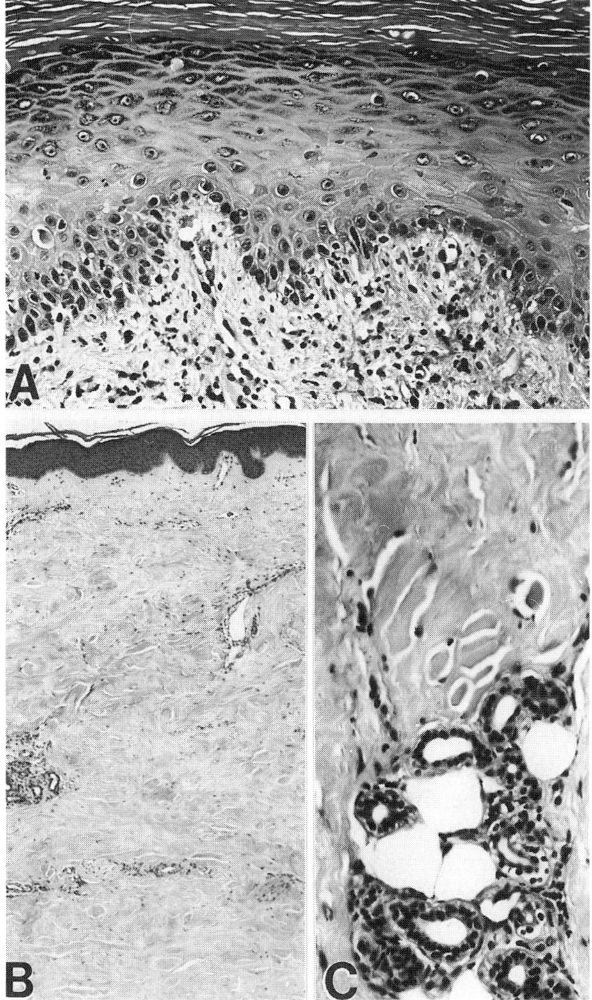

Figure 4 Chronic GVHD: epidermal and dermal types. A. Epidermal (lichen planus–like) chronic GVHD. Note the diffuse lymphocytic infiltrate within the superficial dermis, with infiltration and destruction of the basal-cell layer, epidermal hyperplasia, and increased surface keratin production. These alterations contrast sharply with the relatively normal epidermal layer observed in acute GVHD (Fig. 2A). *B*. Dermal chronic GVHD, showing diffuse replacement of normal dermal architecture by pale hyalinized, sclerotic, and thickened bundles of collagen. C. Higher magnification demonstrating characteristic atrophy and entrapment of eccrine sweat glands by the broad, pale bands of abnormal collagen.

and loss of basal-cell melanin into the dermis. The papillary dermis may also show deposition of coarse collagen bundles, a harbinger of deeper dermal sclerosis that may ensue. The epidermal layer is generally hyperplastic, and the stratum corneum is thickened and hyperkeratotic. These changes bear a striking similarity to lichen planus, although the clinical setting and appearance make this diagnosis unlikely.

A major differential diagnostic consideration in hyperplastic epidermal forms of chronic GVHD is lichen planus–like drug eruptions. Such lesions may be disseminated and therefore mimic epidermal forms of chronic GVHD clinically. Histologically, however, lichen planus–like drug eruptions generally contain eosinophils, whereas the inflammatory infiltrates in epidermal forms of chronic GVHD are usually composed solely of mononuclear cells.

Not all epidermal changes observed in chronic GVHD resemble lichen planus, although all show alterations indicative of chronicity. In some lesions, epidermal atrophy may dominate the histological picture, and there may also be thickening of the basement membrane at the dermal-epidermal interface and IgM and C3 deposition by direct immunofluorescence. Such changes thus resemble chronic atrophic interface dermatitis, as is typical of lupus erythematosus. In general, the dermal mucin deposition that is characteristic of lupus erythematosus is lacking in atrophic variants of chronic GVHD. The common denominator, therefore, in all forms of chronic GVHD of the epidermal type is a lichenoid (bandlike) interstitial papillary dermal infiltrate of lymphocytes, satellitosis, and epidermal alterations indicative of chronicity (altered scale formation associated with either hyperplasia or atrophy).

2. Dermal Alterations

The dermal alterations of chronic GVHD often follow a phase of chronic epidermal injury (discussed above) and consist of deep-seated sclerosis remarkably similar to that seen in morphea and progressive systemic sclerosis (Fig. 4B). The alterations begin at the interface of the reticular dermis and subcutaneous fat, where thick bundles of pale, homogeneous collagen are deposited. Early changes are frequently accompanied by a deep dermal perivascular lymphoplasmacytic infiltrate. Over time, the abnormally deposited collagen replaces subcutaneous fat and extends to involve thickened interlobular septa. The overlying reticular dermis is also progressively replaced, with encasement and eventual atrophy of adnexal epithelium (Fig. 4C). When eccrine coils persist, their placement at the normal junction that previously separated reticular dermis from underlying fat is helpful in determining the extent of subcutaneous replacement. The end result is a markedly thickened dermal layer composed of thickened bundles of pale, hyalinized collagen. The adnexae are generally absent in advanced disease, and the overlying epidermis is generally diffusely atrophic.

Not all lesions of acute GVHD progress to chronic forms, nor do all epidermal forms of GVHD evolve to dermal involvement. However, some lesions do advance from acute epidermal to chronic dermal phases, and such evolution is conceptually useful in visualizing the temporal histopathological sequence of this disorder. Figure 5 provides a schematic representation of the potential temporal evolution of GVHD from the most acute angiocentric and epidermotropic phases to stages involving target-cell injury and eventual dermal sclerosis. Each of these stages provides insight into pathogenesis, particularly in view of recent advances in cellular and molecular immunology of this and related inflammatory disorders of skin.

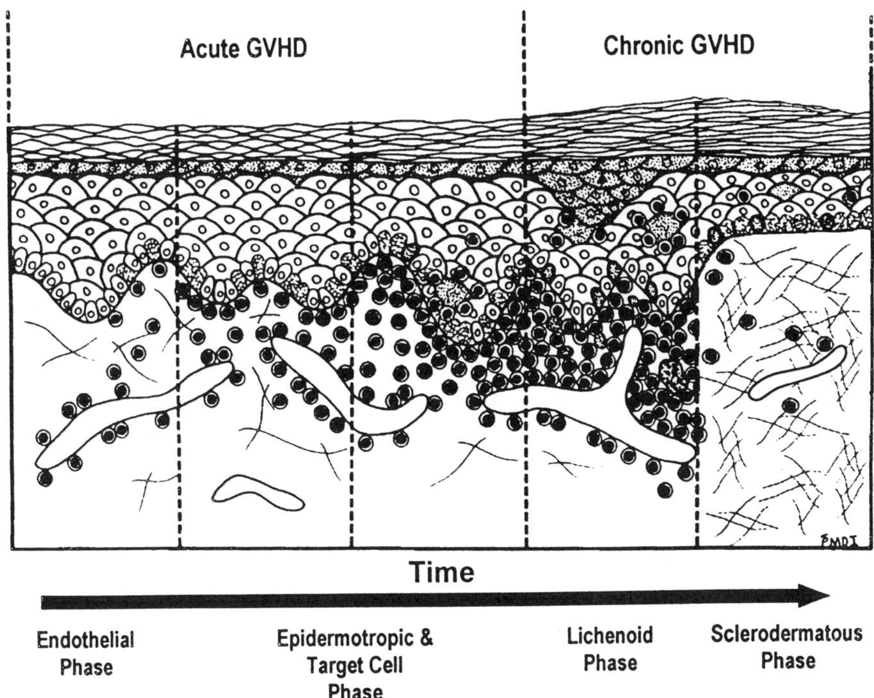

Figure 5 Schematic representation of possible natural evolution of acute and chronic GVHD. Although not all lesions so transform, some progress from acute endothelial, epidermotropic, and target phases to more chronic epidermal (lichenoid) and dermal (sclerodermatous) lesions. Specific stages are illustrated as photomicrographs in Figs. 2 to 4. (Modified from Ref. 61.)

II. PATHOBIOLOGY OF CUTANEOUS GVHD

Although acute and chronic GVHD may appear to occur on a continuum in a single individual, they probably represent two different disease processes. Acute GVHD is a cytotoxic attack of donor lymphocytes on host tissues, most dramatically on epithelial cells (gut, liver, skin), which are seen as foreign. Chronic GVHD, on the other hand, involves cytotoxicity and also a derangement of host immune function stimulated by donor lymphocytes, allowing the development of autoimmunity in a permissive genetic background. In situations of GVHD where there is no tissue incompatibility (syngeneic GVHD), the immune dysfunction becomes paramount.

A. Dermal Effector-Cell Trafficking

The cellular pathology of acute cutaneous GVHD initially involves the ability of circulating donor leukocytes ("effector cells") to traffic to target tissue within the host, where cytotoxic changes subsequently occur. Effector cells in acute GVHD are generally regarded to be T lymphocytes, although their precise phenotype remains elusive, and an extensive literature exists also implicating natural killer cells, monocytes/macrophages, and soluble mediators in production of tissue injury. The process whereby effector lymphocytes home to specific tissues requires the ability of effector cells to "recognize" target sites as they circulate and to bind to and migrate within these potentially hostile microenvironments.

A potentially useful and well-studied paradigm for such highly directed cellular homing is found in the cutaneous delayed-type hypersensitivity reaction (DTH). For several decades it has been recognized that T-cell influx into sites of epicutaneous antigen challenge initially involves the postcapillary venule within the superficial dermis (1,2). This observation, left dormant for many years, is now the central theme of an enormous body of data indicating a critical role for recruitment of lymphocytes to the postcapillary venule of the dermal microvasculature in antigen-driven cutaneous inflammation.

The microanatomy of the superficial dermis is critical to understanding the cellular and molecular interactions responsible for target-specific leukocyte homing. Exogenous and endogenous antigenic targets within the epidermal layer are separated from a complex microvascular plexus by a thin layer of type III collagen, called the papillary dermis. The plexus is composed of small anastomosing arterioles and venules that give rise to capillary loops extending within the papillary dermis toward the epidermal layer. The immediate perivascular microenvironment of postcapillary venules contains mast cells, monocyte/macrophages, and dendritic cells (Fig. 6). Ultrastructural studies show an intimate relationship of mast cells to the venules. During the earliest phases (minutes to hours) of cutaneous inflammation, there are prominent alterations involving the postcapillary venule and the cells that surround it. The changes consist of degranulation of perivenular mast cells and these changes in endothelium: a) prominence of endothelial cytoplasmic filaments; b) endothelial bulging into the venular lumen; and c) gap formation between adjacent endothelial cells. The endothelial alterations, initially believed to be solely the result of liberation of histamine from mast cells and termed "histamine effect," occur at timepoints that correlate with the earliest recruitment of leukocytes to affected venules.

Today it is known that this "endothelial activation" involves complicated and precisely orchestrated molecular signals that produce the efficient display of adhesion molecules, promoting leukocyte binding to the lumenal endothelial surface. Such molecules are expressed in a cascade, with the earliest (e.g. P- selectin) appearing within minutes and mediating the weakest binding which only slows circulating leukocytes to slow "roll" along the endothelial membrane. Display of subsequent molecules may either serve to favor adhesion of specific subpopulations of effector cells (e.g. E-selectin), or to strengthen leukocyte- endothelial binding and promote diapedesis—e.g., vascular-cell adhesion molecule-1 (VCAM-1), intercellular adhesion molecule-1 (ICAM-1), and platelet endothelial cell adhesion molecule-1 (PECAM-1). Reciprocal ligands on effector cells may be either constitutively expressed by certain subpopulations (e.g., as in lymphocyte function associated antigen-1, or LFA-1, the ligand for ICAM-1) (3,4), or progressively upregulated during the binding process (5,6). Mast-cell degranulation may facilitate the display of these binding cascades, since mast cells liberate secretory substances that either induce or alter distribution of endothelial adhesion molecules (histamine for P-selectin; tumor necrosis factor α for E-selectin, ICAM-1, and VCAM-1).

The provocative stimuli for mast-cell degranulation in early inflammation are potentially of critical importance in understanding what triggers initial effector-cell binding to microvenular endothelium. In experimental DTH reactions, it appears that antigen-specific antibody molecules that function like IgE may be generated

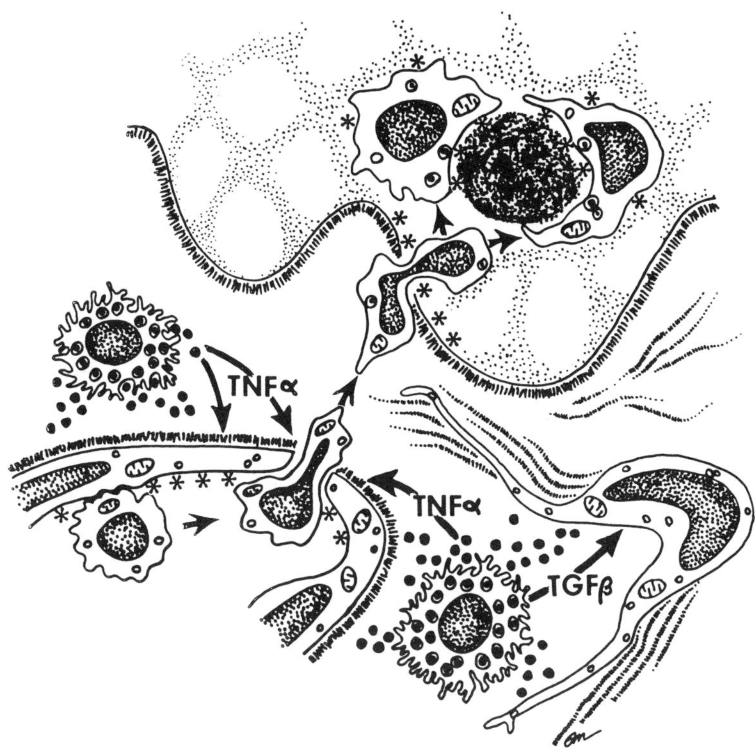

Figure 6 Schematic diagram of hypothetical TNFα/TGFβ pathways in acute and chronic GVHD. Early mast cell degranulation (left) results in release of histamine and TNF-α, which initiates early expression of endothelial glycoproteins (*) important in early leukocyte adhesion. Adherent leukocytes then migrate across the vessel wall and undergo directed migration to the epidermal layer via as yet undetermined chemotactic/chemokinetic signals. Once in the epidermal layer, effector lymphocytes bind to different strata by adhesive interactions with basement membrane keratinocyte surface proteins (*) and ultimately localize about target cells (dark cell undergoing degenerative changes). Mast-cell degranulation may also results in cytokine release (TNF-α, TGF-β) capable of activation of dermal dendrocytes and fibroblasts, resulting in increased expression of factor XIIIa and mRNA for collagen type I, respectively. Thus, mast cells may play an important role in both acute and chronic phases of GVHD.

during sensitization (7). Challenge with epicutaneous antigen provokes mast-cell degranulation by local cross-linking of these antibodies on mast-cell membranes, setting into motion an endothelial adhesion cascade that results in recruitment of specific memory T cells. Mast-cell degranulating properties have also been identified in supernatants of allostimulated T cells (8). In human GVHD, early expression of endothelial adhesion molecules (e.g., E-selectin) potentially induced by mast-cell cytokines, also has been documented (9). Moreover, the potential importance of mast cells to the early inflammatory phases of GVHD is emphasized by ultrastructural studies indicating that degranulation of these cells consistently precedes effector cell influx. In keeping with this observation, cutaneous GVHD lesions are delayed when genetically mast-cell–deficient animals serve as transplant recipients. Disease eventually occurs only when granulated mast cells develop, either from donor stem cells or due to microenvironmental factors that are as yet unclear (10).

B. Epidermal Effector-Cell Trafficking

Once effector leukocytes have effectively identified and infiltrated the mesenchyme of target organs, they then must complete their voyage into the epidermal layer, where putative antigens are concentrated. Navigation into the epidermal layer, a process referred to as "epidermotropism," is likely to involve molecular interactions equally or more complicated than what has already transpired within the underlying dermis. The first adhesive events between effector leukocytes and epidermal cells are likely to involve the basal-cell layer and the basement membrane zone, which defines the boundary between epidermis and superficial dermis. In human and experimental GVHD, many cells infiltrating the epidermal layer are often localized in close proximity to the basement membrane zone. These T cells, lymphokine activated killer cells, and alloreactive cytotoxic cells, but not B cells, express the $\alpha 3\beta 1$ membrane integrin which is a receptor for the basement membrane ligand epiligrin (11). This molecule is synthesized by basal keratinocytes and is expressed primarily in the lamina lucida of the basement membrane. Such binding interactions between specific subsets of T cells and basal epidermal cells are therefore likely to influence early epidermotropic migration and adhesion in GVHD.

Binding of T cells to the suprabasal epidermal layers is likely to be mediated by additional interactions between leukocytes and keratinocytes, including well-established LFA-1/ICAM-1 adhesion. Unlike endothelial cells, keratinocytes do not constitutively express ICAM-1 and therefore must be induced by early migrant T cells via elaboration of cytokines and lymphokines, such as γ-interferon (INF- γ). Both ICAM-1 and HLA-DR are upregulated on epidermal cells by INF-γ, and both are prominently displayed during the epidermotropic phases of GVHD (12). Recently, by analogy with the trafficking patterns of intestinal intraepithelial T cells and malignant lymphocytes of cutaneous T-cell lymphoma, it has been suggested that leukocytes may also bind to epidermal cells via hetrophilic adhesion between keratinocyte E-cadherin and the lymphocyte integrin, $\alpha E\beta 7$ (13,14). This possibility deserves further scrutiny in the setting of naturally occurring and experimental GVHD.

C. Effector–Target-Cell Interaction

Once effector lymphocytes have completed their highly directed journey from peripheral circulation to specific microvascular beds and finally to microanatomical compartments where target cells reside, direct effector–target-cell interactions are believed to produce cytotoxicity. The mechanism(s) of this cellular killing remain elusive.

The two constant features of injury in both acute and chronic forms of epidermal GVHD are cytotoxic changes in basal keratinocytes and eosinophilic degeneration (necrosis or apoptosis) of individual keratinocytes. Direct toxicity of chemotherapeutic drugs or radiation is a possible cause of keratinocyte degeneration and necrosis when the individual has been pretreated for bone marrow transplantation, and it may be difficult to distinguish such toxicity from early GVHD. Even as late as 1 month posttreatment, the epidermis may show alterations compatible with stem cell injury and loss of regenerative capacity (15,16). However, the cytotoxic changes are present also in nonirradiated animal models for GVHD, raising important questions about mechanisms of injury in these animals.

Damage to the various tissues by the immune system can occur via multiple specific and nonspecific mechanisms. The specific mechanisms are the best understood. They are (a) antibody and complement-mediated cytotoxicity, with directed attack by specific antibodies, producing immune complexes and stimulating the complement cascade, with resulting tissue destruction (classic antibody- mediated injury has not been shown to play a role in cutaneous GVHD); (b) directed attack by cytotoxic T cells recognizing histocompatibility antigens and foreign antigens on the surfaces of targeted cells; (c) Nonspecific mechanisms, including attack by natural killer cells (large granular lymphocytes), which, once activated, kill in a nonrestricted fashion; and (d) nonspecific damage by mediators of inflammation and cytotoxic cytokines such as TNF-α. Because cutaneous involvement is present in 90 to 100% of individuals with both acute and chronic GVHD, the skin is a useful organ system for studies of the various mechanisms of injury.

One of the most puzzling observations in both acute and chronic cutaneous GVHD is that the amount of damage to the epidermis is out of proportion to the inflammatory infiltrate, which is sparse. Clearly, there are increased numbers of lymphocytes in the epidermis and surrounding dermal vessels in GVHD. Studies of populations of the cells infiltrating the skin are complicated by the problem of identifying those cells that are directly attacking epithelial cells versus those secreting factors that may help cytotoxic cells kill their targets. Also, in human GVHD, patients have almost always been treated with cyclosporine to prevent GVHD; the effects of this immunosuppressant on the histopathology of cutaneous eruptions is unclear. As a result, the literature describing effector cytotoxic cells in cutaneous GVHD is contradictory and confusing. The most obvious form of cytotoxicity is thought to be *satellitosis*, in which targeted keratinocytes are surrounded, contacted, and killed by lymphocytes.

Three donor-cell populations probably interact to produce acute cutaneous GVHD. They are natural and lymphokine-activated killer cells and cytotoxic T cells. All are part of a larger category of cells called cytotoxic lymphocytes (CTL).

1. Natural Killer Cells (Large Granular Lymphocytes) and Lymphokine- Activated Killer Cells

Cells bearing markers for natural killer cells have been identified as possible effector cells infiltrating organs of mice with acute GVHD; they have been found closely associated with dead or dying epithelial cells in skin, liver, and colon (17,18). These cells are donor in origin and can mediate cytotoxicity in the absence of class I or II on target cells.

2. Cytotoxic T Cells

Mature donor CD8$^+$ cytotoxic T cells have also been shown to play an important role in acute GVHD. Cytotoxic T cells kill via recognition of self-MHC (class I) molecules and processed foreign antigens expressed on the surface of a targeted cell, typically a virally infected cell or a tumor cell. Hess and coworkers (19) have shown that the presence of CD8$^+$ cytotoxic T cells is correlated with the onset of the acute phase of syngeneic GVHD in rats, and that these cells recognize a public determinant of class II histocompatibility antigens. The histological changes in mucosa of the tongue shows CD4$^-$CD8$^+$ lymphocytes infiltrating mucosa, with prominent epithelial cell destruction and satellitosis.

A useful murine model for the study of various T-cell donor-lymphocyte subsets in GVHD utilizes highly purified populations of these subsets to generate GVHD across minor histocompatibility loci, the experimental model most like that of allogeneic bone marrow transplantation in humans (20,21). In multiple different mouse strain combinations, mature $CD8^+$ T cells can mediate GVHD without help from donor $CD4^+$ helper lymphocytes. $CD4^+$ lymphocytes can produce GVHD alone also, but only in certain strain combinations, suggesting that genetic factors play an important role in GVHD. In two strain combinations designed to evaluate the histopathology of GVHD mediated by either $CD4^+$ or $CD8^+$ lymphocytes, epidermal cytotoxicity is present in both, indicating that a final common pathway of cytotoxicity may exist for these T-cell subsets. Significantly, dermal fibrosis is evident only in $CD8^+$- mediated disease in these murine models (22). The use of this "Korngold-Sprent" model for murine GVHD has illustrated the complexity of effector lymphocyte pathways as well as the importance of immunohistocompatibility target antigens in initiation and progression of GVHD.

D. Molecular Mechanisms of Target Cell Injury

Although the target molecules responsible for directed cell killing have not been identified, we are beginning to understand more about the potential mechanisms for cytotoxicity in GVHD. Two distinct mechanisms have been defined at the molecular level for cytotoxic cell activity (23–25). Both require stable contact and interdigitation involving large surface areas of both CTL and target cells.

1. Perforins and Granzymes

The first mechanism of killing utilizes a perforin mechanism, which appears to involve exocytosis of cytotoxic granules containing perforin protein and serine esterases (granzymes), which are expressed by cytotoxic T and killer lymphocytes. Perforin has considerable sequence homology to complement components C6 to C9 and presumably spans the target-cell membrane, as does the membrane attack complex of complement, allowing disruption of the target-cell membrane and lysis of the cell. Because isolated cytotoxic granules are able to induce DNA fragmentation and death in target cells only in the presence of Ca^{2+} and perforin protein, it has been suggested that granzymes may gain access to the target cell intracellular milieu via perforin channels. Sale et al. (26,27) examined skin and lip biopsies of patients with chronic GVHD following marrow allograft transplantation; they used immunofluorescence with a mouse monoclonal antibody (TIA-1) to serine esterase–positive membrane granules of human cytotoxic T cells. These investigators determined that 80 to 90% of the cells infiltrating and destroying epidermal cells in these tissues are CD8/TIA-1- positive, whereas very few of the infiltrating cells are Leu-7 (natural killer) positive. Perforin and granzymes have also been identified in Thy1 + dendritic epidermal cells and in purified human gamma-delta T cells (24). The roles of these cells in cutaneous GVHD is unknown.

2. Fas

The other mechanism of cytotoxicity involves the cell death–transducing molecule Fas (APO-1), a member of the TNF-α receptor superfamily; transfection of Fas antigen cDNA to fibroblast cell lines confers susceptibility to cytotoxic activity (28). Therefore, expression of Fas defines target cells for cytotoxic T cells, which lyse them via a mechanism dependent on ligand-receptor binding. This mechanism involves DNA fragmentation in a distinctive ladderlike pattern, reflecting double-stranded DNA breakage between nucleosomes, probably produced by endogenous endonucleases activated by Fas and requiring a metabolically active target cell. Sayama et al. (29) have shown that Fas antigen is expressed on keratinocytes of skin in inflammatory processes such as lichenoid drug reaction, erythema multiforme, contact dermatitis, bullous pemphigoid, pemphigus vulgaris, and herpes zoster; coexpression with ICAM-1 in the lower half of the epidermis is noted in these biopsy specimens. In addition, these investigators have demonstrated that IFN-γ-stimulated cultured human keratinocytes upregulate Fas antigen expression and can undergo apoptotic death mediated by anti-Fas antibody. Whether these two mechanisms, perforin-based and Fas-based killing, can be accomplished by the same cytotoxic T cell is not known (23). It is likely that the dyskeratotic cells observed in the epidermis in GVHD are undergoing apoptosis, but to date, there are no studies of Fas expression or apoptosis in cutaneous GVHD.

E. Cutaneous Cytokine Effects in GVHD

When mature T cells from a bone marrow transplant inoculum recognize allogeneic cutaneous antigens, multiple inflammatory cytokines are induced that may contribute to the manifestations of cutaneous GVHD. The release of these inflammatory cytokines in GVHD has been documented at the protein and mRNA levels, suggesting the concept of GVHD as a "cytokine storm" (30). Therapeutic agents such as cyclosporine, which inhibit cytokine production by lymphocytes, can thereby ameliorate GVHD. Antin and Ferrara (30) have proposed that cytokine dysregulation may explain pathological features of acute GVHD in which tissue damage appears to involve more than direct T-cell mediated cytotoxicity. It is thought that IL-1, IL-2, TNF-α, and IFN-γ are the major cytokines driving cytotoxicity in GVHD (31) and that TGF-β may be important in dermal changes. The time course of cytokine mRNA transcription suggests a hierarchy of cytokine dysregulation in this process.

1. Interleukins (IL-1 and IL-2)

IL-1, a central mediator of inflammation, may function at multiple levels in the cytokine cascade of GVHD. Like TNF-α, it induces expression of E-selectin and ICAM-1 on dermal vascular endothelial cells, and it is important in the activation of T cells to enhance an immune response. Unlike most other cells, however, the keratinocyte does not respond to IL-1 by upregulation of ICAM-1, thought to be important in epidermotropism of lymphocytes. Clearly there are other mechanisms (IFN-γ) by which this can occur in GVHD.

IL-1 mRNA transcription is upregulated early by several hundred-fold in GVHD target organs, including the skin (32,33). IL-1 continues to increase over the following weeks, and GVHD in a mouse model, described below, can be ameliorated dramatically by the administration of IL-1 receptor antagonist (34).

Surprisingly, IL-2—secreted by macrophages, stimulatory to T lymphocytes, and implicated in many cutaneous inflammatory disorders—is upregulated only in the spleen during the first week after bone marrow transplantation in a murine model for GVHD due to minor histocompatibility loci (32). In this study, utilizing a quantitative polymerase chain reaction technique, the authors noted that the relatively minor increase in IL-2 mRNA in the skin is consistent with the presence of a sparse lymphocytic infiltrate in early GVHD. They suggest that cytotoxicity may be due to other cytokines and to natural killer cells (32). In keeping with this hypothesis, anti–IL-2 receptor antibodies are variably effective on the manifestations and course of GVHD. Ferrara et al. (33) showed amelioration of experimental acute GVHD by in vivo administration of IL-2 receptor antibodies. However, depending on when administered, they may actually exacerbate GVHD (31).

2. IFN-γ

This cytokine increases the in vitro expression of MHC antigens on keratinocytes (12), which may enhance their recognition by donor cytotoxic lymphocytes in MCH- incompatible transplantation. Similarly, IFN-γ causes upregulation of cell adhesion molecules such as ICAM-1 on keratinocytes, enabling binding by LFA-1, the corresponding recognition molecule on lymphocytes. IFN-γ also upregulates mRNA and protein expression of the leukocyte adhesion molecule ICAM-1, on dermal endothelial cells, presumably initiating the first steps in targeting of effector lymphocytes to the skin in the endothelial phase of GVHD.

3. TNF-α

Although the levels of TNF-α mRNA transcripts in the skin are upregulated by only 4- to 6-fold in GVHD in the study by Abhyankar et al. (32), this cytokine has been implicated as a major contributor to cytotoxicity in GVHD. Circulating levels of TNF-α protein are high and correlate with the severity and course of cutaneous GVHD. Piguet et al. (35,36) have shown that neutralizing antibodies against TNF-α administered to mice with acute GVHD will reduce mortality and morbidity of disease, whereas TNF-α itself administered to normal mice will reproduce some of the clinical and pathological features of GVHD. As mentioned previously, mast cells degranulate in early GVHD, releasing TNF-α, a cytokine with pleiotropic effects including promotion of endothelial-leukocyte adhesion (37), induction of apoptosis, and promotion of collagen synthesis. The effects of TNF-α on keratinocytes are diverse, from upregulation of ICAM-1 expression to direct cytotoxicity. Although TNF-α can produce apoptotic cell death with characteristic laddered DNA degradation in certain sensitive cells, it is not known if it causes a necrotic or an apoptotic type of cell death in keratinocytes. TNF-α also upregulates mRNA production and protein expression of endothelial cell molecules such as ICAM-1 and E-selectin, and it may play an important role in the endothelial phase of cutaneous GVHD.

4. TGF-β

Transforming growth factor β (TGF-β) has been shown to play an important role in wound healing and tissue remodeling. It stimulates proliferation of fibroblasts, production of protease inhibitors, and inhibits matrix proteinases, collectively leading to increased stabilized dermal matrix. Release of TNF-α and TGF-β by mast cells can upregulate collagen I mRNA expression by fibroblasts (38). In addition, cutaneous mast cells have recently been shown to express basic fibroblast factor, a polypeptide also important in tissue remodeling (39). Therefore, degranulation of mast cells in early GVHD can be linked with molecular events in the extracellular matrix, potentially leading to dermal fibrosis, as may occur in chronic GVHD (see "Mechanisms of Mesenchymal Activation," below).

The potential local sources of these cytokines and growth factors in cutaneous

GVHD are multiple. Macrophages, tissue histiocytes, lymphocytes, and mast cells can produce cytokines. It has only recently been appreciated that keratinocytes can also release immunologically active cytokines and so are participants as well as targets in various cutaneous inflammatory processes. In fact, removal of the stratum corneum and disruption of the epidermal barrier by tape stripping will activate keratinocytes to produce mRNA for ICAM-1, TNF-α, IFN-γ, IL-8, and IL-10 (40). In addition, IL-1 and IL-2 receptors are found in large quantities in epidermis of inflamed skin (41).

F. Mechanisms of Mesenchymal Activation

As GVHD progresses, cytotoxic injury to the epidermis is accompanied by fibrosis in the underlying dermis. Although benign cutaneous inflammatory processes can produce some dermal fibrosis (usually superficial and mild), the fibrosis in chronic cutaneous GVHD is out of proportion to the amount of lymphocytic infiltrate present. Abnormal responses of mast cells and fibroblasts are important also, although much less is known about the roles these cells play in chronic cutaneous GVHD.

Mast cells are bone marrow–derived cells that are distributed in a potentially strategic perivascular location, where their secretion products can rapidly affect dermal vessels. Mast cells have been described classically as mediators of anaphylactic and allergic responses via IgE cross-linking by antigen and discharge of their mast-cell granules, which contain histamine and other potent biologically active factors. Mast cells clearly have other more subtle functions as well. The involvement of mast cells in fibrosis is supported by many independent observations of increased numbers of mast cells in the following conditions: around wounds, in tumors such as growing edges of keloids, carcinoid, hemangiomas, neurofibromas, and mastocytosis; in bleomycin fibrosis, toxic oil syndrome, eosinophilic fasciitis, pulmonary fibrosis, radiation-induced fibrosis, venous stasis, parasitic disease, synovitis of rheumatoid arthritis, early progressive systemic sclerosis, and GVHD (42–45). Often in these conditions, the mast cells are degranulated, suggesting activation. We have shown that mast-cell degranulation precedes GVHD target-cell injury in two different combinations of irradiated murine strains with minor histocompatibility differences, and as described earlier, onset of GVHD can be delayed in allogeneic bone marrow transplantation to mast-cell-deficient B6WWv mice. The onset of GVHD in these animals can be correlated with appearance of granulated mast cells (10). TNF-α and TGF-β release as a consequence of mast-cell degranulation in mice has recently been linked to induction of collagen type I mRNA in dermal fibroblasts (38). In humans, we have shown that mast-cell TNF-α may be linked to increased numbers of dendritic dermal cells expressing the coagulation factor FXIIIa (46), and dendritic stromal cells increase dramatically during early phases of experimental murine GVHD (G.F.M., unpublished observation). Therefore, mast cells may not only play an important role in the endothelial cell phase of acute GVHD but may also trigger stromal alterations integral to the development of chronic GVHD (Fig. 6).

G. Autoimmunity and Chronic GVHD

The striking similarities of chronic cutaneous GVHD to autoimmune disorders such as lupus erythematosus and progressive systemic sclerosis has prompted a search for common pathogenic features. GVHD affects hematopoiesis and lymphopoiesis as a result of immunosuppression and immunodeficiency. Multiple abnormalities have been documented: a deficiency in IL-2 secreting cells; a decrease in other lymphokines such as colony stimulating factors, which may be necessary for hematopoiesis; and, most importantly, a decrease in the functional repertoire of T cells. This may reflect inability of injured thymic epithelium to produce differentiation factors necessary for normal T-cell development (47). Therefore, abnormal recovering immune functions provide a setting for the development of autoimmune processes in the recipient.

The abnormal immune functions described above are important in the development of antibodies to self antigens in chronic GVHD. Autoantibodies directed against histones, DNA, and the small nuclear ribonucleoprotein particles (snRNPs) are found in connective tissue diseases (lupus erythematosus, scleroderma, chronic progressive polyarthritis, primary biliary cirrhosis, and mixed connective tissue disease) (48). These autoantibodies can also be found arising spontaneously in patients with chronic GVHD (49), in normal individuals (50), and in certain mouse strains with chronic GVHD induced by P → F1 transplantation (51). As in the various autoimmune diseases, the autoantibodies appear to involve only selected antigen-antibody systems. The chronic GVHD and the specificities of autoantibodies induced in nonirradiated, nonautoimmune mice resemble the clinical, histopathological, and serological features of systemic lupus erythematosus (SLE) and scleroderma, suggesting that GVHD has features of SLE- or sclerodermalike autoimmunity. As in systemic lupus, autoantibodies to DNA and to proteins in complexes with nucleic acids (histones and small nuclear ribonucleoprotein polypeptides, snRNPs) are consistent features. Gleichman and coworkers (52) showed the presence of autoantibodies to DNA by *Crithidia* assay and to nuclear antigens, thymocytes, and red blood cells by immunofluorescence in nonirradiated (C57BL/10 × DBA/2) F1 hybrid mice, which developed GVHD after injections with lymphoid cells of DBA/2 donor mice. Similarly, Portanova and coworkers (53) identified selective production of autoantibodies to DNA in DBA/2 → (C57BL/6 × DBA/2) F1 mice with GVHD. An initial polyclonal stimulation of IgM and IgG-secreting B cells appears to precede the later antigen-specific stimulation (54). Gelpi and coworkers (55) studied the molecular basis of autonantibody specificity in a murine model for GVHD: when unirradiated (BALB/c × A/J) F1 mice are injected with lymphoid cells from the parental A/J strain, they develop glomerulonephritis, forefoot edema, alopecia, splenomegaly, and lymphadenopathy compatible with chronic GVHD. Forty percent of these mice also develop antinuclear antibodies to the U1 and U3 snRNPs. The epitope recognition of the 70-kDa and A polypeptide components of the U1 snRNP on Western blot analysis with ANA-positive mouse sera is similar to that of mixed connective tissue disease in humans, whereas the epitope recognition of the 34- kDa fibrillarin protein of the U3 snRNP is specific for scleroderma. Although these mice are identical genetically, not all develop the autoantibodies, as in the human manifestation of an autoimmune disease such as lupus or scleroderma, suggesting a process with several stimuli (permissive genetic background, environmental stimulus such as GVHD, and perhaps a random immunological event such as somatic mutation, which does not occur in all animals). In summary, autoantibody production in chronic GVHD resembles that in SLE and scleroderma; is mainly to DNA, histones, and less commonly to specific components of the U1 and U3 snRNPs; and may reflect an idiosyncratic or random immunological process.

Establishing that autoantibodies in chronic GVHD are pathogenic has been problematic, as it has been in autoimmune disease. Because the main target of chronic cutaneous GVHD is the basal layer of keratinocytes, investigators have looked for antibodies to the dermal-epidermal junction (DEJ) and to keratinocytes. In patients with chronic cutaneous GVHD, 86% have IgM deposits at the DEJ compared with their own pretransplantation biopsies, with posttransplantation biopsies in patients without chronic cutaneous GVHD, and with healthy bone marrow donors (56). In 2 of 4 patients with chronic cutaneous GVHD, Saurat et al. (57) found antibodies to epidermal basal cells. In certain mice undergoing chronic GVHD due to H-2 incompatibility, antibodies are found along the basement membrane zone, and these autoantibodies correlate with severe nephrotic syndrome and immune complex glomerulonephritis (58).

In mouse models for GVHD involving class II incompatibilities and in autoimmune mouse strains with similar cutaneous histopathological findings, the presence of antibodies to nuclear antigens such as double-stranded DNA, histones, extractable nuclear antigens, snRNPs, and ribosomal P protein have not been shown to correlate with tissue injury in other organs such as the kidney. Therefore, the direct role of injury by specific autoantibodies in chronic cutaneous GVHD is unclear. These autoantibodies may be markers for the immune dysfunction allowing cytotoxic lymphocytes to produce epidermal target cell injury in these P → F1 models for cutaneous GVHD, but they may not be pathogenic themselves.

III. FUTURE DIRECTIONS

It is clear from the discussion above that the pathobiology of cutaneous GVHD is even more problematic than its diagnostic pathology. And yet, enormous strides have been made in the development of experimental systems for exploration of this important disorder. The development of murine models relevant to human allotransplantation has permitted dissection of the immunogenetics that determine the identities and functions of effector cells as they produce highly characteristic lesions in target keratinocytes. The burgeoning interest concerning programmed cell death, or apoptosis, presents a novel opportunity to examine the phenomenon as an explanation for target-cell injury of GVHD. Limitations due to lack of complete analogy between murine and human skin can be overcome by using in vivo models of human inflammatory skin disease. For example, it has recently been demonstrated that human skin xenotransplanted onto mice with severe combined immune deficiency syndrome (SCID mice) is functionally responsive to many of the proinflammatory cytokines released during acute GVHD. Moreover, we have recently demonstrated the presence of an inflammatory infiltrate at the level of the superficial dermal microvasculature when mast cells are degranulated in these human xenografts in a manner similar to that observed in early acute GVHD (59,60). Finally, we have recently developed an assay whereby human lymphocytes migrate within human xenografts within the SCID mouse chimeras, resulting in effector cell–target-epidermal-cell interactions that faithfully reproduce lichen planus–like GVHD. Such approaches hold enormous promise for design of future studies that will elucidate precise mechanisms of effector–target-cell interaction in cutaneous GVHD as well as provide a basis for defining immunogenetic strategies for disease prevention.

ACKNOWLEDGMENT

This work was supported by grant CA40538 from the National Cancer Institute of the NIH.

REFERENCES

1. Dvorak HF, Mihm MC, Dvorak AM. Morphology of delayed-type hypersensitivity reaction in man. J Invest Dermatol 1976; 67:391–401.
2. Dvorak AM, Mihm MC, Dvorak HF. Morphology of delayed-typed hypersensitivity reactions in man: II. Ultrastructural alteration affecting the microvasculature and the tissue mast cells. Lab Invest 1976; 1976:179–191.
3. Springer TA. Adhesion receptors of the immune system. Nature 1990; 346:425–434.
4. Springer TA. Traffic signals for lymphocyte recirculation and leukocyte emigration: The multistep paradigm. Cell 1994; 76:301–314.
5. Lasky LA. Selectins: Interpreters of cell-specific carbohydrate information during inflammation. Science 1992; 258:964–969.
6. Picker LJ. Control of lymphocyte homing. Curr Opin Immunol 1994; 6:349–405.
7. Askenase PW. Delayed-type hypersensitivity recruitment of T-cell subsets via antigen-specific non-IgE factors or IgE antibodies: Relevance to asthma, autoimmunity and immune responses to tumors and parasites. Chem Immunol 1992; 54:166–211.
8. Levi-Schaffer F, Mekori YA, Segal V, Claman HN. Histamine release from mouse and rat mast cells cultured with supernatants from chronic murine graft-vs- host splenocytes. Cell Immunol 1990; 127:146–158.
9. Shen N, Ffrench P, Guyotat D, Ffrench M, et al. Expression of adhesion molecules in endothelial cells during allogeneic bone marrow transplantation. Eur J Haematol 1994; 52:296–301.
10. Murphy GF, Sueki H, Teusche C, et al. Role of mast cells in early epithelial target cell injury in experimental acute graft-vs-host disease. J Invest Dermatol 1994; 102:451–461.
11. Wayner EA, Gil SG, Murphy GF, et al. Epiligrin, a component of epithelial basement membranes, is an adhesive ligand for $\alpha3\beta1$ positive T lymphocytes. J Cell Biol 1993; 121:1141–1152.
12. Volc-Platzer B, Stingl G. Cutaneous graft-versus-host disease. In: Burakoff SJ, Deeg HJ, Ferrara J, Atkinson K, eds. Graft-vs.-Host Disease. New York: Marcel Dekker, 1990:245–254.
13. Simonitsch I, Volc-Platzer B, Mosberger I, Radaszkicwicz T. Expression of monoclonal antibody HML-1-defined α E β 7 integrin in cutaneous T cell lymphoma. Am J Pathol 1994; 145:1148–1158.
14. Cepek KL. Adhesion between epithelial cells and T lymphocytes mediated by E-cadherin and $\alpha E\beta 7$ integrin. Nature 1994; 372:190–193.
15. Shulman HM, Sale GE. Pathology of acute and chronic cutaneous GVHD. In: Sale GE, Shulman WM, eds. The Pathology of Bone Marrow Transplantation. New York: 1984:40–76.
16. LeBoit PE. Subacute radiation dermatitis: A histologic imitator of acute cutaneous graft-versus-host disease. J Am Acad Dermatol 1989; 20:236–241.

17. Guillén FJ, Ferrara J, Hancock WW, et al. Acute cutaneous graft-versus- host disease to minor histocompatibility antigens in a murine model: Evidence that large granular lymphocytes are effector cells in the immune response. Lab Invest 1986; 55:35–42.
18. Ferrara JL, Guillén FJ, van Dijken PJ, et al. Evidence that large granular lymphocytes of donor origin mediate acute graft-versus-host disease. Transplantation 1989; 47:50–54.
19. Hess AD. Syngeneic graft-vs-host disease. In Burakoff SJ, Deeg HJ, Ferrara J, Atkinson K, eds. Graft-vs-Host Disease. New York: Marcel Dekker, 1990:95–107.
20. Korngold R, Sprent J. Lethal graft-vs-host disease following bone marrow transplantation across minor histocompatibility barriers in mice: Prevention by removing mature T cells from marrow. J Exp Med 1978; 148:1687–1698.
21. Korngold R. Biology of graft-versus-host disease. Am J Pediatr Hematol/Oncol 1993; 15:18–27.
22. Murphy GF, Witaker D, Sprent J, Korngold R. Characterization of target injury of murine acute graft-versus-host disease directed to multiple minor histocompatibility antigens elicited by either $CD4^+$ or $CD8^+$ effector cells. Am J Pathol 1991; 138:983–990.
23. Kägi D, Vignaux F, Ledermann B, et al. Fas and perforin pathways as major mechanisms of T cell-mediated cytotoxicity. Science 1994; 265:528–530.
24. Berke G. The binding and lysis of target cells by cytotoxic lymphocytes: Molecular and cellular aspects. Annu Rev Immunol 1994; 12:735–773.
25. Squier MKT, Cohen JJ. Cell-mediated cytotoxic mechanisms. Curr Opin Immunol 1994; 6:447–452.
26. Sale GE, Anderson P, Browne M, Myerson D. Evidence of cytotoxic T-cell destruction of epidermal cells in human graft-versus-host disease: Immunohistology with monoclonal antibody TIA-1. Arch Pathol Lab Med 1992; 116:622–625.
27. Sale GE, Beauchamp M, Myerson D. Immunohistologic staining of cytotoxic T and NK cells in formalin-fixed paraffin-embedded tissue using microwave TIA-1 antigen retrieval. Transplantation 1994; 57:287–289.
28. Itoh N, Yonehara S, Ishii A, et al. The polypeptide encoded by the cDNA for human cell surface antigen Fas can mediate apoptosis. Cell 1991; 66:233–243.
29. Sayama K, Yonehara S, Watanabe Y, Miki Y. Expression of Fas antigen on keratinocytes in vivo and induction of apoptosis in cultured keratinocytes. J Invest Dermatol 1994; 103:330–334.
30. Antin JH, Ferrara JLM. Cytokine dysregulation and acute graft-versus-host disease. Blood 1992; 80:2964–2968.
31. Jadus MR, Wepsic HT. The role of cytokines in graft-vs-host reactions and disease. Bone Marrow Transplant 1992; 10:1–14.
32. Abhyanker S, Gilliland DG, Ferrara JL. Interleukin-1 is a critical effector molecule during cytokine dysregulation in graft-vs-host disease to minor histocompatibility antigens. Transplantation 1993; 56:1518–1523.
33. Ferrara JLM, Abhyankar S, Gilliland DG. Cytokine storm of graft-vs-host disease: A critical effector role for interleukin-1. Transplant Proc 1993; 25:1216–1217.
34. McCarthy PL, Abhyankar S, Neben S, et al. Inhibition of interleukin-1 receptor antagonist prevents graft-vs-host disease. Blood 1991; 78:1915–1918.
35. Piguet PF, Grau GE, Allet B, Vassalli P. Tumor necrosis factor/cochectin is an effector of skin and gut lesions of the acute phase of graft-versus-host disease. J Exp Med 1987; 166:1280–1289.
36. Piguet PF. Tumor necrosis factor and graft-vs-host disease. In: Burakoff SJ, Deeg HJ, Ferrara J, Atkinson K, eds. Graft-vs-Host Disease. New York: Marcel Dekker, 1990: 255–276.

37. Walsh LJ, Murphy GF. Role of adhesion molecules in cutaneous inflammation and neoplasia (review). J Cutan Pathol 1992; 19:161–171.
38. Gordon JR, Galli SJ. Promotion of mouse fibroblast collagen gene expression by mast cells stimulated via the FcεRI: Role for mast cell-derived transforming growth factor β and tumor necrosis factor α. J Exp Med 1994; 180:2027–2037.
39. Reed JA, Albino AP, McNutt NS. Human cutaneous mast cells express basic fibroblast growth factor. Lab Invest 1995; 72:215–222.
40. Nickoloff BJ, Naidu Y. Pertubation of epidermal barrier function correlates with initiation of cytokine cascade in human skin. J Am Acad Dermatol 1994; 30:535–546.
41. Groves RW, Sherman L. Mizutani H, et al. Detection of interleukin-1 receptors in human epidermis: Induction of the type II receptor after organ culture and in psoriasis. Am J Pathol 1994; 145:1048–1056.
42. Claman HN. Mast cells, T cells and abnormal fibrosis. Immunol Today 1985; 6:192–196.
43. Claman HN. Mast cells and fibrosis: The relevance to scleroderma. Rheum Dis Clinic North Am 1990; 16:141–151.
44. Choi KL, Claman HN. Mast cells in murine graft-versus-host disease: A model of immunologically induced fibrosis. Immunol Ser 1989; 46:641–651.
45. Hawkins RA, Claman HN, Clark RAF, Steigerwald JC. Increased dermal mast cell populations in progressive systemic sclerosis: A link in chronic fibrosis? Ann Intern Med 1985; 102:182–186.
46. Sueki H, Whitaker D, Buchsbaum M, Murphy GF. Novel interactions between dermal dendrocytes and mast cells in human skin. Implications for hemostasis and matrix repair (see comments). Lab Invest 1993; 69:160–172.
47. Hakim FT, Shearer GM. Immunologic and hematopoietic deficiencies of graft- vs.-host disease. In: Burakoff SJ, Deeg HJ, Ferrara J, Atkinson K, eds. Graft-vs- Host Disease. New York: Marcel Dekker, 1990: 133–160.
48. Hardin JA, Mimori T. Autoantibodies to ribonucleoproteins. Clin Rheum Dis 1985; 11: 485–505.
49. Wesierski-Gadek J, Penner E, Hitchman E, et al. Nucleolar proteins B23 and C23 as target antigens in chronic graft-vs-host disease. Blood 1992; 79:1081–1086.
50. Calvancio NJ. The humoral response in autoimmunity. Dermatol Clin 1993; 11:379–389.
51. Rolink AG, Strasser A, Melcher F. Autoimmune diseases induced by graft-vs- host disease. In: Burakoff SJ, Deeg HJ, Ferrara J, Atkinson K, eds. Graft-vs-Host Disease. New York: Marcel Dekker, 1990: 161–175.
52. Gleichmann E, Van Elven EH, Van der Veen JPW. A systemic lupus erythematosus (SLE)-like disease in mice induced by abnormal T-B cell cooperation: Preferential fomation of autoantibodies characteristic of SLE. Eur J Immunol 1982; 12:152–159.
53. Portanova JP, Claman HN, Kotzin BL. Autoimmunization in murine graft- versus-host disease. I. Selective production of antibodies to histones and DNA. J Immunol 1985; 135:3850–3856.
54. Aoki I, Aoki A, Otani M, et al. A correlation between IgG class antibody production and glomerulonephritis in the murine chronic graft-versus-host reaction. Clin Immunol Immunopathol 1992; 63:34–38.
55. Gelpi C, Rodriquez-Sanchez JL, Martinez MA, et al. Murine graft-versus-host disease: A model for study of mechanisms that generate autoantibodies to ribonucleoproteins. J Immunol 1989; 140:4160–4166.
56. Tsoi MS, Storb R, Jones E, et al. Deposition of IgM and complement at the dermoepidermal junction in acute and chronic cutaneous graft-vs-host disease in man. J Immunol 1978; 120:1485–1492.

57. Saurat JH, Didier-Jean L, Gluckman E, Bussel A. Graft-versus-host reaction and licken planus-like eruption in man. Br J Dermatol 1975; 92:591–592.
58. van Elven EH, Agterberg J, Sadal S, Gleichmann E. Diseases caused by reactions of T lymphocytes to incompatible structures of the major histocompatibility complex. J Immunol 1981; 126:1684–1691.
59. Christofidou-Solomidou M, Albelda SM, Murphy GF. Cutaneous inflammation is inducible by degranulation of human mast cells. Lab Invest 1995; 72:46A.
60. Christofidou-Solomidou M, Murphy GF, Albelda SM. E-selectin blockade inhibits cutaneous inflammation induced by mast cell degranulation. Lab Invest 1995; 72:47A.
61. Murphy GF. *Dermatopathology*. Philadelphia, W.B. Saunders Co.

12

Graft-Versus-Host Disease of the Liver

James M. Crawford
Brigham and Women's Hospital and Harvard Medical School
Boston, Massachusetts

I. INTRODUCTION

Bone marrow transplantation subjects the liver to numerous potential insults. The patterns of damage fall into the broad categories of toxic injury, infection, recurrence of disease, and immunologically mediated injury (1), (Table 1). Liver toxicity generally is attributable to the cytoreductive therapy used during induction for bone marrow transplantation and may take the form of a generalized impairment of liver function in the immediate posttransplantation period (2), or as venoocclusive disease or nodular regenerative hyperplasia in the weeks following transplantation (3,4). Systemic infection involving the liver or infection by hepatotropic viruses are ever-present threats. Emerging from this morass of potential problems is the clinical syndrome of graft-versus-host disease (GVHD), featuring, to varying degrees, skin rashes, diarrhea and weight loss, and cholestatic liver dysfunction. In this chapter, the hepatic features are addressed.

II. CLINICAL SYNDROMES

The conditions necessary for the development of GVHD (infusion of immunocompetent cells, histocompatibility differences between donor and recipient, and inability of the recipient to destroy donor cells) are met most frequently in the setting of allogeneic bone marrow transplantation, with the likelihood of developing GVHD increasing with the degree of histoincompatibility between donor and recipient (5). Hepatic GVHD also may occur following transplantation of organs containing abundant lymphoid tissue, particularly the small intestine (6–8). GVHD has been separated into acute and chronic forms, with acute GVHD usually developing within 7 to 50 days after marrow transplantation and chronic GVHD evolving 100 or more days after transplantation (9).

Table 1 Differential Diagnosis of Hepatic Dysfunction in Bone Marrow Transplantation Patients

Timing	Common causes	Less common causes
Pretransplant	Viral hepatitis Malignancy	Drug toxicity Venoocclusive disease Opportunistic infections Biliary tract disease
Day 0–25	Venoocclusive disease Drug toxicity	Acute GVHD Opportunistic infections Nodular regenerative hyperplasia Total parenteral nutrition toxicity Cholestasis of sepsis Acalculous cholecystitis
Day 25–100	Acute GVHD Venoocclusive disease Opportunistic infections Drug toxicity	Total parenteral nutrition toxicity Nodular regenerative hyperplasia
Day > 100	Chronic GVHD Viral hepatitis (hepatotropic)	Opportunistic infections Drug toxicity Epstein-Barr virus–induced lymphoproliferative disorder

Source: Ref. 1.

A. Acute Graft-Versus-Host Disease

Although GVHD-related liver dysfunction may develop within days, more commonly abnormalities are encountered 2 to 4 weeks after transplantation. Onset is heralded by a gradual rise in serum levels of both direct and indirect bilirubin and in serum alkaline phosphatase and transaminases (SGOT/AST, SGPT/ALT). These elevations may be mild or may exceed 40 mg/dL (684 μmol/L) for bilirubin and reach 10 to 20 times normal values for serum enzymes. γ-Glutamyl transpeptidase may be elevated even if other enzymes remain in the normal range. Hepatomegaly may occur, usually without pain. In the more severe cases, clinically evident jaundice and icterus develop. The incidence of acute GVHD ranges from 10% to more than 80% of bone marrow recipients, depending on the degree of histoincompatibility, number of T cells in the graft, patient's age (incidence increases with age), and immunoprophylactic regimen (5). Clinical symptomatology attributable partly to hepatic dysfunction includes fatigue, easy bruising, and onset of confusion.

The severity of acute GVHD is graded according to the extent of organ involvement (2,10,11). In mild GVHD (grade 1), symptoms are limited to the skin; hepatic involvement is subclinical, with serum bilirubin <3 mg/dL. In moderate GVHD (grade 2), skin rash, diarrhea, and jaundice are evident, and serum bilirubin is in the 3- to 6-mg/dL range. With severe GVHD (grade 3), generalized erythroderma and severe diarrhea predominate. Jaundice is more marked, with serum bilirubin values in excess of 6 mg/dL. With the progression of disease to life-threatening grade 4 GVHD, coagulopathy and a bleeding diathesis develop, along with hepatic failure with ascites and encephalopathy. Such signs of liver failure are rare in the absence of liver damage from antecedent causes. Survival is directly related to the clinical severity, and the proximate causes of death are multifactorial.

B. Chronic Graft-Versus-Host Disease

Chronic GVHD is conventionally defined as a syndrome arising after day 100 and may arise de novo after a disease-free interval following an episode of acute GVHD (quiescent) or as a continuous extension of acute GVHD (progressive) (5). Since the syndrome may develop as early as 40 to 50 days after transplantation, the time frames for acute and chronic GVHD can overlap. Unlike acute GVHD, in which skin, gut, and liver symptoms predominate, chronic GVHD is a blend of autoimmune syndromes involving a much wider range of organ systems. Damage occurs to the skin (systemic sclerosis), ductal epithelia of the salivary and lacrimal glands (Sjögren's syndrome), intestines, liver, lymph nodes, lungs, musculoskeletal system, and mucous membranes of the mouth.

The incidence of chronic GVHD in allogeneic bone marrow transplant recipients ranges from 30 to 60%, with the occurrence of acute GVHD increasing the probability of chronic GVHD. This syndrome is the most common cause of cholestatic liver disease (elevated alkaline phosphatase and hyperbilirubinemia) in long-term survivors of bone marrow transplantation and may occur in the absence of extrahepatic GVHD (12). However, since such laboratory findings are nonspecific, other causes such as drug injury (e.g., trimethoprim-sulfamethoxazole, azathioprine, cyclosporine), infiltrative liver disease (fungus, recurrent tumor), and extrahepatic biliary disease (stones, infection) must also be considered. Since the immune system appears to be affected in all transplant patients, they are highly susceptible to bacterial, viral, fungal, and opportunistic infections. In particular, chronic GVHD and viral hepatitis may coexist in these patients, and liver biopsy may be necessary to distinguish between these etiologies (see below).

Limited chronic GVHD consists of localized skin disease and/or mild liver dysfunction (elevated serum bilirubin and alkaline phosphatase). The designation of severe chronic GVHD is reserved for patients with generalized skin involvement, or localized skin involvement or liver dysfunction with one of the following: severe chronic hepatitis (confirmed by histology, see below); eye, mucosalivary, or mucosal involvement; or disease involvement of other target organs (13).

III. PATHOLOGY

The morphological diagnosis of GVHD in the liver is based, first, on identifying a constellation of nonspecific alterations, of which bile duct lesions and portal inflammation with mononuclear cells are the most characteristic features (Table 2), and second on excluding other causes of liver damage.

A. Acute Graft-Versus-Host Disease

The sine qua non of acute GVHD is selective epithelial damage of target organs (skin, intestine, and liver) (14). In the liver, the most characteristic lesion is direct attack of donor lymphocytes on bile duct epithelial cells (15–17). The bile ducts

Table 2 Key Histological Features of Hepatic GVHD

Disease condition	Key features
Acute GVHD	Bile ducts
	Lymphocytic infiltrates
	Nuclear pleomorphism and pyknosis
	Cytoplasmic swelling and eosinophilia
	Segmental duct disruption and loss
	Portal tracts
	Inflammation: mild, mononuclear
	Piecemeal necrosis[a]
	Parenchyma
	Hepatocyte necrosis (acidophil bodies)
	Lobular disarray
	Ballooning degeneration of hepatocytes
	Centrilobular cholestasis
Chronic GVHD	Bile ducts
	Lymphocytic infiltrates
	Nuclear pleomorphism and pyknosis
	Cytoplasmic eosinophilia
	Disruption of epithelial continuity
	Segmental duct disruption and loss; paucity of bile ducts
	Portal tracts
	Inflammation: variable, mononuclear
	Piecemeal necrosis[a]
	Fibrosis (advanced cases)
	Parenchyma
	Minimal evidence of hepatocyte necrosis
	Cholestasis

[a]Piecemeal necrosis is defined as necrosis of hepatocytes at the margins of portal tracts, with accompanying inflammation.
Source: Refs. 15 and 16.

most frequently involved are of small caliber (18). Lymphocytic infiltrates are seen surrounding, invading, and disrupting the walls of interlobular bile ducts (Fig. 1A). Lymphocytic attack is accompanied by necrosis of duct epithelial cells, evident as cytoplasmic vacuolization, nuclear pleomorphism or loss of nuclei, and sloughing of cells into the bile duct lumen (19). By electron microscopy, lymphocytes are found to be in close point contact with the bile duct epithelial cells (20,21). Residual duct epithelial cells may become attenuated to the point of appearing squamous around a portion of the duct circumference (Fig. 1B). This "withered" appearance of the ductal epithelium is to be distinguished from the heaped-up, reactive duct epithelial cells commonly encountered in viral hepatitis, particularly with infection by hepatitis C virus (22). Because these patients are usually pancytopenic, the degree of bile duct and portal tract inflammation may be quite minimal, despite obvious damage to bile ducts.

In keeping with the generalized attack on epithelial cells, necrosis of hepatocytes also may occur, giving rise to a hepatitis-like picture. The histological pattern of hepatocellular ballooning, intralobular lymphocytic infiltration, and eosinophilic degeneration of hepatocytes (apoptosis, Fig. 1C) may be confused with viral infections such as cytomegalovirus (CMV) and herpes, both of which occur in BMT patients (16). Immunostaining for peptide antigens or in situ hybridization for viral genomic material may be used to exclude the presence of viruses within tissue sections (23,24). Hepatocellular cholestasis may be observed in both acute and chronic GVHD.

An additional feature of GVHD is so-called endothelialitis, in which portal vein radicles and terminal hepatic venules exhibit attachment of lymphocytes to the endothelium, with damage to the endothelium (Fig. 1D). This particular feature is a relatively specific but less sensitive marker for GVHD (15), being observed relatively infrequently and generally only in more severe cases (24). Endothelialitis can be observed in other conditions, such as alcoholic and viral hepatitis (and solid-organ transplant rejection). However, the usual vascular lesion in these conditions is a subendothelial collection of lymphoid cells associated with hepatocellular necrosis (15), as opposed to the attachment of lymphoid cells to the lumenal endothelium seen in GVHD (9). The absence of hepatocellular necrosis in the immediate vicinity of venular endothelialitis is more characteristic of GVHD.

B. Chronic Graft-Versus-Host Disease

Chronic GVHD is chiefly characterized by portal infiltration by lymphocytes without or with plasma cells (Fig. 2A) and damage to interlobular bile ducts (19). These bile ducts are generally of small size, <45 μm in diameter (25). Although bile duct epithelial degeneration resembling that of acute GVHD may be observed, more commonly damaged bile duct epithelial cells appear eosinophilic and "coagulated" when compared to healthy neighboring cells (Fig. 2B). As with acute GVHD, lymphocytes are seen in close point contact with bile duct epithelial cells (20). Loss of bile ducts is a relatively late phenomenon in chronic GVHD, although it has been observed as early as 1 month after BMT (24,26). Regardless of the time frame, bile duct loss may lead to a vanishing bile duct syndrome or outright cirrhosis (27–29) (Fig. 2C). With rare exception (30), extrahepatic biliary injury is absent (31). Degenerative changes in the epithelium of intrahepatic periductal glands has been described (32).

Unlike the case in acute GVHD, hepatocellular involvement is minimal. The loss of interlobular bile ducts gives rise to progressive hepatocellular cholestasis. In the more advanced stages of chronic GVHD, hepatocellular cholestasis may be so severe as to lead to degeneration of hepatocytes, particularly along the portal tract margins (Fig. 2D). Venous endothelialitis is not a prominent feature of chronic GVHD. Noncaseating granulomas of the portal tract are encountered only rarely.

Several studies (15,16) have attempted to distinguished the morphological changes of GVHD from other conditions affecting the liver of bone marrow transplantation patients. However, no alterations specific to GVHD have so far been documented. Extensive bile duct damage with minimal portal inflammatory changes

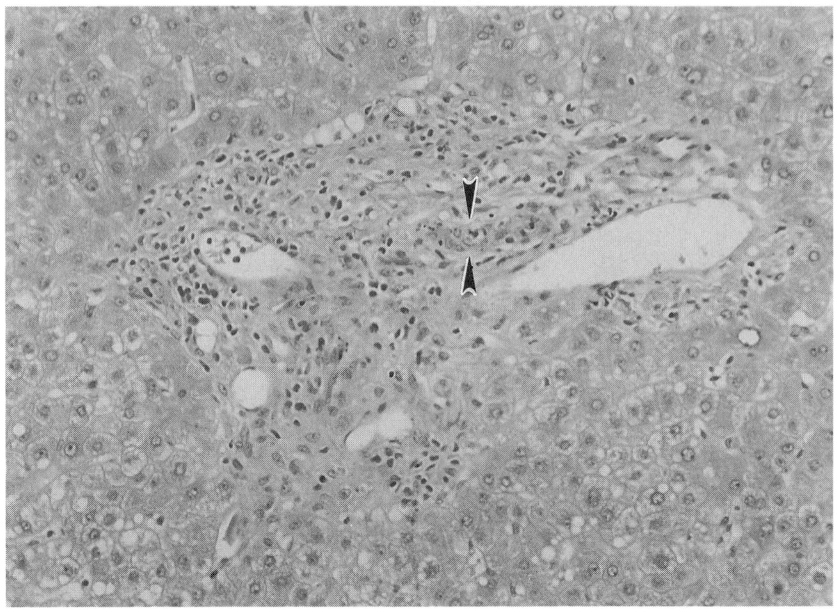

(A)

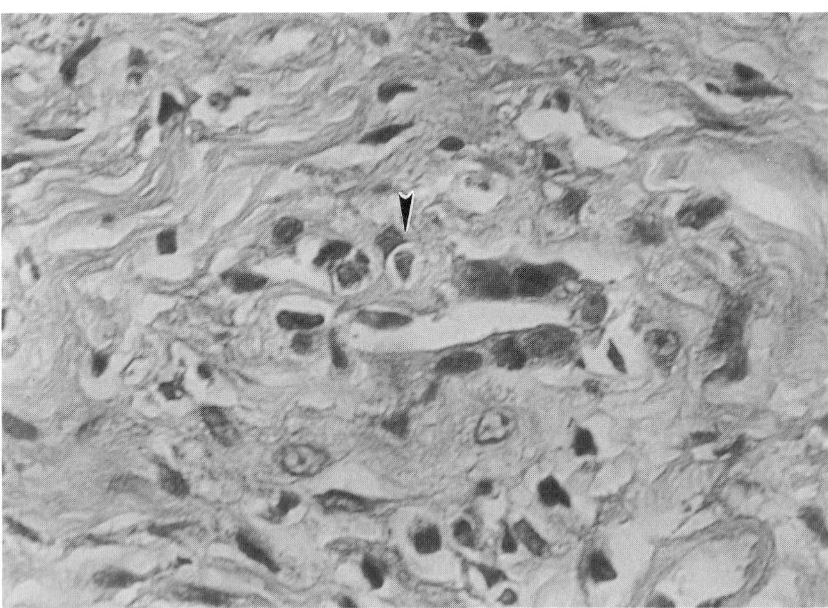

(B)

Figure 1 Acute hepatic GVHD. A. Portal tract. A mild lymphocytic infiltrate is present in an expanded portal tract; the bile duct is more difficult to identify (arrowheads). Original magnification, ×300. B. Interlobular bile duct. A portion of the bile duct has undergone destruction, and intraepithelial lymphocytes are present (arrowhead). Residual bile duct epithelial cells are attentuated and have a low cuboidal to squamous appearance. Original magnification, ×1000.

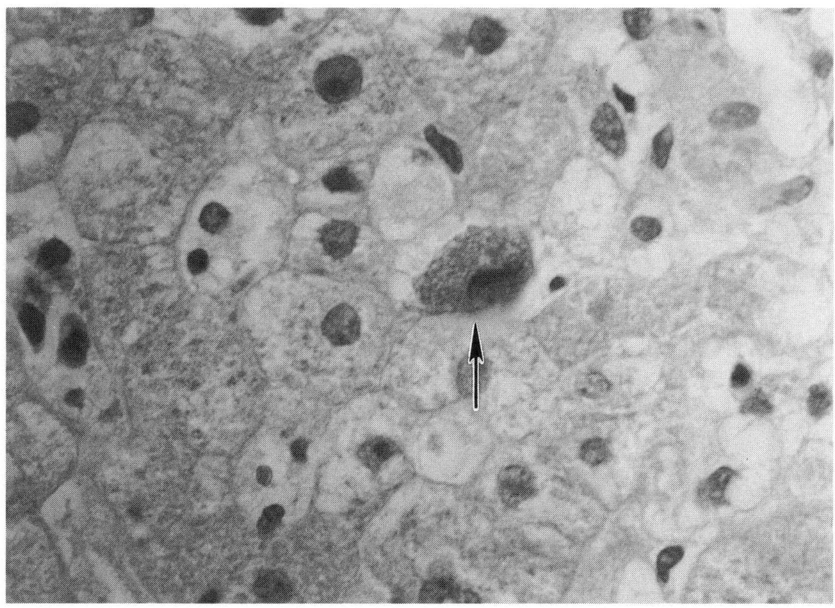

(C)

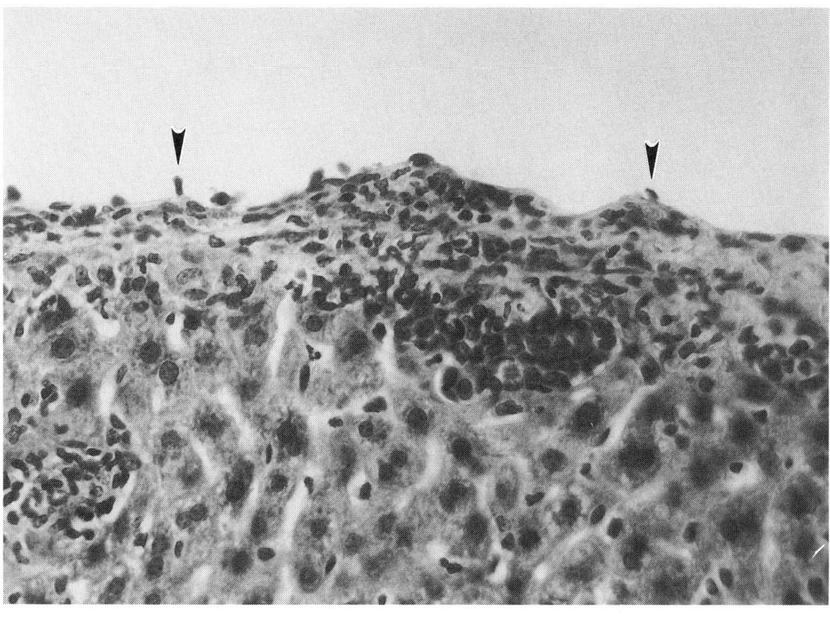

(D)

C. Hepatitis-like features. A hepatocyte is undergoing focal necrosis (arrow). Original magnification, ×1000. D. Endothelialitis. A terminal hepatic vein exhibits lumenal attachment of lymphocytes (arrowheads), and subendothelial lymphocytic infiltrates. Original magnification, ×1000.

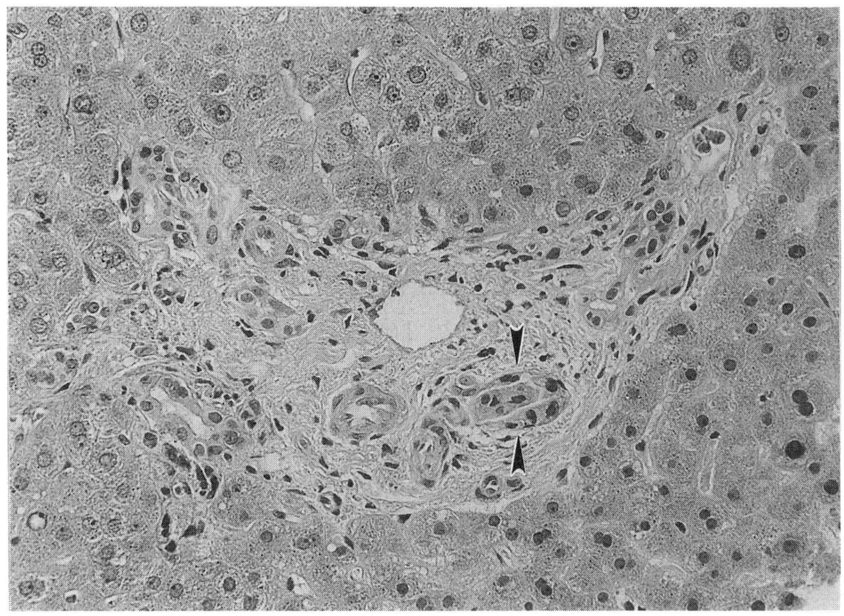

(A)

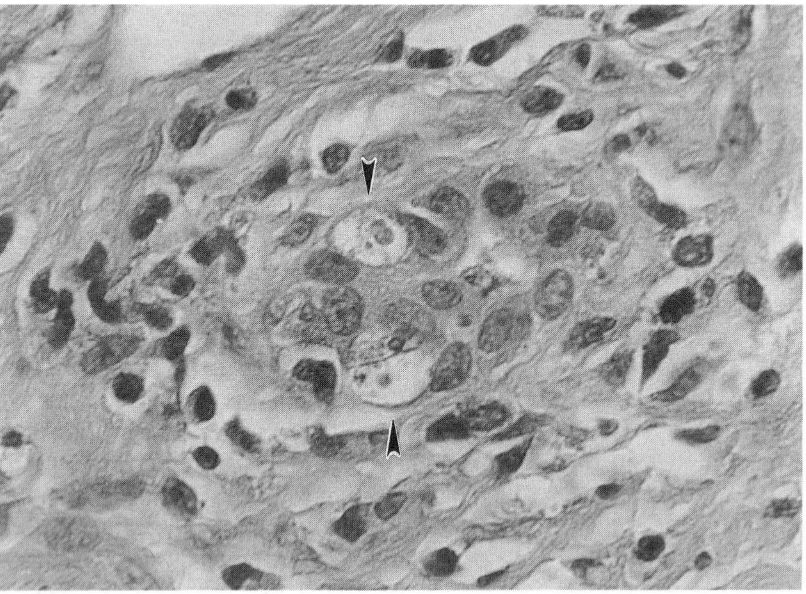

(B)

Figure 2 Chronic hepatic GVHD. A. Portal tract. The portal tract is expanded, and scattered lymphocytes are present. The bile duct appears damaged (arrowheads), similar to acute GVHD (Fig. 1A). Original magnification, ×300. B. Interlobular bile duct. The epithelial cells of the bile duct are undergoing necrosis (arrowheads) or are reactive in appearance. Mononuclear cells are present in the vicinity of the bile duct. Original magnification, ×1000.

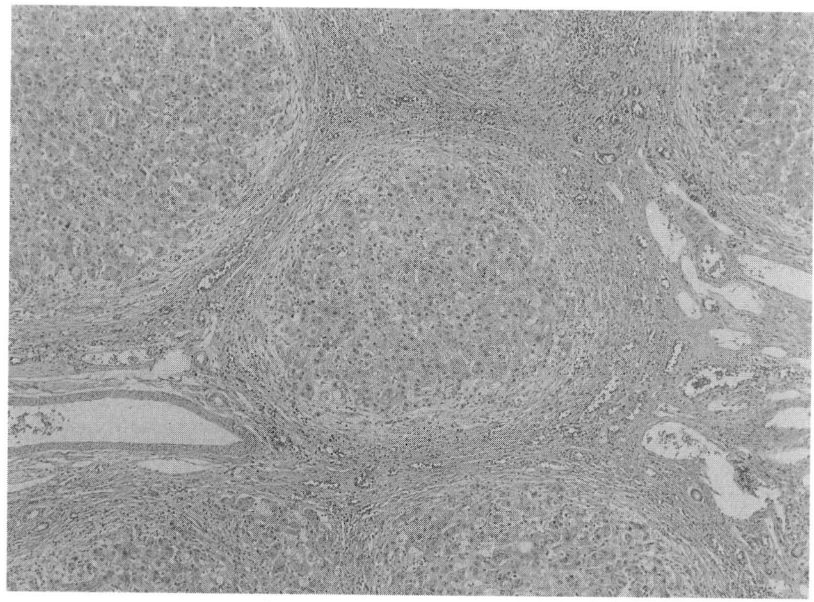

(C)

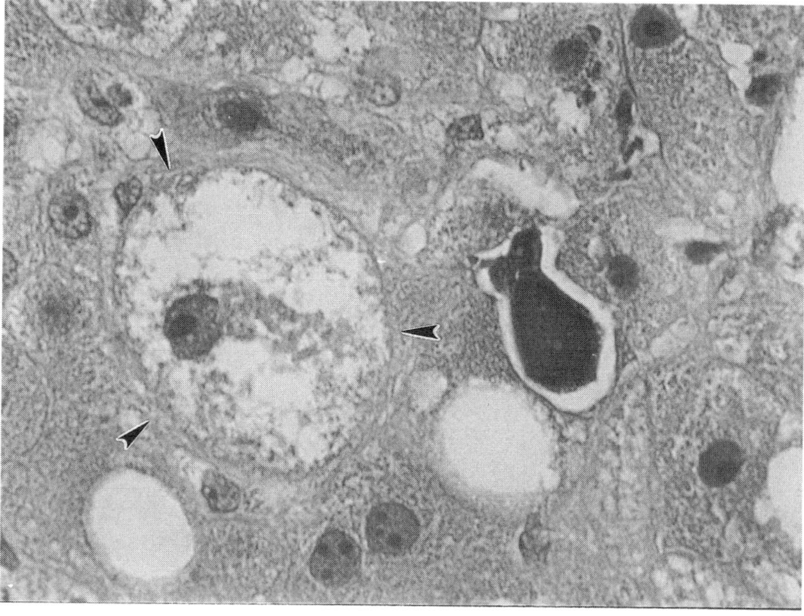

(D)

C. Cirrhosis arising in the setting of chronic GVHD. Long-term loss of intrahepatic bile ducts has led to progressive hepatic damage, eventuating in cirrhosis. Original magnification, ×100. D. Cholestatic changes of hepatocytes in chronic GVHD. A hepatocyte exhibits ballooning degeneration (arrowheads), and a prominent bile canalicular plug of inspissated material is present. Original magnification, ×1000.

has been described as the most characteristic morphological finding in both acute and chronic GVHD. However, features of GVHD vary greatly in severity from one portal tract to another, and damage to interlobular and septal bile ducts is segmental (15,16,33). This variability can make interpretation of liver biopsies quite difficult. The diagnosis of GVHD is reinforced by demonstrating the inflammatory cells in the liver to be of donor origin by molecular techniques (24).

IV. PATHOGENESIS

Despite the often subordinate role of the liver in the clinical symptomatology of GVHD, the liver is one of the major sites of involvement in both the acute and chronic forms of GVHD (34). Unfortunately, although hepatic disease in both humans and experimental animals is reproducibly encountered (15,35,36), insights into the mechanisms producing hepatic GVHD have been difficult to obtain. Investigative efforts have focused primarily on the generation of bile duct lesions in chronic GVHD, as these are most characteristic of this disorder (24). The mechanisms by which hepatocytes are attacked in acute GVHD remain largely unexplored. Current concepts are reviewed in this section, as outlined in Table 3; the more general immunobiology of GVHD is covered extensively elsewhere in this volume.

A. Antigenicity of the Host Liver

Two processes are inherent in immunologically mediated events: (a) identification of antigens as foreign by immunologically competent cells and (b) reaction to those antigens. One must ask, therefore, which antigens in the host liver are recognized as foreign. While the specific antigens are unknown, a major role has been proposed

Table 3 Current Concepts of the Pathogenesis of Hepatic GVHD

Alloreactive mechanism	Proposed contribution
Host-liver antigenicity	MHC class I antigens
	Constituitive expression on all cell types
	MHC class II antigens
	Neoexpression on bile duct cells and endothelium in GVHD
	Non-MHC antigens
	Role undefined
Immunological effector cells	Antigen-presenting cells
	Kupffer cells (donor origin)
	Endothelium (host origin)
	Bile duct epithelial cells (host origin)
	Lymphocytes (donor origin)
	T cells: $CD4^+$ directed against MHC class I
	T cells: $CD8^+$ directed against MHC class II
	Monocytes/Macrophages (donor origin)
Immunomodulation	Lymphokines and monokines
	Role undefined

for the major histocompatibility complex (MHC) system of HLA antigens. In the normal liver, MHC class I antigens are constituitively expressed on the cells lining the vascular sinusoids (i.e., endothelial cells and the tissue-resident macrophages, or Kupffer cells), bile duct epithelial cells, and to a lesser extent on hepatocytes (37). MHC class II antigens are expressed only by Kupffer cells and by dendritic antigen-presenting cells in the portal tracts. Normal bile duct epithelial cells and large-vessel endothelial cells express few or no detectable MHC class II antigens (38).

A consistent observation in both acute and chronic GVHD is the aberrant expression of MHC class II antigens by bile duct epithelial cells and the endothelial cells of hepatic arteries, veins, and sinusoids as compared to normal livers or those of bone marrow transplant patients without hepatic GVHD (24,39–42). Increased bile duct MHC class II antigen expression also has been noted in liver allograft rejection. In both disease conditions, the upregulation occurs in temporal association with the onset of immunological damage to the bile ducts and appears to be mediated by inflammatory cytokines (e.g., TNF and γ-interferon, see below). Thus, the concept has arisen that unique biliary epithelial peptides might be expressed with the MHC class II molecules, rendering bile ducts vulnerable to immunological attack (40,43,44).

However, it is not established that aberrant MHC class II antigen expression is the cause or result of inflammation caused by donor immunologically competent cells. In fact, it is not even clear that allogeneic differences in MHC class II antigens play a role in hepatic GVHD. While class II MHC disparities are among the most potent inducers of alloimmune responses to other organs (e.g., heart and kidney) during GVHD or graft rejection (45,46), in the case of liver allografts, there appear to be no significant effects of class II MHC disparities on the incidence of vanishing bile duct syndrome or liver allograft rejection following liver transplantation (45). In murine models of GVHD, isolated class II MHC differences lead to portal tract and bile duct lymphocytic infiltrates but are insufficient to induce destructive bile duct lesions (33). When MHC class I disparities are present, MHC class II alloantigen differences provide neither a direct nor additive stimulus for the generation of destructive bile duct lesions. Thus, the issue has been raised as to whether the liver is either an immunologically privileged site or a site in which there is a relative "indifference" to the MHC class II antigens (45,46).

Alloantigen expression responsible for hepatic GVHD instead appears to be multifactorial, at least in murine hepatic GVHD. Class I MHC, class II MHC, or non-MHC-encoded antigenic differences between donor and recipient are sufficient to generate lymphocytic infiltrates around and in the walls of interlobular bile ducts, so characteristic of hepatic GVHD (33). However, frank destruction of bile ducts is most dramatically apparent in hepatic GVHD elicited by isolated class I MHC differences. Despite the uncertainty in the specific hepatic antigens subject to attack, we can conclude that allogeneic disparities are of paramount importance, given the conspicuous absence of hepatic GVHD in the unfortunate liver transplant patients who develop systemic GVHD from donor lymphocytes contained within the organ graft (47–49).

The possibility of temporal evolution of immunological reaction to different antigens also must be considered. Class I MHC antigen differences occur ab initio, given the constitutive expression of class I molecules on the biliary epithelium.

Thus, early in the course of GVHD, immunological response may occur only to class I MHC antigens or to non-MHC-encoded antigens. Later in the course of GVHD, ample class II MHC expression is encountered on bile duct epithelium and the vascular endothelium. The large number of class II MHC–restricted effector cells (discussed below) observed in the later cholangitic lesions of a variety of allograft models suggests that class II MHC–restricted responses to the biliary and vascular antigens may play a more substantive role in established hepatic GVHD (33).

Finally, the wide variation in the incidence of GVHD, and the occasional occurrence of GVHD in instances in which the donor and patient exhibit an exact match, has raised the issue of whether foreign antigenic influences, particularly viruses, are operative (50,51). For example, an association of herpes infection with an increased incidence of GVHD has led to speculation that latent viruses might act as antigenic targets for donor immune surveillance in some cases of GVHD (52). Alternatively, immunological imbalances produced by cytoreductive induction therapy prior to bone marrow transplantation may underlie the occurrence of GVHD in recipients of marrow from HLA-identical siblings (9).

B. Immunologic Effector Cells

1. Resident Antigen-Presenting Cells

While effector lymphocytes are the most notable inflammatory cells entering the liver during GVHD, the interplay between effector cells and antigen-presenting cells must be considered, beginning with the resident macrophages in the liver, Kupffer cells. The life span of these adherent sinusoidal cells is estimated to be between 7 days and 3 months (53), and it is expected, but not proven, that host Kupffer cells would be abrogated by induction therapy prior to bone marrow transplantation. Kupffer cells are migratory cells, and repopulation of the host liver by circulating donor monocytes is observed both in bone marrow transplant patients (24) and in liver transplant patients whose (donor) livers are repopulated by host monocytes (54). This replacement can occur within 1 month of transplantation and is persistent (24). The newly acquired Kupffer cells of allophenotype are postulated to act as antigen-presenting cells, and thereby may be involved in the immunological establishment of GVHD.

Host endothelial cells are not replaced during bone marrow transplantation. However, experimental studies have documented processing and presentation of antigens by host endothelial cells (55). This finding, plus the observation that expression of MHC class II antigens is upregulated on host endothelial cells during hepatic GVHD (24), raises the possibility that host endothelial cells also may process and display host antigens, thus presenting them to alloreactive T lymphocytes as an early event in the triggering of GVHD. Endothelial cells also may be a target of alloreactive attack. Whether the dendritic cells of portal tracts are of host or donor origin and play a role in alloantigen presentation remains unknown.

2. Lymphocytes

T lymphocytes dominate the inflammatory infiltrates of hepatic GVHD (24), in accordance with the concept that T cells of donor origin react against recipient histocompatibility antigens (5,56). In particular, $CD4^+$ (helper/inducer) and $CD8^+$ (cytolytic) T cells seem to play the major role (43,57,58). B lymphocytes are few and only present in cases where lymphoid follicular aggregates have been found. Natural killer (NK) cells have only occasionally been demonstrated. Among the T cells, CD8$^+$ lymphocytes are increased relative to the distribution of lymphocytes found in the livers of bone marrow transplantation patients without hepatic GVHD (59). Helper/inducer (CD4$^+$) T cells are capable of responding to antigens presented by sinusoidal lining cells (endothelial and Kupffer cells) (55).

Class II MHC antigens are essential for the presentation of foreign or self antigens and the activation of CD4$^+$ cells, whereas class I MHC antigens are required for the cytolytic activity of CD8$^+$ cells (60). Thus, it is not surprising that in murine models, GVHD arising from class II MHC differences is mediated by CD4$^+$ donor T cells, whereas GVHD directed at class I MHC differences appears to be mediated by CD8$^+$ donor T cells (56,61,62). In most instances, CD4$^+$ donor T cells are capable of generating only inflammatory infiltrates and not bile duct destruction (56). However, in selected murine strain combinations, CD4$^+$ helper T-cell responses alone are sufficient to generate bile duct destruction (33). Whether such bile duct lesions are mediated directly by cytokines secreted by these alloreactive T cells or indirectly by activation of other non-T-cell-mediated mechanisms is unclear (61).

When the murine host is both MHC class I- plus II-different, a sequence of interdependent immune reactions evolves (63). Injection of donor CD4$^+$ cells alone into recipients leads to mononuclear infiltrates in portal tracts and bile ducts but not to destruction of bile duct epithelial cells. Injection of donor CD4$^+$ cells followed by injection of host CD8$^+$ cells leads to similar changes. In contrast, injection of donor CD4$^+$ followed by donor CD8$^+$ cells precipitates destructive injury to bile ducts. Thus, initial inflammatory reactions may be mediated by alloreactive CD4$^+$ cells, but progression to cytodestruction requires activation of alloreactive CD8$^+$ cells. Cytolytic activity is then perpetuated and extended by the local release of lymphokines capable of enhancing the expression of class I and II MHC antigens on host cells (60). Supporting this proposed sequence of events is the observation that mononuclear inflammatory cells isolated from the livers of mice with GVHD show increased homing to the liver when these cells are injected into normal animals expressing the same MHC differences (36). Notably, the homing mechanism is toward minor histocompatibility antigens expressed by the host biliary epithelial cells.

Collectively, these studies suggest that hepatic GVHD is initiated by alloreaction to host antigens, but progression of hepatic GVHD relates to continuous changes in the microenvironment rather than continued exposure to fixed antigenic differences (60). Activation of host cytodestructive mechanisms also may play a role in the perpetuation of the disease (56).

We cannot conclude that alloreactive CD4$^+$ and CD8$^+$ cells are the sole mechanisms for bile duct damage in GVHD (60). On the one hand, the CD4$^+$ and CD8$^+$ cells used in experimental studies are not pure cell populations. Suppressor cell subsets are present in both the CD4$^+$ (ostensibly helper/inducer) and CD8$^+$ (ostensibly cytotoxic) cell preparations. On the other hand, other cell types, such as CD22$^+$ cells and CD45RO$^+$ cells (which respond to recall stimulation), have yet to be explored (60). NK cells have no MHC restrictions, but they have been described in the cellular milieu of murine GVHD (43). Finally, histologically similar patterns of destructive bile duct lesions can be generated by diverse T-effector mechanisms directed at MHC or non-MHC-encoded antigen differences (33).

3. Monocytes and Macrophages

Phenotypic analysis of infiltrating inflammatory cells in GVHD has focused primarily on lymphocytes, as detailed in the previous section. However, an evolving hypothesis invokes a role of macrophages primed by gut-derived endotoxin (lipopolysaccharide, LPS) in the pathogenesis of acute GVHD. A key feature of the hypothesis is the failure of hepatic clearance of LPS from splanchnic blood in the setting of intestinal injury, resulting in spillover of LPS into the systemic circulation and generalized triggering of macrophages. We must ask, therefore, whether LPS-induced septic shock induces hepatic changes similar to those of acute GVHD and whether cells of monocyte/macrophage lineage are found in the inflammatory infiltrates of hepatic acute GVHD.

The fixed macrophages of the liver, Kupffer cells (of either host or donor origin), play a key role in clearing LPS released into the splanchnic circulation following gut injury. Hepatic exposure to LPS results in Kupffer cell activation, platelet aggregation, intravenous thrombosis, and neutrophil infiltration (64). Kupffer cells, in turn, release a whole spectrum of protein and lipid mediators, including TNF- α, interleukin-1, interleukin-6, and eicosanoids (65). Some LPS is taken up by hepatocytes, most likely following initial clearance and modification by Kupffer cells (65,66). From a histological standpoint, LPS exposure to experimental animals usually leads to focal hepatocellular necrosis and a predominantly neutrophilic infiltration; some monocytes are present (64,65). Portal tracts per se are not substantially affected following acute exposure. In human liver biopsies from septic patients, the predominant features are cholestasis and a periductal infiltrate of neutrophils. It would appear, therefore, that the liver in septic shock does not bear much resemblance to the liver affected by acute GVHD.

With regard to the second question, monocytes do appear to be present in hepatic GVHD. Donor lymphocytes are found to predominate in the inflammatory infiltrates of both acute and chronic hepatic GVHD (24,67), but cells of myeloid/histiocytic lineage also are abundant when specific immunotyping studies are performed (24). Interestingly, these cells are of donor origin, and murine studies indicate that such monocytes appear to home to the liver (24,36). Moreover, donor monocytes accumulate preferentially in hepatic portal spaces and in close proximity to interlobular bile ducts (36), supporting the hypothesis that sensitized monocytes may play a role in bile duct destruction by lymphocytes. However, hepatic monocytes do not necessarily enhance local immunological function, since murine livers affected with acute GVHD contain monocytes that exhibit defective proliferation when stimulated by LPS; coculture with splenic cells also inhibits monocyte proliferation following LPS-exposure (35,68).

Thus, evidence to support or refute a role of monocytes and macrophages in promoting hepatic GVHD is not yet available. While monocytes are clearly present during both human and experimental GVHD, their function remains unclear. Human studies are not yet available to enable evaluation of the potential role of LPS in the pathogenesis of hepatic GVHD.

3. Immunomodulation: Cytokines and Monokines

Cytokines facilitate cell-to-cell communication and modulate immune responses in the local microenvironment (60). They promote the expression of class II MHC antigens, enhance target antigen presentation, activate neutrophils and T and B cells, modulate the expression of intercellular adhesion molecules, and may also promote tissue damage by direct action. Cytokines, particularly lymphokines produced locally during the immune response, almost certainly play a role in the immunomodulation of hepatic GVHD. Likely cytokine effects are the upregulation of MHC class II expression and modulation of the expression of intercellular adhesion molecules (43,60).

The nature and interrelationships of cytokine-mediated events have been difficult to clarify, particularly since cytokines are continuous variables with counterbalancing actions within the microenvironment, so that their net contributions are difficult to identify. Possibilities for cytokine action have recently been reviewed (60) and can be summarized as follows. First, local secretion of lymphokines by activated T lymphocytes can induce autoreactive cells that promote tissue injury. Conversely, they can stimulate natural suppressor cells that promote immunosuppression. Second, macrophages or Kupffer cells (of host or donor origin) activated by T-cell lymphokines may themselves secrete monokines that are immunosuppressive (35,68). Third, bile acids (which will accumulate systemically in the setting of cholestasis) may play a role, as they can inhibit the release of one potent cytokine, tumor necrosis factor (TNF), from mononuclear cells (69). Finally, intercellular adhesion molecule-1 (ICAM-1), which is found on interlobular bile ducts and proliferating bile ductules in other bile duct destructive diseases (70), is inducible by proinflammatory cytokines. Both TNF and γ-interferon can induce the expression of class II MHC antigens and ICAM-1 on bile duct epithelia (60). Furthermore, monoclonal antibodies to lymphocyte-function-associated antigen 1, which binds to ICAM-1, have been shown to prevent GVHD in mice (71).

Thus, there are indications that cytokines play a major role in the evolution of hepatic GVHD (72), and their influence on general immunological function is well documented (37). Nevertheless, data on the direct effects of cytokines on liver function and histology are sketchy. Lipopolysaccharide-induced release of interleukin-6 from Kupffer cells can have a profound effect on hepatocellular function, as evidenced by a marked inhibition in hepatic bile salt uptake (73). In addition, TNF-α release by Kupffer cells, which occurs during hepatic GVHD (74), also is associated with cholestatic jaundice (75). It is clear that much investigative work is needed before the exact mechanisms of cytokine-induced hepatic injury are elucidated.

V. DIAGNOSIS AND MANAGEMENT

A. Differential Diagnosis

The clinical abnormalities arising from hepatic GVHD (described earlier) are quite nonspecific. The chief conditions to be distinguished from hepatic GVHD are drug effects, including cytoreductive therapy, infectious processes (viral, bacterial, and fungal), the effects of parenteral alimentation, extrahepatic obstruction, and posttransplant lymphoproliferative disorders (see Table 1).

In the acute situation (< 100 days posttransplant), perhaps the most important pertinent information is whether there are symptoms and signs of graft-versus-host reaction in the skin and gastrointestinal tract (15,26). Specific indicators of hepatic GVHD are largely absent. The development of ascites and hepatomegaly would favor drug toxicity or venoocclusive disease more than GVHD. Viral serologies are helpful in excluding infection by hepatotropic viruses. Hepatic infection by nonhepatotropic viruses, such as herpes or cytomegalovirus, or by fungi, such *Candida*, may be exceedingly difficult to exclude clinically, although negative viral serologies are reassuring.

In the chronic situation (>100 days posttransplant), evidence of GVHD-induced hepatic damage (e.g., persistent low-grade elevation of serum transaminases and alkaline phosphatase) may occur with or without clinically manifest GVHD in other systems (e.g., skin, gut, and mucous membranes) (5) or may lag behind the evolution of disease in other organs (28). A prominent feature of chronic hepatic GVHD is cholestasis, which occurs in 80% of patients. The cholestasis is characterized by increases in the levels of serum alkaline phosphatase, aminotransferases, and bilirubin (76). Assuming that acute decompensation from opportunistic infection is not a concern, one must frequently resort to liver biopsy to satisfactorily exclude other causes of hepatic disease.

B. The Role of Liver Biopsy

Although the differential diagnosis for acute liver disease after bone marrow transplantation is broad, hemodynamic instability of the more severely affected patients often precludes the use of liver needle biopsy. Fine-needle aspiration biopsy, which carries a much lower risk of bleeding complications, has been used to assess the degree of inflammatory reaction in acute GVHD (67) but this procedure provides only minimal information. Overall, liver biopsies in the acute situation are not widely used. Since hepatic improvement may lag behind that of the skin and gut during treatment of acute GVHD, liver biopsy may be used to rule out other possible causes of liver disease, such as concurrent CMV infection (14).

Liver needle biopsies are an important clinical adjunct in evaluating chronic hepatic disease following bone marrow transplantation. Although there is considerable overlap between the histological changes caused by different disease processes, the key features of hepatic GVHD described earlier serve as important discriminators (15,16). Specifically, the findings of extensive bile duct damage involving >50% of bile ducts with minimal inflammatory changes, or evidence of bile duct loss, is highly suggestive of GVHD (14). Although observed less frequently, the presence of endothelialitis of portal or central veins is even more predictive of GVHD. Parenchymal inflammation and hepatocyte necrosis, cholestasis, and secondary bile duct proliferation may be observed, but they are not satisfactory discriminators between GVHD and other etiologies (such as drug toxicity, hepatotropic and nonhepatotropic viral infection, and bile duct obstruction). Moreover, GVHD may be accompanied by other processes producing similar histological changes, such as viral hepatitis or drug toxicity. Confident exclusion of viral causes may require in situ hybridization techniques using specific antiviral probes (24), techniques that are not routinely used.

Avoidance of false-positive diagnoses requires both careful correlation with clinical data and appropriate caution in invoking GVHD as the solitary diagnosis. Given the common occurrence of bile damage or loss in hepatic GVHD, false-negative diagnoses are less of a problem than false positivity. However, the patchy distribution of the bile duct lesion may lead to its absence in needle biopsy specimens from patients with milder forms of the disease (77). Finally, pretransplant biopsies on all patients with preexisting liver disease will help to reduce the likelihood of misinterpreting prior liver disease as newly evolving GVHD. The value of nuclear magnetic resonance spectroscopy as an adjunct to liver biopsy (78) remains unclear.

C. Clinical Management

The overall prognosis of patients with acute GVHD correlates directly with the severity of the clinical disease. Severe hepatic compromise, as described earlier, plays a major role in the multisystemic failure encountered in fatal cases of acute GVHD. The treatment of acute GVHD is covered elsewhere in this volume; management of the deficiencies in hepatic function (e.g., in hepatic synthesis of clotting factors) is supportive in nature (79).

In the case of chronic GVHD, hepatic dysfunction from progressive chronic hepatitis or cirrhosis may eventuate in hepatic failure, with ensuing demise. Since chronic GVHD is also a systemic condition, systemic therapy will presumably have a favorable impact on hepatic function. At the present time, only one treatment modality may have specific relevance to the liver. Given that bile duct destruction is a prominent feature of chronic hepatic GVHD, attention has recently been given to the long-term maintenance of adequate hepatic bile flow (76). The exogenous bile salt ursodeoxycholate (also called ursodiol), is more hydrophilic than the predominant bile salts (cholate and chenodeoxycholate) normally present in the human enterohepatic circulation. When taken orally, this supplemental bile salt promotes enhanced biliary fluid secretion in normal subjects and helps to maintain bile salt secretion and bile flow in individuals with cholestatic syndromes (80). This reasoning prompted Fried and coworkers (81) to treat patients with chronic hepatic GVHD unresponsive to immunosuppressive therapy for 6 weeks with 10 to 15 mg/kg per day of ursodiol. Serum levels of alkaline phosphatase, aminotransferases, and bilirubin improved while on therapy but returned to previous abnormal levels upon cessation of therapy. Symptomatology from cholestasis (e.g., pruritus) did not improve during treatment, but no adverse effects were encountered. As the study did not provide information on whether long-term maintenance on ursodiol altered the natural history of chronic hepatic GVHD, the ultimate utility of this form of therapy remains unknown.

Although liver transplantation is an important therapy for the treatment of end-stage cholestatic liver disorders, there is as yet no consensus that chronic hepatic GVHD is an indication for liver transplantation (82). This approach has been utilized in isolated instances (83).

D. Long-Term Sequelae

Acute GVHD is a potentially reversible or at least controllable multisystemic illness provided that prompt therapy is instituted upon its detection (84). In addition to generalized hepatic dysfunction, extensive bile duct destruction can generate a so-called "vanishing bile duct syndrome," which is the most severe form of acute liver GVHD (26). Assuming survival of the acute condition, evolution into chronic GVHD is a worrisome problem. Although the debilitation caused by chronic GVHD is multisystemic, the most ominous long-term hepatic condition is progressive fibrosis eventuating in cirrhosis, which has been reported in a few instances (27–29). The life-threatening problems with esophageal bleeding and hepatic encephalopathy are much like those encountered with cirrhosis from other causes.

VI. CONCLUSION

Hepatic involvement with GVHD has a major clinical impact in both acute and chronic situations. Severe acute hepatic GVHD contributes to multisystem decompensation, and in this setting the mortality rate is high. Chronic hepatic GVHD may lead to a progressive cholestatic syndrome, with associated morbidity and potential mortality from end-stage liver disease. In both settings, exclusion of other potential causes of liver disease on clinical grounds may be exceedingly difficult. Liver biopsy, particularly in the chronically affected patient, is an important diagnostic tool. Immunosuppressive therapy generally leads to improvement in hepatic dysfunction, and oral bile salt therapy has been advocated as an adjunct for symptomatic treatment of cholestasis. Progress in understanding the pathogenesis of hepatic GVHD has been slow. Particular issues are (a) determining which hepatic antigens are the primary targets of immunologic attack and the mechanisms for their presentation to immunologically competent cells; (b) unraveling the interplay between subclasses of lymphocytes; (c) evaluating the role of activation of host immunological mechanisms; and (d) elucidating the role of cytokines. Armed with such insights, it may be possible in the future to design more effective therapeutic interventions for hepatic GVHD.

ACKNOWLEDGMENT

This work was supported in part by NIH grant DK-39512.

REFERENCES

1. Crawford JM, Ferrell LD. The liver in transplantation, in Rustgi VK, Van Thiel DH, eds. The Liver in Systemic Diseases. New York: Raven Press, 1993:337–364.
2. McDonald GB, Shulman HM, Wolford JL, et al. Liver disease after human marrow transplantation. Semin Liver Dis 1987; 7:210–229.
3. Snover DC, Weisdorf S, Bloomer J, et al. Nodular regenerative hyperplasia of the liver following bone marrow transplantation. Hepatology 1989; 9:443–448.
4. Shulman HM, Fisher LB, Schoch HG, et al. Venoocclusive disease of the liver after marrow transplantation: Histological correlates of clinical signs and symptoms. Hepatology 1994; 19:1171–1181.
5. Ferrara JLM, Deeg HJ. Mechanisms of disease: Graft-versus-host disease. N Engl J Med 1991; 324:667–674.
6. Grant D, Zhong R, Gunn H, et al. Graft-versus-host disease associated with intestinal transplantation in the rat: Host immune function and general histology. Transplantation 1989; 48:545–549.
7. Velio P, Bertoglio C, Bardella MT, et al. Histologic findings after orthotopic small bowel transplantation alone or with the liver. Transplant Proc 1994; 26:1632–1633.
8. Wallander J, Scheynius A, Läckgren G, et al. Immunomorphology of graft-versus-host disease after small bowel transplantation in the rat. Scand J Immunol 1990; 32:93–101.
9. Snover DC. Acute and chronic graft-versus-host disease: Histopathological evidence for two distinct pathogenetic mechanisms. Human Pathol 1984: 15:202–205.

10. Deeg HJ, Cottler-Fox M. Clinical spectrum and pathophysiology of acute graft-vs-host disease, in Burakoff SJ, Deeg HJ, Ferrara J, et al, eds. Graft-vs-Host Disease: Immunology, Pathophysiology, and Treatment. New York: Marcel Dekker, 1990:311–335.
11. Wick MR, Moore SB, Gastineau DA, et al. Immunologic, clinical, and pathologic aspects of human graft-versus-host disease. Mayo Clin Proc 1983; 58:603–612.
12. Gholson CF, Yau JC, LeMaistre CF, et al. Steroid-responsive chronic hepatic graft-versus-host disease without extrahepatic graft-versus-host disease. Am J Gastroenterol 1989; 84:1306–1309.
13. Shulman HM, Sullivan KM, Weiden PL. Chronic graft-versus-host syndrome in man: A long-term clinicopathologic study of 20 Seattle patients. Am J Med 1980; 69:204–217.
14. Snover DC. The pathology of acute graft-vs-host disease, in Burakoff SJ, Deeg HJ, Ferrara J, et al, eds. Graft-vs-Host Disease: Immunology, Pathophysiology, and Treatment. New York: Marcel Dekker, 1990:337–353.
15. Snover DC, Weisdorf SA, Ramsay NK, et al. Hepatic graft versus host disease: A study of the predictive value of liver biopsy in diagnosis. Hepatology 1984; 4:123–130.
16. Shulman HM, Sharma P, Amos D, et al. A coded histologic study of hepatic graft-versus-host disease after human bone marrow transplantation. Hepatology 1988; 8:463–470.
17. Nonomura A, Koizumi H, Yoshida K, et al. Histological changes of bile duct in experimental graft-versus-host disease across minor histocompatibility barriers: I. Light microscopic and immunocytochemical observations. Acta Pathol Jpn 1987; 37:763–773.
18. Tanaka M, Umihara J, Chiba S, et al. Intrahepatic bile duct injury following bone marrow transplantation. Acta Pathol Jpn 1986; 36:1793–1806.
19. Desmet VJ. Vanishing bile duct disorders, in Boyer JL, Ockner RK, eds. Progress in Liver Diseases: vol X. Philadelphia: Saunders, 1992:89–122.
20. Bernuau D, Gisselbrecht C, Devergie A, et al. Histological and ultrastructural appearance of the liver during graft-versus-host disease complicating bone marrow transplantation. Transplantation 1980; 29:236.
21. Nonomura A, Kono N, Yoshida K, et al. Histological changes of bile duct in experimental graft-versus-host disease across minor histocompatibility barriers: II. Electron microscopic observations. Liver 1988; 8:32–41.
22. Bach N, Thung SN, Schaffner F. The histological features of chronic hepatitis C and autoimmune chronic hepatitis: A comparative analysis. Hepatology 1992; 15:572–577.
23. Brainard JA, Greenson JK, Vesy CJ, et al. Detection of cytomegalovirus in liver transplant biopsies: A comparison of light microscopy, immunohistochemistry, duplex PCR, and nested PCR. Transplantation 1994; 57:1753–1757.
24. Andersen CB, Horn T, Sehested M, et al. Graft-versus-host disease: Liver morphology and pheno/genotypes of inflammatory cells and target cells in sex- mismatched allogeneic bone marrow transplant patients. Transplant Proc 1993; 25:1250–1254.
25. Vierling JM. Immune disorders of the liver and bile duct. Gastroenterol Clin North Am 1992; 21:427–449.
26. Yeh KH, Hsieh HC, Tang JL, et al. Severe isolated acute hepatic graft- versus-host disease with vanishing bile duct syndrome. Bone Marrow Transplant 1994; 14:319–321.
27. Yau JC, Zaner AR, Srigley JR, et al. Chronic graft-versus-host disease complicated by micronodular cirrhosis and esophageal varices. Transplantation 1986; 41:129–130.
28. Knapp AB, Crawford JM, Rappeport JM, et al. Cirrhosis as a consequence of graft-versus-host disease. Gastroenterology 1987; 92:513–519.
29. Stechschulte DJ Jr., Fishback JL, Emami A, et al. Secondary biliary cirrhosis as a consequence of graft-versus-host disease. Gastroenterology 1990; 98:223–225.
30. Geubel AP, Cnudde A, Ferrant A, et al. Diffuse biliary tract involvement mimicking primary sclerosing cholangitis after bone marrow transplantation. J Hepatol 1990; 10: 23–28.

31. Vierling JM, Ruderman WB, Jaffee BD, et al. Hepatic lesions in murine chronic graft-versus-host disease to minor histocompatibility antigens: A reproducible model of non-suppurative destructive cholangitis. Transplantation 1989; 48:717–718.
32. Nakanuma Y, Terada T, Ohtake S, et al. Intrahepatic periductal glands in graft-versus-host disease. Acta Pathol Jpn 1988; 38:281–289.
33. Williams FH, Thiele DL. The role of major histocompatibility complex and non-major histocompatibility complex encoded antigens in generation of bile duct lesions during hepatic graft-vs-host responses mediated by helper or cytotoxic T cells. Hepatology 1994; 19:980–988.
34. Shulman HM, Sullivan KM, Weiden PL, et al. Chronic graft-versus-host syndrome in man: A long-term clinicopathologic study of 20 Seattle patients. Am J Med 1980; 69:217.
35. Howell CD, Yoder TD, Vierling JM. Suppressor function of hepatic mononuclear inflammatory cells during murine chronic graft-versus-host disease: I. Macrophage-enriched cells mediate suppression in the liver. Cell Immunol 1991; 132:256–268.
36. Howell CD, Yoder T, Claman HN, et al. Hepatic homing of mononuclear inflammatory cells isolated during murine chronic graft-versus-host disease. J Immunol 1989; 143:483.
37. Vierling JM, Hu K. Immunologic mechanisms of hepatobiliary injury, in Kaplowitz N, ed. Liver and Biliary Diseases. Baltimore: Williams & Wilkins, 1992:48–69.
38. Suitters AJ, Lampert IA. Class II antigen induction in the liver of rats with graft-versus-host disease. Transplantation 1984; 38:194–196.
39. Siegert W, Stemerowicz R, Hopf U. Antimitochondrial antibodies in patients with chronic graft-versus-host disease. Bone Marrow Transplant 1992; 10:221–227.
40. Nonomura A, Yoshida K, Kono N, et al. Histological changes of bile duct in experimental graft-versus-host disease across minor histocompatibility barriers: III. Immunoelectron microscopic observations. Acta Pathol Jpn 1988; 38:269–280.
41. Demetris AJ, Lasky S, Van Thiel DH, et al. Induction of DR/IA antigens in human liver allografts: An immunocytochemical and clinicopathologic analysis of twenty failed grafts. Transplantation 1985; 40:504–509.
42. Hubscher SG, Adams DH, Elias E. Changes in the expression of major histocompatibility complex class II antigens in liver allograft rejection. J Pathol 1990; 162:165–171.
43. Tanaka M, Umihara J, Shimmoto K, et al. The pathogenesis of graft-versus-host reaction in the intrahepatic bile duct: An immunohistochemical study. Acta Pathol 1989; 39:655.
44. Takacs L, Scende B, Rot A, et al. Expression of MHC class II antigens on the bile duct epithelium in experimental graft versus host disease. Clin Exp Immunol 1985; 60:456.
45. Donaldson P, Underhill J, Doherty D, et al. Influence of human leukocyte antigen matching on liver allograft survival and rejection: "The dualistic effect." Hepatology 1993; 17:1008–1015.
46. Calne RY, White HJO, Yoffa DE, et al. Prolonged survival of liver transplants in the pig. Br Med J 1967; 4:645–648.
47. Cattral MS, Langnas AN, Wisecarver JL, et al. Survival of graft-versus-host disease in a liver transplant recipient. Transplantation 1994; 57:1271–1274.
48. Burdick JF, Vogelsang GB, Smith WJ, et al. Severe graft-versus-host disease in a liver-transplant recipient. N Engl J Med 1988; 318:689–691.
49. Collins RH Jr, Cooper B, Nikaein A, et al. Graft-versus-host disease in a liver transplant recipient. Ann Intern Med 1992; 116:391–392.
50. Chen P-M, Tzeng C-H, Fan FS, et al. Bone marrow transplantation in Taiwan: Low incidence of acute GVHD in patients with hematologic malignancies and severe aplastic anemia. Bone Marrow Transplant 1994; 13:709–711.
51. Fujii Y, Kaku K, Tanaka M, et al. Hepatitis C virus infection and liver disease after allogeneic bone marrow transplantation. Bone Marrow Transplant 1994; 13:523–526.

52. Appleton AL, Sviland L. Pathogenesis of GVHD: Role of herpes viruses. Bone Marrow Transplant 1993; 11:349–355.
53. Kuiper J, Brouwer A, Knook DL, van Berkel TJC. Kupffer and sinusoidal endothelial cells. In: Arias IM, et al, eds. The Liver: Biology and Pathobiology: vol 3. New York: Raven Press, 1994.
54. Demetris AJ, Murase N, Fujisaki S, et al. Hematolymphoid cell trafficking, microchimerism, and GVH reactions after liver, bone marrow, and heart transplantation. Transplant Proc 1993; 25:3337–3344.
55. Rubinstein D, Roska AK, Lipsky PE. Antigen presentation by liver sinusoidal lining cells after antigen exposure in vivo. J Immunol 1987; 138:1377–1382.
56. Saitoh T, Fujiwara M, Asakura H. L3T4$^+$ T cells induce hepatic lesions resembling primary biliary cirrhosis in mice with graft-versus-host reactions due to major histocompatibility complex class II disparity. Clin Immunol Immunopathol 1991; 59:449–461.
57. Cray C, Levy RB. CD8$^+$ and CD4$^+$ T cells contribute to the exacerbation of class I MHC disparate graft-versus-host reaction by concurrent murine cytomegalovirus infection. Clin Immunol Immunopathol 1993; 67:84–90.
58. Jansen J, Hanks S, Akard L, et al. Selective T cell depletion with CD8-conjugated magnetic beads in the prevention of graft-versus-host disease after allogeneic bone marrow transplantation. Bone Marrow Transplant 1995; 15:271–278.
59. Dilly SA, Slane JP. An immunohistological study of human hepatic graft-versus-host disease. Clin Exp Immunol 1985; 62:545–553.
60. Czaja AJ. Chronic graft-versus-host disease and primary biliary cirrhosis: Sorting the puzzle pieces. Lab Invest 1994; 70:589–592.
61. Korngold R, Sprent J. Surface markers of T cells causing lethal graft-versus-host disease to class I vs class II H-2 differences. J Immunol 1985; 135:3004–3010.
62. Eigenbrodt ML, Eigenbrodt EH, Thiele DL. Histologic similarity of murine colonic graft-versus-host disease (GVHD) to human colonic GVHD and inflammatory bowel disease. Am J Pathol 1990; 137:1065–1076.
63. Suzuki K, Narita T, Yui R, et al. Mechanism of the induction of autoimmune disease by graft-versus-host reaction: Role of CD8$^+$ cells in the development of hepatic and ductal lesions induced by CD4$^+$ cells in MHC class I plus II-different host. Lab Invest 1994; 70:609–619.
64. Fox ES, Thomas P, Broitman SA. Hepatic mechanisms for clearance and detoxification of bacterial endotoxins. J Nutr Biochem 1990; 1:620–628.
65. Spitzer JA, Mayer AMS. Hepatic neutrophil influx: Eicosanoid and superoxide formation in endotoxemia. J Surg Res 1993; 55:60–67.
66. Fox ES, Broitman SA, Thomas P. Bacterial endotoxins and the liver. Lab Invest 1990; 63:733–741.
67. Leskinen R, Volin L, Taskinen E, et al. Monitoring of bone marrow transplant recipient liver by fine-needle aspiration biopsy. Transplantation 1989; 48:969–974.
68. Howell CD, Yoder TY, Vierling JM. Suppressor function of liver mononuclear cells isolated during murine chronic graft-versus-host disease: II. Role of prostaglandins and interferon-gamma. Cell Immunol 1992; 140:54–66.
69. Greve JW, Gouma DJ, Buurman WA. Bile acids inhibit endotoxin-induced release of tumor necrosis factor by monocytes: An in vitro study. Hepatology 1989; 10:454–458.
70. Van de Water K, Gershwin ME. Primary biliary cirrhosis: Cells, sera, and soluble factors. Mayo Clin Proc 1993; 68:1128–1130.
71. Shiohara T, Moriya N, Gotoh C, et al. Locally administered monoclonal antibodies to lymphocyte function-associated antigen-1 and to L3T4 prevent cutaneous graft-versus-host disease. J Immunol 1988; 7:2261–2267.
72. Ferrara JLM. A paradigm shift for graft-versus-host disease. Bone Marrow Transplant 1994; 14:183–4.

73. Green RM, Whiting JF, Rosenbluth AB, et al. Interleukin-6 inhibits hepatocyte taurocholate uptake and sodium-potassium-adenosinetriphosphatase activity. Am J Physiol Gastrointest Liver Physiol 1994; 267:G1094–G1100.
74. Remberger M, Ringden O, Markling L. TNFα levels are increased during bone marrow transplantation conditioning in patients who develop acute GVHD. Bone Marrow Transplant 1995; 15:99–104.
75. Jones A, Selby PJ, Viner C, et al. Tumour necrosis factor, cholestatic jaundice, and chronic liver disease. Gut 1990; 31:938–939.
76. Rubin RA, Kowalski TE, Khandelwal M, et al. Ursodiol for hepatobiliary disorders. Ann Intern Med 1994; 121:207–218.
77. Sloane JP, Farthing MJG, Powles RL. Histopathological changes in the liver after allogeneic bone marrow transplantation. J Clin Pathol 1980; 33:344–350.
78. Blatter DD, Crawford JM, Ferrara JLM. Nuclear magnetic resonance of hepatic graft-versus-host disease in mice. Transplantation 1990; 50:1011–1018.
79. Sherlock S. Fulminant hepatic failure. Adv Intern Med 1993; 38:245–267.
80. Jazrawi RP, De Caestecker JS, Goggin PM, et al. Kinetics of hepatic bile acid handling in cholestatic liver disease: Effect of ursodeoxycholic acid. Gastroenterology 1994; 106: 134–142.
81. Fried RH, Murakami CS, Fisher LD, et al. Ursodeoxycholic acid treatment of refractory chronic graft-versus-host disease of the liver. Ann Intern Med 1992; 116:624–629.
82. Bismuth H. Consensus statement on indications for liver transplantation: Paris, June 22–23, 1993. Hepatology 1994; 20:63S–68S.
83. Rhodes DF, Lee WM, Wingard JR, et al. Orthotopic liver transplantation for graft-versus-host disease following bone marrow transplantation. Gastroenterology 1990; 99: 536–538.
84. Ramsay NKC, Kersey JH, Robinson LL, et al. A randomized study of the prevention of acute graft-versus-host disease. N Engl J Med 1982; 306:392–397.

13

Intestinal Graft-Versus-Host Disease

Allan Mowat
University of Glasgow
Glasgow, Scotland

I. INTRODUCTION

Early studies of graft-versus-host reaction (GVHR) quickly identified intestinal damage as an important component of host disease (1). Most animals with severe GVHR developed diarrhea, and this feature remains one of the characteristic signs of GVHD in both humans and experimental animals. Nevertheless, there is not yet a clear understanding of the mechanisms responsible for intestinal damage. Partly this reflects a failure to discriminate between intestinal alterations that are true consequences of GVHR and those that are artifacts of irradiation or infection. Furthermore, the mucosal features vary markedly with time, even within a single experimental model, and it is unwise to extrapolate from the intestinal changes found in the dying (or even dead) animals studied by many authors. Finally, it should be remembered that the intestine is not only the largest lymphoid tissue in the body but, as part of the mucosal immune system, represents a distinct component of the host immune response. Therefore, measurements of systemic immune responsiveness in animals with GVHR may not reflect events within the intestine.

This chapter reviews the intestinal pathology that characterizes GVHD both in experimental animals and under clinical conditions before discussing the mechanisms responsible for the intestinal damage in experimental GVHR.

II. THE INTESTINE AND ITS IMMUNE SYSTEM

A. Epithelial Pathophysiology

The gut-associated lymphoid tissues (GALT) are not only the largest immune compartment in the body but also contain populations of lymphoid cells whose origin and function are distinct from cells in other tissues (for reviews, see Refs. 2, 3, and 4). Furthermore, this enormous population is in intimate contact with a specialized epithelial layer, whose function is essential for the survival of the animal (Fig. 1). Both the epithelial and lymphoid cells in the gut are constantly changing, and it follows that local immune responses can produce rapid and profound changes in intestinal structure and function (Fig. 2). In this section, we review aspects of intestinal immunology and physiology which are important for understanding enteropathy in GVHR.

The principal function of the small intestine is the digestion and absorption of food material. These activities are performed by a wide range of enzymes found principally on the microvilli which comprise the "brush border" on the luminal surface of columnar enterocytes. Any form of insult that compromises the production and function of these cells will inevitably have profound consequences for the well-being of the host. The functional unit of the small intestine is the villus (Figs. 1 and 2), which comprises a cylinder consisting of sheets of enterocytes. The profusion of these fingerlike processes greatly increases the surface area of epithelial cells available for digestive functions. Atrophy or disruption of this villus architecture is an important cause of intestinal failure. As described below, GVHR is one of the most potent means of producing this type of intestinal pathology.

The enterocytes that form the villus move upward in continuous sheets from their origin in the crypts of Lieberkuhn, where a self-renewing population of stem cells normally balances loss of effete enterocytes from the villus tip (Figs. 1 and 2). In the steady state in normal animals, around 10 new cells are produced in each crypt per hour and the migration of enterocytes from the crypt to the villus tip takes 2 to 3 days. However, when epithelial cell damage or increased cell loss occurs, both the production of new cells by the crypts and their subsequent migration can be rapidly and dramatically increased. In this way, secondary alterations in epithelial cell renewal form the principal means of repairing damage to mature enterocytes. In addition, certain stimuli can have direct effects on crypt-cell turnover. Although these repair mechanisms probably evolved as a means of eliminating parasites which have attached to the epithelium, similar effects also occur in GVHR.

Villus atrophy frequently occurs in association with these alterations in crypt-cell kinetics, but increased production of new epithelial cells can itself interfere with intestinal function. When enterocytes leave the crypts, they are immature with no microvilli and poorly developed enzymes. However, as the cells enter the villus compartment, they differentiate rapidly and acquire the ability to digest and absorb foods. Conditions that enhance crypt cell turnover or enterocyte migration result in the appearance of a large number of recently produced, immature cells on the part of the villus normally covered by mature cells. As a result, there is an effective decrease in absorptive surface area.

The features discussed above illustrate how pathogenic insults can alter intestinal function either by direct damage to villus enterocytes or by interfering with the dynamic balance between epithelial-cell renewal and differentiation. One further potential means of causing intestinal damage is to disrupt the tissues which underly the epithelium. The three-dimensional structure of the villus is highly dependent on the integrity of its basement membrane and associated ground substance. In addition, these mesenchymal structures play an important role in maintaining epithelial function. Thus, inflammatory insults that harm these elements are likely to have profound effects on epithelial behavior. Finally, the epithelium is invested closely

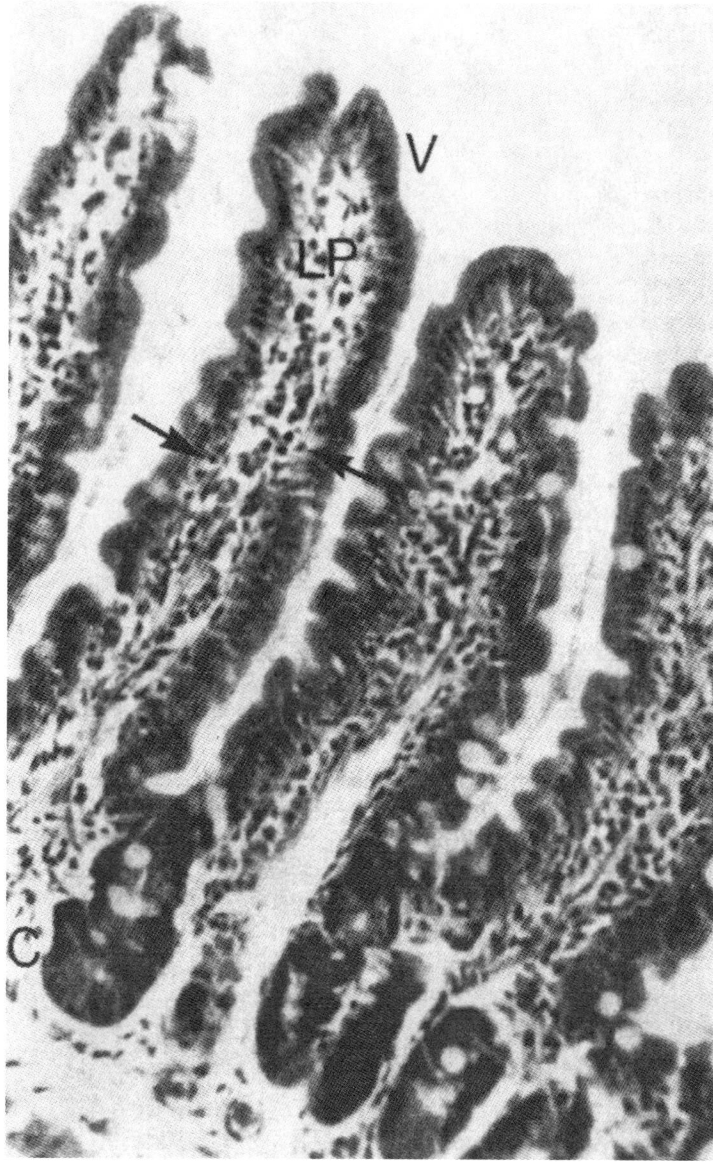

Figure 1 The appearance of the normal small intestine. The villus (V) is clothed by a layer of columnar epithelial cells that arise from dividing cells in the crypts (C). The lamina propria (LP) is separated from the epithelium by a basement membrane and contains a wide variety of lymphoid cells. Intraepithelial lymphocytes (arrows) are found between the epithelial cells. H&E, ×500.

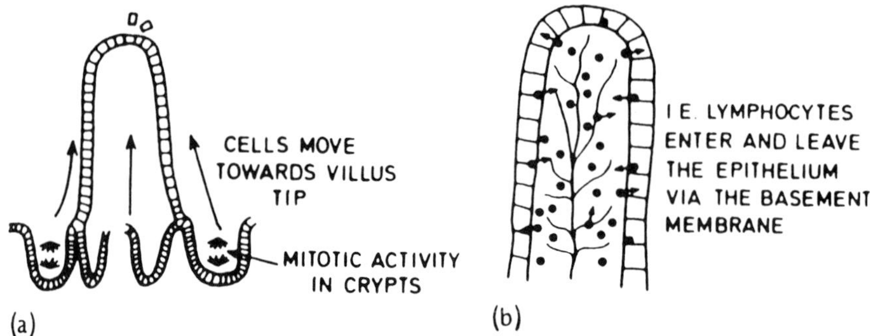

Figure 2 The villus/crypt unit as a dynamic structure. Enterocyte loss from the villus tip is normally balanced by continual upward movement of new cells produced in the crypts. Lymphocytes move constantly in and out of the epithelium.

by a complex network of blood vessels as well as autonomic and peptidergic nerves, and the normal function of these elements is essential for intestinal integrity.

B. Mucosal Lymphoid Cells

The preceding section has highlighted the dynamic relationships between different epithelial and stromal components which are involved in maintaining the health of the intestine. To this must be added the effects of the large numbers of lymphoid cells found within the mucosa.

The most cursory microscopic examination reveals that the lamina propria, which underlies the epithelium contains a wide variety of lymphoid and myeloid cells (Fig. 1). Many of these cell types are identical to those found in peripheral lymphoid tissues, with macrophages, eosinophils, and basophils particularly well represented in the mucosa. In addition, there are numerous B lymphocytes, T lymphocytes, plasma cells, and mast cells, but many of these appear to be distinct from their peripheral counterparts. The predominance of IgA-producing B cells in the intestine is well known, and up to 90% of plasma cells within the mucosa are committed to IgA synthesis. These cells are also derived from a distinct population of precursors within the GALT.

Mucosal T cells may also form a discrete population of lymphocytes and are found within two separate compartments. Those in the lamina propria have a $CD4^+$:$CD8^+$ ratio of 2 : 1, and are generally believed to contain a large number of functional helper T cells (3–5). Interestingly, lamina propria T cells congregate close to the crypts and are thus in an ideal position to modulate crypt cell behavior. Some 15 to 20% of cells in the intestinal epithelium are also lymphocytes, making this unique population of lymphocytes the largest in the immune system. Virtually all intraepithelial lymphocytes (IEL) are $CD3^+$ T cells, but over 80% are $CD8^+$ and there are <10% $CD4^+$ T cells. They express a unique integrin molecule ($\alpha^E\beta_7$) and there are no B cells, plasma cells or macrophages within the epithelium, emphasizing how different this population is from the lymphoid cells found in the adjacent lamina propria (6–8). In humans, the vast majority of IEL normally carry the $\alpha\beta$ T-cell receptor (TcR), but in some species, including mice, a substantial proportion may be $\gamma\delta$ T cells (9,10). The number of $\gamma\delta$ IEL is also expanded in humans with celiac disease (11). The dominant population of CD8$^+$ IEL has many unusual properties, with a low expression of markers found on all other peripheral CD8$^+$ T cells, including CD2, CD5, CD28, and Thy1. Of particular note, a large proportion of CD8$^+$ IEL (up to 60%) express a homodimeric CD8$\alpha\alpha$ molecule, in contrast to the CD8$\alpha\beta$ heterodimer found on other T cells (10,12). Recent studies show that the majority of IEL represent the progeny of oligoclonal expansion that occurs in response to local antigen, and it has been suggested that many if not all these cells are extrathymically derived in ontogeny (9,13,14). IEL lie between epithelial cells on the basement membrane and may migrate in and out of this compartment (Fig. 3). Their close proximity to the enterocytes suggests that IEL could play an important role in the pathogenesis of epithelial damage. Although this is supported by the increased number of IEL found in immunologically based disorders such as celiac disease and GVHR (see below), their functions remain unclear. Most IEL show marked nonspecific cytolytic activity when their TcR is cross-linked in vitro, but true antigen-specific cytotoxic T lymphocyte (CTL) activity is limited to a small subset of classical CD8$\beta^+\alpha\beta$TcR-T cells (7,10,15,16,17). They can also secrete lymphokines such as IL5 and γ-IFN in vitro but show little or no proliferative activity to antigen or T-cell mitogens (15,16). Therefore, the contribution of IEL to local immune responses is unknown.

Mucosal mast cells (MMC) are a further population of intestinal effector cells that differ from the equivalent cells in the periphery and are important in GVHR. MMC occur predominantly in the lamina propria and differ from classic connective tissue mast cells in staining pattern, chemical content, and response to mast-cell

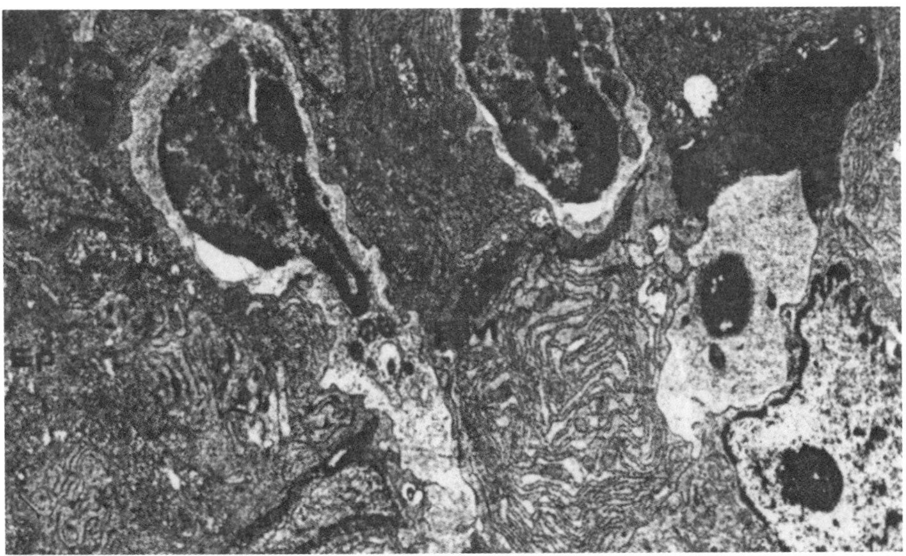

Figure 3 Electron microscopic appearance of two intraepithelial lymphocytes, one of which is crossing into the epithelium through the basement membrane (BM). ×16,000. Ep = epithelial cell nucleus.

activators (17,18). They contain little or no histamine and secrete a serine protease (mast-cell protease II) which is antigenically different from that found in peripheral mast cells (19). The differentiation and function of MMC are highly dependent on T lymphocytes, and MMC hyperplasia is a characteristic feature of cell-mediated responses to intestinal parasite infections (17,20). Their exact role in other intestinal immune responses remains to be clarified.

The interaction between these distinct populations of local immune effector cells and the epithelial elements of the gut are critical to understanding how GVHR can produce intestinal pathology and is an important focus of later sections.

III. INTESTINAL GVHR IN EXPERIMENTAL ANIMALS

A. Occurrence

The runting disease found in the earliest studies of tolerance to allogeneic cells in neonatal mice was accompanied by diarrhea (21,22). Subsequent studies of "graft-versus-host" disease also noted the presence of diarrhea (23), and since then, this sign has provided one of the most important indicators of both clinical and experimental GVHD.

B. Clinical Features

As noted above, diarrhea is the cardinal sign of intestinal GVHR and is seen in most animals with severe disease. Several mechanisms may account for this feature (Table 1). First, damage to enterocytes produces deficiency of several of the epithelial cell enzymes required for absorption of sugars (24,25). The resulting increased amounts of intact sugar left undigested in the lumen lead to osmotic water loss. Second, the damaged small intestine has a large number of immature of abnormal enterocytes (see below), and this may lead to decreased reabsorption of ions and water by the epithelium. This has not been examined directly in GVHR, but such choleralike effects have been observed in IgE-mediated intestinal damage (26) and can be responsible for considerable water loss. Colonic damage in GVHR could also potentially interfere with normal water absorption mechanisms, but it has not been studied in detail. Finally, the damaged epithelium may become hyperpermeable to serum and tissue proteins, with a concomitant loss of water. A protein-losing enteropathy of this type is evidenced by low serum proteins and increased intestinal loss of intravenously injected chromium 51 in mice with severe GVHR (27). There is also

Table 1 Possible Mechanisms for Diarrhea in Intestinal GVHR

Small intestine
Disaccharidase deficiency in epithelium due to enterocyte damage → luminal sugars + osmotic water loss
Increased proportion of immature enterocytes → enzyme deficiency + abnormal water transport
Protein + water exudation through hyperpermeable epithelium
Large intestine
Damage to colonic enterocytes → water reabsorption

increased fecal loss of the serum protein α_1-antitrypsin in human GVHD (28), and irradiated mice with acute GVHR have increased intestinal loss of the tracer material ^{125}I-PVP from serum (29).

The profound metabolic consequences of the diarrheal loss of fluid, ions, and protein are complicated by the malabsorption of all essential nutrients. This is caused by the loss of mature, absorptive surface area due to villus atrophy and by deficiencies in epithelial-cell enzymes. A further effect of GVHR on intestinal function is to increase the permeability of the epithelium to materials within the lumen. Increased uptake of large, orally administered molecules such as proteins and sugars is a nonspecific consequence of several forms of intestinal inflammation, including GVHR (30, Strobel S: personal communication). Animals with GVHR also have evidence of increased serum levels of endotoxin, presumably derived from intestinal bacteria (31). Together, the diarrhea, malabsorption, and altered intestinal permeability account for much of the morbidity and mortality in GVHR.

C. Distribution of Intestinal Pathology

As will be discussed, human GVHD can affect the entire gastrointestinal tract, sparing few sites from the mouth to the rectum and causing lesions in several of the associated exocrine glands, including the pancreas and salivary glands. There is less information of this kind from studies of experimental GVHR. The colon and ileum appear to be the worst-affected areas of the bowel in acute GVHD in humans (32), and one early study reported that the ileum was the most seriously damaged site in neonatal mice with acute GVHR (33). Colonic disease has also been reported in mice with GVHR (27); it may even occur before pathology in other parts of the intestine (34). Sclerodermalike lesions have been found in the esophagus and tongue of rats undergoing a chronic form of GVHR across minor histocompatibility differences (35), but in general, these aspects of intestinal GVHR in experimental animals have not been documented in detail.

IV. NATURE OF THE INTESTINAL PATHOLOGY

A. Epithelial Damage

1. Evolution of Enteropathy

Initial studies of homologous disease in mice noted severe intestinal inflammation, with macroscopic ulceration of the ileum and colon associated with focal degeneration of the crypts (22,36). Later, more detailed studies found intestinal dilatation and bloody exudates during acute GVHR in mice. These changes were accompanied by severe villus atrophy, crypt necrosis, and increased extrusion of necrotic cells from the villus tip (27,33,37,38). Most research on human GVHD has also emphasized this destructive pattern of intestinal damage, and it is widely assumed that the pathology is simply due to a direct cytotoxic attack on mature villus enterocytes. That this is not the case can be demonstrated by examining the evolution of intestinal damage in more detail. This shows that the enteropathy evolves through distinct phases, each of which seems to reflect the effects of distinct immune mediators on crypt stem cells (Table 2). These phases are as follows. First, *proliferation*: This is characterized by increased epithelial cell turnover, crypt hypertrophy, and infiltration of the mucosa by lymphoid cells. This type of pathology is not accompanied by

Table 2 Pathological Stages of Intestinal GVHR in Experimental Animals

Early Proliferative
Increased crypt cell mitotic activity
Crypt lengthening (± villus lengthening)
Increased density of intraepithelial lymphocytes, mucosal mast cells
Destructive
Villus atrophy
Continued crypt hyperplasia →↓ crypt cell turnover
Crypt stem cell apoptosis → necrosis
Loss of mucosal lymphoid cells
Atrophic
Mucosal thinning
Normal/short villi
Crypt hypoplasia
Absence of local lymphoid cells

villus atrophy or damage to mature enterocytes (Fig. 4) and may be the only evidence of gut disease in mature, immunocompetent hosts. It also represents the early phase of damage in more severe models of GVHR. Second, *destruction*: Depending on the model system, a second phase of enteropathy may ensue, in which continuing and intense crypt hyperplasia is accompanied by the rapid onset of villus damage. Shortly thereafter, there is a sudden cessation in crypt-cell proliferation, associated with apoptosis of stem cells, and the mucosa shows evidence of the necrosis familiar from clinical studies. This may lead to complete intestinal destruction, but occasionally sufficient crypts may survive to allow regeneration. These destructive changes are accompanied by the loss of lymphoid infiltrates and the appearance of the inflammatory cells more typical of necrosis (Fig. 5). Third, *atrophy*: A further, unusual form of enteropathy has been observed under some circumstances. This lesion is characterized by thinning and shortening of both villi and crypts as well as a complete absence of lymphoid cells. It may occur as an end-stage event after destructive enteropathy has resolved or may be the only manifestation of intestinal GVHR.

2. Crypt Cell Pathology

Crypt cells are the principal target of small-intestinal GVHR irrespective of the type of enteropathy. Focal necrosis and degeneration of individual crypts has long been recognized in models of severe GVHR, and this is a highly characteristic feature of the terminal stages of intestinal damage. However, even in early studies, these destructive changes were often associated with histological evidence of crypt lengthening and increased mitotic activity (27,33). Wall et al. (37) then showed that the uptake of ^{3}H-TdR was greatly enhanced in crypts of both the jejunum and ileum of newborn mice with GVHR. As this hyperplasia was always accompanied by marked villus atrophy, it was concluded that the increased crypt cell mitotic activity was an attempt to repair the loss of mature enterocytes. Nevertheless, these studies examined intestinal pathology at only one time point in animals that were already acutely ill. It was not until 1977 that elegant studies by Elson et al. (39) demonstrated that

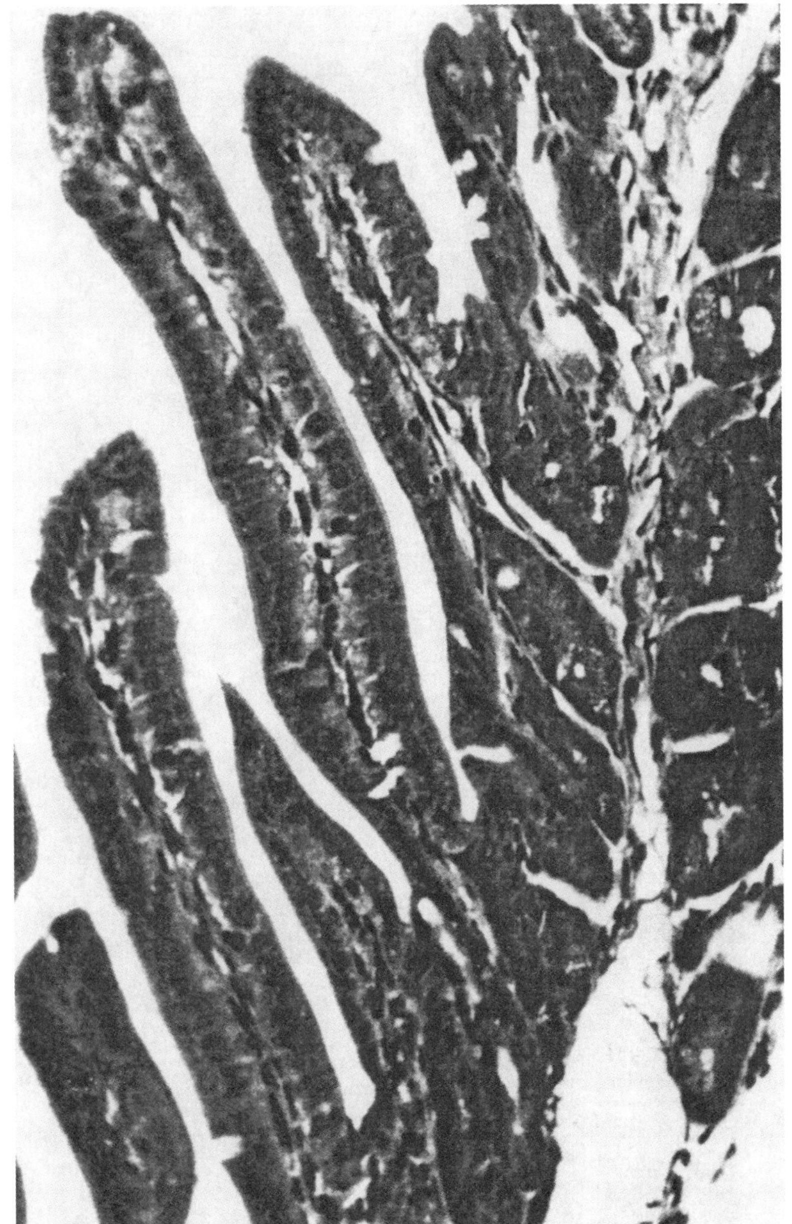

Figure 4 Proliferative enteropathy in murine graft-versus-host reaction. There is crypt lengthening and increased numbers of mucosal lymphoid cells but no villus atrophy or enterocyte damage. HPE, ×320.

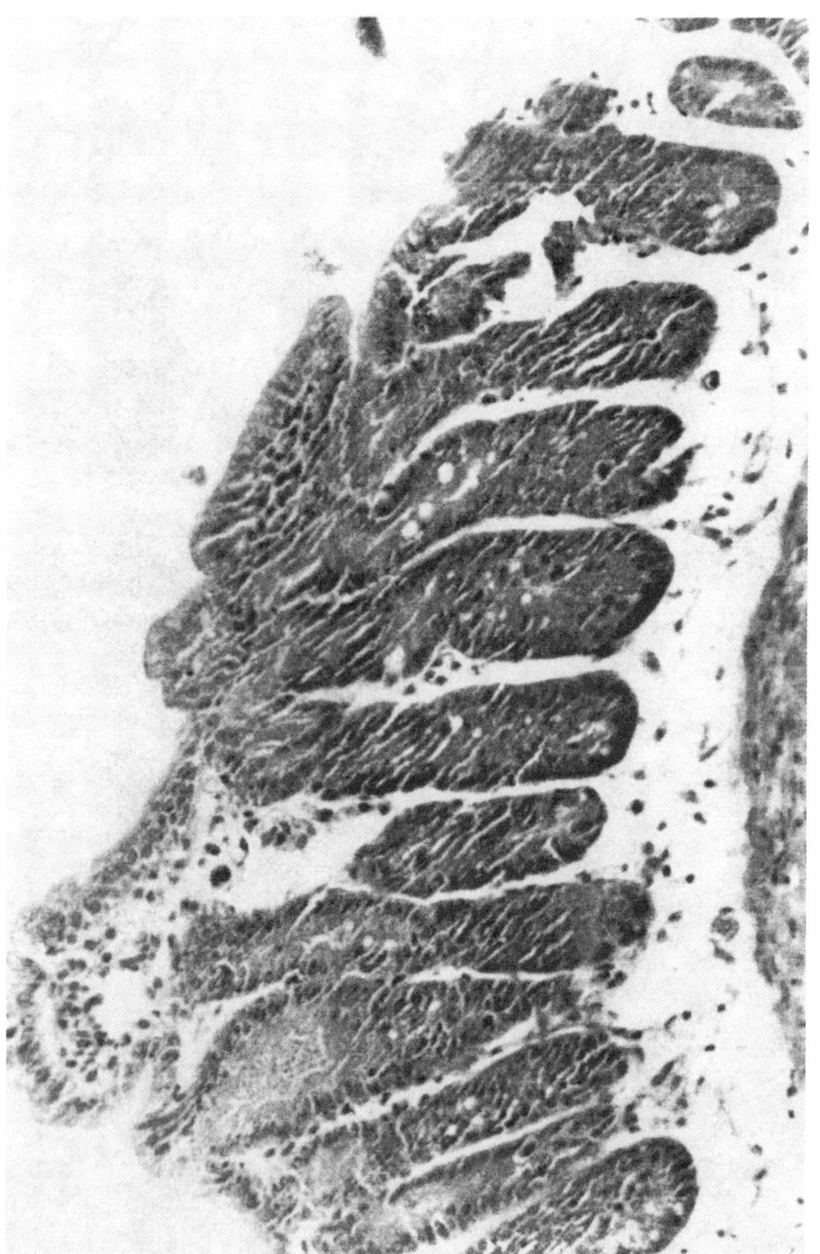

Figure 5 Destructive enteropathy in murine GVHR. Many crypts remain long and hyperplastic, but there is also necrosis of individual enterocytes and severe villus atrophy. The mucosa is devoid of lymphoid cells. HPE, ×320.

crypt hyperplasia could occur in the absence of detectable villus atrophy and so suggested that stimulation of crypt-cell production rate (CCPR) might be a direct consequence of GVHR. These conclusions were supported by subsequent work using a sensitive stathmokinetic technique to measure epithelial-cell turnover and villus/crypt architecture throughout the course of a GVHR in neonatal (CBA × BALB/c)F_1 mice. This showed that there was an increase in CCPR in the jejunum during the first 5 to 7 days of GVHR, and this preceded any evidence of villus atrophy (40). Nevertheless, significant villus damage did occur in this model, and so it remained possible that an earlier, undetected phase of villus atrophy had been the initial stimulus to crypt-cell proliferation. This criticism was addressed in a subsequent time-course study of intestinal GVHR in slightly older mice of the same strain (41). Under these conditions, there was a significant increase in CCPR within 2 to 3 days of inducing the GVHR. This progressed until the peak of the GVHR during the second week and then resolved completely (Fig. 6). It is important to note that these animals never had villus atrophy and, in fact, conventional histoglogy revealed no evidence of any damage to mature enterocytes whatsoever. We have made similar observations of crypt hyperplasia in the absence of villus atrophy during many subsequent studies of intestinal GVHR in mature, unirradiated mice. Identical findings have also been reported in rats with GVHR (42). Stimulation of the CCPR is undoubtedly the principal consequence of GVHR under these circumstances.

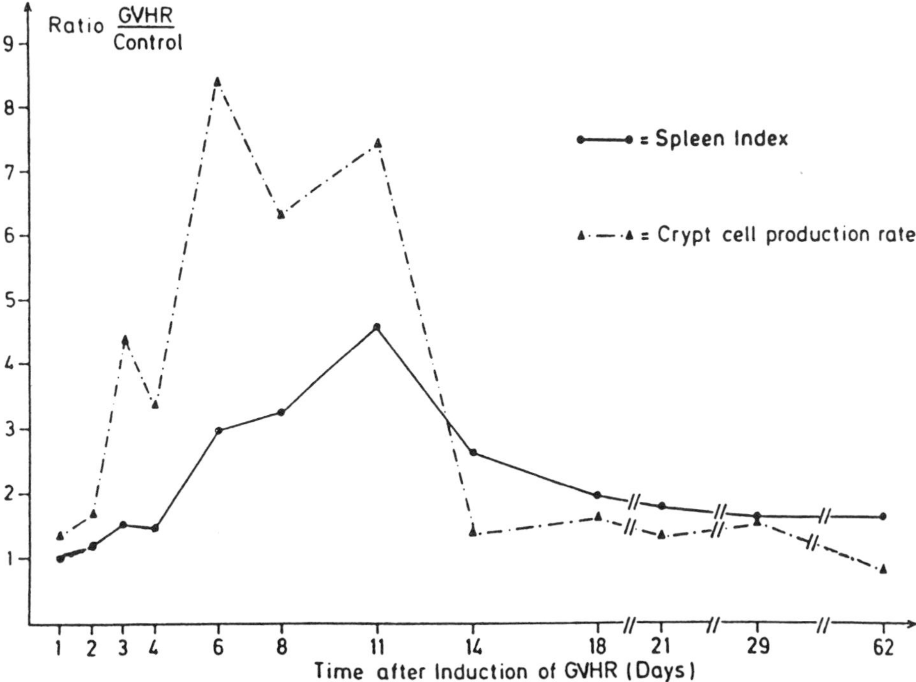

Figure 6 Progress of crypt hyperplasia in proliferative GVHR. Crypt cell production rate in jejunum of 6- to 7-day-old (CBA × BALB/c)F_1 mice with GVHR, expressed as a ratio to that in controls. The CCPR develops in parallel with the splenomegaly in the same animals.

Subsequent alterations in crypt-cell proliferation depend on the model under study. In mild, proliferative forms of disease, the mitotic activity returns to normal and the intestine shows no other evidence of damage (41). Destructive forms of GVHR are associated with prolonged crypt hyperplasia, which may continue for some months after resolution of other aspects of intestinal pathology (43). In the most severe cases of intestinal GVHR, there is a sudden cessation of crypt-cell proliferative activity, associated with the appearance of apoptosis of basal crypt enterocytes (27,33,38,44,45,46,47).

Enhanced proliferation is not the only direct effect of GVHR on the biology of intestinal epithelial cells and their precursors (Table 3). The migration of enterocytes from the crypts up the villus is also markedly increased in mice with GVHR (25,37). This reflects a greater upward pressure arising from the enlarged crypt-cell population, rather than increased cell loss, as crypt hyperplasia early in GVHR frequently produces villus lengthening, indicating an absolute increase in the number of villus enterocytes (our unpublished observations). As discussed above, one consequence of the more rapid appearance of recently formed enterocytes on the villus is that the proportion of cells with mature enzyme function will be decreased. This has been confirmed in GVHR, where jejunal lactase and aminopeptidase activities do not develop until much higher up the villus than normal (37). Interestingly, however, the increased production of immature cells is balanced partly by a concomitant enhancement in the rate of differentiation of new enterocytes. Sucrase activity is enhanced in GVHR, and it has been noted that the architecture of the small intestine in neonatal mice with GVHR has a more "adult" appearance than that of age-matched controls (24). In addition, Lund et al. (37) showed that enzyme differentiation in individual cells actually occurred more rapidly in GVHR than in normal mice. Thus, the immunological insult of the GVHR not only alters the mitotic activity of enterocytes but also modifies the subsequent differentiation of these cells.

Enhanced expression of class II MHC molecules by the epithelium is a further effect of GVHR on enterocyte differentiation. Class II MHC molecules are expressed in the cytoplasm and on the surface of small-bowel villus enterocytes in most species (48,49). However, in normal animals, this is usually at a low level and is restricted to mature epithelial cells, with none being found on normal crypt cells. However, the pattern of class II MHC expression is altered dramatically in the intestine of rodents and humans with acute GVHR. Villus enterocytes have markedly increased levels of MHC expression, and this phenomenon now involves the entire epithelium, including the crypts (50). In addition, the intestinal epithelium of GVHR animals begins to express class II MHC products not normally found on enterocytes, such as I-E in mice (51). These observations are similar to those in

Table 3 Effects of GVHR on Behavior of Intestinal Crypt Cells

Increased proliferation rate
Enhanced migration on to villus
More rapid differentiation of enzymes
Induction of expression of Class II MCH molecules
Ultimately, suppression of proliferation + necrosis

other tissues during GVHR and in other forms of intestinal inflammation, including celiac disease, parasitic infections, inflammatory bowel disease, and in cytokine-knockout mice (50,52,53). Intestinal class II MHC expression in murine GVHR appears within the first few days of inducing GVHR and peaks before villus atrophy is detected (47). However, the appearance of class II MHC molecules on crypt cells is not directly related to the alterations in mitotic activity, as class II MHC expression does not continue to increase as the CCPR rises later in GVHR (47). There is also no clear evidence of a gradient of class II MHC expression along the villus-crypt axis (51). These findings suggest that immune mediators such as γ-interferon (γ-IFN) may influence MHC gene expression by both mature and immature epithelial cells. The in vivo consequences of the enhanced class II expression by enterocytes are unknown. However, epithelial cells from humans with IBD and mice with GVHR have an enhanced capacity to present antigen to T cells (47,54), suggesting that class II MHC–expressing enterocytes could help sustain the activation of donor T cells in the mucosa in GVHR.

3. Evolution of Villus Damage

The findings discussed above indicate that the primary effects of a GVHR on the intestine are to modify the behavior of crypt cells. Nevertheless, villus atrophy remains the best recognized feature of intestinal GVHR; in many cases, there can be complete loss of the normal villus architecture (Fig. 5). As noted earlier, many workers have made the implicit assumption that villus damage represents the primary lesion of intestinal GVHR and that crypt hyperplasia is a secondary event. However, villus atrophy occurs only in severe forms of GVHR, such as those found in neonatal or irradiated hosts or in certain unirradiated adults. It is preceded by a particularly intense period of crypt hyperplasia, which reaches its peak shortly before villus atrophy can be demonstrated. The villus atrophy may develop because very intense crypt hyperplasia creates a hyperdynamic, unstable mucosa, which cannot maintain the usual column of mature enterocytes. An additional factor is that the stem-cell apoptosis described above may lead to a failure to repopulate the villus. This latter possibility was suggested by studies of GVHR in irradiated (CBA $\times$ BALB/c)F_1 mice in which significant crypt hyperplasia occurred within 1 to 2 days of inducing the GVHR, rising to very high levels by 3 to 4 days (46). Villus atrophy appeared only on day 5 and was accompanied by a sudden cessation in crypt-cell mitotic activity, rather than the further rise in CCPR that would be anticipated if crypt-cell turnover were merely responding to epithelial-cell damage. Thereafter, progressive mucosal destruction occurred, with evidence of crypt necrosis and ulceration. We have subsequently observed a similar association between inhibition of CCPR and the appearance of villus atrophy in other models of acute GVHR in mice.

In our own and others' hands, there is little evidence of direct damage to mature villus enterocytes even in advanced GVHR (37). Minor changes such as the cytoplasmic vacuolation reported by some workers (27,33,55), are unlikely to account for the major structural abnormalities found in villus atrophy and may simply reflect the alterations in differentiation and migration described above.

In summary, the intestinal epithelium provides an important target for the pathogenic effects of GVHR, and most evidence seems to favor the idea that crypt cells are the principal focus of this attack. Initially, the immune stimulus produces a proliferative enteropathy characterized by increased crypt-cell proliferation, migration and differentiation, but with few effects on mature enterocytes (Table 2). In severe cases, this early phase intensifies rapidly and progresses to a destructive disorder associated with cessation of crypt-cell mitotic activity and crypt necrosis. Only at this stage does villus atrophy and damage to mature enterocytes appear, and we propose that these events are secondary to the alterations in crypt-cell turnover and function.

B. Pathology of Nonepithelial Structures in Intestinal GVHR

Direct damage to the functioning epithelial tissues of the gut has obvious and important consequences for the host, but many components of the extracellular matrix (ECM) and underlying tissues are also involved in maintaining the integrity of the intestine. Although there have been no detailed studies of the effects of GVHR on, e.g., intestinal basement membrane (BM) or local microvascalature, damage to these tissues can be seen readily in animals with acute GVHR. Thickening of the basement membrane occurs early in GVHR, but later the BM and underlying ECM appears to disintegrate as villus atrophy develops (unpublished observations). Damage to local blood vessels may also be important in intestinal GVHR. Swelling of the intestinal vascular endothelium has been noted in irradiated mice with severe GVHR (47), and hemorrhagic exudates are present during the terminal stages of intestinal GVHR (33,55). We have found that mice dying of GVHR have evidence of segmental ischemia (unpublished observations), while TNF-α, one of the mediators implicated in intestinal GVHR, is a well-known mediator of vascular pathology. Thus, immune-mediated destruction or occlusion of the local blood supply may contribute significantly to the failure of intestinal function in GVHR.

C. Effects of GVHR on Intestinal Lymphoid Cells

1. General

One of the most characteristic features of GVHR is its ability to disrupt the structure and function of the immune system. It would be surprising, therefore, if a lymphoid organ as large as the gut were to escape this damage. In parallel with their assessment of epithelial pathology, initial studies on intestinal GVHR emphasized atrophy of Peyer's patches (PP) and depletion of mucosal lymphoid cells (22,23,33,56). Loss of lymphoid elements undoubtedly occurs in the terminal phase of intestinal GVHR (Fig. 5) and is found frequently on examination of humans with acute GVHD (see below). Nevertheless, these findings are again biased by studying late stages of severe disease using nonquantitative methods. Some microscopic studies did report that early, acute GVHR in mice was associated with infiltration of the mucosa by lymphoblasts (27,55), but the nature and origin of these cells was not determined. Subsequent work showed marked infiltration of the lamina propria by T lymphocytes, which correlated with the severity of mucosal damage in different models of murine GVHR (44,57). Interestingly, the majority of infiltrating T cells are found near the crypts, the major targets of the GVHR. Both donor and host T cells can be found in the infiltrate, but infiltration of the gut by donor T cells and the epithelial damage can both be prevented by local irradiation of the PP, suggesting that these cells are derived from intestinal rather than peripheral lymphoid tissues (57). These results are consistent with the hypothesis that intestinal GVHR reflects local activation of donor T lymphoblasts within the draining lymphoid tissues.

2. Intraepithelial Lymphocytes

A characteristic component of the lymphocytic infiltration of the gut in GVHR is an increased proportion of intraepithelial lymphocytes. Indeed, counts of IEL have proved to be an important quantitative means of assessing intestinal GVHR. An increased IEL count is one of the earliest detectable signs of intestinal GVHR, occurring within 24 hr of inducing GVHR in neonatal or irradiated mice and continuing to rise in parallel with the other proliferative features of GVHR, such as crypt hyperplasia and splenomegaly (41,46). Although this increase in IEL involves both crypt and villus epithelium, it has been suggested that the enhanced number of IEL in crypt epithelium precedes that in the villus compartment (47). This finding is reminiscent of the pattern of IEL hyperplasia that occurs during the evolution of the mucosal lesion in human celiac disease, where a relative increase in the number of crypt IEL is the earliest feature of the local immune response to gluten antigen (58,59). It is tempting to believe that these findings reflect a primary role for crypt IEL in the immunopathogenesis of enteropathy.

The subsequent behavior of IEL depends on the type of intestinal GVHR (Fig. 7). Whereas the IEL count falls to normal levels after the peak of the GVHR in mice undergoing an entirely proliferative enteropathy, a GVHR that causes villus atrophy and mucosal destruction is associated with almost complete loss of IEL (Fig. 7) (41,46).

The nature and origin of the increased number in IEL in GVHR is of obvious interest for determining their possible role in mucosal pathology. As noted above, the vast majority of normal IEL are $CD8^+$ T cells, and this remains the case during GVHR (44,47 and our unpublished observations). These cells retain the low Thy 1 expression characteristic of murine IEL (44), but as the GVHR evolves, a larger proportion of IEL begins to express the $\alpha\beta$ form of the CD8 molecule (44,47) (Table 3). This change is accompanied by the appearance of increased numbers of $\alpha\beta$ TcR-expressing T cells among IEL (Table 3) (12). The vast majority of the IEL recruited during the proliferative phase of GVHR is of host origin, but in the destructive disease, an increased number of donor-derived $CD8^+$ IEL partly balances the marked loss of host IEL (47). These changes parallel the onset of crypt cell apoptosis, suggesting that the elimination of host IEL and destruction of crypt stem cells are both consequences of the donor antihost response in severe disease. The donor IEL that appear in GVHR are mostly conventional $CD8^+$ $\alpha\beta TcR^+$ T cells and appear to derive via the thoracic duct and bloodstream from lymphoblast precursors stimulated by host alloantigens in the Peyer's patches (13,44,57).

The reasons for the early infiltration by host-derived IEL are unknown, but it has been suggested that they may be potentially autoreactive $CD8^+$ T cells that recognize self antigens expressed at abnormally high levels on the damaged epithelium. According to this hypothesis, CTL activity by these IEL may contribute to the intestinal damage (47). This remains to be proven, and it is equally possible that the infiltration by host IEL is part of a generalized, nonspecific, recruitment of inflammatory cells that occurs in the mucosa during GVHR. Alternatively, alterations in the epithelial microenvironment resulting from GVHR may enhance the

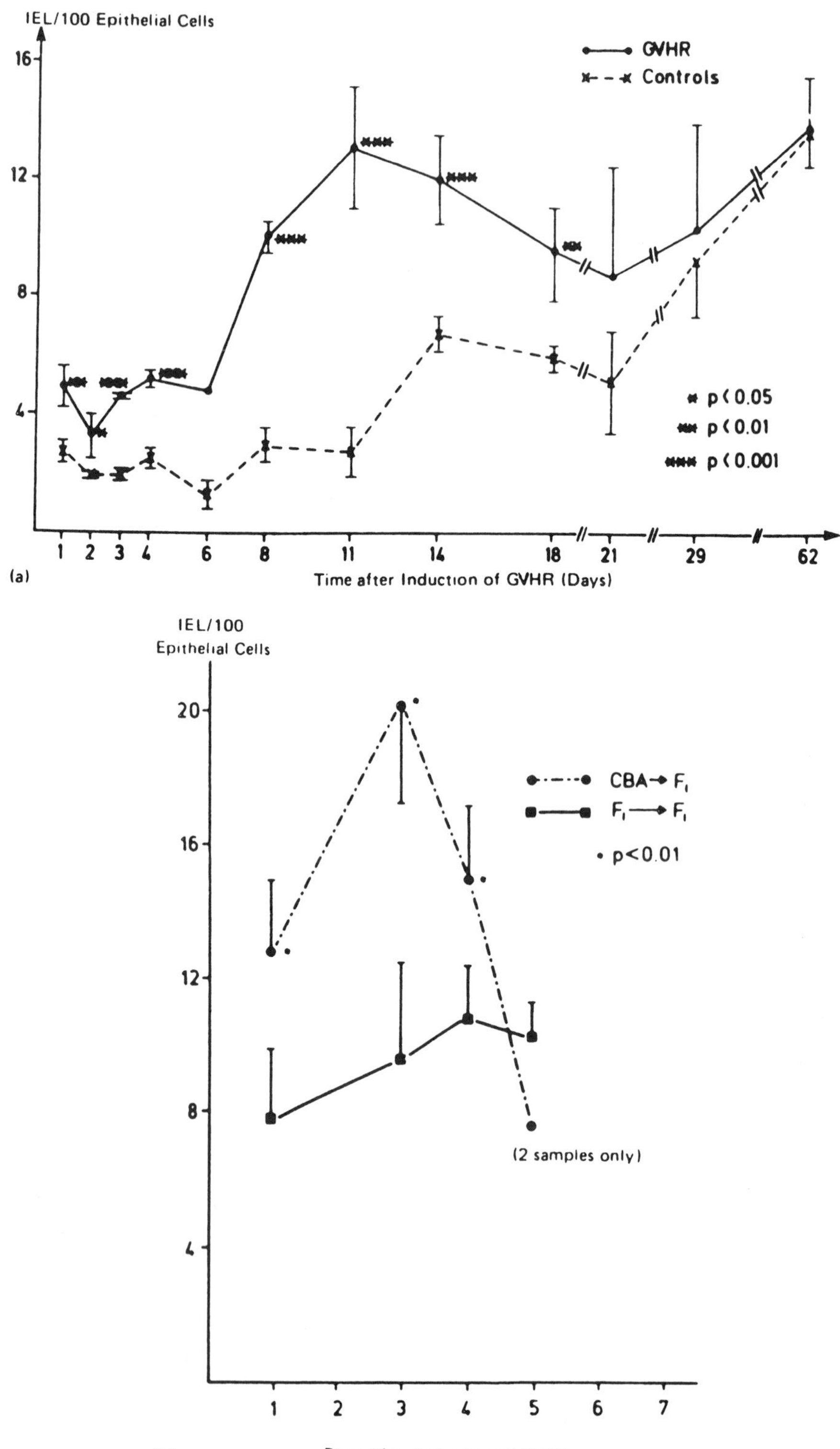

Figure 7 Behavior of intraepithelial lymphocyte populations in different forms of intestinal GVHR. IEL counts increase rapidly in both proliferative (A) and destructive (B)

local extrathymic differentiation of host IEL T cells in situ, an idea supported by the increase in mitotic activity found among IEL in GVHR (60).

3. Other Lymphoid Cells

The biphasic increases and decreases in IEL and lamina propria T lymphoblasts are accompanied by parallel changes in other mucosal lymphoid cells. Increased numbers of class II MHC-expressing accessory cells are found in the lamina propria early in GVHR (51) and the density of MHC expression is higher. Subsequently, there is marked depletion of IA^+ macrophages and dendritic cells in established GVHR (44). Similar effects on IgA-producing plasma cells in the lamina propria have been observed, with substantial loss of these cells occurring in severe murine GVHR (61), preceded by a phase of enhanced IgA production and hyperplasia of IgA plasma cells (62). It is important to note that the depletion of both these cell types late in GVHR could compromise local defense mechanisms and hence contribute to the evolution of intestinal damage.

Hyperplasia of mucosal mast cells is a further indicator of the proliferative consequences of intestinal GVHR. Several studies have reported an increase in MMC in rodent GVHR (41,44,57,63). In parallel, there is an increase in serum levels of interleukin-3 (IL-3) (64), while the intestine and serum show increased levels of the mucosal mast cell specific protease II (63,65). The time course of MMC hyperplasia and release of protease parallels other proliferative changes of GVHR, but does not seem to reduce to the same extent as other indices of host inflammation during the destructive phase of GVHR (65).

4. Organized Lymphoid Tissues

The organized tissues of the gut associated lymphoid tissues (GALT) are also involved in the intestinal phase of GVHR and show a similar biphasic pattern of damage. As we have noted, depletion and atrophy of Peyer's patches is a characteristic feature of late, acute GVHR and, of course, this may contribute to depletion of mucosal lymphocytes. However, the presence of a proliferative GVHR accelerates the development of PP in isografts of fetal small intestine implanted under the kidney capsule of mice (66), indicating that the depletion of PP may be preceded by initial lymphoid hyperplasia. The crypts supplying the dome epithelium of PP share the biphasic pattern of crypt hyperplasia and atrophy found elsewhere during intestinal GVHR (67).

In conclusion, the pattern of damage to intestinal lymphoid components parallels that found in the associated epithelium. As in other peripheral lymphoid organs, there is an early period of infiltration by donor T lymphoblasts and an associated proliferation of many host-derived immune cells. In mild forms of GVHR, this proliferation may be the only abnormality; but in acute, destructive models of GVHR, there is progression to the lymphoid depletion often thought to be the principal feature of GVHR.

---

enteropathy. However, the IEL counts remain increased for some time in the proliferative GVHR in unirradiated (CBAxBALB/c)F_1 mice, while IEL disappear rapidly as GVHR progresses in irradiated F_1 hosts given CBA donor cells (B).

V. MECHANISMS OF INTESTINAL GVHR

Intestinal GVHR shows the same requirement for T cells as GVHR in other sites, being inhibited by elimination of mature T cells from the donor inoculum (34) and by administration of cyclosporin A (42). Although there are also many similarities between the mechanisms responsible for systemic and intestinal GVHD, there are several important differences. In this review, we first address the cellular and genetic factors that determine the induction of intestinal GVHR, before discussing local and systemic effector mechanisms.

A. Cellular and Genetic Basis of Intestinal GVHR

For many years, the focus of research in GVHR was to identify the phenotype and genetic restriction of the T cells responsible for the immunopathology. As will be clear from other chapters in this volume, much of the resulting information is somewhat devalued by the recognition that the function of T-cell populations is not necessarily determined by their phenotype. It is also now feasible to study individual effector mechanisms directly. Nevertheless, the evidence from the earlier studies revealed some important features of the pathogenesis of intestinal GVHR and formed the basis of the more functional experiments to be discussed below.

1. Intestinal GVHR Across MHC Differences

Most work on intestinal GVHR emphasized the relatively greater contribution of $CD4^+$ T cells to the disease. In our own experience, both $CD8^-$ and $CD8^+$ T cells were required to induce fully developed enteropathy in either proliferative or destructive models of fully allogeneic GVHR in mice (Fig. 8). However, $CD8^-$ T cells could alone cause complete hyperplasia of IEL in adult, unirradiated mice with proliferative GVHR as well as significant villus atrophy and crypt hyperplasia in either adult or neonatal hosts. In contrast, although purified $CD8^+$ T cells produced some villus atrophy and crypt hyperplasia in destructive GVHR, this population was incapable alone of inducing hyperplasia of IEL or crypts in adult hosts (68) (Fig. 8). In analogous studies of three different models of destructive GVHR in (C3H × DBA/2)F_1 mice, Guy-Grand et al. (44) also found that both $CD4^+$ and $CD8^+$ T cells could produce some degree of intestinal pathology. However, $CD4^+$ T cells were much more efficient than $CD8^+$ T cells at inducing crypt hyperplasia, class II MHC expression by crypts, and mucosal infiltration by donor lymphoblasts in irradiated hosts. Interestingly though, only $CD8^+$ T cells induced significant enteropathy in unirradiated adults and were more efficient than $CD4^+$ T cells in newborn hosts (44). Colonic GVHR can also be induced in BDF_1 hosts using either $CD4^+$ or $CD8^+$ T cells of DBA/2 origin, but, again, $CD4^+$ cells are much more effective (34).

The genetic requirements for intestinal GVHR in experimental mice underline the predominant role of $CD4^+$ T cells, as a number of groups have shown that a class II MHC incompatibility is alone sufficient for the induction of both proliferative and destructive enteropathy (29,44,68,69). Using both allogeneic and mutant MHC molecules as targets, it has been confirmed that the cells responsible for the class II MHC-restricted intestinal GVHR are $CD4^+$ T cells (44,69). The ability of isolated class I MHC disparities to induce intestinal GVHR is less certain. Some studies have reported that no enteropathy occurs in congenic mice differing only at the class I MHC locus, even if very sensitive techniques are used to measure intesti-

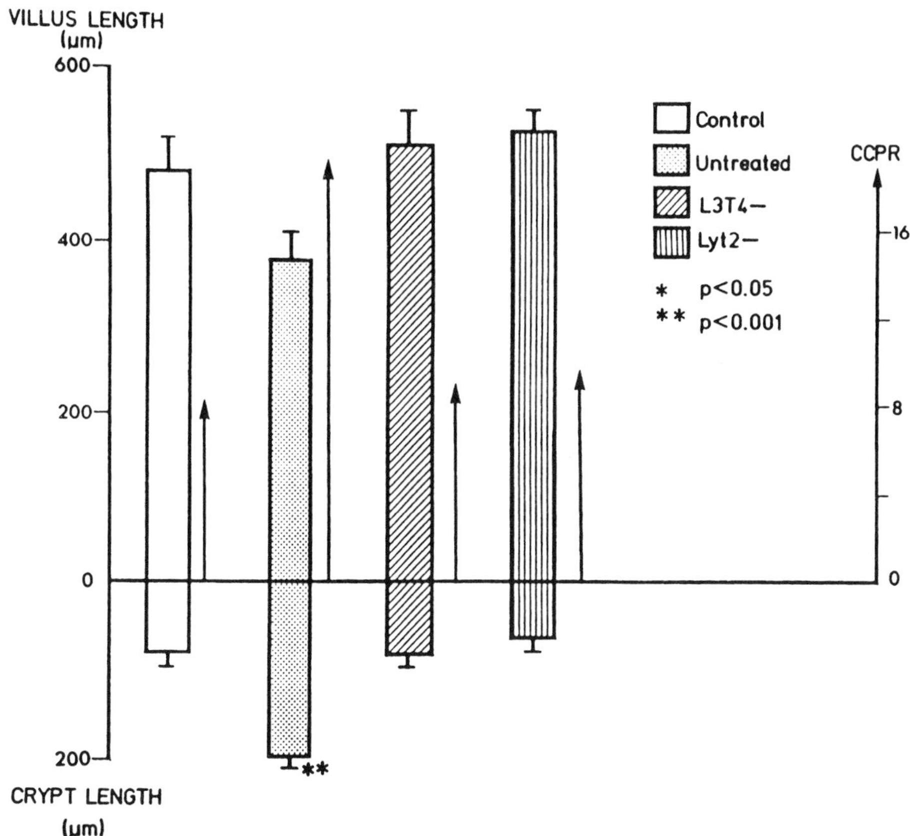

Figure 8 Requirement for both CD8$^+$ and CD4$^+$ donor T cells in the induction of intestinal GVHR in (CBA × BALB/c)F_1 mice. Villus and crypt lengths and CCPR in jejunum of mice given unseparated, CD4- or CD8-depleted donor cells.

nal damage and in models which produce significant systemic disease (29,68). However, if sufficient donor T cells are transferred into class I MHC disparate congenic recipients, intestinal GVHR can be produced in irradiated hosts (44). In addition, purified CD8$^+$ T cells can induce villus atrophy and crypt hyperplasia in irradiated recipients carrying the highly stimulatory H- 2K^{bm1} class I MHC alloantigen (69). However, in the latter study, the acute intestinal GVHR induced by class I MHC antigens was much less severe than that induced by purified CD4$^+$ T cells stimulated by the I- A^{bm12} mutant class II alloantigen. Moreover, the K^{bm1} antigen is unusual among class I MHC molecules in its ability to stimulate intestinal GVHR, as other class I mutations were without effect in this system. Of additional interest from this work was the finding that class I MHC-disparate recipients that underwent acute intestinal GVHR after transfer of CD8$^+$ T cells went on to develop the unusual atrophic form of enteropathy described above.

Together, these studies show that although both major subsets of T lymphocytes can induce intestinal GVHR, class II MHC-restricted CD4$^+$ T cells are much more potent than their class I MHC-restricted counterparts. Nevertheless, as in many other forms of cell-mediated immunity, activation of both CD4$^+$ and CD8$^+$

T cells may usually be required to generate the full range of effector responses necessary for the development of enteropathy in GVHR. In addition, the two subsets may each be responsible for individual aspects of the pathology, with $CD4^+$ T cells appearing to be of particular importance in recruiting local inflammatory cells such as IEL.

2. Intestinal GVHR Induced by Minor Histocompatibility Differences

Few studies have examined intestinal GVHR induced by minor histocompatibility differences in experimental animals. Mild crypt hyperplasia and villus edema has been reported in irradiated, minor antigen incompatible (DBA/2 × B10.D2)F_1 mice with GVHR induced by unseparated donor lymphocytes (55). In addition, there are anecdotal reports of diarrhea in other models of GVHR directed at minor histocompatibility differences. Although systemic GVHR can be induced across minor histoincompatibility antigens by both $CD4^+$ and $CD8^+$ T cells (70,71), only $CD4^+$ T cells have been found to produce enteropathy across minor histocompatibility differences (71).

B. Effector Mechanisms in Intestinal GVHR

1. Nature of the Local Cell-Mediated Immune Response

Much of the initial interest in the mechanisms of intestinal GVHR focused on the possible role of cytotoxic T cells in the epithelial pathology. As we have discussed, class I MHC-restricted $CD8^+$ T cells may be required to induce full-blown intestinal GVHR. Furthermore, the most severe forms of intestinal pathology tend to occur in experimental models of GVHR in which class I MHC-restricted antihost CTL are generated (43,46,72,73). A possible role for CTL is supported further by the finding that $CD8^+$ T cells dominate the population of donor T lymphoblasts found in the thoracic duct and intestinal lamina propria of mice with acute GVHR directed at full MHC differences (44). In addition, the increased population of intraepithelial T cells in GVHR contains a large proportion of $CD8^+$ T cells with the surface phenotype, cytoplasmic granules and potent spontaneous lytic functions characteristics of activated CTL (13,44,47). IEL of this type are capable of lytic activity against enterocytes (17) and, as we have noted, it has been proposed that autoreactive CTL reactivity by IEL may contribute to epithelial pathology in GVHR (47). However, several pieces of evidence argue against an essential role for CTL in the pathogenesis of intestinal GVHR. First, the elimination of actively cytotoxic donor cells using the lysosomotropic agent L-leucyl- leucine-O-methyl ester has no effect on the induction of colonic GVHR, even under conditions where systemic disease is inhibited (34).

The experiments carried out in our own laboratory also indicated that CTL were not required for small intestinal damage in GVHR. In these studies, crypt hyperplasia and increased IEL counts occurred in adult, unirradiated F_1 hosts in the absence of antihost CTL in the gut or other lymphoid tissues (74). The evolution of the intestinal alterations paralleled exactly the development of splenomegaly, a feature which probably reflects the nonspecific, proliferative consequences of GVHR (41). Identical intestinal changes occurred in parental-strain mice made chimeric for F_1 bone marrow cells, despite the fact that the intestinal epithelium of these animals remains syngeneic to the parental donor T cells. Conversely, F_1 mice made chimeric for donor BM had no evidence of intestinal GVHR after injection of donor T cells (75). Further experiments showed that class II MHC-disparate BM cells of F_1 origin could induce intestinal GVHR in parental animals. These findings indicated that the crypt hyperplasia and increased IEL counts could not be due to a direct attack by donor CTL on the intestinal tissue itself but rather was secondary to recognition of recirculating Ia^+ "passenger leucocytes" of BM origin. Although an earlier study did not find intestinal GVHR in $F_1 \rightarrow$ parent BM chimeras (76), this report was poorly documented and the "bystander effect" of GVHR that we observed in BM chimeras was confirmed by an alternative type of experiment. Here, pieces of fetal small intestine of parental type were implanted under the kidney capsule of adult F_1 hybrid mice. After some weeks, grafts of this kind develop relatively normal intestinal architecture of donor type (77) but are infiltrated by recirculating BM-derived cells of host origin. When a GVHR was induced in the F_1 hosts by injection of parental lymphocytes, the donor-type grafts showed increases in IEL count, CCPR, and crypt length similar to those found in the host jejunum (39,66). We and others have shown that T-cell infiltration, villus atrophy, crypt hyperplasia, and crypt-cell necrosis can all also occur as bystander phenomena in fetal intestine of donor type implanted in mice with destructive GVHR (Fig. 9) (38,46,57). Finally, there is no strict correlation between CTL activity and intestinal damage in experimental models of GVHR (69,72). These experiments show that the gut itself does not need to present an allogeneic stimulus to the alloreactive donor cells and suggest that the alterations such as crypt hyperplasia are due to nonspecific soluble mediators released during a DTH response directed at BM-derived cells.

2. Role of Soluble Mediators

More recent studies have provided direct support for this hypothesis and have identified some of the mediators involved. Three approaches have been used to explore the role of cytokines in the enteropathy of GVHR.

a. Production of Cytokines During GVHR. Due to the technical difficulties involved, cytokine production within the intestine itself has not been documented adequately in GVHR. A single report has shown that mucosal lymphocytes from mice with acute GVHR produce IL-2, IL-3, and γ-IFN, but the association between cytokine levels and intestinal pathology was not examined in this case (44).

In common with other groups, we have found that murine GVHR is accompanied by increased production of a wide range of different cytokines in peripheral lymphoid organs, including, IL-1, IL-2, IL-3, IL-4, IL-5, IL-10, γ-IFN, and TNF-α (78–84) (Fig. 10 and unpublished observations). The exact pattern of cytokines produced depends on the experimental model under examination and often cannot be correlated directly with discrete components of intestinal pathology. However, one consistent finding is that the crypt-cell hyperplasia early in GVHR is accompanied by increasing levels of γ-IFN production, which peak at the time of maximal proliferation in the mucosa (Fig. 10) (82). γ-IFN production then falls rapidly, even in models in which the enteropathy continues to progress to villus atrophy. Conversely, TNF-α production is not a consistent feature of GVHR; when it occurs, it is associated with the late, destructive phase of disease (Fig. 10) (82). The levels of TNF-α may vary considerably, even within the same disease model, probably reflecting the requirement for several independent factors to trigger the release of this cytokine (see below).

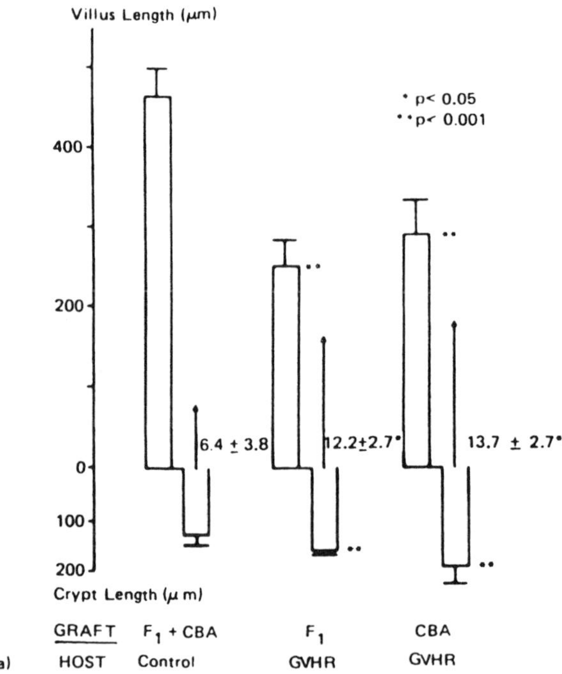

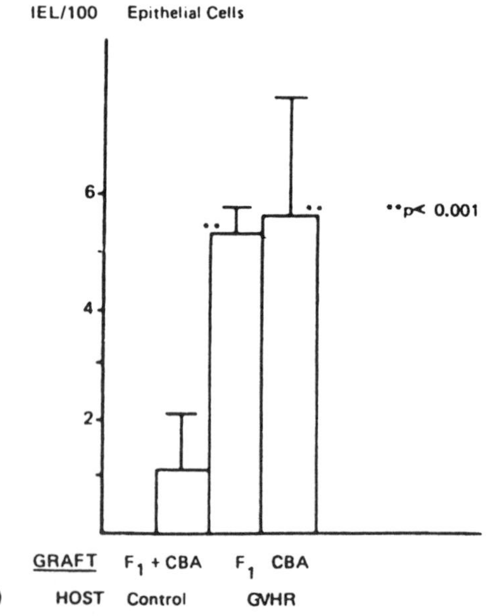

Figure 9 Intestinal GVHR occurs as a "bystander phenomenon." Mucosal architecture (A) and IEL counts (B) in grafts of fetal $(CBA \times BALB/c)F_1$ or CBA small intestine implanted in irradiated $(CBA \times BALB/c)F_1$ mice given CBA donor cells. Villus atrophy, as well as increases in CCPR, crypt length, and IEL count occur irrespective of whether the gut grafts are syngeneic to the donor.

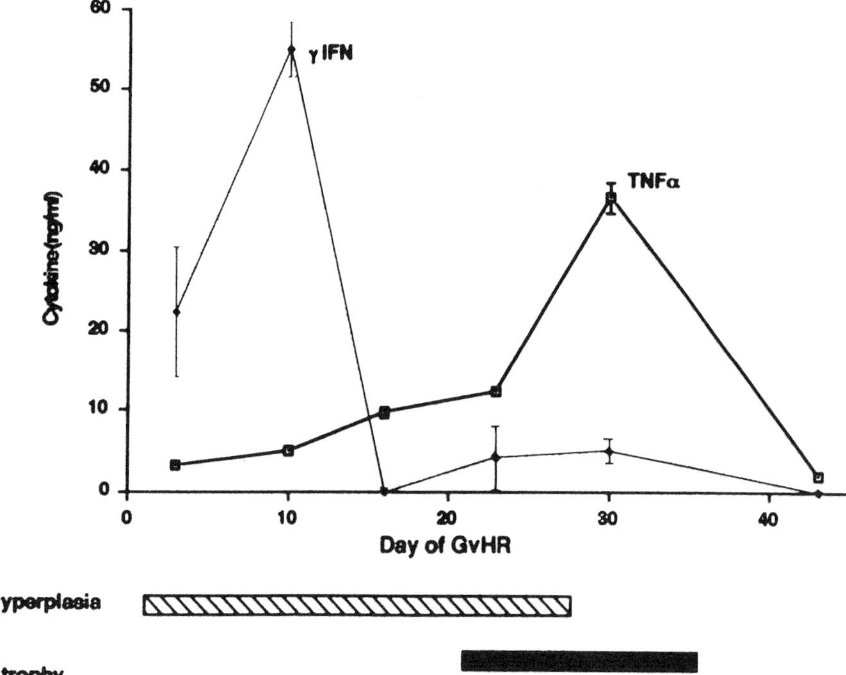

Figure 10 Correlation between γ interferon and tumor necrosis factor α production and intestinal pathology in acute GVHR. During the early proliferation period, there is a rapid rise in splenic γIFN production which parallels the development of crypt–hyperplasia. At this time, there is no TNFα production, but this appears as villus atrophy and mucosal destruction progresses.

Transforming growth factor β (TGF-β) is an important autocrine and paracrine mediator of epithelial-cell proliferation. It is produced by normal enterocytes and, as a product of activated T lymphocytes and macrophages (mϕ), also has many immunoregulatory properties (85). TGF-β therefore offers a potential link between immune activation and epithelial pathology in disorders like GVHR. TGF-β is expressed constitutively by villus epithelial cells in mouse small intestine (Fig. 11A), but during the proliferative phase of intestinal GVHR, enterocyte TGF-β expression falls dramatically (Fig. 11B). Thereafter, as the epithelial pathology and crypt hyperplasia resolve, TGF-β expression returns to normal or above normal levels (Fig. 11C). Thus local TGF-β production correlates inversely with the mitotic activity of epithelial cells in intestinal GVHR. This could reflect a primary effect of the GVHR on TGF-β production, resulting in altered proliferative activity. Alternatively, as discussed below, the alterations in the expression of TGF-β could be a homeostatic response by epithelial cells to the proliferative consequences of GVHR.

b. Effects of Inhibiting Cytokine Function on Intestinal GVHR. The presence of a cytokine does not necessarily mean that the mediator plays a primary pathogenic role in tissue pathology. This can best be determined by inhibiting the production or effector functions of the cytokine in vivo.

Experiments of this type have confirmed the central importance of γ-IFN in

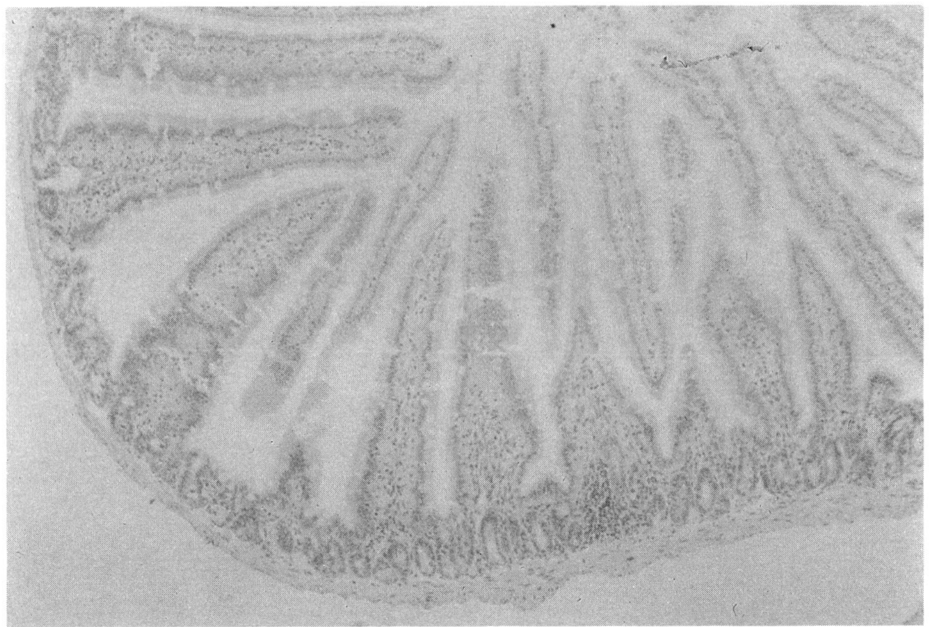

(A)

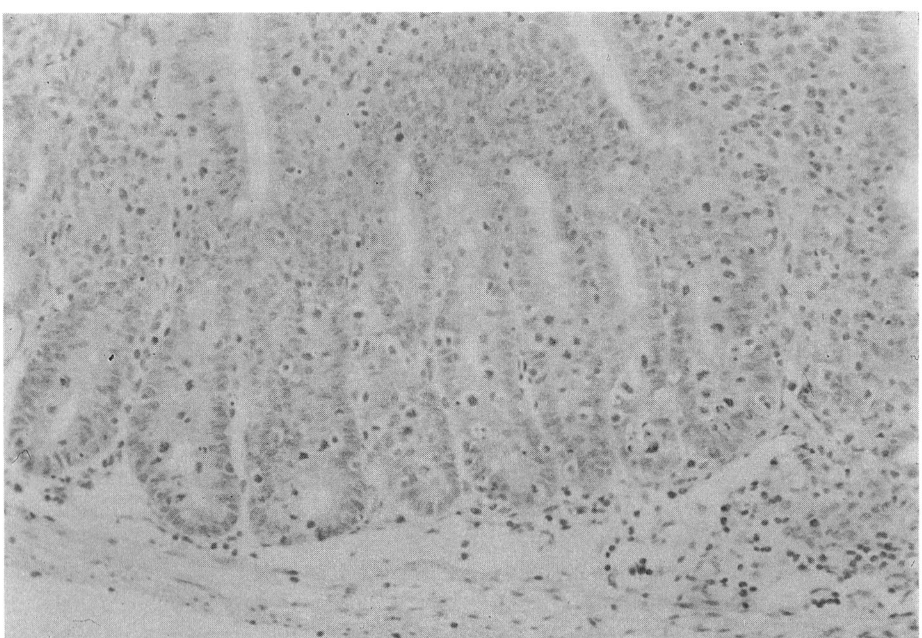

(B)

Figure 11 Modulation of epithelial expression of TGFβ during intestinal GVHR. (A) Normal small intestine expresses substantial amounts of TGFβ1 in mature enterocytes on the villus, but not in the crypt. (B) During the proliferative phase of acute GVHR, the enhanced crypt cell mitotic activity is associated with loss of epithelial TGFβ1 expression. (C) As the pathology in intestinal GVHR repairs, TGFβb expression returns to normal or above normal levels. (Immunoperoxidase $\times 250$).

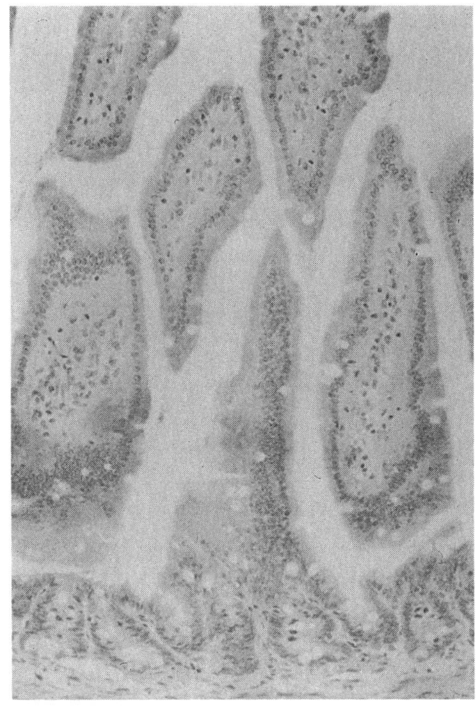

(C)

intestinal GVHR, as treatment of mice with monoclonal anti-γ-IFN antibody prevents all aspects of enteropathy. These include the proliferative lesion characterized by crypt hyperplasia and increased IEL counts in unirradiated (CBA × BALB/c)F_1 mice as well as the crypt hyperplasia and villus atrophy found in destructive models of disease (86). Interestingly, anti-γ- IFN antibody has much less ability to modify systemic components of GVHR, including splenomegaly, weight loss, and antihost CTL activity.

Analogous depletion strategies have also indicated an involvement of IL-1 and IL-4 in intestinal GVHR. Treatment of mice with polyclonal anti-IL-1α antibody inhibited the development of crypt hyperplasia and increased IEL counts in GVHR and, as with γ-IFN, the systemic manifestations of disease were less dependent on the presence of IL-1 (81). Rather more suprisingly, IL-4 also appears to be necessary for the enteropathy of GVHR, as administration of either anti-IL-4 antibody or a soluble form of the IL-4 receptor (IL-4R) prevented crypt hyperplasia, crypt hypertrophy, and IEL hyperplasia in a dose-dependent fashion (87). Depletion of IL-4 did not influence the progress of destructive enteropathy and had only a minor effect on the systemic manifestations of GVHR, with a minor reduction in splenomegaly in GVHR but no effect on NK-cell activation or antihost CTL activity. From these results, it appears that IL-4 may play a selective role in the early proliferative phase of GVHR-associated enteropathy.

Studies of this type have provided rather equivocal evidence on whether TNF-α has a pathogenic role in intestinal GVHR. Early work suggested that all the consequences of destructive intestinal GVHR in irradiated mice could be prevented by administration of a polyclonal anti-TNF-α antibody (45). Although these results would be consistent with the production of this cytokine late in GVHR, they have not been documented further. Indeed, we have been unable to influence any aspect of intestinal GVHR by administering a number of different polyclonal or monoclonal anti-TNF antibodies or by treatment with a soluble, blocking form of the mouse TNF receptor fused to human IgG (unpublished observations). Together, these findings suggest that if TNF-α is involved in intestinal GVHR, it may not be a primary causal mediator of the disease. As discussed below, this may reflect the fact that TNF-α is released in GVHR only when host factors such as bacterial LPS are present in sufficinet quantities.

A further mϕ-derived mediator whose role in intestinal GVHR has been studied by in vivo depletion is IFN-α. IFN-α/β is itself enteropathic in mice (see below), but its depletion has no effect on the development of intestinal pathology in GVHR, despite the fact that this protocol abolishes other, systemic aspects of disease in the same animals (Garside P: unpublished observations). Thus, IFN-α/β may play an accessory but nonessential effector role in the enteropathy of GVHR.

Depletion of TGF-β in vivo with anti-TGF-β antibody enhances many of the intestinal and systemic features of proliferative GVHR, including crypt hyperplasia, increased IEL counts (Fig. 12), splenomegaly, and NK-cell activation (Garside et al: unpublished observations). Although it is not known whether the primary effect of depleting TGF-β is on the immune system or the intestine, these findings indicate that endogenous production of this cytokine may normally play a homeostatic role in regulating the epithelial manifestations of GVHR.

c. Induction of Enteropathy by Administration of Cytokines. The ways in which a cytokine contributes to intestinal pathology can be addressed by exploring the effects on the intestine of administering purified exogenous cytokine to normal animals. Parenteral administration of nontoxic doses of recombinant γ-IFN induces a proliferative enteropathy in mouse small intestine. Significant crypt hypertrophy and hyperplasia are found after a single dose of intraperitoneal γ-IFN, and these become more marked if the cytokine is given continuously over a period of days by osmotic pump (Fig. 13) or if it is derived from a growing tumor mass in vivo (88). γ-IFN alone is unable to induce villus atrophy in normal animals, but it will act in synergy to cause significant villus damage when given with TNF-α (Fig. 13). Despite these effects on mucosal architecture, γ-IFN does not alter populations of local lymphoid cells such as IEL or MMC (unpublished observations).

In contrast to the conflicting effects of depleting TNF-α, administration of this mediator consistently produces severe intestinal damage in normal animals. Both villus atrophy and crypt hyperplasia occur after injection of TNF-α, with enterocyte damage and villus shortening being seen within 1 hr after a single injection (89). As noted above, the enteropathic effects of TNF-α are enhanced by coadministration of γ-IFN. Mucosal necrosis is a further feature of the TNF-induced lesion, which, overall, is reminiscent of the terminal stages of severe intestinal GVHR. An additional, unusual property of TNF-α is its ability to activate MMC (Fig. 14).

IL-1 and IFN-α/β also produce enteropathy similar to that found in GVHR. Treatment of mice with the interferon inducer polyinosinic:polycytydylic acid (polyI:C), exacerbates the intestinal and systemic consequences of murine GVHR, and administration of polyI:C itself induces crypt hyperplasia and villus atrophy in normal animals (39). The enteropathic effects of polyI:C can be reproduced by

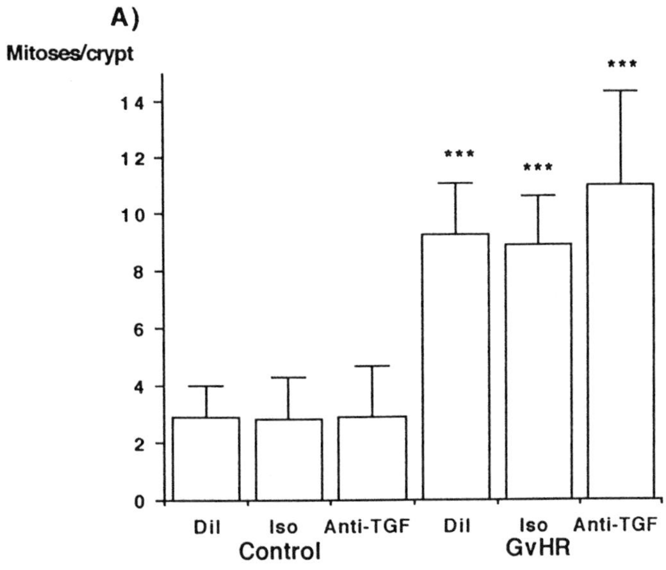

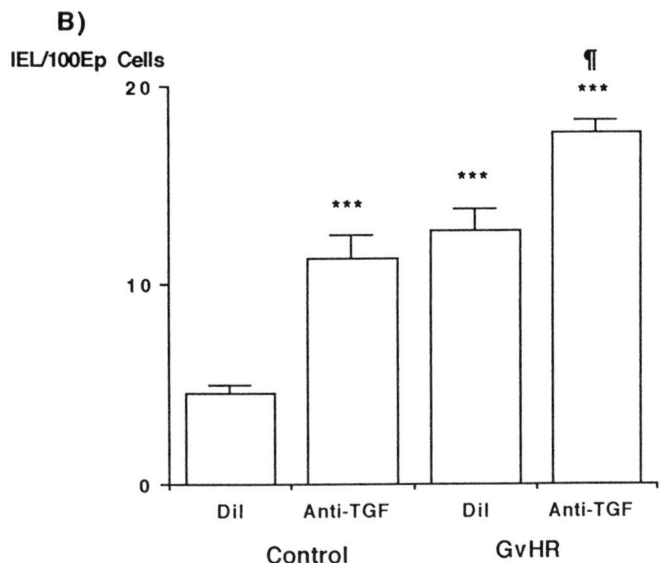

Figure 12 Endogenous TGFβ production normally inhibits intestinal immunopathology in GVHR. In vivo depletion of TGFβ enhances the crypt hyperplasis (A) and lymphocytic infiltration of the epithelium (B) which occur in (CBA × BALB/c)F1 mice with GVHR.

injection of purified IFN-α/β, with the initial effect appearing to be stimulation of crypt hyperplasia (90). This contrasts with the pattern of pathology induced by TNF-α. Finally, IL-1α provokes full enteropathy in normal animals, with intense crypt hyperplasia, villus atrophy, focal necrosis, and increased IEL counts (81). Interestingly, of the cytokines examined, IL-1 is the only one that produces recruitment of IEL in normal animals.

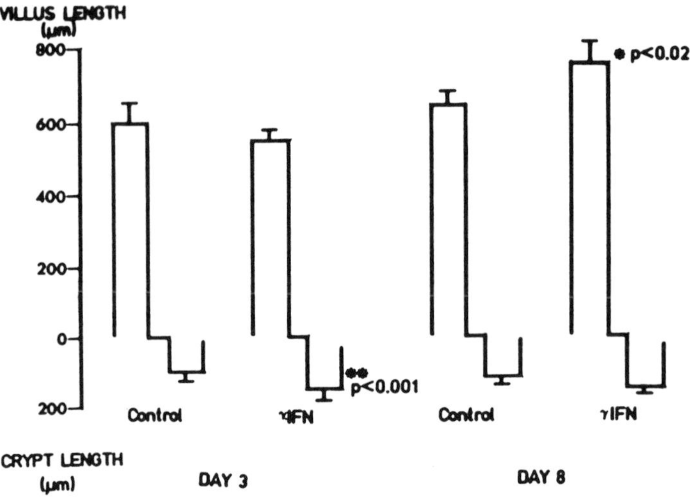

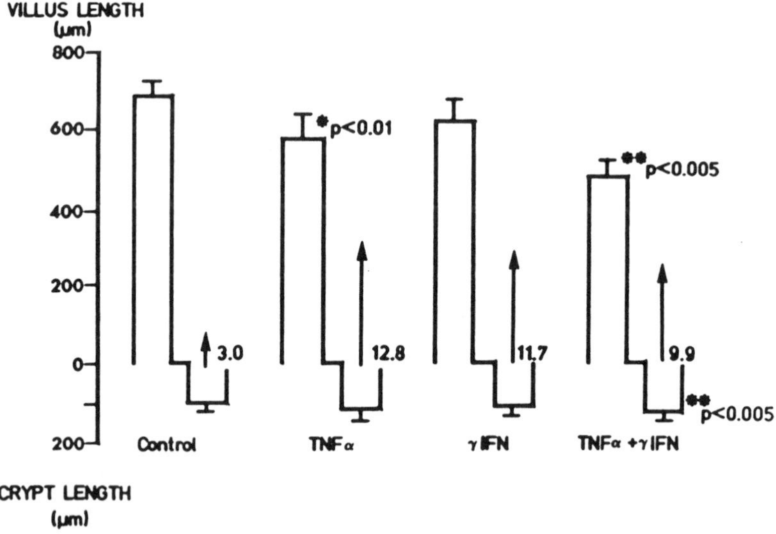

Figure 13 Induction of intestinal pathology by systemic administration of γ-IFN or TNF-α. Continuous intraperitoneal administration of γ-IFN by osmotic mini-pump produces significant crypt hyperplasia in the jejunum, which becomes less marked with time. Villus atrophy is not found and indeed chronic treatment with γ-IFN stimulates villus lengthening (top). A single injection of γ-IFN or TNF-α produces mild crypt hypertrophy 24 hours later, but not significant villus damage. However, the two cytokines together produce synergistic changes in crypt and villus lengths (bottom).

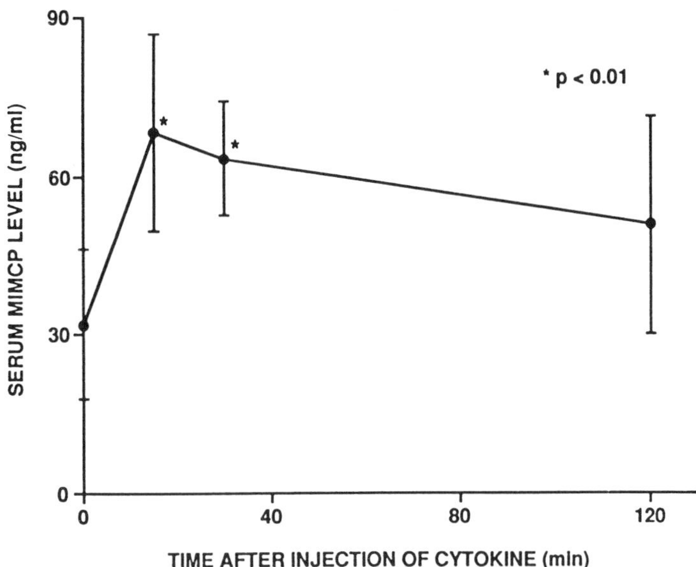

Figure 14 Administration of TNF-α rapidly induces release of mucosal mast cell protease (MMCP) in the serum of normal mice.

Together, these studies support the association between γ-IFN and proliferative intestinal pathology, while TNF-α and other, macrophage-derived products may be important for the later stages of enteropathy.

In view of its immunosuppressive properties and of the effects of in vivo depletion, it is not surprising that administration of TGF-β inhibits the proliferative manifestations of GVHR both in the intestine and elsewhere (Garside et al: unpublished observations). That the effects of TGF-β on the intestinal epithelium are not simply due to downregulation of the immune response in GVHR is suggested by the fact that TGF-β also inhibits crypt-cell turnover in normal mice. Again, these results support the concept that TGF-β is an endogenous regulatory mediator which is part of the host response to epithelial insult in conditions like GVHR.

3. Mechanisms of Cytokine-Induced Intestinal Pathology

The ways in which cytokines can produce intestinal pathology in GVHR are not known with certainty but could reflect direct effects on enterocytes or indirect actions on nonspecific effector cells.

a. Direct Interactions Between Cytokines and Intestinal Epithelial Cells. There is now ample evidence that enterocytes possess receptors for many cytokines and that epithelial cell function can be influenced directly by cytokines. In addition, enterocytes are themselves capable of producing a range of cytokines with the potential both to modity the immune response and to influence epithelial function, including IL-1, IL-6, IL-8, TNF-α, and TGF-β (91–94). Thus, direct interactions between cytokines and epithelial cells offer the potential for both paracrine and autocrine regulation of local immunopathology.

γ-IFN upregulates the expression of a number of surface proteins on purified enterocytes in vitro, including class I and II MHC molecules, adhesion molecules, and the polymeric immunoglobulin receptor (Fig. 15) (95). γ-IFN also decreases the ability of enterocyte monolayers to secrete Cl^- anions and to maintain an intact barrier, as measured by electrical resistance between their apical and basolateral surfaces or by their permeability to low-molecular-weight markers (96–98). Abnormalities of these important functions in vivo could produce many of the characteristic features of intestinal GVHR including diarrhea, malabsorption, and increased epithelial permeability. However, in contrast to its proposed role in enteropathy and to its predominantly hyperplastic effects in vivo, γ-IFN is usually profoundly cytostatic to enterocytes in vitro (99). Similar findings have been made in the skin, where the proliferation of isolated keratinocytes is inhibited by γ-IFN, but local injection of the cytokine induces epidermal hyperplasia in vivo (100). These results confirm the potential for γ- IFN to interact directly with enterocytes but also underline that its overall effect in intestinal GVHR is likely to involve a number of different cell types.

Few other individual cytokines have been shown to have direct effects on the proliferation of enterocytes in vitro. TGF-β has well-documented cytostatic effects on a wide range of cells of epithelial origin (85), and we have found that IL-1 stimulates mitosis of a crypt stem cell line in vitro (81). TNF-α can also enhance the proliferation of this cell line, but its effects are dependent on the stage of the cell

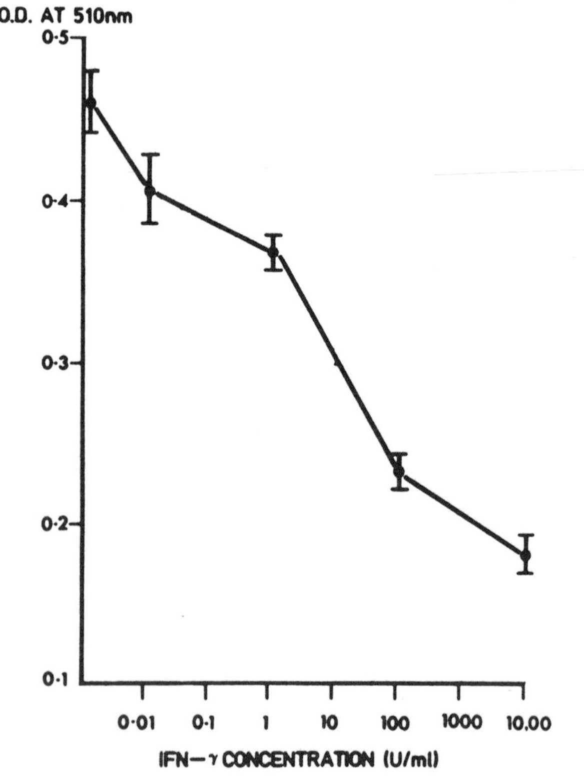

Figure 15 γ-IFN is directly cytostatic to crypt stem cells in vitro. The RIE epithelial cell line shows a dose-dependent inhibition of growth in the presence of recombinant γ-IFN.

cycle at which the epithelial cell is exposed to TNF-α (99). TNF-α has other important direct effects on enterocytes, including cytotoxicity (Fig. 16); enhanced expression of MHC molecules (Fig. 16), secretory component, and adhesion molecules; as well as altering the barrier and secretion functions of epithelial monolayers (101,102). It also induces the production of enterocyte-derived cytokines, such as IL-6 and IL-8 (91,93). Nevertheless, it is important to note that many of the effects of TNF-α are minor unless γ-IFN is also used or unless the epithelial cells have been subjected to other insults, such as serum deprivation or inhibition of protein synthesis. These findings are compatible with the in vivo evidence that TNF-α is involved only late in intestinal GVHR, requiring the presence of other mediators both for its production and functional effects.

Although lacking major effects on epithelial proliferation, IL-1 and IL-6 can stimulate the release of inflammatory cytokines from enterocytes in vitro (91). IL-4 also enhances epithelial expression of MHC and adhesion molecules in vitro as well as interfering with ion secretion and transepithelial migration of neutrophils (103). Although these findings have yet to be confirmed, they are compatible with the ability of depleting IL-4 in vivo to inhibit intestinal GVHR (see above) and with the fact that human intestinal epithelial cells express at least one component of the IL-4 receptor (Ritter M: personal communication).

b. Indirect Effects of Cytokines in Intestinal GVHR. Although the results discussed above support the possibility that many cytokines may interact directly with enterocytes, there is also ample evidence that at least part of their role in enteropathy is to recruit and activate a number of inflammatory and/or mesenchymal cells.

Macrophages

Release of cytokines and other inflammatory mediatoras by γ-IFN-activated macrophages appears to be central to many aspects of intestinal GVHR. Activation of mϕ has long been known to be a feature of systemic GVHR and depletion of mϕ in vivo by administration of silica or liposomes containing the lysosomal toxin CL 1,2 MDP reduces the intestinal consequences of GVHR in mice (Table 4). The way in which activated mϕ may contribute to enteropathy has not been clarified fully, but, as we have discussed, GVHR in mice is associated with increased levels of mϕ-derived cytokines such as IL-1 and TNF-α. In addition, there is enhanced production of nitric oxide (NO) (Garside P: unpublished observations) and specific inhibition of mϕ-dependent NO produciton by treatment with L-N^G-monomethyl arginine (L-NMMA) prevents crypt hyperplasia and increased IEL counts in GVHR (104). These findings are consistent with other studies suggesting that the systemic consequences of GVHR are due to the effector functions of mϕ that have been primed initially by γ- IFN and then activated fully by other stimuli such as bacterial LPS (see below). The direct relevance of this hypothesis for intestinal GVHR has yet to be proven by correlating mucosal mϕ function with cytokine release and epithelial pathology in GVHR. However, our studies indicate that activated mϕ can influence crypt stem-cell growth in vitro, and this partly reflects the action of soluble mediators such as NO (99). Local mϕ could also interact with epithelial cells either directly by membrane-membrane contact or via the effects of their cytokines and/or other inflammatory mediators on mesenchymal cells. These possibilities require further investigation.

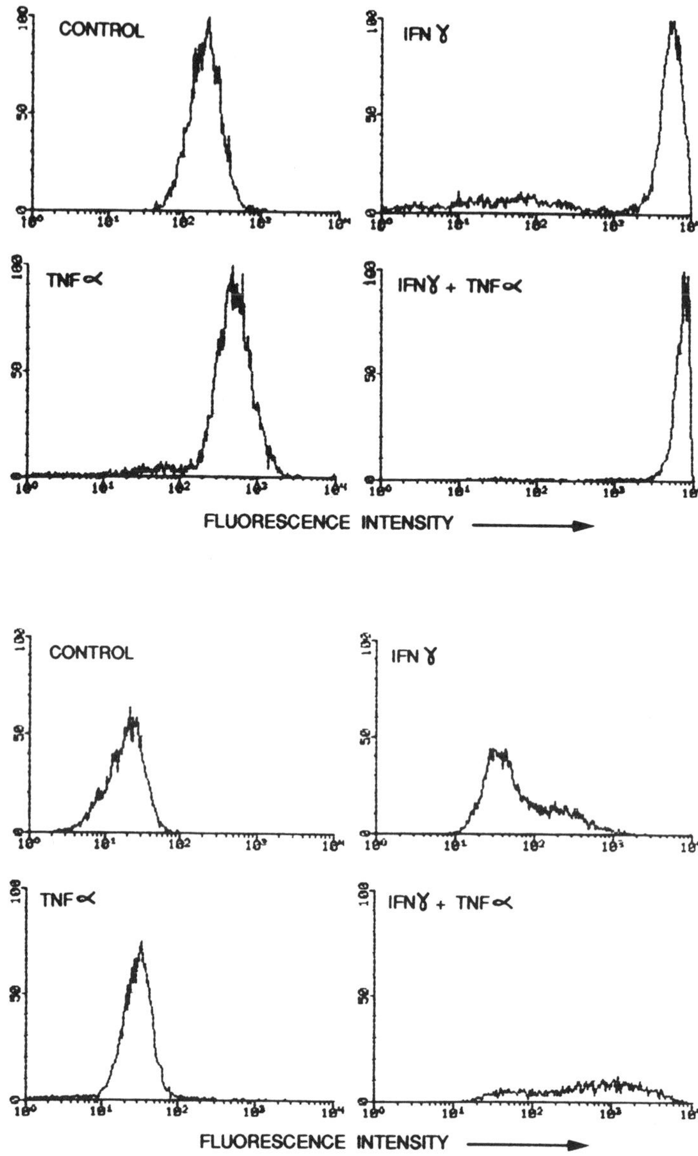

Figure 16 Induction of MHC expression on crypt stem cells by treatment with γIFN and/or TNFα in vitro. Both cytokines alone produce increased levels of class I MHC antigens by RIE cells after 48 hours of culture and produce maximal expression when added together (Top). Although RIE cells do not normally express class II MHC antigens, treatment with γIFN alone produces some increase in expression and addition of both cytokines together induces the appearance of class II MHC on most cells (Bottom).

Table 4 Effects of Macrophage Depletion on Intestinal GVHR. (CBAxBALB/c)F_1 Mice Were Depleted of Macrophages 1 Day Before Induction of GVHR by Intravenous Injection of Liposomes Containing the Lysosomotropic Agent CL1,2 MDP. On Day 8 of GVHR, These Mice Had Significantly Less Crypt Lengthening in the Jejunum Compared With Untreated GVHR Mice (*$p < 0.02$ vs control; +$p < 0.02$ vs GVHR)

Group	CL1,2 MDP Lips	Crypt Length
Control	−	103.6 ± 4.1μm
Control	+	98.1 ± 7.9μm
GvHR	−	125.6 ± 10.8μm
GvHR	+	106.0 ± 10.8μm

It should also be noted that mϕ could play an important role in the induction phase of intestinal GVHR, both as alloantigenic stimulator cells and as sources of the IL-12 required for costimulating production of γ-IFN (see below).

Natural Killer Cells

Enhanced NK-cell activity by peripheral lymphocytes is a feature of the early proliferative phase of experimental GVHR (74,105,106). It parallels splenomegaly and γ-IFN production and is dependent on the production of IL-12 during the initiation of disease (Williamson E: unpublished observations). The systemic NK-cell activation is accompanied by enhanced NK cell function by IEL isolated from the small intestine (74). This parallels other features of proliferative enteropathy in unirradiated adult mice with GVHR and is preceded by a systemic antihost DTH response (107). That mucosal NK cells are an important nonspecific effector mechanism in intestinal GVHR is supported by the fact that treatment of mice with anti-asialo G_{M1} (AsG_{M1}) antibody prevents the crypt hyperplasia normally found in GVHR (108) and after administration of the nonspecific mediators IFN-α/β (90). Interestingly, some IEL express AsG_{M1} (109) and control mice treated with anti-AsG_{M1} antibody have somewhat lower IEL counts than normal mice (108). Thus, $As_{GM1}{}^{+}$ IEL may be involved directly in the pathogenesis of intestinal GVHR.

Table 5 Behavior of IEL Populations During Proliferative Graft-vs.-host reaction. There is an Increased Density of Total IEL, Which Consists of Enhanced Proportions of αβ T cells Expressing the CD8αβ Heterodimer

	Control	GVHR
αβ T cells	43%	54%
$CD8^+$	80%	87.5%
$CD8\beta^+$	24%	35%
$CD8\alpha\alpha^+$:$CD8\beta^+$	2.3:1	1.5:1

The effects of anti-AsG_{M1} on intestinal GVHR have been examined only in a model that produced hyperplasia in the absence of villus atrophy. Nevertheless, rapid and marked activation of NK cells also occurs as part of the proliferative phase of models of GVHR that progress to villus atrophy (46). In addition, the NK-cell-dependent enteropathy induced by IFN-α/β involves both villus atrophy and crypt hyperplasia (90), while depletion of NK cells is also extremely effective in preventing systemic disease in severe, destructive forms of GVHR (110,111).

The ways in which NK cells can influence intestinal pathology are unknown but could reflect their ability to produce cytokines. In particular, NK cells are now recognized to be major sources of γ-IFN in vivo, and it is tempting to speculate that their central role in intestinal GVHR is to produce γ-IFN in response to mϕ-derived IL-12, as has been suggested in a number of infectious diseases (112).

Mucosal Mast Cells

As discussed above, hyperplasia of mucosal mast cells is a histological feature of many experimental models of GVHR and probably reflects recruitment by IL-3. The hyperplasia of MMC in rodent GVHR is accompanied by increased levels of the MMC-specific protease II in the serum and intestinal mucosa (63,65). Protease release occurs in both destructive and proliferative enteropathy, although as MMC are radiosensitive, MMC protease levels do not increase as dramatically during GVHR in irradiated hosts (63). Although the natural substrate of MMC-specific protease II appears to be the type IV collagen found in the intestinal basement membrane (113), it seems unlikely that MMC play a primary role in the pathogenesis of intestinal GVHR. As we have noted, hyperplasia of MMC is not a significant feature of GVHR in irradiated hosts, despite the more severe enteropathy that occurs under these circumstances (63). More importantly, intestinal GVHR is, if anything, more severe in W/W^v mice that have a congenital lack of all mast cells, including MMC (65). The recruitment of MMC thus appears to be a nonessential consequence of cytokine release in GVHR, although mediators from these cells may obviously help explain the altered intestinal permeability found in GVHR.

4. Other Immune Mechanisms

This review has concentrated on the role of T lymphocytes and T-dependent effector mechanisms in intestinal GVHR. There are no studies of the role of antibodies in the pathogenesis of intestinal GVHR, but the production of alloantibodies does not correlate with the analogous enteropathy found in rejecting allografts of gut (114). However, it is interesting to note that the spontaneous enteropathy that develops in mice with genetically engineered lack of IL-2, IL-10, or the $\alpha\beta$ TcR has some similarities to intestinal GVHR and is thought to be due to antibody-dependent mechanisms (52). The overlap between these models of pathology deserves further attention.

C. Host Factors in Intestinal GVHR

Several host factors other than the capacity of tissue antigens to activate donor T cells influence the development of intestinal GVHR in experimental animals.

1. Intestinal Microflora

a. Bacteria. The beneficial effect of bowel decontamination on survival after clinical BMT has been well documented, but the effects of the intestinal flora on organ-specific consequences of experimental GVHR are less clear. Several workers have reported that germ-free mice or mice with a gut flora consisting entirely of anaerobes have markedly less mortality due to acute GVHR than conventional animals. In parallel, removal of aerobic gut flora prevents much of the liver and gut damage normally associated with severe GVHR (115,116). If these animals are subsequently returned to conventional conditions or associated with gram-negative aerobes, mortality and tissue damage due to GVHR reappear. Administration of *E. coli* or purified LPS exacerbates systemic GVHR in irradiated mice, while passive immunization with antibody to *E. coli* has a moderately, beneficial effect (117,118). Together, these findings suggest that gram-negative aerobes in the gut flora are critical for the pathogenesis of systemic GVHR. Nevertheless, it should be noted that the beneficial effects of the germ-free state are frequently transient, with final mortality rates and pathology ultimately being similar to those in conventional hosts (31,115,116). Furthermore, the reported effects of exogenous LPS or passive immunization with anti-*E. coli* antibody were generally small and restricted to GVHR across minor histocompatibility antigen differences (117,118).

These apparently paradoxical findings on the influence of intestinal bacteria may reflect the rather variable effects of mϕ-derived mediators whose production can be regulated by bacterial lipopolysaccharide. Increased levels of endotoxin are found during GVHR (31,119), probably resulting from enhanced uptake through the intestinal epithelium, which has been damaged by the initial T-lymphocyte response. The progressive increase in serum LPS in GVHR correlates with the full activation of mϕ that are presumed to have been primed by the early surge in γ-IFN production. Combined stimulation by γ-IFN and LPS then results in release of mediators such as TNF-α and NO (119; Nestel F, Lapp WS: personal communication). However, as discussed above, these mediators may have rather different involvements in GVHR; although NO seems to be critical for the disease, TNF-α may not be esential for tissue damage to occur. It may be that stimulation of TNF-α release by mϕ may require levels of LPS that occur only in hosts with severe GVHR and with particular types of gut flora. Given these conditions, the resulting release of TNF-α may exacerbate the lesions of terminal GVHR, including bone marrow aplasia, cachexia, and destruction of epithelia via stem-cell apoptosis. In contrast, however, the production of NO (and perhaps other mediators such as IL-1 or IFN-α/β) by primed mϕ may be less dependent on additional stimulation by LPS; hence these mediators may play a more critical role in the primary pathogenesis of GVHR.

The role of local infection in intestinal GVHR is particularly contentious. Early studies suggested that the characteristic necrotic lesions of established GVHR were due to local abscesses, which had formed due to mucosal penetration of organisms (116). However, as discussed, crypt hyperplasia, villus atrophy, and lymphocytic infiltration occur in sterile, antigen-free grafts of small intestine implanted under the kidney capsule of mice with GVHR (39,46,66). Thus, although it may undoubtedly occur, local infection is not necessary for the development of GVHR-specific lesions within the intestine. However, direct bacterial infection of the mucosa could undoubtedly contribute to the intestinal lesion. Sepsis induces epithelial hyperplasia in the gut (120) and focal necrosis is a characteristic feature of severe GVHR, particularly in the colon. This is associated with local abscess formation, and it is likely that there is enhanced adhesion to and invasion of the mucosa due to initial alterations in the epithelial barrier caused by the early T-lymphocyte-mediated immune response.

These results indicate that local bacterial infection may determine tissue pathology in acute GVHR and highlight the possible applications of bacterial decontamination in preventing the worst consequences of the disease. One attractive way of achieving this might be the use of selective decontamination antibiotic regimes that target LPS-producing gram-negative bacteria, leaving intact other components of the gut flora that may have beneficial effects on intestinal physiology.

b. *Viral Infection*

There are no studies on the role of local viruses in intestinal GVHR in experimental animals. However, Coxsackie virus A1 has been shown to cause intestinal damage after human BMT (121), while the studies of Grundy et al. (122) have highlighted the synergistic ability of CMV to cause severe lung disease in experimental GVHR. These potential complicating effects of both bacterial and viral infections are particularly serious considerations in view of the local and systemic immune deficiences that can occur in GVHR.

2. Endogenous Host Factors

The influence of host factors in intestinal GVHR is illustrated by the varying spectrum of disease seen in different types of host using the same donor-host strain combination. Intestinal pathology is much more severe when the hosts used are irradiated, athymic, or very immature, with destructive GVHR evolving very rapidly under these conditions (46,72,123). This may reflect an absence of host T cells thought to be capable of resisting the proliferation of alloreactive donor T cells (124). Alternatively, the intestine of compromised hosts may be unusually susceptible to the effects of GVHR. Irradiation has particularly profound effects on the function and renewal of the intestinal epithelium, while rapid alterations in mucosal architecture occur during the early neonatal period. In common with GVHR, the major maturational changes affect crypt cell function and a synergistic effect on intestinal damage can readily be imagined. Thus, the more severe intestinal GVHR in compromised hosts may be due to factors both within the immune system and the gut.

VI. CLINICAL ASPECTS OF INTESTINAL GRAFT-VERSUS-HOST DISEASE

A. Incidence and Clinical Features of Acute GVHD

Intestinal pathology is one of the most frequent nonlymphoid features of acute GVHD in humans, occurring at the same time as or shortly after the onset of skin GVHD. Gastrointestinal disturbances were recognized in the earliest series of allogeneic bone marrow transplants, and the resulting clinicopathological features have been reviewed extensively by previous authors (125–128). Since the general use of cyclosporine, barrier nursing, and marrow purging, the incidence and severity of intestinal GVHD have decreased. In addition, advances in clinical practice have improved the treatment of the metabolic and infective consequences of intestinal damage. For these reasons, we summarize here only the principal features of the disorder; for more detailed accounts of the clinical manifestations and grading of the condition, the reader is referred to previous detailed reviews of the topic (32,125–128).

The exact incidence of acute intestinal GVHD is difficult to assess, as its symptoms and pathological features often overlap with other conditions that can complicate allogeneic BMT. The presenting features are frequently nonspecific, including nausea, anorexia, abdominal pain, and diarrhea. The last is the most characteristic and, in severe cases, can account for >2 L fluid loss per day. It may be choleric or steatorrheic in nature, reflecting the wide spectrum of epithelial damage that can occurs in GVHD and its ability to affect all parts of the GI tract. Rectal bleeding may also occur, particularly in cases with colonic involvement; rarely, severe hemorrhage from the stomach, small intestine, or colon may be a terminal event. Other major complications include intestinal perforation, obstruction, and paralytic ileus, but these are now rarely seen in carefully monitored patients.

B. Distribution of Intestional Pathology

All parts of the GI tract from the mouth to rectum may be involved in acute GVHD. However, clinically significant damage is most frequent in the small and large intestine, with the esophagus being relatively spared. Although many workers have emphasized the frequency of colonic pathology as represented by damage to the rectum, this may simply reflect the accessibility of this site for biopsy purposes rather than a true difference in incidence. The animal work discussed above shows that small-intestinal pathology is an almost universal component of experimental GVHR, and those clinical studies which have examined the upper GI tract have revealed that gastritis and small-intestinal damage occur frequently in the absence of discernible rectal changes (126). Intestinal GVHD is undoubtedly more aggressive in the lower small intestine, cecum, and colon, probably reflecting the distribution of bacterial flora, but mild damage to the upper GI tract may be overlooked unless detailed histological analysis is performed.

C. Pathological Features of Enteropathy in Acute GVHD

The possibility that clinical intestinal GVHD evolves from proliferative to destructive enteropathy has not been addressed fully, mainly because it is impossible to follow developing pathology under clinical conditions. Most human material inevitably comes postmortem or from biopsy of patients with severe disease; the picture is therefore biased toward the terminal phase of enteropathy. Under these conditions, villus atrophy is a predominant feature in the small intestine, with ulceration and mucosal degeneration being seen in other sites. In parallel, there is increased expression of class II MHC antigens on enterocytes and increased lymphocytic infiltration of the mucosa, particularly the crypt epithelium and lamina propria (129). However, depletion of local lymphoid populations and deficiency of secretory IgA is a characteristic feature of many patients with acute GVHD (130,131). Although these morphological features are reminiscent of the terminal phase of intestinal GVHR in animals, it is not known if the fully established lesion is preceded by the crypt hyperplasia seen in experimental GVHR. Hyperplastic crypts have been identified in clinical GVHD, but these are frequently found in association with other manifestations of advanced enteropathy, and the temporal relationship between crypt hyperplasia and villus atrophy has not been established.

The understanding of clinical intestinal GVHD has also been influenced by the fact that the histopathological hallmark of the condition has long been considered to be necrosis of individual epithelial cells. This occurs throughout the length of the

GI tract and is similar to the pattern seen in the skin. Typically, the epithelial destruction is seen in the crypts or the equivalent region of the epithelium responsible for regeneration. Many writers have ascribed this feature to abscess formation resulting from localized penetration by bacterial flora. However, careful inspection suggests that a more likely explanation is apoptosis of regenerating stem cells, as would be predicted from the animal studies discussed above. In the small and large intestines, crypt cell damage in GVHD is typified by karyorrhectic nuclear disintegration, with ballooning of the cytoplasm and, ultimately, complete loss of crypts from large areas of the mucosa. Again, we would argue that these features are similar to those found in animals with end-stage intestinal GVHR, and they are consistent with the direct immunologically mediated damage to dividing stem cells discussed above. However, a direct role for cytokines has not been established in clinical intestinal GVHD, and its immunological basis remains to be confirmed.

D. Differential Diagnosis of Acute Intestinal GVHD

The histological diagnosis of intestinal GVHD may present a number of difficulties. Many of its features, particularly late in the disease, are relatively nonspecific in appearance and may be confused with other conditions likely to be present in BMT recipients. The most significant of these are infection and the effects of radiation or chemotherapy. Infection of the GI tract by viruses such as CMV and HIV or by *Cryptosporidium* may produce allmost identical patterns of pathology to that seen in GVHD (126,132). Differentiation between these conditions may be extremely difficult, especially as they may co-exist in individual patients. Although the mucosal damage may present some similarities, bacterial infection and other forms of nonspecific enterocolitis are usually easier to distinguish from GVHD. Radiation and cytoreductive chemotherapy can cause villus atrophy, crypt-cell necrosis, and mucosal ulceration and may complicate the diagnosis of GVHD in the early period after BMT. However, in GVHD, the epithelial-cell pathology is more characteristically limited to individual cells within the crypt region, whereas cytoreductive treatment tends to produce diffuse epithelial damage at all levels of the mucosa.

E. Intestinal Pathology in Chronic GVHD

Intestinal involvement has never been a frequent component of chronic GVHD and, with the use of effective immunosuppression, is now seen only rarely. The squamous epithelium of the esophagus may show sclerodermalike inflammation, fibrosis, and desquamation similar to that found in chronic cutaneous GVHD. The remainder of the GI tract is usually unaffected, with the occasional findings of mucosal fibrosis, stenosis, and ulceration more likely to reflect persisting acute GVHD rather than true chronic disease. There may also be reduced numbers of plasma cells and other lymphoid populations in the mucosa and GALT, but this parallels the changes in other lymphoid tissues and is unlikely to indicate local immumopathology.

VII. CONCLUSIONS AND WIDER IMPLICATIONS

A. GVHR as a Model for Enteropathy

This review has highlighted the effects that the T-lymphocyte-mediated immune response in GVHR can have on the small intestine. As we have shown, several aspects of the mucosal pathology can be used as sensitive indices to measure the evolving local immune response. These observations have a number of important implications of a wider nature. First, the fact that it is possible to generate a range of different immune effector functions using a GVHR means that intestinal GVHR can be used to perform qualitative and quantitative assessments of the immunopathological potential of T lymphocytes and other lymphoid effector mechanisms. Second, the pattern of intestinal pathology in GVHR reproduces that found in several naturally occurring enteropathies that cause villus atrophy, crypt hyperplasia, and increased numbers of MMC and IEL and which are associated with local CMI reactions (133). These include gluten-sensitive enteropathy (celiac disease), cow's milk protein intolerance, several parasitic infections, and Crohn's disease. Indeed, clinicopathological studies over the last few years have shown that the evolution of mucosal pathology in gluten-sensitive enteropathy is remarkably similar to that seen in intestinal GVHR (58,59). Thus, in patients with latent celiac disease or during the early period after challenge with gluten, the mucosa shows lymphocytic infiltration of the epithelium, followed by crypt hyperplasia and, latterly, villus atrophy. These findings support the view that the intestinal mucosa responds to T-cell-mediated immune insults in an identical manner, irrespective of the original antigenic stimulus. Intestinal GVHR offers a flexible model for studying the pathogenesis of such enteropathies under experimental conditions in an intact animal.

B. Immunopathogenesis of T-Lymphocyte-Mediated Enteropathy

A hypothetical basis for the immunopathogenesis of these disorders is illustrated in Figs. 17 and 18. The observations discussed in this chapter show that dividing stem cells are the principal target of the immune response in GVHR. The initial effect on these cells is a stimulation of proliferation, followed either by a return to normal levels or by death via apoptosis. These changes produce distinct morphological phases of enteropathy, characterized respectively by crypt hypertrophy and hyperplasia, followed by a period in which villus atrophy accompanies persistent crypt hypertrophy. Finally, crypt loss, villus ablation, and mucosal necrosis occur (Fig. 17). These pathological features are accompanied by distinctive immunological events, with the early proliferative enteropathy being preceded by infiltration of the epithelium by T lymphocytes and being associated with the production of large amounts of γ-IFN (Fig. 17). A number of effects of this cytokine are then crucial for the progress of the disease, including activation of NK cells and priming of mϕ. In addition, γ-IFN is likely to have direct effects on enterocytes, such as modulation of crypt-cell turnover and differentiation, enhanced MHC expression, and alterations in epithelial barrier functions. The resulting enhanced uptake of bacterial LPS may allow further activation of γ-IFN-primed mϕ, with release of inflammatory cytokines such as NO, IL-1, IFN-α/β, TNF-α, and TGF-β. These mϕ-derived mediators may contribute to the evolving enteropathy in two ways. First, they may exacerbate the crypt-cell pathology, either by their effects on proliferation or by causing stem-cell necrosis and apoptosis. In addition, many can act on the stromal components of the mucosa, including fibroblasts and endothelial cells. These effects accelerate the enteropathy, causing increased vascular permeability, thrombosis, influx of further inflammatory cells, and interference with synthesis of the extracellular matrix of the villus/crypt unit. The catalytic effects of enzymes produced by

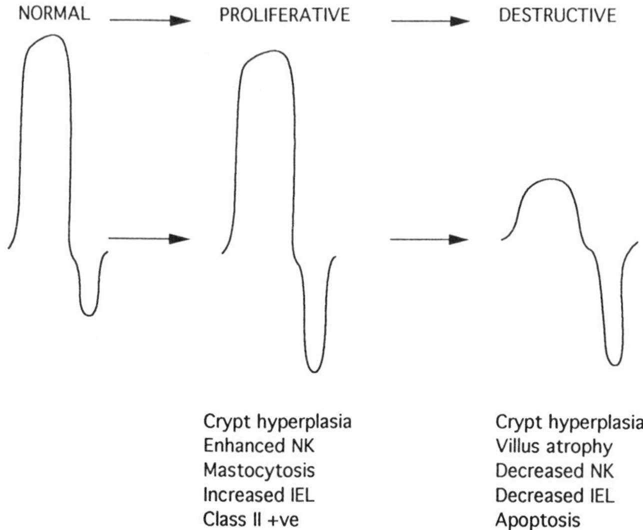

Figure 17 Schematic representation of evolving intestinal GvHR. Early proliferative GvHR is characterised by crypt hyperplasia, γIFN production, recruitment of IEL and non-specific activation of host cells, as indicated by NK cell activation and splenomegaly. Subsequently, villus atrophy develps due to a combination of continued dysregulation of epithelial cell turnover and damage to the intestinal stroma. This destructive phase may be accompanied by the appearance of anti-host CTL and the production of toxic cytokines such TNFα. In some cases, a final phase ensues, in which the anti-host immune response destroys crypt stem cells and ablates intestinal repair.

the activated mϕ, such as metalloproteianases, are likely to contribute further to degradation of the ECM. Villus atrophy is the primary consequence of these effects on mucosal infrastructure, but ultimately mucosal necrosis and autolysis may ensue, particularly if there is also a failure of epithelial repair due to apoptotic loss of crypt stem cells.

mϕ may also be important for the initiation of GVHR-associated enteropathy, both as alloantigenic stimulus and as a source of IL-12, which may be critical for the activation of γ-IFN-producing $CD4^+$ T cells as well as $CD8^+$ T cells and NK cells. NK cells activated by mϕ-derived IL-12 may then be the predominant sources of γ-IFN at this early stage. This γ- IFN will further activate mϕ and T cells, with resulting positive feedback effects on NK cells via IL-12, IFN, and IL-2. Together, the complex cellular interactions underlying intestinal GVHR emphasize why this disorder may develop so rapidly and highlight the need to inhibit it in its early stages. Understanding how individual mediators may be associated with distinct pathological features may help the development of better therapeutic and preventative strategies.

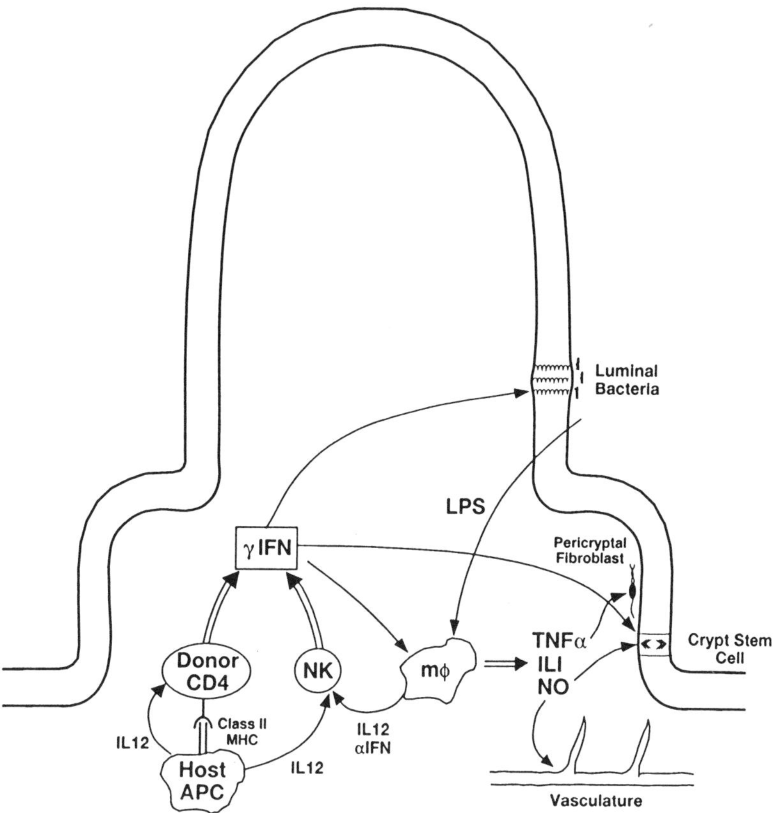

Figure 18 Mechanisms of intestinal immunopathology mediated by $CD4^+$ T lymphocytes in GvHR. Donor $CD4^+$ T cells initiate the response by production of γIFN. Together with its direct effects on crypt stem cells, γIFN activates non-specific effector cells such as mϕ, whose soluble products continue the evolving stem cell damage (see text for details).

ACKNOWLEDGMENTS

The work quoted in this chapter was supported by the Medical Research Council (U.K.) and the Coeliac Trust.

REFERENCES

1. See Ref. 21.
2. See Ref. 48.
3. Mowat AM. The cellular basis of gastrointestinal immunity. In: Marsh NN, ed. Immunopathology of the Small Intestine. New York: Wiley, 1987:41–72.
4. Parrott DMV. The structure and organisation of lymphoid tissue in the gut. In: Brostoff J, Challacombe SJ, eds. Food Allergy and Intolerance. London: Bailliére Tindall, 1987:3-26.
5. James SP, Zeitz M. Human gastrointestinal mucosal T cells. In: Ogra PL, Mestecky J,

Lamm ME, Strober W, et al, eds. Handbook of Mucosal Immunology. Boca Raton, FL: CRC Press, 1994; 275–286.

6. Ferguson A. Intraepithelial lymphocytes of the small intestine. Gut 1977; 18:921.
7. Ernst PB, Befus AD, Bienenstock J. Leukocytes in the intestinal epithelium: An unusual immunological compartment. Immunol Today 1985; 6:50–55.
8. Kilshaw PJ, Murant SJ. Expression and regulation of B_7 (Bp) integrins on mouse lymphocytes: relevance to the mucosal immune system. Eur J Immunol 1991; 21:2591–2597.
9. Poussier P, Julius M. Thymus independent T cell development and selection in the intestinal epithelium. Annu Rev Immunol 1994; 12:521–533.
10. Lefrancois L. Basic aspects of intraepithelial lymphocyte immunobiology. In: In Ogra PL, Mestecky J, Lamm ME, Strober W, et al, eds. Handbook of Mucosal Immunology. Boca Raton, FL: CRC Press, 1994:287–298.
11. Halstensen TS, Scott H, Brandtzaeg P. Intraepithelial T cells of the $TcR\gamma/\delta^+$ $CD8^-$ and $V_\delta 1/J_\delta 1^+$ phenotypes are increased in coeliac disease. Scand J Immunol 1989; 30: 665–672.
12. Guy-Grand D, Cerf-Bensussan N, Malissen B, et al. Two gut intraepithelial $CD8^+$ lymphocyte populations with different T cell receptors; A role for the gut epithelium in T cell differentiation. J Exp Med 1991; 173:471–481.
13. Guy-Grand D, Malassis-Seris M, Briottet C, Vassalli P. Cytotoxic differentiation of mouse gut thymodependent and independent intraepithelial T lynphocytes is induced locally: Correlation between functional assays, presence of perforin and granzyme transcripts, and cytoplasmic granules. J Exp Med 1991; 173:1549–1552.
14. Gross GG, Schwartz VL, Stevens C, et al. Distribution of dominant T cell receptor β chains in human intestinal mucosa. J Exp Med 1994; 180:1337–1344.
15. Ernst PB, Clark DA, Rosenthal KL, et al. Detection and characterisation of cytotoxic T lymphocyte precursors in the murine intestinal intraepithelial leucocyte population. J Immunol 1986; 136:2121–2126.
16. Sydora BC, Mixter PF, Holcombe HR, et al. Intestinal intraepithelial lymphocytes are activated and cytolytic but do not proliferate as well as other T cells in response to mitogenic signals. J Immunol 1993; 150:2179–2191.
17. Jarrett EEE, Haig DM. Mucosal mast cells in vivo and in vitro. Immunol Today 1984; 5:115–119.
17. Chardes T, Buzoni-Gatel D, Lepage A, et al. Toxoplasma gondii oral infection induces specific cytotoxic $CD8\alpha/\beta^+$ $Thyl^+$ gut intraepithelial lymphocytes, lytic for parasite-infected enterocytes. J Immunol 1994; 153:4596–4603.
18. Befus AD, Pearce F, Bienenstock J. Intestinal mast cells in pathology and host resistance. In: Brostoff J, Challacombe SJ, eds. Food Allergy and Intolerance. London: Baillière Tindall, 1987: 88–102.
19. Woodbury RG, Gruzenski GM, Lagunoff D. Immunofluorescent localisation of a serine protease in rat small intestine. Proc Natl Acad Sci USA 1978; 75:2785–2789.
20. Miller HRP. The protective mucosal response against gastrointestinal nematodes in ruminants and laboratory animals. Vet Immunol Immunopathol 1984; 6:176–259.
21. Billingham RE, Brent L, Medawar PB. Acquired tolerance of skin homografts. Ann NY Acad Sci 1955; 59:409–498.
22. Billingham RE. The biology of graft-versus-host reactions. Harvey Lectures 1967; 62: 21–79.
23. Simonsen M. Graft versus host reactions: Their natural history and applicability as tools of research. Prog Allergy 1962; 6:349–467.
24. Hedberg CA, Reiser S, Reilly RW. Intestinal phase of the runting syndrome in mice: II. Observations on nutrient absorption and certain disaccharidase abnormalities. Transplantation 1968; 6:104–110.

25. Lund EK, Bruce MG, Smith MW, Ferguson A. Selective effects of graft- versus-host reaction on disaccharidase expression by mouse jejunal enterocytes. Clin Sci 1986; 71: 189–198.
26. Perdue MH, Chung M, Gall DG. Effect of intestinal anaphylaxis on gut function in the rat. Gastroenterology 1984; 86:391-397.
27. Cornelius EA. Protein-losing enteropathy in the graft-versus-host reaction. Transplantation 1970; 9:247–252.
28. Weisdorf SA, Salati LM, Longsdorf JA, et al. Graft-versus-host disease of the intestine: A protein losing enteropathy characterised by fecal α_1-antitrypsin. Gastroenterology 1983; 85:1076–1081.
29. Piguet P-F. GvHR elecited by products of class I or class II loci of the MHC: Analysis of the response of mouse T lymphocytes to products of class I and class II loci of the MHC in correlation with GvHR-induced mortality, medullary aplasia and enteropathy. J Immunol 1985; 135:1637–1643.
30. Turner MW, Boulton P, Shields JG, et al. Intestinal hypersensitivity reactions in the rat: I. Uptake of intact protein, permeability to sugars and their correlation with mucosal mast cell activation. Immunology 1988; 63:119–124.
31. Walker RI. The contribution of intestinal endotoxin to mortality in hosts with compromised resistance: A review. Exp Haematol 1978; 6:172–184.
32. Slavin RE, Woodruff JM. The pathology of bone-marrow transplantation. In: Sommers SC, ed. Pathology Annual. New York: Appleton-Century-Crofts, 1974:291–344.
33. Reilly RW, Kirsner JB. Runt intestinal disease. Lab Invest 1965; 14:102–107.
34. Thiele DL, Eigenbrodt ML, Bryde SE, et al. Intestinal graft-versus-host disease is initiated by donor T cells distinct from classic cytotoxic T lymphocytes. J Clin Invest 1989; 84:1947–1956.
35. Beschorner WE, Tutschka PJ, Santos GW. Chronic graft-versus-host disease in the rat radiation chimera: I. Clinical features, haematology, histology and immunopathology in long-term chimeras. Transplantation 1982; 33:393–399.
36. Gorer PA, Boyse EA. Pathological changes in F_1 hybrid mice following transplantation of spleen cells from donors of the parental strains. Immunology 1959; 2:182–193.
37. Wall AJ, Rosenberg JL, Reilly RW. Small intestinal injury in the immunologically runted mouse: Morphologic and autoradiographic studies. J Lab Clin Med 1971; 78: 833–834.
38. van Bekkum DW, Knaan S. Role of bacterial microflora in development of intestinal lesions from GvHR. J Natl Cancer Inst 1977; 58:787–790.
39. Elson CO, Reilly RW, Rosenberg IH. Small intestinal injury in the GvHr: An innocent bystander phenomenon. Gastroenterology 1977; 72:886–889.
40. MacDonald TT, Ferguson A. Hypersensitivity reactions in the small intestine: III. The effects of allograft rejection and of GvHD on epithelial cell kinetics. Cell Tiss Kinet 1977; 10:301–312.
41. Mowat AM, Ferguson A. Intraepithelial lymphocyte count and crypt hyperplasia measure the mucosal component of the graft-versus-host reaction in mouse small intestine. Gastroenterology 1982; 83:417–423.
42. Cummins AG, Munro GH, Miller HRP, Ferguson A. Effect of cyclosporin A treatment on the enteropathy of graft-versus-host reaction in the rat: A quantitative study of intestinal morphology, epithelial cell kinetics and mucosal immune activity. Immunol Cell Biol 1989; 67:153–160.
43. Mowat AM, Felstein MV. Experimental studies of immunologically mediated enteropathy: V. Destructive enteropathy during an acute graft-versus-host reaction in adult BFD_1 mice. Clin Exp Immunol 1990; 79:279–284.
44. Guy-Grand D and Vassalli P. Gut injury in mouse graft-versus-host reaction: Study of its occurrence and mechanisms. J Clin Invest 1986; 77:1584–1595.

45. Piguet P-F, Grau GE, Allet B, Vassalli P. Tumor necrosis factor/cachectin is an effector of skin and gut lesions of the acute phase of graft-versus-host disease. J Exp Med 1987; 166:1280–1289.
46. Mowat AM, Felstein MV, Borland A, Parrott DMV. Experimental studies of immunologically mediated enteropathy: Delayed type hypersensitivity is responsible for the proliferative and destructive enteropathy in irradiated mice with graft-versus-host reaction. Gut 1988; 29:949–956.
47. Tsuzuki T, Yoshikai Y, Ito M, et al. Kinetics of intestinal intraepithelial lymphocytes during acute graft-versus-host disease in mice. Eur J Immunol 1994; 24:709–715.
48. Mayrhofer G. Physiology of the intestinal immune system. In: Newby TJ, Stokes TR, eds. Local Immune Responses of the Gut. Boca Raton, FL: CRC Press, 1984: 1–96.
49. Bland PW. MHC class II expression by the gut epithelium. Immunol Today 1988; 9: 174–178.
50. Barclay AN, Mason DW. Introduction of Ia antigen in rat epidermal cells and gut epithelium by immunological stimuli. J Exp Med 1982;156:1665–1676.
51. Bland PW, Whiting CV. Induction of MHC class II gene products in rat intestinal epithelium during graft-versus-host disease and effects on the immune function of the epithelium. Immunology 1992; 75:366–367.
52. Strober W, Ehrhardt RO. Chronic intestinal inflammation: An unexpected outcome in cytokine or T cell receptor mutant mice. Cell 1993; 75:203–205.
53. Arnaud-Battandier F, Cerf-Bensussan N, Amsellem R, Schmitz J. Increased HLA-DR expression by enterocytes in children with coeliac disease. Gastroenterology 1986; 19: 1206–1212.
54. Mayer L, Eisenhardt D. Lack of induction of suppressor T cells by intestinal epithelial cells from patients with inflammatory bowel disease. J Clin Invest 1990; 86:1255–1260.
55. Rappaport H, Khalil A, Halle-Pannenko O, et al. Histopathologic sequence of events in adult mice undergoing lethal graft-versus-host reaction developed across H-2 and/ or non-H-2 histocompatibility barriers. Am J Pathol 1979; 96:121–142.
56. Nowell PC, Cole LJ. Lymphoid pathology in homologous disease of mice. Transplant Bull 1959; 6:435.
57. Guy-Grand D, Griscelli C, Vassalli P. The mouse gut T-lymphocyte, a novel type of T-cell: Nature, origin and traffic in mice in normal and graft-versus-host conditions. J Exp Med 1978; 148:1661–1677.
58. Marsh MN. Grains of truth: Evolutionary changes in small intestinal mucosa in response to environmental antigen challenge. Gut 1990; 31:111–114.
59. Marsh MN. Correlative aspects of mucosal pathology across the spectrum of gluten sensitivity. In Geighery C, O'Farrelly C, eds. Gastrointestinal Immunology and Gluten-Sensitive Disease. Dublin: Oak Tree Press, 1994:145–157.
60. Ferguson A. Models of immunologically driven small intestinal damage. In Marsh MN, ed. Immunopathology of the Small Intestine. Chichester, England: Wiley, 1987: 225–252.
61. Gold JA, Kosek J, Wanek N, Baur S. Duodenal immunoglobulin deficiency in graft-versus-host disease (GVHD) mice. J Immunol 1976; 117:471–476.
62. Watret K. Ph.D. thesis. University of Edinburgh, 1990.
63. Cummins AG, Munro GH, Huntley JE, et al. Separate effects of irradiation and of graft-versus-host reaction on rat mucosal mast cells. Gut 1989; 30:355–360.
64. Crapper RM, Schrader JW. Evidence for the in vivo production and release into the serum of a T cell lymphokine, persisting-cell stimulating factor (PSF), during graft-versus-host reactions. Immunology 1986; 57:553–558.
65. Newlands GJ, Mowat MA, Felstein MV, Miller HRP. Role of mucosal mast cells in

intestinal graft-versus-host reaction in mice. Int Arch Allergy Appl Immunol 1990; 98: 308–313.
66. Mowat AM, Ferguson A. Hypersensitivity reactions in the small intestine: 6. Pathogenesis of the graft-versus-host reaction in the small intestinal mucosa of the mouse. Transplantation 1981; 32:238–243.
67. Klein RM, Clancy J, Sheridan K. Acute lethal graft-versus-host disease stimulates cellular proliferation in Peyer's patches and follicle associated ileal epithelium of adult rats. Virchows Arch B 1984; 47:303–311.
68. Mowat AM, Borland A, Parrott DMV. Hypersensitivity reactions in the small intestine: 7. The intestinal phase of murine graft-versus-host reaction is induced by Lyt 2^- T cells activated by I-A alloantigens. Transplantation 1986; 4:192–198.
69. Mowat AM, Sprent J. Induction of intestinal graft-versus-host reactions across mutant major histocompatibility antigens by T lymphocyte subsets in mice. Transplantation 1989; 47:857–863.
70. Korngold R, Sprent J. Variable capacity of L3T4$^+$ T cells to cause lethal graft-versus-host disease across minor histocompatibility barriers in mice. J Exp Med 1987; 165: 1552–1564.
71. Murphy GF, Whitaker D, Sprent J, Korngold R. Characterization of target injury of murine acute graft-versus-host disease directed to multiple minor histocompatibility antigens elicited by either CD4$^+$ or CD8$^+$ effector cells. AM J Pathol 1991; 138:983–990.
72. Felstein MV, Mowat AM. Experimental studies of immunologically mediated enteropathy: IV. Correlation between immune effector mechanisms and type of enteropathy during a graft-versus-host reaction in neonatal mice of different ages. Clin Exp Immunol 1988; 72:108.
73. Felstein MV, Mowat AM. Experimental studies of immunologically mediated enteropathy: VI. Inhibition of acute intestinal graft-versus-host reaction in mice by 2'-deoxyguanosine. Scand J Immunol 1990; 32:461–469.
74. Borland A, Mowat AM, Parrott DMV. Augmentation of intestinal and peripheral natural killer cell activity during the graft-versus-host reaction in mice. Transplantation 1983; 36:513–519.
75. Mowat AM. Ia$^+$ bone marrow derived cells are the stimulus for the intestinal phase of murine graft-versus-host reaction. Transplantation 1986; 42:141–144.
76. Cornelius EA, Martinez C, Yunis EJ, Good RA. Haematological and pathological changes induced in tolerant mice by the injection of syngeneic lymphoid cells. Transplantation 1968; 6:33–44.
77. Ferguson A, Parrott DMV. Growth and development of antigen-free grafts of foetal mouse intestine. J Pathol 1972; 106:95–101.
78. Allen RD, Staley TA, Sidman CL. Differential cytokine expression in acute and chronic murine graft-versus-host disease. Eur J Immunol 1993; 23:333–337.
79. Smith SR, Terminelli C, Kenworthy-Bott L, Phillips DL. A study of cytokine production in acute graft-versus-host disease. Cell Immunol 1991; 134:336–348.
80. Fowler DH, Kurasawa K, Husebekk A, et al. Cells of T_H2 cytokine phenotype prevent LPS-induced lethality during murine graft-versus-host reaction: Regulation of cytokine and CD8$^+$ lymphoid engraftment. J Immunol 1994; 152:1004–1013.
81. Mowat AM, Hutton AK, Garside P, Steel MA. A role for interleukin-1α in immunologically mediated enteropathy. Immunology 1993; 80:110–115.
82. Garside P, Reid S, Steel M, Mowat AM. Differential cytokine production associated with distinct phases of murine graft-versus-host reaction. Immunology 1994; 82:211–214.
82. Cleveland MG, Annable CR, Klimpel GR. In vivo and in vitro production of IFN-β and IFN-γ during graft vs host disease. J Immunol 1988; 141:3349–3356.

83. Clancy J, Goral J, Kovacs EJ. Expression of cytokine genes (TNF-α, TGF-β and IFN-γ) in acute lethal graft versus host disease. Prog Leuk Biol 1990; 10B:165–170.
84. Kelso A. Frequency analysis of lymphokine-secreting CD4$^+$ and CD8$^+$ T cells activated in a graft-versus-host reaction. J Immunol 1990; 145:2167–2176.
85. Roberts AB, Sporn MB. Physiological actions and clinical applications of transforming growth factor-β (TGF-β). Growth Factors 1993; 8:1–9.
86. Mowat AM. Antibodies to γ-interferon prevent immunologically mediated intestinal damage in murine graft-versus-host reaction. Immunol 1989; 68:18–23.
87. Mowat AM, Widmer MB. A role for interleukin 4 in immunologically mediated enteropathy. Clin Exp Immunol 1995; 99:65–69.
88. Lollini P-L, D'Errico A, DeGiovanni C et al. Systemic effects of cytokines released by gene-transduced tumour cells: Marked hyperplasia induced in glands of small bowel by γ-interferon transfectants through host's lymphocytes. Int J Cancer 1995; 61:425–430.
89. Garside P, Bunce C, Tomlinson RC, et al. Analysis of the enteropathic effects of tumour necrosis factor α. Cytokine 1994; 5:24–30.
90. Garside P, Felstein MV, Green EA, Mowat AM. The role of interferon α/β in the induction of intestinal pathology in mice. Immunology 1991; 74:279–283.
91. McGee DW, Bambert T, Vitkus SJD, McGhee JR. A synerigistic relationship between TNF-α, IL-1β and TGF-1β on IL-6 secretion by the IEC-6 intestinal epithelial cell line. Immunology 1995; 86:6–11.
92. Shirota K, LeDuy L, Yuan S, Jothy S. Interleukin-6 and its receptor are expressed in human intestinal epithelial cells. Virchows Arch 1990; 58:303–308.
93. Schuerer-Maly CC, Eckmann L, Kagnoff MF, et al. Colonic epithelial cell lines as a source of interleukin-8: Stimulation by inflammatory cytokines and bacterial lipopolysaccharide. Immunology 1994; 81:85–92.
94. McGee DW, Beagley KW, Aicher WK, McGhee, JR. Transforming growth factor-β induces intestinal epithelial cells to secrete interleukin-6. Immunology 1992; 77:7.
95. Kaiserlian D, Rigal D, Abello J, Revillard J-P. Expression, function and regulation of the intercellular adhesion molecule-1 (ICAM-1) on human intestinal epithelial cell lines. Eur J Immunol 1991; 21:2415–2421.
96. Madara JL, Stafford J. Interferon-γ directly affects barrier function of cultered intestinal epithelial monolayers. J Clin Invest 1989; 83:724–727.
97. Adams RB, Planchon SM, Roche JK. IFN-γ modulation of epithelial barrier function: Time course, reversibility, and site of cytokine binding. J Immunol 1993; 150:2356–2363.
98. Planchon SM, Martins CAP, Guerrant RL, Roche JK. Regulation of intestinal epithelial barrier function by TGF-β1: Evidence for its role in abrogating the effect of a T cell cytokine. J Immunol 1994; 153:3730–3739.
99. Hutton AK. Ph.D. thesis. University of Glasgow, 1994.
100. Prinz JC, Gross B, Vollmer S, et al. T cell clones from psoriasis skin lesions can promote keratinocyte proliferation in vitro via secreted products. Eur J Immunol 1994; 24:593–598.
101. Kvale D, Lovhaug D, Sollid LM, Brandtzaeg P. Tumor necrosis factor-α up-regulates expression of secretory component, the epithelial receptor for polymeric Ig. J Immunol 1988; 140:3086–3089.
102. Kandil HM, Berschneider HM, Argenzio RA. Tumour necrosis factor α changes procine intestinal ion transport through a paracrine mechanism involving prostaglandins. Gut 1994; 35:934–940.
103. Colgan SP, Resnick MB, Parkos CA, et al. IL-4 directly modulates function of a model human intestinal epithelium. J Immunol 1994; 153:2122–2129.
104. Garside P, Hutton AK, Severn A, Lien FY, Mowat AM. Nitric oxide mediates intestinal pathology in graft-vs-host disease. Eur J Immunol 1992; 22:2141–2145.

104. Roy C, Ghayur T, Kongshavn PAL, Lapp WS. Natural killer activity by spleen lymph node and thymus cells during the graft-versus-host reaction. Transplantation 1982; 34: 144–146.
106. Kubota E, Ishikawa H, Saito K. Modulation of F_1 cytotoxic potentials by GvHR: Host and donor-derived cytotoxic lymphocytes arise in the unirradiated F_1 host spleens under the condition of GvHR-associated immunosuppression. J Immunol 1983; 131: 1142–1148.
107. Mowat AM, Borland A, Parrott DMV. Augmentation of natural killer cell activity by anti-host delayed-type hypersensitivity during the graft-versus-host reaction in mice. Scand J Immunol 1985; 22:389–399.
108. Mowat AM, Felstein MV. Experimental studies of immunologically mediated enteropathy: II. Role of natural killer cells in the intestinal phase of murine graft-versus-host reaction. Immunology 1987; 68:179–183.
109. Carman PS, Ernst PB, Rosenthal KL et al. Intraepithelial leukocytes contain a unique subpopulation of NK-like cytotoxic cells active in the defence of gut epithelium to enteric murine coronavirus. J Immunol 1986; 136:1548–1553.
110. Charley MR, Mikhael A, Bennett M, et al. Prevention of lethal, minor-determinate graft-host disease in mice by the in vivo administration of anti-asialo GM_1. J Immunol 1983; 131:2101–2103.
111. Varkila K. Depletion of asialo-GM1$^+$ cells from the F_1 recipient mice prior to irradiation and transfusion of parental spleen cells prevents mortality to acute graft-versus-host disease and induction of anti-host specific cytotoxic T cells. Clin Exp Immunol 1987; 69:652–659.
112. Trinchieri G. Interleukin-12: A proinflammatory cytokine with immunoregulatory functions that bridge innate resistance and antigen-specific adaptive immunity. Annu Rev Immunol 1995; 13:251-276.
113. Woodbury RG, Neurath H. Purification of an atypical mast cell protease and its levels in developing rats. Biochemistry 1978; 17:4298–4304.
114. Elves MW, Ferguson A. The humoral immune response to allografts of foetal small intestine in mice. Br J Exp Pathol 1975; 56:454–458.
115. Jones JM, Wilson R, Bealmear PM. Mortality and gross pathology of secondary disease in germfree mouse radiation chimeras. Radiat Res 1971; 45:577–588.
116. van Bekkum DW, Roodenburg J, Heidt PJ, van der Waalt D. Mitigation of secondary disease of allogeneic mouse radiation chimeras by modification of the intestinal microflora. J Natl Cancer Inst 1974; 52:401.
117. Moore RH, Lampert IA, Chia Y, et al. Influence of endotoxin on graft-versus-host disease after bone morrow transplantation across major histocompatibility barriers in mice. Transplantation 1987; 43:731–736.
118. Moore RH, Lampert IA, Chia Y, et al. Effect of immunization with Escherichia coli J5 on graft-versus-host disease induced by minor histocompatibilty antigens in mice. Transplantation 1987; 44:249–253.
119. Nestel FP, Price KS, Seemayer TA, Lapp WS. Macrophage priming and lipopolysaccharide-triggered release of tumour necrosis factor α during graft-versus-host disease. J Exp Med 1992; 175:405–413.
120. Rafferty JF, Noguchi Y, Fischer JE, Hasselgren PO. Sepsis in rats stimulates cellular proliferation in the mucosa of the small intestine. Gastroenterology 1994; 107:121–127.
121. Buckner CD, Clift RA, Sanders JE, et al. Protective environment for marrow transplant recipients: A prospective study. Ann Intern Med 1978; 89:893–901.
122. Grundy JE, Shanley JD, Shearer GM. Augmentation of graft-versus-host reaction by cytomegalovirus infection resulting in interstitial pneumonitis. Transplantation 1985; 39:548–553.

123. Mowat AM, Felstein MV, Baca ME. Experimental studies of immunologically mediated enteropathy: III. Severe and progressive enteropathy during a graft-versus-host reaction in athymic mice. Immunology 1987; 61:185–188.
124. Bellgrau D, Wilson DB. Immunological studies of T-cell receptors:I. Specifically induced resistance to graft-versus-host disease in rats mediated by host T-cell immunity to alloreactive parental T cells. J Exp Med 1978; 148:103–114.
125. Slavin RE, Santos GW. The graft-versus-host reaction in man after bone marrow transplantation: Pathology, pathogenesis, clinical features and implications. Clin Immunol Immunopathol 1973; 1:472–498.
126. Snover DC. The pathology of acute graft-versus-host disease. In: Burakoff SJ, Deeg HJ, Ferrara J, Atkinson K, eds. Graft-vs-Host Disease. New York: Marcel Dekker, 1990:337–353.
127. McDonald GB, Shulman HM, Sullivan KM, Spencer GD. Intestinal and hepatic complications of human bone marrow transplantation. Gastroenterology 1986; 90:460–477, 770–784.
128. McDonald GB, Sale GE. The human gastrointestinal track after allogeneic bone marrow transplantation. In: Sale GE, Shulman HM, eds. The Pathology of Bone Marrow Transplantation. New York: Masson, 1984:77–103.
129. Nakhleh RE, Snover DC, Weisdorf S, Platt JL. Immunopathology of graft-versus-host disease in the upper gastrointestinal tract. Transplantation 1989; 48:61–65.
130. Abedi MR, Hammarstrom L, Ringden O, Smith CIE. Development of IgA deficiency after bone marrow transplantation: The influence of acute and chronic graft-verus-host disease. Transplantation 1990; 50:415–421.
131. Cunningham-Rundles C, Brandeis WE, Safai B, et al. Selective IgA deficiency and circulating immune complexes containing bovine proteins in a child with chronic graft-versus-host disease. Am J Med 1979; 67:883–890.
132. Cummins AG, Labrooy JT, Stanley DP, et al. Quantitative histological study of enteropathy associated with HIV infection. Gut 1990; 31:317–321.
133. Mowat AM. The immunopathogenesis of food sensitive enteropathies. In: Newby TJ, Stokes CR, eds. Local Immune Responses of the Gut. Boca Raton, FL: CRC Press, 1984:199–225.

14

Graft Versus Leukemia

Robert L. Truitt, Bryon D. Johnson, Cathleen M. McCabe, and Michael B. Weiler
Medical College of Wisconsin
Milwaukee, Wisconsin

I. INTRODUCTION

Approximately 85% of all allogeneic bone marrow transplants (BMT) are done as a treatment for leukemias and lymphomas that are resistant to conventional chemoradiotherapy (1). Initially the eradication of leukemia after clinical BMT was attributed to the effects of high-dose chemotherapy and radiation given pretransplant. However, studies in animal models and subsequent clinical experience in humans have shown that immunocompetent donor cells contribute to the antileukemic effect of bone marrow transplantation. This immunological component is called the "graft-vs-leukemia" (GVL) effect (2,3). The precise relationship between the GVL effect and graft-vs-host disease (GVHD) is controversial (2–6). It has been postulated that either distinct and, therefore, separable immune effector cells are responsible for GVL and GVH reactions or the same effector cells with differing thresholds of reactivity mediate the preferential killing of leukemia.

GVHD represents an immunological conflict between donor and host manifested by an attack of donor T cells against alloantigens of the host. Several excellent reviews of GVHD have been published (e.g., Refs. 7 to 10), and others are contained in this volume. In recent years, much attention has been focused on the role of T cells and inflammatory cytokines in GVH pathophysiology (8,11–13). This has led to the hypothesis that donor T cells, regardless of their $CD4^+$ or $CD8^+$ phenotype, are activated in a GVH reaction to produce specific cytokines, which trigger the production of additional cytokines by other cell types including donor NK cells and other donor or host-derived cells. This "cytokine cascade" contributes significantly to the pathology of GVHD. Cytotoxic T lymphocytes (CTL) may play a minimal role in GVH pathology unless they secrete lymphokines or undergo antigen-driven proliferation in situ (6,12). The pretransplant conditioning also affects cytokine patterns and exacerbates GVHD (11,14).

Although the pathophysiology of GVHD in complex, recent experimental studies have demonstrated that it is possible to harness the GVH reaction and enhance the beneficial GVL reaction. Some examples include ex vivo depletion of GVH-reactive T cells (15–18), in vivo elimination of GVH-reactive T cells (19–21), in vivo elimination of NK cells (22), in vivo inhibition of $CD3^+$ T cells (23,24), manipulation of $CD4^+$ subsets (25), use of high-dose IL-2 (26), use of IL-4 plus IL-2 to shift functional Th-subsets (27), and combination of ex vivo T-cell depleted (TCD) and lymphokine therapy (28).

Until recently, evidence for a GVL effect in human BMT has been indirect and derived mostly from anecdotal reports of leukemia remissions and retrospective statistical analyses of the risk of leukemia relapse (2,29). The importance of the immunological component was not fully appreciated until TCD became widely used to prevent GVHD (30). Recently, direct evidence for a GVL effect in humans has been provided by Kolb (31), Drobyski (32), Hertenstein (33), Antin (34), and Goldman (35), among others, who showed that infusion of donor leukocytes induced long-lasting cytogenetic and molecular remissions in patients with chronic myelogenous leukemia (CML) who had relapsed post-BMT.

In this chapter we review the general principles of GVL reactivity and present data from our recent experimental studies on manipulation of GVH reactivity without loss of the GVL effect. Using animal models, we show that GVL and GVH reactions are multicompartmental, dynamic, and highly interactive. Based on both clinical and experimental data, we propose that the fundamental question is no longer whether GVL reactivity is separable for GVHD but rather how we most effectively separate them for the benefit of the patient.

II. GENERAL PRINCIPLES OF GVL REACTIVITY

A. Principle #1: There Are Multiple GVL Effector-Cell Populations

At a minimum, GVL reactivity requires the presence of functional effector cells and tumor cells susceptible to the effector cells. Based on extensive experimental and clinical data, GVL effector cells can be broadly divided into two major groups as shown in Fig. 1. Some recognize cell surface molecules that are unique to or preferentially expressed on leukemia cells, and others recognize structures expressed on both normal and neoplastic host cells. The former are "leukemia-specific" and the latter "allospecific." Cells in each category have been identified in both experimental and clinical studies, but their relative importance to GVL reactivity is controversial and may depend upon the nature of the leukemia (see Principle #3, below).

Goulmy and colleagues (36) analyzed CTL derived from recipients of HLA-identical BMT at different times posttransplant for reactivity against the patients' own leukemia as well as normal lymphocytes (PHA lymphoblasts). They identified three functionally different types of clones: (a) clones directed at host specific minor histocompatibility antigens (miHA) expressed on both normal and neoplastic cells, (b) clones recognizing only normal host lymphocytes, and (c) clones that appeared to be leukemia-specific (i.e., they did not kill normal host cells used in the assays). These results are similar to those reported previously from our laboratory, using murine models of allogeneic BMT (6,37). Thus, in humans as in mice, antihost and antileukemia reactivity may be mediated by overlapping as well as distinct subsets

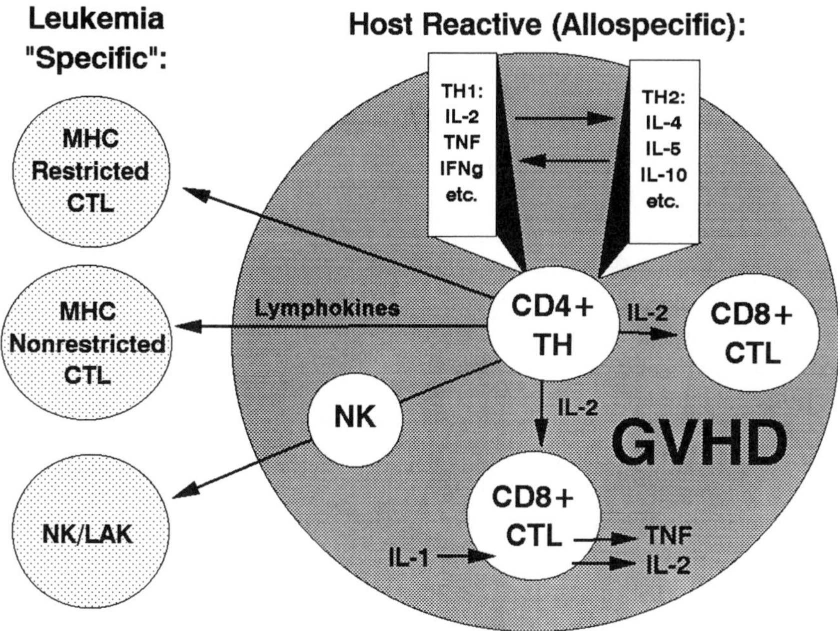

Figure 1 Conceptual model of relationship between GVL and GVH effector cells. T cells that recognize host alloantigens trigger GVH reactivity. In addition to the number of T cells in the graft, the incidence and intensity of GVHD depends upon the antigen specificity and functional properties of the activated T cells. The relative contribution of $CD4^+$ and $CD8^+$ T cells is influenced by the immunogenetic relationship between the donor and host. The presumed targets for alloreactive T cells in the context of MHC-matched allogeneic BMT are miHA, self peptides that occupy the antigen-binding groves of the MHC molecules. Allospecific $CD4^+$ T cells can be divided into subsets based on the spectrum of cytokines they secrete, and these cytokines are known to be cross-regulatory (e.g., γ-IFN downregulates Th2 cells and IL-4 and IL-10 down-regulate Th1 cells). Th1 cytokines appear to be the major contributors to tissue damage and to activation of secondary GVH effector mechnisms. Cytolytic activity by $CD8^+$ T cells in vitro does not necessarily predict ability to cause GVHD in vivo. On a clonal level, GVH potential of $CD8^+$ T cells may have to do with their ability to secrete certain cytokines or to undergo Th-independent clonal expansion in situ. NK cells also contribute to GVH pathology but play a relatively minor role in comparison to T cells.

T cells that recognize and react against host alloantigens contribute to the GVL effect and are referred to as allospecific or GVH-associated GVL effector cells. In addition, there are multiple other GVL effector populations that, if not leukemia-specific, at least mediate preferential leukemia kill. Leukemia "specific" effector cells include T cells that recognize leukemia-associated peptides in an MHC-restricted manner via their $\alpha\beta$TCR as well as MHC-nonrestricted $\gamma\delta TCR^+$ T cells and NK/LAK cells. The cell surface molecules recognized by these GVL effector cells may be present exclusively or expressed preferentially by neoplastic host cells and not normal host cells. GVL-specific effectors may be dependent upon allospecific Th-cells for essential lymphokines to activate and/or stimulate their proliferation. Some redundancy in the type of effector cells contributing to GVL reactivity after allogeneic BMT may be desirable given the many levels at which leukemia cells are known to escape immunological recognition and destruction. (Used with permission: Biol of Blood and Marrow Transplant 1995; 1:61.)

of T cells. It is incorrect, however, to equate lysis of host cells in vitro with ability to cause GVHD in vivo (see Principle #2, below). In point of fact, some investigators have speculated that CTL may play a relatively minor role in the pathophysiology of GVHD (11).

1. $\alpha\beta$TCR$^+$ T Cells as GVL Effector Cells

The preponderance of experimental data indicates that T cells are the primary mediators of GVL reactivity following allogeneic BMT. Pan T-cell depletion with MoAb and complement (C′) ex vivo eliminates GVL reactivity in murine models of BMT in mice (15–18,38) as well as humans (2,29,30), but equivalent results are not always obtained in studies that use antibodies specific for different T-cell epitopes. For example, in recent studies, OKunewick et al. (17) reported that ex vivo depletion with anti-CD3 and anti-CD5 MoAbs resulted in contrasting results in a murine model of MHC-matched BMT. Selective depletion of CD3$^+$ T cells was accompanied by decreased GVHD as well as GVL reactivity. In contrast, depletion of CD5$^+$ T cells had no effect on the rates of leukemia relapse or GVHD, but it significantly increased graft failure. Although CD3 and CD5 are both pan-T-cell antigens, they are expressed on T cells at various stages of differentiation. Thus, experimental evidence suggests that T subsets may exist that preferentially provide GVL reactivity. A similar variable effect with different pan-TCD strategies on leukemia relapse has been observed at the clinical level (30). At the Medical College of Wisconsin, a MoAb directed at $\alpha\beta$ T-cell receptor ($\alpha\beta$TCR$^+$) T cells has been used successfully to prevent GVHD without significantly increasing the risk of relapse after unrelated BMT (39,40), whereas some other T-depletion methods have been less successful in preserving the GVL effect (30).

Both CD4$^+$ and CD8$^+$ T cells have been shown to contribute to GVL reactivity in animal models (15,16,18,41). CD8$^+$ cells appear to be the primary mediators of GVL reactivity in most models, while CD4$^+$ are indirect effectors. CD4$^+$ T cells may enhance the GVL reaction by inducing clonal expansion of CD8$^+$ CTL through secretion of interleukin-2 (IL-2) or by activating secondary effector mechanisms. Quantitative assessments of the level of GVL reactivity provided by different effector subpopulations has not been done; most experimental studies provide only qualitative or semiquantitative evaluations. Under experimental conditions, cloned CD8$^+$ T cells are able to mediate a GVL effect in the absence of CD4$^+$ T cells or exogenous growth factors (6). The ability of CD8$^+$ T cells to mediate T-helper-independent GVL reactivity may depend upon their ability to undergo antigen-driven proliferation and/or produce cytokines (42). The relative importance of CD4$^+$ and CD8$^+$ T cells to GVL reactivity depends upon the genetic relationship between donor and host as well as the nature of the target antigens expressed by neoplastic cells. In general, CD4$^+$ T cells are restricted to recognition of peptides presented in the context of class II major histocompatibility complex (MHC) molecules, while CD8$^+$ T cells recognize peptides and class I MHC molecules (43). Exceptions, however, have been observed (e.g., Ref. 44).

The increased risk of leukemia relapse associated with T-cell depletion provides indirect evidence that T cells are essential to GVL reactivity after BMT in humans (2,29,30). Sosman et al. (45) generated $\alpha\beta$TCR$^+$CD4$^+$ T-cell clones that killed allogeneic acute lymphocytic leukemia (ALL) cells but not normal lymphoblasts from the same patient. Occasionally, these "leukemia-specific" T-cell lines killed nonleukemic cells from certain unrelated donors through unidentified cross-reactive determinants. More recently, Falkenberg and colleagues (46) derived CTL lines and clones from the peripheral blood of HLA-genotypically identical siblings of patients with leukemia by stimulation of the donor cells with irradiated leukemic cells from the patient. Both HLA class I-and II-restricted CTL were obtained. In 5 of 7 patients, the CTL showed specific lysis of leukemic cells from the patient but not normal lymphoblasts (46).

The vast majority of CTL (90%) generated between HLA-identical individuals show exclusive lysis of nonleukemic targets following primary stimulation in vitro with nonleukemic cells (47). At the same time, a substantial number of putatively leukemia-specific clones can be detected upon stimulation with leukemic cells (47). In vivo priming may increase the ability to detect antileukemia reactive T cells. The frequency of CTL precursor in patients following allogeneic BMT has been estimated by Jiang and colleagues using limiting dilution analysis (48). While donor cells tested before BMT failed to generate CTL against the patients' leukemia, a low frequency of CTL directed against the patients' CML was detected in all patients. The frequency of leukemia-specific CTL was significantly lower than the frequency of CTL directed against the recipient's PHA-transformed pretransplant lymphocytes, suggesting that only a subpopulation of donor lymphocytes has antileukemia reactivity.

MHC-restricted $\alpha\beta TCR^+$ CTL specific for miHA antigens on recipient tissues are potential effectors for GVL reactivity. The antileukemic reactivity of miHA-specific CTL clones against circulating lymphocytic and myeloid leukemia cells was examined by van der Harst and colleagues (49). They found that miHA specificities were present on leukemia cells and could serve as targets for HLA class I-restricted CTL. CTL specific for miHA have been shown to participate in the GVL effect in several murine models of MHC-matched BMT (e.g., Ref. 6).

2. $\gamma\delta TCR^+$ T Cells as GVL Effector Cells

$CD3^+$ cells that express the $\gamma\delta$TCR represent a unique subset of T cells that mediate MHC-unrestricted killing of virus-infected and tumor target cells (50,51), but mycobacterial antigens appear to stimulate both human and murine $\gamma\delta$ T cells in an MHC-restricted fashion (51). In a series of studies, Fisch and colleagues (52–55) characterized the lytic activity of $\gamma\delta$ T cells and showed that they recognized a heat-shock protein (hsp60) expressed on the surface of tumor cells and cross-reactive with an antigen found in mycobacterial extracts. HSPs chaperon antigenic peptides within cells, and immunization with HSPs extracted from tumor cells can elicit tumor specific T-cell immunity, including class I MHC-restricted CTL responses (56). HSPs may act like "superantigens" to facilitate interaction between lytic effector cells and tumor cells, resulting in what appears to be "leukemia-specific" killing in an MHC-nonrestricted manner. Similar cells may contribute to GVL reactivity post-BMT. Although there is no direct clinical evidence for this, there is experimental data to support an antilymphoma effect of human $\gamma\delta$ T cells in vivo (57).

3. NK and LAK Cells as GVL Effectors

Natural killer (NK) cells are cytolytic cells capable of mediating MHC-nonrestricted lysis of leukemia cells in vitro. NK cells are among the earliest cells to reappear after both autologous and allogeneic BMT (58,59). NK cells are a diverse population; at least some of them recognize distinct specificities controlled by genes linked to the MHC (60). Although precursors of lymphokine-activated killer (LAK) cells derive primarily from large granular lymphocytes of the NK lineage, activated MHC-nonrestricted killer cells of both T ($CD3^+$) and NK ($CD56^+$) lineages may participate in the antitumor effect after allogeneic BMT (61). Hauch et al. (62) examined PBMC from a series of patients transplanted for CML and observed lytic activity as early as 3 weeks posttransplant. Lytic activity to fully allogeneic and host-derived CML targets appeared to be mediated by $CD16^+$ and $CD56^+$ cells but not by $CD3^+$ cells. When donor and recipient NK cells were tested in parallel against host-derived CML targets, their relative lytic activity was correlated. In patients who failed to generate any lytic activity against host-derived CML targets, there was a significant increase in the risk of leukemia relapse as compared to patients with lytic activity (62). In a similar study, Mackinnon and colleagues found that LAK activity was inducible in recipients of both TCD and T-cell-replete donor marrow and in recipients with or without GVHD (61). The antileukemia effects of NK/LAK cells may be mediated by release of lymphokines that act directly or indirectly on tumor cells.

In animal models, LAK cells can be adoptively transferred for a graft-versus-tumor effect without causing GVHD (63); in one murine model, GVL activity post-BMT appeared to depend more on the donors NK/LAK cell activity than on the presence or absence of GVH-inducing T cells (64). As described later in this chapter, we have observed that NK cells contribute to GVL reactivity early after transplantation of MHC-matched BM but also to GVH-associated immunodeficiency.

Several patients with advanced lymphoma have responded to therapy with high-dose IL-2 with and without coadministration of LAK cells, demonstrating the antileukemia potential of these cells (65,66). Anti-CD3 MoAb can be used to activate human T cells in the presence of IL-2 to induce proliferation and cytotoxicity (67,68). Lum and colleagues (69) demonstrated that anti-CD3 MoAb and IL-2 induced MHC-nonrestricted CTL in normal and tumor-bearing patients. Such cells could be used for adoptive immunotherapy after autologous or perhaps even allogeneic BMT under certain circumstances.

4. Other Potential GVL Effector Cells

Autologous BMT has achieved some success in the treatment of hematological malignancies and solid tumors, but the magnitude of the antitumor reaction appears to be limited. In an attempt to augment antitumor reactivity, Hess and colleagues (70) devised a strategy to induce autologous (or syngeneic) GVHD in transplanted animals. Autologous GVHD is mediated by autoreactive T cells directed against a public determinant of the MHC class II molecules. It is caused by the failure of central (thymic) regulatory mechanisms that restrict self-recognition (71,72). These normal mechanisms are inhibited by irradiation and cyclosporine treatment, resulting in release of autoreactive cells into the periphery. Studies in animal models of autologous GVHD have shown that the effector cells recognize MHC class II expressed by tumor cells (73). Autologous GVHD is being investigated clinically for potential augmented antitumor effects (74).

GVHD perturbs thymic education (75), and autoreactive cells have been described in peripheral tissues following allogeneic BMT (76). Mechanisms of T-cell repertoire selection may be altered during GVHD, allowing "forbidden T-cell clones" to escape into the periphery. These "self-reactive" cells are thought to cause or contribute to the development of chronic GVHD, but they may also provide a level of immune surveillance against reemergence of leukemia cells that survive the initial immunological confrontation or are sequestered in immunologically privileged tissues. It is noteworthy that chronic GVHD is the single most significant clinical factor that correlates with decreased leukemia relapse after allogeneic BMT (2,29,77).

Finally, it is important to remember that cytotoxicity is not the only biological property that may result in GVL reactivity. Lytic as well as nonlytic GVL effector cells may secrete cytokines that kill leukemia cells, activate other secondary effector cells, induce differentiation of leukemia cells, or retard growth through cytostatic mechanisms. In this regard, the relatively long period (often measured in months) between infusion of donor leukocytes and induction of a remission may be significant (31–35). It remains to be determined whether the disappearance of malignant cells is due to direct killing or creation of an immunological environment that no longer supports survival of the host leukemia.

B. Principle #2: The Antigen-Specificity and Functional Properties of Responding Cells Determine Whether the GVL Effect Is Separable from GVH Disease

The question of whether GVL reactivity is separable from GVHD has challenged experimental and clinical investigators since the earliest experimental report of Barnes and colleagues (78). Early studies in animal models demonstrated that the pathologic effects leading the GVH syndrome can be dissociated from the beneficial antileukemia effects (79). Similar evidence in humans, however, evolved more slowly (80). Anecdotal case reports and retrospective statistical studies provided the initial evidence for a relationship between GVHD and the risk of leukemia relapse (2,29). In an analysis of transplants reported to the International Bone Marrow Transplant Registry (IBMTR) for patients receiving HLA-identical sibling BMT for "early" leukemia—ALL and acute myelogenous leukemia (AML) in first remission; chronic myelogenous leukemia (CML) in chronic phase—at least three graft-related antileukemia effects were identified:

- An antileukemia effect associated with GVHD
- An antileukemia effect of allogeneic marrow grafts that is independent of clinically evident GVHD
- An antileukemia effect that is independent of GVHD, but altered by depletion of T-cells.

The biological basis for these effects is not entirely clear, but the observations lend support to the concept that distinct as well as overlapping populations of effector cells mediate GVL and GVH reactivity; a conclusion supported by clonal analysis of CTL in vitro (36). GVH-associated GVL reactivity contributes more to the cure of ALL than AML or CML, but GVHD-independent GVL reactivity appears to be greater in CML and AML than in ALL (29,81).

Our understanding of the biological basis and complexity of immunological reactions leading to GVHD has undergone significant change in recent years (82). Cytotoxic T cells, once considered the sine qua non of GVHD, are being supplanted by cytokines and inflammatory cells as the critical effectors of GVHD (7–12). Self-reactive T cells are now recognized as contributing to the GVH syndrome (70,74,75). With respect to GVL reactivity, we maintain that the antigen-specificity and functional activity of the responding cells (T as well as non-T cells; allo- as well as autoreactive; cytokine secreting as well as cytolytic; etc.) determines whether GVL reactivity is separable from GVH reactivity in both clinical and experimental BMT. Various strategies designed to minimize GVHD affect the different ways. Furthermore, the cells and cytokines involved in GVL and GVH reactivity are highly interactive and dynamic, making attempts to modulate GVH reactivity without loss of GVL reactivity challenging but not impossible. The general principles of GVH reactivity can be summed up as follows:

- GVH reactivity is triggered by T-cell activation.
- The relative contribution of $CD4^+$ and $CD8^+$ T-cells to GVHD depends on the immunogenetic relationship between donor and host.
- The capacity to provoke a lethal GVH reaction depends on the functional properties of the responding T-cell clones.
- Inflammatory processes, non-T cells, and environmental factors contribute to the pathophysiology of GVHD.

The essential role for T-cell activation in triggering GVHD (in an autologous as well as allogeneic setting) is well founded and is not reviewed here. Our discussion focuses on the role of T cells in MHC-matched allogeneic BMT, recognizing that similar but not necessarily identical mechanisms contribute to GVHD in the setting of MHC class I and/or II disparities.

Data from animal models indicate that the T-cell subsets involved in GVH reactivity following MHC-matched BMT vary based on the immunogenetic relationship between donor and host. In comparing several MHC-matched donor:host combinations, Korngold (83) found that $CD8^+$ T cells contributed to GVHD in every combination tested but that $CD4^+$ T cells were involved in only a few combinations. However, $CD4^+$ T cells exacerbate CD8-mediated GVHD in a dose-dependent manner (84). Our own data indicate that $CD4^+$ cells are the primary mediators of GVHD in B10.BR → AKR chimeras in which there is a superantigen (Mls-1^a) disparity in the GVH direction (15); $CD8^+$ T cells do not cause lethal GVHD in the absence of help from $CD4^+$ cells or unless they are presensitized to host alloantigens (discussed below). Hamilton (85) also has reported that $CD4^+$ T cells can mediate GVHD. Clearly, the success of selective T-subset depletion as a strategy to limit GVHD will depend in large part upon our ability to predict whether particular donor T subsets capable of causing GVHD are activated in a particular donor:host pair. Initial results using selective CD8 TCD in HLA-matched BMT in humans are encouraging, with a low incidence and severity of GVHD reported (86). Although this suggests that miHA GVHD may be similar to that of most mouse models (CD8-mediated), it is important to keep in mind that pharmacological immunosuppression (cyclosporine) was also used in that study and may have affected GVH-causing $CD4^+$ T cells. Furthermore, $CD4^+$ T cells may play a more important role in GVHD following BMT from haplotype mismatched related and/or HLA-matched unrelated donors (87,88).

The mechanism by which $CD8^+$ T cells mediate GVHD to miHAs is not clear, but cytoxicity alone does not appear to correlate with ability to cause GVHD (6). Cytokine secreting $CD8^+$ T cells have been identified during GVHD (89). Subpopulations of $CD8^+$ CTL may secrete cytokines (such as IL-2) and drive their own proliferation in an autocrine or paracrine fashion (90), resulting in their accumulation in target tissues, where they can cause extensive damage through direct lytic activity or cytokine secretion. It has been proposed that local secretion of cytokines such as γ-interferon (γIFN) by $CD8^+$ CTL may be more important in antiviral immunity than direct lytic activity (91). In murine systems, Ly6 expression has been used to discriminate cytokine secreting $CD8^+$ CTL from nonsecreting CTL (90). The implications of these data for human BMT is clear—detection of lytic activity against host target cells in vitro is not sufficient to identify a CTL clone as "GVH"-reactive, but simply "antihost" reactive.

$CD4^+$ cells secrete cytokines that drive clonal expansion of $CD8^+$ CTL. Roopenian (92) has proposed that some miHA loci may actually be complex genetic units in which separate genes, encoding products that activate $CD8^+$ CTL and $CD4^+$ Th cells, respectively, are so closely linked that they give the illusion of segregating as a single genetic unit. Alternatively, environmental antigens, such as microbes and viruses, may stimulate $CD4^+$ T cells to secrete IL-2 and induce clonal expansion of miHA-activated $CD8^+$ T cells, thereby exacerbating GVH reactivity. This may explain in part why GVHD is diminished under gnotobiotic conditions (93,94).

Antigen-activated $CD4^+$ T cells are a major source of cytokines that contribute to GVHD (8), and there is evidence that the presence of proliferating, noncytolytic T cells specific for host miHAs, rather than CTLs, correlates with the incidence of severe acute GVHD (95,96). In an analysis of GVH mortality induced by noncytolytic $CD4^+$ T-cell clones specific for miHAs, Miconnet et al. (97) reported a correlation between the capacity to induce GVHD, mediate DTH, and release high levels of TNF. They concluded that GVH mortality induced by $CD4^+$ T-cell clones resulted from an inflammatory process associated with TNF production. These cells may be regulated by $CD3^+$ double negative T cells (see Principle #4, below) (98).

Cytokines secreted by alloactivated $CD4^+$ cells belonging to the Th1 subset (e.g., IL-2, γ-IFN, TNF, etc.) are critical to the development of GVHD (8,11,12), and cytokine secreting $CD8^+$ CTL have been described as having a Th1-like cytokine profile, although their lytic activity and cytokine profile can be modified in the presence of Th2 cytokines (99). Th2 cells and their cytokines have been reported to suppress GVHD (27). Wall and Sheehan (100) have proposed an interaction between T cells and natural suppressor cells involving γ-IFN and TNF that leads to GVH-associated immune deficiency and death. NK cells also are involved in GVH-associated pathology and immune deficiency (22). Thus, there is a complex network of cells and cytokines that ultimately contribute to the clinical manifestations of GVHD. Some but not all of these immunological reactions are involved in the elimination of leukemia cells. Continuing advances in our understanding of the basic biology of GVHD should lead to the development and implementation of new strategies to avoid or minimize GVHD without loss of GVL reactivity by specifically targeting GVH while sparing GVL effector mechanisms (101).

C. Principle #3: Immunological Characteristics of the Leukemia Affect Susceptibility to GVL Effector Cells

As noted at the beginning of this chapter, GVL reactivity requires, at a minimum, functional effector cells and susceptible tumor cells. GVL reactivity may be absent or suboptimal due to any of a number of qualitative and quantitative elements such as those listed in Table 1. The leukemia cells may not be susceptible to some or all of the GVL effector cells described above because they lack appropriate target peptides—either leukemia-associated or minor histocompatibility antigen (miHA). Putative leukemia-associated peptides or miHA may not be sufficiently immunogenic or may not be presented appropriately to immunocompetent donor cells (for example, because of a deficiency in MHC-restricting elements). The tumor cells may lack the appropriate costimulatory molecules necessary to induce a response, or they may secrete factors (cytokines) that actively suppress antitumor immune responses. The quantity of T cells or non-T effector cells may be below the threshold necessary for a clinical response as a result of TCD or other manipulations of the donor marrow or because of the degree of genotypic identity between donor and recipient.

There is substantial evidence that the immunological characteristics of the leukemia affect GVL reactivity at each of these levels. For example, when a genetically identical donor (monozygotic twin) is used to minimize GVH reactivity, the relative risk of leukemia relapse in significantly higher (2,29), suggesting that allogeneic disparity increases the GVL effect. This may occur by a direct mechanism through the expression of alloantigens that serve as appropriate targets for GVL effector cells or through indirect mechanisms such as the activation of cells which provide essential cofactors to GVL reactive cells (such as IL-2, IL-12, etc.).

In transplants for chronic phase CML done at the Medical College of Wisconsin, Drobyski and colleagues (102) have observed a significant decrease in the risk of leukemia relapse for CML patients given TCD marrow from matched unrelated donors as compared to matched siblings. With a median follow-up of greater than 2 years, the relative risk of relapse in 27 recipients of unrelated BMT was 8%(CI_{95} 0-28) as compared to 47%(CI_{95} 23-71) for 15 recipients of sibling BMT ($p < 0.002$). These patients had the same disease, received the same conditioning regimen, and were given the same posttransplant immunosuppression. The donor marrows were depleted with the same $\alpha\beta$TCR-specific monoclonal antibody (MoAb) + C′ (39,103). The major difference between the groups was the genetic relationship between donor and host. Of significant note is the fact that most of the CML patients receiving TCD HLA-matched sibling marrow could be salvaged following relapse by infusion of donor leukocytes (32). This suggests that while donor cells had a capacity to react against the host leukemia, the initial reaction was not sufficient to eliminate the leukemia. Aizawa et al. (104) evaluated the role of MHC and miHA antigens in experimental GVL and GVH reactivity against several radiation-induced leukemias. They reported that GVL reactivity could be consistently

Table 1 Immunological Factors Contributing to Leukemia Relapse Post-BMT

Susceptibility of leukemia to effector cells
Suboptimal reaction to GVL effector cells
Quantitative deficiency
Low killing efficiency
GVH-associated immune suppression
Premature establishment of donor:host tolerance
Mixed donor:host chimerism ("microchimerism")

induced after MHC-incompatible allogeneic BMT, whereas the intensity of the GVL effect induced in MHC-compatible donor:host combinations varied among different leukemias. The intensity of the GVL effect correlated with the induction of lethal GVHD (104).

The success in using delayed leukocyte infusions for the treatment of CML relative to acute leukemias suggests that myeloid leukemias may be highly susceptible to T-cell mediated GVL reactivity (105). A strong inverse correlation between GVHD and leukemia relapse in AML and CML has been reported in several clinical studies (2,29), and AML and CML exhibit the greatest risk of relapse following TCD BMT (29,30,106). Korngold et al. (107) observed a syngeneic GVL response mediated by both $CD4^+$ and $CD8^+$ T-cells in an experimental model of myeloid leukemia. This supports the expression of a leukemia-specific antigen(s) on the myeloid leukemia cell line, which apparently involves both MHC class I and II restricted peptides, since both $CD4^+$ and $CD8^+$ T-cells are activated. In the context of allogeneic MHC-matched BMT, the authors speculate that miHA-specific $CD4^+$ T cells might provide help to leukemia-specific $CD4^+$ and $CD8^+$ GVL effector cells. Thus, in this experimental model, both the leukemia and the immunogenetic relationship between donor and host affected the nature and number of cells contributing to the GVL reaction. Only donor $CD4^+$ T-cells mediated a GVL effect without induction of clinically evident GVHD in an MHC-matched allogeneic combination (107).

While evaluating the response of normal donor lymphocytes against allogeneic leukemia cells using limiting dilution techniques, Delain and colleagues (108) reported considerable variability of CTL precursor frequency. The variability appeared to depend upon the leukemic population itself, since the CTL frequency was comparable among the normal allogeneic donors tested for each leukemia. There was a strong correlation between the proliferative response of alloactivated lymphocytes and the percentage of leukemia cells expressing class II HLA-DR molecules, and anti-class II MHC MoAb inhibited lymphocyte proliferation in mixed lymphocyte-tumor cells cultures (108). These data suggest that allogeneic T cells may not mount an effective T-cell response against DR^- leukemia. Alloreactive CTL may be induced but not clonally expanded in the absence of sufficient allo-class II-induced T-cell help. That is, the allospecific GVL response may not be absent but suboptimal.

Sondel and colleagues have evaluated human lymphocytes for antileukemic reactivity using an in vitro system (45). Although it was often difficult to detect T cells from leukemia patients in remission that specifically recognized their autologous leukemia, T cells that preferentially recognized allogeneic leukemia cells but not normal lymphoblasts from the same patient could be readily detected. These techniques were applied to allogeneic CML cells known to express a leukemia specific protein, the p210 BCR-ABL fusion protein controlled by the Ph^1 chromosome, in an attempt to determine whether leukemia-specific T cells are generated in an allogeneic setting (109). Allogeneic $CD3^+$ T-cell clones (predominantly $CD4^+$) that mediated selective cytotoxicity of Ph^{1+} leukemic cells were isolated; however, with prolonged culture, the clones began to kill Ph^{1-} B-cell lines from the same CML patient, indicating that the T-cell clones were selectively, not exclusively, lytic for Ph^{1+} cells (109). These investigators speculated that adhesion structures on the Ph^{1+} CML cells initially allowed for better interactions with CTL clones, resulting in selective killing as compared to Ph^{1-} cells, but that the CTL function was subsequently qualitatively or quantitatively modified to permit killing of both Ph^{1+} and Ph^{1-} target cells (109). These experiments suggest that even when a leukemia-specific peptide (such as the BCR-ABL fusion protein) is expressed, T cells generated in an allogeneic setting may be allospecific and leukemia-preferential rather than exclusively leukemia-specific.

van der Harst and colleagues (49) evaluated the antileukemic reactivity of miHA-specific CTL against circulating lymphocytic and myeloid leukemia cells. Although miHA specificities HA-1 through HA-5 and H-Y were present, leukemic cells of lymphoid origin were found to be less susceptible to lysis by miHA-specific CTLs and clones when compared to IL-2 stimulated normal lymphocytes. The mechanism responsible for the decreased susceptibility to lysis appeared to be impaired expression of the LFA-1 adhesion molecule, since expression of the HLA restriction element (HLA-A2) on leukemic blasts was normal (49).

Adhesion molecules are critical for efficient CTL:target-cell interactions (110). Expression or induction of adhesion molecules such as LFA-1/ICAM-1 or LFA-3/CD2 can enhance the susceptibility of leukemia or lymphoma cells to cell mediated lysis (111,112). Oblakowski et al. (113) showed that MHC-unrestricted $CD2^+$ LAK cells are able to preferentially inhibit the growth of leukemic myeloblasts, in part because of the differential expression of CD54 adhesion molecules by normal and malignant myeloid cells. Furthermore, erythrocytes that express LFA-3, the ligand for CD2, competitively inhibit killing of normal but not malignant cells. Thus, some antileukemia effector cells, and possibly GVL reactive cells, may not be specific for malignant cells but mediate preferential lysis. The absence of essential adhesion molecules on the tumor cells may limit GVL reactivity. Immunoregulatory cytokines, such as IFN-α, which is often used in conjunction with delayed leukocyte infusions (31–35), may upregulate the expression of important adhesion molecules, thereby augmenting the GVL effect (105).

Perreault and colleagues (114) used mouse models to examine the expression of miHA by normal and neoplastic cells of lymphoid and myeloid lineage to determine if they could trigger lysis by CTL. Cell-mediated lympholysis assays showed that mouse leukemia cells of both lymphoid and myeloid lineages were sensitive to CTL directed against "immunodominant" but not "immunorecessive" miHA. At a molecular level, leukemic cells were found to express only immunodominant miHA and to have decreased density of MHC class I–restricting elements. In vivo resistance to leukemia correlated with susceptibility of the leukemia cells to miHA-specific CTL in vitro. Thus, some but not all miHA can serve as appropriate targets for antileukemia reactivity. Minor histocompatibility antigens are known to be hierarchical (115,116), and immunodominant miHAs have been identified (116,117). The biological basis for immunodominant and immunorecessive miHAs is not known but may relate to peptide competition for presentation by MHC molecules. The absence of a sufficient number of "dominant" miHA or their restricting elements could limit GVL reactivity.

D. Principle #4: GVL Effector Cells Are Subject to Immunoregulatory Control

GVL effector cells, like all immunocompetent cells, are subject to both positive and negative immunoregulatory control mechanisms. Activation and clonal expansion of $CD8^+$ CTL precursors capable of recognizing leukemia-specific or miHA antigens requires both antigen-presenting cells and T-cell help. Optimum immunological reactivity may occur only when both $CD4^+$ and $CD8^+$ T cells are activated. Absence of one component or the other may result in diminished reactivity. T-helper-independent CTL have been described, but they also require appropriate presentation of antigen by regulatory ("accessory") cells for activation.

GVHD is associated with severe immunodeficiency and perturbation of T-cell repertoire development (75,118). In murine models of BMT, potent regulatory cells that suppress T-cell responses are prominent in the early post-BMT period and are accentuated in the setting of GVHD (119–121). These cells are dependent upon γ-IFN (122) and induce macrophages to secrete tumor necrosis factor-α (TNF-α) as part of a regulatory circuit central to GVHD pathophysiology (100). They appear to be similar to "classical" natural suppressor (NS) cells that are important in hematopoietic regulation (123,124). NS cells consist of hematopoietic stem cells (125) as well as $\alpha\beta TCR^+$ $CD4^-$ $CD8^-$ or "double negative" (DN) T cells (126) and may also express NK markers (127). Down regulation of immune cells has significant implications for survival after allogeneic BMT for the treatment of leukemia if GVL reactivity is impaired and may account in part for the paradoxical situation in which patients relapse despite severe acute GVHD. The effect of GVH-induced immunosuppression on GVL reactivity has received little attention.

Self-tolerance is a central tenant of immunology. In the context of allogeneic BMT, development of mutual tolerance is beneficial. However, the onset of donor: host tolerance may increase the risk of relapse by allowing host leukemia cells to persist. The factors that determine when and whether tolerance develops after allogeneic BMT in humans are not known, but studies in animal models suggest that T-cell depletion may accelerate the development of tolerance (128).

Induction of tolerance to the host is not always accompanied by loss of GVL reactivity. For example, Sykes and colleagues (26,129,130) used high-dose IL-2, with and without TCD syngeneic BMT, to prevent GVHD without loss of GVL reactivity in an MHC-mismatched donor:host combination. The mechanism appears to be selective inhibition of donor $CD4^+$ T cells (26,130). $CD8^+$ T cells, which mediate the GVL effect, do not cause GVHD and are not inhibited by IL-2 treatment. The precise mechanism for selective inhibition of CD4-mediated GVHD is not known, but $CD3^+$ $CD4^-$ $CD8^-$ T-cells may play a role (131). The ability of IL-2, an important factor in clonal expansion of alloactivated T cells, to induce tolerance seems paradoxical, but the timing of IL-2 administration is critical, since it must be given within the first 5 days post-BMT; administration at later times exacerbates GVHD (129,130).

We have observed that early treatment with high-dose IL-2 treatment augments the activity of NS-like cells in MHC-matched B10.BR → AKR chimeras (R. Truitt, unpublished data). These cells appear to affect naive T cells preferentially as compared to alloactivated T cells. Early administration of IL-2 may induce NS-like activity before GVH-reactive T cells manifest any damage. If T cells are activated, then NS activity may be perturbed, leading to a state of immune deficiency, as reported by Wall and Sheehan (100). Thus, NS cells are capable of preventing as well as contributing to the GVH syndrome. It is also worth noting that the failure of donor leukocytes to cause GVHD when infused 21 days after allogeneic BMT in our murine model (132,133) coincides with the disappearance of NS activity in the spleens of the recipients (B. Johnson, unpublished data). Furthermore, NS activity is stabilized after in vivo administration of anti-CD3 $F(ab')_2$ MoAb to prevent GVHD in B10.BR → AKR chimeras (134). Thus, data from several experimental models suggest that perturbation of NS activity post-BMT may contribute to GVHD, while enhancement or stabilization of activity may prevent GVHD.

We have shown, in a murine model of MHC-matched BMT, that complete donor T-cell engraftment is necessary for an effective GVL reaction but also increases the risk of GVHD (14,128). In these animal studies, mixed donor:host T-cell chimerism was associated with decreased GVHD and increased susceptibility to leukemia. TCD increases the risk of mixed chimerism in both humans (135–137) and mice (15,22,128). Lawler et al. (135) reported that the proportion of patients with mixed chimerism can exceed 80% after TCD BMT. Mackinnon et al. (138) looked at the relationship between mixed T-cell chimerism and minimal residual disease in 32 CML patients after TCD BMT. At a median follow-up of 12 months, molecular evidence of minimal residual disease was present in 82% (18/22) of patients with mixed T-cell chimerism but only 30% (3/10) of patients with full donor T-cell chimerism. Of patients with mixed chimerism, 9 had relapsed at 12 months as compared to only 1 patient with full donor chimerism.

The importance of donor cells in maintaining a remission after BMT is evident in CML patients who relapsed posttransplant and were subsequently infused with donor leukocytes (31–35,105). Repeated infusions of donor leukocytes induced complete hematologic, cytogenetic, and molecular remissions. None of the patients had developed severe GVHD prior to relapse, and all were predominantly host chimeras. Host-type hematopoietic cells disappeared after the donor leukocyte infusions, and the patients remained in complete remission for as long as followed. The precise mechanism by which leukemia is eradicated by delayed infusion of donor leukocytes is not known (105). Both quantitative and qualitative factors may have limited the initial GVL reactivity, resulting in relapse. Alternatively, immunoregulatory mechanisms mediating donor:host tolerance may have been induced before all leukemia cells are destroyed. An initial suboptimal GVL response may be due to premature development of donor:host tolerance, active immunosuppression, too few GVL effector cells, or a combination of these and other unidentified mechanisms.

III. EXPERIMENTAL APPROACHES TO THE SEPARATION OF GVL AND GVH REACTIVITY

Reviewed in this section are some of the recent experimental strategies used in our laboratory to minimize GVHD without loss of GVL reactivity in two murine models: B10.BR ($H\text{-}2^k$) donor cells into AKR ($H\text{-}2^k$) hosts, a model of MHC-matched BMT that simulates the use of an HLA-matched unrelated donor in which there are multiple miHA disparities and a positive MLR response in the GVH direction, and SJL ($H\text{-}2^s$) donor cells into $(SJLxAKR)F_1$ ($H\text{-}2^{s/k}$) hosts, a model of single haplotype mismatched BMT.

A. Depletion of Immunocompetent Donor Cells Prior to BMT

1. Relative Contributions of CD4⁺ and CD8⁺ T Cells to GVHD and GVL Reactivity

In MHC-matched B10.BR → AKR chimeras the incidence and intensity of GVHD is directly related to the concentration of $CD4^+$ T-cells in the marrow inoculum (Fig. 2). Increasing the number of $CD4^+$ while keeping the $CD8^+$ cells constant results in rapid loss of body weight and early death from GVHD. Change in body weight is an objective indicator of GVH status in murine models of BMT (139). Complete CD4 depletion allows for the infusion of as many as 50 × 10^6 donor spleen cells without GVH-associated mortality (R. Truitt, unpublished data). In earlier studies, we had shown that $CD8^+$T cells are the proximal mediators of GVL reactivity in this donor:host combination (6) and that optimum GVL reactivity required both $CD4^+$ and $CD8^+$ T-cells (15). To examine this further, irradiated recipients were given BM plus escalating numbers of spleen cells containing only $CD8^+$ T cells (the donor mice were depleted of $CD4^+$ cells using MoAb in vivo).

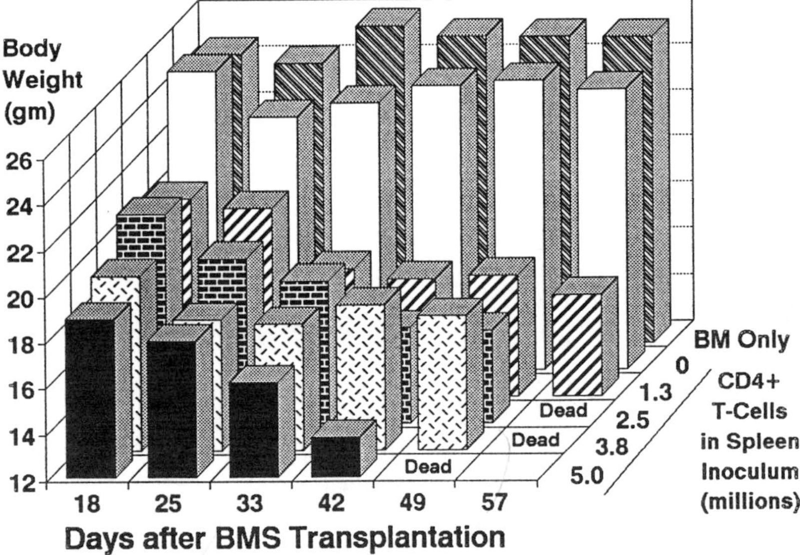

Figure 2 Effect of $CD4^+$ T-cells on GVL/GVH reactivity in MHC-matched B10.BR → AKR chimeras. Normal and CD4TCD spleen cells were mixed in various proportions to adjust the number of donor $CD4^+$ cells to that shown and injected IV into lethally irradiated (11 Gy TBI) AKR hosts. The total number of BM (10^7) and spleen cells transplanted (25 × 10^6) as well as the $CD8^+$ T-cell content (5 × 10^6) remained constant. Six mice in each group were transplanted, then challenged with 10,000 AKR-leukemia cells on day +4. Incidence and intensity of GVHD, as indicated by body weight loss and survival, was directly related to the number of $CD4^+$ T-cells given. GVL reactivity was observed in all groups except the group receiving CD4TCD spleen cells (0 $CD4^+$) in which 4 of 6 mice died from leukemia. BMO controls were not given leukemia.

Despite a 10-fold increase in transplanted CD8$^+$ T cells over our previous study (15), there was not increase in leukemia-free survival (R. Truitt, unpublished data). The magnitude of CD8$^+$ and NK mediated GVL effect was limited, and CD4$^+$ help was required to achieve maximal GVL reactivity after transplantation of MHC-matched cells. GVL reactivity can be detected in recipients of CD4TCD cells as well as pan-T-cell deficient BM only when the leukemia burden is minimal. Increasing the genetic disparity between donor and host (e.g., a haplotype mismatch in the GVH direction) can compensate for suboptimal T-cell content of the marrow graft (R. Truitt, unpublished data), but at an increased risk of GVHD.

In the B10.BR → AKR model of matched unrelated BMT, naive CD8$^+$ B10.BR cells do not cause significant GVH-associated mortality except in the presence of CD4$^+$ T-cells (15). However, CD8$^+$ T cells sensitized to host alloantigens mediate lethal GVHD even in the absence of CD4$^+$ help (Fig. 3). Presumably, presensitization of the donor to host alloantigen results in activation and expansion of CD8$^+$ T-cell clones capable of causing lethal GVHD. We have shown at a clonal level that some but not all CD8$^+$ CTL are capable of causing lethal GVHD in this model (6,140). The kinetics of mortality and GVH-associated loss of body weight following transplantation of CD4$^-$ CD8$^+$ spleen cells, however, is distinctly different from that seen with CD4$^+$ CD8$^-$ cells (data not shown). In this model, the early phase of body weight loss and mortality appears to be CD4-mediated, while later phases are CD8-mediated. This is supported by the results of studies using anti-CD8 and anti-CD4 MoAb to deplete donor cells in vivo post-BMT (see Figs. 7B and 7C below).

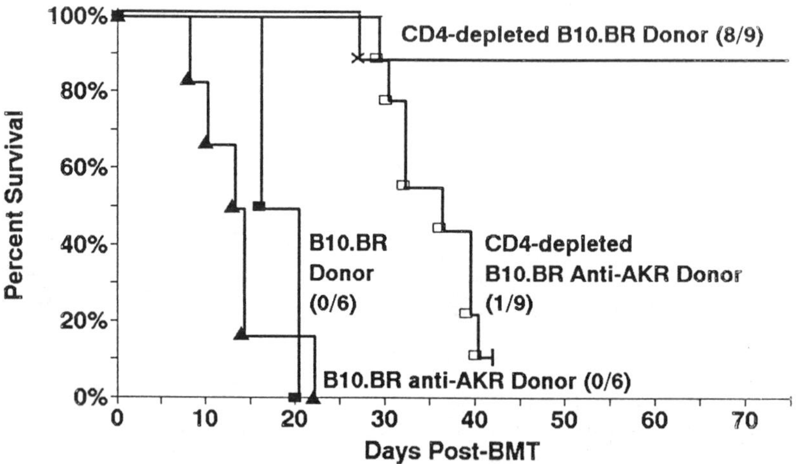

Figure 3 Donor CD8$^+$ T-cells do not cause lethal GVHD in MHC-matched B10.BR→AKR chimeras in the absence of CD4$^+$ help unless presensitized to host alloantigens. Irradiated (9 Gy) AKR hosts were given 10^7 BM plus 30 × 10^6 spleen cells from naive B10.BR donors (■, ×) or donors presensitized to host alloantigens by two weekly injections of AKR spleen cells IP (days −14 and −8) (▲, □). For depletion of CD4$^+$ T-cells, donor mice were injected with anti-CD4 ascites MoAb on days −6, −4 and −2 (×, □). The proportion of mice alive at termination of the experiment is shown in parenthesis.

2. Manipulation of CD4$^+$ T-Cell Subsets to Prevent GVHD Without Loss of the GVL Effect

During studies on the role of CD4$^+$ T cells in GVHD, we serendipitously observed that bone marrow plus added spleen (BMS) cells taken from donors that had been depleted of CD4$^+$ T-cells, then allowed to repopulate their spleens with newly immigrating thymocytes failed to cause GVHD when transplanted into susceptible hosts (25). To examine this phenomenon further, B10.BR donors were depleted of peripheral CD4 cells using anti-CD4 MoAb in vivo (clone GK-1.5) and allowed to repopulate. Their BM and spleens were then collected and processed for transplantation into irradiated AKR recipients ("repopulated CD4"). As controls, host mice were given donor cells completely depleted of CD4$^+$ cells ("CD4TCD control"; 0.2% CD4$^+$) or a mixture of CD4TCD BMS cells plus normal B10.BR BMS cells ("control mixture") that contained the same number of CD4$^+$ (7%) and CD8$^+$ (11%) cells as the repopulated experimental group. Experimental and control mice were challenged with 1000 AKR-leukemia cells 4 days after transplant to assess their GVL reactivity. Survival results are shown in Fig. 4. GVHD failed to develop after transplantation of CD4TCD BMS cells, and most of the recipients died with progressive leukemia. In contrast, there was a significant ($p = 0.03$) improvement in GVH- and leukemia-free survival when CD4-repopulated BMS cells were given (Fig. 4). The majority of AKR hosts given the control mixture of BMS cells also survived leukemia-free, but they developed clinically evident GVHD. The lack of GVHD in the experimental group was indicated by decreased body weight loss (data not shown), the absence of GVH-associated splenic atrophy (Fig. 5A), and a significant restoration of B-cell lymphopoiesis in comparison to mice given comparable numbers of "normal" CD4$^+$ T-cells (Fig. 5B). Similar results were observed with donors depleted of Thy-1.2$^+$ T cells and allowed to repopulate for 10 days (R. Truitt, unpublished data).

The biological basis for this phenomenon is not clear. CD4$^+$ cells that have recently emigrated from the thymus and repopulated peripheral lymphoid tissues may be anergic or highly susceptible to peripheral tolerance, although Fathman and colleagues (141) found that recent thymic emigrant CD4$^+$ T cells were able to mediate GVH reactivity against miHA. Data from other laboratories indicate a skewing of Th1 and Th2 subsets following so-called "partial" CD4 depletion (142,143). In vivo depletion and repopulation of CD4$^+$ cells may result in the predominance of CD4 T-cells with "altered" cytokine profiles in peripheral lymphoid tissues, since newly emigrating CD4$^+$ thymocytes appear to be the Th0 type (144). The spectrum of cytokines secreted by alloactivated CD4$^+$ T cells in vivo may affect GVH reactivity. For example, Fowler et al. (27) have shown that treatment of the donor with IL-4 and IL-2 can activate Th2-type CD4$^+$ T cells that suppress lethal GVHD. Alternatively, newly emigrating CD4$^+$ T-cells may not recognize alloantigens as efficiently as those that have undergone "peripheral selection." This is supported by preliminary studies in our laboratory indicating a decreased response in mixed lymphocyte reaction (MLR) assays after CD4-depletion and repopulation (C. McCabe, unpublished results). Regardless of the mechanism, manipulation of CD4$^+$ T cell subsets offers a promising new approach for controlling or limiting GVH reactivity, perhaps without loss of the GVL effect (145).

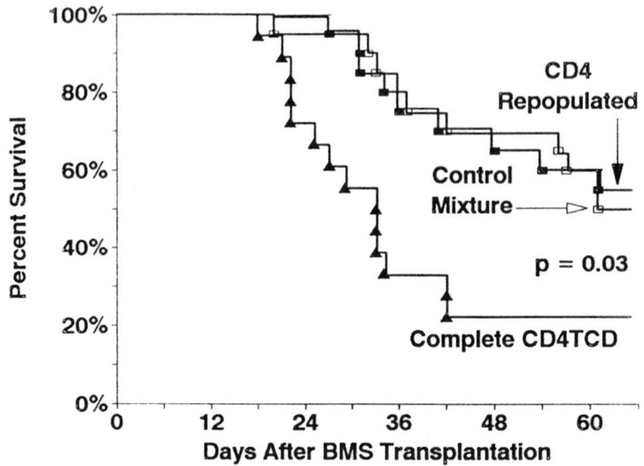

Figure 4 GVL reactivity is retained in the absence of clinical GVHD when $CD4^+$ T-cells repopulating the donor (B10.BR) spleen after complete CD4-depletion are transplanted into AKR hosts. Donor B10.BR mice were completely depleted with anti-CD4 MoAb, then allowed to repopulate their peripheral tissues with $CD4^+$ T cells newly emigrating from the thymus. At the time of donor tissue collection, the spleens of CD4-depleted/repopulated donors contained 7% $CD4^+$ and 11% $CD8^+$ T-cells. Irradiated AKR hosts (9 Gy) were transplanted with 10^7 BM plus 25×10^6 spleen cells from the CD4-repopulated B10.BR donors on day 0 ($n = 20$). A GVH-negative control group (Complete CD4TCD; $n = 18$) received BMS cells from B10.BR donors that were completely depleted of $CD4^+$ T cells but not allowed time to repopulate (0.2% $CD4^+$ cells). A GVH-positive control group (control mixture; $n = 20$) received a mixture of BM plus spleen cells from normal B10.BR donors and completely CD4-depleted donors that was mixed in proportions matching the CD4 content of the CD4-repopulated group (i.e., 7% $CD4^+$ and 11% $CD8^+$). CD4 T-cells in this group, however, were not recent thymic emigrants. Deaths in the complete CD4TCD group were due to leukemia, and deaths in the group given the control mixture were attributed to GVHD. Leukemia-free survival was significantly higher ($p = 0.03$) for the CD4-repopulated groups as compared to chimeras given completely CD4TCD cells, but some deaths were due to leukemia progression. This suggests that while GVL reactivity persisted in the absence of clinical GVHD, it may have been quantitatively diminished, perhaps as a result of the loss of T-cell help for $CD8^+$ and NK effector cells.

3. Role of NK Cells in GVH and GVL Reactivity

T cells are not the only cells which contribute to GVHD. We have used an allele specific MoAb (anti-NK-1.1) to show that donor NK cells contribute to both GVH (Table 2) and GVL (Table 3) reactions in B10.BR → AKR chimeras. NK depletion had a beneficial effect on GVHD and survival, but it was dependent on the intensity of the GVH reaction (Table 2). There was no significant effect of donor NK depletion on survival when GVHD was severe in the MHC-matched B10.BR → AKR combination (Table 2) or when full MHC-mismatched donor cells were transplanted (22). However, as shown in Table 2, donor NK depletion increased survival of AKR hosts with mild-to-moderate GVHD. Since depletion of $CD4^+$ donor T cells prior to transplant results in complete elimination of clinical GVHD in B10.BR → AKR

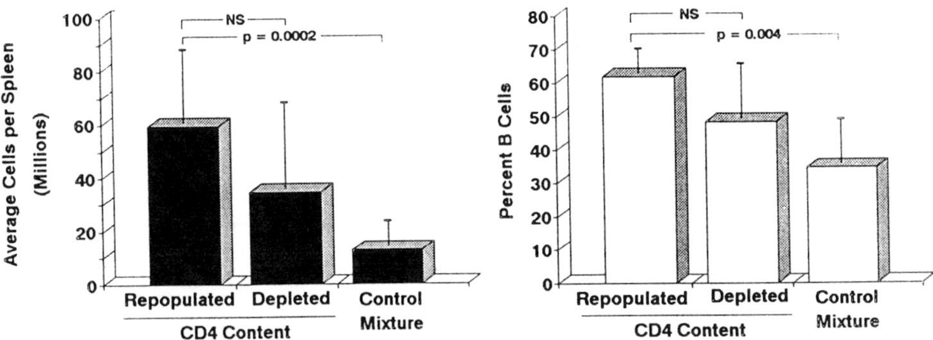

Figure 5 Splenic atrophy with few B cells is indicative of GVHD in B10.BR → AKR chimeras (control mixture), but spleens from AKR recipients of CD4-depleted/repopulated B10.BR BMS cells (from Fig. 4) were significantly larger and had a significantly higher B-cell content (CD4-repopulated). Their spleens were not different from those of the GVH-negative control group (CD4-depleted). Number of spleens analyzed: CD4 repopulated = 8; CD4-depleted = 4; control mixture = 10.

chimeras, NK depletion provided no additional benefit when combined with CD4 depletion (22). Pretransplant depletion of either donor $CD8^+$ cells or donor NK-1.1^+ cells reduced GVH-associated mortality, but the use of both CD8 and NK depletion offered no improvement over either alone (22). However, in contrast to CD8 depletion, donor NK depletion did not compromise the rapid and complete establishment of donor T-cell chimerism nor the ability of chimeras to mount an effective GVL reaction when challenged at 21 days post-BMT. These observations

Table 2 In Vivo Depletion with Anti-NK-1.1 MoAb Prevents GVH-Related Mortality in B10.BR → AKR Chimeras

Tissue[a]	Anti-NK-1.1 treated[b]	*N*	Mortality at 70 days	Median survival time, days	*P* value[c]
BM	No	20	5%	>70	NS
BM	Yes	20	0%	>70	
BMS-5	No	42	44%	>70	0.06
BMS-5	Yes	42	22%	>70	
BMS-10	No	48	57%	45	0.013
BMS-10	Yes	48	33%	>70	
BMS-20	No	23	76%	39	NS
BMS-20	Yes	23	71%	33	

[a]Irradiated AKR hosts (9 Gy) were given BM alone or with 5, 10 or 20 × 10^6 spleen cells (BMS) from MHC-matched B10.BR donors.
[b]Both donors and transplanted hosts were given anti-NK-1.1 MoAb in vivo (22).
[c]In comparison to untreated chimeras using log rank test for survival curves.
Source: Ref. 22.

Table 3 Donor NK-1.1$^+$ Cells Contribute to Early but not Late Phases of GVL Reactivity in B10.BR → AKR Chimeras

BMS-10 chimeras[a]	Leukemia challenge	Day	% Survival to 60 days, # chimeras	P value[b]
Untreated	150–900	3	80% (12/15)	0.04
NK-depleted	150–900	3	13% (2/15)	
Untreated[c]	50,000	21	50% (6/12)[d]	0.02
NK-depleted[c]	50,000	21	92% (13/14)	

[a]Irradiated AKR hosts were given BM plus 10 × 10^6 spleen cells from untreated B10.BR donors or from donor mice depleted of NK-1.1$^+$ cells with MoAb prior to transplantation, then challenged with AKR-leukemia on the day indicated.
[b]*P* value calculated by chi-square analysis.
[c]Reported in Ref. 22.
[d]Deaths attributed to GVHD, not leukemia.

support the hypothesis of a three-compartment model of GVHD in the B10.BR → AKR donor:host combination, involving CD4$^+$, CD8$^+$, and NK-1.1$^+$ cells. Ferrara et al. (146) have proposed a two-compartment CD8 → NK model in which CD4$^+$ T cells play a minimal role. Immunogenetic relationships (e.g., presence or absence of a strong CD4-activation signal such as Mls-1^a or MHC class II) apparently dictate the relative importance of CD4$^+$ and CD8$^+$ T cells in different donor-host combinations.

Our initial report indicated that depletion of NK cells did not adversely affect GVL reactivity (22). However, the results of subsequent experiments indicate that NK cells are involved in early GVL reactivity, while later phases of GVL reactivity are T cell–dominated (Table 3). MHC-matched B10.BR → AKR chimeras were challenged with AKR leukemia cells at 3 and 21 days after transplantation of NK-depleted BMS cells to determine whether GVL reactivity was compromised (Table 3). The majority of chimeras challenged with a low dose of AKR leukemia (150 to 900 cells) 3 days after transplantation of NK-depleted BMS cells relapsed, whereas 80% of the nondepleted chimeras survived leukemia-free (p = 0.04). In contrast, 92% of the B10.BR → AKR chimeras given NK-depleted donor cells survived a supralethal challenge dose of 50,000 leukemia cells at 21 days posttransplant. The higher mortality rate (p = 0.02) in recipients of spleen cells from normal (non-NK-depleted) donors following leukemia challenge on day 21 was due to GVHD, not leukemia (Table 3). This is consistent with the data in Table 2 showing that NK cells contribute to GVH-associated mortality. Based on the results of these and other experiments, we speculate that NK cells contribute to the GVL effect early post-BMT, whereas T cells are more critical to the GVL effect at later times. A contribution of NK cells to early GVL reactivity was evident only when low numbers of T cells were transplanted (i.e., the GVL response is normally T-cell-dominated) and when the leukemia challenge dose was minimal (R. Truitt, unpublished data). These studies indicate that the GVL effect associated with allogeneic BMT is a dynamic immunological phenomenon in which the effector may change over time.

We have observed that GVH reactivity in a haplotype-mismatched P/F1 combination [SJL → (SJLxARK)F_1] was also dominated by $CD4^+$ T-cells (147). In leukemia-bearing F_1 hosts, transplantation of CD8-depleted donor cells resulted in a less intense GVH reaction but significant mortality (Fig. 6). On the other hand, CD4-depletion resulted in substantial long-term leukemia-free survival (Fig. 6). NK 1.1 depletion had no effect on GVHD and survival in this P → F_1 model (data not shown), perhaps because of the strong T-cell-dominated GVH reaction to MHC molecules encoded by the disparate haplotype.

The data described in this section indicate that it is possible to use selective depletion of T-cell subsets and NK cells to minimize GVHD without complete loss of GVL reactivity in both MHC-matched and haplotype mismatched settings. With the exception of the CD8-depletion studies of Champlin and colleagues (86) noted earlier, T-subset depletion has not been tested in the clinical setting. Given the disparate results obtained with various experimental models using different leukemias and donor:host combinations and the heterogeneity of the human patient population, there is a significant need for the development of reliable techniques to identify GVL and GVH effector cells prior to BMT.

B. Use of MoAbs in Vivo to Manipulate GVH Reactivity Post-BMT

1. Comparison of Anti-Thy1.2, Anti-CD8 and Anti-CD4 MoAbs Post-BMT for Prevention and Treatment of GVHD in MHC-Matched Chimeras

MoAbs can be used to induce donor:host tolerance in vivo (148). We initiated a series of studies comparing the efficacy of MoAbs with specificity for Thy-1.2^+ (clone 30-H12), $CD8^+$ (clone 2.43) and $CD4^+$ (clone GK 1.5) T-cells in the B10.BR → AKR model of MHC-matched BMT. All are rat IgG_{2b} antibodies that deplete T cells in vivo. Whole antibody was given as a single bolus injection IP on day 0 for GVH prevention or on day 8 for GVH treatment. The mice were observed for

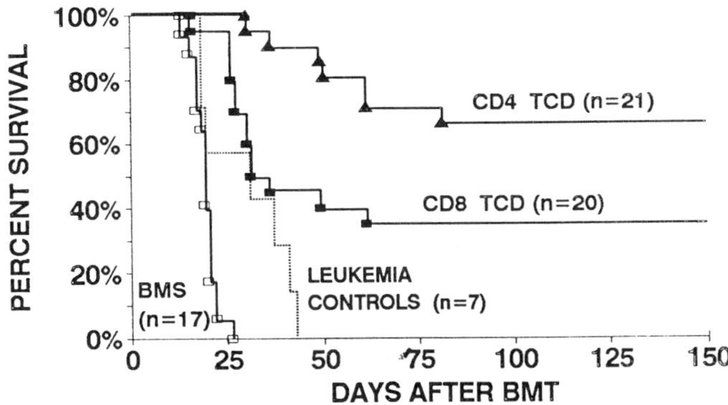

Figure 6 Effect of CD4 and CD8 T-cell depletion on GVL/GVH reactivity in a haplotype mismatched donor:host combination. Lethally irradiated (SJL × AKR)F_1 (H-$2^{s/k}$) hosts (11 Gy) were given 1000 AKR-leukemia cells on day −1, then transplanted with SJL (H-2^s) BM (10^7) and spleen cells (10^7) 1 day later. SJL donors were untreated (□, BMS) or depleted pretransplant of CD4 (▲) and CD8 (■) cells by injection of T-subset-specific MoAbs. Normal (SJL × AKR)F_1 mice were used as leukemia controls (dotted line).

clinical appearance, body weight change, and survival. The body weight results are summarized in Fig. 7. Loss of body weight is an objective and accurate indicator of GVH disease in these chimeras. Control AKR mice received BMS cells but no MoAb (BMS or GVH$^+$ controls) or donor BM without added spleen cells (BMO or GVH$^-$ controls). Untreated BMS controls show persistent body weight loss, leading ultimately to death of most chimeras, whereas BMO controls are GVH-free and survive long-term (control groups in Fig. 7A to C).

A single dose of anti-Thy1.2 MoAb effectively prevented clinical GVHD in B10.BR → AKR chimeras (Fig. 7A) as documented by the absence of body-weight loss in comparison to untreated BMS controls. Anti-CD8 MoAb (Fig. 7B) had a moderating effect on GVH-associated body-weight loss beyond the first 2 weeks posttransplant, but did not prevent all clinical symptoms. In contrast, anti-CD4 MoAb (Fig. 7C) prevented wasting and clinically evident GVHD during the first 15 days post-BMT, but GVHD rapidly developed in these mice subsequently. This suggests that early GVHD is CD4-mediated, while CD8 cells contribute significantly to GVHD at a later time in this model. None of the antibodies (anti-Thy1.2, anti-CD8, anti-CD4) were effective in the treatment of GVHD when given as a single injection on day 8, although more intense depletion therapy may be effective (B. Johnson, unpublished data).

Control and experimental mice from GVH-prevention experiments in Fig. 7 were randomly killed and their spleens collected for flow cytometric analysis between 40 and 45 days post-BMT. Important results are shown in Fig. 8. Lymphoid atrophy is characteristic of GVHD in this model (GVH$^+$ BMS Controls, Figure 8D). The spleens of mice treated with whole anti-Thy1.2 MoAb were not different from the GVH$^-$ BMO controls (cf. Fig. 8A and 8D). Treated mice appeared clinically healthy and showed positive body weight gain (Fig. 7A). In contrast, the spleens of chimeras given a single infusion of anti-CD8 and anti-CD4 MoAb (Fig. 8A) were smaller and barely distinguishable from those of GVH$^+$ controls (Fig. 8D). GVH reactivity is known to diminish B-cell lymphopoiesis (149), but the B-cell content of spleens from chimeras treated with anti-Thy1.2 MoAb was within the range of BMO controls (cf. Figs. 8C and 8F). The percentage of B cells in the spleens of chimeras treated with anti-CD8 and anti-CD4 MoAb was below that of BMO controls but above that of untreated BMS controls (cf. Figs. 8C and 8F). In a separate set of experiments, we observed that multiple infusions of anti-CD4 MoAb post-BMT was able to modulate GVHD, but anti-CD8 was less effective (B. Johnson, unpublished data).

In this experimental model, complete donor T-cell engraftment and elimination of residual host T cells (as well as any leukemia cells) is dependent on the presence of immunocompetent donor T cells in the transplant inoculum (14,15). In their absence, the mice become mixed T-cell chimeras (i.e., the proportion of donor T cells in the spleen is <0.8). Graft rejection is not a problem in this model because of minimal host-vs-graft reactivity. Persistent mixed chimerism is correlated with an increased risk of leukemia relapse (128). As shown in Fig. 8B, none of the chimeras treated with anti-Thy-1.2 MoAb and examined by flow cytometry analysis were fully donor-engrafted at 41 days posttransplant. The predominant T-cell population was of host origin, indicating that alloreactive T cells in the donor BMS inoculum had failed to eliminate residual host T cells in the sublethally irradiated recipients. Donor T-cell chimerism was complete or nearly complete in the majority of chime-

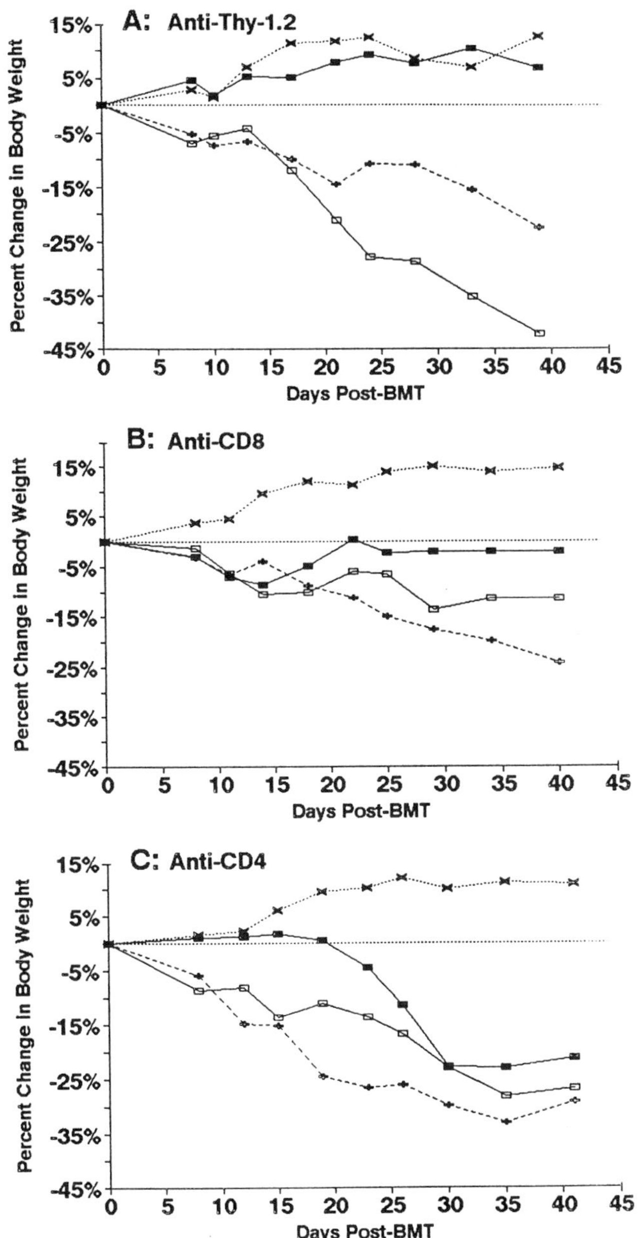

Figure 7 Use of T-cell-specific MoAbs to modulate GVH reactivity in vivo following MHC-matched BMT. Irradiated AKR hosts (9 Gy) were transplanted with B10.BR 10^7 BM only (×) or BM plus 20 × 10^6 spleen cells (+, □, ■) on day 0 and randomized to receive no further treatment or T-cell-specific MoAb posttransplant. Untreated GVH-negative (BM only) (×) and GVH-positive (BMS cells) (+) controls were included in each experiment. Experimental mice were given a single infusion of 100 μL of ascites MoAb for GVH prevention on day 0 (■) or for GVH treatment on day +8 (□). Experimental chimeras were treated with anti-Thy-1.2 MoAb in panel A, anti-CD8 MoAb in panel B, and anti-CD4 MoAb in panel C. Data are presented as the average percent body weight change for 3 to 6 chimeras per group. GVHD is indicated by a decline in body weight with time.

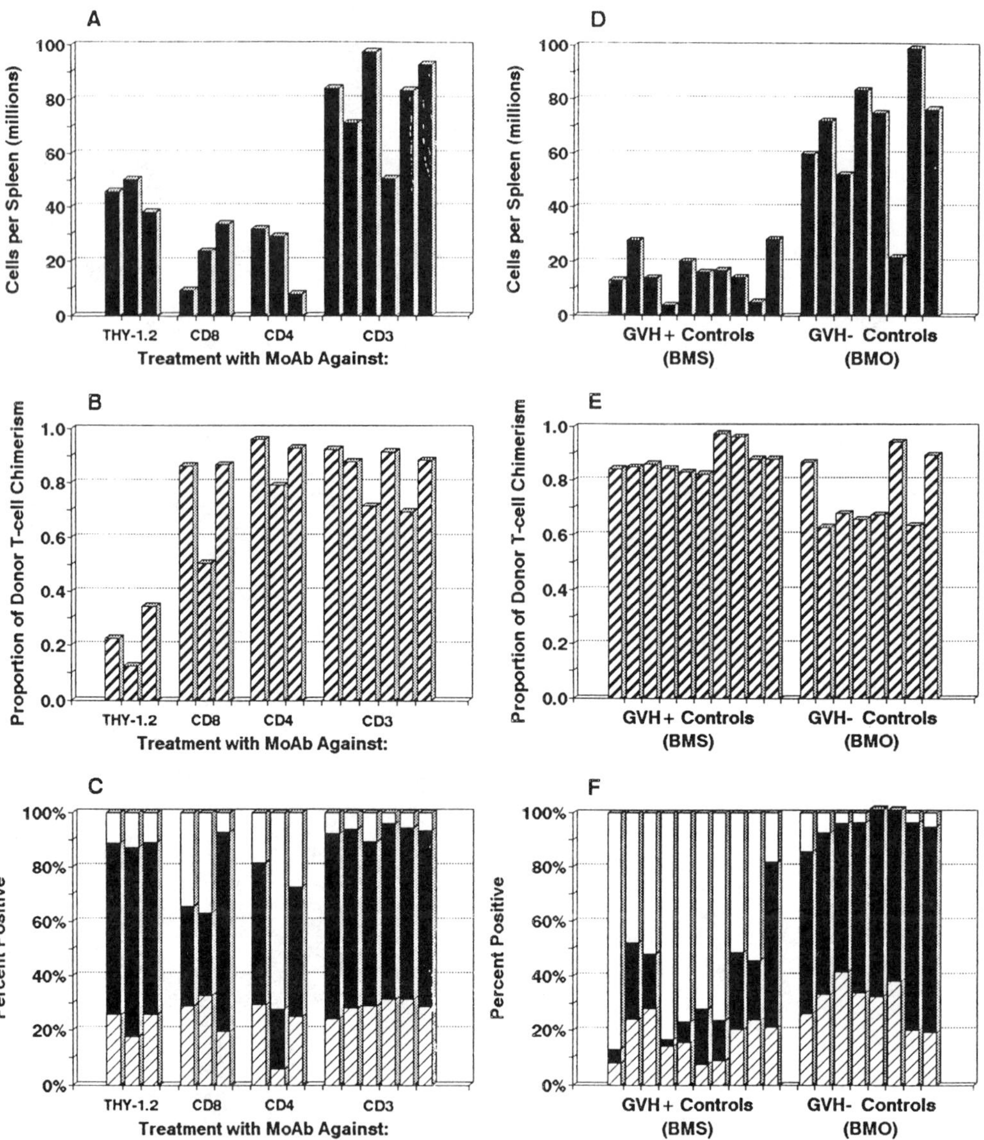

Figure 8 Immune recovery and T-cell chimerism in B10.BR → AKR chimeras treated post-BMT with MoAb for GVH prophylaxis. Chimeras given MoAb on day 0 in Fig. 7 were killed 40 to 45 days posttransplant and their spleens examined by flow cytometry. For comparison, data on similar chimeras treated with anti-CD3 $F(ab')_2$ MoAb fragments (days 0–8 in Fig. 10) are included. Data for experimental (antibody-treated) chimeras are presented in panels A to C; data for untreated GVH-negative (BMO) and GVH-positive (BMS) controls are shown in panels D to F. Each bar represents an individual chimera. Panels A and D: Viable nucleated cells per spleen. Panels B and E: Proportion of donor T-cells in the spleen calculated using the formula % Thy-1.2$^+$/(Thy-1.2$^+$ + Thy-1.1$^+$). Donor T-cell proportions >0.8 are considered evidence of "complete" T-cell engraftment based on the lower 99% confidence interval for normal B10.BR spleens (14). Panels C and F: Flow cytometric analysis of chimeric spleens for T-cells (CD4$^+$ + CD8$^+$) (striped bars), B-cells (Ly5$^+$) (solid bars), and "other" cells (not T- or B-cells) (open bars). T-cell data includes both donor (Thy-1.2$^+$) and host (Thy-1.1$^+$) cells in the proportion indicated in panels B and E.

ras treated with anti-CD8 or anti-CD4 MoAb, indicating that some alloreactive cells persisted after antibody treatment. More extensive depletion with anti-CD4 or anti-CD8 MoAb decreases GVHD, but increases the risk of mixed chimerism and susceptibility to leukemia (B. Johnson, unpublished data).

Collectively, the data presented in Fig. 7 and 8 indicate that some GVH reactivity persisted in anti-CD8 and anti-CD4 treated chimeras but not in mice treated with anti-Thy1.2 antibody. The kinetics of GVHD onset, prevention or resolution appear to differ with the type and specificity of antibody used. Studies on the effect of T-subset depletion posttransplant on GVL reactivity are in progress.

2. Effect of Anti-CD3 F(ab′)$_2$ Fragments on Prevention and Treatment of GVHD in MHC-Matched Chimeras

In addition to the antibodies described above, we evaluated a CD3-specific MoAb (clone 145 2C11) for its ability to prevent and treat GVHD in MHC-matched B10.BR → AKR chimeras. Clone 145 2C11 produces a hamster IgG which recognizes the ϵ-chain of the murine TCR complex (150) and was chosen on the basis of reports by others that it prevents GVHD in MHC-mismatched chimeras (20). Intact anti-CD3 IgG induces a rapid and lethal acute syndrome in recipients of T-replete BMT (134), which is identical to the anti-CD3-induced "cytokine syndrome" described in normal mice (151). Use of anti-CD3 F(ab′)$_2$ fragments eliminates the cytokine syndrome (152), induces a selective T-helper dysfunction in vivo (153), and modulates GVHD after MHC-mismatched murine BMT (20). Therefore, only nonmitogenic F(ab′)$_2$ fragments of the anti-CD3 MoAb were used in these studies. No one has evaluated anti-CD3 F(ab′)$_2$ antibody in an MHC-matched BMT model for its effect on GVL reactivity.

Irradiated AKR hosts were transplanted with BM plus spleen cells (BMS) from B10.BR donors and given F(ab′)$_2$ fragments between days 0 and 8 for GVH-prophylaxis and days 8 and 16 for GVH therapy. Body weight gain/loss was used as an objective indicator of GVH status, as shown in Fig. 9. Clinical symptoms of GVHD did not develop in chimeras treated with anti-CD3 F(ab′)$_2$ MoAb prophylactically, and their body weight gain paralleled that of the BM controls during the first 20 to 25 days. The effects of anti-CD3 F(ab′)$_2$ MoAb were dose-dependent (data not shown). When given in sufficient quantity, the antibody completely abrogated clinical symptoms of GVHD and resulted in long-term GVH-free survival (134). Chimeras treated with F(ab′)$_2$ fragments for prevention of GVH had normal-sized spleens with normal B-cell content and were complete donor T-cell chimeras when killed (Fig. 8A–C). Treated chimeras often could not be distinguished from BM controls (Fig. 8D–F). Untreated BMS controls wasted away with debilitating and ultimately fatal GVHD (Figs. 8D–F and 9). The antibody-treated chimeras consistently showed a transient decline in body weight approximately 25 to 40 days post-BMT (Fig. 9). We attributed this to the effects of secondary GVH effector cells (probably alloactivated CD8$^+$ CTL, although this remains to be proven). The decline in body weight during this period was reproducible but did not occur when antibody treatment was extended into the third or fourth week post-BMT (134).

To determine whether anti-CD3 F(ab′)$_2$ antibody could stop and/or reverse an ongoing GVH reaction, antibody treatment was not started until 8 days post-BMT (50 μg of antibody every other day [qe2d] between days 8 to 16) (Fig. 9). Chimeras in which administration of the antibody was delayed for 8 days showed a decline in

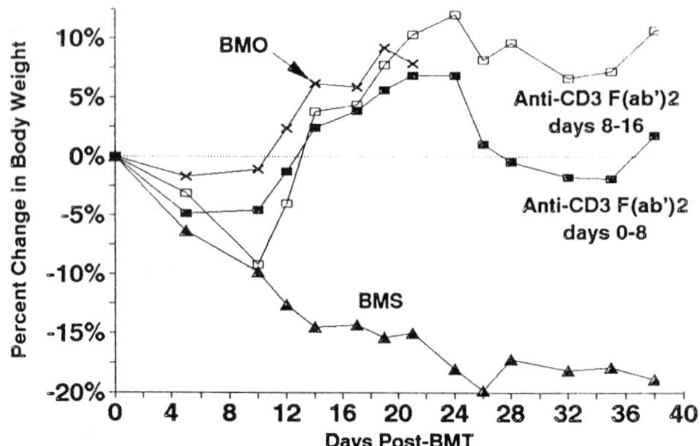

Figure 9 Anti-CD3 F(ab$'$)$_2$ MoAb can be used in vivo to prevent as well as treat established GVHD following MHC-matched allogeneic BMT. Irradiated AKR hosts (9 Gy) were given 10^7 BM only or BM plus 20 $\times$ 10^6 spleen cells from normal MHC-matched B10.BR donors on day 0, then randomized to receive no further treatment ($\times$, ▲) or 50 μg of anti-CD3 F(ab$'$)$_2$ MoAB (IP) every other day between days 0 and 8 for GVH-prevention (■) and days 8 and 16 for GVH-treatment (□). Data are shown as the change in body weight with time. Some mice (including all BMO controls) were sacrificed at +21 days for flow cytometric analysis of their tissues. Group size = 3 to 5 mice.

body weight during the peritransplant period (comparable to that of the BMS controls); however, anti-CD3 F(ab$'$)$_2$ antibody was able to halt and, in most mice, reverse clinical symptoms of GVHD as evidenced by increased body weight gain (Fig. 9). Clinical symptoms of GVHD could be reversed when antibody was delayed until 10, 14 or even 18 days posttransplant (134). Although some chimeras showed clinical symptoms associated with mild GVHD (diarrhea and alopecia), therapeutic administration of anti-CD3 F(ab$'$)$_2$ MoAb resulted in a significant improvement in survival (Fig. 10). These long-term survivors, however, had a significant decline in spleen size and B-cell lymphopoiesis (data not shown). Thus, it may not be possible to completely reverse all of the pathological effects of severe GVHD once secondary effector mechanisms are induced.

In contrast to anti-CD3 F(ab$'$)$_2$ MoAb, antibodies to CD8 and CD4 molecules were not effective in either the prevention or treatment of GVHD when given as F(ab$'$)$_2$ fragments (data not shown). In fact, when given between days 8 and 16, the clinical appearance and weight losses usually exceeded those of the untreated BMS controls (R. Truitt, unpublished data).

3. Effect of Prophylactic and Therapeutic Use of Anti-CD3 F(ab$'$)$_2$ MoAb on GVL Reactivity

Because anti-CD3 F(ab$'$)$_2$ fragments effectively prevented and reversed symptoms of GVHD, we examined their effect on GVL reactivity in MHC-matched B10.BR → AKR chimeras (134). Leukemia-bearing AKR hosts given B10.BR BMS cells and treated with anti-CD3 F(ab$'$)$_2$ antibody in five doses, starting on the day of the transplant, relapsed with leukemia between days 28 and 54 (134). The mice did not show any significant diarrhea, alopecia, scaly skin, periorbital or ear involvement typical of GVHD. Thus, GVHD was prevented, but the beneficial GVL effect

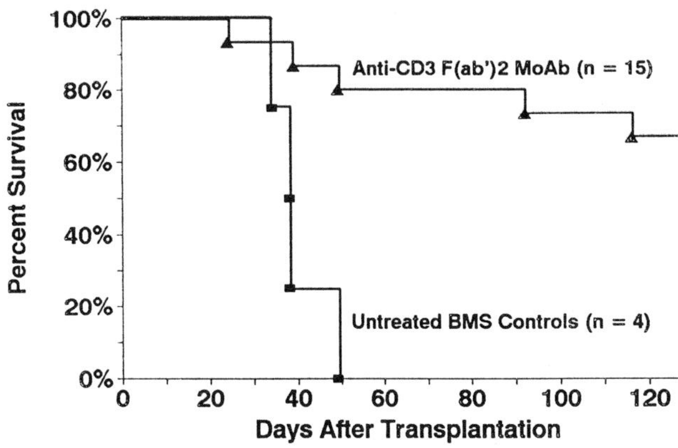

Figure 10 Therapeutic use of anti-CD3 $F(ab')_2$ MoAb results in long-term survival of B10.BR → AKR chimeras. Irradiated AKR hosts (9 Gy) were given 10^7 BM and 20×10^6 spleen cells from normal MHC-matched B10.BR donors on day 0, then randomized to receive no further treatment (■) or 10 μg of anti-CD3 $F(ab')_2$ Moab (IP) qe2d between days 10 to 18 ($n = 3$), 14 to 22 ($n = 6$), and 18 to 26 ($n = 6$). Data from all antibody-treated chimeras ($n = 15$) have been combined into one survival curve (▲).

was significantly diminished. In contrast, chimeras given the same total amount of anti-CD3 $F(ab')_2$ antibody in three doses (days 0, 2, and 4) did not develop clinically significant GVHD and survived leukemia-free. Examination of their spleens indicated that they were complete donor T-cell chimeras with normal-sized spleens and B-cell content (134). Leukemic mice given a single infusion of antibody (50 μg on day 0) also survived beyond 60 days and were leukemia-free (134). The kinetics of their body weight changes paralleled those of untreated BMS controls but was less severe. In contrast to the BMS controls, which were extremely sick, these treated chimeras appeared relatively healthy at termination of the experiment. However, flow cytometric analysis showed that they had undergone some GVH reactivity, as indicated by the small size of their spleens and the presence of few B cells (134). They were completely engrafted with donor T cells and leukemia-free. Anti-CD3 $F(ab')_2$ antibody is more effective at depleting T cells when given over several days rather than as a single bolus (i.e., $10\ \mu g \times 5 > 16.7\ \mu g \times 3 > 50\ \mu g \times 1$) (134). Thus, the intensity of the immunosuppressive regimen had a significant influence on clinical outcome—leukemia-free survival with ($50\ \mu g \times 1$) or without ($16.7\ \mu g \times 3$) GVHD versus leukemia relapse in the absence of GVH-associated GVL reactivity ($10\ \mu g \times 5$) (134).

BMO controls treated with anti-CD3 $F(ab')_2$ fragments relapsed within 34 days post-BMT (data not shown) (134). Anti-CD3 $F(ab')_2$ treatment prolonged survival of BMO controls approximately 2 weeks beyond untreated BMO controls, but did not "cure" the mice. BMS control mice did not relapse with leukemia but developed severe, often fatal GVHD (134).

To further explore the effect of anti-CD3 $F(ab')_2$ on GVL/GVH reactivity, we examined the consequences of delaying the immunosuppressive regimen for 8 days (134). We speculated that allowing donor T cells to recognize and react to alloantigens on normal and leukemic AKR tissues for 8 days would result in a more effective

Table 4 Minimum Lethal Dose of AKR-Leukemia in B10.BR → AKR Chimeras With and Without Anti-CD3 $F(ab')_2$ MoAb Treatment[a]

B10.BR BM cells	B10.BR spleen cells	Anti-CD3 $F(ab')_2$ treatment[b]	Minimum lethal dose of AKR-leukemia[c]
Yes	Yes	None	>100,000
Yes	Yes	Days 8–16	87,000
Yes	Yes	Days 0–8	35,000
Yes	No	Days 0–8	<1000
Yes	No	Days 8–16	<1000
Yes	No	None	<1000

[a]Irradiated AKR hosts were injected with various doses of AKR-leukemia (1000 to 100,000 in 0.5 $\log_{10}$ increments) on day − 1 and transplanted with B10.BR BM plus 20 × 10^6 spleen cells on day 0.
[b]Anti-CD3 $F(ab')_2$ MoAb (10 μg per dose) was given IP every other day for 5 injections starting on day 0 for GVH prevention and day 8 for GVH therapy.
[c]Minimum lethal dose was calculated from the leukemia-dose response regression curves as described in Ref. 134.

GVL reaction, but GVHD could still be prevented, since earlier experiments had established that anti-CD3 $F(ab')_2$ fragments given between days 8 and 16 were able to reverse clinically evident GVHD (Fig. 9). BMS control mice developed GVHD, and most died within 30 days. BM control mice did not develop GVHD; however, all chimeras given anti-CD3 $F(ab')_2$ (either days 0 to 8 or days 8 to 16) relapsed within 30 days. In the experimental groups, none of the mice developed GVHD, but most of the mice given BMS cells and treated with anti-CD3 $F(ab')_2$ between days 0 to 8 relapsed. In contrast, none of the mice treated with anti-CD3 $F(ab')_2$ between 8 and 16 days developed leukemia.

Quantitative analysis of the GVL effect using leukemia dose-response assays revealed that prophylactic as well as therapeutic use of anti-CD3 $F(ab')_2$ MoAb resulted in diminished GVL reactivity as compared to untreated chimeras (Table 4). However, GVL reactivity remained significantly higher in GVH-negative antibody-treated BMS chimeras as compared to the GVH-negative antibody-treated BMO controls. These results indicate that GVHD can be regulated without loss of the GVL effect through the use of MoAb administered after allogeneic BMT but that ill-timed or excessive administration of antibody may lead to relapse. This has significant implications for the design of clinical strategies using MoAb in vivo.

C. Use of Delayed Leukocyte Infusions to Break Donor:Host Tolerance and Induce GVL Reactivity Without GVHD

B10.BR → AKR and SJL → SAKF1 murine models of BMT were used to test strategies for avoiding GVHD while still providing a GVL effect by delayed donor leukocyte infusions (DLI) (132,133). These studies were initiated to help identify the critical factors and mechanisms that might be operative in the successful use of delayed leukocyte infusions as a treatment for relapse post-BMT in CML patients. AKR hosts transplanted with 10^7 B10.BR BM plus 30 × 10^6 spleen cells became complete donor chimeras but died with severe GVHD. When the spleen cell infusion was delayed until at least 21 days post-BMT, few mice showed signs of clinical GVHD, and 96% survived long-term (132,133). Importantly, the infused cells induced complete donor T-cell chimerism by 21 days after infusion and the cells mounted an in vivo antileukemic reaction. In the haplotype mismatched BMT model, $SAKF_1$ hosts that received SJL spleen cell infusions posttransplant also did not develop GVHD (133). GVL reactivity persisted in the MHC-matched DLI chimeras long-term, but the magnitude of the GVL effect was greater when haplotype mismatched donor cells were infused (133).

In MHC-matched chimeras, infusion of cells before 21 days was associated with an increasing probability of developing GVHD (133). It was not clear, however, whether lower doses could be administered earlier without causing GVHD. Therefore, we evaluated the use of a lower but constant dose or incrementally increasing doses of spleen cells beginning the first week post BMT. Earlier administration may be important in elimination of residual leukemia cells, since both experimental and clinical data indicate that DLI is less effective when the disease is in an advanced stage (e.g., CML in blast crisis and acute leukemias). Results are shown in Fig. 11.

Delayed infusion of 30×10^6 donor spleen cells to B10.BR → AKR chimeras on day 21 failed to cause any significant GVH-associated mortality (Fig. 11). How-

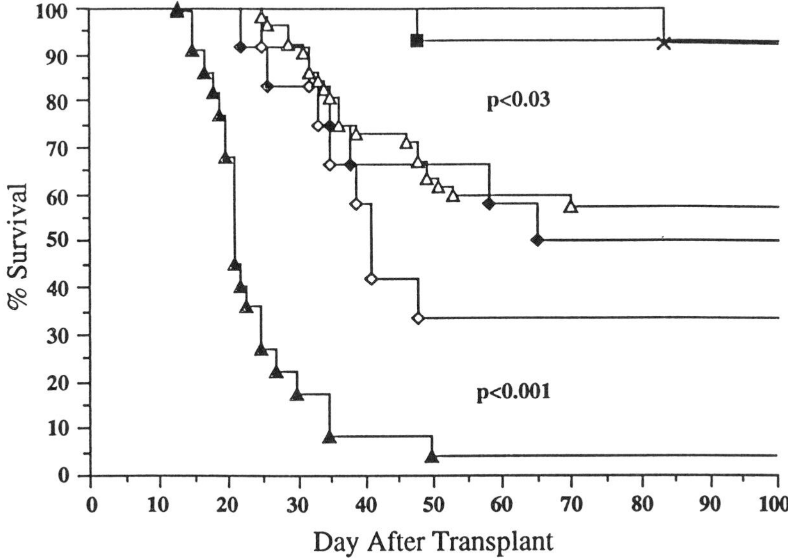

Figure 11 Delayed infusion of donor leukocytes avoids lethal GVHD in MHC-matched B10.BR → AKR chimeras. Irradiated AKR hosts (9 Gy) were given B10.BR BM (10^7) on day 0, then infused with donor spleen cells at various times and doses post-BMT. Control mice were given BM only (■, $n = 17$) or BM plus 30×10^6 spleen cells (▲, $n = 22$) on day 0. Experimental groups were given BM on day 0 and infused with spleen cells as follows: × = 30×10^6 cells on days +21, +28 and +35 ($n = 12$); ◆ = 10×10^6 cells on days +7, +14, and +21 ($n = 12$); △ = 5, 10, and 20×10^6 cells on days +7, +14, and +21, respectively ($n = 52$); or ◇ = 10, 20, and 30×10^6 cells on days +7, +14, and +21, respectively ($n = 12$).

ever, when the same total spleen cell dose was infused over a 3-week period beginning on day 7 ($10^7 + 10^7 + 10^7$), there was significant GVH mortality ($p < 0.03$). Incremental increases in the weekly inoculum starting on day 7 (5, 10, and 20 $\times 10^6$ or 10, 20, and 30 $\times 10^6$) also resulted in significant GVH-related mortality. In contrast, when the initial inoculum was delayed until 21 days post-BMT, a total of 90×10^6 spleen cells could be infused without any mortality. It is important to note, however, that although infusion of donor spleen cells starting on day 7 did not result in optimum GVH-free survival, the survival rates were significantly greater ($p < 0.001$) than when spleen cells were given on the day of BMT (day 0) (Fig. 11).

The GVH reactivity of spleen cell from donors presensitized to host alloantigens was also diminished when infused 21 days post-BMT, but not completely (133). The kinetics of body-weight loss shifted from an early to a late time period. This shift was similar to that observed when anti-CD4 MoAb was used post-BMT to deplete donor T cells (Fig. 7C), suggesting to us that $CD4^+$ T cells may have been preferentially affected. To examine this, limiting dilution analysis assays were used to quantify the number of functional IL-2 secreting (Th) cells and CTL following delayed leukocyte infusion (133). The results showed that Th activity was suppressed but that CTL activity remained largely intact (132). Thus, posttransplant immunotherapy with normal or presensitized donor cells may be an effective way to eliminate residual disease or to treat leukemia relapse without inducing significant GVHD.

IV. SUMMARY

The GVL effect is a dramatic example of immunological reactivity against leukemia. Once controversial and limited to the realm of animal models, the successful use of delayed leukocyte infusions to induce remissions after leukemia relapse post-BMT has provided direct evidence for a GVL effect in humans and demonstrated our ability to harness the reaction for the benefit of patients. Analysis of leukemia-reactive cells has shown in humans, as originally identified in murine systems, that multiple GVL effector-cell populations exist. Whether individual clones or subpopulations of GVL effector cells can be successfully manipulated to provide a clinical GVL effect without GVHD remains to be demonstrated, but the results of experimental studies are encouraging. Furthermore, our understanding of the complex interactions between cells and cytokines in GVHD has increased dramatically in recent years, and innovative new strategies for separating the pathological consequences of GVH reactivity from the beneficial antitumor effects are being developed. Some have entered clinical trial. There is a critical need, however, for the further development of reagents that specifically target GVH-inducing cells or cytokines while sparing GVL effector mechanisms, for reliable in vitro assays to predict GVL and GVH reactivity in the clinical setting, for a better understanding of the biology of miHA as they relate to GVL/GVH reactivity, for greater insight into donor:host tolerance and immunoregulatory systems that affect GVL reactivity, and for elucidation of molecular mechanism(s) by which leukemia cells are targeted for and escape from immunological destruction.

ACKNOWLEDGMENTS

This chapter is dedicated to the memory of the late Mortimer M. Bortin, MD, cofounder of the International Bone Marrow Transplant Registry and a pioneer in the study of graft-versus-leukemia reactions.

Work presented in this chapter was supported by USPHS grant No. CA39854 from the National Cancer Institute, a grant from the Midwest Athletes Against Childhood Cancer (MACC) Fund (Milwaukee, WI), and the Cancer Center of the Medical College of Wisconsin. C.M. was supported by Institutional Research Grant #170 from the American Cancer Society.

The authors are grateful to Carrie Hanke, Laura McOlash, and Nancy Eisenberg for providing technical assistance and to Jeffrey Bluestone, University of Chicago, for providing the 145 2C11 hybridoma.

REFERENCES

1. Bortin MM, Horowitz MM, Rimm AA. Increasing utilization of allogeneic bone marrow transplantation: Results of the 1988–1990 survey. Ann Intern Med 1992; 116:505.
2. Horowitz MM, Truitt RL. Graft-versus-leukemia effects of bone marrow transplantation. In: Atkinson K, ed. Clinical Bone Marrow Transplantation. Cambridge, England: Cambridge University Press, 1994; 704–714.
3. Truitt RL, Johnson BJ. Graft-versus-host disease and the graft-versus-leukemia effect: Lessons from allogeneic bone marrow transplantation. In: Spitzer T, Mazumder A, eds. Immunotherapy and Bone Marrow Transplantation. Armonk, NY: Futura, 1995; 1–33.
4. Gale RP, Champlin RE. How does bone-marrow transplantation cure leukemia? Lancet 1984; 2:28.
5. Champlin R. Graft-versus-leukemia without graft-versus-host disease: An elusive goal of bone marrow transplantation. Semin Hematol 1992; 29:46.
6. Truitt RL, LeFever AV, Shih CY, et al. Graft-vs-leukemia effect. In Burakoff SJ, Deeg HJ, Ferrara J, Atkinson K, eds. Graft-vs-Host Disease: Immunology, Pathophysiology, and Treatment. New York: Marcel Dekker. 1990: 177–204.
7. Ferrara JLM, Deeg HJ. Graft-versus-host disease. N Eng J Med 1991; 324:667.
8. Jadus MR, Wepsic HT. The role of cytokines in graft-versus-host reactions and disease. Bone Marrow Transplant 1992; 10:1.
9. Korngold, R. Biology of graft-vs-host disease. Am J Pediatr Hematol Oncol 1993; 15: 18.
10. Kelemen E, Szebeni J, Petrányi GyG. Graft-versus-host disease in BMT: Experimental, laboratory and clinical contributions of the last few years. Int Arch Allergy Immunol 1993; 102:309.
11. Antin JH, Ferrara JLM. Cytokine dysregulation and acute graft-versus-host disease. Blood 1992; 80:2964.
12. Ferrara JLM. Cytokines other than growth factors in bone marrow transplantation. Curr Opin Oncol 1994; 6:127.
13. Allen RD, Staley TA, Sidman CL. Differential cytokine expression in acute and chronic murine GVHD. Eur J Immunol 1993; 23:333.
14. Truitt RL, Atasoylu AA. Impact of pretransplant conditioning and donor T cells on chimerism, graft-versus-host disease, graft-versus-leukemia reactivity, and tolerance after bone marrow transplantation. Blood 1991; 77:2515.
15. Truitt RL, Atasoylu AA. Contribution of $CD4^+$ and $CD8^+$ T cells to graft-vs-host disease and graft-vs-leukemia reactivity after transplantation of MHC-compatible bone marrow. Bone Marrow Transplant 1991; 8:51.
16. OKunewick JP, Kociban DL, Machen LL, Buffo MJ. The role of CD4 and CD8 T-cells in the graft-versus-leukemia response in Rauscher murine leukemia. Bone Marrow Transplant 1991; 8:445.
17. OKunewick JP, Kochiban DL, Machen LL, Buffo MJ. Comparison of the effects of

CD3 and CD5 donor T cell depletion on graft-versus-leukemia in a murine model for MHC-matched unrelated-donor transplantation. Bone Marrow Transplant 1994; 13:11.
18. Weiss L, Weigensberg M, Morecki S, et al. Characterization of effector cells of graft vs leukemia following allogeneic bone marrow transplantation in mice inoculated with murine B-cell leukemia. Cancer Immunol Immunother 1990; 31:236.
19. Mysliwietz J, Thierfelder S. Antilymphocytic antibodies and marrow transplantation: XII. Suppression of GVHD by T-cell-modulating and depleting antimouse CD3 antibody is most effective when preinjected in the marrow recipient. Blood 1992; 80:2661.
20. Blazar BR, Taylor PA, Vallera DA. In vivo or in vitro anti-CD3ϵ chain MoAb therapy for the prevention of lethal murine GVHD across the MHC barrier in mice. J Immunol 1994; 152:3665.
21. Truitt RL, Johnson BD, Eisenberg N, McCabe C. Use of T-cell specific MoAbs to manipulate GVH and GVL reactions after BMT in mice. J Immunother 1994; 14:369.
22. Johnson BD, Truitt RL. A decrease in graft-vs-host disease without loss of graft-vs-leukemia reactivity after MHC matched bone marrow transplantation by selective depletion of donor NK cells in vivo. Transplantation 1992; 54:104.
23. Blazar BR, Taylor PA, Snover DC, et al. Nonmitogenic anti-CD3 $F(ab')_2$ fragments inhibit lethal murine graft-versus-host disease induced across the MHC barrier. J Immunol 1993; 150:265.
24. Truitt RL, Johnson BD, McCabe CM. Effect of anti-CD3 $F(ab')_2$ MoAb on GVH and GVL reactivity when given in vivo after MHC-matched BMT. J Cell Biochem 1994; 18B:78.
25. McCabe CM, Truitt RL. Manipulation of CD4 T-cell subsets to avoid GVH disease without loss of antileukemic reactivity. Proceedings of the Midwest Autumn Immunology Conference, Chicago, IL, November 1993.
26. Sykes M, Abraham VS, Harty MW, et al. IL-2 reduces GVHD and preserves a GVL effect by selectively inhibiting $CD4^+$ T cell activity. J Immunol 1993; 150:197.
27. Fowler DH, Kurasawa K, Husebekk A, et al. Cells of Th2 cytokine phenotype prevent LPS-induced lethality during murine GVH reactions. J Immunol 1994; 152:1004.
28. Weiss L, Lubin I, Factorowich I, et al. Effective graft-versus-leukemia effects independent of graft-versus-host disease after T cell-depleted allogeneic bone marrow transplantation in a murine model of B cell leukemia/lymphoma: Role of cell therapy and recombinant IL-2. J Immunol 1994; 153:2562.
29. Horowitz MM, Gale RP, Sondel PM, et al. Graft-versus-leukemia after bone marrow transplantation. Blood 1990; 75:555.
30. Marmont AM, Horowitz MM, Gale RP, et al. T-cell depletion of HLA-identical transplants in leukemia. Blood 1991; 78:2120.
31. Kolb HJ, Mittermüller J, Clemm C, et al. Donor leukocyte transfusions for treatment of recurrent CML in marrow transplant patients. Blood 1990; 76:2462.
32. Drobyski WD, Keever CA, Roth MS, et al. Salvage immunotherapy using donor leukocyte infusions as treatment for relapsed chronic myelogenous leukemia after allogeneic bone marrow transplantation: Efficacy and toxicity of a defined T-cell dose. Blood 1990; 82:2310.
33. Hertenstein B, Wiesneth M, Novotny J, et al. Interferon-α and donor buffy coat transfusions for treatment of relapsed chroic myeloid leukemia after allogeneic bone marrow transplantation. Transplantation 1993; 56:1114.
34. Porter DL, Roth MS, McGarigle C, et al. Induction of GVHD as immunotherapy for relapsed chronic myeloid leukemia. N Engl J Med 1994; 330:100.
35. van Rhee R, Lin F, Cullis JO, et al. Relapse of chronic myeloid leukemia after allogeneic bone marrow transplant: The case for giving donor leukocyte transfusions before the onset of hematologic relapse. Blood 1994; 83:3377.
36. van Lochem E, de Gast B, Goulmy E. In vitro separation of host specific graft-versus-

host and graft-versus-leukemia cytotoxic T cell activities. Bone Marrow Transplant 1992; 10:181.
37. Truitt RL, Shih C, LeFever AV, et al. Characterization of alloimmunization-induced T-lymphocytes reactive against AKR leukemia in vitro and correlation with graft-vs-leukemia activity in vivo. J Immunol 1983; 131:2050.
38. Aizawa S and Sado T. Graft-versus-leukemia effect in MHC-compatible and -incompatible allogeneic bone marrow transplantation of radiation-induced, leukemia-bearing mice. Transplantation 1991; 52:885.
39. Ash RC, Casper JT, Chitambar CR, et al. Successful allogeneic transplantation of T-cell-depleted bone marrow from closely HLA-matched unrelated donors. N Engl J Med 1990; 322:485.
40. Casper J, Camitta B, Truitt R, et al. Unrelated bone marrow donor transplants for children with leukemia or myelodysplasia. Blood 1995; 85:2354.
41. Korngold R, Leighton C, Manser T. Graft-versus-myeloid leukemia responses following syngeneic and allogeneic bone marrow transplantation. Transplantation 1994; 58: 278.
42. Klarnet JP, Matis LA, Kern DE, et al. Antigen-driven T cell clones can proliferate in vivo, eradicate disseminated leukemia, and provide specific immunologic memory. J Immunol 1987; 138:4012.
43. Swain SL. T-cell subsets and the recognition of MHC class. Immunol Rev 1983; 74: 129.
44. McKisic MD, Lancki DW, Fitch FW. Cytolytic activity of murine $CD4^+$ T cell clones correlates with γ-IFN production in mouse strains having a BALB/c background. J Immunol 1993; 150:3793.
45. Sosman JA, Oettel KR, Smith SD, et al. Specific recognition of human leukemic cells by allogeneic T cells: II. Evidence for HLA-D restricted determinants on leukemic cells that are crossreactive with determinants present on unrelated non-leukemic cells. Blood 1990; 75:2005.
46. Falkenburg JHF, Faber LM, van den Elshout M, et al. Generation of donor-derived antileukemic cytotoxic T-lymphocyte responses for treatment of relapsed leukemia after allogeneic HLA-identical bone marrow transplantation. J Immunother 1993; 14:305.
47. Hoffmann T, Theobald M, Bunjes D, et al. Frequency of bone marrow T cells responding to HLA-identical non-leukemic and leukemic stimulator cells. Bone Marrow Transplant 1993; 12:1.
48. Jiang YZ, Kanfer EJ, Macdonald D, et al. Graft-versus-leukaemia following allogeneic bone marrow transplantation: Emergence of cytotoxic T lymphocytes reacting to host leukaemia cells. Bone Marrow Transplant 1991; 8:253.
49. van der Harst D, Goulmy E, Falkenburg JHF, et al. Recognition of minor histocompatibility antigens on lymphocytic and myeloid leukemic cells by cytotoxic T-cell clones. Blood 1994; 83:1060.
50. Haas W, Pereira P, Tonegawa S. Gamma/delta cells. Annu Rev Immunol 1993; 11: 637.
51. Havran WL, Boismenu R. Activation and function of $\gamma\delta$ T cells. Curr Opin Immunol 1994; 6:442.
52. Fisch P, Malkovska M, Braakman E, et al. γ/δ T cell clones and natural killer cell clones mediate distinct patterns of non-major histocompatibility complex-restricted cytolysis. J Exp Med 1990; 171:1567.
53. Fisch P, Malkovsky M, Kovats S, et al. Recognition by human $V\gamma9/V\delta2$ T cells of a GroEL homolog on Daudi Burkitt's lymphoma cells. Science 1990; 250:1269.
54. Fisch P, Oettel K, Fudim N, et al. MHC-unrestricted cytotoxic and proliferative responses of two distinct human γ/δ T-cell subsets to Daudi cells. J Immunol 1992; 148: 2315.

55. Kaur I, Voss SD, Gupta RS, et al. Human peripheral $\gamma\delta$ T cells recognize hsp60 molecules on Daudi Burkitt's lymphoma cells. J Immunol 1993; 150:2046.
56. Blachere NE, Udono H, Janetzki S, et al. Heat shock protein vaccines against cancer. J Immunother 1993; 14:352.
57. Malkovska V, Cigel FK, Armstrong N, et al. Antilymphoma activity of human $\gamma\delta$ T-cells in mice with severe combined immune deficiency. Cancer Res 1992; 52:5610.
58. Rooney CM, Wimperis JZ, Brenner MK, et al. Natural killer cell activity following T-cell depleted allogeneic bone marrow transplantation. Br J Haematol 1986; 62:413.
59. Niederwiesser D, Gastl G, Rumpold H, et al. Rapid reappearance of large granular lymphocytes (LGL) with concomitant reconstitution of natural killer (NK) activity after human marrow transplantation (BMT). Br J Haematol 1987; 65:301.
60. Bellone G, Valiante NM, Viale O, et al. Regulation of hematopoiesis in vitro by alloreactive natural killer cell clones. J Exp Med 1993; 177:1117.
61. Mackinnon S, Hows JM, Goldman JM. Induction of in vitro graft-versus-leukemia activity following bone marrow transplantation for chronic myeloid leukemia. Blood 1990; 76:2037.
62. Hauch M, Gazzola MV, Small T, et al. Anti-leukemia potential of interleukin-2 activated natural killer cells after bone marrow transplantation for chronic myelogenous leukemia. Blood 1990; 75:2250.
63. Toshitani A, Taniguchi K, Himeno K, et al. Adoptive transfer of H-2-incompatible lymphokine-activated killer (LAK) cells: An approach for successful cancer immunotherapy free from graft-versus-host disease (GVHD) using murine models. Cell Immunol 1988; 115:373.
64. Uharek L, Glass B, Gaska T, et al. Natural killer cells as effector cells of graft-versus-leukemia activity in a murine transplantation model. Bone Marrow Transplant 1993; 12:S57.
65. Rosenberg SA, Lotze MT, Muul LM, et al. A progress report on the treatment of 157 patients with advanced cancer using lymphokine-activated killer cells and interleukin-2 or high-dose interleukin-2 alone. N Engl J Med 1987; 316:889.
66. Allison MAK, Jones SE, McGuffey P. Phase II trial of outpatient interleukin-2 in malignant lymphoma, chronic lymphocytic leukemia, and selected solid tumors. J Clin Oncol 1989; 7:75.
67. Mackinnon S. Graft-versus-leukemia reactions following bone marrow transplantation for chronic myeloid leukemia. Prog Clin Biol Res 1992; 377:113.
68. Nishimura T, Nakamura Y, Takeuchi Y, et al. Generation, propagation, and targeting of human $CD4^+$ helper/killer T cells induced by anti-CD3 monoclonal antibody plus recombinant IL-2: An efficient strategy for adoptive tumor immunotherapy. J Immunol 1992; 148:285.
69. Ueda M, Hoshi ID, Dan M, et al. Preclinical studies for adoptive immunotherapy in bone marrow transplantation: Generation of anti-CD3 activated cytotoxic T cells from normal and autologous bone marrow transplant candidates. Transplantation 1993; 56: 351.
70. Hess AD, Horwitz L, Beschorner WE, Santos GW. Development of graft-versus-host disease-like syndrome in cyclosporine-treated rats after syngeneic bone marrow transplantation: I. Development of cytotoxic T-lymphocytes with apparent polyclonal anti-Ia specificity, including autoreactivity. J Exp Med 1985; 161:718.
71. Shinozawa T, Beschorner WE, Hess AD. Prolonged administration of cyclosporine and the thymus: Irreversible immunopathologic changes associated with autologous pseudo-graft-vs-host disease. Transplantation 1990; 50:106.
72. Beschorner WE, Ren H, Phillip J, et al. Recovery of thymic microenvironment after cyclosporine prevents syngeneic graft-vs-host disease. Transplantation 1991; 52:668.
73. Geller R, Esa A, Benhomer W, et al. Successful in vitro graft-versus-tumor effect

against an Ia-bearing tumor using cyclosporine induced syngeneic graft-versus-host disease in the rat. Blood 1989; 74:1165.
74. Yeager AM, Vogelsang GB, Jones RJ, et al. Cyclosporine-induced graft-versus-host disease after autologous bone marrow transplantation for acute myeloid leukemia. Leuk Lymph 1993; 11:215.
75. Holländer GA, Widmer B, Burakoff SJ. Loss of normal thymic repertoire selection and persistence of autoreactive T cells in graft vs host disease. J Immunol 1994; 152: 1609.
76. Parkman R. Graft-versus-host disease: An alternate hypothesis. Immunol Today 1989; 10:362.
77. Barrett AJ, Locatelli F, Treleaven JG, et al. Second transplants for leukaemic relapse after bone marrow transplantation: High early mortality but favorable effect of chronic GVHD on continued remission. Br J Haematol 1991; 79:567.
78. Barnes DWH, Corp MJ, Loutit JF, et al. Treatment of murine leukemia with x-rays and homologous bone marrow. Br Med J 1956; 2:626.
79. Bortin MM, Truitt RL, Rimm AA, Bach FH. Graft versus leukemia reactivity induced by alloimmunisation without augmentation of graft versus host reactivity. Nature 1979; 281:490.
80. Sullivan KM, Weiden PL, Storb R, et al. Influence of acute and chronic graft-versus-host disease on relapse and survival after bone marrow transplantation from HLA-identical siblings as treatment of acute and chronic leukemia. Blood 1989; 73:1720.
81. Marmont AM. The graft versus leukemia (GVL) effect after allogeneic bone marrow transplantation for chronic myelogenous leukemia (CML). Leuk Lymph 1993; 11(S1): 221.
82. Vogelsang GB, Hess AD. Graft-versus-host disease: New directions for a persistent problem. Blood 1994; 84:2061.
83. Korngold R, Sprent J. Variable capacity of L3T4$^+$ T cells to cause lethal graft-versus-host disease across minor histocompatibility barriers in mice. J Exp Med 1987; 165: 1552.
84. Korngold R. Lethal graft-versus-host disease in mice directed to multiple minor histocompatibility antigens: Features of CD8$^+$ and CD4$^+$ T cell responses. Bone Marrow Transplant 1992; 9:355.
85. Hamilton BL. L3T4-positive T cells participate in the induction of graft-vs-host disease in response to minor histocompatibility antigens. J Immunol 1987; 139:2511.
86. Champlin R, Giralt S, Przepiorka D, et al. Selective depletion of CD8-positive T-lymphocytes for allogeneic bone marrow transplantation: Engraftment, graft-versus-host disease and graft-versus-leukemia. Prog Clin Biol Res 1992; 377:385.
87. Mickelson EM, Anasetti C, Yoon Choo S, et al. Role of the mixed lymphocyte culture reaction in predicting acute graft-versus-host disease after marrow transplants from haploidentical and unrelated donors. Transplant Proc 1993; 25:1239.
88. Batchelor JR, Schwarer AP, Jiang YZ, et al. Helper T lymphocytes precursor frequencies predict risks of GVH disease in bone marrow transplantation. Transplant Proc 1993; 25:1237.
89. Kelso A. Frequency analysis of lymphokine-secreting CD4$^+$ and CD8$^+$ T cells activated in a graft-versus-host reaction. J Immunol 1990; 145:2167.
90. Kung JT, Castillo M, Heard P, et al. Subpopulations of CD8$^+$ cytotoxic T-cell precursors collaborate in the absence of conventional CD4$^+$ helper T cells. J Immunol 1991; 146:1783.
91. Ruby J, Ramshaw I. The antiviral activity of immune CD8$^+$ T cells is dependent on interferon-gamma. Lymphokine Cytokine Res 1991; 10:353.
92. Roopenian DC. What are minor histocompatibility loci? A new look at an old question. Immunol Today 1992; 13:7.

93. Beelen DW, Haralambie E, Brandt H, et al. Evidence that sustained growth suppression of intestinal anaerobic bacteria reduces the risk of acute graft-versus-host disease after sibling marrow transplantation. Blood 1992; 80:2668.
94. Vossen JM, Heidt PJ. Gnotobiotic measures for the prevention of acute graft-vs-host disease. In: Burakoff SJ, Deeg HJ, Ferrara J, Atkinson K, eds. Graft-vs-Host Disease: Immunology, Pathophysiology, and Treatment. New York: Marcel Dekker, 1990; 403: 423.
95. Van Els CACM, Bakker A, Awinderman AH, et al. Effector mechanisms in graft-versus-host disease in response to minor histocompatibility antigens: I. Absence of correlation with cytotoxic effector cells. Transplantation 1990; 50:62.
96. Van Els CACM, Bakker A, Zwinderman AH, et al. Effector mechanisms in graft-versus-host disease in response to minor histocompatibility antigens: II. Evidence of a possible involvement of proliferative T cells. Transplantation 1990; 50:67.
97. Miconnet I, Huchet R, Bonardelle D, et al. Graft-versus-host mortality induced by noncytolytic $CD4^+$ T cell clones specific for non-H-2 antigens. J Immunol 1990; 145: 2123.
98. Pritchard LL, Huchet R, Bruley-Rosset M, et al. Induction and suppression of delayed-type hypersensitivity to non-MHC antigens during lethal graft-versus-host reaction. J Immunol 1992; 149:45.
99. Le Gros G, Erard F. Non-cytotoxic, IL-4, IL-5, IL-10 producing $CD8^+$ T cells: Their activation and effector functions. Curr Opin Immunol 1994; 6:453.
100. Wall DA, Sheehan KCF. The role of TNF and IFNγ in graft-versus-host disease and related immunodeficiency. Transplantation 1994; 57:273.
101. Sykes M. Novel approaches to the control of graft versus host disease. Cur Opin Immunol 1993; 5:774.
102. Hessner MJ, Endean DJ, Casper JT, et al. Use of unrelated marrow grafts compensates for reduced graft-versus-leukemia reactivity after T-cell-depleted allogeneic bone marrow transplantation for chronic myelogenous leukemia. Blood 1995; 86:3987.
103. Truitt RL, Ash RC. Manipulation of T-cell content in transplanted human bone marrow: Effect on GVH and GVL reactions. Prog Clin Biol Res 1987; 244:409.
104. Aizawa S, Sado T, Kamisaku H, et al. Graft-versus-leukemia effect in allogeneic bone marrow transplantation in mice against several radiation-induced leukemias. Bone Marrow Transplant 1994; 13:109.
105. Antin JH. Graft-versus-leukemia: No longer an epiphenomenon. Blood 1993; 82:2273.
106. Goldman JM, Gale RP, Horowitz MM, et al. Bone marrow transplantation for chronic myelogenous leukemia in chronic phase: Increased risk for relapse associated with T-cell depletion. Ann Intern Med 1988; 108:806.
107. Korngold R, Leighton C, Manser T. Graft-versus-myeloid leukemia responses following syngeneic and allogeneic bone marrow transplantation. Transplantation 1994; 58: 278.
108. Delain M, Tiberghien P, Racadot E, et al. Variability of the alloreactive T-cell response to human leukemia blasts. Leukemia 1994; 8:642.
109. Oettel KR, Wesly OH, Albertini MR, et al. Allogeneic T-cell clones able to selectively destroy Philadelphia chromosome-bearing (Ph^{1+}) human leukemia lines can also recognize Ph^{1-} cells from the same patient. Blood 1994; 83:3390.
110. Krensky AM, Sanchez-Madrid F, Robbins E, et al. The functional significance, distribution, and structure of LFA-1, LFA-2, and LFA-3: Cell surface antigens associated with CTL-target interactions. J Immunol 1983; 131:611.
111. Jansen JH, Van deı Harst D, Wientjens GJHM, et al. Induction of LFA-1 and ICAM-1 on hairy cell leukemia is accompanied by enhanced susceptibility to T-cell but not to LAK-cell cytotoxicity. Blood 1992; 80:478.
112. Khanna R, Burrows SR, Suhrbier A, et al. EBV peptide epitope sensitization restores

human cytotoxic T cell recognition of Burkitt's lymphoma cells: Evidence for a critical role for ICAM-2. J Immunol 1993; 150:5154.

113. Oblakowski P, Bello-Fernandez C, Reittie JE, et al. Possible mechanism of selective killing of myeloid leukemic blast cells by lymphokine-activated killer cells. Blood 1991; 77:1996.

114. Pion S, Fontaine P, Baron C, et al. Immunodominant minor histocompatibility antigens expressed by mouse leukemic cells can serve as effective targets for T cell immunotherapy. J Clin Invest 1995; 95:1561.

115. Wettstein PJ, Bailey DW. Immunodominance in the immune response to multiple histocompatibility antigens. Immunogenetics 1982; 16:47.

116. Korngold R, Wettstein PJ. Immunodominance in the graft-vs-host disease T cell response to minor histocompatibility antigens. J Immunol 1990; 145:4079.

117. Van Els CACM, Pool J, Blokland E, et al. Human minor histocompatibility antigens: Immunodominance and population frequencies. Immunogenetics 1992; 35:161.

118. Martin PJ, Hansen JA, Storb R, Thomas ED: Human marrow transplantation: An immunological perspective. Adv Immunol 1987; 40:379.

119. Wall DA, Hamberg SD, Reynolds DS, et al. Immunodeficiency in graft-versus-host disease: I. Mechanisms of immune suppression. J Immunol 1988; 140:2970.

120. Holda JH, Maier T, Claman HN. Murine graft-versus-host disease across minor barriers: Immunosuppressive aspects of natural suppressor cells. Immunol Rev 1985; 88:87.

121. Wall DA, Hamberg SD, Ferrara JLM, Abbas AK. Immunodeficiency in graft-versus-host disease: II. Effects of GVHD-induced suppressor cells on $CD4^+$ T cell clones. J Immunol 1989; 143:74.

122. Holda JH, Maier T, Claman HN. Evidence that IFNγ is responsible for natural suppressor activity in graft-versus-host disease, spleen and normal bone marrow. Transplantation 1988; 45:772.

123. Strober S. Natural suppressor cells, neonatal tolerance and total lymphoid irradiation: Exploring obscure relationships. Ann Rev Immunol 1984; 2:219.

124. Claman HN, Holda JH, Maier T. Natural suppressor cell systems. Prog Immunol 1986; 6:1035.

125. Saffran DC, Parsons MF, Singhal SK. Separation of allostimulatory and natural suppressor/stem cell functions of murine bone marrow—implications for bone marrow transplantation. Transplantation 1991; 52:680.

126. Strober S, Dejbachsh-Jones S, Van Vlasselaer P, et al. Cloned natural suppressor cell lines express the $CD3^+$ $CD4^-$ $CD8^-$ surface phenotype and the α,β heterdimer of the T cell antigen receptor. J Immunol 1989; 143:1118.

127. Sykes M. Unusual T cell populations in adult bone marrow: prevalence of $CD3^+$ $CD4^-$ $CD8^-$ and $\alpha\beta TCR^+$ NK-1.1$^+$ cells. J Immunol 145; 3209, 1990.

128. Truitt RL, Horowitz MM, Atasoylu AA, et al. Graft-versus-leukemia effect of allogeneic bone marrow transplantation: Clinical and experimental aspects of late leukemia relapse. In: Stewart THM, ed. Cellular Immune Mechanisms and Tumor Dormancy. Boca Raton, FL: CRC Press, 1992:111–128.

129. Sykes M, Romick ML, Sachs DH. Interleukin 2 prevents graft-versus-host disease while preserving the graft-versus-leukemia effect of allogeneic T cells. Proc Natl Acad Sci USA 1990; 87:5633.

130. Sykes M, Harty MW, Szot GL, Pearson DA. Interleukin-2 inhibits graft-versus-host disease-promoting activity of $CD4^+$ cells while preserving CD4- and CD8-mediated graft-versus-leukemia effects. Blood 1994; 83:2560.

131. Abraham VS, Sachs DH, Sykes M. The mechanism of protection from GVHD mortality by IL-2: III. Early reductions in donor T cell subsets and expansion of a $CD3^+$ $CD4^-CD8^-$ cell population. J Immunol 1992; 148:3746.

132. Johnson BD, Drobyski WD, Truitt RL. Delayed infusion of normal donor cells after

MHC-matched bone marrow transplantation provides an antileukemia reaction without graft-versus-host disease. Bone Marrow Transplant 1993; 11:329.
133. Johnson BD, Truitt RL. Delayed infusion of immunocompetent donor cells after bone marrow transplantation breaks graft-host tolerance and allows for persistent antileukemic reactivity without severe graft-vs-host disease. Blood 1995; 85:3302.
134. Johnson BJ, McCabe C, Hanke CA, Truitt RL. Use of anti-CD3ε $F(ab')_2$ fragments in vivo to modulate graft-vs-host disease without loss of graft-vs-leukemia reactivity after MHC-matched bone marrow transplantation. J Immunol 1995; 154:5542.
135. Lawler SD, Harris H, Millar J, et al. Cytogenetic follow-up studies of recipients of T-cell depleted allogeneic bone marrow. Br J Haematol 1987; 65:143.
136. Lawler M, Humphries P, McCann SR. Evaluation of mixed chimerism by in vitro amplification of dinucleotide repeat sequences using the polymerase chain reaction. Blood 1991; 77:2504.
137. Offit K, Burns JP, Cunningham I, et al. Cytogenetic analysis of chimerism and leukemia relapse in chronic myelogenous leukemia patients after T cell-depleted bone marrow transplantation. Blood 1990; 75:1346.
138. Mackinnon S, Barnett L, Heller G, O'Reilly RJ. Minimal residual disease is more common in patients who have mixed T-cell chimerism after bone marrow transplantation for chronic myelogenous leukemia. Blood 1994; 83:3409.
139. Fontaine P, Perreault C. Diagnosis of graft-versus-host disease in mice transplanted across minor histocompatibility barriers. Transplantation 1990; 49:1177.
140. LeFever AV, Truitt RL, Shih CY. Reactivity of in vitro expanded alloimmune CTL and Qa-1 specific CTL against AKR leukemia in vivo. Transplantation 1985; 40:531.
141. Charlton B, Meltzer J, Fathman CG. $CD4^+/HSA^+$ thymocytes cause graft-versus-host disease across non-major histocompatibility complex incompatibilities. Eur J Immunol 1994; 24:1706.
142. Cowdery JS, Tolaymat N, Weber SP. The effect of partial in vivo depletion of CD4 T cells by monoclonal antibody: Evidence that incomplete depletion increases IgG production and augments in vitro thymic-dependent antibody responses. Transplantation 1991; 51:1072.
143. Field EH, Rouse TM, Fleming AL, et al. Altered IFNγ and IL-4 pattern lymphokine secretion in mice partially depleted of CD4 T cells by anti-CD4 monoclonal antibody. J Immunol 1992; 149:1131.
144. O'Garra A, Murphy K. Role of cytokines in determining T-lymphocyte function. Curr Opin Immunol 1994; 6:458.
145. Sykes M. Novel approaches to the control of graft versus host disease. Curr Opin Immunol 1993; 5:774.
146. Ferrara J, Marion A, Murphy G, Burakoff S. Acute graft-versus-host disease: Pathogenesis and prevention with a monoclonal antibody in vivo. Transplant Proc 1987; 19: 2662.
147. Truitt RL, McCabe CM, Weiler MB, Johnson BD. Contribution of $CD4^+$, $CD8^+$, and NK-1.1$^+$ cells to antileukemia (GVL) and antihost (GVH) reactions after allogeneic bone marrow transplantation. J Cell Biochem 1993; 17D:118.
148. Waldman H. Manipulation of T-cell responses with monoclonal antibodies. Annu Rev Immunol 1989; 7:407.
149. Schreiber KL, Forman J. The effect of chronic graft-versus-host disease on B cell development. Transplantation 1993; 55:597.
150. Leo O, Foo M, Sachs DH, et al. Identification of a MoAb specific for a murine T3 polypeptide. Proc Natl Acad Sci USA 1987; 84:1374.
151. Ferran C, Sheehan K, Dy M, et al. Cytokine-related syndrome following injection of anti-CD3 MoAb: further evidence for transient in vivo T cell activation. Eur J Immunol 1990; 20:509.

152. Hirsch R, Bluestone JA, DeNenno L, Gress RE. Anti-CD3 $F(ab')_2$ fragments are immunosuppressive in vivo without evoking either the strong humoral response or morbidity associated with whole mAb. Transplantation 1990; 49:1117.
153. Hirsch R, Archibald J, Gress RE. Differential T cell hyporesponsiveness induced by in vivo administration of intact or $F(ab')_2$ fragments of anti-CD3 MoAb: $F(ab')_2$ fragments induce a selective T helper dysfunction. J Immunol 1991; 147:2088.

15

Lung Injuries Associated with Graft-Versus-Host Reactions

David K. Madtes and Stephen W. Crawford

Fred Hutchinson Cancer Research Center and University of Washington Seattle, Washington

I. INTRODUCTION

Pulmonary disease occurs in 40 to 60% of patients after marrow transplantation and contributes significantly to the morbidity and mortality (1,2). The incidence of pulmonary complications varies with the type of transplant, conditioning regimen, underlying disease and age of the patient (2,3). The noninfectious pulmonary processes described in the posttransplant period include idiopathic pneumonitis, hemorrhagic alveolitis, obliterative bronchiolitis and lymphocytic bronchitis, and alveolitis. The role of graft-versus-host disease (GVHD) in the pathogenesis of these complications has been the subject of considerable debate. Unlike GVHD of the skin, liver, and intestine, which displays well- characterized histopathological alterations that have been attributed in part to selective T- lymphocyte–mediated epithelial destruction, a direct association between lung damage and alloreactivity in marrow recipients has been more obscure. Although a variety of pulmonary complications have been described in the literature as manifestations of GVH reactions (GVHR), these associations are primarily based on the simultaneous occurrence of pulmonary abnormalities with GVHD and the absence of a specific pulmonary pathogen. Identification of specific immunologically mediated mechanisms responsible for the observed pulmonary pathology are lacking. However, animal models of alloreactivity may provide insight into potential causal relationships.

Unquestionably, the demonstration of "pulmonary GVHD" would provide an etiological link between two major complications of allogeneic marrow transplantation and could have important therapeutic implications, including an indication for immunosuppressive therapy in the treatment of posttransplant pneumopathies. In this chapter we focus on noninfectious pulmonary complications that can occur in the presence of GVHD. We describe the clinical presentation, incidence, and risk factors for these pulmonary abnormalities as they pertain to allogeneic marrow transplantation. Furthermore, we examine the pathogenesis of these respiratory complications within the context of cell-mediated and inflammatory cytokine-directed lung injury

II. IDIOPATHIC PNEUMONITIS

Idiopathic pneumonitis (IP) is an important clinical entity involving diffuse lung injury that occurs after marrow transplantation and for which no infectious etiology can be identified. This syndrome is defined by the following criteria: (a) evidence of widespread alveolar injury as manifest by multilobar infiltrates on chest x-ray or computed tomography as well as clinical symptoms and signs of pneumonia and evidence of abnormal respiratory physiology, such as hypoxemia or restrictive impairment on pulmonary function testing, and (b) absence of active lower respiratory tract infection as documented by negative bronchoalveolar lavage, lung biopsy, or autopsy, including stains and cultures for bacteria, fungi, and viruses (4). The cumulative incidence of IP ranges from 3 to 7% after allogeneic transplant for severe aplastic anemia (5,6), from 7 to 17% after allogeneic transplant for malignancy (2,3,7,8), and 6% after autologous transplantation (9). The median time of onset is 21 days, with a range of 1 to 117 days after marrow transplant (9). The case fatality rate associated with IP is 60 to 82%, with up to 69% of patients dying of respiratory failure (2,8).

A. Pathology

The histological patterns identified in IP are primarily of two major types: interstitial pneumonitis and diffuse alveolar damage. In a case series review of 43 open lung biopsies for diffuse noninfectious pulmonary infiltrates, interstitial pneumonitis—as characterized by mononuclear cell interstitial infiltration with varying degrees of fibrosis, intact alveolar epithelium, and absence of hyaline membranes—was identified in 59% of cases (10). Diffuse alveolar damage—characterized by alveolar epithelial degeneration, hyaline membrane formation, interstitial edema, sparse interstitial mononuclear inflammatory infiltrate, and variable fibrosis—occurred in 37% of cases (10). Other histological abnormalities were bronchopneumonia without identification of a specific pathogen in 5% of cases and bronchiolitis obliterans in 2% of cases. These various histological patterns are thought to represent a continuum of responses to lung injury rather than an evolving response, since the histological findings remained consistent over time, from open lung biopsy to autopsy (11).

B. Risks of Idiopathic Pneumonitis

It is probable that the risks for IP are distinct from those for diffuse infectious pneumonias. Meyers (2) and Wingard (8) evaluated the risks for IP separately. Only transplant for malignancy rather than aplastic anemia was associated with IP in the Johns Hopkins experience (8). Meyers (2) reported the same association, as well as increasing age as a risk. The effect of total body irradiation (TBI) as a risk for IP was noted among patients with aplastic anemia. The risk appears lower among recipients of fractionated (as opposed to single-dose) TBI (2) as well as lower-dose rates of TBI (3). TBI in addition to previous thoracic irradiation appears to increase the incidence of IP among patients with lymphoma (12).

There are few data regarding the risk of IP associated with acute GVHD. Weiner reported that patients who developed moderate to severe acute GVHD had a relative risk of 1.6 for developing IP compared to patients with mild or no GVHD (3). Similarly, acute GVHD was associated with a relative risk of 3.5 (5) and 6.4 (2) for subsequent development of IP in allogeneic recipients undergoing marrow transplant for severe aplastic anemia. Of note, recipients of syngeneic transplants for hematologic malignancy developed less IP than did patients who received HLA-identical sibling transplants despite similar cytoreductive regimens (4). The risk of developing IP for these syngeneic recipients was no different than that for HLA-identical sibling transplants without GVHD and that for autologous marrow recipients (4). These observations support the concept that GVHD is a significant risk factor for IP. There are, however, no data to substantiate that idiopathic pneumonitis is a pulmonary manifestation of GVHD.

C. Potential Mechanisms of Lung Injury in GVH Reactions

Potential etiologies for IP following marrow transplant include chemoradiation damage, unrecognized infection, nonspecific injury from uncontrolled intravascular inflammation, direct immunological effector mechanisms, or a combination of these processes. These lung injuries likely result both from direct cell-mediated damage and nonspecific effector mechanisms (cytokines, natural killer cells). Evidence of direct cell-mediated injury in the pathogenesis of noninfectious pneumonitis has been demonstrated in a major histocompatibility complex (MHC)-compatible murine model of allogeneic marrow transplantation. Transplantation of T lymphocytes across a minor histocompatibility barrier enhances the pulmonary toxicity induced by conditioning with TBI (13). The resultant mononuclear interstitial pneumonitis is characterized by focal thickening of alveolar septa, perivenular infiltrates, and lumenal accumulation of macrophages, lymphocytes, and cellular debris. These histopathological features are similar to those described after allogeneic transplant in irradiated mice (14) and rats (15). The specific lymphocyte effector populations responsible for this cell-mediated lung injury are uncertain; however, CD_4^+ and $CD8^+$ cells (16) as well as natural killer cells (17,18) have been implicated. In this murine model, the lung appears to be a sensitive target for the combined effects of radiation and the GVHR.

In a rat model, the GVHR may be capable of producing lung toxicity. Infusion of parental lymphoid cells into nonirradiated F_1 hybrid rats results in acute systemic GVHD including noninfectious pneumonitis and lymphoid bronchitis (19). The pulmonary lesions produced consist of mononuclear cell infiltration into alveolar septa and perivascular regions similar to that seen in acute lung allograft rejection. Because this model did not utilize irradiation, chemotherapy, or immunosuppressive agents and since overt pulmonary infections were excluded by culture and histology, the only apparent etiology for the interstitial pneumonitis was the alloreaction. Likewise, adoptive immunotherapy utilizing lymphokine-activated killer (LAK) cells and recombinant interleukin-2 (IL-2) has been shown to induce lung injury, as manifest by a capillary leak syndrome in both mice (20) and humans (21).

1. Cell-Mediated Immunity and Lung Injury

Cytotoxic T-lymphocyte–mediated lung injury occurs following lung or heart lung transplantation in which recipient T lymphocytes become sensitized to donor histocompatibility antigens. The demonstration of donor- specific alloreactivity by T lymphocytes recovered by bronchoalveolar lavage (BAL) of heart-lung transplant recipients provides support for immunologically mediated lung injury after clinical transplantation and appears to signal acute allograft rejection (22). Because pulmonary parenchymal cells (endothelial and epithelial cells) express class I, class II, and minor histocompatibility antigens, they can serve as targets for these cytotoxic T lymphocytes, resulting in direct cell-mediated damage. Activation of T lymphocytes in the lung may be accomplished by dendritic cells, located beneath the airway epithelium, which function as antigen-presenting cells. In the presence of macrophages or inflammatory cytokines such as IL-1, dendritic cells become potent immunostimulatory cells for allogeneic T lymphocytes. Thus cytokines released in the injured lung may initiate dendritic cell differentiation into antigen-presenting cells that modulate T-cell-mediated lung injury (23).

2. Cytokines and Lung Injury

In addition to direct cell-mediated damage, the lung injury observed in idiopathic pneumonitis is likely the consequence of "networks" of multiple inflammatory cytokines. A large body of data indicates that cytokines such as tumor necrosis factor-α (TNF-α), IL-1, IL-6, and interferon-γ (IFN-γ) are present in the acutely injured lung (e.g., adult respiratory distress syndrome, lung allograft rejection) and may modulate the inflammatory and fibroproliferative responses to lung injury. It is therefore reasonable to speculate that one or more of these cytokines may play a role in the pathogenesis of IP. Furthermore, the expression of these cytokines appears to be increased in association with systemic GVHD. This raises the possibility that IP may represent a pulmonary GVHR mediated, at least in part, by one or more cytokines.

a. Tumor Necrosis Factor-α. TNF-α is a T-lymphocyte and mononuclear-phagocyte–derived cytokine with pleiotropic effects on a spectrum of inflammatory and immunological responses. Although low levels of TNF-α may participate in physiological homeostasis, increased levels of TNF-α expression have been implicated in the pathogenesis of a number of diseases, including GVHD (24); adult respiratory distress syndrome (ARDS) (25–28); lung, heart, kidney, and liver allograft rejection (29,30); and septic shock (31–33). The immunoregulatory properties of TNF-α include the ability to augment cytolytic activity of natural killer (NK) cells (34), enhance lymphocyte expression of MHC class II antigens and IL-2 receptors (35), and stimulate T-lymphocyte proliferation and production of IFN-γ (35). In addition, TNF-α may be a significant mediator of proximal nonspecific inflammation through leukocyte chemotaxis (36), increased endothelial expression of leukocyte adhesion molecules (ICAM) (37), and induction of IL-1 production by T lymphocytes (38) and mononuclear phagocytes (39,40).

Several lines of investigation implicate TNF-α in the pathogenesis of acute GVHD. Infusion of TNF-α in mice produces a systemic response that mimics the manifestations of GVHD, including fever, cachexia, diarrhea, and severe intestinal injury with epithelial cell necrosis (41). In a murine model of acute GVHD, administration of neutralizing antibody to TNF-α inhibits the development of cutaneous and intestinal lesions (24). Likewise, monoclonal or polyclonal antibodies to TNF-α ameliorate the GVH reaction in newborn mice (42). In the murine model of allogeneic marrow transplant, prophylactic administration of polyclonal antibody to TNF-α reduces GVHD-related mortality (43).

In humans, increased serum TNF-α levels following marrow transplant are associated with an increased incidence of acute GVHD (43–45). Preliminary data suggest that the prophylactic use of monoclonal antibody to TNF-α may reduce the incidence of acute GVHD in high-risk patients (43). Interestingly, anti-TNF-α monoclonal antibody produced significant although transient improvement in patients with severe acute GVHD (46).

TNF-α also appears to be a proximal mediator of nonspecific lung inflammation. Infusion of TNF-α in rats (47,48) or guinea pigs (49,50) produces noncardiogenic pulmonary edema within 8 hr, leading to respiratory insufficiency and death. In vitro TNF-α increases pulmonary artery endothelial cell permeability (51). Administration of monoclonal antibody to TNF-α in a baboon model of gram-negative sepsis blocks the development of pulmonary edema, suggesting that TNF- α is a proximal mediator of pulmonary injury in this setting (52). In humans, TNF-α levels in BAL fluid are significantly increased in patients with early severe ARDS compared to those at risk for developing ARDS, prior to the onset of ARDS, or later in the course of severe ARDS (25–27). Of note, TNF-α levels in serum do not correlate with those in the BAL fluid and are not significantly different among ARDS patients, those at risk for ARDS, or normal controls (26,53). Together these data suggest that TNF-α is an early participant in the inflammatory phase of the response to acute lung injury.

Currently there are insufficient data to define a role for TNF-α in the pathogenesis of IP after marrow transplant. Holler et al. (54) observed that TNF-α serum levels in marrow transplant recipients who developed interstitial pneumonitis were increased compared to those in transplant recipients who had an uneventful course. In this study maximal serum TNF-α levels preceded the clinical manifestations of pneumonitis by 24 to 54 days. The authors speculated that these increased serum cytokine levels prior to the onset of clinical pneumonitis might be indicative of local activation of pulmonary macrophages. However, given the lack of correlation between serum TNF-α levels and the development of ARDS, the significance of elevated serum TNF-α levels preceding the onset of idiopathic pneumonitis is uncertain, especially with the long lag period that is observed. Clarification of the cytokine alterations in the alveolar compartment at the time of noninfectious lung injury will come from the measurement of TNF-α levels in the alveolar lining fluid of patients at risk for as well as of those who develop IP.

b. Interleukin-1. IL-1 may function as a proximal mediator of GVHD through direct cell-mediated mechanisms as well as via nonspecific inflammatory pathways. IL-1 is the product of both inflammatory effector cells (such as mononuclear phagocytes, neutrophils, and B lymphocytes) as well as pulmonary parenchymal cells (including fibroblasts and smooth muscle and endothelial cells), and serves as a costimulatory factor for T lymphocytes responding to alloantigens and enhances NK and LAK cell activity. As an inflammatory cytokine, IL-1 augments leukocyte adhesion through increased ELAM and ICAM-1 expression on endothelial cells (37), promotes neutrophil chemotaxis by inducing IL-8 expression (55), stimulates endothelial cell secretion of procoagulant activity (56,57) and IL-6 (58), and upregulates endothelial expression of platelet activating factor (59), an established mediator of acute lung injury (60).

A number of in vivo observations support a central role for IL-1 in the efferent phase of GVHD. In a murine model, IL-1 mRNA and protein levels are increased in the skin of animals that develop GVHD to minor histocompatibility antigens (61). In clinical marrow transplantation, increased IL-1α mRNA and protein levels are present in the leukocytes and plasma of allogeneic recipients with acute GVHD (62,63). Interestingly, IL-1 receptor antagonist, a specific competitive inhibitor of both IL-1α and IL-1β, reduces GVHD-related mortality when administered to mice prophylactically or therapeutically (61,64).

IL-1 may be an inflammatory mediator of acute lung injury. Infusion of IL-1 into rabbits produces an acute lung injury characterized by pulmonary leukostasis, venular endothelial cell injury, and perivascular as well as interstitial edema (65). Expression of IL-1 appears to be upregulated in patients with acute lung injury. IL-1β immunoreactive protein levels are elevated in the BAL fluid of patients with early severe ARDS compared to patients at risk for ARDS or with late severe ARDS (27) and compared to normal controls (66). Furthermore, alveolar macrophages of ARDS patients release increased amounts of IL-1β compared to those recovered from patients with infectious pneumonia or normal controls (67). Thus, enhanced IL-1β production by pulmonary secretory effector cells and increased IL-1β concentration in the alveolar lining fluid of patients with early severe ARDS implicate this cytokine as a proximal mediator of acute lung injury. However, as with TNF-α, serum or plasma IL-1β levels do not correlate with those in the BAL fluid or with the presence of ARDS (27,66).

IL-1β may also participate in the pathogenesis of acute lung injury in idiopathic pneumonitis after bone marrow transplantation. Currently, there are no data addressing this question. IL-1 content in the alveolar lining fluid of IP patients should be examined as a first step to determine a role of this cytokine in the pathogenesis of IP after marrow transplantation.

c. *Interleukin-6.* IL-6, a pleotropic cytokine that mediates a number of physiological and immune responses, may play a role in GVHD. It functions as a soluble accessory factor in direct cell-mediated damage. Specifically, IL-6 induces cytotoxic T-lymphocyte (CTL) precursor responsiveness to IL-2 and, in conjunction with IL-1, stimulates IL-2 secretion by CTL precursors (68). In addition, IL-6 enhances LAK-cell secretion of TNF-β and expression of TNF receptors (69). Other immunoregulatory properties of IL-6 include induction of terminal B lymphocyte differentiation (70) and stimulation of immunoglobulin production by plasma cells. Cellular sources of IL-6 include mononuclear phagocytes, T lymphocytes, fibroblasts, smooth muscle cells, and epithelial and endothelial cells.

There is growing evidence to support a regulatory role of IL-6 in the pathogenesis of host versus graft (HVG) reactions in organ allograft rejection. In a murine model of the HVG reaction between host T and donor B lymphocytes, IL-6 levels in the serum were increased in allogeneic recipient animals (71). Of note, the hypergammaglobulin production by cultured spleen cells of these HVG mice was inhibited by anti IL-6 antibody or IL-6 receptor blocking antibody, implying a direct role for this cytokine in the allosensitization response. Similarly, in another murine model of HVG disease, IL-6 levels were elevated within sponge allografts containing donor lymphocytes simultaneous to the appearance of allosensitized cytotoxic T lymphocytes within the graft (72). In a murine model of renal allograft rejection, allograft infiltrating mononuclear cells produced a greater amount of IL-6 compared to peripheral blood monocytes recovered from the same animal (73). Finally, increased IL-6 expression was demonstrated in allograft lung RNA, bronchoalveolar lavage fluid, and lung homogenates of rats that developed acute lung allograft rejection (74). Interestingly, there was no correlation between plasma IL-6 levels and those of the allograft lung or with the presence of acute lung allograft rejection, suggesting that IL-6 expression was compartmentalized to the injured lung. As these examples indicate, increased IL-6 expression is associated with acute allograft rejection; however, the role played by this cytokine in the pathogenesis of the HVG reaction remains uncertain.

Increased IL-6 levels have also been reported in association with GVHD following bone marrow transplantation. Using a logistic regression model, Symington et al. demonstrated a correlation between elevated serum IL-6 levels and the onset of acute GVHD within 3 days of the cytokine peak (75). Likewise, peripheral blood monocyte IL-6 mRNA levels, as determined by semiquantitative RT-PCR, were increased in allograft recipients with acute or extensive chronic GVHD (62,63). These data implicate IL-6 in the cytokine response associated with GVHD after allogeneic marrow transplant. Based on its biological properties, IL-6 could indirectly modulate the GVH response by stimulating immune cell activation or, alternatively, it could act through nonspecific mechanisms to mediate disease directly.

IL-6 may also participate in the pathogenesis of inflammatory lung disease. Elevated IL-6 levels have been identified in the bronchoalveolar lavage fluid of patients with such inflammatory pulmonary disorders as idiopathic pulmonary fibrosis and hypersensitivity pneumonitis (76). As observed in the rat model of lung allograft rejection, there was no correlation between serum IL-6 levels and those found in the BAL fluid, suggesting that IL-6 is produced in the alveolar compartment rather than extravasated from the peripheral circulation. The role of IL-6 in the pathogenesis of inflammatory lung diseases or acute lung allograft rejection remains to be determined. Based upon the administration of IL-6 to tumor-bearing mice, there may be little or no direct pulmonary toxicity produced by this cytokine (77).

Likewise, a role for IL-6 in idiopathic pneumonitis associated with GVHD after bone marrow transplantation has yet to be defined. In an analysis of serial serum sets from 22 allogeneic marrow recipients, Symington et al. demonstrated elevated IL-6 levels temporally related to the onset of bilateral pulmonary infiltrates in three patients, all of whom had either no or only grade I GVHD (75). This report did not distinguish between infectious versus idiopathic interstitial pneumonitis. Furthermore, there was no analysis of IL-6 content in the alveolar lining fluid. Since there is no apparent correlation between serum IL-6 levels and either acute HVG reaction (74) or inflammatory lung disorders (76), the significance of increased serum IL-6 levels in these three allogeneic recipients with diffuse pulmonary infiltrates is uncertain. Moreover, while IL-6 may participate in lung injury after marrow transplantation, there are no data to substantiate a role for IL-6 in the pathogenesis of IP associated with acute GVHD.

d. Interferon-γ. Interferon-γ (IFN-γ) is an immunomodulatory and proinflammatory cytokine secreted by T lymphocytes and natural killer (NK) cells. The biological properties of IFN-γ include regulation of class I and II major histocompatibility antigen expression (78–80), promotion of IL-2–dependent growth and maturation of cytotoxic T-lymphocyte precursors (81), enhancement of NK cell cytotoxicity (82), stimulation of B lymphocyte growth and differentiation (83), induction of TNF-α and IL-1 secretion by macrophages (83), and modulation of procoagulant, permeability, and adhesive properties of endothelial cells (83). Several different lines of evidence support a role for IFN-γ in the pathogenesis of GVHD. In murine models of acute GVHD, splenocytes recovered from GVH mice express increased steady-state mRNA levels of IFN-γ compared to controls (84) and produce significantly higher levels of this cytokine in response to concanavalin A stimulation than do syngeneic spleen cells (85). Using an in vitro human skin explant model, IFN-γ as well as TNF-α have been implicated as producing epithelial cell damage histologically similar to that seen in cutaneous GVHD, because this epithelial cell damage was prevented by the use of neutralizing antibody against either IFN-γ or TNF-α (86). The results of this study suggest a role for both IFN-γ and TNF-α in the pathogenesis of GVH reactions and indicate that these cytokines can act independently or synergistically to cause direct cellular damage.

IFN-γ has also been shown to participate in the pathogenesis of GVHD using in vivo systems. In a murine model of the GVH reaction, treatment of allograft recipients with IFN-γ antibody prior to the induction of GVHR abrogated virtually all of the enteropathy, including villus atrophy and crypt hyperplasia, observed in untreated animals that developed GVHD (87). Similarly, infusion of soluble IFN-γ receptor ameliorated weight loss, elevation of the acute-phase reactant serum amyloid protein (SAP), and mortality associated with acute GVHD in another murine model (83). Moreover, the administration of neutralizing antibody against IFN-γ has been demonstrated to suppress acute organ allograft rejection (88,89).

Two possible mechanisms by which IFN-γ may modulate GVH related cell destruction are (a) through a direct effect on epithelial cells, increasing the expression of class II MHC antigens and rendering these cells susceptible to the cytolytic activity of other immune effector cells, or (b) through an indirect effect, stimulating immune effector cells such as NK cells or macrophages, which directly damage epithelium by lytic attack or by releasing other inflammatory cytokines such as TNF-α or IL-1.

There is only indirect evidence implicating IFN-γ in the pathogenesis of clinical GVHD. IFN-γ mRNA and protein have been detected in the leukocytes and serum, respectively, of allogeneic recipients with acute GVHD (62). Furthermore, Niederwieser et al. have demonstrated significantly increased serum IFN-γ levels as early as 4 days prior to the clinical onset of grade 2 or greater acute GVHD compared to allogeneic recipients with uncomplicated marrow transplants (90). Although the expression of IFN-γ is increased in the setting of clinical GVHD, the biological significance of this upregulation has yet to be determined.

There are no data regarding IFN-γ in the pathogenesis of nontransplant acute lung injury. However, increased levels of IFN-α have been identified in the bronchoalveolar lavage fluid recovered from patients with early severe ARDS compared to that of patients at risk or with early mild ARDS (27). There was no correlation between IFN-α levels in the BAL fluid with those in the plasma or between plasma IFN-γ levels and the presence of ARDS.

IFN-γ was not detected in the BAL fluid or serum of allogeneic recipients with non-CMV-related interstitial pneumonitis, irrespective of the presence of GVHD

(91). Although IFN-γ levels in the BAL fluid may have been decreased relative to those at the alveolar surface because of the dilution of alveolar lining fluid with saline introduced at lavage, this cytokine was detected in comparable samples recovered from normal subjects as well as allogeneic recipients without interstitial pneumonitis. Thus, the absence of measurable IFN-γ in the BAL fluid and serum of these patients argues against a crucial role for this cytokine in the pathogenesis of noninfectious interstitial pneumonitis associated with GVHD after bone marrow transplantation.

III. HEMORRHAGIC ALVEOLITIS

In a subset of bone marrow recipients, IP is accompanied by pulmonary hemorrhage or hemorrhagic alveolitis. In a necropsy series, Sloan identified acute hemorrhagic pulmonary edema (AHPE) in 16% of 32 patients (92). Eighty percent of the patients who developed AHPE had received a non-HLA-identical allograft and had previous GVHD. The pulmonary lesions were characterized by intraalveolar and interstitial exudation of edema fluid, fibrin, and erythrocytes, and no specific pathogens were detected. Each of these patients died of acute respiratory failure after the onset of a syndrome characterized by fever, skin rash, fluid retention, uremia, low serum albumin concentration, low central venous pressure, and pulmonary edema.

In an autopsy review of 37 allogeneic bone marrow recipients at the Johns Hopkins Hospital, Wojno et al. identified 15 cases of terminal pulmonary hemorrhage with no evidence of systemic infection (93). Pulmonary hemorrhage was listed as the cause of death in 59% of those patients with grade 2 or greater GVHD as opposed to 25% of those with no or mild GVHD and 20% of autologous marrow recipients. Likewise, terminal pulmonary hemorrhage occurred in association with total body irradiation (TBI) as a component of the preparative regimen. Analysis of variance demonstrated that acute GVHD and TBI were independently related to pulmonary hemorrhage. Varying degrees of pulmonary hemorrhage were observed in all the cases of significant acute GVHD compared to only 50% in the group with mild or no GVHD. Of note, there was no significant difference in the incidence of interstitial pneumonitis between these two groups. Furthermore, terminal platelet counts were no different between patients with acute GVHD compared to those without or between patients who died of terminal pulmonary hemorrhage versus those who died of other causes. The authors speculated that endothelial cell injury mediated by acute GVHD was responsible for pulmonary hemorrhage in these patients; however, direct evidence to support an alloreactive mechanism of lung injury was not identified.

A. Pathogenesis of Hemorrhagic Alveolitis

Hemorrhagic alveolitis has been reported in a murine model of acute GVHD (14). When irradiated (CBA × B10)F1 hybrid mice were infused with parental bone marrow cells together with T lymphocytes, they developed a lethal GVHR at 15 days characterized by intestinal and epidermal alterations, weight loss, and loss of hypodermic fat. Recipients of B10 parental T lymphocytes developed an alveolitis during the acute phase of this lethal GVHR. The alveolitis was characterized by (a) alveolar hemorrhage, (b) accumulation of platelet microthrombi and neutrophils within alveolar capillaries, (c) infiltration of the endothelium by mononuclear cells, and (d) alterations in type II alveolar epithelial cells with increased numbers of mitotic figures. Electron microscopic characterization of the alveolitis was remarkable for endothelial cell damage, loss of lamellar bodies in type II epithelial cells, and interstitial edema. The alveolitis was accompanied by a vasculitis consisting of infiltration of the large veins and arteries by mononuclear cells. There was no evidence of bacterial or viral infection to account for these pulmonary abnormalities. In addition, alveolitis was not observed in irradiated recipients of T-lymphocyte-depleted bone marrow cells. Thus, in this murine model, hemorrhagic alveolitis appeared to be a strain-specific manifestation of the GVH reaction, since F1 recipients of B10 but not CBA parental T lymphocytes developed this complication.

TNF-α may be partly responsible for the hemorrhagic alveolitis seen in this murine model of acute GVHD. This conclusion is supported by three observations. First, the lungs of recipients of parental T lymphocytes showed a 10- fold increase in TNF-α mRNA transcripts compared to recipients of bone marrow cells without T lymphocytes. Second, bronchoalveolar lavage cells recovered from recipients of B10 parental T lymphocytes secreted increased amounts of TNF-α in vitro compared to the amounts secreted by control mice (5 to 20 U/mL versus 0 to 10 U/mL, respectively). Finally, administration of TNF-α–neutralizing antibody prevented alveolar hemorrhage in recipients of B10 parental T lymphocytes but did not eliminate the vasculitis or platelet microthrombi formation. Based on these observations, one would conclude that hemorrhagic alveolitis is associated with lethal acute GVHD in this murine model and that the lung injury is mediated, at least in part, through the induction of TNF-α.

In addition to nonspecific cytokine-mediated endothelial cell injury, hemorrhagic alveolitis may also be the consequence of direct cell-mediated damage to pulmonary endothelium. An association between endothelial cell injury and acute GVHD has been described in both hepatic (94) and skin GVHR (95). Vascular injury in skin GVHD is characterized histologically by intimal and perivascular lymphocytic infiltrates, perivascular edema, and endothelial cell swelling and sloughing (95). A number of studies support the concept of cell-mediated endothelial injury. Human umbilical vein endothelial cells are capable of directly stimulating allogeneic responses in mixed lymphocyte-endothelial cell cultures (96). Moreover, immune-mediated endothelial cell injury has been produced in vitro with allogeneic splenocytes recovered from rats with acute GVHD (97). Human microvascular endothelial cells express HLA class I and II molecules in situ as demonstrated by immunohistochemistry (98). The expression of endothelial cell HLA class I antigen in vitro is independently induced by IFN-γ and TNF-α (99,100). Likewise, IFN-γ stimulates surface expression of class II MHC antigens in human umbilical vein endothelial cells (101). Presumably, cytokines that induce HLA antigen expression on the endothelial cell surface may enhance susceptibility of these cells to cytotoxic T-lymphocyte-mediated lysis.

IV. AIRFLOW OBSTRUCTIVE DISEASE

Obstructive airways disease as a sequela to marrow transplantation was first recognized in 1982 (102,103), and within the next 5 years, a total of 36 recipients of allogeneic marrow transplants with severe obstructive airways disease were described (1,104–111). All patients were recipients of allogeneic transplants, had clinical evidence of chronic GVHD, and presented with respiratory symptoms of cough, wheeze, or dyspnea within 1.5 to 10 months after marrow transplantation. Lung function tests revealed diminished FEV_1/FVC in all those tested. Chest radiographs only occasionally revealed infiltrates. The case-fatality rate in these 36 cases was over 50%, despite aggressive treatments with corticosteroids, bronchodilators, and, in many cases, azathioprine. Only 3 patients (8%) demonstrated slowly improved lung function, usually over 6 to 24 months (106).

Bronchiolitis was the predominant but not invariable pathological finding among allogeneic marrow transplant recipients with new-onset symptomatic obstructive airways disease. Evidence of parenchymal lung injury also was present (106). Small airway involvement with bronchiolitis, occasionally with fibrinous obliteration of the lumen, was evident in 16 of 21 (76%), with or without associated interstitial pneumonia, fibrosis, or diffuse alveolar damage. In 5 cases (24%), only bronchitis or interstitial pneumonia was noted. The inflammatory cellular infiltrates vary in relative proportions of neutrophils and lymphocytes and tend to be peribronchiolar. Two distinct patterns of lung inflammation have been identified by BAL in allogeneic recipients with new onset of airflow obstruction in the setting of GVHD. Of 12 patients evaluated for obstructive impairment, St. John et al. found that 42% had a neutrophil-predominant (neutrophil percentage = 20 ± 6%) while 25% had a lymphocyte-predominant (lymphocyte percentage = 36 ± 12%) lavage (112). Pulmonary pathogens were not identified in any patient and tobacco use was minimal or none. These data imply that airflow obstruction in allogeneic recipients with GVHD may represent a heterogeneous group of disorders arising from distinctly different causes.

Pulmonary infection has been identified in half of the cases examined histopathologically. Infectious agents included bacteria, fungus, *Pneumocystis*, and viruses. Although some of these infections may have been causally related to the bronchiolitis, more likely they were the consequence of the immune deficiency associated with chronic GVHD and represent coincident or terminal events.

Thirty-five allogeneic marrow recipients transplanted at a single center with new-onset obstructive airways disease were reviewed to further define the clinical presentation (113). The onset of obstructive airways disease (defined as a decline in the FEV_1 and FEV_1/FVC to less than 70% of predicted values compared to normal baseline) was between 50 and 150 days after marrow transplantation in 40% and between 150 and 500 days in almost all others (54%). Chronic GVHD was present in 74% of patients. Chest radiographs were usually normal on presentation (80%). Most patients had pulmonary symptoms (80%), including cough (60%), dyspnea (51%), and wheezing or "flu" symptoms (23% each). Physical examination was frequently unrevealing. Only 40% had wheeze and fewer (14%) had crackles. The study confirmed that infections were common, occuring more than 100 days after marrow transplantation in over half of the cases. Sinusitis was the most common infection.

Airways obstructive disease is not limited solely to allogeneic transplants. Two cases of fatal bronchiolitis (demonstrated by open lung biopsy) associated with autologous marrow transplantation have features that distinguish them from the cases occurring after allogeneic transplantation (114). Both of these cases occurred in the absence of GVHD, and both patients had been transplanted as treatment for lymphoma after extensive courses of conventional chemotherapy and local thoracic irradiation. As in other cases, onset of wheezing, dyspnea and cough was 3 and 9 months after marrow transplantation; but in contrast to previous reports among allogeneic marrow transplant recipients, pulmonary function testing revealed no decrease in FEV_1/FVC suggestive of obstructive airways disease. However, both FEV_1 and FVC declined compared to pretransplant values and an increase in the residual volume suggested small airway obstruction.

A. Prevalence and Risk Factors for Airflow Obstruction

The estimated incidence of airflow obstruction is 10 to 11% of long-term survivors of bone marrow transplantation with chronic GVHD (106,110). The incidence after autologous marrow transplantation appears to be much lower, but it is not zero.

The prevalence of chronic GVHD strongly suggested that this immune reaction is a risk factor for new-onset obstructive airways disease after allogeneic marrow transplantation. In a review of 281 marrow recipients who returned for pulmonary function tests after 1 year, Clark et al. (115) found that only 1 of 75 patients without chronic GVHD had a decrement in the FEV_1/FVC greater than 15% at 1 year compared to baseline. In contrast 11% (16 of 143) of patients with chronic GVHD had new-onset obstructive airways disease by this definition ($p = 0.0002$). Other risk factors were increasing age and the use of methotrexate for immunosuppression to prevent GVHD. The effect of methotrexate appeared in multivariate analysis to be synergistic with the presence of chronic GVHD on worsening airflow obstructive disease. The role of methotrexate in inducing or augmenting obstructive airways disease in this setting is unexplained. Recent data suggest that cyclosporine for GVHD prophylaxis may significantly decrease the incidence of airflow obstruction associated with chronic GVHD (116).

The putative role of low serum IgG levels as a risk factor for obstructive airways disease is less well established. A review of 549 marrow transplant recipients treated at the Johns Hopkins Oncology Center over a period of 9 years revealed that obliterative bronchiolitis occurring more than 120 days after marrow transplantation was seen only among patients with both chronic GVHD and reduced IgG levels (117). The incidence of obliterative bronchiolitis was 5% among 120- day survivors with low IgG levels compared with none of those with normal levels ($p = 0.04$). The interpretation of these data is difficult, since the diagnoses were on the basis of histopathological findings at autopsy, not physiological airflow obstruction. The 2% incidence is substantially lower and the method of identifying cases different than reported elsewhere, making comparisons difficult.

B. Pathogenesis

The pathogenesis of new-onset airflow obstructive disease in patients with chronic GVHD may be related to host bronchiolar epithelial cells that serve as targets for donor CTL (118). The hypothesis that a CTL response contributes to obstructive airways disease after marrow transplantation is supported indirectly by the finding that bronchiolar epithelial cells can express MHC class II antigens on their surfaces and could be targets for HLA-unrestricted CTL responses. Expression of class II antigen can be induced in lung cells by IFN-γ as well as in lung injury experimentally induced with bleomycin and in idiopathic pulmonary fibrosis (119–121). Augmented MHC class I and II antigen expression has been noted on lung endothelial and epithelial cells from lung transplant recipients with obliterative bronchiolitis (122). Results of MHC antigen expression in the lungs of marrow transplant recipients have not been published. In preliminary studies at our center, expression of class II antigen was noted in the several lung tissue samples examined after marrow transplantation, but this finding did not appear related to the presence of GVHD (J. G. Clark and G. E. Sale, unpublished results.)

Airway involvement is usually not seen in GVHD reactions induced in animal models. However, Stein-Streilein et al. did create a GVHR in the lungs of F_1 hybrid hamsters by intratracheal inoculation of parental lymph node cells (123). Evidence of trafficking of inoculated lymph node cells across the bronchial epithelium was demonstrated, and the pulmonary inflammatory response was due to contact of inoculated cells with host histocompatibility antigens. The GVHR in this hamster model was characterized by an intense mononuclear inflammatory infiltration in the alveolar spaces and interstitium. Also, there was a marked and distinctive perivascular infiltration. This response is in contrast to the peribronchial infiltration reported in patients with bronchiolitis after marrow transplantation.

There are no direct data to support that obstructive airways disease after marrow transplantation is a pulmonary GVHD reaction. Although it is an attractive theory for the pathogenesis of bronchiolitis, evidence of bronchiolar epithelial-directed CTL response by donor lymphocytes has not been established. Alternatively, inflammatory cytokines could play a role in the bronchiolar injury; however, data to support this concept are currently lacking. Other explanations for small airway inflammation after marrow transplantation include recurrent aspiration of oral material due to esophagitis associated with GVHD or unrecognized viral infection. The varied histopathologies, BAL cell differentials and apparent clinical courses, frequency of associated pulmonary infection, and occurrence after autologous marrow transplantation together suggest that new-onset obstructive airways disease after marrow transplantation is not a single entity but rather a response to multiple inciting events.

V. LYMPHOCYTIC BRONCHITIS AND ALVEOLITIS

A. Lymphocytic Bronchitis

Lymphocytic bronchitis, histologically defined as the lymphocytic infiltration of large airway mucosa accompanied by necrosis of individual epithelial cells, has been proposed as a pulmonary manifestation of GVHD. In an autopsy review, Beschorner et al. reported a 60% incidence of lymphocytic bronchitis in allogeneic recipients with grade 2 or greater GVHD, compared to an 8% incidence in those patients with no or grade I GVHD (124). These authors concluded that lymphocytic bronchitis was a manifestation of GVHD for three reasons: (a) lymphocytic bronchitis had a histological appearance similar to that of GVH reactions in the intestine; (b) in this study, lymphocytic bronchitis was present in the majority of patients with grade 2 or greater GVHD of other organ systems; and (c) in 80% of cases, pulmonary symptoms appeared within 1 to 32 days (median 5 days) of the onset of grade 2 or greater GVHD. Of concern, however, is the fact that acute bronchitis or bronchopneumonia was identified in 73% of these cases of lymphocytic bronchitis compared to a 25% incidence in allogeneic recipients who did not develop this abnormality. The authors postulated that damage to mucociliary transport mechanisms resulted in lower respiratory tract inflammation; however, this interpretation is controversial.

An association between lymphocytic bronchitis and GVHD has not been substantiated by other investigators. Hackman et al., in their review of 128 autopsies—including 84 allogeneic recipients, 7 autograft recipients, 7 syngeneic recipients and 30 nontransplant patients—identified histologic changes consistent with lymphocytic bronchitis in 20% of the cases (125). However, there was no significant correlation between the airway abnormality and the presence of acute GVHD in other organs. Furthermore, lymphocytic bronchitis was identified in 30% of trauma victims maintained on mechanical ventilation for at least 48 hrs prior to death and in 38% of non-transplant patients who died of viral pneumonia. Likewise, in a review of biopsy and autopsy lung tissue from 54 marrow recipients, Connor et al. found no correlation between lymphocytic bronchitis and GVHD (126).

Two different animal models have been utilized to investigate an association between lymphocytic bronchitis and GVHD. Stein-Streilein et al. observed that acute GVHD—manifest by splenomegaly, lymphadenopathy, and thymic atrophy following the intravenous or intracutaneous inoculation of hyperimmune parental cells into F_1 hybrid hamsters—was not accompanied by lymphocytic infiltration of the airway mucosa or airway epithelial cell necrosis (123). In a canine model of GVHD, lymphocytic bronchitis was present in 22% of allogeneic recipients compared to 12% of autologous recipients (127). Chi square analysis failed to demonstrate a significant correlation between lymphocytic bronchitis and either the origin of the infused marrow or the presence of GVHD involving two or more organs. Furthermore, binary logistic regression analysis showed that lymphocytic bronchitis was not significantly associated with GVHD of the skin, liver, or bowel. Based on the results of these animal models together with the above clinical studies, it is reasonable to conclude that lymphocytic bronchitis represents nonspecific large airway inflammation rather than a pulmonary manifestation of GVHD.

B. Lymphocytic Alveolitis

Lymphocytic alveolitis following bone marrow transplantation is characterized by dyspnea, nonproductive cough, abnormal chest radiography featuring localized or diffuse interstitial infiltrates, the presence of more than 15% lymphocytes with a minimum of 25×10^3 lymphocytes per milliliter in the bronchoalveolar lavage and the absence of pulmonary pathogens. Leblond et al. identified lymphocytic alveolitis in 10% of allogeneic recipients of HLA-identical marrow, all of whom had chronic GVHD (128). This disorder occurred relatively late after transplant, with a median onset of 210 days. All patients had a T-lymphocytic alveolitis consisting primarily of $CD8^+$ cells that were approximately equally divided between cytotoxic (D44 and S6F1) and immunomodulatory (CD57) phenotypes. Lung biopsy specimens of two patients were remarkable for lymphocytic interstitial pneumonitis and moderate alveolar septal fibrosis. Notably, epithelial cell necrosis and exocrine gland destruction were absent. The majority of cases (86%) responded to corticosteroid therapy and no case progressed to obliterative bronchiolitis. Similar patients were reported by Perreault et al. with respect to the BAL features, histology, and response to corticosteroids (129).

T-lymphocytic alveolitis is not unique to allogeneic marrow transplantation and has been observed as a virus-associated as well as idiopathic disorder in nontransplant patients (130). The pathogenesis of this inflammatory process remains to be elucidated. However, the abundance of $CD8^+$ T-lymphocytes within the alveolar lumen and infiltrating alveolar septa suggest a direct cell-mediated injury involving one or more cellular constituents of the alveolus. The increased expression of HLA class II antigen by alveolar epithelium in these patients suggests that these cells may be performing an accessory function in this disorder (130). Although it is tempting to speculate that lymphocytic alveolitis in allogeneic recipients with GVHD is a pulmonary GVH reaction, the absence of lymphocyte-associated epithelial cell destruction—comparable to that observed in GVHD of the skin, liver or intestine—leaves the question unresolved. Alternatively, T lymphocytes that accumulate in the alveolar compartment could release one or more inflammatory cytokines. However, data that substantiate cytokine secretion in lymphocytic alveolitis have not been reported. Moreover, since lymphocytic alveolitis occurs in association with a variety of non-transplant-related conditions, it may represent a nonspecific chronic inflammatory response localized primarily to the alveolus.

VI. CONCLUSION

Is the lung a target organ for GVHD? The data clearly document a statistical association between the occurrence of noninfectious pulmonary complications and GVHD. In addition, there exists an association between increased inflammatory cytokine expression and transplant-related complications, including GVHD. Moreover, expression of these cytokines is upregulated in acutely injured lungs of nontransplant patients. Animal models of transplantation suggest that both T-lymphocyte-mediated alloreactivity and inflammatory cytokines play roles in the pathogenesis of acute lung injury in allogeneic recipients. However, evidence of either cytokine or T-lymphocyte-directed acute lung injury in patients with GVHD is lacking.

Thus, the most conservative and reasonable interpretation of the data is that "GVHD-associated lung injuries" are transplant-related complications that encompass a spectrum of pulmonary abnormalities including idiopathic pneumonitis and obliterative bronchiolitis. But there is insufficient evidence to conclude that the lung is a target organ for GVHD in bone marrow transplant patients. Specifically, the hallmark of GVHD, lymphocyte-mediated epithelial cell necrosis, has not been demonstrated. In the absence of this characteristic histopathology, evidence of cell-mediated and cytokine-directed mechanisms within the airways and alveolar compartment are required to demonstrate alloreactivity.

REFERENCES

1. Krowka MJ, Rosenow EC, Hoagland HC. Pulmonary complications of bone marrow transplantation. Chest 1985; 87:237–246.
2. Meyers JD, Flournoy N, Thomas ED. Nonbacterial pneumonia after allogeneic marrow transplantation: A review of ten years' experience. Rev Infect Dis 1982; 4:1119–1132.
3. Weiner RS, Bortin MM, Gale RP, et al. Interstitial pneumonitis after bone marrow transplantation. Ann Intern Med 1986; 104:168–175.

4. Clark JG, Hansen JA, Hertz MI, et al. Idiopathic pneumonia syndrome following bone marrow transplantation. Am Rev Respir Dis 1993; 147:1601–1606.
5. Crawford SW, Longton G, Storb R. Acute graft-versus-host disease and the risks for idiopathic pneumonia after marrow transplantation for severe aplastic anemia. Bone Marrow Transplant 1993; 12:225–231.
6. Weiner RS, Horowitz MM, Gale RP, et al. Risk factors for interstitial pneumonia following bone marrow transplantation for severe aplastic anemia. Br J Haematol 1989; 71:535–543.
7. Grañena A, Carreras E, Rozman C, et al. Interstitial pneumonitis after BMT: 15 years experience in a single institution. Bone Marrow Transplant 1993; 11:453–458.
8. Wingard JR, Mellits ED, Sostrin MB, et al. Interstitial pneumonitis after allogeneic bone marrow transplantation: Nine-year experience at a single institution. Medicine 1988; 67:175–186.
9. Kantrow SP, Hackman RC, Boeckh M, et al. Idiopathic pneumonia syndrome after bone marrow transplantation. Am Rev Respir Dis 1994; 149:A1030.
10. Sale GE, Shulman HM, Hackman RC. Pathology of bone marrow transplantation. In: Forman SJ, Blume KG, Thomas ED, eds. Bone Marrow Transplantation. Boston: Blackwell, 1994:200.
11. Crawford SW, Hackman RC, Clark JG. Open lung biopsy diagnosis of diffuse pulmonary infiltrates after marrow transplantation. Chest 1988; 94:949–953.
12. Pecego R, Hill R, Appelbaum FR, et al. Interstitial pneumonitis following autologous bone marrow transplantation. Transplantation 1986; 42:515–517.
13. Down JD, Mauch P, Warhol M, et al. The effect of donor T lymphocytes and total-body irradiation on hemopoietic engraftment and pulmonary toxicity following experimental allogeneic bone marrow transplantation. Transplantation 1992; 54:802–808.
14. Piguet PF, Grau GE, Collart MA, et al. Pneumopathies of the graft-versus-host reaction: Alveolitis associated with an increased level of tumor necrosis factor mRNA and chronic interstitial pneumonitis. Lab Invest 1989; 61:37–45.
15. Varekamp AE. Interstitial pneumonitis following bone marrow transplantation: Studies in the Brown Norway rat (thesis). The Netherlands: University of Leiden, 1990.
16. Korngold R, Sprent J. Variable capacity of L3T4^{+} T cells to cause lethal graft versus host disease across minor histocompatibility barriers in mice. J Exp Med 1987; 165: 1552–1564.
17, Ferrara JLM, Guillen FJ, Van Dijken PJ, et al. Evidence that large granular lymphocytes of donor origin mediate acute graft-versus-host disease. Transplantation 1989; 47:50–54.
18. Ghayur T, Seemayer TA, Lapp WS. Prevention of murine graft-versus-host disease by inducing and eliminating ASGM1^{+} cells of donor origin. Transplantation 1988; 45: 586–590.
19. Workman DL, Clancy Jr. Interstitial pneumonitis and lymphocytic bronchiolitis/ bronchitis as a direct result of acute lethal graft-versus-host disease duplicate the histopathology of lung allograft rejection. Transplantation 1994; 58:207–213.
20. Rosenberg SA, Lotze MT, Muul LM, et al. Observation on the systemic administration of autologous lymphokine- activated killer cells and recombinant interleukin-2 to patients with metastatic cancer. N Engl J Med 1985; 313:1485–1492.
21. Rosenstein M, Ettinghausen SE, Rosenberg SA. Extravasation of intravascular fluid mediated by the systemic administration of recombinant interleukin 2. J Immunol 1986; 137:1735–1742.
22. Rabinowich H, Zeevi A, Paradis IL, et al. Proliferative responses of bronchoalveolar lavage lymphocytes from heart-lung transplant patients. Transplantation 1990; 49: 115–121.

23. Toews GB. Pulmonary dendritic cells: Sentinels of lung-associated lymphoid tissues. Am J Respir Cell Mol Biol 1991; 4:204–205.
24. Piguet P-F, Grau GE, Allet B, Vassalli P. Tumor necrosis factor/cachectin is an effector of skin and gut lesions of the acute phase of graft-vs-host disease. J Exp Med 1987; 166:1280–1289.
25. Millar AB, Singer M, Meager A, et al. Tumour necrosis factor in bronchopulmonary secretions of patients with adult respiratory distress syndrome. Lancet 1989; 2:712–714.
26. Hyers TM, Tricomi SM, Dettenmeier PA, Fowler AA. Tumor necrosis factor levels in serum and bronchoalveolar lavage fluid of patients with the adult respiratory distress syndrome. Am Rev Respir Dis 1991; 144:268–271.
27. Suter PM, Suter S, Girardin E, Roux-Lombard P, et al. High bronchoalveolar levels of tumor necrosis factor and its inhibitors, interleukin-1, interferon, and elastase, in patients with adult respiratory distress syndrome after trauma, shock, or sepsis. Am Rev Respir Dis 1992; 145:1016–1022.
28. Van Nhieu JT, Misset B, Lebargy F, et al. Expression of tumor necrosis factor-α gene in alveolar macrophages from patients with the adult respiratory distress syndrome. Am Rev Respir Dis 1993; 147:1585–1589.
29. Lin H, Chensue SW, Strieter RM, et al. Antibodies against tumor necrosis factor prolong cardiac allograft survival in the rat. J Heart Lung Transplant 1992; 11:330–335.
30. Imagawa DK, Millis JM, Olthoff KM, et al. The role of tumor necrosis factor in allograft rejection. Transplantation 1990; 50:219–225.
31. Beutler B, Cerami A. Cachectin and tumour necrosis factor as two sides of the same biological coin. Nature 1986; 320:584–588.
32. Beutler B. Tumor necrosis, cachexia, shock, and inflammation: A common mediator. Ann Rev Biochem 1988; 57:505–518.
33. Sherry B, Cerami A. Cachectin/tumor necrosis factor exerts endocrine, paracrine, and autocrine control of inflammatory responses. J Cell Biol 1988; 107:1269–1277.
34. Ostensen ME, Thiele DL, Lipsky PE. Tumor necrosis factor-α enhances cytolytic activity of human natural killer cells. J Immunol 1987; 138:4185–4191.
35. Scheurich P, Thoma B, Ücer U, Pfizenmaier K. Immunoregulatory activity of recombinant human tumor necrosis factor (TNF)-α: Induction of the receptors of human T cells and TNF-α-mediated enhancement of T cell responses. J Immunol 1987; 138: 1786–1790.
36. Ming WJ, Bersani L, Mantovani A. Tumor necrosis factor is chemotactic for monocytes and polymorphonuclear leukocytes. J Immunol 1987; 138:1469–1474.
37. Pober JS, Lapierre LA, Stolpen AH, et al. Activation of cultured human endothelial cells by recombinant lymphotoxin: Comparison with tumor necrosis factor and interleukin 1 species. J Immunol 1987; 138:3319–3324.
38. Zucali JR, Elfenbein GJ, Barth KC, Dinarello CA. Effects of human interleukin 1 and human tumor necrosis factor on human T lymphocyte colony formation. J Clin Invest 1987; 80:772–777.
39. Turner M, Chantry D, Buchan G, et al. Regulation of expression of human IL-1α and IL-1β genes. J Immunol 1989; 143:3556–3561.
40. Danis VA, Kulesz AJ, Nelson DS, Brooks PM. Cytokine regulation of human monocyte interleukin-1 (IL-1) production in vitro: Enhancement of IL-1 production by interferon (IFN) gamma, tumor necrosis factor-alpha, IL-2 and IL-1, and inhibition by IFN-alpha. Clin Exp Immunol 1990; 80:435–443.
41. Remick DG, Kunkel SL. Pathophysiologic alterations induced by tumor necrosis factor. Int Rev Exp Pathol 1993; 34B:7–25.
42. Shalaby MR, Fendly B, Sheehan KC, et al. Prevention of the graft-versus-host reaction

in newborn mice by antibodies to tumor necrosis factor-alpha. Transplantation 1989; 47:1057–1061.

43. Holler E, Kolb HJ, Hintermeier-Knabe R, et al. Role of tumor necrosis factor alpha in acute graft-versus-host disease and complications following allogeneic bone marrow transplantation. Transplant Proc 1993; 25:1234–1236.
44. Symington FW, Pepe MS, Chen AB, Deliganis A. Serum tumor necrosis factor alpha associated with acute graft- versus-host disease in humans. Transplantation 1990; 50: 518–521.
45. Holler E, Hintermeier-Knabe R, Kolb HJ, et al. Low incidence of transplant-related complications in patients with chronic release of tumor necrosis factor-alpha before admission to bone marrow transplantation: A clinical correlate of cytokine desensitization. Pathobiology 1991; 59:171–175.
46. Hervé P, Flesch M, Tiberghien J, et al. Phase I-II trial of a monoclonal anti-tumor necrosis factor α antibody for the treatment of refractory severe acute graft-versus-host disease. Blood 1992; 79:3362–3368.
47. Tracey KJ, Beutler B, Lowry SF, et al. Shock and tissue injury induced by recombinant human cachectin. Science 1986; 234:470–474.
48. Ferrari-Baliviera E, Mealy K, Smith RJ, Wilmore DW. Tumor necrosis factor induces adult respiratory distress syndrome in rats. Arch Surg 1989; 124:1400–1405.
49. Stephens KE, Ishizaka A, Larrick JW, Raffin TA. Tumor necrosis factor causes increased pulmonary permeability and edema. Am Rev Respir Dis 1988; 137:1364–1370.
50. Lilly CM, Sandhu JS, Ishizaka A, et al. Pentoxifylline prevents tumor necrosis factor-induced lung injury. Am Rev Respir Dis 1989; 139:1361–1368.
51. Horvath CJ, Ferro TJ, Jesmok G, Malik AB. Recombinant tumor necrosis factor increases pulmonary vascular permeability independent of neutrophils. Proc Natl Acad Sci USA 1988; 85:9219–9223.
52. Tracey KJ, Fong Y, Hesse DG, et al. Anti-cachectin/TNF monoclonal antibodies prevent septic shock during lethal bacteraemia. Nature 1987; 330:662–664.
53. Roten R, Markert M, Feihl F, et al. Plasma levels of tumor necrosis factor in the adult respiratory distress syndrome. Am Rev Respir Dis 1991; 143:590–592.
54. Holler E, Kolb HJ, Möller A, et al. Increased serum levels of tumor necrosis factor α precede major complications of bone marrow transplantation. Blood 1990; 75:1011–1016.
55. Strieter RM, Kunkel SL, Showell HJ, et al. Endothelial cell gene expression of a neutrophil chemotactic factor by TNF-α, LPS, and IL-1β. Science 1989; 243:1467–1469.
56. Bevilacqua MP, Pober JS, Majeau GR, et al. Interleukin 1 (IL-1) induces biosynthesis and cell surface expression of procoagulant activity in human vascular endothelial cells. J Exp Med 1984; 160:618–623.
57. Dejana E, Breviario F, Erroi A, et al. Modulation of endothelial cell functions by different molecular species of interleukin 1. Blood 1987; 69:695–699.
58. Sironi M, Breviario F, Proserpio P, et al. IL-1 stimulates IL-6 production in endothelial cells. J Immunol 1989; 142:549–553.
59. Bussolino F, Breviario F, Tetta C, et al. Interleukin 1 stimulates platelet-activating factor production in cultured human endothelial cells. J Clin Invest 1986; 77:2027–2033.
60. McManus LM, Pinckard RN. Kinetics of acetyl glyceryl ether phosphorylcholine (AGEPC)-induced acute lung alterations in the rabbit. Am J Pathol 1985; 121:55–68.
61. Abhyankar S, Gilliland DG, Ferrara JLM. Interleukin-1 is a critical effector molecule during cytokine dysregulation in graft versus host disease to minor histocompatibility antigens. Transplantation 1993; 56:1518–1523.

62. Parkman R, Lenarsky C, Barrantes B, et al. Cytokines versus cytotoxic T lymphocytes (CTL) in the pathogenesis of acute graft-versus-host disease (GVHD). J Cell Biochem 1992; 16a:186.
63. Tanaka J, Imamura M, Kasai M, et al. Cytokine gene expression in peripheral blood mononuclear cells during graft-versus-host disease after allogeneic bone marrow transplantation. Br J Haematol 1993; 85:558–565.
64. McCarthy PL Jr, Abhyankar S, Neben S, et al. Inhibition of interleukin-1 by an interleukin-1 receptor antagonist prevents graft-versus-host disease. Blood 1991; 78: 1915–1918.
65. Goldblum SE, Jay M, Yoneda K, et al. Monokine-induced acute lung injury in rabbits. J Appl Physiol 1987; 63:2093–2100.
66. Siler TM, Swierkosz JE, Hyers TM, et al. Immunoreactive interleukin-1 bronchoalveolar lavage fluid of high-risk patients and patients with the adult respiratory distress syndrome. Exp Lung Res 1989; 15:881–894.
67. Jacobs RF, Tabor DR, Burks AW, Campbell GD. Elevated interleukin-1 release by human alveolar macrophages during the adult respiratory distress syndrome. Am Rev Respir Dis 1989; 140:1686–1692.
68. Renauld J-C, Vink A, Van Snick J. Accessory signals in murine cytolytic T cell responses: Dual requirement for IL-1 and IL-6. J Immunol 1989; 143:1894–1898.
69. Dett CA, Gatanaga M, Ininns EK, Cappuccini F, et al. Enhancement of lymphokine-activated T killer cell tumor necrosis factor receptor mRNA transcription, tumor necrosis factor receptor membrane expression, and tumor necrosis factor/lymphotoxin release by IL-1β, IL-4, and IL-6 in vitro. J Immunol 1991; 146:1522–1526.
70. Muraguchi A, Hirano T, Tang B, et al. The essential role of B cell stimulatory factor 2 (BSF-2/IL-6) for the terminal differentiation of B cells. J Exp Med 1988; 167:332–344.
71. Vandenabeele P, Abramowicz D, Berus D, et al. Increased IL-6 production and IL-6 mediated Ig secretion in murine host-vs-graft disease. J Immunol 1993; 150:4179–4187.
72. Ford HR, Hoffman RA, Tweardy DJ, et al. Evidence that production of interleukin 6 within the rejecting allograft coincides with cytotoxic T lymphocyte development. Transplantation 1991; 51:656–661.
73. Hamashima T, Yoshimura N, Oka T. Graft-infiltrating cells produce much more B-cell stimulating factor 2 compared with spleen, peripheral blood, and regional lymphnode cells. Transplant Proc 1991; 23:174–175.
74. Rolfe MW, Kunkel SL, Demeester SR, et al. Expression of interleukin-6 in association with rat lung reimplantation and allograft rejection. Am Rev Respir Dis 1993; 147: 1010–1016.
75. Symington FW, Symington BE, Liu PY, et al. The relationship of serum IL-6 levels to acute graft-versus-host disease and hepatorenal disease after human bone marrow transplantation. Transplantation 1992; 54:457–462.
76. Jones KP, Reynolds SP, Capper SJ, et al. Measurement of interleukin-6 bronchoalveolar lavage fluid by radioimmunoassay: Differences between patients with interstitial lung disease and control subjects. Clin Exp Immunol 1991; 83:30–34.
77. Mulé JJ, McIntosh JK, Jablons DM, Rosenberg SA. Antitumor activity of recombinant interleukin 6 in mice. J Exp Med 1990; 171:629–636.
78. Lapierre LA, Fiers W, Pober JS. Three distinct classes of regulatory cytokines control endothelial cell MHC antigen expression. J Exp Med 1988; 167:794–804.
79. Arenzana-Seisdedos F, Mogensen SC, Vuillier F, et al. Autocrine secretion of tumor necrosis factor under the influence of interferon-γ amplifies HLA-DR gene induction in human monocytes. Proc Natl Acad Sci USA 1988; 85:6087–6091.
80. Pfizenmaier K, Scheurich P, Schlüter C, Krönke M. Tumor necrosis factor enhances HLA-A,B,C and HLA-DR gene expression in human tumor cells. J Immunol 1987; 138:975–980.

81. Farrar WL, Johnson HM, Farrar JJ. Regulation of the production of immune interferon and cytotoxic T lymphocytes by interleukin 2. J Immunol 1981; 26:1120–1125.
82. Bandyopadhyay S, Miller DS, Matsumoto-Kobayashi M, et al. Effects of interferons and interleukin 2 on natural killing of cytomegalovirus-infected fibroblasts. Clin Exp Immunol 1987; 67:372–382.
83. Ozmen L, Fountoulakis M, Gentz R, Garotta G. Immunomodulation with soluble IFN-γ receptor: Preliminary study. Int Rev Exp Pathol 1993; 34B:137–147.
84. Allen RD, Staley TA, Sidman CL. Differential cytokine expression in acute and chronic murine graft-versus-host disease. Eur J Immunol 1993; 23:333–337.
85. Smith SR, Terminelli C, Kenworthy-Bott L, Phillips DL. A study of cytokine-production in acute graft-vs-host disease. Cell Immunol 1991; 134:336–348.
86. Dickinson AM, Sviland L, Dunn J, et al. Demonstration of direct involvement of cytokines in graft-versus-host reactions using an in vitro human skin explant model. Bone Marrow Transplant 1991; 7:209–216.
87. Mowat AM. Antibodies to IFN-γ prevent immunologically mediated intestinal damage in murine graft-versus-host reaction. Immunology 1989; 68:18–23.
88. Landolfo S, Cofano F, Giovarelli M, et al. Inhibition of interferon-gamma may suppress allograft reactivity by T lymphocytes in vitro and in vivo. Science 1985; 229:176–179.
89. Didlake RH, Kim EK, Sheehan K, et al. Effect of combined anti-gamma interferon antibody and cyclosporine therapy on cardiac allograft survival in the rat. Transplantation 1988; 45:222–223.
90. Niederwieser D, Herold M, Woloszczuk W, et al. Endogenous IFN-gamma during human bone marrow transplantation: Analysis of serum levels of interferon and interferon-dependent secondary messages. Transplantation 1990; 50:620–625.
91. Slavin MA, Dobbs S, Crawford S, Bowden RA. Interleukin-2, interferon-γ and natural killer cell activity in bronchoalveolar lavage fluid from marrow transplant recipients with cytomegalovirus pneumonia. Bone Marrow Transplant 1993; 11:113–118.
92. Sloane JP, Depledge MH, Powles RL, et al. Histopathology of the lung after bone marrow transplantation. J Clin Pathol 1983; 36:546–554.
93. Wojno KJ, Vogelsang GB, Beschorner WE, Santos GW. Pulmonary hemorrhage as a cause of death in allogeneic bone marrow recipients with severe acute graft-versus-host disease. Transplantation 1994; 57:88–92.
94. Snover DC, Weisdorf SA, Ramsay NK, et al. Hepatic graft versus host disease: A study of the predictive value of liver biopsy in diagnosis. Hepatology 1984; 4:123–130.
95. Dumler JS, Beschorner WE, Farmer ER, et al. Endothelial-cell injury in cutaneous acute graft-versus-host disease. Am J Pathol 1989; 135:1097–1103.
96. Hirschberg H, Evensen SA, Henriksen T, Thorsby E. The human mixed lymphocyte-endothelium culture interaction. Transplantation 1975; 19:495–504.
97. Beschorner WE, Shinn CA, Hess AD, et al. Immune-related injury to endothelium associated with acute graft-versus-host disease in the rat. Transplant Proc 1989; 21: 3025–3027.
98. Baldwin WM III, Claas FHJ, van Es LA, van Rood JJ. Distribution of endothelial-monocyte and HLA antigens on renal vascular endothelium. Transplant Proc 1981; 13:103–107.
99. Collins T, Lapierre L, Fiers W, Strominger JL, Pober JS. Recombinant tumor necrosis factor increases mRNA levels and surface expression of HLA-A,B antigens in vascular endothelial cells and dermal fibroblasts in vitro. Proc Natl Acad Sci USA 1986; 83: 446–450.
100. Cotran RS. New roles for the endothelium in inflammation and immunity. AM J Pathol 1987; 129:407–413.
101. Pober JS, Gimbrone MA Jr, Cotran RS, et al. Ia expression by vascular endothelium

is inducible by activated T cells and by human γ interferon. J Exp Med 1983; 157: 1339–1353.
102. Link H, Reinhard U, Niethammer D, et al. Obstructive ventilation disorder as a severe complication of chronic graft-versus-host disease after bone marrow transplantation. Exp Hematol 1982; 10:92–93.
103. Roca J, Granena A, Rodriquez-Roison R, et al. Fatal airway disease in an adult with chronic graft-versus-host disease. Thorax 1982; 37:77–78.
104. Atkinson K, Bryant D, Biggs J, et al. Obstructive airways disease: A rare but serious manifestation of chronic graft-versus-host disease after allogeneic bone marrow transplantation in humans. Transplant Proc 1984; 16:1030–1033.
105. Bradstock KF, Coles R, Despar P, et al. Fatal obstructive airways disease after bone marrow transplantation. Transplant Proc 1984; 16:1034–1036.
106. Chan CK, Hyland RH, Hutcheon MA, et al. Small-airways disease in recipients of allogeneic bone marrow transplants: An analysis of 11 cases and a review of the literature. Medicine 1987; 66:327–340.
107. Johnson FL, Stokes DC, Ruggerio M, et al. Chronic obstructive airways disease after bone marrow transplantation. J Pediatr 1984; 105:370–376.
108. Kurzrock R, Zander A, Kanojia M, et al. Obstructive lung disease after allogeneic marrow transplantation. Transplantation 1984; 37:156–160.
109. Ostrow D, Buskard N, Hill RS, Vickars L, Churg A. Bronchiolitis obliterans complicating bone marrow transplantation. Chest 1985; 87:828–830.
110. Ralph DD, Springmeyer SC, Sullivan KM, et al. Rapidly progressive air-flow obstruction in marrow transplant recipients: Possible association between obliterative bronchiolitis and chronic graft-versus-host disease. Am Rev Respir Dis 1984; 129:641–644.
111. Wyatt SE, Nunn P, Hows JM, et al. Airways obstruction associated with graft-versus-host disease after bone marrow transplantation. Thorax 1984; 39:887–894.
112. St John RC, Gadek JE, Tutschka PJ, et al. Analysis of airflow obstruction by bronchoalveolar lavage following bone marrow transplantation: Implications for pathogenesis and treatment. Chest 1990; 98:600–607.
113. Clark JG, Crawford SW, Madtes DK, Sullivan KM. The clinical presentation and course of obstructive lung disease after allogeneic marrow transplantation. Ann Intern Med 1989; 111:368–376.
114. Paz HL, Crilley P, Patchefsky A, Schiffman RL, Brodsky I. Bronchiolitis obliterans after autologous bone marrow transplantation. Chest 1992; 101:775–778.
115. Clark JG, Schwartz DA, Flournoy N, et al. Risk factors for airflow obstruction in recipients of bone marrow transplants. Ann Intern Med 1987; 107:648–656.
116. Payne L, Chan CK, Fyles G, et al. Cyclosporine as possible prophylaxis for obstruction airways disease after allogeneic bone marrow transplantation. Chest 1993; 104: 114–118.
117. Holland HK, Wingard JR, Beschorner WE, et al. Bronchiolitis obliterans in bone marrow transplantation and its relationship to chronic graft-v-host disease and low serum IgG. Blood 1988; 72:621–627.
118. Sullivan KM, Storb R. Bone marrow transplantation and graft-versus-host disease. In: Brent L, Sells RA, eds. Organ Transplantation: Current Clinical and Immunological Concepts. London: Bailliére, 1989:91–118.
119. Fuchs HJ, Czarniecki CW, Chiu HH, et al. Interferon-gamma increases the alveolar macrophage Ia antigen expression despite oral administration of dexamethasone to rats. Am J Respir Cell Mol Biol 1989; 1:525–532.
120. Kallenberg CG, Schilizzi BM, Beaumont F, et al. Expression of class II major histocompatibility complex antigens on alveolar epithelium in interstitial lung disease: Relevance to pathogenesis of idiopathic pulmonary fibrosis. J Clin Pathol 1987; 40:725–733.

121. Stuhar D, Greif J, Harbeck RJ. Class II antigens of the major histocompatibility complex are increased in lungs of bleomycin-treated rats. Immunol Lett 1990; 26(2): 197–201.
122. Taylor PM, Rose ML, Yacoub MH. Expression of MHC antigens in normal human lungs and transplanted lungs with obliterative bronchiolitis. Transplantation 1989; 48: 506–510.
123. Stein-Streilein J, Lipscomb MF, Hart DA, Darden A. Graft-versus-host reaction in the lung. Transplantation 1981; 32:38–44.
124. Beschorner WE, Saral R, Hutchins GM, et al. Lymphocytic bronchitis associated with graft-versus-host disease in recipients of bone-marrow transplants. N Engl J Med 1978; 299:1030–1036.
125. Hackman RC, Sale GE. Large airway inflammation as a possible manifestation of a pulmonary graft-versus-host reaction in bone marrow allograft recipients. Lab Invest 1981; 44:26A.
126. Connor RE, Ramsay NKC, McGlave P, et al. Pulmonary pathology in bone marrow transplant recipients. Lab Invest 1982; 46:3P.
127. O'Brien KD, Hackman RC, Sale GE, et al. Lymphocytic bronchitis unrelated to acute graft-versus-host disease in canine marrow graft recipients. Transplantation 1984; 37: 233–238.
128. Leblond V, Zouabi H, Sutton L, et al. Late $CD8^+$ lymphocytic alveolitis after allogeneic bone marrow transplantation and chronic graft-versus-host disease. Am J Respir Crit Care Med 1994; 150:1056–1061.
129. Perreault C, Cousineau S, d'Angelo G, et al. Lymphoid interstitial pneumonia after allogeneic bone marrow transplantation. Cancer 1985; 55:1–9.
130. Kradin RL, Divertie MB, Colvin RB, et al. Usual interstital pneumonitis is a T-cell alveolitis. Clin Immunol Immunopathol 1986; 40:224–235.

16

The Effect of GVHD on the Hematopoietic System

Derek N. J. Hart and David B. Fearnley
Christchurch Hospital
Christchurch, New Zealand

I. INTRODUCTION

Clinical graft-versus-host disease (GVHD) following allogeneic bone marrow transplantation (BMT) is recognized as producing two distinct clinical syndromes: acute GVH, generally occurring within 50 days of BMT (1,2) and chronic GVH, which may occur after this and continue for years post-BMT (3,4). The two differ in many respects in terms of pathogenesis, reflecting the complexity of the immunological response, which follows the artificial event of infusing a new bone marrow (BM) stem-cell-derived immune system into a histoincompatible host. Most experience pertains to allogeneic HLA-matched sibling BMT (e.g., Refs. 5 and 6), but the increasing use of extended family-and volunteer-matched transplants has emphasized the complexity and importance of GVH responses (7,8). Much effort of late has been expended to distinguish and amplify any graft versus (host) leukemia (GVL) effect (9,10) from the otherwise destructive effects of GVHD on BMT recipients. This chapter reviews the effect of GVHD on the hematopoietic system, one of the less obvious organs at risk for a GVH response.

Acute GVH primarily affects skin, liver, gut, and the reconstitution and function of the recipient's now donor-derived immune system. Chronic GVH also affects these organs, but proper emphasis has been placed on the marked dysfunction of the immune response and the connective tissue changes present within most organ systems. The hematopoietic system, at least in terms of myelopoiesis, is not normally regarded as a target for GVH because it is derived from the donor. As such, it is compatible with immunologically active donor cells infused at the time of transplantation and, following engraftment, might be expected to give rise to a histocompatible immune system. Nonetheless, the antigenic differences in the host environment do influence the emerging immune system and dysfunction results because the immune system is operating within a different host. These aspects are described elsewhere in this volume. The presumption that donor graft hematopoiesis proceeds uneventfully within the host, protected from the effects of GVH, is not justified for several reasons. Most importantly, there are experimental data to show that donor hematopoiesis is affected by GVHD, albeit in a rather subtle fashion. Furthermore, as we will discuss, new biological data regarding the molecular mechanisms of hematopoiesis and immune responses make it clear that GVHD will influence graft hematopoiesis, within a new histoincompatible environment.

To examine the theoretical mechanisms for a GVH effect on hematopoiesis is useful, as it assists the interpretation of experimental and clinical data with the prospect of directing further useful experimentation (see Table 1).

The *first* formality to consider is the tissue antigens, which hematopoetic stem cells (HSC) and their subsequent progeny express, that might allow them to become targets for an immune response. Clearly conventional major histocompatibility complex (MHC) antigens and minor histocompatibility antigens (mHA) are fully syngeneic with the donor HSC-derived lymphoid system. However, the graft-derived lymphoid cells may recognize the HSC or their progenitors either because tolerance of self is lost or generated inadequately in the host or the new host environment provides exogenous antigens recognized as foreign peptides in the context of self MHC (11–13). It is, for example, conceivable that specific BM stroma-derived peptides sensitize the graft hematopoietic system to “allogeneic” recognition.

The *second* and perhaps most readily appreciated mechanism whereby GVHD may disrupt hematopoiesis is via one of many indirect effects on HSC. These may include (a) damage to essential stromal cells that support hematopoiesis within the marrow microenvironment (14); (b) endothelial cell damage influencing stem-cell and other cell trafficking; (c) dysregulation of other essential support cells, e.g., the recently described $CD3^+$, $CD8^+$ MHC class II dim TCR^-cell (15); and (d) the effects of cytokines, notably the cytokine storm of GVH (16), both directly and indirectly via their influence on the endogenous hematopoietic growth factor production.

A *third* concern, a very real one clinically, is that any GVH immune reaction

Table 1 Mechanisms of GVHD-Induced Damage to Donor Hematopoiesis

1. Direct donor HSC or committed lineage progenitor damage by recognition of host-acquired alloantigens. This might result from the infusion of autologous mature T lymphocytes at grafting or the failure to tolerize emerging donor T lymphocytes effectively.
2. Amplification of residual alloimmune response.
3. Indirect effects on donor HSC resulting from:
   a. Damage to recipient BM stroma (including obvious fibrosis in cGVHD)
   b. Cellular dysregulation of supporting and inhibitory cell populations
   c. The cytokine storm
4. Stem-cell exhaustion
5. Autologous hematopoietic cell reactions
   a. Self-targeted T lymphocytes (autologous cGVHD)
   b. Self-targeted antibody-mediated reactions (particularly in cGVHD)

may independently amplify a residual host versus graft (HVG) response to reject donor hematopoietic cells, leading to late graft failure (17).

A *fourth* possibility, made more real by recent data indicating a finite life for stem cells, is the possibility that the excessive hematopoietic drive in GVH exhausts stem cells. *Fifth*, there is data to suggest that hematopoiesis is susceptible to autologous immune responses during GVH. These may be relatively nonspecific, e.g., the effects of activated natural killer (NK) cells (18), or specific, e.g., the autoimmune responses more common in chronic GVHD (3); of course, they may include some autoimmune T-cell responses to HSC akin to those generated in autologous GVH (19–21). The phenomenon of autologous GVH, which is discussed in more detail further on, is clear evidence that dysregulation within a completely compatible individual will generate strong autoimmune responses.

Although the outcomes of the processes described above are all likely to be detrimental to the function of the transplanted HSC graft, it is conceivable that the GVH response may also have a counterbalancing beneficial effect. Thus it is clear that donor marrow T-cell depletion increases graft failure (17). The role of donor T lymphocytes in facilitating stem-cell engraftment may relate to blockage of recipient immune responses that survive conditioning or the absence of T-lymphocyte cytokine production. Recent data argue for at least some GVH effect directed against residual immunologically active host cells (22).

Impaired graft function has not been reported with great frequency in either acute or chronic GVHD (23,24). Changes in blood count or marrow cellularity are relatively imprecise indicators of marrow function, and it is easy to see how a relatively minor effect on hematopoiesis secondary to GVHD could be overlooked in the clinical situation. Indeed, in the context of GVHD post-BMT, the potential causes for a deterioration in the peripheral blood counts or a return to transfusion dependence are legion without postulating a specific GVHD effect. Such an association might have been more obvious in the first BMTs, when therapy for GVHD prophylaxis was less established. Indeed, seminal descriptions of GVHD do contain reference to occasional patients with pancytopenia or hypoplasia of the BM (2,25), and late graft failure (potentially a more extreme version of the same problem) was a problem in a small series of young patients given no GVHD prophylaxis who developed hyperacute GVHD after BMT (26). An effect on hematopoiesis was clearly evident with 4 of 16 patients failing to engraft, 2 of these being late failures. Furthermore, the potential susceptibility of the hematopoietic system to immune attack is dramatically illustrated in the lethal consequences of transfusion-associated GVHD (27) and the efficacy of donor lymphocyte transfusions in irradiating large leukaemic cell loads when CML relapse follows allogeneic BMT (28,29). With modern GVH prophylaxis, the effects of GVH on hematopoiesis in HLA histocompatible sibling allografts appears to be minimal; nonetheless, as HLA-matched unrelated donor transplantation becomes widely applied, more GVH effects on hematopoiesis are likely to be revealed.

The apparent lack of a clinically important effect of GVHD on hematopoiesis has limited research interest in this area, but the more detailed analysis required to document a subtle effect and elucidate the mechanisms is perhaps more appropriately addressed in animal models. We will review the hematopoietic system as a potential acute GVHD target, discussing the experimental and clinical data available with a view to interpreting the potential role of the different mechanisms postulated above. Although the effect of acute GVHD on the specific immune system, i.e., the lymphoid series is reviewed in Chapt. 00, we will draw on some essential findings in the area as well, while necessarily mentioning certain lessons from the GVL effects reviewed in Chapt. 00. As mentioned, chronic GVHD may involve different mechanisms, and its effect on hematopoiesis will be considered separately.

II. THE HEMATOPOIETIC SYSTEM AS A TARGET ORGAN

Normal adult hematopoiesis takes place in the BM and the progeny of the myeloid series exit into the bloodstream. Lymphoid progenitors traffic via the bloodstream into the thymus and the other lymphoid tissues, notably the spleen and lymph nodes (LN). Circulating blood also provides a vehicle for moving HSC and progenitors between marrow sites and, in conjunction with the lymphatic system, for recirculating lymphoid cells between the different parts of the immune system. Antigen-presenting cells (APC), notably dendritic cells (DC), are produced from hematopoietic precursors and circulate via the bloodstream to the tissues where, once exposed to antigen, they migrate via the lymphatics to the central immune system to initiate a primary T-lymphocyte immune response (30). Subsequently, other cell types are recruited to elaborate a full immune response. The cell growth, differentiation, trafficking, and function of the progency of the HSC require a complex set of molecular interactions, all of them potential targets for disruption by GVHD. These potential cellular and antigenic targets whereby a GVHD response might damage hematopoiesis directly (i.e., mechanisms 1 to 3 of Table 1) are discussed below.

A. Stem Cells

The pluripotent HSC capable of fully reconstituting both the hematopoietic and lymphoid systems has now been identified, at least in mice (31,32). It remains contentious whether these HSC contribute to a stromal cell population as well as to the recognized hematopoietic lineages. HSC express MHC antigens, and studies in mice imply that they are readily recognized and eliminated by both $CD8^+$ and $CD4^+$ cells recognizing class I and class II respectively (33,34). Although the most primitive pluripotent hematopoietic progenitors in humans are generally held to be $CD34^+$ HLA-DR^- (35,36), it seems that their immediate progeny are HLA-DR^+, providing sufficient target for MHC mismatched GVHD to eradicate functional hematopoiesis (27,28). Recent evidence suggests that mHA are genetically polymorphic peptides derived from a variety of tissue/cell proteins (12). These are recognized by T lymphocytes after presentation in the context of MHC molecules. The mHA may have a relatively restricted tissue distribution; however, at least some mHA are present on BM (37).

Specific CTL cells capable of recognizing and eradicating hematopoietic progenitor cells have been described in allogeneic systems (38). The MHC antigens and mHA on HSC and hematopoietic progenitors are obviously targets for rejection of the graft but do not provide, in conventional terms, a target for the histocompatible isologous T lymphocyte GVHD response. Nonetheless it is conceivable that the stem cell may be exposed to peptides or larger allogeneic host-derived protein fragments that are exchanged or presented via MHC molecules as targets for recognition by the nontolerized T-lymphocyte progeny of the hematopoietic graft. Exchange of peptides in MHC molecules is documented (although its significance in human systems is not fully explored) (39), making this a real possibility. Perhaps even more relevant are recent observations that $CD34^+$ human BM mononuclear cells are capable of initiating primary T-lymphocyte responses (40), suggesting that APC function, including costimulator activity, is derived early in hematopoiesis.

B. Lineage-Committed Progenitors

These cells express MHC molecules and minor histocompatibility antigens, as above. However, as commitment to a lineage occurs, a unique set of gene regulation and protein expression results. This may conceivably be accompanied by a relatively selective microenvironment and, theoretically, tissue-restricted mHA could be expressed; but again, providing tolerance is maintained, these should not be GVHD targets. However, lineage-specific derived host molecules might be presented. For example, a theoretical nonfunctional mutation in host erythropoietin might well be presented on developing erythroid cells via MHC molecules as a target for an "acquired" allogeneic GVHD response.

C. Bone Marrow Stroma

Normal hematopoiesis requires an appropriate microenvironment (14). Dexter et al. (41) and others have established beyond doubt that the stroma provides the essential microenvironment, providing growth factor and other support for hematopoiesis. While it is generally assumed that the complex mixture of extracellular matrix and constituent cells survives the chemical or irradiation conditions of a BMT without being indirectly compromised, this assumption should now be challenged. The supporting stromal cells are generally thought to be fibroblasts, adipocytes, and endothelial cells (host-derived) as well as lymphoid and macrophagelike (donor-derived) cells. The latter two cell types are clearly derived from the HSC, but the former represent a real allogeneic target for a GVHD response. The fibroblast stromal cell has been suggested to have a HSC origin, and with time the host stromal cells may be replaced following BMT (42).

High-dose irradiation, busulphan, or recurrent courses of chemotherapy may all damage the stroma. Sites of high-dose local irradiation fail to support hematopoiesis (43). Compromising stromal function clinically by repeated high-dose chemotherapy conditioning may result in progressively longer engraftment times with sequential autologous stem-cell transplantation. Thus if stroma is a target for allogeneic GVHD responses directed against host-derived fibroblasts, adipocytes, and endothelial cells, GVHD might be expected to impair hematopoiesis. As fibroblasts provide targets for MHC restricted responses to other minor antigens (37), there is every reason to suspect that this could be a real phenomenon.

This possibility was appreciated early (44) and some limited evidence for this was provided in experiments showing that femurs subjected to allogeneic GVH reaction could not support autologous hematopoiesis (45). Others have specifically excluded a contribution from stromal cells in GVH-induced marrow aplasia (34).

Direct cytotoxicity of allogeneic T lymphocytes against human host-derived stromal cells has been demonstrated (43). Further indirect effects on human stroma have been described in which cytomegalovirus (CMV) infection of stromal cells has been documented (46,47). The viral infection may damage the stroma directly or make it a target for viral directed cytotoxic activity.

D. Endothelium

The trafficking of HSC and their differentiated myeloid and lymphoid progeny requires recognition of molecular ligands on specialized endothelium with BM, LN, and endothelium at other sites (48). The endothelial cells lining the marrow sinuses are thought to influence the cellular traffic between the intra- and extravascular compartments of the marrow (49). As endothelial cells are of host origin, they will express allogeneic mHA and, furthermore, they have significant antigen-presenting function (50). Endothelial cells are proven susceptible targets for cellular and antibody-mediated immune damage. GVHD responses directed at endothelial cells may impede cell trafficking and disrupt circulation of HSC, if not the egress and appropriate localization of their progeny. Methods for isolating BM endothelial cells have evolved, and these could be tested as GVH targets (51). Damage to endothelium in lymphoid tissues may contribute to GVH effects on the immune system.

E. Thymic Stroma

The complexities of T-lymphocyte differentiation from BM-derived progenitors arriving in the thymus and the production of tolerant single positive CD4 or CD8, MHC class I and II restricted T lymphocytes that egress into the circulation are reviewed elsewhere (52). We make three points in relation to these events in allogeneic BMT. First, damage to the host thymic epithelium may interfere with T-lymphocyte selection. Such damage may result from BMT conditioning, but in GVHD responses, specific T-lymphocyte blasts have been documented to enter the thymus in mice (53). Second, delivery of BM-derived thymic DC to tolerize thymocytes may be impaired—this has not been examined as yet. Third, damage to the stroma and vasculature may affect delivery of autoantigens from recipient tissues to the thymus, frustrating new tolerance to the host. The result may be the evolution of T-lymphocyte clones reactive with MHC and host "allogeneic" peptides, including minor histocompatibility antigens. Indeed in mice, after allogeneic BMT, clonal deletion of BM-derived T lymphocytes did not occur in GVHD (53) and the authors concluded that GVH in the thymus did abrogate thymic stromal elements essential to induction of tolerance. It has also been argued that stress-induced steroid elevation leads to thymic involution (54).

F. Antigen-Presenting Cells

A GVHD response requires donor T lymphocytes to recognize antigenic peptides restricted by MHC class I and II molecules. Some host APC survive conditioning (55), and direct antigen presentation may be involved in initiating GVHD. Engraftment of donor-derived APC (DC) has been shown to be detectable within 1 to 2 weeks of reinfusion (56), and indirect antigen presentation of host antigens might be expected to amplify a GVHD response. The ways in which these different mechanisms may affect the subtleties of the subsequent T-lymphocyte immune response are not fully understood. It is conceivable that autologous GVHD responses, particularly those directed against MHC class II antigens, delete APC in GVHD, thereby contributing to the immunodeficiency of GVHD.

III. ANIMAL MODELS

Given these possible influences of GVH on hematopoiesis, do animal models of GVH allow some conclusions as to their relative importance? Some experimental systems have provided at least a few insights. Induction of GVHD in animals allows a detailed analysis of hematopoietic function that would be difficult to achieve in clinical practice. Not all of these models parallel clinical BMT conditions, and it is vital to appreciate the variables in the model under review, in particular whether the effects on the host or donor hematopoietic systems are being studied.

A. Murine

The mouse model common to many experiments transfers spleen or LN ± BM cells from one of two homozygous parental (P) donors into irradiated ($P_1 \times P_2$) F_1 recipients and generates one-way GVH with no allogeneic response directed against the donor (33). In the absence of donor BM, classic runting disease GVHD develops associated with BM aplasia. The situation is exactly analogous to that occurring in transfusion-associated GVHD. When donor BM is given (in the mouse this contains relatively few T lymphocytes) plus a calculated dose of splenic cells, purified T lymphocytes, or T lymphocyte subsets, BM engraftment with variable GVHD ensues, similar to the clinical situation. The type and severity of the resultant GVHD are influenced by the degree of histoincompatibility (e.g., total MHC incompatibility, class I or class II mismatch, or mHA mismatches), as well as the T lymphocyte subset and dose, the dose of irradiation used, and the conditions under which the mice are kept. The results inevitably vary according to the mouse strain combination used.

1. MHC Mismatched

GVHD induced across MHC barriers is most severe when the donor and recipient differ at both class I and class II loci. In general, in murine models, GVHD caused by class I differences alone requires a relatively higher T-cell dose for its initiation and runs a milder clinical course compared to GVHD induced by class II differences (33). If host rather than donor BM is infused along with the appropriate T-cell population, lethal marrow aplasia usually occurs in both class I and class II mismatches (57,58). In both instances the effect on donor BM reconstitution in the host is more subtly affected by GVHD. In early experiments, P lymphoid cells infused into MHC-incompatible ($P_1 \times P_2$) F_1 recipients generated lethal GVHD. There are considerable data available on the kinetics of the GVH effect on host BM in *unirradiated* P_1 or P_2 donor to ($P_1 \times P_2$) F_1 recipients across class I and class II disparities. GVHD was induced by a limited number of donor spleen cells, and donor engraftment resulted from HSC present in the donor spleen cells. In this system the recipient lymphohematopoietic system is the most sensitive target of GVHD in that it is affected by spleen cell doses that do not apparently damage other target organs. When donor-cell infusions did not contain HSC (e.g., using LN rather than spleen cells), there was no repopulation of the hematopoietic system and the GVHD was lethal, again demonstrating the specificity of the effect in host cells. For a comprehensive review of this system, see Hakim and Shearer (59).

Early observations in irradiated recipients showed that erythropoietic tissue was at risk (60), and application of the colony forming unit-spleen (CFU-S) assay in pioneering experiments (61) established that recipients with GVH lacked HSC by day 5 in spleen and day 7 in marrow. The animals were not rescued by further infusions of incompatible host stem cells. However, if the GVH reaction was controlled by a further 800-rad total body irradiation (TBI) dose, both recipient and donor marrow rescued a proportion of the animals. The failure of recipient BM to protect was most likely explained as being due to ongoing GVHD. The failure of donor BM to salvage the animals was interpreted to be due to "irreparable injury to certain tissues in addition to the hematopoietic elements"—i.e., the stroma.

This was further investigated by Hirabayashi (45), who induced GVHD by infusion of alloreactive P_1 LN cells into ($P_1 \times P_2$) F_1 mice from which the femur was removed subsequently and implanted subcutaneously into syngeneic mice at different times after the transfer of LN cells. The number of CFU-S in the femur (repopulated from the second host) correlated inversely with the number of GVH-inducing LN cells infused. Femurs removed from days 7 to 14 after LN-cell infusion (at which the control mice were developing GVH) had dramatically lower CFU-S numbers than femurs removed in the first 7 days after the GVH inducing infusion—i.e., before GVH had occurred. The possibility of stromal damage was again raised as an explanation for the results.

A recent series of experiments using $CD4^+$ cells to induce GVHD in lightly irradiated single class II locus–disparate hosts studied the relative contribution of bystander effects (cytokine-mediated) and direct CTL activity (34). Lightly irradiated (600 cGY) (B6 × bm12) F_1 hosts were infused with B6 CD4 cells. After an initial (10 to 20×) reduction in marrow cellularity (due to irradiation), the cellularity steadily increased (in a similar fashion to irradiated-only control mice), but between days 7 and 16, there was an abrupt reduction in marrow cellularity due to GVHD. Relatively small numbers of donor CD4 cells were able to cause marrow aplasia, with similar effects noted on splenic hematopoiesis. BM CFU-S in the recipients of donor lymphocytes were reduced 300-fold relative to control irradiated mice, and the absence of HSC was inferred by the failure of residual cells to repopulate lethally irradiated F_1 mice. When class II–deficient knockout mice were used as recipients, no atrophy of host marrow occurred, again demonstrating the specificity of the reaction.

In contrast, donor BM cells infused with CD4 cells were able to engraft and protect mice from the hematopoietic failure, and there was no evidence that donor hematopoiesis suffered as a result of the GVH response. Indeed, the number of donor BM cells recovered from tibias of host mice was very similar in mice infused with either donor-strain BM alone or BM and CD4 cells. The authors conclude that the GVH effect on host hematopoietic cells was mediated by $CD4^+$ CTL alone, as no evidence of humeral factors and no adverse effects on host stroma or cytokine support of donor BM were implicated. Although the $CD4^+$ CTL effects were obviously potent in vivo, their CTL activity was not very great in vitro.

The murine model of BMT in lethally irradiated mice across MHC barriers has recently been used to test a novel immunosuppresive agent. Wallace et al. (62) used CTLA-4lg, a fusion peptide capable of blocking the B7 family (CD80 and CD86) costimulatory signals required for T-cell activation, to control GVHD in mice transplanted with MHC-mismatched marrow and spleen. Control and treated mice showed reduction in RBC, WBC, and platelets at day 15 compared to mice transplanted with syngeneic marrow (and spleen cells). After this time point, mice not treated with CTLA-4lg died (median survival time (MST), 21 days) of GVHD, whereas CTLA-4lg–treated mice survived much longer (MST 57 to 85 days), with some long-term survivors. However the hematological parameters measured above remained depressed compared to controls and did not recover to the normal range in the time period studied. In control experiments, CTLA-4lg did not affect syngeneic engraftment. This could simply reflect problems inherent in stem cells engrafting across MHC barriers (41) but may also indicate that donor hematopoiesis is affected by non-CD28-mediated pathways of GVHD.

2. Minor Histocompatibility Differences

BMT across mHA disparities in mice in the absence of immunosuppression is an instructive model due to the increased survival observed. The potential for purified donor T-lymphocyte subsets to mediate GVHD in BMT across mHA disparities has also been investigated (63). The severity of the GVH reaction varies with the strain combination and T-lymphocyte dose used. $CD8^+$ T-lymphocyte-induced GVH in 6/6 strain combinations were tested, and when mice had been previously sensitized for a single mHA, the $CD8^+$ cells generated CTL activity without any requirement for $CD4^+$ helper cells. Although adding $CD4^+$ cells increased the GVHD potential of these cells, purified $CD4^+$ lymphocytes induced GVHD in only 2/6 strains. Neither the CD8 or CD4 T lymphocyte subsets appeared to target host BM inasmuch as there was no significant shortening in the mean survival time whether donor, *host*, or a mixture of both BM cells were infused. Using these endpoints, only a very significant—i.e., lethal—effect on host marrow would be evident in this system. It is also possible that in mice, either the tissue distribution or immunodominance of mHA antigens or the inefficient recognition and killing of allogeneic lymphocytes allows host stem cells to survive unscathed (64).

Whether GVH affects donor BM function in the host has recently been addressed in a crucial set of experiments by van Dijken et al. (65), using an established model involving transplantation of B10.BR (H-2^k) BM and T lymphocytes into CBA/J(H-2^k) MHC-compatible, mHA-incompatible recipients. The effects of GVH on donor marrow were examined in some detail. Peripheral blood counts in all transplanted mice normalized by 1 month. Despite this, there was a significant diminution in the stem-cell component (CFU-S), and GVHD caused an additional decrease in the number of donor stem cells. Increased numbers of cycling stem cells and splenic hematopoiesis help to support the peripheral blood counts, but the occurrence of GVH suppresses splenic hematopoiesis. BMT reduced CFU-S numbers and stem-cell self-renewal capacity for 5 months, and GVH caused a further reduction. The authors speculated on the influence of GVH on the microenvironment, especially in the spleen, to explain these effects.

Particularly relevant to this discussion are data suggesting that GVH in mice may depend on the microbiological background of the donor. This suggests that lymphoctes sensitized by self MHC and peptide (microorganism-derived) react with recipient tissues. This emphasizes the possibility that donor stem cells may acquire new antigen peptides in a recipient capable of targeting self-directed lymphocyte responses.

One conclusion that clearly emerges from mouse studies is that when host hematopoietic cells are direct targets of allogeneic responses, the effects on stem cells are profound. The bystander effects that have been documented on histocompatible donor BM appear to be more subtle. While limited evidence suggests that GVH involving BM stroma may well be a potential problem, no good model has been developed as yet to clarify this. Present mouse models of BMT have used short-term endpoints (primarily mortality) and do not allow any conclusions about potential long-term effects to be drawn.

3. Autologous/Syngeneic GVHD

Several factors are critical for the induction of autologous GVHD (21). The combination of TBI and cyclosporin-A (CSP-A) followed by CSP-A withdrawal engenders a modified GVHD state with mild skin GVHD as the predominant effect. The acute phase of autologous GVHD is often short-lived, and the process progresses to a state more closely resembling chronic GVHD, with the skin being primarily affected. TBI has an important role, perhaps by a direct thymic effect and also in suppressing host peripheral autoregulatory tolerance mechanisms. Thymectomized animals or animals whose thymus was shielded during TBI do not develop the syndrome. Further immune perturbation with CSP-A is required to induce autologous GVHD in most animals. These conditions seem to result in both the development of autoreactive T cells and the loss of normal mechanisms for regulation of autoreactive T cells (66). These autoreactive T cells appear to recognize public determinants of MHC class II molecules [as shown by blocking experiments (67,68)]. Most reactivity is directed to the skin and no effects on hematopoiesis have been reported to date.

Of particular interest are experiments showing that allogeneic GVHD may include an autologous component. Cells from hosts with established GVHD (caused by MHC-mismatched donor stem cells) infused into irradiated donor-strain recipients led to the development of GVHD manifestations in the donor-strain recipients (69). This potential mechanism for autologous recognition and subsequent damage of donor-derived cells has interesting parallels in the autologous responses thought to play a part in aplastic anemia.

Also of interest is evidence provided from a rat model suggesting that donor dendritic cells contribute APC activity to the GVH response, indicating that indirect presentation of host antigen is important (70).

B. Other Animal Models

1. Dogs

The outbred canine model of BMT pioneered in Seattle contributed much to the investigation of GVHD, but no significant effect of GVHD on hematopoiesis has been reported. In the early dog BMT studies, where GVHD was first identified as "secondary" disease, it was noted that donor marrow engrafted and that dogs dying of GVHD did so with a cellular marrow, although some GVH deaths were associated with neutropenia, presumably sepsis-related.

The dog model has been used to explore mechanisms of BMT graft failure/rejection (reviewed in Chapt. 00). Recipient pretreatment with anti-MHC class II monoclonal antibody allows engraftment of complete DLA-mismatched marrow in up to 50% of unrelated dogs, compared to less than 10% of historical controls (71). This may relate to suppression of residual recipient APC activity. More recent experiments (22) have identified a graft-enhancing effect of donor T lymphocytes with recipient cytotoxic specificity. Autologously transplanted dogs treated with a different anti–class II monoclonal antibody on days 0 to 4 posttransplant develop late graft failure (72). This may indicate that another class II bearing accessory cell populations may play an important part in marrow engraftment and may also therefore be another important target for GVHD across MHC barriers.

2. Monkeys and Baboons

Limited experimental BMT programs have made use of cynomolgus monkeys and baboons. These experimental reports do not describe the hematopoietic system as a major GVH target.

IV. CLINICAL EFFECTS OF GVH ON HEMATOPOIESIS

Clinical data imply that the major and minor histocompatibility antigens on human HSC are significant targets for allogeneic immune responses. Although the clinical situations involving rejection of BM grafts, transfusion-associated GVHD, and graft-versus-leukemia (GVL) are not central to this chapter, some features are pertinent to the discussion.

A. Graft Rejection

It is now clear that BM graft failure in allogeneic BMT in humans is associated at least in some instances with a residual recipient immune-response target on the donor BM. In a now classic study, specific cytotoxic cells recognizing a single HLA incompatibility were associated with graft rejection (73). In allogeneic BMT using cyclo/TBI conditioning, the risk of graft failure is quite low, generally < 1%. If a similar transplant is performed with T-depleted marrow, the risk of graft rejection ranges from 10 to 30% (74). It is generally held that a certain degree of GVH reactivity capable of eliminating the residual host T/NK cells that survive conditioning has a protective effect for the newly engrafting marrow (75). It is also possible that a subset of donor T cells augment engraftment of the donor BM, and a CD3 negative cell with these properties in vitro has recently been described (15).

It is not surprising that with the greater antigen disparities involved in unrelated HLA-matched BMT, the incidence of graft rejection is increased (7,8). Again, T-lymphocyte depletion increases graft rejection, presumably by similar mechanisms. It has not been easy to assay T-lymphocyte responses to even these antigenic differences, but investigations have defined the susceptibility of mHAs on HSC and committed hemopoietic progenitors (38).

B. Transfusion-Associated GVHD

This clinical syndrome mimics the effects seen in the models of MHC-mismatched GVHD in mice that do not transfer HSC and emphasizes once again that certain HLA incompatibilities stimulate strong allogeneic anti-HSC responses. The transfer of viable immunologically competent lymphoid cells in blood into either immunocompromised patients or perhaps patients whose natural immunological defenses against such cells are limited by chance HLA compatibility results in transfusion-associated GVHD (27). It is believed to result from the transfer of cells that are homozygous for one of the recipients HLA haplotypes (76), meaning potential for the GVH reactivity is far greater than the potential for HVG reactions. Statistically it is highly likely that there is a significant class I or class II difference (or both) that acts as a significant antigenic target. The clinical features of transfusion associated GVHD resemble BMT associated GVHD, but in addition a profound effect on the allogeneic host BM is seen. The resulting hypoplasia or aplasia of the host BM is rarely influenced by therapy (27) and contributes significantly to high mortality. In at least one case of transfusion-associated GVHD following CML granulocyte transfusions, donor myeloid engraftment was documented (77), indicating that the aplasia was mediated in an entirely host specific manner and the BM stroma and cytokine milieu were able to support (donor) hematopoiesis.

C. Graft Versus Residual Host BM/Graft Versus Leukemia Effect

Attempts to manipulate GVHD to generate a significant GVL response have shown that although GVH is undoubtedly antileukemic, GVHD may be disassociated from an additional specific antileukemic response (78,79). In vitro there are now data to suggest that leukemia-specific responses are possible. This, of course, does not mitigate against an additional nonspecific antileukemic effect—e.g., from the GVHD-generated cytokine storm (16), described below. If (a) host BM/leukemia survives myeloablative conditioning, (b) there is a sufficiently immunogenic incompatibility in the GVH direction, and (c) postgraft immunosuppression does not eliminate the GVH, a graft anti-host marrow/leukemia effect should be observed.

A major point of significance of this is that, in the case of leukemias, a GVH effect directed against residual host marrow would, ipso facto, provide a degree of GVL effect provided that the host leukemic cells retain the same MHC/mHA phenotype as the host BM. It has been shown that lymphocytic and myeloid leukemia cells are positive for mHA (80,81) and that they are susceptible to lysis by mHA-specific CTL.

These effects are most clinically obvious in the use of donor lymphocyte infusions as adoptive immunotherapy for CML patients who have relapsed after allogeneic BMT (28,29). These infusions induce a high rate of complete remissions (demonstrable at the molecular level) but also often cause GVHD that may be severe. The GVH and GVL effects often occur together, but either may occur in apparent isolation. Marrow aplasia may result (potentially either as a GVH or specific GVL effect) and seems to be more frequent when the relapse is hematologically evident (i.e., the marrow is mainly host-derived) than when it is only detectable by molecular or cytogenetic methods (mixed BM chimerism). Infusion of donor stem cells without any prior conditioning in those circumstances may repopulate the marrow to normal levels. In our experience with this situation, donor BM promptly engrafted in the aplastic marrow despite concomitant GVH at other sites, suggesting that the BM microenvironment (stromal and cytokines) is not necessarily severely affected by these processes.

D. Graft-Versus-Host Disease Effects on Donor BM Hematopoiesis ("Graft-Versus-Graft" Effect)

The problem of graft failure in unmodified acute GVH was described earlier (26). Few studies on the effect of GVH on hematopoiesis after allogeneic BMT with GVHD prophylaxis have been reported. Atkinson et al. (24) noted that following allogeneic sibling-matched BMT, most recipients' BM was hypocellular for the first 14 to 42 days. At 84 days, 48% had hypocellular marrows, but most surviving BMT were considered normocellular at 6 to 12 months. Platelet counts were at the lower limit of normal at 1 year. Examination of committed progenitors—i.e., CFU-GM and BFU-E—showed that these returned to normal by day 21 and no differences were noted between patients with and without acute GVHD.

Poor marrow function as indicated by a reduction in peripheral blood counts of <40% of maximal preceding values posttransplant was reported in 24 (14%) of 171 recipients of an allogeneic HLA-matched BMT (23). A multivariate analysis showed that acute GVHD (grade II or more) was a major risk factor ($p = 0.001$) for developing poor graft function. Hematopoietic recovery was strongly associated with resolution of acute GVHD and of infections.

The limited clinical evidence for this "graft-versus-graft" phenomenon is reviewed in terms of the possible mechanisms elucidated earlier.

1. There is no evidence to date that donor BM hematopoietic elements acquire novel antigenic specificities from the host. However, the reader is reminded that donor APC do process recipient antigen to generate allospecific GVHD and presumably GVL responses. The subtlety of the specific GVL response described above may be matched by a donor antidonor stem cell *plus acquired host antigen* response; however, this mechanism might be expected to affect only a small proportion of stem cells that acquire host antigens. There is no evidence for hematopoietic lineage-restricted GVHD directed responses, although numerous cases of selective lineage engraftment have been documented.

2. The possibility that GVHD may influence hematopoiesis via an effect on BM stroma has been investigated in humans. There is a GVH response directed against host-derived stromal cells. It has been shown that stromal cells (as represented by adherent cells in long-term BM culture) are susceptible to cell-mediated lysis by alloantigen- or lymphokine-activated mononuclear cells (43). The murine data mentioned earlier support this possibility. While damage to host stromal cells is an attractive hypothesis to explain some of the effects seen on donor hematopoiesis, it is not really clear to what extent this is relevant clinically. Stromal damage by other agents, radiotherapy, and chemotherapy are likely to be more relevant.

Rampant destruction of host stem cells by GVH can coexist with donor stem engraftment, as occurs in GVL-induced immunotherapy of CML, suggesting that host stromal cells are not necessarily directly involved in GVH. This may be explained by differential expression of mHA, but further work in this area is justified, particularly in relation to matched unrelated donor transplants.

Even without stromal damage, the marrow microenvironment is likely to be altered by other factors associated with GVHD, especially in the clinical situation where infections and drugs other than chemotherapy may all have significant effects. The fact that BM stromal cells have been shown to be susceptible to infection by organisms such as cytomegalovirus, which interferes with their ability to support hematopoiesis, adds further complexity to the situation (46).

The major dysregulation of hematopoiesis that might be wrought by the profound cellular dysregulation and cytokine storm are addressed in the subsequent sections.

3. Donor stem-cell graft rejection is a common phenomenon, as documented

above. There is no good evidence that it is triggered by GVH, and the minimal data quoted earlier argue against such a mechanism.

4. There has been limited study of the clinical phenomenon of stem-cell exhaustion. Evidence from animal experiments (65) discussed above suggests that ongoing GVHD increases cycling of stem cells, but whether or not this is likely to have significant consequences in the lifetime of the host unknown.

5. In contrast to the situations described above, if the donor marrow and HSC are to be directly damaged by a GVHD effect, some element of autologous recognition must be present, as seems to occur in autologous or syngeneic GVHD. Autologous and syngeneic GVHD have been recognized for some time. In most reports, the skin was the main target organ, although more extensive disease involving liver and sometimes the gut has been described (82,93). The effect on BM has not been reported, however, nor has it been actively sought, and detailed analysis of marrow function in these patients is not available. Early clinical trials have suggested promising results in patients who have developed autologous GVHD as part of an antileukemic protocol (84). It is relevant at this point to introduce the concept of the autoimmune response, which is a common feature of GVHD. Clearly, autoimmune mechanisms are thought to play a role in spontaneous aplastic anemia, and autoimmune responses targeted on stem cells or lineage-committed progenitors may mediate rejection of syngeneic marrow grafts in aplastic anemia (85).

V. EFFECTOR CELLS AND CYTOKINE MEDIATORS

If the effects of GVHD on hematopoiesis are difficult to describe, then detailing which of the hematopoietic-derived cells, both specific and nonspecific, are involved and what cytokines contribute is currently impossible. Nonetheless, some clear areas for investigation may be identified.

A. Effector Cells

1. T Lymphocytes

The T lymphocyte is undoubtedly the prime mediator of specific responses. Cytotoxic T lymphocytes (CTL) with specific activity against mHA have been used to examine the tissue distribution of mHA. mHA are present on normal hematopoietic cells and leukemic cells (80,86). It has also been shown that CTL recognizing mHA can inhibit hematopoietic progenitor cell growth in a manner dependent on cell-to-cell contact. No evidence that cytokines acting independently of cell-cell interactions inhibited hematopoietic progenitor cell growth was seen (demonstrated in the HVG direction). Host mHA-specific CTL can often be detected in host blood in the early phase of hematopoietic reconstitution but may not correlate with the incidence of GVHD (87). Others have found host mHA-specific CTL only in patients with severe, acute GVHD (aGVHD) and also demonstrated their specificity to host, not donor cells via lysis of host hematopoietic cells and leukemic cells (81). CTL clones capable of lysing either both host PBC and leukemic cells or host PBC/leukemic cells only have been described. Some mHA are constitutively expressed on a wide range of tissues, whereas others are found on hematopoietically derived cells (37). This provides two possible explanations for a GVL effect occurring in the absence of GVH—namely, the recognition of truly leukemia-specific antigens by effector cells or a GVH effect limited by differential mHA expression to cells of host hematopoietic origin.

As CTL-mediated cell lysis appears to be mediated by perforin and fas ligand-dependent T-cell mechanisms in a target-specific manner, it is perhaps not surprising that GVH destruction of host/leukemic tissue can probably occur side by side with apparently unaffected donor hematopoiesis.

CD4 cytotoxic cells are also involved (88). Likewise the role of CD4$^+$, Th1, and Th2 cells in recruiting other immune responses will have to be considered.

2. NK Cells

NK cells have traditionally been characterized as lymphoid cells capable of mediating non-HMC-restricted lysis of target cells. The fact that NK cells can reject BM grafts and are the effector cells that produce hematopoietic hybrid resistance (89) shows not only that they are capable of recognizing and destroying BM cells but that they may do so in a relatively specific manner. This apparent specificity seems to be related to self class I. It now appears that NK cells have the ability to recognize class I/peptide complexes, possibly via conformational changes in class I structure induced by peptide binding (90). It is postulated that the NK ability to recognize self class I leads to a negative signal that inhibits their effector function (90,91). However viral infections or other events (possibly GVHD) may cause conformational changes in class I antigens, allowing NK cells to cause cytotoxicity and cytokine release.

Theoretically, donor hematopoietic cells should be largely spared from the direct effects of NK-mediated cytotoxicity in GVHD, although resting NK cells have been reported to mediate syngeneic graft failure in human BMT (92). NK cells may also have either a supportive or inhibitory role in regulating hematopoiesis, depending on the conditions in which the BM cells are growing (18) and the activation state of the NK cells. Activated NK cells have been shown to enhance hematopoiesis of syngeneic (but not allogeneic) BM cells in rat (93). There may be NK cell subsets with distinct effects on hematopoiesis (18). While donor NK cells may suppress GVHD in a mouse model (18,94), they also seem to be important effectors in GVHD (95) and are important sources of inflammatory cytokines such as IL-1 and TNF, whose potential effects at hematopoiesis are discussed below. Phenotyping data suggest that large granular lymphocytes (LGL) are directly associated with the lesions of GVHD (96).

3. Monocytes

Monocytes are important in the efferent phase of GVHD, primarily as a source of cytokines (16). Endotoxin stimulation of activated monocytes amplifies the production of inflammatory cytokines. Monocyte migration is a potential mechanism for increasing levels of inflammatory cytokines in the BM, as a consequence either of local activation or of subsequent trafficking (97).

B. Cytokines

Current understanding of the pathogenesis of GVHD centers on a biphasic model of GVHD. The afferent phase is mediated by donor T lymphocytes that recognize host antigens that are presented on either recipient APC (direct) or donor APC (indirect) and then proliferate. The afferent phase expands by activating (via T-lymphocyte release of cytokines) monocytes, NK cells, B lymphocytes, and other cell types. The efferent phase is mediated by the effector cells, as mentioned, and by the production of cytokines (and possibly other factors) that result in target-organ damage. Virtually all of the cytokines are produced in the efferent response, but TNF and IL-1 have been shown to play particularly important roles in GVHD.

The effects of cytokines on hematopoiesis is inevitably complex and variable (98), differing according to the BM population and experimental conditions used. The cytokines may mediate indirect effects via up- or downregulation of other cytokines and cytokine receptors.

Cytokine production during GVHD has been extensively investigated as described elsewhere in this volume. In addressing the salient effects each cytokine may have on hematopoiesis (this subject is now represented by an immense body of literature) and attempting to relate this to GVHD, some basic principles are essential. Systemic levels of cytokines indicate their presence, but the concentration or even the failure to detect a cytokine may not be relevant. Local cellular production may be more relevant, and most cytokines are thought to be active at short range. We and others have made extensive use of reverse transcriptase polymerase chain reaction (RT-PCR) to analyze cytokine production. The limitations of this assay should be recognized and the presence of secreted functional cytokine protein documented wherever possible. Cytokine inhibitors also exist, either as direct competitors, e.g., IL-1Ra, (uncommon) or in the form of secreted soluble receptors (common). Finally, the complexity of cytokine regulation and their plethora of effects makes it sensible to be cautious in drawing direct cause-and-effect relationships. Inevitably the best means of assessing the effect of a cytokine is to block its action with a specific inhibitor or to make use of cytokine gene knockout mice.

There is no evidence to suggest that failure to secrete adequate levels of hematopoietic growth factors is a problem during GVHD. The T-helper cells, NK cells, and monocytes activated during GVHD may be expected to produce any or all of the currently known cytokines. Most of these (e.g., IL-3, IL-6, IL-9, GM-CSF, G-CSF) are stimulatory for hematopoietic progenitor cells or their progeny. These cytokines can synergize with each other or cytokines such as IL-4, IL-7, and IL-11 to enhance stem-cell or lineage-committed progenitor proliferation. For other cytokines, the ability to directly influence GVHD (i.e., IL-12 effects on T and NK cells and TNF production or IL-10 having inhibitory effects on monocyte/macrophage function and inflammation) may be more relevant avenues for influencing GVHD-affected hematopoiesis. The potential effects these and the other more recently described cytokines (IL-13, IL-15) may have on GVHD/hematopoiesis still await fuller exploration.

The role of cytokines in GVHD has been reviewed previously (99) and a schema has been proposed whereby a sequential cytokine cascade accounts for the different phases of GVHD. The authors concluded that the cytokines produced early in GVHD were likely to cause hematopoietic cell proliferation but noted that potential mechanisms existed for impairment of marrow function (direct inhibition, fibrosis, or stem-cell depletion). In discussing the cytokines, we shall briefly describe their known activities and levels in GVH responses and then cover their potential effects on hematopoiesis in vitro and in vivo.

1. IL-1

IL-1 is a polypeptide that exists in two structurally related forms, IL-1α and IL-1β, either of which can bind to the two receptors with differing affinities. IL-1 is the primary mediator of the acute-phase response. It is also an important regulator of hematopoiesis (100,101) and has a radioprotective effect. IL-1 contributes to a number of immune interactions. Thus IL-1 may induce early progenitors into cell cycle. Indirect effects of IL-1 also include synergy with TNF and IL-6 in activating T and B lymphocytes; increase of G, GM, M-CSF, IL-3, and IL-6 (101); increased IL-1R on HSC (102); possibly mobilization of stem cells; opposing the inhibitory effect of TNFβ (103); and increased GM-CSF and IL-3 receptors on BM cells (104).

In a mHA-disparate experimental model of GVHD, quantitative PCR showed a 600-fold increase in IL-1 mRNA in target organs (skin and spleen) (105). Inhibition of IL-1 via an IL-1ra has been shown to be useful in preventing GVHD (106). Animals treated with IL-1ra showed no detrimental effect on hematopoiesis; indeed prevention of the systemic effects of GVHD appeared to enhance hematopoietic engraftment as judged by day 12 CFU-S. The net effect of IL-1 on hematopoiesis in GVHD is probably positive. Indeed, pretreatment of mouse hosts with IL-1 prior to allogeneic BMT appeared to accelerate multilineage recovery and engraftment of allogeneic marrow (107). Ongoing GVHD may cause hematopoietic tissue to be exposed to increased cytokine levels for prolonged periods. In mice given rhIL-1 β for 10 days, differential effects were seen in the BM and spleen (108). BM erythroid progenitors were reduced, whereas granulocytic cells were increased. In the spleen, erythroid progenitors increased and CFU-GM were markedly increased. The conclusion was that the IL-1 could lead to inhibition or stimulation of HOC, depending on the microenvironment. Weekly addition of IL-1 to long-term BM cultures resulted in an initial stimulation of CFU-GM, apparently mediated by increased stromal cell CSFs, especially G-CSF. After 4 weeks, CFU-GM numbers diminished—an effect thought to be mediated by prostaglandin inhibitors (109).

The type II IL-1 receptor (IL-1RII) has no known signaling function and has been proposed as a regulatory "decoy" receptor for IL-1 (110). However, its relevance to GVHD and hematopoiesis is as yet unknown.

A small number of clinical trials using IL-1 have been performed, which allow some inferences to be drawn about its in vivo effects. A phase 1 trial studying the effect of rIL-1 following autologous BMT has recently been reported (111). Infusion of rIL-1 post-BMT was associated with an enhancement of neutrophil recovery to >500. Platelet recovery was not affected and no other hematologic toxicity was reported. Other investigators suggest a possible protective effect on chemotherapy-induced myelosuppression.

2. TNF

The genes for both TNF-α and TNF-β are located close together with the MHC of human chromosome 6. Both TNF-α and TNF-β bind to the same receptors. There are two types of receptor of similar affinity, and these are widely distributed and readily inducible.

The main activities of TNF include induction of other cyctokine gene and receptor expression; recruitment and activation of lymphocytes, monocytes, and neutrophils in inflammatory response; upregulation of both MHC class I and II expression; and augmented cytotocity of T, NK, and LAK cells (112). In vitro experiments show that human DC initiating a primary allogeneic response activate T-lymphocyte TNF and TNF receptor expression in an essential autocrine stimulation loop (113).

The major part played by TNF in GVHD has been documented in a number of models. Anti-TNF-α antibody has shown promise in suppressing the damage caused by GVHD (114) in both animal models and clinical practice.

A number of TNF-mediated effects on hematopoiesis have been documented, including induction of cell-cycle-specific arrest in multipotent HSC (115). A short-term stimulatory potentiation of GM-CSF and IL-2 effect on purified CD34$^+$ cells has been noted (116), in contrast to the effect of TNF on CSF-stimulated low-density BM cells. In subsequent experiments, this potential for early hematopoiesis was followed after 10 to 12 days by largely inhibitory effects on granulocytic development and enhancement of monocytoid development (117). In LTBMC, TNF appeared to cause inhibitory effects on nonadherent cells, partly balanced by stromal changes that later led to exhaustion of hematopoiesis (118). Administration of rh-TNF to mice causes dose-dependent suppression of mononuclear cells in BM colony forming unit-granulocyte, erythroid, macrophage, megakaryocyte (CFU-GEMM) (119). Similar inhibitory effects on CFU-GM and BFU-E for TNF-α have been reported using both BM and purified CD34$^+$ cells suggesting the effect is not mediated via accessory cells (120). Inhibitory and stimulatory signals provided by TNF to hematopoietic progenitor cells may in part be due to differential signaling through the p55 and p75 TNF receptors (121). Of course multiple additional indirect effects of TNF on hematopoiesis are likely via induction of cytokine genes via transcription factors such as NF-GMa and NF-KB (122). TNF-α has been shown to at least partly mediate an inhibitory effect on donor and unrelated BM growth exhibited by supernatants from cultured residual host CD3$^+$ cells obtained from BMT patients following conditioning (chemotherapy and TBI) (123). Supernatants from cells obtained prior to conditioning did not show this effect. Overall, it is highly likely that TNF will be identified as a major contributor to any changes in hematopoiesis attributed to GVHD.

3. IL-2

IL-2 is important in the initial afferent phase of GVHD, and its potential role in tolerance should not be forgotten. The activated T lymphocytes in GVH release IL-2 and IL-2R are induced on these and other leukocytes. Most HSC do not express IL-2 receptors and generally do not proliferate in response to IL-2. However, IL-2 stimulates the release of IL-3, IL-5, GM-CSF, and TNF-α as well as IFN-γ; therefore secondary effects on hematopoiesis are likely. During clinical IL-2 infusions, increased levels of cytokines that stimulate hematopoiesis have been documented, as well as neutrophilia, and the clinical use of IL-2 has been complicated by thrombocytopenia, but this may be due to a consumptive effect mediated by TNF (124). Attempts to control GVHD using antibodies to IL-2r have been modestly successful and during this no major hematological complications were reported (125).

4. Interferon Gamma (IFN-γ)

Interferon gamma (IFN-γ) is important in the induction phase of GVHD, where it is able to activate monocytes, DC, upregulate MHC class I and II antigens, and induce costimulator activity (126). It may play an important role in the effector phase and has been reported to increase mHA targets on epidermal cells for the GVH response (81). Some highly relevant effects of IFN-γ on hematopoiesis have been reported, including its ability to inhibit proliferation of CD34$^+$/38$^-$ stem cells but not the more mature 34$^+$/38$^+$ population of progenitors (127). It is also capable of synergizing with IL-3 or GM-CSF in inducing CD34 proliferation (128, 129). It also tends to favor the maturation of CFU-M over CFU-G (130) colonies and has been shown to inhibit myelopoiesis in unseparated BM. Clinical use of IFN-γ in chronic granulomatous disease had modest effects on myelopoiesis. The use of IFN-α clinically is, of course, well known to be myelosuppressive.

5. IL-3

This cytokine, produced during activation of the immune response, is stimulatory for hematopoietic progenitor cells and its progeny. Levels are increased in GVHD. Any effect of this on hematopoiesis is likely to be beneficial.

6. IL-4

The production of IL-4 by Th2 cells was associated initially with B-lymphocyte growth and differentiation. Its action on T lymphocytes and the induction of CTL is a more recent observation. The addition of IL-4 to early hematopoietic cells probably influences myeloid differentiation as well, and it has been shown to contribute to the production of allostimulatory cells from cord blood and BM. Potentially this could, in turn, have profound effects on an evolving GVH response. Recent data detail IL-4 and SCF synergizing to stimulate primative progenitors in long-term cultures of bone marrow (131).

7. IL-5

Traditionally associated with eosinophilic responses, this cytokine is produced during GVH responses (99). The eosinophilia seen in chronic GVH is attributed to this cytokine.

8. IL-6

As another monocyte/macrophage-produced cytokine involved in inflammatory responses, IL-6 may be an important player in GVH. In humans, circulating IL-6 is readily detected during inflammatory responses. It may stimulate B lymphocytes and assist developing CTL responses, thereby encouraging the GVHD effector phase. Its effects on BM are probably stimulatory, with effects reported on megakaryocyte and platelet growth (132).

9. IL-7

This cytokine reacts with a receptor that shares a common γ chain with the IL-2 and IL-4 receptors. Its main reported effect is on pre-B cells. However it has effects on LAK induction, and a role in thymic T lymphocyte differentiation is suggested. Again, any influence on T-cell tolerance is relevant to GVHD. A recent publication (133) suggesting that IL-2, IL-4, and IL-7 signaling via the common IL-2γc chain receptor can overcome the anergy resulting from lack of T-lymphocyte costimulation is highly relevant.

10. IL-8

The chemokine IL-8 acts as a neutrophil chemoattractant and has other proinflammatory effects. It is comitogenic for keratinocytes (134) and its effect on marrow stroma may be relevant.

11. IL-9

Preferentially expressed in $CD4^+$ T lymphocytes, IL-9 has phenotypic activity. In the presence of erythropoietin, it supports the formation of BFU-E (135).

12. IL-10

This cytokine has profound regulatory properties in immune responses. Notably, it downregulates costimulator activity and has been shown to inhibit DC CD80 and CD86 expression (136). It suppresses other macrophage activity. Direct effects on hematopoiesis are not reported.

13. IL-11

Produced by mesenchymal cells, any increase due to GVH is likely to be beneficial to platelet production.

14. IL-12

This cytokine, which consists of two chains, stimulates IFN-γ production notably from NK cells (137). It is thought to be a powerful mediator of Th1 responses and information on its role in GVH is eagerly awaited, although it may be predicted to have an important role in the afferent phase of GVHD. Influences on hematopoiesis remain to be clarified.

15. IL-13

This T-cell-derived cytokine was isolated as a CD28 responsive cDNA. It shares the γ chain with IL-2, IL-4, and IL-7. Effects in GVH are inevitable but await clarification. It also inhibits the proliferation of normal and leukemic B-cell progenitors (138). Its effects on mature B cells and monocytes are similar to those of IL-4.

16. IL-14

High-molecular-weight B-cell growth factor remains an unknown quantity in the context of GVHD.

17. IL-15

The cDNA for IL-15 was recently cloned and the costimulatory properties of the molecule on T lymphocytes (139) will inevitably link it to GVH responses.

18. Hematopoietic Growth Factors

The reader is probably very familiar with the contributions of stem-cell factor (SCF), GM-CSF, G-CSF, M-CSF, and other cytokines to myelopoiesis. The function of erythropoietin in regulating the latter phases of erythroid differentiation (140) and thrombopoietin, which appears to have similar effects on platelet production (141), are well defined. Lymphopoiesis and the differentiation and growth of DC are likewise controlled by cytokines and growth factors, although their growth in vitro has been more problematic.

Levels of hematopoietic growth factors are not, it seems, greatly influenced by GVHD. Administration of cytokines to assist hematopoiesis after BMT has been widely reported. G-CSF accelerates neutrophil recovery (142). Erythropoietin improves hemoglobin levels and reduces transfusion requirements (140). M-CSF has been used post-BMT (143). IL-3 has been used alone and fused to GM-CSF in PIXY 123 (144). These have not been reported to affect GVHD. The use of GM-CSF, however, bears closer examination. Therapetic administration or endogenous increases induced by activation of T lymphocytes and mononuclear cells during GVH might be predicted to drive DC differentiation and activation (145), exacerbating GVH responses, although evidence of this has not been seen in clinical trials (142). It is interesting that the use of GM-CSF after allogeneic BMT had a negative influence on outcome, although the reasons for this are not entirely clear. The recent evidence that GM-CSF can protect leukemic cells from apoptosis by upregulating bcl-2 may be relevant (146).

19. Chemokines

A number of small (8 to 10-kDa) inducible, secreted proinflammatory cytokines have been divided on the basis of their conserved four-cysteine motifs into the α (c-x-c) or β (c-c) families. They are involved in a variety of immunoregulatory functions, acting primarily as chemoattractants and activators of specific leukocytes.

The increased secretion of these compounds in GVH is to be anticipated, as are direct and indirect effects on hematopoiesis. These may be as diverse as altering collagen production in fibroblasts potentially influencing BM stroma or direct effects on suppression of HSC activity, as reported for MIP-1α.

20. Other Cytokines

Substances such as TGF-β and MIP-1α, which have been regarded as having a negative effect on hematopoiesis (140,141,147,148), have now been shown to be capable of bidirectional modulation of hematopoietic progenitor cell growth (149). As with other cytokines discussed, the relative contribution of each of these potential effects is as yet unclear. The beneficial effects of TGF-β depend upon its correct regulation, and the interesting finding that its dysregulated production or systemic administration lead to features such as fibrosis and recurrent infections (150) hints at a potential role, especially in chronic GVHD. If proven to be important in GVHD, dysregulated TGFβ production will be an important candidate for negative effects on hematopoiesis. The current interest in the use of MIP-1α as an inhibitor of leukemic cell growth indicates that substances potentially liberated in GVHD may contribute to the GVL effect (151).

The role that oncostatin M, leukemia inhibitory factor (LIF), and similar molecules may play in this situation awaits elucidation.

C. Other Mechanisms

Enhanced nitric oxide (NO) production has been documented in rats with GVHD. Cytokines such as IL-1, TNF, and INF-γ can stimulate expression of inducible nitric oxide synthase (NOS); therefore NO could potentially be a common pathway for these effects of these cytokines in GVH. In a mHA-disparate GVHD model, the effect of inhibiting NO production has been studied using L-NMA (an inhibitor of NO synthase). L-MNA alone had no effect on normal mouse BM as judged by CU-GM function (152). In mice with GVHD treated with L-NMA, reduced BM cellularity, reduced extramedullary hematopoiesis, and reduced CFU-GM numbers were seen compared to control animals with GVHD not given L-NMA. L-NMA did not appear to exacerbate GVH, indicating that NO was not providing important immunosuppressive activity. Assessment of T-lymphocyte chimerism showed impaired donor T-lymphocyte repopulation after L-LMA treatment. While this experiment was done in only a single mouse strain combination and perhaps should be confirmed in other models, it does illustrate that previously unknown mechanisms may have an effect on donor BM in GVHD. In the meantime the significance of the apparent beneficial effect of NO on alloengraftment remains speculative.

D. Chronic GVHD

It may be that any subtle GVHD effect on hematopoiesis may become more obvious over time and therefore may be more easily appreciated in chronic GVHD (cGVHD), especially when it follows acute GVHD. Even in milder forms of cGVHD, other processes may contribute to an effect on hematopoiesis. The anemia of chronic disease, infection, the effects of malabsorption, the effects of fibrotic changes in interstitial tissues, and the autoimmune responses are influences that are more evident in chronic GVHD (cGVHD). Fibrosis is a hallmark of cGVHD and a case of BM fibrosis associated with cGVHD has been reported (153).

The number of hematopoietic progenitor cells in blood and BM are reduced in cGVHD (24). A number of effects on BM have been documented in association with cGVHD, including hypocellularity, megaloblastic change, plasmacytosis, and eosinophilia, but their etiology is not clear cut. The relative frequency with which abnormal blood counts are seen in cGVHD (3) suggests that an adverse effect on hematopoiesis may not be uncommon.

Autoimmune phenomena are common in cGVHD and may be responsible for a number of these cytopenias, with antiplatelet antibodies being detectable in over 50% of cases. Allotyping of antiplatelet or antineutrophil antibodies arising in cGVHD show that these can be true (i.e., antidonor) autoantibodies (154,155). Whether the cases where autoantibodies are not detected are due to other mechanisms (such as a lineage-specific effect on megakaryocytes) is not clear. Increased levels of IL-3 have been found in extensive chronic GVHD (156), and it is arguable that this may represent a part of a compensatory mechanism to maintain peripheral blood counts.

Nutritional deficiency secondary to GVHD of the gut or liver and the anemia of chronic disease may occur but are perhaps best regarded as "secondary" effects of GVHD on hematopoiesis.

While BM appears to be affected relatively frequently and in occasional cases quite profoundly, the cGVHD effect on marrow does not at present constitute a defined clinical syndrome. Because impaired long-term marrow function may also be seen after autologous BMT (an effect not as yet attributed to autologous GVHD) and because of the profound immunosuppression of cGVHD, predisposing patients to infections with potential adverse effects on BM, and the fact that treatment may also impair marrow function, it is very difficult to define a subgroup of patients with cGVHD in whom impaired marrow function can be directly attributed to GVHD. This may partly be the reason why such an effect is not recognized.

Additionally, if acute or chronic GVHD does affect stem-cell reserve (as indicated above), it may be that the late manifestations of this will not be fully revealed until very long term follow-up is available on a larger number of patients.

VII. CONCLUSIONS

There is good reason to consider the effects of GVHD on the hematopoietic system. HSC seem particularly sensitive to GVH (or HvG) effects when there is allogeneic recognition of either MHC or mHA differences between the host and the graft. This effect appears to be very specific. There is no evidence that donor stem cells acquire host antigens to become targets for GVHD. Likewise, there is little evidence to suggest that GVHD contributes to graft failure, even in matched unrelated donor transplants.

There is evidence that donor BM may be affected by acute GVHD and the possibility of stromal cell damage is identified as an area for further investigation, particularly if GVL responses using donor lymphocytes are to be applied more widely. Nonetheless, this is currently not identified as a major clinical problem.

The cytokine storm of a GVHD undoubtedly accounts for many aspects of the acute GVHD syndrome (16). It is not really possible to derive a net effect of the potential GVHD cytokine environment on hematopoiesis. The degree to which the cytokine environment of the BM may be perturbed in GVHD is not really known. Even if it is altered by local effects against residual host tissue or GVL effects, this effect may be patchy throughout the marrow, and some areas may be relatively unaffected. Since donor hematopoietic function does seem to be altered by GVHD and cytokines appeal as the most likely mediators of this effect, it is probably fair to say that disruption of the normal carefully controlled cytokine-mediated pathways of hematopoiesis could be responsible for phenomena such as increased stem-cell cycling and reduction in stem-cell reserve seen in GVHD, as the HSC receive the conflicting and contradictory signals one may expect in a disorder mediated by a dysregulated cytokine "storm." Potentially, future experiments with cytokine-deficient knockout mice may clarify the roles of individual cytokines in GVHD.

The concept of stem-cell exhaustion is now proven in certain experimental models, and this may contribute to the reduction of HSC noted in GVHD.

Autologous responses noted as autologous GVH when T lymphocytes respond to self antigen inappropriately is a real phenomenon. To date it does not appear to affect the hematopoietic compartment, but parallels with aplastic anemia are acknowledged. More obvious autoantibody responses are seen in cGVHD.

In chronic GVHD, there are more mechanisms for end-organ damage and it is apparent that cGVHD can cause profound effects on hematopoiesis in individual patients. A more generalized effect on hematopoiesis probably exists but is again difficult to quantitate.

Possibly the lack of a reliably recognizable clinical effect on hematopoiesis may be due to the overall effect of the cytokine environment of GVHD being a rough balance of inhibitory and stimulatory factors. In some individuals, where either the net balance is more inhibitory or the newly engrafting marrow is perturbed by the contradictory signals or has its stem-cell compartment reduced by continuous cycling, the effects may be more apparent.

As will be apparent to the reader, it is premature to discuss therapeutic intervention in this area. Therapy appropriate to acute or chronic GVHD as a whole should be given with standard hematological support and treatment of precipitating factors.

ACKNOWLEDGEMENT

The authors wish to acknowledge the editors' contributions to the manuscript and the input of their colleagues in the Haematology/Immunology Research Laboratory. We thank Mrs. Susan Banks for careful preparation of the manuscript.

REFERENCES

1. Graw RG, Herzig GP, Rogentine GN, et al. Graft versus host reaction complicating HLA matched bone marrow transplantation. Lancet 1970; 2:1053.
2. Glucksberg H, Storb R, Fefer A, et al. Clinical manifestations of graft versus host disease in human recipients of marrow from HL-A matched sibling donors. Transplantation 1974; 18:295.

3. Shulman HM, Sullivan KM, Weiden PL et al. Chronic graft versus host syndrome in man: A long term clinicopathologic study of 20 Seattle patients. Am J Med 1980; 69: 204.
4. Atkinson K, Horowitz HM, Gale RP, et al. Consensus among bone marrow transplanters for diagnosis, grading and treatment of chronic graft versus host diseases. Bone Marrow Transplant 1989; 4:247.
5. Nash RA, Pepe MS, Storb R, et al. Acute graft versus host disease: Analysis of risk factors after allogeneic marrow transplantation and prophylaxis with cyclosporine and methotrexate. Blood 1992; 80:1838.
6. Ochs LA, Miller WJ, Filipovich AH, et al. Predictive factors for chronic graft-versus-host disease after histocompatible sibling donor bone marrow transplantation. Bone Marrow Transplant 1994; 13:455.
7. Beatty PG, Hansen JA, Longton GM, et al. Marrow transplantation from HLA-matched unrelated donors for treatment of hematological malignancies. Transplantation 1991; 51:443.
8. Kernan N, Bartsch G, Ash R, et al. Analysis of 462 transplantations, from unrelated donors facilitated by the National Marrow Donor Program. N Engl J Med 1993; 328: 593.
9. Odorn LF, August CS, Gilkins JH, et al. Remission of relapsed leukaemia during a graft versus host reaction: A graft versus leukaemia reaction in man? Lancet 1978; 2: 537.
10. Sullivan KM, Storb R, Buckner CD, et al. Graft versus host disease as adoptive immunotherapy in patients with advanced haematological neoplasms. N Engl J Med 1989; 320:828.
11. Goulmy E, Gratana JW, Blokland E, et al. A minor transplantation antigen detected by MHC restricted cytotoxic T lymphocytes during graft versus host disease. Nature 1983; 302:159.
12. Perreault C, Decany F, Brochu S, et al. Minor histocompatibility antigens. Blood 1990; 76:1269.
13. Goulmy E, Voogt P, van Els L, et al. The role of minor histocompatibility antigens in GVHD and rejection: A mini review. Bone Marrow Transplant 1991; 7:(suppl 1)49.
14. Torok-Storb B, Holmberg L. Role of marrow microenvironment in engraftment and maintenance of allogeneic hematopoietic stem cells. Bone Marrow Transplant 1994; 14 (suppl 4):s71.
15. Kaufman CL, Colson YL, Uren S, et al. Phenotypic characterization of a novel bone marrow-depleted cell that facilitates engraftment of allogeneic bone marrow stem cells. Blood 1994; 84:2436.
16. Ferrara J. Paradigm shift for graft versus host disease. Bone Marrow Transplant 1994; 14:183.
17. Hows JM. Mechanisms of graft failure after human marrow transplantation: A review. Immunol Lett 1991; 29:77.
18. Murphy WJ, Reynolds CS, Tigerghien P, Longo DL. Natural killer cells and bone marrow transplantation (review). J Natl Cancer Inst 1993; 85:1475.
19. Gluckman E, Devergie A, Sohier J, Sacret St. Graft versus host disease in recipients of syngeneic bone marrow. Lancet 1980; 1:253.
20. Thien SW, Goldman JM, Galton DG. Acute "graft versus host disease" after autologous grafting for chronic granulocytic leukaemia. Ann Intern Med 1981; 94:210.
21. Glazier A, Tutschka PJ, Farmer ER, Santos GW. Graft versus host disease in cyclosporin-A treated rats after syngeneic and autologus bone marrow reconstitution. J Exp Med 1983; 158:1.
22. Schwarzinger I, Raff RF, Flowers M, et al. Recipient specific donor cytotoxic T

lymphocytes enhance engraftment of unrelated DLA non-identical canine marrow. Bone Marrow Transplant 1994; 13:303.
23. Peravalo J, Bacigalupo A, Pittaluga PA, et al. Poor graft function associated with graft versus host disease after allogeneic bone marrow transplantation. Bone Marrow Transplant 1987; 2:279.
24. Atkinson K, Norrie S, Chan P, et al. Haematopoietic progenitor cells function after HLA-identical sibling BMT; influence of chronic graft versus host disease. Int J Cell Cloning 1986; 4:203.
25. Storb R, Deeg JH, Anasetti C, et al. Pathophysiology of marrow graft failure: A review of the Seattle data. In: Gale 0000, Champlin 0000, eds. Bone Marrow Transplantation: Current Controversies. New York: Liss, 1999 19–30.
26. Sullivan KM, Deeg HJ, Sanders J, et al. Hyperacute graft vs host disease in patients not given immunosuppression after allogeneic marrow transplantation. Blood 1986; 67:1172.
27. Desforges JF, Anderson KC, Weinstein HJ. Transfusion associated graft versus host disease. N Engl J Med 1990; 323:315.
28. Porter D, Roth M, McGarigle C, et al. Induction of graft versus host disease as immunotherapy for relapsed chronic myeloid leukaemia. N Engl J Med 1994; 330:100.
29. van Rhee F, Feng L, Cullis JO, et al. Relapse of chronic myeloid leukaemia after allogeneic bone marrow transplantation: The case for giving donor leukocyte infusions before onset of haematological relapse. Blood 1994; 83:3377.
30. Williams LA, Egner W, Hart DNJ. Isolation and function of human dendritic cells. In Jeon KW, ed. International Review of Cytology. San Diego, CA: Academic Press, 1994; 153:41.
31. Sutherland HJ, Eaves HJ, Eaves CJ, et al. Characterization and partial purification of human marrow cells capable of initiating long term haematopoiesis in vitro. Blood 1989; 74:1563.
32. Baum CM, Weissman IL, Tsukamoto AS, et al. Isolation of a candidate human hematopoietic stem cell population. Proc Natl Acad Sci USA 1992; 89:2804.
33. Korngold R. Lethal graft versus host disease in mice directed to multiple minor histocompatibility antigens: Features of $CD8^+$ and $CD4^+$ T cell responses. Bone Marrow Transplant 1992; 9:355.
34. Sprent J, Surh CD, Agus D, et al. Profound atrophy of the bone marrow reflecting major histocompatibility complex class II-restricted destruction of stem cells by $CD4^+$ cells. J Exp Med 1994; 180:307.
35. Huang S, Terstappen LWMM. Formation of hematopoietic microenvironment and hematopoietic stem cells from single human bone marrow stem cells. Nature 1992; 360:745.
36. Deeg HJ, Huss R. Major histocompatibility complex class II molecules, haemopoiesis and the marrow microenvironment (review). Bone Marrow Transplant 1993; 12: 425.
37. de Bueger M, Bakker A, Van Rood J, et al. Tissue distribution of human minor histocompatibility antigens: Ubiquitous versus restricted tissue distribution indicates heterogeneity among human cytotoxic T lymphocyte defined non MHC antigens. J Immunol 1992; 149:1788.
38. Voogt RJ, Fibbe WG, Marijt W, et al. Rejection of bone marrow graft by recipient derived cytotoxic T lymphocytes. Lancet 1990; 335:131.
39. Lanzavecchia A, Watts C. Peptide partners call the tune. Nature 1994; 371:198.
40. Egner W, Hart DNJ. The phenotype of freshly isolated and cultured human bone marrow allostimulatory cells: Possible heterogeneity in bone marrow dendritic cell populations. Immunology 1995. In press.

41. Dexter YTM, Allen TD, Lajtha LG. Conditions controlling the proliferation of HSC in vitro. J Cell Physiol 1971; 91:335.
42. Keating A, Singer J, Killen P, et al. Donor origin of the in vitro hematopoietic microenvironment after marrow transplantation in man. Nature 1982; 298:280.
43. Tarok-Storb B, Simmons P, Przepiorka D. Impairment of haemopoiesis in human allografts. Transplant Proc 1987; 19(6, suppl 7):33.
44. Kitamura Y, Kawata T, Suda O, Ezum K. Changed differentiation pattern of parental colony-forming cells in F_1 hybrid mice suffering from graft versus host disease. Transplantation 1970; 10:455.
45. Hirabayashi N. Studies on graft versus host (GVH) reactions. 1: Impairment of hemopoietic stroma in mice suffering from GVH disease. Exp Hematol 1981; 9:101.
46. Steinberg HN, Anderson J Jr, Lim B, Chatis PM. Cytomegalovirus infection of the BS-1 human stroma cell line: Effect on murine haemopoiesis. Virology 1993; 196:427.
47. Simmons P, Kaishansky K, Torok-Storb B. Mechanisms of cytomegalovirus-mediated myelosuppression: Pertubation of stromal cell function versus direct infection of myeloid cells. Proc Natl Acad Sci USA 1990; 87:1386.
48. Tavassoli M, Hardy CL. Molecular basis of homing of intravenously transplanted stem cells to the marrow. Blood 1990; 76:1059.
49. Tavassoli M. The marrow blood barrier. Br J Haematol 1979; 41:297.
50. Geppert T, Lipsky P. Antigen presentation by interferon gamma treated endothelial cells and fibroblasts: Differential ability to function as antigen presenting cells despite comparable la expression. J Immunol 1991; 135:3750.
51. Masek LC, Sweetenham JW. Isolation and culture of endothelial cells from human bone marrow. Br J Haematol 1994; 88:855.
52. Shortman K. Cellular aspects of early Tcell development. Curr Opin Immunol 1992; 4: 140.
53. Fukushi N, Anase H, Wang B, et al. Thymus: A direct target organ in graft versus host reaction after allogeneic bone marrow transplantation that results in abrogation of induction of self tolerance. Proc Natl Acad Sci USA 1990; 87:6301.
54. Heirn LR, Martinez C, Good RA. Cause of homologous disease. Nature 1967; 214:26.
55. Perreault C, Pelletier M, Landry D, Auger M. Study of Langerhans cells after allogeneic bone marrow transplantation. Blood 1984; 63:807.
56. Hart DNJ, Fabre JW. Demonstration and characterization of la-positive dendritic cells in the interstitial connective tissues of rat heart and other tissues, but not brain. J Exp Med 1981; 153:347.
57. Sprent J, Schaeffer M, Korngold R. Role of T cell subsets in lethal GVHD directed to class I versus class II H-2 differences: II. Protective effective of $L3T4^+$ cells in anti-class II GVHD. J Immunol 1990; 144:2946.
58. Sprent J, Schaeffer M, Gao EK, Korngold R. Role of T cell subsets in lethal GVHD directed to class I versus class II H-2 differences: 1. $L3T4^+$ cells can either augment or retard GVHD elicited by Lyt-2 cells in class I different hosts. J Exp Med 1988; 167: 566.
59. Hakim FT, Shearer GM. Immunological and hematopoietic deficiencies of graft-vs-host disease. In Burakoff SJ, Deeg HJ, Ferrara J, Atkinson K, eds. Graft-vs-Host Disease. New York: Marcel Dekker, 1990.
60. Garver RM, Cole LJ. Anaemia and leukopenia after injection of parental strain blood in F1 hybrid mice previously treated with sub-lethal irradiation. Int J Radiat Biol 1960; 2:309.
61. Davis WE, Cole LJ. Suppression of hemopoietic colony forming units in mice by graft versus host reactions. Transplantation 1967; 5:60.
62. Wallace PM, Johnson JS, Macmaster JF, et al. CTLA-4lg treatment ameliorates the lethality of murine G-V-H-D across MHC barriers. Transplantation 1994; 58:602.

63. Korngold R, Sprent J. Variable capacity of L3T4$^+$ T cells to cause GVHD across minor histocompatibility barriers in mice. J Exp Med 1987; 165:1552.
64. Korngold R. Pathophysiology of GVHD directed to minor histocompatibility antigens. Bone Marrow Transplant 1991; 7:835.
65. Van Dijken PJ, Wimpersis J, Crawford JM, Ferrara JLM. Effect of GVHD in haematopoiesis after BMT in mice. Blood 1991; 78:2773.
66. Vogelsang G, Hess A. Graft versus host disease: New directions for a persistent problem. Blood 1994; 84:2061.
67. Hess AD, Horwitz LR, Laulis MK. Cyclosporine induced syngeneic graft versus host disease: Recognition of self MHC class II antigens in vivo. Transplant Proc 1993; 25: 1218.
68. Hess A, Horwitz L, Bescharier W, Santos G. Development of GVH like syndrome in cylosporine A treated rats after syngeneic bone marrow transplantation: 1. Development of cytotoxic T lymphocytes with apparent polyclonal anti la specificity including autoreactivity. J Exp Med 1985; 161:718.
69. Hess AD, Vogelsang GB, Silankis M, et al. Syngeneic graft versus host disease (GVHD) after allogeneic bone marrow transplantation and cyclosporine treatment. Transplant Proc 1988; 20:487.
70. Perreault C, Allard A, Brochu S, et al. Studies of immunologic tolerance to host minor histocompatibility antigens following allogeneic bone marrow transplantation in mice. Bone Marrow Transplant 1990; 6:127.
71. Deeg J, Sale G, Storb R, et al. Engraftment of DLA-non identical bone marrow facilitated by recipient treatment with anti class II monoclonal antibody and methotrexate. Transplantation 1987; 44:340.
72. Greinix HT, Ladiges WC, Graham TC, et al. Late graft failure of autologous grafts in lethally irradiated dogs given anti class II monoclonal antibody. Blood 1991; 78:2131.
73. Bunges D, Heit W, Arnold R, et al. Evidence for the involvement of host derived OKT8 positive T cells in the rejection of T depleted HLA identical bone marrow grafts. Transplantation 1987; 43:501.
74. Martin PJ, Hansen JA, Buckner CD, et al. Effects of in vitro depletion of T cells in HLA identical allogeneic marrow grafts. Blood 1985; 66:664.
75. Martin PJ. Determinants of engraftment after allogeneic marrow transplantation (editorial). Blood 1992; 79:1647.
76. Marcus JN, Krushall MS, Westphal R. HLA homozygous donors and transfusion associated graft versus host disease. N Engl J Med 1989; 322:1004.
77. Lowenthal RM, Grossman L, Goldman JM, et al. Granulocyte transfusions in treatment of infections in patients with acute leukaemia and aplastic anaemia. Lancet 1975; 1:353.
78. Mehta J. Graft-versus-leukaemia reactions in clinical bone marrow transplantation. Leuk Lymph 1993; 10:427.
79. Antin J. Graft versus leukaemia: No longer an epiphenomenon. Blood 1993; 82:2273.
80. van der Harst D, Goulmy E, Falkenberg JH, et al. Recognition of minor histocompatibility antigens on lymphocytic and myeloid leukaemic cells by cytotoxic T cell clones. Blood 1994; 83:1060.
81. Niederweiser D, Grassenger M, Arbock J, et al. Correlation of minor histocompatibility antigen-specific cytotoxic and lymphocytes with graft versus host disease status and analyses of tissue distribution of their target antigens. Blood 1993; 81:2200.
82. Talbot DC, Poules RL, Sloane JP, et al. Cyclosporine induced graft versus host disease following autologous BMT in AML. Bone Marrow Transplant 1990; 6:17.
83. Einsele H, Ehninger G, Schneider EM, et al. High frequency of graft versus host like syndromes following syngeneic bone marrow transplantation. Transplantation 1988; 45:579.

84. Yeager A, Vogelsang G, Jones R, et al. Cyclosporine induced graft versus host disease after autologous bone marrow transplantation for acute myeloid leukaemia. Leuk Lymph 1993; 11:215.
85. Appelbaum F, Cheever M, Fefer A, et al. Recurrence of aplastic anaemia following cyclophosphamide and syngeneic bone marrow transplantation: Evidence for two mechanisms of graft failure. Blood 1985; 65:553.
86. Falkenberg JH, Goselink HM, van der Harst D, et al. Growth inhibition of allogeneic leukaemic precursor cells by minor histocompatibility antigen specific cytotoxic T lymphocytes. J Exp Med 1991; 174:
87. de Bueger M, Bakker A, Bontkes H, et al. High frequency of cytotoxic T cell precursors against minor histocompatibility antigens after HLA-identical BMT: Absence of correlation with GVHD. Bone Marrow Transplant 1993; 11:363.
88. Eb P, Gross D, Troxler M, et al. $CD4^+$ T cell mediated killing of MHC class II positive APCS: 1. Characterization of target cell recognition by in vivo or in vitro activated $CD4^+$ killer T cells. J Immunol 1990; 144:790.
89. Kiessling R, Hochman PS, Haller O, et al. Evidence for a similar or common mechanism for natural killer cell activity and resistance to haemopoietic grafts. Eur J Immunol 1977; 7:655.
90. Trinchieri G. Recognition of major histocompatibility complex class I antigens by natural killer cells (commentary). J Exp Med 1994; 180:417.
91. Bellone G, Valiante NM, Viale O, et al. Regulation of haematopoiesis in vitro by alloreactive natural killer cell clones. J Exp Med 1991; 177:1117.
92. Goss GD, Wittmer MA, Bezwoda WR, et al. Effect of natural killer cells on syngeneic bone marrow: In vitro and in vivo studies demonstrating graft failure due to NK cells in an identical twin treated by bone marrow transplantation. Blood 1985; 66:1043.
93. Rolstad B, Benestad HB. Spontaneous alloreactivity of natural killer (NK) and lymphokine activated killer (LAK) cells from athymic rats against normal haemic cells: NK cells stimulate syngeneic but inhibit allogeneic haemopoiesis. Immunology 1991; 74:86.
94. Murphy WJ, Bennett M, Kumor V, et al. Donor-type activated natural killer cells provide marrow engraftment and B cell development during allogeneic BMT. J Immunol 1992; 148:2953.
95. Johnson BD, Truitt RC. A decrease in graft versus host disease without loss of graft versus leukemia reactivity after MHC matched bone marrow transplantation by selective depletion of donor NK cells in vivo. Transplantation 1992; 54:104.
96. Guillen FJ, Ferrara J, Hancock W, et al. Acute cutaneous graft versus host disease to minor histocompatibility antigens in a murine model: Evidence that large granular lymhocytes are the effector cells in the immune response. Lab Invest 1986; 55:35.
97. Rowbottom AW, Riches PG, Downie L, Hobbs JR. Monitoring cytokine production in peripheral blood during active graft versus host disease following allogeneic bone marrow transplantation. Bone Marrow Transplant 1993; 12:635.
98. Metcalf D. Hematopoietic regulators: Redundancy of subtlety. Blood 1993; 8:3515.
99. Jadus MR, Wespic HT. The role of cytokines in graft versus host reactions and disease (review). Bone Marrow Transplant 1992; 10:1.
100. Grown J, Jakubowski A, Gabrilove J. Interleukin-1 biological effects in human hematopoiesis. Leuk Lymph 1993; 9:433.
101. Fibbe WE, Wellenze R. The role of interleukin-1 in hematopoiesis (review). Acta Haematol 1991; 86:148.
102. Dubois CM, Ruscetti FW, Keller JR, et al. In vivo interleukin-1 (IL-1) administration indirectly promotes type II IL-1 receptor expression on haematopoietic bone marrow cells: Novel mechanism for the haematopoietic effects of IL-1. Blood 1991; 78:2841.
103. Ruscetti F, Dubois C, Jacobsen SE, Keller JR. Transforming growth factor beta and

interleukin-1: A paradigm for opposing regulation of haemopoiesis (review)., Bailliére's Clin Haematol 1992; 5:702.
104. Hestdal K, Jacobsen SE, Ruscetti FW. et al. In vivo effect of interleukin-1 alpha on haemopoiesis: Role of colony stimulating factor receptor modulation. Blood 1992; 80: 2486.
105. Abhyankar S, Gilliand DG, Ferrara JLM. Interleukin-1 is a critical effector molecule during cytokine dysregulation in graft versus host disease to minor histocompatibility antigens. Transplantation 1993; 56:1518.
106. McCarthy PL Jr, Abhyankars S, Neben S, et al. Inhibition of interleukin 1 by an interleukin 1 receptor antagonist prevents graft versus host disease. Blood 1991; 78: 1915.
107. Tiberghien P, Laithier V, Mabed M, et al. Interleukin-1 administration before lethal irradiation and allogeneic bone marrow transplantation: Early transient increase of peripheral granulocytes and successful engraftment and platelet recovery. Blood 1993; 81:1933.
108. de Haan G, Dontje B, Lueffler M, Nijhof W. Microenvironmentally dependent effects on murine haemopoiesis by a prolonged interleukin-1 treatment. Br J Haematol 1993; 55:15.
109. Marley S, Reilley I, Russell N. Interleukin-1 has positive and negative regulatory effects in human long term bone marrow culture. Exp Haematol 1994; 20:75.
110. Colotta F, Dower S, Sims J, Mantovani A. The type II "decoy" receptor: A novel regulatory pathway for interleukin-1. Immunol Today 1994; 15:562.
111. Nemunaitis J, Appelbaum FR, Lilleby K, et al. Phase I study of recombinant interleukin-1 beta in patients undergoing autologous bone marrow transplant for acute myelogenous leukaemia. Blood 1994; 83:3473.
112. Coze CM. Glossary of cytokines. Bailliére's Clin Haematol 1994; 7:1.
113. McKenzie JL, Calder VC, Starling GC, Hart DNJ. Role of tumor necrosis factor α in dendritic cell mediated primary mixed leukocyte reactions. Bone Marrow Transplant 1995. In press.
114. Herve P, Flesch M, Tiberghein P. Phase I-II trial of a monoclonal anti-TNFα antibody for the treatment of refractory severe GVHD. Blood 1992; 81:1193.
115. Warren DJ, Slordal L, Moore MA. Tumor necrosis factor induces cell cycle arrest in multipotential haematopoietic stem cells: A possible radioprotective mechanism. Eur J Haematol 1990; 45:158.
116. Caux C, Saeland S, Farre L, et al. Tumor necrosis factor-alpha strongly potentiates interleukin-3 and granulocyte-macrophage stimulating factor–induced proliferation of human CD34$^+$ haematopoietic progenitor cells. Blood 1990; 75:2292.
117. Caux C, Favre L, Saeland S, et al. Potentiation of early haematopoiesis by TNF alpha is followed by inhibition of granulopoietic differentiation and proliferation. Blood 1991; 78:635.
118. Khoury E, Lemoine P, Baillov C, et al. TNF alpha in human long term bone marrow cultures: Distinct effects on non-adherent and adherent progenitors. Exp Haematol 1992; 20:991.
119. Warzocha K, Robak T, Korycka A, et al. The influence of recombinant human TNF alpha, alone and in combination with cyclophosphamide or methotreaxate on leukaemia L1210 and normal haematopoiesis in mice. Arch Immunol Ther Exp 1991; 39:587.
120. Ferrajoli A, Talpaz M, Kurzrock R, Estrov Z. Analysis of the effects of tumor necrosis factor inhibitors on human haematopoiesis. Stem Cells 1993; 11:112.
121. Rusten LS, Jacobsen FW, Lesslauer W, et al. Bifunctional effects of tumor necrosis factor-alpha (TNF-alpha) on the growth of mature and primitive human haemopoietic progenitor cells: Involvement of p55 and -75 TNF receptors. Blood 1994; 83:3152.
122. Shannon MF, Pell LM, Lenardo MJ, et al. A novel tumor necrosis factor-responsive

transcription factor which recognizes a regulatory element in haemopoietic growth factor genes. Mol Cell Biol 1990; 10:2950.
123. Vinci G, Chouaib S, Autran B, Vernant JP. Evidence that residual host cells surviving conditioning regimen to allogeneic bone marrow transplantation inhibit donor haematopoiesis in vitro—The role of TNF-alpha. Transplantation 1991; 52:406.
124. Brenner MK. Haematological applications of IL-2 and other immunostimulatory cytokines. Bailliére's Clin Haematol 1994; 7:115.
125. Anasetti C, Hansen SA, Waldman TA, et al. Treatment of graft versus host disease with humanized anti-Tac: An antibody that binds to the interleukin-2 receptor. Blood 1994; 84:1320.
126. Demayer G, Demayer-Guignard J. Interferon-γ: Current opinion. Immunology 1992; 4:321.
127. Snoek HW, van Bockstaele DR, Nys G, et al. Interferon gamma selectively inhibits very primature $CD34^{++}$ $CD38^{-}$ and not more mature $CD34^{+}$ $CD38^{+}$ human haematopoietic progenitor cells. J Exp Med 1994; 180:1177.
128. Kawano Y, Takaue Y, Kirao A, et al. Synergistic effect of recombinant human interferon-gamma and interleukin-3 on the growth of immature human haematopoietic progenitors. Blood 1991; 77:2118.
129. Caux C, Moreau I, Saeland S, Banchereau J. Interferon-gamma enhances factor dependent myeloid proliferation of human $CD34^{+}$ haematopoietic progenitor cells. Blood 1992; 79:2628.
130. Snoek HW, Lardon F, Lenjoy M, et al. Interferon-gamma and interleukin 4 reciprocally regulate the production of monocytes/macrophages and neutrophils through a direct effect on committed monopotential bone marrow progenitor cells. Eur J Immunol 1993; 25:1072.
131. Keller U, Aman M, Derigs G, et al. Human interleukin-4 enhances stromal cell-dependent hematopoiesis: Costimulation with stem cell factor. Blood 1994; 84:2189.
132. Han ZC, Caen JP. Cytokines acting as committed haematopoietic progenitors. Bailliére's Clin Haematol 1994; 7:65.
133. Boussiotis V, Barber D, Nakari T, et al. Prevention of T cell anergy by signalling through the γc chain of the IL-2 receptor. Science 1994; 266:1039.
134. Kreuger G, Jorgensen C, Miller C, et al. Effects of IL-8 on epidermal proliferation. J Invest Dermatol 1990; 94:545.
135. Bourette R, Royet J, Mauchinova A, et al. Murine interleukin-9 stimulates the proliferation of mouse erythroid progenitor cells and favor the erythroid differentiation of multipotent FDCP-mix cells. Exp Haematol 1992; 20:868.
136. Ding L, Linsley P, Huang L, et al. IL-10 inhibits macrophage co-stimulatory activity by selectively inhibiting the upregulation of B7 expression. J Immunol 1993; 151:1224.
137. Trinchieri G, Scott P. The role of interleukin-12 in the immune response, disease and therapy. Immunol Today 1994; 15:455.
138. Renard N, Duvert V, Banchereau J, Saeland S. Interleukin-13 inhibits the proliferation of normal and leukemic human B-cell precursors. Blood 1994; 84:2253.
139. Carson W, Giri J, Lindeman M, et al. Interleukin (IL) 15 is a novel cytokine that activates human natural killer cells via components of the IL-2 receptor. J Exp Med 1994; 180:1395.
140. Vannucchi AM, Bosi A, Grossi A, et al. The use of epo in the treatment of post bone marrow transplantation anaemia (review). Int J Artif Organs 1993; 16:8.
141. McDonald TP. Thrombopoietin: Its biology, clinical aspects and possibilities (review). Am J Pediatr Hematol Oncol 1992; 14:8.
142. Harmenberg J, Hoglund M, Heustrom-Lindberg E. G- and GM-CSF in oncology and oncological haematology. Eur J Haematol 1994; 152:1.
143. Masaoka T, Suibata H, Ohno R, et al. Double bind test of human urinary M-CSF for

allogeneic and syngeneic bone marrow transplant: effectiveness of treatment and two year follow up for relapse of leukaemia. Br J Haematol 1990; 76: 501.

144. Vadhan Raj S. Pixy 321 (GM-CSF/IL-3 fusion protein) biology and early clinical development (review). Stem Cells 1994; 12:253.
145. Caux C, Yong-Jun Liu, Banchereau J. Recent advances in the study of dendritic cells and follicular dendritic cells. Immunol Today 1995; 16:2.
146. Bradbury D, Zhu YM, Russell N. Regulation of Bcl-2 expression and aptoptosis in acute myeloblastic leukaemia cells by GM-CSF. Leukaemia 1994; 8:786.
147. Keller JR, Sing GK, Ellingsworth LR, Ruscetti FW. Transforming growth factor B, possible roles in the regulation of normal and leukaemic haematopoietic cell growth. J Cell Biotech 1989; 39:175.
148. Broxmeyer HE. Suppressor cytokines and regulation of myelopoiesis. Am J Pediatr Hematol Oncol 1992; 14:22.
149. Keller JR, Bartelmez SH, Sitnicka E, et al. Distinct and overlapping direct effects of macrophage inflammatory protein-1α and transforming growth factor β on haematopoietic progenitor/stem cell growth. Blood 1994; 84:2175.
150. Wahl SM. Transforming growth factor β: The good, the bad and the ugly. J Exp Med 1994; 180:1587.
151. Ferrajoli A, Talpaz M, Zipf T, et al. Inhibition of AML progenitor proliferation by macrophage inflammatory protein 1α. Leukaemia 1994; 8:798.
152. Drobyski WR, Keever CA, Hanson GA, et al. Inhibition of nitric oxide production is associated with enhanced weight loss, decreased survival and impaired alloengraftment in mice undergoing graft versus host disease after bone marrow transplantation. Blood 1994; 84:2363.
153. Atkinson K, Dodds A, Concammon A, Biggs JC. Late onset of transfusion dependent anaemia with thrombocythopaenia secondary to marrow fibrosis and hypoplasia associated with chronic GVHD. Bone Marrow Transplant 1987; 2:44.
154. Minchinton RM, Waters AH. The occurrence and significance of neutrophil antibodies. Br J Haematol 1984; 56:251.
155. Koeppler H, Goldman JH. Autoimmune neutropenia after allogeneic bone marrow transplant unresponsive to conventional immunosuppression but resolving promptly after splenectomy. Eur J Haematol 1988; 41:182.
156. Valent P, Sillaber KC, Scherver R, et al. Detection of circulating endogenous IL-3 in extensive chronic graft versus host disease. Bone Marrow Transplant 1992; 9:331.

17

Graft-Versus-Host Disease as a Th1-Type Process: Regulation by Donor Cells of Th2 Cytokine Phenotype

Daniel H. Fowler and Ronald E. Gress

National Cancer Institute
National Institutes of Health
Bethesda, Maryland

I. INTRODUCTION

Graft-versus-host disease (GVHD) represents a major barrier for allogeneic bone marrow transplantation (allo-BMT). Alloreactive donor T lymphocytes are necessary for the generation of GVHD; indeed, clinical GVHD can be prevented by extensive T-cell depletion (TCD) of the marrow inoculum (1). However, because of an increase in leukemia relapse and graft rejection associated with TCD-allo-BMT (2), strategies to administer functional donor T-cell populations that mediate graft-versus-leukemia (GVL) effects and abrogate marrow graft rejection post-BMT without significant GVHD are potentially clinically important. Successful dissection of the beneficial from the deleterious effects of donor T cells will be dependent upon identifying T-cell populations that mediate each effect and an ability to regulate such T cells in vivo.

Recently, observations from both murine models and clinical studies have led to a more complete understanding of the role of donor T cells in the pathogenesis of GVHD. The GVH alloreaction is complex and includes both cellular ($CD4^+$ and $CD8^+$T lymphocytes, NK cells, and cells of monocyte/macrophage lineage) and cytokine (from both T lymphocytes and accessory cells) components. One important emerging theme is that while donor T lymphocytes are essential for the generation of GVHD, the pathology is in large part mediated by distal, non-T-cell immune processes such as the secretion of multiple inflammatory products from cells of monocyte/macrophage lineage.

Such advances in understanding the pathogenesis of GVHD has occurred concomitant with an expansion of knowledge from related fields of immunology regarding the critical role of various T-cell subsets in the regulation of systemic in vivo immune responses. One important development has been the description of a functional dichotomy among CD4-expressing T cells characterized by differential cytokine secretion profiles; such $CD4^+$ T cell subsets have been designated Th1 and Th2 (3). The nature of the $CD4^+$ T-cell cytokine response to antigenic stimulation influences more distal immune responses such as CTL generation, macrophage activation, and the production of molecules that mediate the inflammatory response. In general, Th1-type responses (initiated by $CD4^+$ T cell production of IL-2 and IFN-γ, but not IL-4 or IL-10) promote cell-mediated immunity (CMI) and enhance systemic inflammatory responses, whereas Th2-type responses (initiated by $CD4^+$ T cell production of IL-4 and IL-10, but not IL-2 or INF-γ) inhibit certain aspects of CMI and reduce the production of inflammatory mediators.

II. Th1/Th2 FUNCTIONAL SUBSETS IN VITRO AND IN VIVO

The "Th1/Th2 paradigm" is based on Mosmann's description in 1986 of a dichotomy of cytokine production with in vitro-generated murine $CD4^+$ T-cell clones (3). Certain clones produced exclusively IL-2 and IFN-γ (Th1-type cytokines), whereas other clones produced exclusively IL-4 (a Th2-type cytokine). Extension of these observations was associated with the discovery of new cytokines—such as IL-10 (4,5)—and the demonstration that Th1 and Th2 clones are cross-regulatory in vitro [Th1 production of IFN-γ regulates Th2 clones (6), whereas Th2 production of IL-10 regulates Th1 clones (7)]. As discussed below, such Th1/Th2 regulation also appears to exist in vivo: multiple murine parasitic (8,9) and neoplastic (10,11) models have illustrated that the Th1/Th2 balance in vivo helps determine the extent to which systemic inflammatory responses and cell-mediated immunity develop (defined by resistance to infection or tumor challenge).

Figure 1 illustrates the basic components of Th1- and Th2-type in vivo immune responses. When considering systemic immune responses, it is important to identify both the initiating, afferent $CD4^+$ T cell cytokine phenotype and the more distal cellular and soluble mediator components.

A. Th1- and Th2-type Subsets Arise from a Common Precursor (Fig. 1, #1)

The development of $CD4^+$ T cells of either Th1 or Th2 cytokine phenotype occurs via a common precursor $CD4^+$ T cell ("Th0") that is undifferentiated for cytokine production [secreting predominately only IL-2 (12), or a combination of Th1- and Th2-type cytokines (13)]. Locksley et al. (14) have shown that in vivo-derived Th1- and Th2-type anti-Leishmania $CD4^+$ T cells express identical T-cell receptors, suggesting that the dichotomous functional subsets arise from a common precursor; this study also emphasizes that the antigenic microenvironment (and not different antigenic epitopes) determines the cytokine phenotype of a given response. Others (12,15,16) have shown that various Th0 clones can develop into either Th1 or Th2 subsets, depending on which cytokines are present when the Th0 cells are stimulated with antigen. These observations further illustrate the intrinsic pliability of the immune response: the $CD4^+$ T cell cytokine response to antigenic stimulation can follow one of two distinct pathways of cytokine differentiation, depending on the specific context of antigen presentation. Variables affecting the pathway of cytokine differentiation may include the type of antigen-presenting cell [APC; for example,

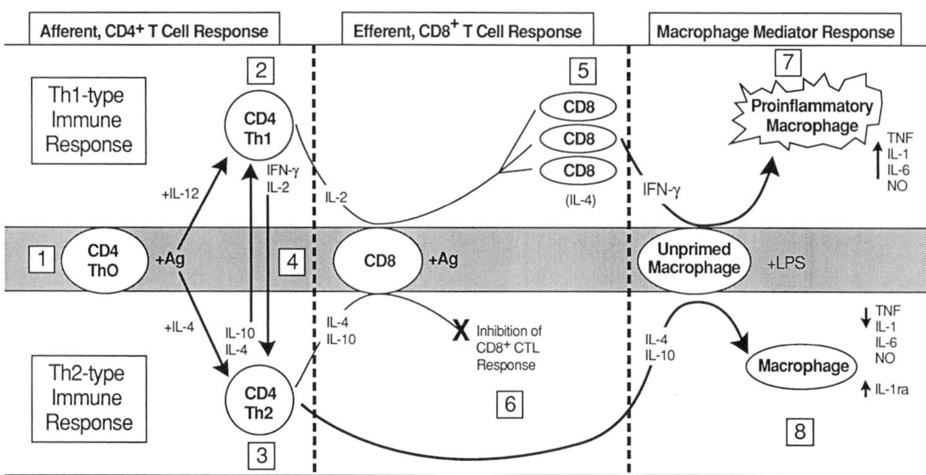

Figure 1 Comparison of in vivo immune responses of Th1- or Th2 type: *Point #1*: Both Th1- and Th2-type CD4$^+$ T cells originate from a common precursor CD4$^+$ T cell ("Th0"). *Point #2*: Specific factors (in particular, IL-12) promote Th0- ⇒ Th1-type differentiation. *Point #3*: Specific factors (in particular, IL-4) promote Th0- ⇒ Th2-type differentiation. *Point #4*: Th1- and Th2-type CD4$^+$ T cells are cross- regulatory. *Point #5*: A Th1-type CD4$^+$ T cell response (in particular, IL-2 production) promotes CD8$^+$ CTL generation. *Point #6*: A Th2-type CD4$^+$ T cell response regulates CD8$^+$ CTL generation. *Point #7*: A CD4-Th1/CD8-CTL response results in macrophage activation. *Point #8*: A CD4-Th2 response regulates macrophage activation.

preferential expansion of Th2 cells when B cells are used as APC (17)], the presence of APC costimulatory molecules [for example, the stimulation of Th1-type cells, but not Th2-type cells, with APC lacking costimulatory factors results in long-term T-cell unresponsiveness (18,19)], and perhaps most importantly, the presence of specific cytokines in the microenvironment where antigenic stimulation is initiated (see below).

B. Promotion of a Th1-Type Immune Response: Role of IL-12 (Fig. 1, #2)

The differentiation of antigen-specific, cytokine-uncommitted Th0-type CD4$^+$ T cells to the Th1-type pathway appears to occur primarily through the influence of specific cytokines present in the antigenic microenvironment. Although the Th1-type cytokine IFN-γ is known to inhibit Th2 development (6), IL-12 (produced predominately by macrophages) has recently been identified as a cytokine capable of inducing a Th0⇒Th1 differentiation. Importantly, this Th1-induction phenomenon observed with IL-12 has been demonstrated not only for in vitro systems (5,20,21) but also in various in vivo studies. Studies utilizing neutralizing antibody to IL-12 indicate that IL-12 may be obligatory for the generation of a Th1-type response in vivo (22); other studies have shown that IL-12 is produced endogenously in mice who develop a cell-mediated immune response to parasite challenge (23), and that the adjutant administration of IL-12 in the context of parasite inoculation results in a $CD4^+$ cytokine response of Th1-type in hosts who otherwise generate Th2-type responses (8). In sum, these studies indicate that the presence of IL-12 during a given antigenic exposure appears to generate a Th1-type response (enhanced CMI, with resultant resistance to infection or tumor) in animals that otherwise might develop Th2-type responses to that antigen.

C. Promotion of a Th2-Type Immune Response: Role of IL-4 (Fig. 1, #3)

Exposure of Th0-type cells to IL-4 during the initiation of antigenic exposure has been shown (12,15,16,24,25) to induce differentiation toward a Th2 cytokine phenotype (secretion of IL-4 and IL-10, but not IL-2 and IFN-γ). The observation that in vivo–derived Th2-type cells express elevated levels of the IL-4 receptor (26) suggests that IL-4 may drive Th2 processes in an autocrine manner. The importance of IL-4 in the generation of Th2-type immune responses in vivo has been confirmed by studies utilizing mice genetically rendered deficient in IL-4 production ("IL-4 knockout mice"): such mice are unable to generate Th2-type responses to antigenic challenge (27).

D. Cross-Regulation of $CD4^+$ Th1/Th2 Subsets

As previously outlined, the cross-regulatory nature of Th1- and Th2-type $CD4^+$ T cell subsets was initially observed in studies of murine in vitro–generated clones (4), recently, the existence of similar cross-regulatory $CD4^+$ T-cell subsets has been described in humans (28,29). Importantly, such Th1/Th2 cross-regulation also appears to exist in vivo; for example, in a murine *Leishmania major* model, the administration of neutralizing antibody to IL-4 during a Th2-type response to parasite challenge can result in a Th1-type response, with the subsequent generation of cell-mediated immunity and resistance to infection (30). Murine models of candidiasis (31) and *Leishmania* (32) have also provided evidence for in vivo Th1/Th2 regulation at the cellular level (the administration of Th1-type clones enhanced CMI, whereas Th2-type clones diminished CMI and resulted in persistence of infection). Most recently, Prurie et al. (9), utilizing purified Th1- and Th2-type cells generated in vivo during the generation of an immune response to *Leishmania*, have directly illustrated that cells of Th1- and Th2-type cross-regulate in vivo. As that study illustrates, the Th1/Th2 nature of the initial $CD4^+$ T cell cytokine response to antigen determines the type of systemic immunity generated: skewing toward a Th1-type response resulted in a cell-mediated, inflammatory reaction (and resistance to infection), whereas a Th2-type response resulted in a lack of cell-mediated immunity (and progressive parasitic disease).

E. $CD4^+$, Th1-Type Responses Generate $CD8^+$ Cytotoxic T Lymphocytes (CTL) (Fig. 1, #5)

The role of Th1-type $CD4^+$ T cells in the development of the systemic immune response is mediated in part through the promotion of a $CD8^+$ CTL response. Although IL-2–producing ("helper-independent") $CD8^+$ T cell clones have been described (3,34), IL-2 production from the Th1-type CD4$^+$ subset is a critical factor in the initiation of CD8$^+$ T cell responses (35). Such generated CD8$^+$ CTL not only mediate direct lysis of cellular targets (36) but also secrete large amounts of IFN-γ, which initiates a complex inflammatory cascade. Indeed, it has been demonstrated that CD8$^+$ T cells (in addition to CD4$^+$ Th1-type cells) are a major source of IFN-γ during in vivo immune responses (37). The importance of both the lytic and cytokine components of the CD8$^+$ CTL response was recently illustrated in a murine transgenic model of fulminant hepatitis (38): the in vivo administration of CD8$^+$ CTL resulted in an initial specific, piecemeal killing of target tissues (CTL lytic phase), which subsequently progressed to a nonspecific inflammatory response characterized by activation of cytokine secretion by CD8$^+$ T cells (IFN-γ) and cells of monocyte/macrophage lineage (TNF-α). Further appreciation of the importance of CD8$^+$-derived cytokine secretion in the development of CMI stems from the observation that INF-γ production (and not target lysis) best correlates with the antitumor efficacy of CD8$^+$ tumor-infiltrating lymphocytes (39).

F. CD4$^+$, Th2-Type Responses Regulate CD8$^+$ CTL Generation (Fig. 1, #6)

Whereas a Th1-type CD4$^+$ T cell response generates CD8$^+$ CTL, a Th2-type afferent CD4$^+$ response appears to regulate CTL generation. Indeed, stimulation of CD8$^+$ T cells in the presence of Th2 cytokines (in particular, IL-4) appears to generate CD8$^+$ (40) or CD3$^+$CD4$^-$CD8$^-$ (41) cells themselves capable of IL-4 production. As such, there appears to be a diversity of cytokine phenotype in both CD4$^+$ and CD8$^+$ T-cell populations. Although these studies suggest that IL-4 exposure during the generation of CD8$^+$ responses may result in CTL with altered cytokine profiles, IL-4 is well known as a growth factor capable of amplifying ongoing CTL responses (42). The timing of exposure of CD8$^+$ T cells to IL-4 thus may be significant: IL-4 exposure at the precursor CTL phase may regulate CTL generation, whereas IL-4 appears to augment existing CTL responses. In vivo, an afferent CD4$^+$ T cell response of Th2-type appears to abrogate the generation of an adequate CD8$^+$ T cell response to viral infection (43); such inhibition of CD8$^+$ CTL generation translates into a reduction in the macrophage inflammatory cascade, with a resultant deficiency in cell-mediated immunity. As such, regulation of CD8$^+$ T cell generation appears to represent a key mechanism for the negative regulatory influence of CD4$^+$, Th2-type cells or Th2-type cytokines in the development of cell-mediated immune responses.

G. A Th1-Type Response Results in Macrophage Activation (Fig. 1, #7)

As discussed, the in vivo manifestation of a Th1-type CD4$^+$ T-cell response is in part mediated by IFN-γ secretion from CD8$^+$ CTL, which in turn leads to activation of macrophage cytokine production. IFN-γ appears to be essential for priming of the macrophage system for release of multiple inflammatory mediators (including TNF-α, IL-1, IL-6, and nitric oxide) (44,45). Although the importance fo this inflammatory cascade to the development of CMI against infectious pathogens (46) and tumors (39,47) has been demonstrated, a vigorous or unopposed (9) Th1-type response appears to be the basis for multiple pathological conditions, including acute fulminant hepatitis (38), intestinal colitis (9,48), and possible GVHD.

H. A Th2-Type Response Regulates Macrophage-Derived Inflammatory Mediators (Fig. 1, #8)

In addition to their differential effects on CD8$^+$ CTL generation, the Th1/Th2 subsets also appear to have opposing effects at the level of the macrophage-derived inflammatory response. Whereas both IL-2 (49) and IFN-γ (44) induce an inflammatory state characterized by macrophage secretion of TNF-α, IL-1, IL-6, and nitric oxide, both IL-4 (50,51) and IL-10 (52–54) have been demonstrated to directly downregulate macrophage production of these mediators. Thus, a Th2-type immune response may regulate the inflammatory cascade by inhibiting the generation of CD8$^+$ T cells capable of IFN-γ production or by the direct inhibitory action of CD4-derived IL-4 and IL-10 on macrophage release of molecules that mediate inflammation. The ability of the Th2-type cytokines IL-4 and IL-10 to regulate this inflammatory cascade in vivo has been demonstrated (55–58). Furthermore, the observations that IL-10 induces monocyte production of the inflammatory inhibitor IL-1 receptor antagonist (59,60) and that IL-4 induces a specific macrophage activation profile (61,62) suggests that Th2-type cells/cytokines may induce an "anti-inflammatory" macrophage profile.

III. ACUTE GVHD AS A CLASSIC Th1-TYPE RESPONSE

The Th1/Th2 CD4$^+$ balance during the generation of immune responses clearly has great influence on the efferent CD8$^+$ T cell response and the subsequent macrophage-mediated inflammatory cascade. Importantly, in vivo experiments have illustrated that shifting of the Th1/Th2 balance can alter the outcome of systemic immune responses. Given this information, it becomes important to consider the pathogenesis of GVHD within the Th1/Th2 framework and to determine whether approaches to alter the Th1/Th2 balance in the setting of allo-BMT might regulate GVHD.

A. The Generation Phase of GVHD Is Characterized by an Afferent, CD4$^+$ T-Cell Response of Th1 Cytokine Phenotype

The importance of the donor anti-host CD4$^+$ T-cell alloreactive response in the generation of GVHD has been previously defined in murine transplantation models (63,64). The afferent helper T-cell response in murine GVHD has been characterized as a Th1-type response, with IL-2 as the predominant cytokine produced early during GVHD. A kinetic study evaluating splenic mRNA expression posttransplant provided data that IL-2 is present early (and transiently) during the GVHD response (65). Direct evidence that IL-2 production during the induction phase of murine GVHD is important for the generation of severe, lethal GVHD is derived from a study showing that early neutralization of IL-2 by monoclonal antibody posttransplant attenuates the severity of GVHD (66). Furthermore, the observation (67) that IL-12 administration stimulates the development of acute GVHD in a murine strain combination that normally develops a Th2-type, autoimmune, chronic GVHD syndrome suggests the critical role of an afferent, Th1-type response in the generation of acute GVHD.

There is also evidence from human studies to suggest that an IL-2 driven, Th1-type response is a key factor in the generation of severe GVHD. Infusion of marrow inocula containing a high precursor frequency of alloreactive T cells capable of IL-2 production upon stimulation with donor cells in vitro correlates with the severity of clinical GVHD (68,69). In addition to providing a potential approach for screening allo-BMT donors, these studies highlight the possible role of IL-2 in the generation of GVHD in the clinical setting. Recent clinical data demonstrating attentuation of GVHD in some patients treated with a humanized form of anti-IL-2 receptor antibody (70,71) further supports the importance of IL-2 and IL-2 receptor stimulation during GVHD.

B. The Efferent Phase of GVHD Includes a $CD8^+$ CTL Component

Although donor $CD4^+$ T cells have been shown to possess CTL activity (72) and to function as effector cells during GVHD in some murine transplant models (63,73,74), $CD8^+$ T cells are also key effector cells contributing to the pathology of GVHD (75,76). Other models illustrate that while $CD4^+$ T cells are the minimum T-cell inocula required to generate GVHR, donor $CD8^+$ T cells seem to be especially important for generating severe GVHR (64). Although $CD8^+$ T cells play an important role in GVHD, the relative contribution of CD8-mediated lysis versus cytokine secretion in GVHD is not known; it is likely that CD8-derived cytokine secretion, primarily IFN-γ, contributes greatly to the pathogenesis of GVHD. Alloreactive $CD8^+$ T-cell clones have been shown to secrete exclusively Th1-type cytokines (predominately IFN-γ) (77), and $CD8^+$ T cells are a significant source of IFN-γ during GVHD (37). It should also be noted that NK cells have been identified as an effector cell of GVHD (78,79); interestingly, the generation of NK activity appears to be induced by Th1-type cytokines [such as IL-2 and IL-12 (80,81)] and perhaps inhibited by Th2-type cytokines (82–85).

The importance of the donor $CD8^+$ T-cell population as an effector of GVHD has been confirmed in human studies. The onset of GVHD in patients post-allo-BMT is associated with a marked increase in the number of peripheral $CD8^+$ T cells of donor origin (86); additionally, an immunopathological evaluation of duodenal biopsies from GVHD patients determined that intestinal infiltrates characteristic of GVHD were predominately made up of $CD8^+$ T cells (87). A recent clinical trial has emphasized the importance of $CD8^+$ T cells in clinical GVHD: recipients of allogeneic marrow depleted of $CD8^+$ T cells developed minimal GVHD (88,89).

C. The Th1-Type, Inflammatory Phase of GVHD

As discussed, Th1-type processes involve not only $CD4^+$ and $CD8^+$ T cell responses but also a phase of monocyte/macrophage activation characterized by the production of inflammatory mediators such as TNF-α, IL-1, IL-6, and nitric oxide. Recent murine and human studies of GVHD suggest that a similar inflammatory process contributes greatly to the pathogenesis of GVHD; this phenomenon has been aptly coined the "cytokine storm" (90) of GVHD. For example, study of cytokine mRNA expression during murine GVHD has illustrated that IL-1 (65) (and not T-cell derived cytokines) represents the major cytokine species at the height of GVHD; subsequent studies using recombinant IL-1 receptor antagonist (91) have shown that reduction of the downstream cytokine cascade can attenuate the severity of GVHD.

The role of TNF-α in the pathology of GVHD has been the subject of much past and recent attention. Murine studies have previously recognized the importance of TNF-α in GVHD, especially in the induction of gastrointestinal lesions of GVHD (92,93). The attenuation of murine GVHD observed with the systemic administration of neutralizing antibodies to TNF-α (94) further suggests the pathological role of this cytokine in GVHD. Recently, Nestel et al. (95) extended these prior observations and proposed a model for TNF-related pathology during GVHD that temporally includes T-cell activation with IFN-γ production, subsequent macrophage priming, and—upon exposure to bacterial-derived lipopolysaccharide (LPS) endotoxin—macrophage release of TNF-α.

Human studies have also implicated TNF-α in the pathogenesis of GVHD. For example, serum TNF-α elevations posttransplant have been shown to correlate with the severity of GVHD (96). Given this information, multiple strategies to interrupt this TNF-α pathway during GVHD are being pursued (97,98). Because of the demonstrated in vitro (52–54) and in vivo (57) regulatory role of IL-10 on LPS-induced TNF-α secretion, and the demonstration that some patients tolerant to their marrow allograft post-BMT have elevated levels of IL-10 expression in vivo (99), attempts to regulate GVHD with IL-10 administration are of particular interest.

In addition to IL-1 and TNF-α, other mediators have been implicated in the pathogenesis of GVHD. For example, the inflammatory product nitric oxide is typically coordinately regulated with TNF-α and is secreted during CMI responses (45,100); recent studies have shown that nitric oxide levels correlate with the severity of murine GVHD (101). Interestingly, Th1-type cytokines [in particular, IFN-γ (50)] are known to enhance nitric oxide production, whereas Th2-type cytokines are potent inhibitors of nitric oxide (54,102,103).

Collectively, current evidence suggests that GVHD represents a systemic Th1-type response: this characterization includes a $CD4^+$ response of Th1-type, resulting in $CD8^+$ CTL generation and an inflammatory cytokine cascade. It should be noted that some murine GVHD models (104) involve strain combinations that result in a chronic, indolent inflammatory process and Th2 cytokine expression consistent with a Th2-type pathological process. Additionally, a murine host-versus-graft disease model (105) illustrates that alloreactive processes of Th2-type can be pathogenic (manifesting as an SLE-like syndrome), thus suggesting that both Th1- and Th2-type pathways may be important considerations for understanding the pathogenesis of the full spectrum of GVHD. However, in both murine and human evaluations, acute GVHD appears to primarily reflect a Th1-type alloreaction.

IV. DONOR CELLS OF Th2 CYTOKINE PHENOTYPE REGULATE THE GENERATION OF GVHD

A. Donor Cells of Th2-Type Regulate LPS-induced, TNF-α-Mediated Lethal GVHR

Nestel et al. have recently identified (95) the role of LPS-induced, TNF-α production in the pathogenesis of GVHD. Utilizing a parent-into-F1 murine model of

GVHR similar to that used by Nestel, the potential regulatory role of donor cells of Th2 cytokine phenotype on LPS-induced lethality during GVHR has been evaluated (106). In this model, GVHR is established by the transfer of 70×10^6 parental C57BL/6 (B6) spleen cells into unirradiated C57BL/6 × C3H (B6C3F1) hosts; on day 7 posttransplant, LPS endotoxin is administered intravenously, and such positive control GVHR recipients develop extreme elevations of serum TNF-α with subsequent lethality.

To generate donor cells of Th2 cytokine phenotype, donor B6 mice were treated in vivo with recombinant cytokines. The combination of recombinant human IL-2 (25,000 Cetus Units) and recombinant murine IL-4 [500 ng; both given three times per day intraperitoneally for 5 days) yielded the most consistent shift toward a Th2 phenotype within the CD4-enriched splenic population (as defined by increased IL-4 and IL-10 production, and decreased IL-2 and INF-γ production). This CD4-enriched, donor-type population of Th2 phenotype was then utilized to evaluate regulation of LPS-induced, TNF-α mediated lethal GVHR.

The results of these investigations are summarized in Table 1. GVHR control mice (Table 1, group 1) showed high levels of both $CD4^+$ and $CD8^+$ donor engraftment, high levels of IFN-γ mRNA expression in vivo, and high levels of serum TNF-α in response to exogenous LPS (resulting in lethality). Thus, the immune response of such GVHR-positive control mice is characteristic of a Th1-type response (as outlined in Fig. 1).

To determine the regulatory role of additional donor cells of Th2 cytokine phenotype, cell mixing experiments were performed (Table 1, group 2): this group received not only the otherwise lethal donor B6 spleen cells but also the CD4-enriched population from donor mice treated with combination IL-2/IL-4. Such recipients of additional donor cells of Th2-type showed comparable levels of $CD4^+$ engraftment as GVHR control mice but had lower levels of $CD8^+$ donor engraftment and lower IFN-γ mRNA expression with a concomitant increase in IL-4 mRNA expression, lower levels of serum TNF-α in response to LPS, and protection from lethality. The administered donor Th2-type cells thus exerted regulatory effects at multiple phases of the Th1-type GVHR immune response.

B. Administration of Th2-Type Donor Cells Regulates the Generation of GVHD in a Transplant Model Utilizing Sublethally Irradiated Mice

In order to study the effects of Th-2-type cells on both GVHD and engraftment, a P1 into P2 model utilizing sublethal host irradiation (B6 into-C3H; 500 cGy) was utilized (107). The major findings from this study are summarized in Table 2. Subtlethally irradiated C3H hosts had an intact rejection response, as evidenced by their ability to reject T-cell–depleted B6 inocula. The addition of T cells to the allogeneic inocula (whole spleen cells) effectively abrogated this HVG rejection response; however, doses of T cells necessary to consistently abrogate rejection resulted in lethal GVHD (average time to lethality of 14.5 days). This model thus emphasizes the bidirectional nature of alloreactions (HVG and GVH) in the setting of BMT, and illustrates the narrow "therapeutic window" that exists for donor T-cell administration. That is, doses of donor T cells that mediate a beneficial effect (abrogation of HVG) often result in severe GVHD. Given this limitation of donor

Table 1 Donor Cells of Th2 Type Regulate LPS-induced, TNF-α–Mediated Lethality During GVHR

	Donor B6 Inocula (B6 ⇒ B6C3F1)		Mean Engraftment (splenic × 10^6)		In Vivo Cytokine Expression[e]		Post-LPS TNF-α	Lethal GVHR
Groups	Untreated Spleen Cells	CD4-Enriched, Th2 Type[a]	$CD4^+$	$CD8^+$	IFN-γ mRNA	IL-4 mRNA	TNF-α[f] (pg/mL)	Post-LPS Lethality[g]
GVHR control	70 × 10^6	none[b]	12.7 (n = 10)	15.1 (n = 10)	11	None	35,536	60/62
Th2 mix	70 × 10^6	15–25 × 10^6	10.6[c] (n = 6)	5.3[d] (n = 6)	4.5	35	7,188	3/41

[a]Th2-type cells were generated by treating B6 mice in vivo (IP, tid, for 5 days) with rhuIL-2 (25,000 Cetus Units) and rmIL-4 (500 ng).
[b]Other control groups (not shown) received additional CD4-enriched cells from untreated B6 mice (no regulation of GVHR was seen in such recipients).
[c]Day 7 $CD4^+$ engraftment (flow cytometric evaluation). No statistical difference (GVHR versus Th2 Mix).
[d]Day 7 $CD8^+$ engraftment (flow cytometric evaluation). $p < 0.001$ (GVHR versus Th2 mix).
[e]Day 7 splenic mRNA expression; avg. of $n = 3$ (GVHR controls) or $n = 5$ (Th2 mix recipients); fold increase compared to untreated controls.
[f]Day 7 serum TNF-α level (90 min postinjection of 25 μg LPS). $p < 0.001$ (GVHR versus Th2 mix)
[g]Lethality post-LPS challenge (day 7 LPS injection, 15 μg).
Source: Ref. 106.

T-cell administration, an ability to regulate donor T-cell effects in vivo might be advantageous clinically.

As Table 2 illustrates, the additional administration of donor cells of Th2 cytokine phenotype effectively reduced GVHD without impairing the engraftment mediated by the whole spleen inocula. The most effective treatment regimen was the administration of the T-cell-containing whole spleen cells on day 0 (just after the sublethal host irradiation), followed by the donor Th2-type cells on day 1 ("Th1 ⇒ Th2 recipients"). Such recipients of Th2-type donor cells had significant reductions in GVHD; compared to recipients of only the day 0 whole spleen inocula, mice receiving additional Th2-type cells on day 1 were more likely to be long-term survivors (survival > 30 days posttransplant; 41% versus 5%, $p < 0.0001$). In contrast, engraftment failure in recipients of the Th2-type inocula (4/33, or 12% of mice rejected the allogeneic inocula) was similar to the rejection rate seen in mice receiving only the whole spleen cell inocla (7/46, or 15% rejected).

In addition to protecting against lethal GVHD, recipients of Th2-type cells also had a reduction in the histopathological lesions characteristic of GVHD. A cohort of mice were sacrificed on day 14 posttransplant, and tissues were semiquantitatively scored for GVHD (0–4 scale, no lesions to severe GVHD). As Table 2 illustrates, compared to the GVHD controls ("Th1 recipients"), the Th1 ⇒ Th2 recipients had a reduction in histologically defined GVHD at all evaluated sites, including liver, small intestine, colon, and thymus. Th2-recipients were particularly spared of the intestinal lesions of GVHD (3/4 mice had no lesions identifiable in the colon or small intestine). In light of the possibility that intestinal lesions promote bacterial invasion and subsequent endotoxin-induced cytokine cascades (95), regulation of intestinal GVHD may have played an important role in the observed reduction in lethal GVHD in recipients of the Th2-type inocula.

Thymic alterations, including loss of thymocyte numbers and a reduction in the $CD4^+CD8^+$ thymocyte precursor population (108), are sensitive indicators of GVHD and are thought to contribute greatly to the manifestations of both acute and chronic GVHD (109). As such, the reduction in GVHD-associated thymic pathology (partial preservation of thymic histology, numbers, and subpopulations) observed in Th1 ⇒ Th2 recipients provided further evidence that Th2-type cells regulated GVHD. Preservation of the $CD4^+CD8^+$ thymocyte precursor population observed in Th2-recipients was particularly marked (Table 2, day-14 analysis; flow cytometric evaluation: <25% $CD4^+CD8^+$ thymocytes in GVHD controls, versus > 90% in Th1 ⇒ Th2 recipients). In spite of the observed protection from thymic damage in this day-14 analysis, long-term survivors of the Th1 ⇒ Th2 regimen were severely immunosuppressed (reduced number and functional activity of splenic T cells). Because immunosuppression is a sensitive indicator of ongoing GVHD, we thus conclude that the administration of the Th2-type cells appeared to regulate primarily early events of GVHD.

This study, by demonstrating that the combination of donor whole spleen (day 0) and Th2-type cells (day 1) resulted in abrogation of graft rejection with subsequent regulation of acute GVHD, illustrates that Th1/Th2 interactions in vivo are important in the transplant setting. The sequential administration of different functional T-cell populations ("Th1 ⇒ Th2") might therefore represent a clinical strategy for increasing the therapeutic index of allogeneic T-cell therapy (i.e., the abrogation of rejection with reduced GVHD).

Table 2 Donor Cells of Th2 Cytokine Phenotype Regulate GVHR Without Impairing Engraftment in Sublethally Irradiated Mice (B6 into-C3H; 500 cGy Host XRT)

	Donor B6 Inocula		Transplantation Readouts (Engraftment/Lethal GVHD)		Histologic Evaluation[f]			Thymic Analysis[g]	
Trx Groups	d 0	d 1	Graft Rejection[d]	Survival[e]	Liver	Small Intestine	Colon	Cell #	CD4$^+$8$^+$ Subset
TCD-BMT	TCD[a]	–	100% (9/9)						
GVHD Controls ("Th1")	Th1[b]	–	15% (7/46)	5% (2/39)	$\frac{11}{16}$	$\frac{11}{16}$	$\frac{10}{16}$	0.7	< 25%
Th1 ⇒ Th2	Th1	Th2-CD4[c]	12% (4/33)	41% (12/29)	$\frac{4}{16}$	$\frac{1}{16}$	$\frac{2}{16}$	14.6	> 90%

[a]This group of C3H mice received 90 × 10^6 T-cell–depleted B6 spleen cells.
[b]The T-cell containing inocula ("Th1") consisted of 90 × 10^6 unseparated B6 whole spleen cells.
[c]B6 mice were treated for 5 days (IP, tid) with rhuIL-2 (25,000 Cetus Units) and rmIL-4 (500 ng), B cells and CD8$^+$ T cells were removed, and 50 to 150 × 10^6 CD4-enriched cells were injected at day 1.
[d]Chimerism determined by flow cytometry at either 14 days (in TCD-BMT group) or after 60 days (for survivors of T-cells containing transplants); rejecting mice had >95% host-type chimerism.
[e]Th1 ⇒ Th2 recipients had an increase in long-term survival (# alive > 30 days post-BMT; $p < 0.0001$).
[f]Day 14 histological analysis; blinded histological scoring (scale 0–4; sum of $n = 4$ for each group).
[g]Day 14 thymic single cell suspension: total thymic cell number, and percentage of "double positive" (CD4$^+$CD8$^+$) thymocyte subpopulation (determined by flow cytometry).
Source: Ref. 107.

C. In Vitro Generated, Allospecific Murine CD4$^+$ T cells of Th1 and Th2 Type: Direct evidence for Th1/Th2 Cross-Regulation in the Transplant Setting

In order to further evaluate the role of Th1- and Th2-type donor cells in the transplant setting, an in vitro culture system to generate alloreactive (B6 anti-B6C3F1) CD4$^+$ T cells of defined cytokine phenotype was developed (110,111). Because of repeated cycles of alloantigen stimulation in vitro during cell expansion, this culture system represents a methodology for enrichment of the alloreactive Th1- or Th2-type populations; as a result, the generated cells secrete cytokines specifically upon antigenic stimulation. The generation of Th1-type CD4$^+$ T cells has permitted investigation of the potential role of alloreactive Th1-type cells in the abrogation of rejection, the mediation of GVL, and further characterization of Th1/Th2 interactions in the allo-BMT setting.

In brief, CD4$^+$ T cells of donor type (B6) were stimulated in a primary in vitro sensitization with irradiated, dendritic cell-enriched splenocytes from host-type mice (B6C3F1 hosts; 20:1 ratio of donor CD4:host dendritic cells). Different coculture conditions were then utilized to generate cells of Th1 or Th2 cytokine phenotype. In this system, serum conditions are of particular importance in determining cytokine phenotype: fetal calf serum (10%) conditions typically resulted in cells of Th1-type, whereas cultures supplemented with syngeneic mouse serum (1%) favored the generation of cells of Th2 phenotype. Additionally, both IL-4 and defined culture media (HL media; Hycor, Inc.) faciliated the growth of Th2-type cultures, whereas IFN-γ enriched for a Th1 cytokine phenotype. The cytokine combination of IL-2, IL-7, IL-1, and IL-6 has been used to optimally propagate both Th1- and Th2-type cultures over extended periods (>6 months; CD4$^+$ harvest and restimulation with fresh host-type dendritic cells performed every 14 to 21 days).

Figure 2 illustrates both the allospecificity and cytokine phenotype of generated CD4$^+$ T cells. This result, obtained by the fifth week in culture (initial B6 anti-F1 sensitization, with subsequent restimulations at week 2 and week 5 of culture), illustrates the dichotomy in allospecific cytokine production generated in parallel cultures. The Th1 culture condition (10% fetal calf serum in RPMI, IFN-γ, and IL-2, IL-7, IL-1, and IL-6) resulted in the F1-specific secretion of both IL-2 and IFN-γ, with an absence of detectable IL-4 and IL-10 secretion. Conversely, the Th2 culture condition (1% syngeneic mouse serum and 2% fetal calf serum in Ventrex-HL media, and IL-2, IL-7, IL-1, and IL-6) resulted in the F1-specific secretion of IL-4 and IL-10, with reduced secretion of IL-2 and IFN-γ.

Both Th1- and Th2-type culture conditions resulted in CD4$^+$ T cells capable of specific cytokine secretion upon antigenic stimulation: that is, cytokine release was observed only when the cultured CD4$^+$ T cells were stimulated against the allogeneic stimulator used in their generation (no cytokine secretion was observed upon stimulation with syngeneic, B6-type cells). This antigen-specific activation also appears to exist in vivo. For example, administration of in vitro-generated Th2-type cells (B6 anti-F1) to a B6C3F1 host resulted in mRNA expression of IL-4 and IL-10 in host tissues, whereas injection of the same cells into syngeneic B6 hosts did not result in Th2-type cytokine expression in vivo. Using the described parent-into-F1, LPS-induced model of lethal GVHR (Sect. IV. A), such in vitro generated B6 anti-F1 CD4$^+$ T cells of Th2 cytokine phenotype potentially downregulated generation of

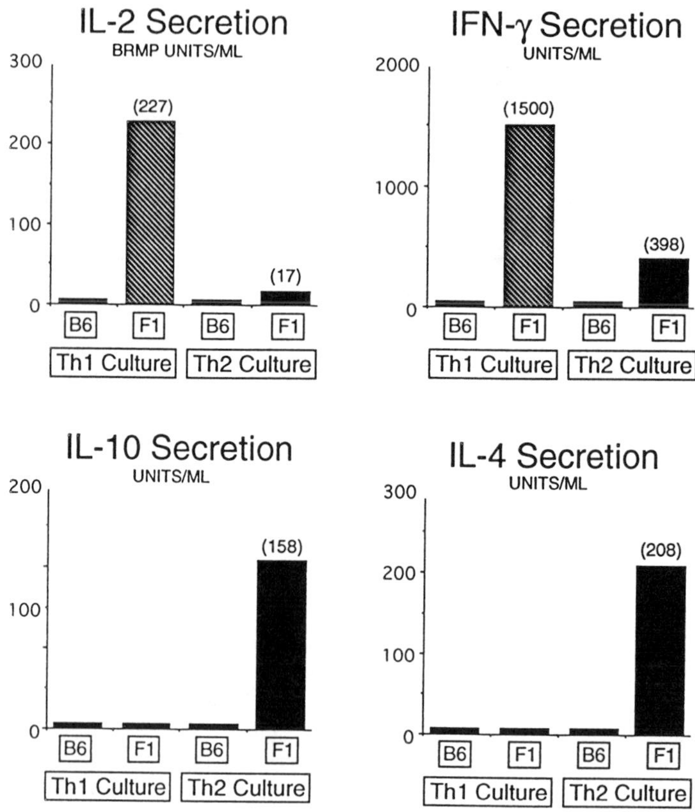

Figure 2 Bulk culture generation of B6 anti-F1 $CD4^+$ T cells of Th1 or Th2 cytokine phenotype. Spleen cells from naive B6 mice were harvested, depleted of B cells and $CD8^+$ T cells (Pierce CD4 negative selection columns; Rockford, IL) and cocultured in 2-mL wells (1×10^6 $CD4^+$ T cells/well) at a 20 : 1 ratio with an irradiated (1000 rad) dendritic cell-enriched (DC) fraction from B6C3F1 mice (obtained by DNase treatment of F1 spleen cells, Percoll gradient fractionation, removal of nonadherent cells, and overnight incubation). The Th1-type culture was generated in RPMI media with 10% fetal calf serum, whereas the Th2-type culture was generated in HL media (Hycor; Irvine, CA) with a combination of 2% fetal calf serum and 1% syngeneic mouse serum. At culture initiation, both Th1- and Th2-type cultures were supplemented with recombinant murine (rm) IL-1α (4 ng/mL) and rmIL-6 (4 ng/mL); subsequently, recombinant human (rhu) IL-2 (50 Cetus Units/mL on day 2, 25 cetus units/mL on days 5 and 8) and rmIL-7 (20 ng/mL on days 2, 5, and 8) were added to both culture conditions. The Th1-type culture additionally received rmIFN-γ (200 units/mL on day 0). Both cultures were harvested on day 14, restimulated with fresh B6C3F1-type DC, and expanded under the same conditions as their initial generation. Three weeks later (week 5 of culture), the $CD4^+$ T cells were harvested and restimulated with fresh F1-type DC; parallel stimulations were performed for the generation of supernatants for ELISA testing (5×10^5 $CD4^+$ T cells/mL; 20 : 1 ratio of B6- or F1-type DC as stimulator). ELISAs were performed using commercially available reagents (PharMingen, San Diego, CA); lower limits of detection (units/mL) for the assay shown were IL-2 (< 2), IL-10 (< 50), IFN-γ (< 84), and IL-4 (< 6).

the graft-versus-host reaction. Th2-mediated regulation of the generation of GVHR has thus been observed with both in vivo-generated donor Th2-type cells (the CD4-enriched population from IL-2/IL-4 treated mice) and in vitro-generated donor antihost Th2-type CD4$^+$ T cells.

Whether such in vitro-generated Th1/Th2 subsets are cross-regulatory for the generation of lethal GVHD has been studied in the setting of a parent-into F1 bone marrow transplantation model [B6-into B6C3F1; lethally irradiated F1 hosts (1050 rad, Cs^{137} source, dose rate of 115 cGy/min)]. In this model, T-cell-depleted B6-type bone marrow was administered alone or in combination with either in vitro generated, CD4$^+$, F1-specific T cells of Th1- or Th2-type. The survival curve in Fig. 3 illustrates that administration of the Th1-type CD4$^+$ T cells resulted in acute lethality characteristic of GVHD (weight loss and diarrhea). In light of the short time to lethality (6 or 7 days posttransplant) and the absence of other T lymphocytes in the marrow inocula, it thus appears that the Th1-type CD4$^+$ inocula may have functioned as an effector cell of GVHD. As mentioned earlier, the ability of CD4$^+$ T cells to function alone as effectors of GVHD has been previously reported (63,73,74). In contrast, the Th2-type anti-F1 cells were nonlethal in this model (such F1 recipients exhibited no clinical symptoms of GVHD). Importantly, the administration of Th2-type anti-F1 cells in combination (1:1 ratio) with the otherwise lethal Th1-type inoculum was protective: such recipients displayed minimal symptoms of GVHD, and have survived more than 6 months posttransplant without clinical sequelae. Thus, this experiment, by utilizing in vitro-generated alloreactive CD4$^+$ T

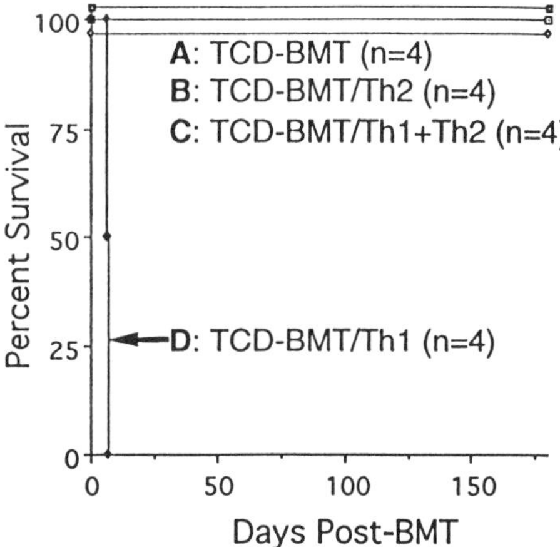

Figure 3 The administration of donor anti-host (B6 anti-F1) CD4$^+$ T cells of Th1-type results in lethal GVHD; Th2-type anti-F1 cells abrogate Th1-mediated lethality. Recipient B6C3F1 mice were lethally irradiated (1050 cGy) and reconstituted with B6-type, T-cell-depleted bone marrow (5×10^6 cells, "group A"). "Group B" received additional donor CD4$^+$ T cells (2.5×10^7; day 0) of Th2 cytokine phenotype (Th2 culture conditions, as described in Fig. 2). Group D received additional donor CD4$^+$ T cells (2.5×10^7; day 0) of Th1 cytokine phenotype (Th1 culture conditions, as described in Fig. 2). Group C received both populations of donor anti-F1 CD4$^+$ T cells (2.5×10^7 cells from each culture, coadministered on day 0).

cells of dichotomous cytokine phenotype, directly illustrates the importance of considering Th1/Th2 interactions in allogeneic bone marrow transplantation.

IV. THE ADMINISTRATION OF DONOR Th2-TYPE CELLS, OR THE Th2-TYPE CYTOKINES IL-4 AND IL-10, TO MICE WITH EXISTING GVHD DOES NOT ATTENTUATE LETHAL GVHD

The possibility that Th2-type cells might regulate established GVHD was also evaluated. In these studies, B6C3F1 mice were lethally irradiated (1050 cGy) and reconstituted with T-cell–depleted B6-type bone marrow (recipients of only this TCD inoculum survived more than 6 months posttransplant without evidence of GVHD). GVHD control mice additionally received 7×10^7 B6-type spleen cells; lethal GVHD was observed in such recipients at approximately 20 to 25 days posttransplant. Utilizing this model, attempts to treat established GVHD by the day 10 administration of either Th2-type cells (in vitro–generalized $CD4^+$ T cells, similar to those illustrated in Fig. 2) or Th2-type cytokines (recombinant murine IL-4, 500 ng, IP, bid; and/or recombinant murine IL-10, 1000 IU, IP, i.p., bid) were unable to delay the onset of lethal GVHD. Indeed, in some experiments, the administration of Th2-type cells or cytokines to mice with ongoing GVHD resulted in an acceleration of lethality. These observations thus illustrate that Th2-type cells are of particular importance during the generation phase of GVHD.

V. CONCLUSIONS

In this chapter, we have outlined the basic features of Th1- and Th2-type immune responses, illustrated that acute GVHD is most characteristic of a Th1-type response, and reviewed our experimental murine results investigating Th1/Th2 interactions in the transplant setting. The pace of research in the Th1/Th2 regulation of immune responses has been phenomenal, and continued basic research advances will certainly enhance our knowledge of the complex regulation of systemic immune responses in vivo. Application of this knowledge to experimental transplantation models and clinical BMT trials will likely allow for an improved regulation of GVHD with a resultant therapeutic benefit.

The observation that purified $CD4^+$ T cells of Th1- or Th2-type are cross-regulatory for GVHD illustrates that optimal "graft engineering" may include functionally distinct T-cell subsets of different cytokine phenotype. It is possible that certain beneficial functions of the allogeneic inocula [such as the abrogation of host-versus-graft mediated rejection or the mediation of graft-versus-leukemia (GVL) effects] are mediated by Th1-type responses. As such, abrogation of GVHD by Th2-type cells may also abrogate some beneficial aspects of the allogeneic T-cell inocula. Indeed, in preliminary experiments, administration of in vitro–generated Th1-type anti-F1 cells was associated with a GVL effect; this Th1-mediated GVL effect was completely abrogated by the concomitant administration of anti-F1 cells of Th2 type. This finding suggests that the timing of administration of functional T-cell populations may be critical for optimal transplantation outcome. That is, because the donor T-cell processes that mediate GVHD, GVL and the abrogation of graft rejection may be of Th1 type, approaches to differentially regulate ongoing

Th1-type responses (such as sequential "Th1 ⇒ Th2" strategies) may be a condition for preservation of the antileukemic and graft facilitation functions of donor T cells while minimizing GVHD in the clinical BMT setting.

The possibility of regulating GVHD by manipulating the Th1/Th2 balance is a clinical strategy worthy of continued research, and preclinical efforts will certainly include evaluation of both Th2-type cells and Th2-type cytokines. As has been observed in a diversity of animal models, Th1/Th2 regulation of immunity is most important at the afferent, generation phase of the immune response; approaches to regulate ongoing immune responses, including established GVHD, are clearly needed. Additional investigations will be required to further elucidate the complex role of Th2 cells and Th2-type cytokines in the prevention and treatment of GVHD before full clinical benefit will likely be realized.

REFERENCES

1. Martin PJ, Hansen JA, Burkner CD, et al. Effects of in vitro depletion of T cells in HLA-identical allogeneic marrow grafts. Blood 1985; 66:664–672.
2. Poynton CH. T cell depletion in bone marrow transplantation. Bone Marrow Transplant 1988; 3:265–279.
3. Mosmann TR, Cherwinski H, Bond MW, et al. Two types of murine helper T cell clone: I. Definition according to profiles of lymphokine activities and secreted proteins. J Immunol 1986; 136:2348–2357.
4. Fiorentino DF, Bond MW, Mosmann TR. Two types of mouse T helper cell: IV. Th2 clones secrete a factor that inhibits cytokine production by Th1 clones. J Exp Med 1989; 170:2081–2095.
5. Moore KW, Vieira P, Fiorentino DF, et al. Homology of cytokine synthesis inhibitory factor (IL-10) to the Epstein-Barr virus gene BCRFI. Science 1990; 248:1230–1234. [Published erratum appears in Science 1990; 250:494].
6. Gajewski TF, Fitch FW. Anti-proliferative effect of IFN-gamma in immune regulation: I. IFN-gamma inhibits the proliferation of Th2 but not Th1 murine helper T lymphocyte clones. J Immunol 1988; 140:4245–4252.
7. Mosmann TR, Moore KW. The role of IL-10 in crossregulation of TH1 and TH2 responses. Immunol Today 1991; 12:A49–A53.
8. Afonso LC, Scharton TM, Vieira LQ, et al. The adjuvant effect of interleukin-12 in a vaccine against Leishmania major. Science 1994; 263:235–237.
9. Powrie F, Correa-Oliveira R, Mauze S, Coffman RL. Regulatory interactions between CD45RBhigh and CD45RBlow $CD4^+$ T cells are important for the balance between protective and pathogeneic cell-mediated immunity. J Exp Med 1994; 179:589–600.
10. Brunda MJ, Luistro L, Warrier RR, et al. Antitumor and antimetastatic activity of interleukin 12 against murine tumors. J Exp Med 1993; 178:1223–1230.
11. Tahara H, Zeh HJ, Storkus WJ, et al. Fibroblasts genetically engineered to secrete interleukin 12 can suppress tumor growth and induce antitumor immunity to a murine melanoma in vivo. Cancer Res 1994; 54:182–189.
12. Sad S, Mosmann TR. Single IL-2-secreting precursor CD4 T cell can develop into either Th1 or Th2 cytokine secretion phenotype. J Immunol 1994; 153:3514–3522.
13. Firestein GS, Roeder WD, Laxer JA, et al. A new murine $CD4^+$ T cell subset with an unrestricted cytokine profile. J Immunol 1989; 143:518–525.
14. Reiner SL, Wang ZE, Hatam F, Scott P, Locksley RM. TH1 and TH2 cell antigen receptors in experimental leishmaniasis. Science 1993; 259:1457–1460.
15. Abehsira-Amar O, Gibert M, Joliy M, et al. IL-4 plays a dominant role in the differential development of Tho into Th1 and Th2 cells. J Immunol 1992; 148:3820–3829.

16. Seder RA, Paul WE, Davis MM, et al. The presence of interleukin 4 during in vitro priming determines the lymphokine-producing potential of $CD4^+$ T cells from T cell receptor transgenic mice. J Exp Med 1992; 176:1091–1098.
17. Gajewski TF, Pinnas M, Wong T, Fitch FW. Murine Th1 and Th2 clones proliferate optimally in response to distinct antigen-presenting cell populations. J Immunol 1991; 146:1750–1758.
18. Quill H, Schwartz RH. Stimulation of normal inducer T cell clones with antigen presented by purified Ia molecules in planar lipid membranes: Specific induction of a long-lived state of proliferative nonresponsiveness. J Immunol 1987; 138:3704–3712.
19. Weaver CT, Hawrylowicz CM, Unanue ER. T helper cell subsets require the expression of distinct costimulatory signals by antigen-presenting cells. Proc Natl Acad Sci USA 1988; 85:8181–8185.
20. Seder RA, Gazzinelli R, Sher A, Paul WE. Interleukin 12 acts directly on $CD4^+$ T cells to enhance priming for interferon gamma production and diminishes interleukin 4 inhibition of such priming. Proc Natl Acad Sci USA 1993; 90:10188–10192.
21. Clerici M, Lucey DR, Berzofsky JA, et al. Restoration of HIV-specific cell-mediated immune responses by interleukin-12 in vitro. Science 1993; 262:1721–1724.
22. McKnight AJ, Zimmer GJ, Fogelman I, et al. Effects of IL-12 on helper T cell-dependent immune responses in vivo. J Immunol 1994; 152:2172–2179.
23. Vieira LQ, Hondowicz BD, Afonso LC, et al. Infection with Leishmania major induces interleukin-12 production in vivo. Immunol Lett 1994; 40:157–161.
24. Le Gros G, Ben-Sasson SZ, Seder R, et al. Generation of interleukin 4 (IL-4) producing cells in vivo and in vitro: IL-2 and IL-4 are required for in vitro generation of IL-4 producing cells. J Exp Med 1990; 172:921–929.
25. Swain SL, Weinberg AD, English M, Huston G. IL-4 directs the development of Th2-like helper effectors. J Immunol 1990; 145:3796–3806.
26. Vella AT, Hulsebosch MD, Pearce EJ. Schistosoma mansoni eggs induce antigen-responsive CD44-hi T helper 2 cells and IL-4- secreting CD44-lo cells. Potential for T helper 2 subset differentiation is evident at the precursor level. J Immunol 1992; 149: 1714–1722.
27. Kopf M, Le Gros G, Bachmann M, et al. Disruption of the murine IL-4 gene blocks Th2 cytokine responses. Nature 1993; 362:245–248.
28. Del Prete G, Maggi E, Romagnani S. Human Th1 and Th2 cells: Functional properties, mechanisms of regulation, and role in disease. Lab Invest 1994; 70:299–306.
29. Romagnani S. Lymphokine production by human T cells in disease states. Annu Rev Immunol 1994; 12:227–257.
30. Sadick MD, Heinzel FP, Holaday BJ, et al. Cure of murine leishmaniasis with anti-interleukin 4 monoclonal antibody: Evidence for a T cell-dependent, interferon gamma-independent mechanism. J Exp Med 1990; 171:115–127.
31. Romani L, Mocci S, Bietta C, Lanfaloni L, et al. Th1 and Th2 cytokine secretion patterns in murine candidiasis: Association of Th1 responses with acquired resistance. Infect Immun 1991; 59:4647–4654.
32. Holaday BJ, Sadick MD, Wang ZE, et al. Reconstitution of Leishmania immunity in severe combined immunodeficient mice using Th1- and Th2-like cell lines. J Immunol 1991; 147:1653–1658.
33. Mizuochi T, Ono S, Malek TR, Singer A. Characterization of two distinct primary T cell populations that secrete interleukin 2 upon recognition of class I or class II major histocompatibility antigens. J Exp Med 1986; 163:603–619.
34. Widmer MB, Bach FH. Antigen-driven helper cell-independent cloned cytolytic T lymphocytes. Nature 1981; 294:750–752.
35. Umlauf SW, Beverly B, Kang SM, et al. Molecular regulation of the IL-2 gene: Rheostatic control of the immune system. Immunol Rev 1993; 133:177–197.

36. Henkart Pa. Lymphocyte-mediated cytotoxicity: Two pathways and multiple effector molecules. Immunity 1994; 1:343–346.
37. Kelso A. Frequency analysis of lymphokine-secreting $CD4^+$ and $CD8^+$ T cells activated in a graft-versus-host reaction. J Immunol 1990; 145:2167–2176.
38. Ando K, Moriyama T, Guidotti LG, et al. Mechanisms of class I restricted immunopathology: A transgenic mouse model of fulminant hepatitis. J Exp Med 1993; 178:1541–1554.
39. Barth RJ Jr, Mule JJ, Spiess PJ, Rosenberg SA. Interferon gamma and tumor necrosis factor have a role in tumor regressions mediated by murine $CD8^+$ tumor-infiltrating lymphocytes. J Exp Med 1991; 173:647–658.
40. Sedar RA, Boulay JL, Finkelman F, et al. $CD8^+$ T cells can be primed in vitro to procedure IL-4. J Immunol 1992; 148:1652–1656.
41. Erard F, Wild MT, Garcia-Sanz JA, Le Gros G. Switch of CD8 T cells to noncytolytic CD8-CD4- cells that make TH2 cytokines and help B cells. Science 1993; 260:1802–1805.
42. Kawakami Y, Haas GP, Lotze MT. Expansion of tumor-infiltrating lymphocytes from human tumors using the T-cell growth factors interleukin-2 and interleukin-4. J Immunother 1993; 14:336–347.
43. Actor JK, Shirai M, Kullberg MC, et al. Helminth infection results in decreased virus-specific $CD8^+$ cytotoxic T-cell and Th1 cytokine responses as well as delayed virus clearance. Proc Natl Acad Sci USA 1993; 90:948–952.
44. Pace JL, Russell SW, LeBlanc PA, Murasko DM. Comparative effects of various classes of mouse interferons on macrophage activation for tumor cell killing. J Immunol 1985; 134:977–981.
45. Nathan C. Mechanisms and modulation of macrophage activation. Behring Inst Mitt 1991; 200–207.
46. Sher A, Gazzinelli RT, Oswald IP, et al. Role of T-cell derived cytokines in the downregulation of immune responses in parasitic and retroviral infection. Immunol Rev 1992; 127:183–204.
47. Nastala CL, Edington HD, McKinney TG, et al. Recombinant IL-12 administration induces tumor regression in association with IFN-gamma production. J Immunol 1994; 153:1697–1706.
48. Kuhn R, Lohler J, Rennick D, et al. Interleukin-10-deficient mice develop chronic enterocolitis (see comments). Cell 1993; 75:263–274.
49. McBride WH, Economou JS, Nayersina R, et al. Influences of interleukins 2 and 4 on tumor necrosis factor production by murine mononuclear phagocytes. Cancer Res 1990; 50:2949–2952.
50. Bogdan C, Nathan C. Modulation of macrophage function by transforming growth factor beta, interleukin-4, and interleukin-10. Ann NY Acad Sci 1993; 685:713–739.
51. Bogdan C, Vodovotz Y, Paik J, et al. Mechanism of suppression of nitric oxide synthase expression by interleukin-4 in primary mouse macrophages. J Leuk Biol 1994; 55:227–233.
52. de Waal Malefyt R, Abrams J, Bennett B, et al. Interleukin 10(IL-10) inhibits cytokine synthesis by human monocytes: An autoregulatory role of IL-10 produced by monocytes. J Exp Med 1991; 174:1209–1220.
53. Wang P, Wu P, Siegel MI, et al. IL-10 inhibits transcription of cytokine genes in human peripheral blood mononuclear cells. J Immunol 1994; 153:811–816.
54. Bogdan C, Vodovotz Y, Nathan C. Macrophage deactivation by interleukin 10. J Exp Med 1991; 174:1549–1555.
55. Powrie F, Menon S, Coffman RL. Interleukin-4 and interleukin-10 synergize to inhibit cell-mediated immunity in vivo. Eur J Immunol 1993; 23:3043–3049.
56. Mulligan MS, Jones ML, Vaporciyan AA, et al. Protective effects of IL-4 and IL-10 against immune complex-induced lung injury. J Immunol 1993; 151:5666–5674.

57. Marchant A, Bruyns C, Vandenabeele P, et al. Interleukin-10 controls interferon-gamma and tumor necrosis factor production during experimental endotoxemia. Eur J Immunol 1994; 24:1167–1171.
58. Howard M, Muchamuel T, Andrade S, Menon S. Interleukin 10 protects mice from lethal endotoxemia. J Exp Med 1993; 177:1205–1208.
59. Jenkins JK, Malyak M, Arend WP. The effects of interleukin-10 on interleukin-1 receptor antagonist and interleukin-1 beta production in human monocytes and neutrophils. Lymph Cy Res 1994; 13:47–54.
60. Cassatella MA, Meda L, Gasperini S, et al. Interleukin 10 (IL-10) upregulates IL-1 receptor antagonist production from lipopolysaccharide-stimulated human polymorphonuclear leukocytes by delaying mRNA degradation. J Exp Med 1994; 179:1695–1699.
61. Stein M, Keshav S, Harris N, Gordon S. Interleukin 4 potently enhances murine marcrophage mannose receptor activity: A marker of alternative immunologic macrophage activation. J Exp Med 1992; 176:287–292.
62. Wong HL, Costa GL, Lotze MT, Wahl SM. Interleukin (IL) 4 differentially regulates monocyte IL-1 family gene expression and synthesis in vitro and in vivo. J Exp Med 1993; 177:775–781.
63. Knorgold R. Lethal graft-versus-host disease in mice directed to multiple minor histocompatibility antigens: Features of $CD8^+$ and $CD4^+$ T cell responses. Bone Marrow Transplant 1992; 9:355–364.
64. Hakim FT, Sharrow SO, Payne S, Shearer GM. Repopulation of host lymphohematopoietic systems by donor cells during graft-versus-host reaction in unirradiated adult F1 mice injected with parental lymphocytes. J Immunol 1991; 146:2108–2115.
65. Ferrara JL, Abhyankar S, Gilliland DG. Cytokine storm of graft-versus-host disease: A critical effector role for interleukin-1. Transplant Proc 1993; 25:1216–1217.
66. Via CS, Finkelman FD. Critical role of interleukin-2 in the development of acute graft-versus-host disease. Int Immunol 1993; 5:565–572.
67. Via CS, Rus V, Gately MK, Finkelman FD. IL-12 stimulates the development of acute graft-versus-host disease in mice that normally would develop chronic, autoimmune graft-versus-host disease. J Immunol 1994; 153:4040–4047.
68. Schwarer AP, Jiang YZ, Brookes PA, et al. Frequency of anti-recipient alloreactive helper T-cell precursors in donor blood and graft-versus-host disease after HLA-identical sibling bone-marrow transplantation. Lancet 1994; 341:203–205.
69. Theobald M, Nierle T, Bunjes D, et al. Host-specific interleukin-2-secreting donor T-cell precursors as predictors of acute graft-versus-host disease in bone marrow transplantation between HLA-identical siblings (see comments). N Engl J Med 1992; 327: 1613–1617.
70. Anasetti C, Hansen JA, Waldmann TA, et al. Treatment of acute graft-versus-host disease with humanized anti-Tac: An antibody that binds to the interleukin-2 receptor. Blood 1994; 84:1320–1327.
71. Waldmann TA. The IL-2/IL-2 receptor system: A target for rational immune intervention. Trends Pharmacol Sci 1993; 14:159–164.
72. Sprent J, Surh CD, Agus D, et al. Profound atrophy of the bone marrow reflecting major histocompatibility complex class II-restricted destruction of stem cells by $CD4^+$ cells. J Exp Med 1994; 180:307–317.
73. Berger M, Wettstein PJ, Korngold R. T cell subsets involved in lethal graft-versus-host disease directed to immunodominant minor histocompatibility antigens. Transplantation 1994; 57:1095–1102.
74. Sakamoto H, Michaelson J, Jones WK, et al. Lymphocytes with a $CD4^+$ $CD8^-$ CD3-phenotype are effectors of experimental cutaneous graft-versus-host disease. Proc Natl Acad Sci USA 1991; 88:10890–10894.

75. Knobloch C, Dennert G. Asialo-GM1-positive T killer cells are generated in F1 mice injected with parental spleen cells. J Immunol 1988; 140:744–749.
76. Korngold R. Biology of graft-vs-host disease. Am J Pediatr Hematol Oncol 1993; 15: 18–27.
77. Fong TA, Mosmann TR. Alloreactive murine $CD8^+$ T cell clones secrete the Th1 pattern of cytokines. J Immunol 1990; 144:1744–1752.
78. Guillen FJ, Ferrara J, Hancock WW, et al. Acute cutaneous graft-versus-host disease to minor histocompatibility antigens in a murine model. Evidence that large granular lymphocytes are effector cells in the immune response. Lab Invest 1986; 55:35–42.
79. Ghayur T, Xenocostas A, Seemayer TA, Lapp WS. Induction, specificity and elimination of asialo-$GM1^+$ graft-versus-host effector cells of donor origin. Scand J Immunol 1991; 34:497–508.
80. Bonnema JD, Rivlin KA, Ting AT, et al: Cytokine-enhanced NK cell-mediated cytotoxicity: Positive modulatory effects of IL-2 and IL-12 on stimulus-dependent granule exocytosis. J Immunol 1994; 152:2098–2104.
81. Naume B, Gately M, Espevik T. A comparative study of IL-12 (cytotoxic lymphocyte maturation factor)-, IL-2-, and IL-7-induced effects of immunomagnetically purified $CD56^+$ NK cells. J Immunol 1992; 148:2429–2436.
82. Paganin C, Matteucci C, Cenzuales S, et al. IL-4 inhibits binding and cytotoxicity of NK cells to vascular endothelium. Cytokine 1994; 6:135–140.
83. Colquhoun SD, Economou JS, Shau H, Golub SH. IL-4 inhibits IL-2 induction of LAK cytotoxicity in lymphocytes from a variety of lymphoid tissues. J Surg Res 1993; 55:486–492.
84. Spagnoli GC, Juretic A, Schultz-Thater E, et al. On the relative roles of interleukin-2 and interleukin-10 in the generation of lymphokine-activated killer cell activity. Cell Immunol 1993; 146:391–405.
85. Holaday BJ, Pompeu MM, Jeronimo S, et al. Potential role for interleukin-10 in the immunosuppression associated with kala azar. J Clin Invest 1993; 92:2626–2632.
86. Fukuda H, Nakamura H, Tominaga N, et al. Marked increase of $CD8^+S6F1^+$ and $CD8^+CD57^+$ cells in patients with graft-versus-host disease after allogeneic bone marrow transplantation. Bone Marrow Transplant 1994; 13:181–185.
87. Roy J, Platt JL, Weisdorf DJ. The immunopathology of upper gastrointestinal acute graft-versus-host disease: Lymphoid cells and endothelial adhesion molecules. Transplantation 1993; 55:572–578.
88. Champlin R, Jansen J, Ho W, et al. Retention of graft-versus-leukemia using selective depletion of CD8-positive T lymphocytes for prevention of graft-versus-host disease following bone marrow transplantation for chronic myelogenous leukemia. Transplant Proc 1991; 23:1695–1696.
89. Champlin R, Gajewski J, Feig S, et al. Selective depletion of CD8 positive T-lymphocytes for prevention of graft-versus-host disease following allogeneic bone marrow transplantation. Transplant Proc 1989; 21:2947–2948.
90. Antin JH, Ferrara JL. Cytokine dysregulation and acute graft-versus-host disease. Blood 1992; 80:2964–2968.
91. Abhyankar S, Gilliland DG, Ferrara JL. Interleukin-1 is a critical effector molecule during cytokine dysregulation in graft versus host disease to minor histocompatibility antigens. Transplantation 1993; 56:1518–1523.
92. Piguet PF, Grau GE, Allet B, Vassalli P. Tumor necrosis factor/cachectin is an effector of skin and gut lesions of the acute phase of graft-vs-host disease. J Exp Med 1987; 166:1280–1289.
93. Guy-Grand D, Vassalli P. Gut injury in mouse graft-versus-host reaction: Study of its occurrence and mechanisms. J Clin Invest 1986; 77:1584–1595.
94. Shalaby MR, Fendly B, Sheehan KC, et al. Prevention of the graft-versus-host reaction

in newborn mice by antibodies to tumor necrosis factor-alpha. Transplantation 1989; 47:1057–1061.
95. Nestel FP, Price KS, Seemayer TA, Lapp WS. Macrophage priming and lipopolysaccharide-triggered release of tumor necrosis factor alpha during graft-versus-host disease. J. Exp Med 1992; 175:405–413.
96. Holler E, Kolb HJ, Moller A, et al. Increased serum levels of tumor necrosis factor alpha precede major complications of bone marrow transplantation (see comments). Blood 1990; 75:1011–1016.
97. Holler E, Kolb HJ, Wilmanns W. Treatment of GVHD—TNF-antibodies and related antagonists. Bone Marrow Transplant 1993; 12(suppl 3):S29–S31.
98. Bianchi M, Tracey K. The role of TNF in complications of marrow transplantation. Marrow Transplant 1994; 57–61.
99. Bacchetta R, Bigler M, Touraine JL, et al. High levels of interleukin 10 production in vivo are associated with tolerance in SCID patients transplanted with HLA mismatched hematopoietic stem cells. J Exp Med 1994; 179:493–502.
100. Nathan CF, Hibbs JB, Jr. Role of nitric oxide synthesis in macrophage antimicrobial activity. Curr Opin Immunol 1991; 3:65–70.
101. Hoffman RA, Langrehr JM, Wren SM, et al. Characterization of the immunosuppressive effects of nitric oxide in graft vs host disease. J Immunol 1993; 151:1508–1518.
102. Oswald IP, Gazzinelli RT, Sher A, James SL. IL-10 synergizes with IL-4 and transforming growth factor-beta to inhibit macrophage cytotoxic activity. J Immunol 1992; 148:3578–3582.
103. Oswald IP, Wynn TA, Sher A, James SL. Interleukin 10 inhibits macrophage microbicidal activity by blocking the endogenous production of tumor necrosis factor alpha required as a costimulatory factor for interferon gamma-induced activation. Proc Natl Acad Sci USA 1992; 89:8676–8680.
104. De Wit D, Van Mechelen M, Zanin C, et al. Preferential activation of Th2 cells in chronic graft-versus-host reaction. J Immunol 1993; 150:361–366.
105. Donckier V, Abramowicz D, Bruyns C, et al. IFN-gamma prevents Th2 cell–mediated pathology after neonatal injection of semiallogenic spleen cells in mice. J Immunol 1994; 153:2361–2368.
106. Fowler DH, Kurasawa K, Husebekk A, et al. Cells of Th2 cytokine phenotype prevent LPS-induced lethality during murine graft-versus-host reaction: Regulation of cytokines and $CD8^+$ lymphoid engraftment. J Immunol 1994; 152:1004–1013.
107. Fowler DH, Kurasawa K, Smith R, et al. Donor CD4-enriched cells of Th2 cytokine phenotype regulate graft-versus-host disease without impairing allogeneic engraftment in sublethally irradiated mice. Blood 1994; 84:3540–3549.
108. Desbarats J, Lapp WS. Thymic selection and thymic major histocompatibility complex class II expression are abnormal in mice undergoing graft-versus-host reactions. J Exp Med 1993; 178:805–814.
109. Kornbluth M, You-Ten E, Desbarats J, et al. T cell subsets in the thymus of graft-versus-host immunosuppresed mice: Sensitivity of the $L3T4^+Lyt\text{-}2^-$subset to cortisone. Transplantation 1991; 51:262–267.
110. Cohen PA, Kim H, Fowler DH, et al. Use of interleukin-7, interleukin-2, and interferon-gamma to propagate $CD4^+$ T cells in culture with maintained antigen specificity. J Immunother 1993; 14:242–252.
111. Cohen PA, Fowler DH, Kim H, et al. Propagation of murine and human T cells with defined antigen specificity and function. *Ciba Foundation Symposium*: No. 187; 179–93. *Vaccines Against Virally Induced Cancers*: Chichester, England: Wiley, 1994.

18

The Role of Endotoxin in the Pathogenesis of Acute Graft-Versus-Host Disease

Frederick Nestel, Krikor Kichian, Kong You-Ten, Julie Desbarats, Kursteen Price, and Wayne S. Lapp

McGill University, Montreal, Quebec, Canada

Premysl Ponka

Lady Davis Institute for Medical Research and Sir Mortimer B. Davis–Jewish General Hospital, Montreal, Quebec, Canada

Thomas A. Seemayer

University of Nebraska Medical Center, Omaha, Nebraska

I. INTRODUCTION

Acute graft-versus-host disease (GVHD) is a frequent complication following the transplantation of allogeneic bone marrow and is responsible for a relatively high rate of morbidity and mortality in such patients. Acute GVHD targets lymphoid organs as well as epithelial tissue of the liver, skin, and gastrointestinal tract. Although considerable evidence suggests that T lymphocytes are important for the initiation of acute GVHD, the mechanism responsible for inflicting the pathological changes to the target organs has not been clearly delineated. Other cell types, including NK cells and macrophages and various cytokines, have been implicated.

In this review, we wish to present studies from our laboratory suggesting that at least three different cell types, several cytokines, and a product of gram-negative organisms in the gut, lipopolysaccharide (LPS), or endotoxin combine to cause the pathological changes that are characteristic of acute GVHD.

In the first section, we will present the mechanism responsible for the pathological changes, including cachexia; in the second section we will demonstrate how the endotoxin pathway may be indirectly responsible for the marked peripheral T-cell immunosuppression that is a hallmark of acute GVHD.

II. ENDOTOXIN AND GVHD PATHOLOGY

A. Macrophage Physiology

A number of observations made in experimental animal models soon after the first bone marrow transplants were performed provided evidence indicating that macrophages (Mϕ) and their secretory products play a central role in the development of acute graft-versus-host disease (GVHD). The significance of these findings could only recently be realized as a result of the characterization of both the physiological mechanisms involved in Mϕ activation and the nature and action of secretory products, including tumor necrosis factor alpha (TNF-α) and nitric oxide (NO), produced by activated Mϕ.

Normal Mϕ are able to produce tumor necrosis factor–alpha (TNF-α) (1) and generate NO (2,3) following activation. These products form an important part of the nonspecific host defense mechanism directed against invading microorganisms. However, injury to surrounding host tissue is an additional potential consequence of TNF-α and NO production, particularly following widespread or excessive Mϕ activation. TNF-α has been shown to mediate weight loss or cachexia, some inflammatory processes, and septic or endotoxic shock (4–7). NO has also been implicated as a mediator in the pathology of endotoxic shock (8,9), and a number of experimental models have demonstrated that NO plays a role in inflammatory or autoimmune disease (10–13).

Mϕ activation occurs following priming by interferon-gamma (IFN-γ) and triggering of the cells by lipopolysaccharide (LPS) (14,15). Quantities of LPS that are insufficient to induce the production and release of TNF-α from normal, unprimed Mϕ trigger IFN-γ primed Mϕ to produce significant quantities of TNF-α (15,16). IFN-γ by itself can activate Mϕ to synthesize NO; however, the level of activation and subsequent production of NO is substantially greater when LPS is provided as a second or triggering signal (17). IFN-γ and LPS, in fact, act synergistically; thus priming of normal Mϕ by greater amounts of IFN-γ results in a significant reduction in the amount of LPS needed to trigger Mϕ production of TNF-α (1,14–16) and synthesis of NO (17). Although IFN-α and IFN-β can also act as priming signals for Mϕ activation, IFN-γ mediates a far greater priming effect on Mϕ for both TNF-α and NO production (17,18).

The first or priming signal involved in Mϕ activation, that is, IFN-γ, is produced by the T-helper 1 (Th1) lineage of $CD4^+$ cells and by natural killer (NK) cells. It has more recently become apparent that interleukin-12 (IL-12), a cytokine produced by Mϕ following interaction with microbial organisms or LPS, is an important mediator in IFN-γ production (reviewed in Ref. 19). IL-12, released from Mϕ that have been exposed to LPS, can act on T cells to initiate the differentiation of Th cells to Th1 and can induce IFN-γ production by Th1 and NK cells.

LPS, the second or triggering signal involved in Mϕ activation, is an integral part of the cell wall of gram-negative bacteria. The intestinal epithelial mucosa acts as an initial obstacle preventing entry of bacteria from the large pool of enteric gram-negative organisms that are normally present in the intestinal tract. In addition, large numbers of Mϕ found in the GI tract, mesenteric lymph nodes, and liver [i.e., Kupffer cells (20,21)] form a second protective barrier against entry. Therefore the translocation of enteric bacteria across the gut epithelium—which is believed to occur at a regular albeit relatively low frequency—does not normally result in widespread septicemia due to the large numbers of phagocytic cells present. An additional protective mechanism mediates the rapid clearance of free LPS that may enter from the GI tract or that is released from the cell wall of killed bacteria. Removal of LPS by phagocytic cells occurs via interaction with LPS-binding protein (LBP) and subsequent binding of the LPS-LBP complex to CD14 on the surface membrane of Mϕ (22).

B. Macrophage Activation During Acute GVHD

One of the characteristic features of GVHD is the severe, prolonged immunosuppression that occurs after transplantation of allogeneic hematopoietic cells (23). Although the alterations in numbers and suppression of T and B lymphocytes that occur in transplant recipients have been extensively studied, the effector cells and mechanisms that mediate acute GVHD, one of the most serious complications of bone marrow transplantation, have not been identified. A paradoxical characteristic of experimental GVHD is the increased Mϕ phagocytic and bactericidal activity (24,25) that occurs in otherwise immunosuppressed transplant recipients. Our studies have focused on this unusual state of nonspecific Mϕ activation in animals undergoing immunosuppression (26). In particular, we have examined the mechanisms underlying Mϕ activation and the release of Mϕ secretory products that we believe are involved in tissue injury and the progression of acute GVHD. The objective of our initial investigations was to determine the nature of the relationship between the state of Mϕ activation and the severity of GVHD. In order to reduce the number of variables that might obscure the basis of the difference between the nonlethal and acute (i.e., lethal) GVHD, we examined nonirradiated C57BL/6xAF1 (B6AF1) animals undergoing GVHD as a result of transplantation with different doses of donor cells, that is, 30×10^6 (nonlethal) or 60×10^6 (acute) B6 lymphoid cells. Experimental animals were studied on day 7 after transplant, when animals in both groups were immunosuppressed, although cachexia or weight loss was not as yet significant, and later on day 14, immediately prior to the onset of mortality in the acute GVHD animals, when the disparity between the two groups in terms of weight loss and the severity of pathological lesions was more apparent.

The results of our studies demonstrate that Mϕ are primed following allogeneic transplantation and that the state of Mϕ activation is in fact greater during acute than during nonlethal GVHD (26). As a result of priming, Mϕ express TNF-α-mediated and NO-mediated cytotoxic effector mechanisms when triggered by bacteria-derived endotoxin or LPS. Mϕ isolated from transplanted animals 12 to 14 days after transplantation could be triggered by 2.5 ng/mL of LPS to express cytotoxic activity against indium 111-labeled L5178Y and P815 tumor cells that are respectively sensitive to TNF-α and NO-mediated killing mechanisms [Table 1 (26)]. The results also indicate that the response of Mϕ to LPS is directly related to the severity of GVHD. Although Mϕ from animals undergoing nonlethal reactions were also primed, they only expressed cytotoxic activity when triggered by much greater amounts of LPS, demonstrating that they were primed to a lesser extent than Mϕ from acute GVHD animals (26).

MDW4 tumor cells—which are resistant to Mϕ-mediated killing (27) but sensitive to the cytostatic effect of Mϕ-derived NO—were not killed. However, their ability to proliferate as measured by [^{3}H]TdR incorporation was inhibited when incubated with Mϕ from acute GVHD animals in the presence of 2.5 ng/mL LPS. In both nonlethal and acute GVHD, Mϕ priming and NO production in response to LPS could be detected on day 7 after transplantation as measured using the Griess reagent. Mϕ priming occurred only transiently in nonlethal GVHD as demonstrated by low-level production of NO in response to LPS on day 14. In contrast, the levels of LPS-triggered NO production increased with time posttransplant in acute GVHD.

Table 1 Macrophage Activation During GVHD

Parameter Measured	Target Cells[a]	Treatment In Vitro	Nonlethal GVHD		Acute GVHD	
MΦ cytotoxic activity	L5178Y	Medium	–		–	
		LPS	+/–		+++	
	P815	Medium	–		–	
		LPS	+/–		+++	
	MDW4	Medium	ND		–	
		LPS	ND		–	
MΦ cytostatic activity	MDW4	Medium	ND		–	
		LPS	ND		+++	
MΦ production of nitric oxide[b]			Day 7	Day 14	Day 7	Day 14
		Medium	–	–	–	–
		LPS	++	+/–	++	+++

[a]Target cells are described in the text.
[b]NO_3^-, by-product of NO measured in MΦ supernatants.

Our in vitro results demonstrating Mϕ priming following transplantation clearly indicated that the mechanisms triggered by LPS should also be detectable in vivo. We therefore examined the response of transplanted animals to injections of normally insignificant amounts of LPS [Table 2 (26)]. Intravenous injection of 10 μg of LPS induced the rapid onset of septic shock, resulting in death within 36 hr of all the acute GVHD animals [Table 2 (26)]. Septic shock was also accompanied by the production of significant amounts of TNF-α detectable in the serum of acute GVHD animals 2 hr after LPS injection IV [Table 2 (26)]. In contrast, IV injection

Table 2 In Vivo Response to LPS in Acute GVHD Mice on Day 7 After Transplantation

Treatment	Parameter Measured	Amount of LPS Injected	Normal B6AF1	Nonlethal GVHD	Acute GVHD
LPS IV	Mortality	0 μg[a]	0/12[b]	0/12[b]	0/12[b]
		10 μg	0/12[b]	6/24[b]	24/24[b]
LPS IV	Serum TNF-α (U/mL) 2 hr after LPS	0 μg[a]	–	–	–
		25 μg[a]	0.5×10^3	1.3×10^3	15×10^3
LPS SC	Cutaneous lesions	0 μg[a]	0/5[c]	ND	0/5[c]
		10 μg	0/5[c]	ND	5/5[c]
		10 μg + rat anti-mTNF-α	ND	ND	1/5[c]

[a]Animals received saline without LPS.
[b]Number of dead animals/total 36 hr after an intravenous injection of LPS.
[c]Number of animals showing positive cutaneous lesions/total within 24 hr after a subcutaneous injection of LPS.

of LPS resulted in the death of only 25% of animals undergoing nonlethal GVHD. In these animals, significant levels of serum TNF-α were not detected; however, Mϕ from these animals did produce NO when triggered by LPS at approximately the same level as Mϕ from acute GVHD animals.

Once again using LPS as an indicator of Mϕ priming, we examined the response to LPS of acute GVHD animals injected subcutaneously (SC) 7 days after transplant. Administration of 10 μg of LPS SC resulted in a Shwartzman-like cutaneous reaction in all transplant recipients, whereas normal mice showed no response. The cutaneous response was significantly reduced in surface area in 1/5 and entirely blocked in the remaining 4/5 animals by the simultaneous injection of anti-TNF-α with the LPS (Table 2) (Nestel et al., manuscript in preparation).

The results demonstrated that during GVHD, Mϕ are primed and produce TNF-α and NO when triggered by LPS. The level of Mϕ priming and production of TNF-α and NO in response to LPS are related to the number of cells transplanted and the time posttransplant. Thus both the sensitivity of animals to LPS and LPS-triggered production and release of secreted products in vitro are greater during acute than during nonlethal GVHD and increase with time posttransplant.

A number of studies have indicated an association between the development of acute GVHD and the presence of the two major mediators of Mϕ activation, IFN-γ and LPS, in transplant recipients. Indeed, a causal relationship between the in vivo presence of LPS and the development of GVHD is indicated by the reduction in severity or prevention of GVHD observed in experimental animals (28–30) and clinical bone marrow transplant recipients (31–33) as a result of the elimination of the gastrointestinal microflora.

Increased production of IFN-γ is also closely associated with the development of acute GVHD (34). During the course of experimental GVHD, T- and B-lymphocyte functions are suppressed (23); however, Mϕ are activated, as demonstrated by an increase in their phagocytic and bactericidal activity (24,25). The characteristic augmentation of Mϕ bactericidal activity can be prevented by treatment with anti-IFN-γ (35). In experimental acute GVHD, the percentage of lymphoid cells expressing IFN-γ mRNA is significantly increased (36,37). The severity of GVHD-associated intestinal lesions is decreased following treatment of animals with anti-IFN-γ (38). Patients receiving bone marrow transplants also have an increased proportion of IFN-γ–producing T cells (39). Indeed a marked increase in serum IFN-γ levels precedes the appearance of clinical symptoms of acute GVHD (34).

The seeming paradox of the increased sensitivity of transplanted animals to LPS (40) accompanied by an augmented bactericidal activity (24,25) can now be explained by the priming effect of IFN-γ on the ability of Mϕ to produce TNF-α and NO (26), which are now recognized as mediators of both antibacterial activity and septic shock (6–9).

The significance of TNF-α production during GVHD has been demonstrated by a number of studies. The symptoms observed in experimental murine acute GVHD—including hunched posture, piloerection and diarrhea—are also characteristic of animals injected with rTNF-α (41). Keratin promoter–driven TNF-α transgenic animals demonstrate both the skin reactions and generalized cachexia observed in acute GVHD (42). Treatment with anti-TNF-α prevents gastrointestinal and skin lesions in an experimental animal model of acute GVHD (43); in patients undergoing acute GVHD, anti-TNF-α therapy reduced the severity of pathological lesions (44). Increased levels of TNF-α have been found in the serum of allogeneic bone marrow transplant recipients (45) and have been correlated with the severity of GVHD (46). More recently it has been demonstrated that increasing the proportion of Th2 cells in the donor innoculum can suppress IFN-γ mRNA and effectively protect recipient animals from LPS-induced septic shock by reducing the amount of TNF-α production (37). These findings strongly suggest that the Th2-derived cytokines, IL-4 and/or IL-10, may prove to be effective therapeutic agents for preventing GVHD by virtue of their downregulating effect on Mϕ.

As is the case for TNF-α production, we have found that the ability of Mϕ to generate NO in response to LPS is directly related to the severity of GVHD (Table 1). It has been observed that during experimental GVHD, serum levels of NO_2 and NO_3 are increased (47) and Mϕ-derived NO can act as mediator of immunosuppression associated with GVHD (48). In addition, treatment with N^G-monomethyl-L-arginine (NMMA), a competitive substrate inhibitor of NO synthase activity, prevents the development of intestinal pathology during GVHD (49).

Our results provide evidence for the activation of Mϕ-mediated mechanisms responsible for acute GVHD. The effectiveness of the intestinal mucosa as a barrier to bacterial entry following transplantation is a key feature in our proposed model of acute GVHD. In the case of excessive priming of Mϕ, following transplantation—as we have described—translocation of even small numbers of gram-negative bacteria could result in a localized gut epithelial tissue injury mediated by TNF-α and NO (26,43,49). The cytostatic effector mechanism mediated by NO may be a particular relevance to acute GVHD in light of the injury to the regenerative cellular compartment of epithelial tissues that is a characteristic pathological finding in acute GVHD.

C. Tissue Endotoxin Levels During Acute GVHD

Up to this stage we have demonstrated that Mϕ are primed in acute GVHD mice, since when they receive a SC injection of LPS they develop a Schwartzman-like reaction, and when injected with LPS IV they die within 24 hr. These results further suggest that priming of Mϕ is not confined only to lymphoid organs but occurs throughout the body. We postulate that the priming is a consequence of the cytokine dysregulation and copious and continuous production of IFN-γ (see Chaps. 7 and 25 on cytokine networks and cytokine inhibitors). The missing link in our hypothesis is the presence of endogenous LPS in the tissues of acute GVHD mice.

We therefore initiated studies using the Pyrotel Limulus Amoebocyte Lysate assay to measure LPS in serum and tissue of animals experiencing GVHD. In these studies we included a syngeneic control (F_1 into F_1) and an allogeneic control to determine whether the simple injection of cells or an allogenic reaction would cause a translocation of LPS from the gut. GVHD was induced in 142 B6AF1 mice by the injection of 60×10^6 B6 spleen and lymph node cells. A minimum of 8 mice were sacrificed on days 4, 8, and 12; on day 16, in each group, 12 to 15 mice were sacrificed.

The results shown in Table 3 demonstrate a detectable amount of LPS in the liver and spleen for up to 10 days in the two control groups, but LPS was not detected in these groups after day 10. In contrast, the GVHD group displayed

Table 3 Maximum Tissue LPS Concentrations During Acute GVHD

Day After GVHD	LPS Concentrations: Liver (ng/organ) S[a]	Liver (ng/organ) G[a]	Spleen (ng/organ) S[a]	Spleen (ng/organ) G[a]	Blood (ng/mL) S[a]	Blood (ng/mL) G[a]
4	1	100	1	100	0	0
8	1	100	0	100	0	0
12	0	100[b]	0	100[b]	0	0
16	0	10,000[b]	0	10,000[b]	0	4

[a]S- B6AF$_1$ recipients received syngeneic cells and did not develop GVHD. G- B6AF$_1$ recipients received B6 parental strain cells and developed GVHD. Animals in the GVHD groups began dying on day 16 and by day 19 over 80% of the animals had died. A minimum of 8 animals were tested in each group on days 4 to 12 and on day 16, 12 to 15 mice were tested in each group.
[b]All of the animals in the group tested positive for LPS in the liver and/or spleen on these days.

considerably more LPS than the control groups as early as day 2 after GVHD induction; by day 10, all of the GVHD mice displayed greater than 100 ng of LPS in the liver, which increased to reach levels of 10 μg by day 16. The spleen also displayed a steady increase in LPS, and by day 16, we detected up to 10 μg of LPS in the spleen. It was of interest that LPS was not detected in the serum until day 16, and that mortality did not occur until LPS was observed in the serum. However, once it did appear, 80% of the animals were dead within 3 days. These results thus demonstrate that LPS does increase in the liver and spleen during acute GVHD and that once LPS is detected in the serum, there is a strong association with mortality. It should be noted that weight loss first started to occur on day 10, with only a slight loss by day 14 (6%); however, between days 14 and 18, weight loss averaged nearly 25% of the preexperimental weight (26) (Price et al., manuscript in preparation).

D. Mechanism of Endotoxin Translocation During Acute GVHD

In a series of earlier studies we identified the mechanism responsible for the early injury to epithelial tissue in all GVHD target organs (50). Ghayur et al. (50), while studying the effector cells in GVHD, were able to demonstrate that the GVHD effector of parental-strain origin was activated early as a result of the initial allogeneic T-cell response. The GVHD effector that caused the initial epithelial-cell injury was shown to be sensitive to antiasialo GM treatment after being activated in the donor and to display NK activity. However, this cell was not a classic NK cell, since it also displayed some allospecificity. We therefore suggested that the activated cell was an NK-like cell (50). Macdonald and Gartner (51) have also demonstrated the importance of an NK-like cell, and Gartner et al. have shown that the NK activity can be eliminated in vitro by removing $\gamma\delta$ T cells (J. G. Gartner, personal communication). We also speculated that the cell may be a $\gamma\delta$ T cell, since it displayed immunological specificity but did not appear to be an $\alpha\beta$ T cell (50). Thus, the initial injury may be caused by an interaction between parental T cells and NK-like cells as early as 6 to 10 days after GVHD induction.

It seems highly likely that macrophages may also contribute to the epithelial lesions of the gut after the initiation of GVHD by an NO-dependent mechanism. Macrophages can act in at least two different ways. If primed Mϕ are triggered, they can release pathological amounts of TNF-α and NO, which could be cytotoxic for epithelial and other cells. In addition, the NO released from Mϕ may exert a cytostatic effect on the rapidly regenerating epithelium of the intestine. Gut epithelial cells arise in the crypts and migrate to the tips of the villi, where they are sloughed. Thus, to maintain an intact epithelial layer, it is important to have a continuous production of epithelial cells. If NO arrests proliferation of the epithelial stem cells in the crypts, it would result in a shedding of epithelial cells without replacement, thus creating a lesion for the translocation of LPS into the gastrointestinal capillaries and the hepatic portal vein in the absence of any direct cytotoxicity.

We propose that the early injury and/or cytostasis of epithelial cells in the GI tract results in a translocation of LPS across the gut wall into the capillaries and lymphatics of the intestine. The blood then collects in the portal vein and is transported to the liver. The liver, which functions to detoxify LPS and export it back into the intestine via the bile (52), eventually becomes saturated with LPS (owing to both the increased amount of LPS and to hepatic injury), resulting in a spillover into the hepatic vein and thus into the systemic circulation. Once LPS reaches the systemic circulation, it is disseminated rapidly to all parts of the body and is thus able to trigger primed Mϕ, which we believe are also dispersed in all parts of the body. The triggering of the primed macrophages results in the release of pathological amounts of TNF-α and NO, resulting in the symptoms of acute GVHD (cachexia, hunched posture, diarrhea) and death of the animal. Once LPS reaches the systemic circulation of a primed animal, death ensues within a matter of hours (26).

III. ENDOTOXIN AND GVHD-INDUCED IMMUNOSUPPRESSION

A. Endotoxin-Mediated Elevation of Glucocorticoid Levels

In addition to having numerous effects on the immune system, endotoxin is well documented to activate the hypothalamic-pituitary-adrenal (HPA) axis. Studies have shown that injection of LPS in humans and animals triggers the HPA axis, resulting in increased levels of adrenal glucocorticoids in the circulation (53,54). We and others have previously demonstrated that mice undergoing GVHD experience severe thymic atrophy, which is prevented by surgical adrenalectomy (55,56), suggesting that GVHD induces the adrenal glands to secrete excessive amounts of glucocorticoids. In order to quantitate the levels of glucocorticoids in the circulation, blood was removed from GVHD mice on different days after GVHD induction and plasma corticosterone levels were measured using a radioimmunoassay. Our results showed that plasma corticosterone levels were elevated in GVHD mice as early as 9 days after GVH induction and persisted as the disease progressed to day 21, whereas the corticosterone levels in control syngeneic mice returned to normal after day 9 (Table 4). Other investigators have reported a similar increase in circulating corticosterone during GVHD (57,58).

The mechanism(s) mediating the secretion of glucocorticoids (i.e., corticoste-

Table 4 Plasma Corticosterone Levels on Different Days After GVHD Induction[a,b,c]

Experimental Group	Plasma Corticosterone Levels (ng/ml mean ± SE)		
	Day 9	Day 16	Day 24
SYN	235.0 ± 47.8	83.4 ± 6.4	88.3 ± 17.5
GVHD	190.0 ± 15.8	141.0 ± 28.5	213.6 ± 37.6

[a]A minumum of 5 mice per group was used.
[b]SYN groups are B6AF1 mice injected with B6AF1 splenic and lymph node cells.
[c]GVHD groups are B6AF1 mice injected with 30 × 10^6 A strain parental splenic and lymph node cells.

rone) in GVHD mice is unknown. We speculate that LPS translocating across the injured gut during GVHD (26) may be involved in the persistent secretion of glucocorticoids into the blood. LPS causes Mϕ to secrete inflammatory cytokines such as IL-1, IL-6, and TNF-α (53). Increasing evidence shows that circulating IL-1 secreted from LPS-activated Mϕ activates the HPA axis by stimulating the hypothalamus to release corticotropin-releasing hormone, which acts on the pituitary to secrete ACTH and, in turn, triggers the secretion of adrenal glucocorticoids (54–62). The activation of the HPA axis in LPS-treated mice is abrogated with an antibody against the IL-1 receptor (59,60), strongly supporting the role of IL-1 as a primary candidate for triggering the HPA axis. The other inflammatory cytokines, TNF-α and IL-6, do not appear to induce glucocorticoid secretion, since antibody against TNF-α injected into LPS-treated mice failed to block the increase in blood glucocorticoid levels (63,64), and glucocorticoid secretion was not attentuated in IL-6–deficient mice treated with LPS (65). It could be argued that lymphokines secreted from T cells activated with IL-1 stimulate the HPA axis. However, this is not the case, since the injection of rIL-1 in nude mice caused an increase in glucocorticoid level similar in magnitude to those in euthymic mice (61), suggesting that T-cell lymphokines have no effect on glucocorticoid secretion. This is further supported by the observations that injection of either rIL-2 or rIFN-γ into normal mice or rats fails to increase glucocorticoids in the circulation (61). Based on these studies and the detection of LPS in the circulation of GVHD mice, we propose that IL-1 secreted by LPS-activated Mϕ in GVHD mice stimulates the HPA axis. In fact, IL-1 transcripts were increased several hundredfold in GVHD target organs for up to 4 weeks after disease induction (66). Moreover, IL-1 secretion from LPS-activated splenic Mϕ of GVHD mice was 100-fold greater than LPS-activated control splenic Mϕ (67).

Our preliminary data also suggest that glucocorticoid secretion in GVHD mice may also be independent of the hypothalamic-pituitary axis (K. E. You-Ten, manuscript in preparation). This raises the possibility that the persistent elevation of plasma glucocorticoids during GVHD may result from direct stimulation of the adrenal glands by IL-1. In support of this proposal are reports showing that IL-1 can directly stimulate the adrenal glands to secrete glucocorticoids, independent of the hypotalamic-pituitary axis (68,69). We propose, therefore, that LPS translocation across the damaged gastrointestinal epithelium of GVHD mice enters the circulation and activates Mϕ to secrete inflammatory cytokines. The prolonged secretion of IL-1 during GVHD can trigger the HPA axis or directly stimulate the adrenal glands, resulting in a persistent increase of glucocorticoids in the circulation of GVHD mice. Thus, the entry of LPS into the circulatory system during GVHD results in elevated glucocorticoid levels.

Glucocorticoids exert a well-documented anti-inflammatory effect, in part via suppression of monocyte and T-cell interleukin secretion (70,71). In addition, glucocorticoids produce a complete suppression of T-cell proliferation in vitro in response to mitogens and TCR ligation (72), suggesting that the elevated levels of circulating glucocorticoids observed during the GVHD may contribute to the GVHD-induced T-cell suppression.

B. T-Cell Immunosuppression

One of the hallmarks of GVHD is a profound suppression of T-cell function as early as 1 week after GVHD induction (23,50). Several mechanisms have been implicated in T-cell suppression, including thymic injury (23,50,73), activation of suppressor cells (74), and production of prostaglandins (75), IFN-γ (76), and NO (48).

GVHD T cells do not proliferate, nor do they produce detectable levels of cytokines, in response to a variety of powerful activation stimuli. Mitogens including concanavalin A and phytohemagglutinin (PHA), a combination of PHA and phorbol myristic acetate (PMA), anti-CD3 antibodies, either alone or in combination with IL-2 or IL-4, and allogeneic cells (77–79) all fail to stimulate T cells from GVHD immunosuppressed mice. In vivo, GVHD T cells are unable to generate self-restricted responses to antigens, and fail to provide help to B cells for Ig production, and to cytotoxic cell precursors for CTL priming (80–83). These T-cell functional defects can be demonstrated in purified $CD4^+$ and $CD8^+$ lymphocyte populations isolated from the spleens of GVHD mice (77), even when cocultured with antigen-presenting cells from normal (non-GVHD) animals (77,78). This complete unresponsiveness is not transferable to cocultured cells, indicating an intrinsic defect in T-cell responsiveness. The T-cell unresponsiveness may involve a defect in TCR-mediated signaling, since T cells from GVHD mice (77) and bone-marrow transplanted patients (84) cannot generate or sustain a normal calcium flux in response to TCR ligation (77,85), although they do respond when treated with ionomycin and PMA. On the other hand, the unresponsive cells express normal cell-surface levels of the TCR and its associated signaling complex (CD3), of the CD4 or CD8 coreceptors, and of the IL-2 receptor (77). This spectrum of dysfunction suggests that the molecular lesion underlying GVHD-induced T-cell unresponsiveness may be a defect upstream of PKC activation in the TCR-mediated signaling pathway.

C. Glucocorticoid-Induced Defects in T-Cell Signaling

We have investigated the molecular basis of the GVHD-induced T-cell signaling defect and the role of glucocorticoids in this defect. Our results demonstrate that p56lck and p59fyn are selectively downregulated in purified spleen and lymph node T cells during GVHD (Fig. 1). p59fyn and p56lck are src family protein tyrosine kinases (PTKs) implicated in early signaling for T-cell activation (86,87). Alternatively spliced variants of fyn are expressed in the brain and in lymphoid tissue

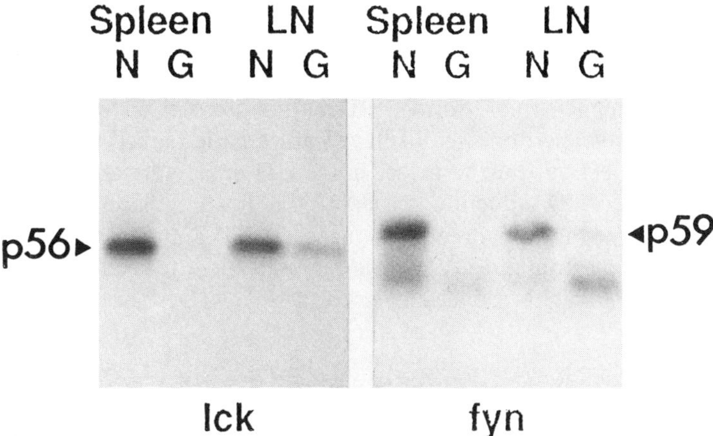

Figure 1 p56^{lck} and p59^{fyn} were downregulated in the T cells of GVHD mice. Lck and fyn immunoblots of T-cell lysates from normal (N) and GVHD (G) mice were prepared from the spleen and lymph nodes (LN) 23 days after GVHD induction. GVHD was induced with 60×10^6 B6 donor cells. T cells from GVHD mice were purified by removing B cells and macrophages from the cell suspensions prepared from spleen and LNs, then T cells were lysed in 1% NP-40 buffer, and 100 μg proteins/lane were resolved by 8% SDS-PAGE and immunoblotted with anti-lck and anti-fyn antisera, generously provided by André Veillette.

(88,89); the lymphoid form is found noncovalently associated with the ε, γ, ζ, and η, chains of the CD3/TCR complex (90), and its activity increases transiently upon TCR stimulation (91). Overexpression of fyn in hybridomas results in increased antigen-induced IL-2 expression (89); in transgenic mice, it produces thymocyte hyperresponsiveness to TCR stimulation (92). Conversely, in fyn-knockout mice and transgenics with kinase-deficient mutant fyn, T-cell activation thresholds, especially in immature cells, are elevated (93,94). Thus, fyn seems to modulate and amplify TCR-mediated signals. Lck is associated with CD4 and CD8 (95,96) and with the IL-2 receptor (97). Lck may be involved in T-cell activation by the early phosphorylation of the TCR-associated signal transduction molecules, notably CD3ζ, upon cross-linking of the TCR with CD4 or CD8 (98). Mutant cell lines lacking expression of lck resemble GVHD-anergized T cells: they are unable to signal through the TCR and fail to induce intracellular calcium mobilization, although they retain the ability to proliferate in response to PMA and ionomycin (99). Thus, the disappearance of T-cell lck and fyn during GVHD may cause an interruption in the TCR-initiated, tyrosine kinase–mediated signaling cascade, resulting in defective T-cell activation.

A marked decrease in T-cell lck and fyn was consistently observed 10 to 15 days after acute GVHD induction, and the reduction was exacerbated progressively over the course of the disease. During chronic GVHD, lck and fyn remained downregulated. The reduction in these PTKs, then, may account for the long-term signaling defect of the GVHD T cells.

Since high levels of glucocorticoids can completely suppress T-cell proliferation in response to TCR-mediated signaling (72) and T cells are refractory to mitogenic signals during GVHD (23,77), when endogenous glucocorticoids are sustained at abnormally high levels [Table 4, (57,58)], we investigated the role of glucocorticoids in the GVHD-induced signaling defect. We have found that the GVHD-induced reduction in lck and fyn could be replicated in normal mice by the injection of exogenous cortisone. Normal (non-GVHD) adrenalectomized animals treated with 2.5 mg cortisone intraperitoneally displayed a dramatic reduction in T-cell lck and fyn 48 hr after injection. Furthermore, in GVHD mice, adrenalectomy performed 10 days prior to GVHD induction prevented the downregulation of T cell lck and fyn that we observed in nonadrenalectomized GVHD animals. Cortisone administered to the adrenalectomized GVH mice reversed the effect of the adrenalectomy and resulted again in highly reduced levels of the PTKs (Desbarats et al., manuscript submitted).

The role of glucocorticoids in the modulation of T-cell signaling may explain the observation first reported more than 30 years ago that adrenalectomy can either exacerbate or alleviate GVHD, depending on the severity of the disease (55,100,101). Adrenalectomized mice experienced higher mortality during acute GVHD induced with high cell doses than did nonadrenalectomized controls (55,100). As discussed, death from acute GVHD results from cytokine-induced septic shock (26), and the lack of adrenal glucocorticoids to negatively regulate cytokine production results in higher mortality. This is analogous to the acute death induced in adrenalectomized mice by oligoclonal T-cell stimuli (such as anti-CD3 antibody or bacterial superantigen), which would not be lethal in animals with an intact HPA axis (102). Paradoxically, in GVHD induced with lower cell doses, adrenalectomized mice experienced a less severe reaction and recovered more fully and earlier than their nonadrenalectomized counterparts (101). These adrenalectomized mice do not undergo glucocorticoid-induced PTK downregulation; thus—despite transient T-cell immunosuppression probably mediated by prostaglandins (75), IFN-γ (76), and NO (48)—they escaped the profound long-term immunosuppression that precludes a rapid recovery. The recovery of immune function in adrenalectomized mice occurs early (Ref. 101 and K. E. You-Ten et al., manuscript in preparation); non-adrenalectomized animals, on the other hand, remain profoundly immunosuppressed for months or years (23,50). Thus, in animals with an intact HPA axis, a T-cell signaling defect consisting of an interruption of the TCR signaling cascade at the level of tyrosine phosphorylation is induced by glucocorticoids and may result in severe, long-term peripheral T-cell unresponsiveness.

IV. ENDOTOXIN AND CYTOKINE PRODUCTION DURING ACUTE GVHD

A. IFN-γ in Target Organs

T cells are severely compromised during acute GVHD, as discussed above, yet Mϕ from GVHD mice display IFN-γ primed characteristics throughout the disease, including an acute sensitivity to LPS, which leads to the production of high levels of IFN-γ and NO (26) (Table 1). For tissue Mϕ to sustain an IFN-γ–primed state and produce TNF-α and NO at target sites, there must be a persistent source of IFN-γ (103), and since INF-γ has a short half-life (103), it must be continuously produced to maintain Mϕ priming.

We investigated whether IFN-γ was produced locally in GVHD target organs.

In this study we examined thymus, lung and salivary gland in which we had previously reported a cellular infiltrate and significant histopathological injury (50,56). As seen in Fig. 2, IFN-γ mRNA was present consistently in the thymus, lung, and salivary gland of acute GVHD mice on day 14. Concomitant with IFN-γ mRNA, inducible nitric oxide synthase (iNOS) mRNA was also detected in these organs, providing evidence for the translation of IFN-γ mRNA into bioactive protein, since the transcription of Mφ and endothelial iNOS is dependent on IFN-γ (104). These data suggest that IFN-γ is produced in many target organs during acute GVHD at the time when T cells are immunosuppressed (Kichian et al., manuscript in preparation).

B. Role of IL-12 in Maintaining Macrophage Priming

Having established that IFN-γ is present in many GVHD target organs on day 14, the critical question that we addressed was the source of the IFN-γ, since T cells are immunosuppressed. Besides T cells, NK cells can also be induced to produce IFN-γ either by IL-2 stimulation or IL-12 in the presence of TNF-α (19). However, T-cell function and production of IL-2 are completely suppressed by day 7 in GVHD mice (105) and therefore would not be expected to play a role in inducing IFN-γ production after the first week of GVHD. On the other hand, Mφ activated with LPS can secrete IL-12, which, in turn, induces NK cells to produce IFN-γ (19). Since NK-cell activity is increased during GVHD in various target organs—including thymus, salivary gland, and lung—at a time when T-cell functions are suppressed (50) and LPS was detected in the serum of acute GVHD mice on day 14 (26) (Table 3), we

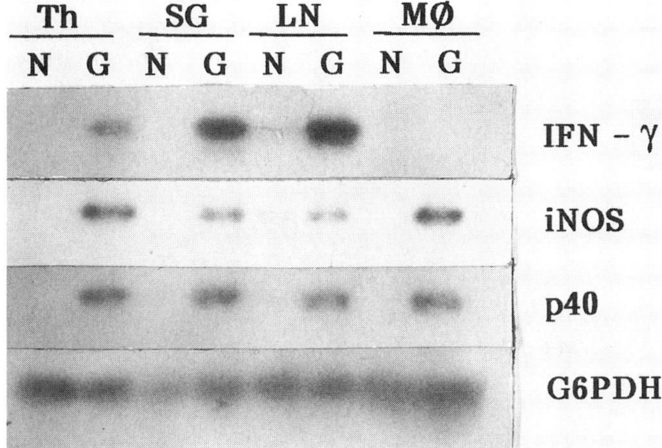

Figure 2 Reverse transcription–polymerase chain reaction (RT-PCR) analysis of IFN-γ iNOS, and p40 mRNA in normal (N) B6AF1 and acute GVHD (G) day 14 target organs. 1-μg samples of total RNA extracted from thymus (Th), submaxillary salivary gland (SG), lung (LN) and purified peritoneal macrophages (MΦ) were reverse transcribed with Moloney murine leukemia virus reverse transcriptase and amplified with *Taq* DNA polymerase. Southern transfers of PCR products were subsequently probed with internal specific oligonucleotides. Data are representative of three experiments. Glucose 6-phosphate dehydrogenase (G6PDH) is the control mRNA.

examined whether IL-12 is produced during the immunosuppressive stages of acute GVHD.

IL-12 is reported to be necessary for the production of IFN-γ by purified NK cells (106) and is shown to induce NK cells to produce IFN-γ in SCID mice (107). LPS induces the expression of the IL-12 p40 peptide in Mϕ which, in the presence of the constitutively expressed p35 subunit, forms the heterodimeric bioactive IL-12 molecule (108). The expression of IL-12 p40 in normal tissue is restricted to lymphoid organs, while p35 has been detected in both lymphoid and nonlymphoid tissue (108). Thus the expression of p40 in thymus, lung, and salivary glands of acute GVHD mice was studied, as we reasoned that Mϕ infiltrating these target sites should express p40 mRNA if they were activated by LPS.

As shown in Fig. 2, p40 mRNA was detected in the thymus, salivary gland, and lung of GVHD mice on day 14 as well as in purified peritoneal Mϕ. In normal mice, p40 mRNA was not detected in any of these organs or in peritoneal Mϕ. The fact that p40 expression coincides with that of IFN-γ in GVHD target tissues supports our claim that IL-12 mediates IFN-γ production by NK cells. In addition, IFN-γ has been shown to potentiate the production of IL-12 by Mϕ already exposed to LPS (107). Therefore, there appears to be a positive feedback interaction between tissue NK cells and Mϕ leading to the production of high levels of IFN-γ at GVHD target sites.

It is of interest to note that IFN-γ mRNA appears early on day 7 in acute GVHD target sites in the absence of p40 expression. In the first week of acute GVHD, T cells are activated, but they are rapidly suppressed thereafter (23). Our results would thus suggest a biphasic mode of IFN-γ production during GVHD: an early phase mediated by activated T cells and/or IL-2 activated NK cells, and a larger phase mediated by LPS through IL-12 activated NK cells. It is the latter LPS-induced IL-12 mediated IFN-γ production that seems to be critical for maintaining Mϕ priming. This later phase of IFN-γ production may be responsible for the release of pathological amounts of TNF-α and NO by tissue Mϕ in the presence of normally nonpathological amounts of LPS (Kichian et al., manuscript in preparation).

V. DISCUSSION

Based on our results, we propose the model illustrated in Fig. 3, which outlines the role of LPS in the pathological events and immunosuppression observed during acute GVHD. Several events contribute to the development of acute GVHD in this model. The initial afferent phase, which occurs during the lymphoproliferative response to alloantigen involves the excessive production of cytokines, including IFN-γ produced by CD4$^+$, CD8$^+$, and/or NK cells. As a result of the interaction with released cytokines, NK or NK-like cells are activated and priming of Mϕ occurs. The next phase involves an initial injury to epithelial tissues, including the epithelium of the gastrointestinal tract, which we suggest is mediated by activated NK or NK-like cells. Following the initial tissue injury, especially to the gut epithelium, increasing amounts of gram-negative bacteria enter the portal circulation and are rapidly taken up and killed by fixed Mϕ in the liver (i.e., Kupffer cells) and splenic Mϕ. LPS derived from the killed gram-negative bacteria then triggers the release of pathophysiological amounts of TNF-α and NO from primed Mϕ, result-

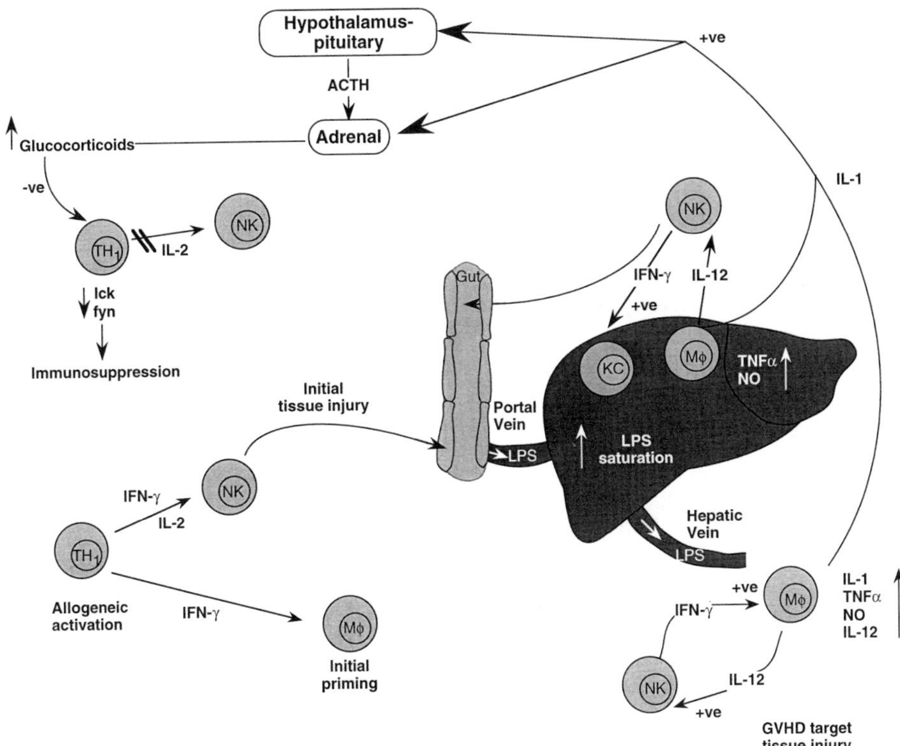

Figure 3 Model outlining the role of endotoxin in the pathogenesis of acute GVHD. T cells are alloactivated and release IFN-γ and IL-2, which activates NK or NK-like cells. IFN-γ also causes initial priming of macrophages (MΦ). The activated NK cells and/or T cells injure the epithelium of the gut, resulting in a translocation of gram-negative organisms and/or endotoxin/LPS into the portal system. The increased LPS level in the liver stimulates primed Kupffer cells (Kc) and MΦ to produce IL-1, TNF-α and NO. IL-1 stimulates the hypothalamus-pituitary-adrenal axis to produce a persistent elevation of glucocorticoids, which acts on T cells to downregulate two important tyrosine kinases, lck and fyn, leading to T-cell immunosuppression. As LPS entry continues, the liver becomes saturated and LPS begins to spill over into the systemic circulation. LPS stimulates MΦ in GVH target tissue to produce IL-12, which, in turn, activates additional NK or NK-like cells, resulting in increased IFNγ synthesis by NK cells. NK cell–derived IFN-γ maintains a strong priming signal for Kc and MΦ. Primed MΦ triggered by LPS release pathological amounts of TNF-α and NO, resulting in the symptoms characteristic of acute GVHD.

ing in cachexia, further tissue injury, shock, and death of the transplant recipient. In addition, IFN-γ production switches from T cells to NK cells as a result of LPS induction of IL-12 synthesis by Mϕ. IL-12 is a potent stimulator of IFN-γ production by NK cells. This pathway functions in a positive feedback loop to maintain a high persistent synthesis of IFN-γ throughout the body and thus maintains Mϕ priming. LPS also indirectly suppresses T-cell activity by downregulating two T-cell tyrosine kinases, lck and fyn. LPS induces IL-1 production which stimulates glucocorticoid synthesis via the HPA axis, which, in turn, may downregulate lck and fyn expression. In summary, LPS can directly or indirectly activate several different cells and cytokines that contribute to the pathological symptoms characteristic of acute GVHD.

It is quite possible that a similar mechanism operates in human bone marrow transplant patients. Some of the clinical symptoms of acute GVHD that are observed in bone marrow transplant recipients can be difficult to distinguish from the effects of the pretransplant radiation conditioning. In the parent-into-F1 experimental model, pretransplant irradiation is unnecessary, since the F1 recipient cannot reject the transplanted parental-strain cells. The mechanism and effects of Mϕ activation that we have characterized in the nonirradiated model of acute GVHD and which are due strictly to the direct or indirect effects of the transplanted cells are particularly relevant to the development of GVHD in irradiated recipients. Among the many effects of tissue irradiation are several important observations related to Mϕ activation. Whole body irradiation results in an increase in Mϕ phagocytic activity (109) and induces expression of Mϕ cytotoxic function (110). Irradiation of the abdomen prior to IV. injection of metastatic tumor cells leads to a reduction in the number of lung metastases, and the effect can be prevented by shielding or removal of the cecum prior to irradiation (111). The induction of the antimetastatic effect of irradiation cannot be elicited in germ-free animals and is reduced with antibiotic therapy, suggesting that transmigration of enteric bacteria across the damaged epithelium of the cecum results in an IFNusion of endotoxin (111). A perhaps equally important observation is that irradiation of Mϕ in vitro causes short term priming as demonstrated by the expression of cytotoxic activity following LPS triggering of the cells (112). TNF-α mRNA and TNF-α production can be induced by irradiation (113). A case report on four bone marrow transplant recipients describes an unusual localization of severe cutaneous lesions localized to fields of prior irradiation (114). In the murine model, we have also shown that irradiation exacerbates cutaneous histological injury (115). The implication of these findings is that radiation therapy as a preconditioning treatment for bone marrow transplantation can itself contribute to the onset of GVHD in the recipient in the model that we outlined above (Fig. 3).

The experimental and clinical results supporting our conclusion that IFN-γ and LPS-induced Mϕ activation leads to the expression of effector mechanisms mediating the development of acute GVHD include the following: prevention of GVHD-related intestinal pathological lesions by treatment with anti-IFN-γ (38); the prevention of pathological lesions and immunosuppression by elimination of NK or NK-like cells (50,116); reduction in the incidence or prevention of acute GVHD and reduction of tissue injury through bacterial decontamination of the intestinal microflora or through the use of germ-free conditions (28–32); reduction in mortality by treatment with an antiserum to lipid A, the common structure found in all bacteria-derived LPS (117); prevention of early enteropathy in experimental GVHD by NMMA (47); prevention of skin and gut pathological lesions and a reduction in mortality by pretreatment with anti-TNF-α (43); reduction in severity of established lesions by anti-TNF-α therapy (44).

It is of interest to note that gut injury and endotoxin entry was implicated in the etiology of wasting disease over 20 years ago (118); however, the mechanism was not elucidated and this observation was not pursued further until recently (26). We believe that endotoxin and the events described in our model are important if not essential for the development of acute GVHD. If we are correct it opens several avenues for the diagnosis, prevention, and/or treatment of acute GVHD that have hitherto not been tested.

ACKNOWLEDGMENTS

This work was supported by grants from the Medical Research Council of Canada (MRC) and the National Cancer Institute of Canada. Julie Desbarats was a recipient of an MRC Studentship and Kursteen Price was the recipient of a studentship award from the Fonds pour la Formation de Chercheurs et l'Aide à la Recherche du Quebec. We thank Drs. André Veillette and Riaz Farookhi for assistance in the tyrosine kinase studies. We thank Ailsa Lee Loy and Rosmarie Siegrist-Johnstone for their careful technical assistance and Christine Pamplin for typing the manuscript.

REFERENCES

1. Mannel DN, Moore RN, Mergenhagen SE. Macrophages as a source of tumoricidal activity (tumor necrotizing factor). Infect Immun 1980; 30:523–530.
2. Stuehr DJ, Nathan CF. Nitric Oxide: A macrophage product responsible for cytostasis and respiratory inhibition in tumor target cells. J Exp Med 1989; 169:1543–1555.
3. Hibbs JB Jr, Taintor RR, Vavrin Z, Rachlin EM. Nitric oxide: A cytotoxic activated macrophage effector molecule. Biochem Biophys Res Commun 1988; 157:87–94.
4. Cerami A, Ikeda Y, Le Trang N, et al. Weight loss associated with an endotoxin-induced mediator from peritoneal macrophages: The role of cachectin (tumor necrosis factor). Immunol Lett 1985; 11:173–177.
5. Torti FM, Dieckmann B, Beutler B, et al. A macrophage product inhibits adipocyte gene expression: An in vitro model of cachexia. Science (Washington DC). 1985; 229: 867–869.
6. Beutler B, Mahoney J, Le Trag N, et al. Purification of cachectin a lipoprotein lipase-suppressing hormone secreted by endotoxin-induced RAW 264.7 cells. J Exp Med 1985; 161:984–995.
7. Beutler BA, Milsark IW, Cerami AC. Passive immunization against cachectin/tumor necrosis factor protects mice from lethal effect of endotoxin. Science 1985; 229:869–871.
8. Kilbourn RG, Gross SG, Jubran A, et al. N^{G}-methyl-L-arginine inhibits tumor necrosis factor-induced hypotension: Implications for the involvement of nitric oxide. Proc Natl Acad Sci USA 1990; 87:3629–3632.
9. Kilbourn RG, Jubran A, Gross SG, et al. Reversal of endotoxin-mediated shock by N^{G}-methyl-L-arginine, an inhibitor of nitric oxide synthesis. Biochem Biophys Res Commun 1990; 172:1132–1138.
10. Macmicking JD, Willenborg DO, Weidemann MJ, et al. Elevated secretion of reactive nitrogen and oxygen intermediates by inflammatory leukocytes in hyperacute experimental autoimmune encephalomyelitis—Enhancement by the soluble products of encephalitogenic T-cells. J Exp Med 1992; 176:303–307.
11. Dawson VL, Dawson TM, London ED, et al. Nitric oxide mediates glutamate neurotoxicity in primary cortical cultures. Proc Natl Acad Sci USA 1991; 88:6368–6371.
12. Kroncke KD, Rodriguez ML, Kolb H, Kolbbachofen V. Cytotoxicity of activated rat macrophages against syngeneic islet cells is arginine-dependent, correlates with citrulline and nitrite concentrations and is identical to lysis by the nitric oxide donor nitroprusside. Diabetologia 1993; 36:17–24.
13. Lopezbelmonte J, Whittle BJR, Moncada S. The actions of nitric oxide donors in the

prevention or induction of injury to the rat gastric mucosa. Br J Pharmacol 1993; 108: 73–78.

14. Pace JL, Russell SW, Torres BA, et al. Recombinant mouse γ interferon induces the priming step in macrophage activation for tumor cell killing. J Immunol 1983; 130: 2011–2013.
15. Gifford GE, Lohmann-Matthes M-L. Gamma interferon priming of mouse and human macrophages for induction of tumor necrosis factor production by bacterial lipopolysaccharide. J Natl Cancer Inst 1987; 78:121–124.
16. Beutler B, Tkacenko V, Milsark I, et al. Effect of γ-interferon on cachectin expression by mononuclear phagocytes: Reversal of the LPS^d (endotoxin resistance) phenotype. J Exp Med 1986, 164:1791–1796.
17. Ding AH, Nathan CF, Stuehr DJ. Release of reactive nitrogen intermediates and reactive oxygen intermediates from mouse peritoneal macrophages: Comparison of activating cytokines and evidence for independent production. J Immunol 1988; 141: 2407–2412.
18. Pace JL, Russell SW, Leblanc PA, Murasko DM. Comparative effects of various classes of mouse interferons on macrophage activation for tumor cell killing. J Immunol 1985; 134:977–981.
19. Brunda MJ. Interleukin-12. J Leuk Biol 1994; 55:280–288.
20. Hume DA, Robinson AP, MacPherson GG, Gordon S. The mononuclear phagocyte system of the mouse defined by immunohistochemical localization of antigen F4/80: Relationship between macrophages, Langerhans cells, reticular cells, and dendritic cells in lymphoid and hematopoeitic organs. J Exp Med 1983; 158:1522–1538.
21. Lee S-H, Starkey PM, Gordon S. Quantitative analysis of total macrophage content in adult mouse tissues: Immunocytochemical studies with monoclonal antibody F4/80. J Exp Med 1985; 161:475–489.
22. Wright SD, Ramos RA, Tobias PS, et al. CD14 a receptor for complexes of lipopolysaccharide (LPS) and LPS binding protein. Science 1990; 249:1431–1433.
23. Lapp WS, Ghayur T, Mendes M, et al. The functional and histological basis for graft-versus-host-induced immunosuppression. Immunol Rev 1985; 88:107–133.
24. Howard JG. Changes in the activity of the reticulo-endothelial system (RES) following the injection of parental spleen cells into F1 hybrid mice. Br J Exp Pathol 1961; 42:72–76.
25. Cooper GN, Howard JG. An effect of the graft-versus-host reaction on resistance to experimental bacteraemia. Br J Exp Pathol 1961; 42:588–591.
26. Nestel FP, Price KS, Seemayer TA, Lapp WS. Macrophage priming and lipopolysaccharide-triggered release of tumor necrosis factor-alpha during graft-versus-host disease. J Exp Med 1992; 175:405–413.
27. Nestel FP, Casson PR, Wiltrout RH, Kerbel RS. Alterations in sensitivity to nonspecific cell-mediated lysis associated with tumor progression: Characterization of activated macrophage and natural killer cell resistant tumor variants. J Natl Cancer Inst 1984; 73:483–491.
28. Van Bekkum DW, Roodenburg J, Heidt PJ, van der Waaij D. Mitigation of secondary disease of allogeneic mouse radiation chimeras by modification of the intestinal microflora. J Natl Cancer Inst 1974; 52:401–404.
29. Jones JW, Wilson R, Bealmear PM. Mortality and gross pathology of secondary disease in germfree mouse radiation chimeras. Radiat Res 1971; 45:577–588.
30. Van Bekkum DW, Knaan S. Role of bacterial microflora in development of intestinal lesions from graft-versus-host reaction. J Natl Cancer Inst 1977; 58:787–789.
31. Beelen DW, Haralambie E, Brandt H, et al. Evidence that sustained growth suppression of intestinal anaerobic bacteria reduces the risk of acute graft-versus-host disease after sibling marrow transplant. Blood 1992; 80:2668–2676.

32. Vossen JM, Heidt PJ, Van Den Berg H, et al. Prevention of infection and graft-versus-host disease by suppression of intestinal microflora in children treated with allogeneic bone marrow transplantation. Eur J Clin Microbiol IFNect Dis 1990; 1:14–23.
33. Storb R, Prentice RL, Buckner DC, et al. Graft-versus-host disease and survival in patients with aplastic anaemia treated by marrow grafts from HLA-identical siblings: Beneficial effect of a protective environment. N Engl J Med 1983; 308:302–307.
34. Niederwieser D, Herold M, Woloszczuk W, et al. Endogenous IFN-gamma during human bone marrow transplantation: Analysis of serum levels of interferon and interferon-dependent secondary messages. Transplantation 1990; 50:620–625.
35. Leist TP, Heuchel R, Zinkernagel RM. Increased bactericidal macrophage activity induced by immunological stimuli is dependent on interferon (IFN)-γ: Interference of anti-IFN-γ but not anti-IFN-α/β with modulation of macrophage activity caused by lymphocytic choriomeningitis infection or systemic graft-vs-host reactions. Eur J Immunol 1988; 18:1295.
36. Troutt AB, Kelso A. Enumeration of lymphokine mRNA-containing cells in vivo in a murine graft-versus-host reaction using the PCR. Proc Natl Acad Sci USA 1992; 89: 5276–5280.
38. Mowat AM. Antibodies to IFN-γ prevent immunologically mediated intestinal damage in murine graft-versus-host reaction. Immunology 1989; 68:18–23.
39. Velardi A, Varese P, Terenzi A, et al. Lymphokine production by T-cell clones after human bone marrow transplantation. Blood 1989; 74:1665–1672.
40. Howard JG. Increased sensitivity to bacterial endotoxin of F1 hybrid mice undergoing graft-versus-host reaction. Nature 1961; 190:1122–1126.
41. Tracey KJ, Wei H, Manogue KR, et al. Cachectin/tumor necrosis factor induces cachexia, anaemia and inflammation. J Exp Med 1988; 167:1211–1227.
42. Cheng J, Turksen K, Yu Q-C, et al. Cachexia and graft-vs-host-disease-type skin changes in keratin promoter-driven TNF-α transgenic mice. Genes Dev 1992; 6:1444–1456.
43. Piguet P-F, Grau GE, Allet B, Vassalli P. Tumor necrosis factor/cachectin is an effector of skin and gut lesions of the acute phase of graft-vs-host disease. J Exp Med 1987; 166:1280–1289.
44. Herve P, Flesch M, Tiberghien P, et al. Phase-I-II trial of a monoclonal anti-tumor necrosis factor-alpha antibody for the treatment of refractory severe acute graft-versus-host disease. Blood 1992; 79:3362–3368.
45. Hirokawa M, Takatsu H, Niitsu H, et al. Serum tumor necrosis factor-α levels in allogeneic bone marrow transplant recipients with acute leukemia. Tohoku J Exp Med 1989; 159:237–244.
46. Holler E, Kolb H, Moller A, et al. Increased serum levels of tumor necrosis factor α precede major complications of bone marrow transplantation. Blood 1990; 75:1011–1106.
47. Langrehr JM, Murase N, Markus PM, et al. Nitric oxide production in host-versus-graft and graft-versus-host reactions in the rat. J Clin Invest 1992; 90:679–683.
48. Hoffman RA, Langrehr JM, Wren SM, et al. Characterization of the immunosuppressive effects of nitric oxide in graft vs host disease. J Immunol 1993; 151:1508–1518.
49. Garside P, Hutton AK, Severn A, et al. Nitric oxide mediates intestinal pathology in graft-vs-host disease. Eur J Immunol 1992; 22:2141.
50. Ghayur T, Seemayer TA, Lapp WS. Histologic correlates of immune functional deficits in graft-versus-host disease. In: Burakoff SJ, Deeg HJ, Ferrara J, Atkinson K, eds. Graft-Versus-Host Disease: New York: Marcel Dekker, 1990; 109–132.
51. McDonald GC, Gartner JG. Prevention of acute lethal graft-versus-host disease in F1 hybrid mice by pretreatment of the graft with anti-NK-1.1 and complement. Transplantation 1992; 54:147–151.

52. Read TE, Harris HW, Grunfield C, et al. Chylomicrons enhance endotoxin excretion in bile. Infect Immun 1993; 61:3495–3502.
53. Tilders FJH, DeRijk RH, Van Dam A-M, et al. Activation of the hypothalamus-pituitary-adrenal axis by bacterial endotoxins: Routes and intermediate signals. Psychoneuroendocrinology 1994; 19:209–232.
54. Bateman A, Singh A, Kral T, Solomon S. The immune-hypothalamic-pituitary-adrenal axis. Endocr Rev 1989; 10:92–112.
55. Heim LR, Martinez CR, Good RA. Cause of homologous disease. Nature 1967; 214: 26–29.
56. Seemayer TA, Lapp WS, Bolande RP. Thymic epithelial injury in graft-versus-host reactions following adrenalectomy. Am J Pathol 1978; 93:325–332.
57. Khairallah M, Spach C, Maitre F, Motta R. Endocrine involvement in minor (non-H-2) graft versus host reaction in mice: Dissociated effect on corticosterone and aldosterone plasma levels. Endocrinology 1988; 123:1949–1954.
58. Hoot GP, Head JR, Griffin ST. Increased free plasma corticosterone and adrenal hyperactivity associated with graft-versus-host disease. Transplantation 1983; 35:478–483.
59. Rivier C, Chizzonite R, Vale W. In the mouse, the activation of the hypothalamic-pituitary-adrenal axis by a lipopolysaccharide (endotoxin) is mediated through interleukin-1. Endocrinology 1989; 125:2800–2805.
60. Schotanus K, Berkenbosch F, Tilders FJH. Human recombinant interleukin-1 receptor antagonist prevents ACTH but not interleukin-6 responses to low doses of bacterial endotoxin in rats. Endocrinology 1993; 33:2461–2468.
61. Besedovsky HO, Del Rey A, Sokin E, Dinarello CA. Immunoregulatory feedback between interleukin-1 and glucocorticoid hormones. Science 1986; 233:652–654.
62. Sapolsky R, Rivier C, Yamamoto G, et al. Interleukin-1 stimulates the secretion of hypothalamic corticotropin-releasing factor. Science 1987; 238:522–524.
63. Dunn AJ. The role of interleukin-1 and tumor necrosis factor in the neurochemical and neuroendocrine responses to endotoxin. Brain Res Bull 1992; 29:807–812.
64. Perlstein RS, Whitnall MH, Abrams JS, et al. Synergistic roles of interleukin-6, interleukin-1 and tumor necrosis factor in the adrenocorticotropin response to bacterial lipopolysaccharide in vivo. Endocrinology 1993; 132:946–952.
65. Fattori E, Cappelletti M, Costa P, et al. Defective inflammatory response in interleukin-6 deficient mice. J Exp Med 1994; 180:1243–1250.
66. Abhyankar S, Gilliland DG, Ferrara JL. Interleukin-1 is a critical effector molecule during cytokine dysregulation in graft versus disease to minor histocompatibility antigens. Transplantation 1993; 56:1518–1523.
67. Smith SR, Terminelli C, Kenworthy-Bott L, Phillips DL. A study of cytokine production in acute graft-vs-host disease. Cell Immunol 1991; 134:336–348.
68. Winter JSD, Cow KW, Perry YS, Greenberg AH. A stimulatory effect of interleukin-1 on adrenocortical cortisol secretion mediated by prostaglandins. Endocrinology 1990; 127:1904–1909.
69. Roh MS, Drazenovich KA, Barbose JJ, et al. Direct stimulation of the adrenal cortex by interleukin-1. Surgery 1987; 102:140–146.
70. Almawi WY, Sewell KL, Hadro ET, et al. Mode of action of the glucocorticosteroids as immunosuppressive agents. Prog Leukocyte Biol 1990; 10A:321.
71. Daynes RA, Araneo BA. Contrasting effects of glucocorticoids on the capacity of T cells to produce the growth factors interleukin-2 and interleukin-4. Eur J Immunol 1989; 19:2319–2325.
72. Nijhuis EWP, Hinloopen B, Odding J, Nagelkerken L. Abrogation of the suppressive effects of dexamethasone by PKC activation or CD28 triggering. Cell Immunol 1994; 156:438–447.

73. Kornbluth M, You-Ten E, Desbarats J, et al. T cell subsets in the thymus of graft-versus-host immunosuppressed mice. Transplantation 1991; 51:262–267.
74. Parthenais E, Lapp WS: Evidence for two types of nonspecific suppressor cells activated by the graft-versus-host reaction in mice. Scand J Immunol 1978; 7:215–220.
75. Lapp WS, Mendes M, Kirchner H, Gemsa D. Prostaglandin synthesis by lymphoid tissue of mice experiencing a graft-versus-host reaction: Relationship to immunosuppression. Cellular Immunology 1980; 50:271–281.
76. Holda JH, Maier T, Claman HN. Evidence that IFN-γ is responsible for natural suppressor activity in GVHD spleen and normal bone marrow. Transplantation 1988; 45:772.
77. Levy RB, Jones M, Cray C. Isolated peripheral T cells from GvHR recipients exhibit defective IL-2R expression, IL-2 production, and proliferation in response to activation stimuli. J Immunol 1990; 145:3998–4005.
78. Tsoi MS, Mori T, Brkic S, et al. Ineffective cellular interaction and interleukin 2 deficiency causing T cell defects in human allogeneic marrow recipients early after grafting and in those with chronic graft-versus-host disease. Transplant Proc 1984; 16: 1470–1472.
79. Klingemann HG, Kohn FR, Phillips GL. Proliferation of peripheral lymphocytes to interleukin-2 and interleukin-4 after marrow transplantation. Eur Cytokine Net 1991; 2:131–136.
80. Moser M, Mizuochi T, Sharrow SO, et al. Graft-vs-host reaction limited to a class II MHC difference results in a selective deficiency in L3T4$^+$ but not in Lyt2$^+$ T helper cell function. J Immunol 1987; 138:1355–1362.
81. Moser M, Sharrow SO, Shearer GM. Role of L3T4$^+$ and Lyt2$^+$ donor cells in graft-versus-host immune deficiency induced across a class I, class II, or whole H-2 difference. J Immunol 1988; 140:2600.
82. Moller G. Suppressive effect of graft-versus-host reaction on immune response to heterologous red cells. Immunology 1971; 20:597–609.
83. Seddik M, Seemayer TA, Lapp WS. The graft-versus-host reaction and immune function: I. T-helper cell immuno-deficiency associated with graft-versus-host induced thymic epithelial cell damage. Transplantation 1984; 37:281–286.
84. Soiffer RJ, Bosserman L, Murray C. Reconstitution of T cell function after CD6-depleted allogeneic bone marrow transplantation. Blood 1990; 75:2076–2084.
85. Guillaume T, Hamdan O, Staquet P, et al. Blunted rise in intracellular calcium in CD4$^+$ T cells in response to mitogen following autologous bone marrow transplantation. Br J Haematol 1993; 84:131–136.
86. Klausner RD, Samelson LE. T cell antigen receptor activation pathways: The tyrosine kinase connection. Cell 1991; 64:875–878.
87. Veillette A, Davidson D. Src-related protein tyrosine kinases and T-cell receptor signalling. Trends Genet 1992; 8:61–66.
88. Cooke MP, Perlmutter RM. Expression of a novel form of the fyn proto-oncogene in hematopoietic cells. New Biol 1989; 1:66–74.
89. Davidson D, Chow LM, Fournel M, Veillette A. Differential regulation of T cell antigen responsiveness by isoforms of the src-related tyrosine protein kinase p59fyn. J Exp Med 1992; 175:1483–1492.
90. Timson Gauen LK, Kong AN, et al. p59fyn tyrosine kinase associates with multiple T-cell receptor subunits through its unique amino-terminal domain. Mol Cell Biol 1992; 12:5438–5446.
91. da Silva AJ, Yamamoto M, Zalvan CH, Rudd CE. Engagement of the TcR/CD3 complex stimulates p59fyn(T) activity: Detection of associated proteins at 72 and 120-130 kD. Mol Immunol 1992; 29:1417–1425.

92. Cooke MP, Abraham KM, Forbush KA, Perlmutter RM. Regulation of T cell receptor signalling by a src family protein-tyrosine kinase ($p59^{fyn}$). Cell 1991; 65:281–291.
93. Appleby MW, Gross JA, Cooke MP, et al. Defective T cell receptor signaling in mice lacking the thymic isoform of p59fyn. Cell 1992; 70:751–753.
94. Stein PL, Lee HM, Rich S, Soriano P. pp59fyn mutant mice display differential signaling in thymocytes and peripheral T cells. Cell 1992; 70:741–750.
95. Turner JM, Brodsky MH, Irving BA, et al. Interaction of the unique N-terminal region of tyrosine kinase p56lck with cytoplasmic domains of CD4 and CD8 is mediated by cysteine motifs. Cell 1990; 60:755–765.
96. Veillette A, Bookman MA, Horak EM, et al. Signal transduction through the CD4 receptor involves the activation of the internal membrane tyrosine-protein kinase p56lck. Nature 1989; 338:257–259.
97. Hatakeyama M, Kono T, Kobayashi N, et al. Interaction of the IL-2 receptor with the src-family kinase p56lck: Identification of novel intermolecular association. Science 1991; 252:1523–1528.
98. Veillette A, Abraham N, Caron L, Davidson D. The lymphocyte-specific tyrosine protein kinase p56lck. Semin Immunol 1991; 3:143–152.
99. Straus DB, Weiss A. Genetic evidence for the involvement of the lck tyrosine kinase in signal transduction through the T cell antigen receptor. Cell 1992; 70:585–593.
100. Heim LR, Good RA, Martinez C. Influence of adrenalectomy on homologous disease. Proc Soc Exp Biol Med 1966; 122:107–111.
101. Kaplan HS, Rosston BH. Studies on a wasting disease induced in F1 hybrid mice injected with parental strain lymphoid cells. Stanford Med Bull 1959; 17:77.
102. Gonzalo JA, Gonzalez-Garcia A, Martinez-A C, Kroemer G. Glucocorticoid-mediated control of the activation and clonal deletion of peripheral T cells in vivo. J Exp Med 1993; 177:1239–1246.
103. Farrar M, Schreiber RD: The molecular cell biology of interferon-γ and its receptor. Annu Rev Immunol 1993; 11:571–611.
104. Nathan C, Xie Q-W: Nitric oxide synthases: Roles, tolls and controls. Cell 1994; 78: 915–918.
105. Via CS: Kinetics of T cell activation in acute and chronic forms of murine graft-versus-host disease. J Immunol 1991; 146:2603–2609.
106. Chan SH, Perussia B, Gupta JW, et al. Induction of interferon γ production by natural killer cell stimulatory factor: Characterization of the responder cells and synergy with other inducers. J Exp Med 1991; 173:869–879.
107. Gazzinelli RT, Hieny S, Wynn TA, et al. Interleukin 12 is required for the T-lymphocyte-independent induction of interferon γ by an intracellular parasite and induces resistance in T-cell-deficient hosts. Proc R Acad Sci 1993; 90:6115–6119.
108. Schoenhaut DS, Chua AO, Wolitzky AG, et al. Cloning and expression of murine IL-12. J Immunol 1992; 148:3433–3440.
109. Swartz RP, Saluk PH. Functional modifications of macrophage activity after sublethal whole-body irradiation (41118). Proc Soc Exp Biol Med 1981; 167:20.
110. Schultz RM, Pavlidis NA, Chirigos MA, Weiss JF. Effects of whole body x-irradiation and cyclosphamide treatment on induction of macrophage tumoricidal function in mice. Cell Immunol 1978; 38:302.
111. Ando K, Peters LJ, Jinnouchi K, Matsumoto T. Inhibition of artificial and spontaneous lung metastases by preirradiation of abdomen: II. Target organ and mechanism. Br J Cancer 1983; 47:73.
112. Lambert LE, Paulnock DM. Modulation of macrophage function by γ-irradiation. Acquisition of the primed cell intermediate stage of the macrophage tumoricidal activation pathway. J Immunol 1987; 139:2834.
113. Hallahan DE, Spriggs DR, Beckett MA, et al. Increased tumor necrosis factor α

mRNA after cellular exposure of ionizing radiation. Proc Natl Acad Sci USA 1989; 86:10104.
114. Socie GE, Gluckman JM, Devergie A, et al. Unusual localization of cutaneous chronic graft-versus-host disease in the radiation fields in four cases. Bone Marrow Transplant 1989; 4:133.
115. Desbarats J, Seemayer TA, Lapp WS. Irradiation of the skin and the systemic graft-versus-host disease synergize to produce cutaneous lesions. Am J Pathol 1994; 144: 883–888.
116. Ghayur T, Xenocostas A, Seemayer TA, Lapp WS. Induction, specificity and elimination of asialo-GM1$^+$ graft-versus-host effector cells of donor origin. Scand J Immunol 1991; 34:497–508.
117. Moore, RH, Lampert IA, Chia Y, et al. Effect of immunization with Escherichia coli J5 on graft-versus-host disease induced by minor histocompatibility antigens in mice. Transplantation (Baltimore) 1987; 44:249.
118. Jutila JW. Etiology of the wasting diseases. J Infect Dis Suppl 1973; 128:599–5103.

19

Clinical Spectrum of Graft-Versus-Host Disease

Olle Ringdén
Karolinska Institute and Huddinge Hospital, Stockholm, Sweden

H. Joachim Deeg
Fred Hutchinson Cancer Research Center and University of Washington Seattle, Washington

I. ACUTE GVHD: INTRODUCTION

Graft-versus-host disease (GVHD), originally termed secondary disease, was first described in murine models. It resembled the syndrome of "runt disease," observed in mice that were neonatally inoculated with allogeneic lymphocytes. These mice showed growth retardation, hypoplasia of lymphatic organs, skin lesion, diarrhea, and hepatic necrosis (1,2). With higher bone marrow cell doses, the disease developed earlier and was more severe (3). Based on the experience in experimental animals, Billingham formulated the essential requirements for induction of GVHD: (a) the marrow graft must contain immunocompetent cells; (b) the host must express minor or major transplantation antigens that are lacking in the marrow donor; and (c) the hosts must be incapable of rejecting the marrow graft (4).

As discussed elsewhere, the immunocompetent cells were contained within a population of small lymphocytes in the marrow, which triggered the development of GVHD (5–8). Early in the course, the invading lymphocytes are mainly CD4 positive, although in later stages CD8 positive cells may be prominent (9,10). Removal of T cells from the donor marrow may completely prevent acute GVHD (11–15). While in inbred murine models of GVHD can be prevented completely with the use of histocompatible donor cells, in clinical transplantation acute GVHD occurs in spite of a suitable matching for the major histocompatibility antigens (HLA) (16). With disparity for the alleles of various loci of the HLA system, there is an increased incident of GVHD (17,18). Furthermore, recipients of bone marrow from phenotypically HLA-identical unrelated donors are reported to experience more GVHD than those from HLA-identical siblings in most (19–21) but not all studies (22–23).

II. IMMUNOLOGY AND PATHOPHYSIOLOGY

The immunopathophysiology of GVHD (see Chap. 00) can be separated into an afferent (sensitizing) phase and an efferent (effector) phase. Donor T cells are responsible for triggering GVHD and proliferate after activation by recipient antigens, expressed on host cells in the form of MHC class I or II antigens, viral antigens, or minor antigenic peptides, including epithelial cell-associated antigens. Antigen-presenting cells such as dendritic cells or macrophages present the antigens to T cells. CD4 positive (helper) T cells recognize antigens in association with HLA class II molecules. Interleukin (IL)-1 produced by monocytes and other factors such as epidermal-cell-derived thymocyte activating factor stimulate the T-helper cells, which in turn release IL-2, which activates cytotoxic CD8 positive T cells, which react with MHC class I positive targets. In addition, natural killer (NK) cells (24) and macrophages appear to participate in the development of GVHD (25), although their role is controversial (26–28). A subset of activated $CD4^+$ cells also produces interferon-gamma (IFN-γ), which enhances the expression of MHC class II on epithelial cells and macrophages, further stimulating T-cell and NK-cell activation. The observation that antibodies to tumor necrosis factor (TNF) prevent GVHD in mice and may delay the appearance of GVHD in humans (29,30) is in agreement with an involvement of IFN in the pathophysiology of GVHD. In fact, as discussed elsewhere, IFN is only one of the cytokines thought to play a pivotal role in the development of GVHD and may indeed be responsible for the observed end-organ damage.

Humoral immune mechanisms may also be involved in GVHD. Several investigators showed depositions of Ig and complement at the dermoepidermal junction during acute and chronic GVHD (31). Furthermore, high numbers of IgG-secreting lymphocytes appeared during acute GVHD in humans (32), and B cells were also demonstrated in the target organ during GVHD in a rat model (33). It is conceivable, of course, that those changes are mediated by a cytokine effect on B cells.

III. RISK FACTORS FOR ACUTE GVHD

GVHD is the most important transplant-related complication adversely affecting outcome (34,35). Therefore it is important to determine risk factors for acute GVHD, because high-risk patients may benefit from special treatment or additional immunoprophylaxis.

A. Histocompatibility

When HLA-identical siblings are used as bone marrow donors, the incidence of moderate to severe acute GVHD (grades II–IV) ranges from less than 10% to 60%, depending on GVHD prophylaxis and other risk factors. A study from Seattle using methotrexate as single-agent prophylaxis showed an incidence of acute GVHD of about 35%, both with HLA genotypically identical or HLA phenotypically identical related donors (17). In another study, the incidence of grades II–IV acute GVHD increased for 60 to 75% with one disparate HLA antigen and up to 90% with two to three HLA-antigen mismatched transplants. Nevertheless, in patients transplanted for leukemia, survival with HLA-identical sibling transplants and transplantation-related donors differing for one HLA antigen was identical, presumably due to an enhanced antileukemia effect (and fewer relapses) with HLA-disparate transplants. Using bone marrow donors with two or three antigen mismatches, however, significantly increased transplant-related mortality. A study from the International Bone Marrow Transplant Registry (IBMTR), including 470 recipients of marrow from alternate (HLA-nonidentical) related donors, showed the risk of acute GVHD to be the same using one-antigen mismatched transplants, HLA-phenotypically matched transplants, or HLA-identical sibling transplants (18). By comparison, the relative risks of acute GVHD after two- and three-antigen mismatched transplants were 3.1 and 4.4, respectively ($p < 0.0001$).

Some reports showed an incidence of grades II–IV acute GVHD of 70% with unrelated donor with no difference between those receiving marrow from HLA-A, -B, and -DR–identical donors and those receiving marrow from donors mismatched at one locus (19–21). However, other studies reported an incidence of 52 and 15% of grades II–IV acute GVHD with HLA-A, -B and -DR–identical related and unrelated donors (22,23), respectively. Figure 1 shows the incidences of GVHD using HLA-identical siblings; HLA-A, -B, and -DR–identical unrelated donors; or one-HLA-locus-mismatched related donors at a single institution.

The relative impact of the various MHC loci on GVHD has not been completely

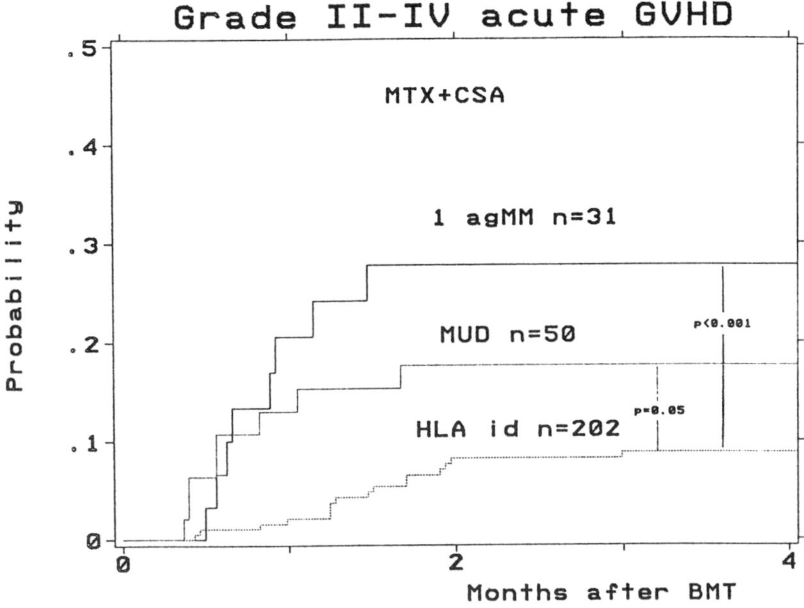

Figure 1 Impact of histocompatibility on the development of acute GVHD. Cumulative incidence and time to grades II–IV acute GVHD in marrow transplant recipients treated with methotrexate (MTX) and cyclosporine (CSA) at Huddinge Hospital. The cumulative incidence of acute GVHD among HLA-identical siblings (HLA id) was 9%. For recipients of HLA-A, -B, and -DR identical bone marrow from unrelated donors (MUD), the cumulative incidence was 18%. Among recipients of bone marrow from related donors with one HLA-A, -B, or -DR antigen mismatch (1 ag mm) the cumulative incidence was 32%.

delineated yet. The DP locus may not be of major importance for acute GVHD. A study from Seattle in HLA-A, -B, -DR, and -DQ–identical recipient/unrelated donor pairs showed an incidence of acute GVHD of 69, 83, and 72% with no, one, or two DP antigen mismatches, respectively (36). The importance of histocompatibility matching for GVHD is discussed in detail in Chap. 22.

B. Graft-Cell Composition

Van Bekkum and de Vries showed in mice that there was a clear correlation between the number of spleen cells (but not marrow cells) transplanted and the incidence and severity of GVHD (1). The addition of donor lymphocytes to the marrow inoculum also facilitates engraftment (37), and it has been argued that it is the development of GVHD that may facilitate engraftment. In patients with severe aplastic anemia, the addition of donor buffy-coat cells after marrow infusion reduced the incidence of graft rejection from 35 to 15% and improved survival from 45 to 70% (38). While buffy-coat cells had little impact on acute GVHD, the incidence of chronic GVHD was increased (39). A high bone marrow cell dose by itself correlated with a low risk of GVHD mortality (40).

T-cell depletion of the bone marrow decreases the risk of GVHD. However, in animal models and clinically, T-cell depletion is associated with an increased risk of graft failure (14,15,40,41). As already stated, the number of donor lymphocytes transplanted may correlate with the probability of acute GVHD (41–43). Clinical studies have also been performed where fixed numbers of T cells were added to T-cell-depleted bone marrow in order to ensure engraftment without increasing the risk of GVHD while maintaining an antileukemic effect (44). An increased incidence of mortality from acute GVHD was also reported in splenectomized patients (45–47). Experimental data may explain this observation. For one, bovine spleen cells were reported to produce peptides that suppress lethal GVHD (48). Furthermore, in murine models, allogeneic T cells reactive to minor MHC antigens become selectively sequestered in the spleen (49).

C. Age and Sex

Older patients have an increased incidence of acute GVHD (34,43,45,50), and the risk of dying from GVHD increases with age (45). One possible reason is that the thymus involutes with age and thereby may become less capable of educating donor-derived T lymphocytes to accept the host environment as self. Also, since colonization of the transplant recipient by bacterial and viral organisms may contribute to GVHD, older age may enhance GVHD by offering a broader range of colonizing organisms. Furthermore, repair processes decline with age, and it is possible that in older patients damaged tissue undergoes repair more slowly; therefore, such tissue may be more vulnerable to GVHD damage than it is in younger individuals.

Some reports show an increased risk for GVHD in recipients of sex-matched marrow (43,51) possibly due to Y-chromosome- associated histocompatibility antigens. Also, use of marrow from a female donor immunized by previous pregnancies (or transfusions) increased the risk of GVHD (52,53). In a study of 2036 recipients of HLA-identical sibling bone marrow performed by the IBMTR, the relative risk of grades II–IV acute GVHD in female donor to male recipient transplants was 2.0

($p < 0.001$) (53). If, in addition, the female donors were previously pregnant or had been transfused, the relative risk increased to 2.9 ($p < 0.0001$). Older patients had an increased risk of GVHD with a relative risk of 1.6 ($p < 0.001$). However, if allosensitized donors were excluded, age was no longer a significant risk factor.

D. Microenvironment

The host environment is of importance for the development of GVHD. Mice raised in a germ-free environment (gnotobiotic) fail to develop GVHD after H-2 incompatible transplants, and mice decontaminated by antibiotics pretransplant or aggressively treated with antibiotics posttransplant have a lower incidence of GVHD than controls (54–56). Patients with aplastic anemia undergoing bone marrow transplantation and treated with skin and gut decontamination with antibiotics and placed in a protective environment, so-called laminar airflow units, also had a reduced incidence of GVHD (57,58). A study from Seattle in patients with aplastic anemia undergoing bone marrow transplantation and treated in a laminar airflow room had a decrease in grades II–IV acute GVHD to 25%, compared to 40% in controls not treated in a protective environment (58). There was also an increase in survival to 85%, compared to 70% in controls. One possible explanation may be that enterobacteria invading GVHD lesions of the intestinal mucosa share antigenic determinants with host epithelial cells and activate alloreactive donor T cells initially primed against host epithelial cells. An alternate explanation may be that bacterial products—e.g., staphylococcal enterotoxin—which can function as "superantigens," stimulate recipient cells nonspecifically or that damage to the intestinal mucosa by chemoradiotherapy may allow endotoxin to enter into the circulation and stimulate cytokine production resulting in enhanced GVHD. A support for the latter hypothesis is that passive immunization with antiendotoxin after bone marrow transplantation in a mouse model protected against GVHD (59).

Some studies from Europe indicate that herpesviruses may play a role in the development of acute and chronic GVHD. Gratama and coworkers reported that moderate to severe acute GVHD was associated with positive Epstein-Barr virus (EBV) serology ($p = 0.002$) in the patient, negative donor EBV serology ($p = 0.005$), and positive donor herpes simplex virus (HSV) serology ($p = 0.003$) (60). Multivariate analyses of 111 consecutive HLA-identical marrow recipients at a single center showed that grades II–IV acute GVHD was correlated to a positive cytomegalovirus (CMV) serology in the recipients ($p < 0.05$) and showed a borderline association with positive donor HSV serology ($p = 0.07$) (61). In a European study of 379 patients undergoing HLA-identical sibling transplantation at 17 centers, 17% of recipients with seropositivity zero to two herpesviruses had grades II–IV acute GVHD as compared to 34% in recipients seropositive for three to four herpesviruses (62). A combination of positive HSV serology in recipient and donor and a strong donor mononuclear cell reactivity to HSV was associated with acute GVHD (63). The mechanism is not clear. However, it has been shown that HSV antigens can induce blast transformation in mixed lymphocyte culture (MLC) between otherwise MLC-nonreactive siblings (64).

High doses of CMV hyperimmune globulin or intravenous immunoglobulin given posttransplant were shown to decrease the risk of acute GVHD (65,66). There may be several reasons. For one, high doses of immunoglobulins may have an immune modulatory effect and therefore may decrease immune reactions associated with GVHD (67). Another possibility is that these antibodies, among other specificities, are directed against bacterial and viral antigens and thereby block antigen determinants that may trigger a GVHD reaction. It is also possible that these immunoglobulins contain antibodies against TNF-α or soluble MHC class I or class II peptides and thereby inhibit GVHD (29,30,68).

E. Prophylaxis

Nonspecific immunosuppression is discussed in detail in Chap. 24.

There is agreement that some form of immunosuppression or modulation is necessary to prevent GVHD. Preclinical studies in random-bred animals show at least 50% of MHC-matched transplant recipients will die from GVHD-related problems if no prophylaxis is given (69). Nevertheless, come clinical studies suggest that a proportion of patients not given GVHD prophylaxis will not develop GVHD, although the vast majority will often present with a hyperacute presentation of GVHD (70,71).

Methotrexate and cyclosporine used as single agents result in comparable incidences of acute GVHD (72). When combined, these agents result in a dramatic decrease in acute GVHD, especially the severe forms of GVHD, and a decline in transplant-related mortality compared to monotherapy using either drug alone (73,74). An IBMTR study suggests that this effect is most relevant in adults; in children, treatment with methotrexate, cyclosporine, or the two drugs combined resulted in similar outcomes (74). In adult HLA-identical siblings treated with methotrexate, the incidence of grades II–IV acute GVHD was 50%, compared to 43% using cyclosporine and 29% when methotrexate and cyclosporine were combined ($p < 0.001$) (74) (see Fig. 2).

F. Blood Group and HLA Alleles

Sparkes and coworkers reported a correlation between blood group MNSs antigens and GVHD after bone marrow transplantation in HLA- identical siblings (75). This has not been confirmed in recent studies.

A correlation between certain HLA alleles and acute GVHD has also been reported (51,76). This has not been confirmed by others; therefore these data must be interpreted with some caution. A study from Seattle indicated that patients with HLA-B18 had a nearly three times higher incidence of GVHD than all other patients (76). In patients with HLA-B8 or HLA-B35, the incidence of GVHD was reduced to about half of that seen in the absence of these alleles. Bross et al., from Johns Hopkins, reported that HLA-Bw21 and Cw4 were significantly correlated with an increased risk of GVHD, while HLA-Aw19 was associated with a decreased risk of GVHD (51). Thus, these questions have not been answered definitively and will probably have to await the results of more complete analyses of patients typed at the molecular level.

IV. CLINICAL DISEASE

Acute GVHD generally develops within the first 2 months of marrow transplantation, with a median onset of about 3 weeks (16,46). Upon withdrawal of cyclosporine, acute GVHD may appear several months after bone marrow trans-

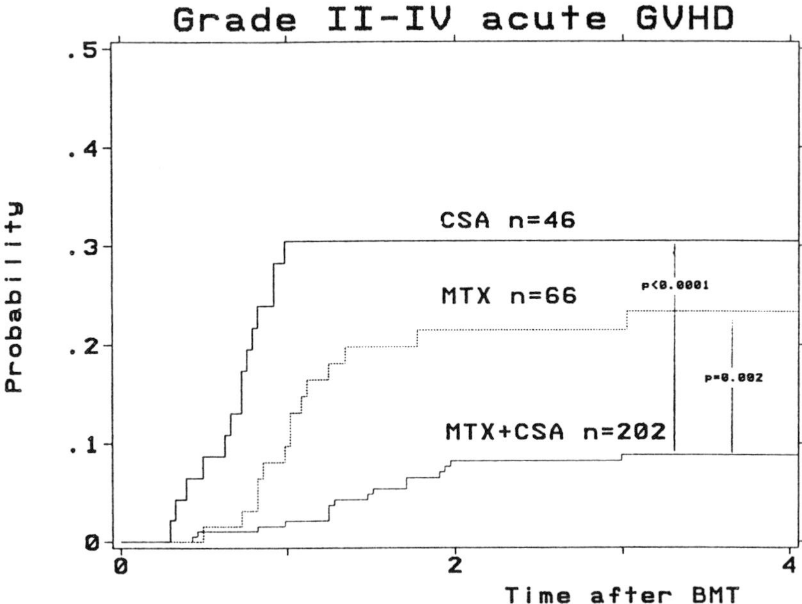

Figure 2 Time to and cumulative incidence of grades II–IV acute GVHD in recipients of bone marrow from HLA-identical sibling donors at Huddinge Hospital. Among patients treated with cyclosporine (CSA) alone, the cumulative incidence of GVHD was 30%. In patients treated with methotrexate (MTX), the cumulative incidence was 23%, and in patients treated with MTX combined with CSA, the cumulative incidence was 9%.

plantation in some patients. In recipients of marrow from HLA-nonidentical donors or patients receiving HLA-identical bone marrow but no GVHD prophylaxis, hyperacute GVHD may appear within a few days of transplantation (70,71). In most cases clinical signs of GVHD are preceded by evidence of marrow engraftment. However, in recipients of HLA- nonidentical bone marrow, hyperacute GVHD may appear before evidence of hemopoietic engraftment and in some patients without it. Presumably donor lymphoid cells, sufficient to trigger GVHD, have engraftment. The presence of GVHD may further suppress hematopoiesis. The main target organs for acute GVHD are skin, gut, liver, and the lymphoid organs (16,77–79). However, involvement of lymphatic organs is not easy to define in humans and is not generally considered in the grading system. Other tissues that may also be involved in acute GVHD include mucous membranes, conjunctivae, exocrine glands, bronchial tree and urinary bladder epithelium.

A. Skin

The first manifestation of acute GVHD is usually a mild skin rash, often involving the palms and soles. Other common sites are the ears, face, chest, and shoulders. In more severe forms of GVHD, the skin of the whole body may be involved (irradiation and drug reactions may mimic acute GVHD). The lesions can remain distinct or become confluent. Usually the rash is pruritic, and some patients experience pruritus before skin lesions are apparent. Many patients complain of burning palms and soles. In some patients, acute GVHD ia associated with fever. In more severe cases, bullae form, and via dermoepidermal separation, large surface areas desquamate, leading to a denudation resembling severe burns. With severe skin disease, there is a significant protein loss and a high risk of infection. Acute GVHD in the skin is generally a clinical diagnosis, but biopsies are sometimes helpful. However, a skin biopsy may not be diagnostic, especially early posttransplant, when histological changes due to chemoradiotherapy cannot be distinguished from those seen with GVHD (80). Drug reactions—induced, for instance, by co- trimoxazole—are also difficult to distinguish from acute GVHD in the skin. Skin changes involve basal vacuolar degeneration or necrosis, dyskeratosis, eosinophilic necrosis of epidermal cells, focal microscopic epidermal-dermal separation, and epidermal loss (81,82).

B. Liver

Acute GVHD of the liver is first manifested by abnormal hepatic function tests, such as elevated s-ALAT, s-ASAT, and bilirubin. GVHD of the liver often develops after skin disease and within 2 to 4 weeks of transplantation. Generally, it starts with a rise of transaminases followed by a gradual rise of both direct and indirect bilirubin. Gamma-glutamyltranspeptidase may also be elevated. However, none of these findings are diagnostic of GVHD. Hepatic (and intestinal) involvement may become manifest concurrently with or following skin involvement. Isolated liver or intestinal involvement without involvement of the skin is infrequent. It is also uncommon to see liver or gut involvement before skin disease is apparent (16,78). In severe forms, ascites and liver enlargement may occur (although this is more typical of venoocclusive disease), and patients rarely complain of pain.

There are many causes of hepatic dysfunctions following bone marrow transplantation. Early posttransplant hepatic dysfunction may be related to chemoradiotherapy used for conditioning. These abnormalities generally normalize spontaneously. Venoocclusive disease of the liver is a vascular complication that usually occurs within a couple of weeks after transplantation. It presents with weight gain, right-upper-quadrant pain, and a rise in bilirubin and transaminases (82,83). Other differential diagnoses of liver dysfunction after marrow or peripheral blood stem-cell transplantation include viral hepatitis, other infections, cyclosporine toxicity, and parenteral nutrition (84). Histologic confirmation of the diagnoses by hepatic biopsy is required in patients with a questionable clinical diagnosis. Liver histology of GVHD is characterized by degeneration and eosinophilic necrosis of paraacinar cells and degeneration and necrosis of the epithelium of small bile ducts, along with focal mononuclear cell infiltrates (84).

C. Gastrointestinal

Symptoms of gastrointestinal GVHD include nausea, vomiting, abdominal pain, and diarrhea, which may be voluminous and associated with cramping (78). Diarrhea may become bloody as the disease progresses. In severe gut GVHD, paralytic ileus may develop (85). The bowel wall is edematous and the lumen is often fluid-filled. Occasionally pneumatosis cystoides intestinalis has been observed. The differential diagnosis has to consider several conditions. Many patients experience diarrhea early after transplantation due to conditioning with chemoradiotherapy. Patients treated with broad-spectrum antibiotics may develop *Clostridium difficile* infection. Other types of bacterial or viral gastroenteritis may appear. To confirm the diagnosis of gastrointestinal GVHD, a rectal or upper GI tract biopsy may be helpful (85). Histological findings of gut GVHD range from single-cell necrosis of epithelial cells to crypt abscesses and mucosal denudation in severe cases. Stenotic lesions may develop.

D. Grading of Acute GVHD

Acute GVHD is generally graded on a five-step scale from 0 to IV, considering involvement of skin, liver, and intestinal tract (16,78) (Fig. 3). Grade 0 indicates no clinical evidence for GVHD. Grade I (mild) GVHD, indicates a localized skin rash, which may disappear without therapy. Grade II represents moderately severe GVHD, such as a skin rash involving most of the body, with bullae and desquamation, or more limited skin disease in association with mild symptoms or findings of either gut or liver involvement. Grade III indicates severe GVHD involving skin, gut, and liver, and grade IV is life-threatening or lethal GVHD involving any or all target organs. However, as discussed at a recent workshop (85A), neither this standard grading system nor several revisions that have been proposed are completely satisfactory. There may have been changes in the clinical spectrum of GVHD associated with changes in transplant procedures, selection of donors, and GVHD prophylaxis. For example, analysis of recent data suggests that persistent nausea with histological evidence of GVHD (esophagus, stomach) should be included as

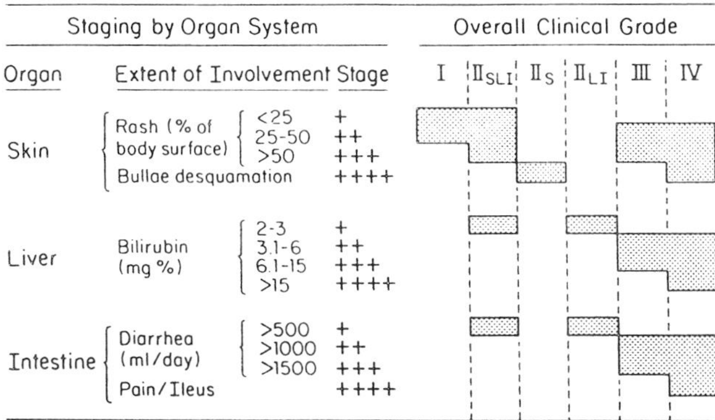

Figure 3 Clinical grading of acute GVHD. Left panel summarizes the staging by organ system; right panel shows the overall clinical grade. With grade I, only the skin can be involved. With more extensive involvement of the skin or involvement of liver and intestinal tract and impairment of the clinical performance status, either alone or in any combination, the overall grade advances from II to IV. Some investigators consider it worthwhile to subdivide the overall grade II into one category, including patients with skin involvement only (II_S), or liver and intestinal involvement without skin involvement (II_{LI}). Patients with grade II_S may have a better prognosis than patients with other grade II diseases. Liver dysfunction also includes transaminase and alkaline phosphatase elevations. However, it appears difficult to correlate the extent of enzyme abnormality with the prognosis of GVHD. Some investigators prefer to grade intestinal involvement according to body weight; + = 10–15; + + = 16–20; + + + = 21–25; and + + + + ≥ 26 mL/kg/day of diarrhea. (From Ref. 79.)

stage 1 GVHD even if there is no diarrhea, pain, etc. (85A). Caution is indicated in the grading of liver and gut also when other non-GVHD problems concurrently afflict the same organs. This is particularly important in assessing responses to therapy. In fact, it has been suggested to grade acute GVHD by response to therapy once prognosis correlates well with response. A simplified grading scheme as discussed at the recent workshop is depicted in Table 1.

V. TREATMENT OF ACUTE GVHD

Treatment of GVHD is discussed in Chap. 24.

Prednisolone, methylprednisolone antithymocyte globulin (ATG), various types of monoclonal antibodies against T cells, cyclosporine, FK506, Psoralen and ultraviolet light (PUVA), anti- IL-2 antibodies, receptor antibodies, thalidomide, and other agents are used (86–92). A study from Seattle in 740 patients with moderate to severe acute GVHD suggested that corticosteroids represent the best initial therapy (93). However, in severe, acute GVHD no treatment is as yet satisfactory, despite attempts with a variety of immunosuppressive agents. Isolated severe GVHD of the liver leading to terminal liver injury may be treated by liver transplantation (94).

VI. GVHD AFTER ORGAN TRANSPLANTATION AND IN OTHER CONDITIONS

GVHD may develop in settings other than allogeneic bone marrow transplantation. GVHD may develop after organ transplantation, especially after transplantation of small intestine, where lymphoid cells from the Peyer's patches react against recipient antigens (95). Passenger leukocytes transferred via the transplanted organ have also been reported to induce GVHD in liver and heart transplant recipients (96,97). Acute GVHD may also be induced by leukocytes contained in transfused blood products given to patients with hematological malignancies, who have been heavily

Table 1 Functional Grading of Acute GVHD

	Organ Involvement		
	Skin	Liver	Gut
Grade[a]			
I	Rash on ≤50% of skin	None	None
II	Rash on >50% of skin	or bilirubin 2–3 mg/day	or diarrhea >500 mL/day[b] or persistent nausea[c]
III–IV	Generalized erythroderma with bullous formation	or bilirubin >3	or diarrhea >1000 mL/day

[a]Criteria for grading given as degree of organ involvement due to GVHD required to confer that grade.
[b]Volume of diarrhea applies to adults. For pediatric patients, the volume of diarrhea should be based on body surface area or possibly weight (see legend to Fig. 3).
[c]Persistent nausea with histological evidence of GVHD in the stomach or duodenum.

immunosuppressed by chemotherapy (98) (Chap. 21). Furthermore, GVHD was described following exchange transfusions in fetuses with hydrops fetalis (99). Some immunodeficient fetuses may develop fatal GVHD (100).

GVHD symptoms and findings may also occur in recipients after syngeneic and autologous marrow transplantation (101,102) (see Chap. 20). In most cases these GVHD-like reactions are limited to the skin, but liver and gut involvement as well as thrombocytopenia may be present. In autologous bone marrow transplant recipients, acute GVHD of the skin may be induced after withdrawal of a short cause of cyclosporine (102) (Chap. 20). This approach is currently being investigated, with the assumption that the induction of a graft-versus-leukemia effect will decrease the probability of leukemic relapse after transplantation (102).

VII. COMPLICATIONS ASSOCIATED WITH ACUTE GVHD

GVHD is associated with severe immunological deficiency (103,104), and treatment with immunosuppressive agents further aggravates immunosuppression (104,105). Not surprisingly, therefore, infections are frequent and often life-threatening (16,45,106,107).

A. Bacterial Infections

During the period of pancytopenia after marrow transplantation, septicemia is common (16,106,108,109). The two most common pathogens are alpha streptococci originating from the oral flora or *Staphylococcus aureus*, which may be associated with intravenous catheters (110,111). Septicemia by gram-negative rods penetrating from the gastrointestinal tract was most common as a cause of septicemia in the early era of marrow transplantation but has become less common with the introduction of gut decontamination and early institution of broad-spectrum antibiotics (108). In one report, 42% of patients experienced bacteremia (108). Gram-positive or -negative bacteria were responsible for 61 and 39% of the septicemias, respectively (106). Even though the incidence was high, fatal infections were rare, and only 12% of the patients died because of bacterial septicemia (113).

After engraftment with the reconstituting immune system, marrow transplant patients are prone to acquire various bacterial infections and develop septicemia, bronchopneumonia, sinusitis, and other manifestations. In particular, patients with acute (and later chronic) GVHD are at an increased risk of such infections (107). Thus, in one analysis, 70% of patients with grades II–IV GVHD were infected, compared to 37% of patients with grades 0–I acute GVHD ($p < 0.0001$). In multivariate analysis, acute GVHD was the strongest factor associated with infection after engraftment. Other significant risk factors were splenectomy and CMV infection. During intestinal GVHD, gram- negative rods from the intestine may give rise to septicemia; with severe GVHD of the skin, staphylococci may penetrate through skin defects and give rise to bacteremia. Bacterial infection is a frequent cause of death in patients with moderate to severe acute GVHD (16,45).

B. Fungal Infections

There is also a substantial risk of invasive fungal infections, the most common pathogens being *Candida albicans, C. parapsilosis, C. glabrata*, and other species and *Aspergillus fumigatus* and other species. The mortality rate in bone marrow transplant patients is around 70% for invasive candidiasis and more than 90% for *Aspergillus* (112). Other less common fungal infections include *Cryptococcus neoformans, Mucor*, and, depending on the geographical location, species of *Coccidioides* and *Histoplasma*.

The incidence of invasive fungal infections in marrow transplant patients has been around 10% (113,114). Often it is difficult to establish an accurate diagnosis without invasive procedures (115). Serological tests are of little value in marrow recipients with a deficient immune system. Antigen tests and colonization from several superficial sites may give an indication but no proof (115). Polymerase chain reaction (PCR) techniques to detect different *Candida* species are under development, but their role is yet to be defined. Because of the difficulties in determining the diagnosis, antifungal treatment is often instituted empirically—for instance, in a patient with high fever of unknown origin, who has not responded to 3 or more days of therapy with broad-spectrum antibacterial antibiotics. The only way to establish the presence of invasive fungal infection is often by biopsies from a deep site or at autopsy. Pulmonary aspergillosis may at times be diagnosed by bronchoalveolar lavage as an alternative to pulmonary biopsy in patients with pulmonary infiltrates. The presence of acute GVHD grades II–IV ($p = 0.005$) and treatment with antithymocyte globulin ($p = 0.0006$) significantly increase the risk of invasive fungal infections (114). Therefore, early treatment with antifungal drugs such as amphotericin B, liposomal amphotericin B, or imidazoles should be considered during fever in patients with severe acute GVHD.

C. Viral Infections

Herpes simplex virus (HSV) is commonly reactivated after marrow transplantation unless acyclovir prophylaxis is administered (116). Patients with high pretransplant HSV IgG titers (> 10.000 ELISA) are especially at risk of developing an infection (117). Epstein-Barr virus (EBV) causes no major infections in marrow transplant recipients, although it is frequently associated with lymphoproliferative disorders developing posttransplant (118). Neither HSV nor EBV infections are associated with acute GVHD.

CMV is a major cause of infection and mortality after marrow transplantation, mainly because of its frequent association with interstitial pneumonitis (119,120). Historically, the incidence of CMV infection after marrow transplantation has been 50% or higher (118–122). With early (preemptive) ganciclovir therapy, infection is prevented in most patients, even those who test positive for CMV antigenemia (see below). Symptoms and findings of CMV infections include, apart from those of interstitial pneumonitis, fever, nausea, vomiting, dysphagia, hepatitis, arthralgias, and occasionally chorioretinitis and encephalitis. In CMV seropositive patients, the risk of reactivation ranges from 62 to 87% (120–122). Several studies have shown a correlation between acute GVHD and CMV infection (120,123,124). For example, CMV infection occurred in 33% of pediatric patients with GVHD, compared to 11% of those without GVHD (124). CMV reactivation and infection with acute GVHD is most probably due to immunosuppression caused by this disorder and the treatment with immunosuppressive drugs (103–105). CMV infection by itself also causes immunosuppression, as evidenced by a slower recovery of lymphocyte mitogenic responses and an increased incidence of bacterial infections in marrow transplant recipients who had a CMV infection (107,125).

Transplant recipients who are seropositive for various herpesviruses pretransplant have a significantly higher incidence of reactivation of the virus if they receive allogeneic marrow as opposed to autologous marrow (126). Cytotoxicity against CMV- infected targets by blood lymphocytes from patients with acute GVHD is significantly reduced 20 to 40 days after transplantation as compared to responses seen in patients without GVHD (127).

The most serious manifestation of CMV infection is interstitial pneumonitis. Clinical as well as experimental studies indicate a correlation between GVHD and CMV interstitial pneumonitis (119,120,128,129). In one study among 100 syngeneic bone marrow transplant recipients, none developed CMV interstitial pneumonitis, compared to 19% among 353 HLA-identical siblings (130). Furthermore, CMV interstitial pneumonitis is less frequent in autologous than in allogeneic marrow transplant recipients (131). Among 197 consecutive marrow transplant recipients, the incidence of CMV interstitial pneumonitis was 26% in patients with grades II–IV acute GVHD, compared to 11% in those with grades 0–I GVHD ($p < 0.001$) (128). The association between acute GVHD and CMV interstitial pneumonitis is also supported by experimental data in mice, which show that CMV infections play a primary role in provoking and accentuating acute GVHD (132).

Improvements in antiviral therapy combining ganciclovir and high- dose immunoglobulin have decreased the morality from CMV pneumonitis to around 50% from the previous 90% (133). However, with early diagnosis of CMV reactivation—using, for instance, PCR and antigenemia testing and early institution with ganciclovir—the incidence of CMV interstitial pneumonitis has decreased significantly (134–146). Therefore, in patients with moderate to severe acute GVHD, it is important to closely follow and diagnose CMV reactivation by PCR, immunofluorescence using antibodies against CMV, or rapid culture techniques. When CMV is demonstrated in blood, antiviral drugs such as ganciclovir or foscarnet should be instituted early to inhibit CMV replication and prevent progression to severe CMV disease, especially pneumonitis (133–137).

D. Nutritional Problems and Supportive Care

GVHD of the gastrointestinal tract may be associated with voluminous diarrhea, nausea, and vomiting, resulting in protein and electrolyte loss. An integral part of therapy is therefore, "gut rest"—i.e., oral intake is stopped and full parenteral nutrition is given. Patients with moderate to severe acute GVHD also have an increased requirement for blood products compared to patients with no or mild disease (138). These patients must also be closely monitored for bacterial, fungal, and viral infections (see above).

E. Secondary Malignancies

The incidence of secondary malignancies in allogeneic bone marrow transplant recipients was calculated to be approximately six times that of the general population (139). Posttransplant lymphoproliferative disorders, leukemia, squamous epithelial tumor, and melanoma were especially common. Posttransplant lymphoproliferative disorders generally occur early after BMT, while many of the other malignancies develop late and are probably influenced by other factors, possibly chronic GVHD.

Treatment of acute GVHD with ATG or anti-T-cell antibodies, HLA nonidentity of donor and recipient, T-cell depletion of the donor marrow, and TBI appear to be the major risk factors for the development of lymphoproliferative disorders (139–143). As many as 90% of these originate in donor cells and are associated with EBV (140). These lymphomas seem to occur less frequently in marrow transplant recipients than in recipients of solid-organ transplants. The reason for this may be the less frequent and, timewise, more restricted use of ATG and monoclonal anti-T-cell antibodies.

VIII. THE IMPACT OF ACUTE GVHD ON SURVIVAL

Due to the high mortality associated with moderate to severe acute GVHD this complication has a profound effect on the prognosis after bone marrow transplantation (16,34,35,45,58). In a study from Seattle in patients transplanted for severe aplastic anemia, survival was 90% in patients with grades 0–I acute GVHD as compared to 60% among those with grades II–III and zero among those with grade IV (58). Death is often caused by infections, hemorrhages, and hepatic failure (16,45).

On the other hand, GVHD has an antileukemia effect (144–150). Weiden et al. reported first that the probability of relapse of leukemia was 2.5 times less in allogeneic marrow recipients with GVHD than in allogeneic recipients without GVHD ($p < 0.01$) or in syngeneic marrow graft recipients (146). In a subsequent Seattle study, Fefer et al. reported that in leukemic patients in second or subsequent remission or relapse at the time of transplant, relapse was observed in 62% of the syngeneic but only in 35% of the allogeneic marrow recipients ($p < 0.0001$) (149). Multicenter studies have also shown that grades II–IV acute GVHD decreases the risk of leukemic relapse (148,150,151). However, the antileukemic effect of acute GVHD seems to be less pronounced than that of chronic GVHD (147,148) (see below). In a study from the IBMTR of 2254 recipients of HLA-identical sibling bone marrow, the relative risk of relapse was 0.68 ($p = 0.03$) in recipients of non-T-cell-depleted allografts with acute GVHD compared to patients without GVHD (148). This effect was most clearly shown in patients with acute lymphoblastic leukemia. The relative risk of relapse was 0.4 in patients with acute GVHD compared to those without GVHD.

However, despite potential benefits of an antileukemic effect of GVHD, GVHD is one of the major obstacles to success after bone marrow transplantation (16,35,45,58). Even if GVHD reduced the risk of leukemic relapse, there is an even higher risk of treatment failure associated with GVHD. Thus, in a report from the IBMTR, the relative risk of relapse or death was 3.73 in HLA- identical siblings with early leukemia, which was significantly higher than among patients without GVHD ($p < 0.00001$) (148). In a single-center study of patients with leukemia, multivariate analyses showed that grades 0–I acute GVHD was the most important factor associated with a favorable patient survival (35). In patients surviving 30 days after transplantation, 5-year survival was 68% among those with grades 0–I acute GVHD compared to 29% among those with grades II–IV acute GVHD ($p < 0.0001$).

With better immunosuppression (T-cell depletion or combinations of immunosuppressive drugs such as cyclosporine and methotrexate), the incidence of GVHD is reduced (11–15,73,74). However, with T-cell depletion, there is an increased risk of leukemic relapse, especially in patients with chronic myeloid leukemia (152–154). Whether intensive pharmacological immunosuppression is associated with an increased probability of relapse is controversial (73,74,154).

To conclude, severe acute GVHD is the most important cause of treatment failure after allogeneic bone marrow transplantation. However, using modern immunosuppression, it can be effectively prevented in most recipients of marrow from HLA-identical siblings. In recipients of HLA-mismatched or unrelated bone marrow, there is an urgent need for more effective immunosuppression. In leukemic marrow recipients, acute GVHD must be moderated to use its antileukemic activity in an optimal way.

IX. CHRONIC CRAFT-VERSUS-HOST-DISEASE: INTRODUCTION

Chronic GVHD was initially reported in the 1970s in the first long-term survivors of HLA-identical sibling transplantation (155–158). This syndrome resembles autoimmune systemic collagen vascular diseases and includes clinical manifestations of dermatitis, keratoconjunctivitis, generalized sicca syndrome, oral mucositis, esophageal and vaginal strictures, liver disease, pulmonary insufficiency, and others (159). Since effective treatment did not exist in the early era, many of these patients developed severe sclerodermalike skin disease progressing to fibrosis and contractures. Untreated gastrointestinal chronic GVHD was often associated with malabsorption and wasting. With immunosuppressive treatment—for instance, with cytotoxic drugs, corticosteroids and cyclosporine—chronic GVHD has changed its clinical appearance. Still, some 30 to 50% of HLA-identical siblings who become long-term survivors develop chronic GVHD (164–167) (Fig. 4). The incidence of chronic GVHD increases with age (160,161). If the disease is extensive, up to 80% of the affected patients will die, in most cases due to infections (159,162), which develop on the basis of severe impaired immune function (103,104). Much insight has been gained from experimental animal models—for instance, rat, mouse, and dog (163–165).

X. IMMUNOPATHOPHYSIOLOGY OF CHRONIC GVHD

This is extensively discussed in Chap. 11. T cells are responsible for the initiation of chronic as well as acute GVHD. They may exert a direct cytotoxic effect on epithelial cells during chronic GVHD. However, there is now strong evidence that epithelial cell injury is also mediated by cytokines such as TNF. IL-1 is overexpressed in skin of mice with GVHD, and it has been shown that soluble IL-1 receptor antagonists may prevent fatal GVHD in mice (166). IL-4 and additional cytokines also appear to be involved.

Epithelial cell damage in skin biopsies is characterized by basal cell degeneration and necrosis (167,168). Initial hyperkeratosis and hypertrophy in the skin is later replaced by epidermal atrophy and dermal fibrosis. T cells from mice with chronic GVHD secrete cytokines that stimulate fibroblast proliferation and collagen synthesis (170). Sweat and salivary glands are destroyed. HLA-DR antigen expression on

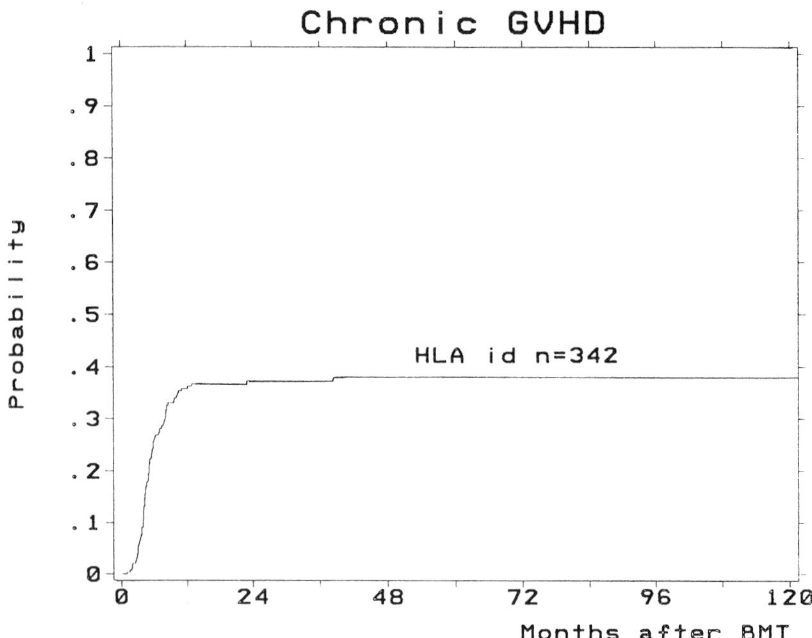

Figure 4 Time to and cumulative incidence of chronic GVHD in 342 recipients of bone marrow from HLA-identical siblings (HLA id) at Huddinge Hospital. The 4-year cumulative incidence of chronic GVHD is 38%.

epithelial cells in skin and gut is upregulated (169). Fibrosis of epithelial tissues has been described in skin, gastrointestinal tract, lungs, liver, vagina, and the hematopoietic system. In chronic GVHD of the liver, small bile duct atypia, necrosis, and hepatocyte damage are typical features.

XI. RISK FACTORS FOR CHRONIC GVHD

A. Acute GVHD

Storb and colleagues showed that in severe aplastic anemia, risk factors for chronic GVHD include prior acute GVHD, increasing patient age, and treatment with viable donor buffy-coat cells after transplantation (160). Multivariate analyses in bone marrow transplant recipients from Stockholm showed that chronic GVHD was associated with donor age above 17 years ($p = 0.003$), infusion of donor buffy-coat cells ($p = 0.003$), and prior grades II–IV acute GVHD ($p = 0.047$) (166).

B. Antiviral Immunity

The role of herpesviruses in the development of chronic GVHD is controversial. Lönnqvist et al. observed that CMV infection frequently preceded the onset of chronic GVHD (171). Subsequently, the Copenhagen group reported that donor CMV serology and not recipient CMV infection after marrow transplantation was correlated with chronic GVHD (172). A study from the IBMTR reported that CMV infection did not predispose to chronic GVHD (162). The role of CMV serology in recipient and donor was not analyzed in that study, where the only significant factor associated with chronic GVHD was preceding acute GVHD. In an analysis by the Nordic bone marrow transplantation group, it was shown in multivariate analyses that older donor age, the use of a female donor for a male recipient, and a donor with positive CMV serology were significantly associated with chronic GVHD (173). A study from Huddinge Hospital specifically addressing the role of herpesvirus immunity in the development of chronic GVHD found that donor seropositivity to three to four herpesviruses ($p < 0.001$) and grades II–IV acute GVHD ($p < 0.02$) were significantly associated with chronic GVHD (174). In an EBMT study of 285 bone marrow transplant patients surviving at least 3 months and reported from 17 teams, the cumulative incidence of chronic GVHD 2 years after transplantation was 32% (175), and the following factors were associated with chronic GVHD: pretransplant recipient seropositivity in combination with donor CMV seropositivity prior to bone marrow transplantation ($p = 0.0006$), previous grades II–IV acute GVHD ($p = 0.001$), and splenectomy ($p = 0.01$). Boström et al. suggested the following hypothesis (175): Latent CMV may be widely spread in various cells in the recipient body—for instance, in monocytes, granulocytes, lymphocytes, and possibly in endothelial cells. Target organs are gut, liver, spleen, salivary glands, and the lymphatic nodules. CMV immune donor cells may react with CMV antigens in those recipient tissues and thereby trigger an immune reaction leading to chronic GVHD. This hypothesis needs to be tested in additional patient populations.

XII. CLINICAL MANIFESTATIONS OF CHRONIC GVHD

A. Incidence and Grading

Of long-term survivors after marrow transplantation, 30 to 50% develop chronic GVHD (159–162) (Fig. 4). Chronic GVHD was reported to occur more frequently in survivors transplanted for aplastic anemia compared to patients with acute leukemia ($p = 0.0018$) (159). This may be related to the fact that patients with aplastic anemia often received donor buffy- coat cells in an attempt to prevent rejection (160). The overall incidence is 40 to 60% in patients with T-cell-replete marrow grafts.

Table 2 shows a classification scheme for chronic GVHD (168). Manifestations may be subclinical or clinical, limited or extensive.

Treatment is not necessary for limited chronic GVHD, which often resolves spontaneously (159). Recurrent infections, weight loss, sicca, mucositis, or other clinical problems were not observed. Extensive chronic GVHD necessitates immunosuppressive treatment; if untreated, it may progress and debilitate the patient by complications such as contractures, malabsorption, blindness, etc. Additional grading systems for extensive disease may be desirable, since this may involve anything from localized skin involvement or liver dysfunction combined with mild sicca syndrome to advanced disease affecting multiple target organs. Because of the complex and dynamic nature of chronic GVHD, the Karnofsky score has often been used to estimate the overall performance status of the patient (176) (Table 3).

Table 2 Classification of Chronic Graft-Versus-Host Disease

Subclinical graft-versus-host disease:
Histologically positive but no clinical symptoms

Clinical limited chronic graft-versus-host disease:
Either or both
– Localized skin involvement
– Hepatic dysfunction (due to chronic GVHD)

Extensive chronic graft-versus-host disease:
Either
– Generalized skin involvement
or
– Localized skin involvement or hepatic dysfunction due to chronic GVHD or both
plus
– Liver histology showing chronic aggressive hepatitis, bridging necrosis, or cirrhosis
or
– Involvement of eye (Schirmer's test with less than 5 mm wetting; or
– Involvement of minor salivary glands or oral mucosa demonstrated on labial biopsy
or
– Involvement of any other target organ (lung, kidney)

Table 3 Karnofsky Score

Percent	Description
100	Normal, no complaints; no evidence of disease.
90	Able to carry on normal activity; minor signs or symptoms of disease.
80	Normal activity with effort; some signs or symptoms of disease.
70	Cares for self and is well but unable to work. Requires infrequent outpatient follow-up and sees MD only once a week.
60	Requires occasional assistance but is able to care for most needs. Visits MD 2 to 3 times a week.
50	Requires considerable assistance and frequent medical care. Daily or alternate-day MD visits are necessary.
40	Disabled and requires special care. If outpatient, requires special MD/RN care; if inpatient, requires little active care (up, out of bed, and in good condition).
30	Severely disabled and hospitalization is indicated, although death is not imminent. Clinical condition is fair.
25	Hospitalization is mandated. Condition is fair to poor but stable.
20	Active supporting treatment in hospital is required. Condition is poor and unstable.
15	Active intensive care is continually required. Condition is critical.
10	Patient is moribund with a fatal process rapidly progressing. Condition is thought to be hypercritical.
5	Patient is moribund. Condition is terminal and irreversible. ("No code" status.)
0	Patient is dead.

B. Onset of Chronic GVHD

Chronic GVHD was initially defined as a GVHD syndrome presenting more than 100 days after marrow transplantation. However, chronic GVHD as determined clinically and histologically has been reported as early as 31 days after marrow transplantation (161). Chronic GVHD is described as *progressive* if it follows as a direct extension of acute GVHD. If a patient had acute GVHD that resolved and chronic GVHD appears after a disease-free interval, the disease is characterized as being *quiescent*. Chronic GVHD may also appear in patients who have not experienced acute GVHD, and is then called *de novo* disease (159). Risk factors for de novo disease are similar to those reported for acute GVHD: age above 20 years, non–T-cell-depleted bone marrow, alloimmune female donors of male recipient, and viable donor buffy-coat infusion (162). Occasionally, chronic GVHD may appear several years after bone marrow transplantation (161,162).

C. Skin Disease

Skin is the most common organ involved by chronic GVHD, which may present as lichenoid papules, areas of local erythema, and hyper- or hypopigmentation. Lichenoid papules can occur anywhere in the skin and may be localized (in limited disease) or generalized (in extensive disease). Areas of hyper- or hypopigmentation can be the sole clinical manifestation of chronic GVHD. In some patients, hyper- and hypopigmentation may develop in different areas. The development of chronic GVHD of the skin may be rapid if prophylactic immunosuppression is discontinued; it may develop more slowly in other patients. Chronic GVHD of the skin may be activated by sunlight. All patients are advised to avoid direct sun exposure and to use UV-blocking creams on exposed areas.

In extensive chronic GVHD, all areas of the skin may become involved; in rare cases, a localized form of subcutaneous fibrosis occurs. With skin progression from induration to sclerosis, facial fixation and contractures develop. Localized fibrosis may resolve spontaneously (159). Alternatively, fibrosis may wax or wane or may be manifest for several years. In severe chronic skin GVHD, bullous eruptions can occur on top of sclerodermalike skin changes and chronic skin ulcers. Wound healing is slow partly due to treatment with corticosteroids and loss of functional skin tissue. Hair follicle involvement may be manifest by focal to diffuse scarring alopecia. Vitiligo with premature graying of the hair or eyelashes may occur. Alopecia is due to subcutaneous fibrosis and destruction of follicles. After the resolution of GVHD, these areas may regenerate. Periungual erythema and dystrophic nails are often seen.

D. Chronic GVHD of the Liver

Chronic GVHD of the liver is manifest by an obstructive jaundice reflecting the bile duct abnormalities. If GVHD of the liver is the only manifestation of chronic GVHD, immunosuppressive treatment may not be necessary (159). Occasionally, however, hepatic disease may progress to cirrhosis with esophageal varices and hepatic failure. The serum alkaline phosphatase may be markedly increased. Transaminases are also increased, although to a much lesser extent than is seen with acute viral hepatitis. The diagnoses of chronic GVHD must be distinguished from other causes of jaundice in marrow transplant recipients, such as venoocclusive disease of the liver, cyclosporine-induced hepatotoxicity, viral hepatitis, and hemolysis. A liver biopsy may be useful. Histological findings in the liver during chronic GVHD are similar to those seen in acute GVHD but more intense, with chronic changes such as fibrosis with hyalinization of portal triads, obliteration of bile ducts, and hepatocellular cholestasis. Progression of chronic GVHD of the liver to cirrhosis and portal hypertension or hepatic failure is rare (see Chap. 12).

E. Oral Mucosa and Gastrointestinal Tract

Oral involvement is common in patients with chronic GVHD. Lichen planus–like striae and plaques, ulcerations, atrophy, erythema, and dryness may be present (177,178). These oral manifestations may be seen on the buccal mucosa, gums, and tongue. An inexperienced physician may mistake the lichenoid changes for oral candidiasis. Patients with ulcers and advanced chronic GVHD in the mouth complain of oral pain. As a part of the sicca syndrome, chronic GVHD also leads to dryness of the mouth, due to involvement of the minor salivary glands and ducts. However, reduction of salivary flow may also be caused by the effect of total body irradiation (178). A lip biopsy may be useful to diagnose chronic GVHD in the mouth. Typical features are lichenoid changes with mononuclear infiltrates of the basal cells and necrosis of individual epithelial cells (179). Salivary glands may show extensive inflammation or fibroses of acini or lymphocytic infiltration, atypia, and necrosis of the ductal epithelium. Untreated, oral chronic GVHD may progress to atrophy and fibrosis, with reduced ability to open the mouth and ensuing malnutrition.

Chronic GVHD of the esophagus has become rare with modern immunosuppression. Manifestations include dysphagia, painful swallowing due to strictures, and severe retrosternal pain. Radiological examination with barium will identify narrowings and strictures (180). Endoscopy shows a characteristic desquamation. Reflux leading to peptic esophagitis may occur and should be treated with antacids or intermittent H2 blockers.

Gastrointestinal involvement is infrequent in chronic GVHD. In occasional patients, gut involvement may be seen, which includes abdominal pain, diarrhea, anorexia, nausea, and vomiting. Histological changes include hypocellularity of the Peyer's patches, with patchy fibrosis of the lamina propia and striking fibrosis of the submucosa and serosa in severe disease (181). Fibrotic strictures of the small intestine can occur but are rare. If obstruction occurs, small bowel resections may be necessary. In severe chronic gastrointestinal GVHD with malabsorption, parenteral nutrition may be needed.

F. Eye Involvement

A common symptom of chronic GVHD is dryness of the eyes, which may be quantitated with a Schirmer's test. Keratoconjunctivitis sicca of the eyes and oral dryness may resemble Sjögren's syndrome. Damage to the lacrimal glands can progress, with appearance of conjunctival ulceration and scarring. The use of artificial tears and shielding with glasses or even patching of the eye to protect the corneal surface may be necessary.

G. Involvement of Other Organs

Airways can also be involved in chronic GVHD (see Chap. 00). Bronchiolitis obliterans, although rare, is highly correlated with chronic GVHD in other organs (182–184). Symptoms include signs of obstructive lung disease, cough, dyspnea and—in advanced cases—pneumothorax. The forced expiratory volume is decreased. The course is often fatal, with death due to respiratory insufficiency. Bronchiolitis obliterans may become manifest after an acute bronchitis or pneumonia.

The sicca syndrome may also lead to gynecologic manifestations, including vaginal strictures and stenosis (185). In addition to immunosuppressive therapy, topical estrogen cream and dilatation may be required. The differential diagnosis includes atrophy due to ovarian failure related to total body irradiation or other components of the conditioning regimen.

Eosinophilia and thrombocytopenia are seen in some patients with extensive chronic GVHD (168). Thrombocytopenia is a poor prognostic sign (186). The bone marrow may be hypoplastic and show fibrosis.

Myasthenia gravis has been observed after transplantation in patients with chronic GVHD mediated by antibodies to the acetylcholine receptor (187). Polymyositis is seen in some patients (188). Histological findings include necrotic fibers, interstitial inflammation, and IgG deposits. Neuropathy associated with subcutaneous fibrosis has also been described in chronic GVHD (169).

A possible association of minimal change nephrotic syndrome and cystitis with chronic GVHD has been reported in some patients (189,190).

XIII. IMMUNODEFICIENCY ASSOCIATED WITH CHRONIC GVHD

A characteristic of chronic GVHD is severe immunodeficiency, which predisposes to recurrent and sometimes fatal infections (103,191). Not only the hematopoietic system but in particular lymph nodes, spleen, and thymus are major target organs for chronic GVHD. Severe and persistent lymphoid hypocellularity and atrophy are associated with chronic GVHD (168).

A. Immunological Aberrations in Chronic GVHD

The most important factor for the recovery of the immune system after bone marrow transplantation is time (104,105). However, a considerable delay is observed in patients with chronic GVHD. For instance, lymphocytes from patients with chronic GVHD show decreased mitogenic response in vitro (103,104). Immunoglobulin levels are low and B-cell responses are deficient (32,103,129,192,193). A lack of helper T-cell activity and presence of suppressor T-cell activity were more frequently found in patients with chronic GVHD than in survivors without chronic GVHD (192). Furthermore, patients with chronic GVHD had CD4 cells and CD8 cells that suppressed immunoglobulin synthesis by normal T and B cells (193,194). Also, nonspecific suppressor cell functions were seen in patients with chronic GVHD (195). In one study, leukocytes from 120 patients were tested for their ability to inhibit mixed lymphocyte culture (MLC) reactivity of their marrow donors to third-party leukocytes. Cells from only 1/40 long-term patients without chronic GVHD showed suppression, compared with cells from 35/80 patients with chronic GVHD

($p < 0.0001$). Therefore it was suggested that aberrations in immune regulatory cells may be the basis for the profound immune deficiency associated with chronic GVHD (196). Approximately three-quarters of the recipients with chronic GVHD had impaired B-cell function, whereas only one-third of the recipients without chronic GVHD had B-cell defects as determined by in vitro immunoglobulin production (192,197,198). Because of detectable antibody titers to tetanus toxoid and diphtheria toxoid, it was suggested that antigen-specific T cells could be transferred via marrow transplants (199). It was also shown that although the antigen-specific B-cell precursor frequency was low, the majority of B-cell defects were primarily due to deficient function and not to low numbers (200).

The generally poor outcome of transplantation and the high frequency of chronic GVHD in older patients is thought to be due to impaired or absent thymic function (201). Circulating autoantibodies are often seen in patients with chronic GVHD (202). Antibodies are directed against double-stranded DNA, smooth muscle, mitochondria, and nucleoli. In some studies, the presence of multiple antibodies correlated with severity of chronic GVHD.

B. Infections

Long-term survivors with chronic GVHD have an increased risk of infection (191,203). Infections in patients with chronic GVHD may be of bacterial, fungal, or viral origin. Infections with encapsulated gram-positive bacteria are common and may cause septicemia, bronchopneumonia, sinusitis, etc. Late interstitial pneumonitis also occurs more frequently in patients with chronic GVHD (204). The etiology may be CMV, *Pneumocystis carinii*, adenovirus, parainfluenza, etc. In one study among 198 patients with extensive chronic GVHD, 28 (14%) developed late interstitial pneumonia (204). CMV was present in 19%, *Pneumocystis carinii* in 19%, varicellae zoster in 10%, and miscellaneous in 29%; no organism was identified in 23%.

There is concern that idiopathic interstitial pneumonia in patients with chronic GVHD may be caused by chronic GVHD involving the lung. Widespread pulmonary fibrosis has been reported as one of the manifestations of chronic GVHD that may respond to treatment with prednisolone and cyclosporine (205). To prevent *Pneumocystis carinii* and bacterial infections, patients with chronic GVHD are given prolonged prophylaxis with co-trimoxazole. Varicellae zoster infections occur in some 50% of bone marrow transplant recipients within the first year after bone marrow transplantation. Patients with chronic GVHD and the presence of nonspecific suppressor cells have an increased risk of developing varicella zoster (203). Varicella zoster infection should be treated with acyclovir to prevent dissemination.

C. Growth and Development in Children with Chronic GVHD

Chronic GVHD can markedly impair growth and development in children. This impairment is above and beyond what may be related to the impact of the conditioning regimen. The chronic nature of GVHD by itself, reduced activity level, and treatment with agents such as steroids interfere with longitudinal growth and sexual maturation. The problem is further aggravated by psychosocial problems that may result from disease effects and lack of rehabilitation (206).

XIV. PROPHYLAXIS AND TREATMENT OF CHRONIC GVHD

Prophylaxis and treatment are discussed elsewhere (Chap. 24). To prevent chronic GVHD, thymosine treatment, prednisolone treatment, or long-term prophylaxis with cyclosporine have been attempted (207–210). Therapy for chronic GVHD includes prednisolone, azathioprine, cyclosporine, and alternate-day prednisone, PUVA, thalidomide, and total lymphoid irradiation (89,91,186,211–214).

XV. IMPACT OF CHRONIC GVHD ON SURVIVAL

Severe chronic GVHD is associated with high mortality, mostly due to infectious complications. Even patients who survive chronic GVHD are often severely disabled. Mild chronic GVHD is associated with improved survival in patients with early leukemia due to a GVL effect, according to a study of more than 2000 patients performed by the IBMTR (148). The antileukemic effect of GVHD was previously shown in studies from Seattle, where chronic GVHD seemed to have a better antileukemic effect than acute GVHD (147). In a study from the IBMTR in patients with early leukemia receiving bone marrow from HLA-identical siblings and non-T-cell- depleted allografts, those with chronic GVHD had a relative risk of relapse of 0.43 compared to patients without GVHD ($p = 0.01$). In this study, chronic GVHD had a strong antileukemic effect in patients with acute and chronic myelocytic leukemia (AML and CML). A study from Seattle involving 1202 patients with leukemia showed that acute and chronic GVHD decreased the risk of relapse in patients with AML, acute lymphocytic leukemia (ALL), and CML transplanted in advanced disease (215). In a study of patients with AML and ALL transplanted in relapse, the probability of posttransplant relapse in those with chronic GVHD was 35%, compared to 74% in patients without GVHD ($p < 0.0001$). Actuarial survival was 62% in patients with chronic GVHD versus 25% in patients without GVHD ($p < 0.0009$). In patients with CML in accelerated phase or blast crisis, the probability of relapse after day 150 was 65% without GVHD and 35% with acute or chronic GVHD or both ($p < 0.02$). Among patients with AML in first remission or CML in chronic phase, (i.e., good-risk situations), GVHD had an adverse effect on survival and no apparent influence on relapse. This is in contrast to findings by the IBMTR, where a clear antileukemic effect of GVHD was seen in patients with early leukemia (148).

In a study of 85 patients from Johns Hopkins, the actuarial survival after onset of chronic GVHD was 42% (213). Factors predictive of death were progressive presentation (chronic GVHD following acute GVHD), lichenoid changes on skin biopsy, and elevation of serum bilirubin. Patients with any combination of two or more of these factors had a projected 6-year survival of 20%.

At Huddinge Hospital, we attempted to induce acute and chronic GVHD in marrow transplant recipients with leukemia by giving individualized GVHD prophylaxis (216). Patients with an anticipated low risk of GVHD were given methotrexate alone. Methotrexate plus cyclosporine was given to patients having a high risk of GVHD. Cyclosporine treatment was discontinued as early as possible after engraftment in the absence of GVHD, and weekly methotrexate was given until 3 months after BMT. Compared to historical controls, the incidence of chronic but not acute

GVHD was increased by individualized GVHD prophylaxis. In multivariate analyses, poor survival was related to high-risk leukemia and absence of chronic GVHD. The relative hazard of relapse in patients without chronic GVHD was 5.66 (p = 0.02). Thus, manipulation of the immunosuppressive regimen aimed at increasing the incidence of chronic GVHD may decrease the probability of relapse in patients with leukemia.

XVI. CONCLUSION

GVHD, both acute and chronic, continues to be a problem after allogeneic marrow (and peripheral blood stem-cell) transplantation. While current prophylaxis regimens have reduced the incidence and severity of GVHD in recipients of HLA-matched related marrow, the incidence remains high in recipients of HLA- nonidentical and unrelated marrow. The clinical appearance of GVHD has changed over the years, in part related to the use of cyclosporine combined with other immunosuppressive agents, in part due to better prophylaxis and therapy for infections. More specific immunosuppressive agents, including cytokines and cytokine inhibitors, are needed. Less toxic conditioning regimens and antileukemic modalities in the form of adoptive immunotherapy may modulate GVHD, yet preserve the anti-leukemic effects to improve long-term survival in marrow recipients with hematological malignancies. In contrast, in marrow transplant recipients with nonmalignant disorders, the most effective prevention of GVHD should be used.

ACKNOWLEDGMENTS

O.R. was supported by grants from the Swedish Cancer Foundation, the Children's Cancer Foundation, the Swedish Medical Research Council, and the Tobias Foundation. H.J.D. was supported by grants CA18029, CA15704, CA18221, and HL36444 from the National Institutes of Health, DHHS, and a grant from the National Marrow Donor Program/Baxter Health Care Division. We thank Sabine Dinse and Bonnie Larson and her colleagues for typing the manuscript.

REFERENCES

1. van Bekkum DW, de Vries JJ. Radiation Chimaeras. London, Logos, 1967.
2. Billingham RE, Brent I. A simple method for inducing tolerance of skin homografts in mice. Transplant Bull 1957; 4:67–71.
3. Santos GE, Cole LJ. Effect of donor and host lymphoid and myeloid tissue injections in healthy x- irradiated mice treated with rat bone marrow. J Natl Cancer Inst 1958; 21:279–293.
4. Billingham RE. The biology of graft-versus-host reactions. In: The Harvey Lectures. New York: Academic Press, 1966:21–78.
5. Gowans JL. The fate of parental strain small lymphocytes in Fl hybrid rats. Ann NY Acad Sci 1962; 99:432–455.
6. Medawar PB. Introduction: Definition of the immunologically competent cell. Ciba Foundation Study Group 1963; 16:1–5.
7. Owens AH Jr, Santos GW. The induction of graft-versus-host disease in mice treated with cyclophosphamide. J Exp Med 1958; 128:277–291.

8. McGregor DD. Bone marrow origin of immunologically competent lymphocytes in the rat. J Exp Med 1968; 127:953–966.
9. Grebe SC, Streilein JW. Graft-versus-host reactions: A review. Adv Immunol 1976; 22:119–221.
10. Renkonen R, Häyry P. Cellular infiltrates in the target organs associated with acute graft-versus-host disease. Bone Marrow Transplant 1987; 2:333–346.
11. Dicke KA, Tridente G, van Bekkum DW. The selective elimination of immunologically competent cells from bone marrow and lymphocytic cell mixtures: 3. In vitro test for detection of immunocompetent cells in fractionated mouse spleen cell suspensions and primate bone marrow suspensions. Transplantation 1969; 8:422–434.
12. Korngold R, Sprent J. T cell subsets and graft-versus-host disease. Transplantation 1987; 44:335–339.
13. Prentice HG, Blacklock HA, Janossy G, et al. Depletion of T lymphocytes in donor marrow prevents significant graft-versus-host disease in matched allogeneic leukaemic marrow transplant recipients. Lancet 1984; 1:472–476.
14. Maraninchi D, Gluckman E, Blaise D, et al. Impact of T-cell depletion on outcome of allogeneic bone-marrow transplantation for standard-risk leukaemias. Lancet 1987; 2: 175–178.
15. Hale G, Cobbold S, Waldmann H. T cell depletion with Campath-1 in allogeneic bone marrow transplantation. Transplantation 1988; 45:753–759.
16. Thomas ED, Storb R, Clift RA, et al. Bone-marrow transplantation (first of two parts). N Engl J Med 1975; 292:832–843.
17. Beatty PG, Clift RA, Mickelson EM, et al. Marrow transplantation from related donors other than HLA-identical siblings. N Engl J Med 1985; 313:765–771.
18. Ash RC, Horowitz MM, Gale RP, et al. Bone marrow transplantation from related donors other than HLA-identical siblings: Effect of T cell depletion. Bone Marrow Transplant 1991; 7:443–452.
19. Beatty PG, Hansen JA, Longton GM, et al. Marrow transplantation from HLA-matched unrelated donors for treatment of hematologic malignancies. Transplantation 1991; 51:443–447.
20. Hows J, Bradley BA, Gore S, et al. Prospective evaluation of unrelated donor bone marrow transplantation: The International Marrow Unrelated Search and Transplant (IMUST) Study. Bone Marrow Transplant 1993; 12:371–380.
21. Kernan NA, Bartsch G, Ash RC, et al. Analysis of 462 transplantations from unrelated donors facilitated by The National Marrow Donor Program. N Engl J Med 1993; 328: 593–602.
22. Marks DI, Cullis JO, Ward KN, et al. Allogeneic bone marrow transplantation from chronic myeloid leukemia using sibling and volunteer unrelated donors: A comparison of complications in the first 2 years. Ann Intern Med 1993; 119:207–214.
23. Ringdén O, Remberger M, Persson U, et al. Similar incidence of graft-versus-host disease using HLA-A, -B and -DR identical unrelated bone marrow donors as with HLA identical siblings. Bone Marrow Transplant. 1995; 15:619–625.
24. Guillen FJ, Ferrara J, Hancock WW, et al. Acute cutaneous graft-versus-host disease to minor histocompatibility antigens in a murine model: Evidence that large granular lymphocytes are effector cells in the immune response. Lab Invest 1986; 55:35–42.
25. Yamashita A, Hattori Y, Mori F, Kosaka A. Acquisition of graft-versus-host reactivity by immature thymocytes in the coexistence of activated macrophages. Transplantation 1982; 33:80–86.
26. Ford WL, Deeg HJ. Bone marrow transplantation, with emphasis on GVH reactions. Transplant Proc 1983; 15:1517–1519.
27. Livnat S, Seigneuret M, Storb R, Prentice RL. Analysis of cytotoxic effector cell function in patients with leukemia or aplastic anemia before and after marrow transplantation. J Immunol 1980; 124:481–490.

28. Dokhelar M-C, Wiels J, Lipinski M, et al. Natural killer cell activity in human bone marrow recipients. Transplantation 1981; 31:61–65.
29. Piguet P-F, Grau GE, Allet B, Vassalli P. Tumor necrosis factor/cachectin is an effector of skin and gut lesions of the acute phase of graft-vs-host disease. J Exp Med 1987; 166:1280–1289.
30. Holler E, Kolb HJ, Möller A, et al. Increased serum levels of TNFα precede major complications of bone marrow transplantation. Blood 1990; 75:1011–1016.
31. Tsoi MS. Immunological mechanisms of graft-versus-host disease in man. Transplantation 1982; 33:459–464.
32. Ringdén O, Witherspoon RP, Storb R, et al. Increased in vitro B-cell IgG secretion during acute graft-versus-host disease and infection: Observations in 50 human marrow transplant recipients. Blood 1980; 55:179–186.
33. Renkonen R, Wangel A, Häyry P. Bone marrow transplantation in the rat: B lymphocyte activation in acute graft-versus-host disease. Transplantation 1986; 41:290–296.
34. Storb R, Thomas ED. Allogeneic bone-marrow transplantation. Immunol Rev 1983; 71:77–102.
35. Ringdén O, Sundberg B, Lönnqvist B, et al. Allogeneic bone marrow transplantation for leukemia: Factors of importance for long-term survival and relapse. Bone Marrow Transplant 1988; 3:281–290.
36. Petersdorf EW, Smith AG, Mickelson EM, et al. The role of HLA-DPB1 disparity in the development of acute graft-versus-host disease following unrelated donor marrow transplantation. Blood 1993; 81:1923–1932.
37. Deeg HJ, Storb R, Weiden PL, et al. Abrogation of resistance to and enhancement of DLA-nonidentical unrelated marrow grafts in lethally irradiated dogs by thoracic duct lymphocytes. Blood 1979; 53:552–557.
38. Storb R, Doney KC, Thomas ED, et al. Marrow transplantation with or without donor buffy coat cells for 65 transfused aplastic anemia patients. Blood 1982; 59:236–246.
39. Niederwieser D, Pepe M, Storb R, et al. Improvement in rejection, engraftment rate and survival without increase in graft-versus-host disease by high marrow cell dose in patients transplanted for aplastic anemia. Br J Haematol 1988; 69:23–28.
40. Ringdén O, Deeg HJ, Beschorner W, Slavin S. Effector cells of graft-versus-host disease, host resistance, and the graft-versus-leukemia effect: Summary of a workshop on bone marrow transplantation. Transplant Proc 1987; 19:2758–2761.
41. Atkinson K, Biggs J, Cooley M, et al. A comparative study of T-cell depleted and non-depleted marrow transplantation for hematological malignancy. Aust NZ J Med 1987; 17:16–23.
42. Ringdén O, Pihlstedt P, Markling L, et al. Prevention of graft-versus-host disease with T cell depletion or cyclosporin and methotrexate: A randomized trail in adult leukemic marrow recipients. Bone Marrow Transplant 1991; 7:221–226.
43. Storb R, Prentice RL, Thomas Ed. Treatment of aplastic anemia by marrow transplantation from HLA identical siblings: Prognostic factors associated with graft versus host disease and survival. J Clin Invest 1977; 59:625–632.
44. de Gast GC, Gratama JW, Verdonck LF, et al. The influence of T cell depletion on recovery of T cell proliferation to herpesviruses and Candida after allogeneic bone marrow transplantation. Transplantation 1989; 48:111–115.
45. Ringdén O, Nilsson B. Death by graft-versus-host disease associated with HLA mismatch, high recipient age, low marrow cell dose, and splenectomy. Transplantation 1985; 40:39–44.
46. Baughan AS, Worsley AM, McCarthy DM, et al. Haematological reconstitution and severity of graft-versus-host disease after bone marrow transplantation for chronic granulocytic leukaemia: The influence of previous splenectomy. Br J Haematol 1984; 56:445–454.

47. Michallet M, Corront B, Bosson JL, et al. Risk factors for GVHD: Study of 157 patients from Bordeaux, Grenoble, Marseille. Bone Marrow Transplant 1988; 3(suppl 1):226.
48. Kiger N, Lenfant M. Prevention of graft-versus-host mortality in mice by preincubation of the graft with highly purified spleen-derived immunosuppressive peptides. Transplantation 1983; 36:243–246.
49. Korngold R, Sprent J. Lethal GVHD across minor histocompatibility barriers: Nature of the effector cells and role of the H-2 complex. Immunol Rev 1983; 71:5–29.
50. Gluckman E, Barrett AJ, Arcese W, et al. Bone marrow transplantation in severe aplastic anemia: A survey of the European Group for Bone Marrow Transplantation (EGBMT). Br J Haematol 1981; 49:165–173.
51. Bross DS, Tutschka PJ, Farmer ER, et al. Predictive factors for acute graft-versus-host disease in patients transplanted with HLA-identical bone marrow. Blood 1984; 63:1265–1270.
52. Atkinson K, Farrell C, Chapman G, et al. Female marrow donors increase the risk of acute graft-versus-host disease: Effect of donor age and parity and analysis of cell subpopulations in the donor marrow inoculum. Br J Haematol 1986; 63:231–239.
53. Gale RP, Bortin MM, van Bekkum DM, et al. Risk factors for acute graft-versus-host disease. Br J Haematol 1987; 67:397–406.
54. van Bekkum DW, Vos O. Treatment of secondary disease in radiation chimeras. Int J Radiat Biol 1961; 3:173–181.
55. Jones JM, Wilson R, Bealmear PM. Mortality and gross pathology of secondary disease in germfree mouse radiation chimeras. Radiat Res 1971; 45:577–588.
56. Heit H, Wilson R, Fliedner TM, Kohne E. Mortality of secondary disease in antibiotic-treated mouse radiation chimeras. In: Heneghan IJ, ed. Germfree Research. New York: Academic Press, 1973:447–483.
57. Vossen JM, Heidt PJ, Guiot HFL, Dooren LJ. Prevention of acute graft-versus-host disease in clinical bone marrow transplantation: Complete versus selective intestinal decontamination. In: Sasaki S, ed. Recent Advances in Germfree Research. Tokyo: Takai University Press, 1981:573–577.
58. Storb R, Prentice RL, Buckner CD, et al. Graft-versus-host disease and survival in patients with aplastic anemia treated by marrow grafts from HLA-identical siblings: Beneficial effect of a protective environment. N Engl J Med 1983; 308:302–307.
59. van Bekkum DW, Knaan S. Role of bacterial microflora in development of intestinal lesions from graft-versus-host reaction: Brief communication. J Natl Cancer Inst 1977; 58:787–789.
60. Gratama JW, Zwaan FE, Stijnen T, et al. Herpes-virus immunity and acute graft-versus-host disease. Lancet 1987; 1:471–474.
61. Boström L, Ringdén O, Sundberg B, et al. Pretransplant herpesvirus serology and acute graft-versus-host disease. Transplantation 1988; 46:548–552.
62. Boström L, Ringdén O, Gratama JW, et al. A role of herpes virus serology for the development of acute graft-versus-host disease. Bone Marrow Transplant 1990; 5:321–326.
63. Boström L, Ringdén O, Frosgren M. Strong donor mononuclear cell reactivity for herpes simplex virus (HSV) antigen in HSV immune donors combined with recipient seropositivity for HSV is associated with acute graft-versus-host disease. Scand J Immunol 1991; 34:45–52.
64. Singal DP, Rawls WE. Effects of herpes simplex virus antigens on human mixed lymphocyte culture. Transplantation 1980; 29:500–502.
65. Winston DJ, Ho WG, Lin C-H, et al. Intravenous immune globulin for prevention of cytomegalovirus infection and interstitial pneumonia after bone marrow transplantation. Ann Intern Med 1987; 106:12–18.

66. Sullivan KM, Kopecky KJ, Jocom J, et al. Immunomodulatory and antimicrobial efficacy of intravenous immunoglobulin in bone marrow transplantation. N Engl J Med 1990; 323:705–712.
67. Kawada K, Terasaki PI. Evidence for immunosuppression by high-dose gammaglobulin. Exp Hematol 1987; 15:133–136.
68. Shimozato T, Iwata M, Tamura N. Suppression of tumor necrosis factor alpha production by human immunoglobulin preparation for intravenous use. Infect Immun 1990; 58:1384–1390.
69. Storb R, Rudolph RH, Kolb HJ, et al. Marrow grafts between DL-A-matched canine littermates. Transplantation 1973; 15:92–100.
70. Lazarus HM, Coccia PF, Herzig RH, et al. Incidence of acute graft-versus-host disease with and without methotrexate prophylaxis in allogeneic bone marrow transplant patients. Blood 1984; 64:215–220.
71. Sullivan KM, Storb R, Witherspoon RP, et al. Deletion of immunosuppressive prophylaxis after marrow transplantation increases hyperacute graft-versus-host disease but does not influence chronic graft-versus-host disease or relapse in patients with advanced leukemia. Clin Transplant 1989; 3:5–11.
72. Ringdén O. Cyclosporine in allogeneic bone marrow transplantation. Transplantation 1986; 42:445–452.
73. Storb R, Deeg HJ, Whitehead J, et al. Methotrexate and cyclosporine compared with cyclosporine alone for prophylaxis of acute graft versus host disease after marrow transplantation for leukemia. N Engl J Med 1986; 314:729–735.
74. Ringdén O, Horowitz MM, Sondel P, et al. Methotrexate, cyclosporine, or both to prevent graft-versus-host disease after HLA-identical sibling bone marrow transplants for early leukemia? Blood 1993; 81:1094–1101.
75. Sparkes RS, Sparkes MC, Crist M, et al. NMSs antigen and graft versus host disease following bone marrow transplantation. Tissue Antigens 1989; 15:212–215.
76. Storb R, Prentice RL, Hansen JA, Thomas ED. Association between HLA-B antigens and acute graft-versus-host disease. Lancet 1983; 2:816–819.
77. Beschorner WE, Tutschka PJ, Farmer ER, Santos GW. Two histopathologic patterns of acute graft-versus-host disease in humans. Exp Hematol 1979; 7:99.
78. Glucksberg H, Storb R, Fefer A, et al. Clinical manifestations of graft-versus-host disease in human recipients of marrow from HL-A-matched sibling donors. Transplantation 1974; 18:295–304.
79. Deeg HJ, Storb R. Graft-versus-host disease: Pathophysiological and clinical aspects. Annu Rev Med 1984; 35:11–24.
80. Sale GE, Lerner KG, Barker EA, et al. The skin biopsy in the diagnosis of acute graft-versus-host disease in man. Am J Pathol 1977; 89:621–635.
81. Sale GE, Shulman HM. The Pathology of Bone Marrow Transplantation. New York: Masson Monographs in Diagnostic Pathology, 1984.
82. Jones RJ, Lee KS, Beschorner WE, et al. Venoocclusive disease of the liver following bone marrow transplantation. Transplantation 1987; 44:778–783.
83. McDonald GB, Sharma P, Matthews DE, et al. Venoocclusive disease of the liver after bone marrow transplantation: Diagnosis, incidence, and predisposing factors. Hepatology 1984; 4:116–122.
84. McDonald GB, Shulman HM, Sullivan KM, Spencer GD. Intestinal and hepatic complications of human bone marrow transplantation: Parts I and II. Gastroenterology 1986; 90:460–477, 770–784.
85. Sale GE, Shulman HM, McDonald GB, Thomas ED. Gastrointestinal graft-versus-host disease in man: A clinicopathologic study of the rectal biopsy. Am J Surg Pathol 1979; 3:291–299.

85A. Przepiorka D, Weisdorf D, Martin P, et al. Meeting Report: Consensus conference on acute GVHD grading. Bone Marrow Transplant. In press.
86. Groth CG, Gahrton G, Lundgren G, et al. Successful treatment with prednisolone of graft-versus-host disease in an allogeneic bone marrow transplant recipient. Scand J Haematol 1979; 22:333–338.
87. Weiden PL, Doney K, Storb R, Thomas ED. Anti-human thymocyte globulin (ATG) for prophylaxis and treatment of graft-versus-host disease in recipients of allogeneic marrow grafts. Transplant Proc 1978; 10:213–216.
88. Fibbe WE, Gratama JW, Teepe RGC, et al. Treatment of active chronic graft versus host disease of the skin with monoclonal antibody OKT3.Pan. Exper Hematol 1985; 13(suppl 17):137.
89. Hymes SR, Morison WL, Farmer ER, et al. Methoxsalen and ultraviolet A radiation in treatment of chronic cutaneous graft-versus-host reaction. J Am Acad Dermatol 1985; 12:30–37.
90. Hervé P, Racadot E, Wijdenes J, et al. Monoclonal anti TNF alpha antibody in the treatment of acute GvHD refractory both to corticosteroids and anti IL-2 R antibody. Bone Marrow Transplant 1991; 7(suppl 2):149.
91. Vogelsang GB, Santos GW, Colvin OM, Chen T. Thalidomide for graft-versus-host disease. Lancet 1988; 1:827.
92. Deeg HJ, Loughran TP Jr, Storb R, et al. Treatment of human acute graft-versus-host disease with antithymocyte globulin and cyclosporine with or without methylprednisolone. Transplantation 1985; 40:162–166.
93. Martin PJ, Hansen JA, Anasetti C, et al. Treatment of acute graft-versus-host disease with anti-CD3 monoclonal antibodies. Am J Kidney Dis 1988; 11:149–152.
94. Marks DI, Dousset B, Robson A, et al. Orthotopic liver transplantation for hepatic GVHD following allogeneic BMT for chronic myeloid leukaemia. Bone Marrow Transplant 1992; 10:463–466.
95. Cohen Z, Silverman R, Levy G, et al. Clinical small intestine transplantation using cyclosporine A and methylprednisolone. Transplant Proc 1987; 19:2588–2590.
96. Burdick JF, Vogelsang GB, Smith WJ, et al. Severe graft-versus-host disease in a liver-transplant recipient. N Engl J Med 1988; 318:689–691.
97. Herman JG, Beschorner WE, Baughman KL, et al. Pseudo-graft-versus-host disease in heart and heart-lung recipients. Transplantation 1988; 46:93–98.
98. Pflieger H. Graft-versus-host disease following blood transfusions. Blut 1983; 46:61–66.
99. Naiman JL, Punnett HH, Lischner HW, et al. Possible graft-versus-host reaction after intrauterine transfusion for Rh erythroblastosis fetalis. N Engl J Med 1969; 281:697–701.
100. Bastien J, Williams R, Ornelas W, et al. Maternal isoimmunization resulting in combined immunodeficiency and fatal graft versus host disease in an infant. Lancet 1984; 1:1435–1437.
101. Rappeport JM, Mihm M, Reinherz EL, et al. Acute graft-vs-host disease in recipients of bone marrow transplants from identical twin donors. Lancet 1979; 2:717–720.
102. Hess AD, Fischer AC. Immune mechanism in cyclosporine-induced syngeneic graft-versus-host disease. Transplantation 1989; 48:895–900.
103. Noel DR, Witherspoon RP, Storb R, et al. Does graft-versus-host disease influence the tempo of immunologic recovery after allogeneic human marrow transplantation? An observation on 56 long-term survivors. Blood 1978; 51:1087–1105.
104. Paulin T, Ringdén O, Nilsson B. Immunological recovery after bone marrow transplantation: Role of age, graft-versus-host disease, prednisolone treatment and infections. Bone Marrow Transplant 1987; 1:317–328.

105. Witherspoon RP, Storb E, Ochs HD, et al. Recovery of antibody production in human allogenic marrow graft recipients: Influence of time posttransplantation, the presence or absence of chronic graft-versus-host disease, and antithymocyte globulin treatment. Blood 1981; 58:360–368.
106. Meyers JD, Thomas ED. Infection complicating bone marrow transplantation. In: Rubin RH, Young LS, eds. Clinical Approach to Infection in the Immunocompromised Host. New York: Plenum Press, 1988:525–556.
107. Paulin T, Ringdén O, Nilsson B, et al. Variables predicting bacterial and fungal infections after allogeneic marrow engraftment. Transplantation 1987; 43:393–398.
108. Winston DJ, Gale RP, Meyer DV, et al. Infectious complications of human bone marrow transplantation. Medicine 1979; 58:1–31.
109. Watson JG. Problems of infection after bone marrow transplantation. J Clin Pathol 1983; 36:683–692.
110. Mattsson T, Heimdahl A, Dahllöf G, et al. Variables predicting oral mucosal lesions in allogenic bone marrow recipients. Head Neck 1991; 13:224–229.
111. Petersen FB, Clift RA, Hickman RO, et al. Hickman catheter complications in marrow transplant recipients. JPEN 1986; 10:58–62.
112. Meyers JD, Atkinson K. Infection in bone marrow transplantation. Clin Haematol 1983; 12:791–811.
113. Clift RA. Candidiasis in the transplant patient. Am J Med 1984; 77:34–38.
114. Tollemar J, Ringdén O, Boström L, et al. Variables predicting deep fungal infections in bone marrow transplant recipients. Bone Marrow Transplant 1989; 4:635–641.
115. Tollemar J, Holmberg K, Ringdén O, Lönnqvist B. Surveillance tests for the diagnosis of invasive fungal infections in bone marrow transplant recipients. Scand J Infect Dis 1989; 21:205–212.
116. Meyers JD, Flournoy N, Thomas ED. Infection with herpes simplex virus and cell-mediated immunity after marrow transplant. J Infect Dis 1980; 142:338–346.
117. Lundgren G, Wilczek H, Lönnqvist B, et al. Acyclovir prophylaxis in bone marrow transplant recipients. Scand J Infect Dis Suppl 1985; 47:137–144.
118. Lange B, Henle W, Meyers JD, et al. Epstein-Barr related serology in marrow transplant recipients. Int J Cancer 1980; 26:151–157.
119. Meyers JD, Flournoy N, Thomas ED. Nonbacterial pneumonia after allogeneic marrow transplantation: A review of ten years' experience. Rev Infect Dis 1982; 4:1119–1132.
120. Meyers JD, Flournoy N, Thomas ED. Risk factors for cytomegalovirus infection after human marrow transplantation. J Infect Dis 1986; 153:478–488.
121. Gratama JW, Middeldorp JM, Sinnige LG, et al. Cytomegalovirus immunity in allogeneic marrow grafting. Transplantation 1985; 40:510–514.
122. Paulin T, Ringdén O, Lönnqvist B, et al. The importance of pre bone marrow transplantation serology in determining subsequent cytomegalovirus infection. Scand J Infect Dis 1986; 18:199–209.
123. Miller W, Flynn P, McCullough J, et al. Cytomegalovirus infection after bone marrow transplantation: An association with acute graft-v-host disease. Blood 1986; 67:1162–1167.
124. Wasserman R, August CS, Plotkin SA. Viral infections in pediatric bone marrow transplant patients. Pediatr Infect Dis J 1988; 7:109–115.
125. Paulin T, Ringdén O, Lönnqvist B. Faster immunological recovery after bone marrow transplantation in patients without cytomegalovirus infection. Transplantation 1985; 39:377–384.
126. Gratama JW, Verdonck LF, van der Linden JA, et al. Cellular immunity to vaccinations and herpesvirus infections after bone marrow transplantation. Transplantation 1986; 41:719–724.

127. Bowden RA, Day LM, Amos DE, Meyers JD. Natural cytotoxic activity against cytomegalovirus-infected target cells following marrow transplantation. Transplantation 1987; 44:504–508.
128. Paulin T, Ringdén O, Ljungman P, Nilsson B. Symptomatic cytomegalovirus infection after bone marrow transplantation. Clin Transplant 1989; 3:279–285.
129. Cordonnier C, Bernaudin J-F, Bierling P, et al. Pulmonary complications occurring after allogeneic bone marrow transplantation: A study of 130 consecutive transplanted patients. Cancer 1986; 58:1047–1054.
130. Appelbaum FR, Meyers JD, Fefer A, et al. Nonbacterial nonfungal pneumonia following marrow transplantation in 100 identical twins. Transplantation 1982; 33:265–268.
131. Pecego R, Hill R, Appelbaum FR, et al. Interstitial pneumonitis following autologous bone marrow transplantation. Transplantation 1986; 42:515–517.
132. Grundy JE, Shanley JD, Shearer GM. Augmentation of graft-versus-host reaction by cytomegalovirus infection resulting in interstitial pneumonitis. Transplantation 1985; 39:548–553.
133. Reed EC, Bowden RA, Dandliker PS, et al. Efficacy of cytomegalovirus immunoglobulin in marrow transplant recipients with cytomegalovirus pneumonia. J Infect Dis 1987; 156:641–645.
134. Goodrich JM, Mori M, Gleaves CA, et al. Early treatment with ganciclovir to prevent cytomegalovirus disease after allogeneic bone marrow transplantation. N Engl J Med 1991; 325:1601–1607.
135. Schmidt GM, Horak DA, Niland JC, et al. A randomized, controlled trial of prophylactic ganciclovir for cytomegalovirus pulmonary infection in recipients of allogeneic bone marrow transplants. N Engl J Med 1991; 324:1005–1011.
136. Einsele H, Steidle M, Vallbracht A, et al. Early occurrence of human cytomegalovirus infection after bone marrow transplantation as demonstrated by the polymerase chain reaction technique. Blood 1991; 77:1104–1110.
137. Ringdén O, Lönnqvist B, Paulin T, et al. Pharmacokinetics, safety and preliminary clinical experiences using foscarnet in the treatment of cytomegalovirus infections in bone marrow and renal transplant recipients. J Antimicrob Chemother 1986; 17:373–387.
138. Pihlstedt P, Paulin T, Sundberg B, et al. Blood transfusion in marrow graft recipients. Ann Hematol 1992; 65:66–70.
139. Witherspoon RP, Deeg HJ, Storb R. Secondary malignancies after marrow transplantation for leukemia or aplastic anemia. Transplantation 1994; 57:1413–1418.
140. Witherspoon RP, Fisher LD, Schoch G, et al. Secondary cancers after bone marrow transplantation for leukemia or aplastic anemia. N Engl J Med 1989; 321:784–789.
141. Martin PJ, Hansen JA, Torok-Storb B, et al. Effects of treating marrow with a CD3-specific immunotoxin for prevention of acute graft-versus-host disease. Bone Marrow Transplant 1988; 3:437–444.
142. Lishner M, Patterson B, Kandel R, et al. Cutaneous and mucosal neoplasms in bone marrow transplant recipients. Cancer 1990; 65:473–476.
143. Socié G, Henry-Amar M, Cosset JM, et al. Increased incidence of solid malignant tumors after bone marrow transplantation for severe aplastic anemia. Blood 1991; 78: 277–279.
144. Bortin MM, Rimm AA, Salzstein EC, Rodey GE. Graft versus leukemia: III. Apparent independent antihost and antileukemic activity of transplanted immunocompetent cells. Transplantation 1973; 16:182–188.
145. Moscovitch M, Slavin S. Anti-tumor effects of allogeneic bone marrow transplantation in (NZB × NZW) F_1 hybrids with spontaneous lymphosarcoma. J Immunol 1984; 132:997–1000.
146. Weiden PL, Flournoy N, Thomas ED, et al. Antileukemic effect of graft-versus-host

disease in human recipients of allogeneic-marrow grafts. N Engl J Med 1979; 300: 1068–1073.
147. Weiden PL, Sullivan KM, Flournoy N, et al. Antileukemic effect of chronic graft-versus-host disease: Contribution to improved survival after allogeneic marrow transplantation. N Engl J Med 1981; 304:1529–1533.
148. Horowitz MM, Gale RP, Sondel PM, et al. Graft- versus-leukemia reactions following bone marrow transplantation in humans. Blood 1989; 75;555–562.
149. Fefer A, Sullivan KM, Weiden P, et al. Graft versus leukemia effect in man: The relapse rate of acute leukemia is lower after allogeneic than syngeneic marrow transplantation. In: Truitt RL, Gale RP, Bortin MM, eds. Cellular Immunotherapy of Cancer. New York: Liss, 1987:401–408.
150. Zwaan FE, Hermans J. Report of the EBMT-Leukaemia Working Party. Exp Hematol 1983; 11(suppl 13):3–6.
151. Barrett AJ, Horowitz MM, Gale RP, et al. Marrow transplantation for acute lymphoblastic leukemia: Factors affecting relapse and survival. Blood 1989; 74:862–871.
152. Apperley JF, Jones L, Hale G, et al. Bone marrow transplantation for patients with chronic myeloid leukaemia: T-cell depletion with Campath-1 reduces the incidence of graft-versus-host disease but may increase the risk of leukaemic relapse. Bone Marrow Transplant 1986; 1:53–66.
153. Goldman JM, Gale RP, Horowitz MM, et al. Bone marrow transplantation for chronic myelogenous leukemia in chronic phase: Increased risk of relapse associated with T-cell depletion. Ann Intern Med 1988; 108:806–814.
154. Aschan J, Ringdén O, Sundberg B, et al. Increased risk of relapse in patients with chronic myelogenous leukemia given T-cell depleted marrow compared to methotrexate combined with cyclosporin or monotherapy for the prevention of graft-versus-host disease. Eur J Haematol 1993; 50:269–274.
155. Saurat JH, Didier-Jean L, Gluckman E, Bussel A. Graft versus host reaction and lichen planus-like eruption in man. Br J Dermatol 1975; 92:591–592.
156. Siimes MA, Johansson E, Rapola J. Scleroderma-like graft-versus-host disease as late consequence of bone-marrow grafting. Lancet 1977; 2:831–832.
157. Hood AF, Soter NA, Rappeport J, Gigli I. Graft-versus-host reaction: Cutaneous manifestations following bone marrow transplantation. Arch Dermatol 1977; 113: 1087–1091.
158. Gratwohl AA, Moutsopopoulos HM, Chused TM. Sjögren-type syndrome after allogeneic bone marrow transplantation. Ann Intern Med 1977; 87:703.
159. Sullivan KM, Shulman HM, Storb R, et al. Chronic graft-versus-host disease in 52 patients: Adverse natural course and successful treatment with combination immunosuppression. Blood 1981; 57:267–276.
160. Storb R, Prentice RL, Sullivan KM, et al. Predictive factors in chronic graft-versus-host disease in patients with aplastic anemia treated by marrow transplantation from HLA-identical siblings. Ann Intern Med 1983; 98:461–466.
161. Ringdén O, Paulin T, Lönnqvist B, Nilsson B. An analysis of factors predisposing to chronic graft-versus-host disease. Exp Hematol 1985; 13:1062–1067.
162. Atkinson K, Horowitz MM, Gale RP, et al. Risk factors for chronic graft-versus-host disease after HLA-identical sibling bone marrow transplantation. Blood 1990; 75: 2459–2464.
163. Hamilton BL, Parkman R. Acute and chronic graft- versus-host disease induced by minor histocompatibility antigens in mice. Transplantation 1983; 36:150–155.
164. Beschorner WE, Tutschka PJ, Santos GW. Chronic graft-versus-host disease in the rat radiation chimera: I. Clinical features, hematology, histology and immunopathology in long-term chimeras. Transplantation 1982; 33:393–399.
165. Atkinson K, Shulman HM, Deeg HJ, et al. Acute and chronic graft-versus-host disease

in dogs given hemopoietic grafts from DLA-nonidentical littermates: Two distinct syndromes. Am J Pathol 1982; 108:196-205.
166. McCarthy PL Jr, Abhyankar S, Neben S, et al. Inhibition of interleukin-1 by an interleukin-1 receptor antagonist prevents graft-versus-host disease. Blood 1991; 78: 1915-1928.
167. Shulman HM, Sale GE, Lerner KG, et al. Chronic cutaneous graft-versus-host disease in man. Am J Pathol 1978; 91:545-570.
168. Shulman HM, Sullivan KM, Weiden P, et al. Chronic graft-versus-host syndrome in man: A long-term clinicopathologic study of 20 Seattle patients. Am J Med 1980; 69: 204-217.
169. Lampert IA, Janossy G, Suitters AJ, et al. Immunological analysis of the skin in graft versus host disease. Clin Exp Immunol 1982; 50:123-131.
170. DeClerck Y, Draper V, Parkman R. Clonal analysis of murine graft-vs-host disease: II. Leukokines that stimulate fibroblast proliferation and collagen synthesis in graft-vs.-host disease. J Immunol 1986; 136:3549-3552.
171. Lönnqvist B, Aschan J, Ljungman P, Ringdén O. Long-term cyclosporin therapy may decrease the risk of chronic graft-versus-host disease. Br J Haematol 1990; 74:547-548.
172. Jacobson N, Andersen HK, Skinhöj P, et al. Correlation between donor cytomegalovirus immunity and chronic graft-versus-host disease after allogeneic bone marrow transplantation. Scand J Haematol 1986; 36:499-506.
173. Jacobsen N, Badsberg JH, Lönnqvist B, et al. Predictive factors for chronic graft-versus-host disease and leukemic relapse after allogeneic bone marrow transplantation. In: Baum SJ, Santos GW, Takaku F, eds. Experimental Hematology Today:1987. New York: Springer-Verlag, 1987:161-164.
174. Boström L, Ringdén O, Sundberg B, et al. Pretransplant herpes virus serology and chronic graft-versus-host disease. Bone Marrow Transplant 1989; 4:547-552.
175. Boström L, Ringdén O, Jacobsen N, et al. A European multicenter study of chronic graft-versus-host disease: The role of cytomegalovirus serology in recipients and donors—Acute graft-versus-host disease, and splenectomy. Transplantation 1990; 49: 1100-1105.
176. Karnofsky DA, Burchenal JH. The clinical evaluation of chemotherapeutic agents in cancer. In: Macleod CM, ed. Evaluation of Chemotherapeutic Agents. New York: Columbia University Press, 1949:191-205.
177. Schubert MM, Sullivan KM, Morton TH, et al. Oral manifestations of chronic graft-vs-host disease. Arch Intern Med 1984; 144:1591-1595.
178. Heimdahl A, Johnson G, Danielsson KH, et al. Oral condition of patients with leukemia and severe aplastic anemia: Follow-up 1 year after bone marrow transplantation. Oral Surg Oral Med Oral Pathol 1985; 60:498-504.
179. Sale GE, Shulman HM, Schubert MM, et al. Oral and ophthalmic pathology of graft versus host disease in man: Predictive value of the lip biopsy. Hum Pathol 1981; 12: 1022-1030.
180. McDonald GB, Sullivan KM, Plumley TF. Radiographic features of esophageal involvement in chronic graft-vs-host disease. Am J Roentgenol 1984; 142:501-506.
181. McDonald GB, Sale GE. The human gastrointestinal tract after allogeneic marrow transplantation in humans. In: Sale GE, Shulman HM, eds. The Pathology of Bone Marrow Transplantation. New York: Masson, 1984:77-103.
182. Roca J, Granena A, Rodriquez-Roison R, et al. Fatal airway disease in an adult with chronic graft- versus-host disease. Thorax 1982; 37:77-78.
183. Wyatt SE, Nunn P, Hows JM, et al. Airways obstruction associated with graft-versus-host disease after bone marrow transplantation. Thorax 1984; 39:887-894.
184. Ralph DD, Springmeyer SC, Sullivan KM, et al. Rapidly progressive air-flow obstruc-

tion in marrow transplant recipients: Possible association between obliterative bronchiolitis and chronic graft-versus- host disease. Am Rev Respir Dis 1984; 129:641–644.
185. Corson SL, Sullivan K, Batzer F, et al. Gynecologic manifestations of chronic graft-versus-host disease. Obstet Gynecol 1982; 60:488–492.
186. Sullivan KM, Witherspoon RP, Storb R, et al. Prednisone and azathioprine compared with prednisone and placebo for treatment of chronic graft-v-host disease: Prognostic influence of prolonged thrombocytopenia after allogeneic marrow transplantation. Blood 1988; 72:546–554.
187. Smith CIE, Aarli JA, Biberfeld P, et al. Myasthenia gravis after bone-marrow transplantation: Evidence of a donor origin. N Engl J Med 1983; 309:1565–1568.
188. Reyes MG, Noronha P, Thomas W Jr, Heredia R. Myositis of chronic graft versus host disease. Neurology 1983; 33:1222–1224.
189. Gomez-Garcia P, Herrera-Arroyo C, Torrez-Gomez A, et al. Renal involvement in chronic graft-versus-host disease: A report of two cases. Bone Marrow Transplant 1988; 3:357–362.
190. Ruutu T, Ruutu M, Volin L, Leskinen R. Severe cystitis as a manifestation of chronic graft-versus- host disease after bone marrow transplantation. Br J Urol 1988; 62:612–613.
191. Atkinson K, Storb R, Prentice RL, et al. Analysis of late infections in 89 long-term survivors of bone marrow transplantation. Blood 1979; 53:720–731.
192. Lum LG, Seigneuret MC, Storb RF, et al. In vitro regulation of immunoglobulin synthesis after marrow transplantation: I. T-cell and B-cell deficiencies in patients with and without chronic graft-versus-host disease. Blood 1981; 58:431–439.
193. Lum LG, Orcutt-Thordarson N, Seigneuret MC, Storb R. The regulation of Ig synthesis after marrow transplantation: IV. T4 and T8 subset function in patients with chronic graft-versus-host disease. J Immunol 1982; 129:113–119.
194. Reinherz EL, Parkman R, Rappeport J, et al. Aberrations of suppressor T cells in human graft-versus-host disease. N Engl J Med 1979; 300:1061–1068.
195. Tsoi MS, Storb R, Dobbs S, Thomas ED. Specific suppressor cells in graft-host tolerance of HLA- identical marrow transplantation. Nature 1981; 292:355–357.
196. Tsoi MS, Storb R, Dobbs S, et al. Specific suppressor cells and immune response to host antigens in long-term human allogeneic marrow recipients: Implications for the mechanisms of graft-host tolerance and chronic graft-versus-host disease. Transplant Proc 1981; 13:237–240.
197. Friedrich W, O'Reilly RJ, Koziner B, et al. T-lymphocyte reconstitution in recipients of bone marrow transplants with and without GVHD: Imbalances of T-cell subpopulations having unique regulatory and cognitive functions. Blood 1982; 59:696–701.
198. Korsmeyer SJ, Elfenbein GJ, Goldman CK, et al. B cell, helper T cell, and suppressor T cell abnormalities contribute to disordered immunoglobulin synthesis in patients following bone marrow transplantation. Transplantation 1982; 33:184–190.
199. Shiobara S, Lum LG, Witherspoon RP, Storb R. Antigen specific antibody responses of lymphocytes to tetanus toxoid after human marrow transplantation. Transplantation 1986; 41:587–592.
200. Jin N-R, Lum LG. IgG anti-tetanus toxoid antibody production induced by Epstein-Barr virus from B cells of human marrow transplant recipients. Cell Immunol 1986; 101:266–273.
201. Atkinson K, Incefy GS, Storb R, et al. Low serum thymic hormone levels in patients with chronic graft- versus-host disease. Blood 1982; 59:1073–1077.
202. Lister J, Messner H, Keystone E, et al. Autoantibody analysis of patients with graft versus host disease. J Clin Lab Immunol 1987; 24:19–23.
203. Atkinson K, Farewell V, Storb R, et al. Analysis of late infections after human bone marrow transplantation: Role of genotypic nonidentity between marrow donor and

recipient and of nonspecific suppressor cells in patients with chronic graft-versus- host disease. Blood 1982; 60:714–720.
204. Sullivan KM, Meyers JD, Flournoy N, et al. Early and late interstitial pneumonia following human bone marrow transplantation. Int J Cell Cloning 1986; 4:107–121.
205. Raschko JW, Cottler-Fox M, Abbondanzo SL, et al. Pulmonary fibrosis after bone marrow transplantation responsive treatment with prednisone and cyclosporine. Bone Marrow Transplant 1989; 4:201–205.
206. Sanders JE. Effects of chronic graft-vs.-host disease on growth and development. In: Burakoff S, Deeg HJ, Ferrara J, Atkinson K, eds. Graft-vs.-Host Disease. New York: Marcel Dekker, 1981.
207. Atkinson K, Storb R, Ochs HD, et al. Thymus transplantation after allogeneic bone marrow graft to prevent chronic graft-versus-host disease in humans. Transplantation 1982; 33:168–173.
208. Witherspoon RP, Sullivan KM, Lum LG, et al. Use of thymic grafts or thymic factors to augment immunologic recovery after bone marrow transplantation: Brief report with 2 to 12 years' follow-up. Bone Marrow Transplant 1988; 3:425–435.
209. Blume KG, Beutler E, Bross KJ, et al. Bone-marrow ablation and allogeneic marrow transplantation in acute leukemia. N Engl J Med 1980; 302:1041–1046.
210. Lindholm A, Zucker W, Ringdén O, Lönnqvist B. Long term cyclosporine treatment in bone marrow transplant recipients. Bone Marrow Transplant 1986; 1(suppl 1):85.
211. Deeg HJ, Ullrich SE. Ultraviolet irradiation for the prevention and treatment of allosensitization and graft-versus-host disease. In: Atkinson K, ed. Clinical Bone Marrow Transplantation: A Reference Textbook. Cambridge, England: Cambridge University Press, 1994:668–675.
212. Sullivan KM, Witherspoon RP, Storb R, et al. Alternating-day cyclosporine and prednisone for treatment of high-risk chronic graft-v-host disease. Blood 1988; 72:555–561.
213. Wingard JR, Piantadosi S, Vogelsang GB, et al. Predictors of death from chronic graft versus host disease after bone marrow transplantation. Blood 1989; 74:1428–1435.
214. Socié G, Devergie A, Cosset JM, et al. Low- dose (one gray) total-lymphoid irradiation of extensive, drug-resistant chronic graft-versus-host disease. Transplantation 1990; 49:657–658.
215. Sullivan KM, Weiden R, Storb RP, et al. Influence of acute and chronic graft-versus-host disease on relapse and survival after bone marrow transplantation from HLA-identical siblings as treatment of acute and chronic leukemia. Blood 1989; 73:1720–1728.
216. Aschan J, Ringdén O, Andström E, et al. Individualized prophylaxis against graft-versus-host disease in leukemic marrow transplant recipients. Bone Marrow Transplant 1994; 14:79–87.

20

The Immunobiology of Syngeneic/ Autologous Graft-versus-Host Disease

Allan D. Hess
Johns Hopkins Oncology Center
Johns Hopkins University School of Medicine
Baltimore, Maryland

I. INTRODUCTION

Graft-versus-host disease (GVHD) occurs after allogeneic bone marrow transplantation (BMT) and is classically thought to be due to the response of donor lymphocytes to foreign histocompatibility antigens of the recipient (1). A GVHD-like syndrome can occur, however, after marrow transplantation performed between identical twins (syngeneic) or after autologous BMT (2–5). The occurrence of an autologous or syngeneic GVHD was met with great skepticism, since it challenged the universal concept that histocompatibility differences between donor and host are absolute requirements for the induction of GVHD, as postulated by Billingham (6). Moreover, the development of GVHD after autologous and syngeneic BMT also raised fundamental questions regarding our understanding of the immunobiology of GVHD, the antigens that induce this reaction, and the reconstitution of self tolerance in the lymphohematopoietic chimera. In fact, it is the disruption of both peripheral and central mechanisms governing self tolerance that leads to autologous/syngeneic GVHD.

Acquisition of tolerance to self antigens is not limited to the developing immune system in the neonate but must also occur after autologous or syngeneic BMT (7). Reconstitution of the immune system after autologous/syngeneic BMT occurs quite rapidly with effective self-nonself recognition and normal T-cell function. Certainly, the developing immune system after BMT (autologous/syngeneic and allogeneic!) is subject to a variety of insults (drugs, infectious agents) that may result in perturbation of the immune system, leading to dysregulation of self-nonself discrimination. Recent studies, in fact, demonstrate that the reconstitution of central and peripheral tolerance mechanisms can be readily disrupted after autologous/ syngeneic BMT, leading to severe autoaggression. Administration of the immunosuppressive drug cyclosporin A (CsA) following autologous or syngeneic BMT results in the induction of a T-lymphocyte-mediated autoimmune syndrome with pathology indistinguishable from GVHD after allogeneic BMT; hence, the autoimmune syndrome induced with CsA was termed syngeneic GVHD (8,9). These observations were indeed surprising and paradoxical, since CsA is the front-line immunosuppressive agent used to prevent solid organ allograft rejection, to prevent GVHD after allogeneic BMT, and to treat a variety of autoimmune diseases (10–13). The finding that, under certain experimental conditions, CsA specifically disrupts the mechanisms that mediate self tolerance challenges our understanding of the immunobiology of a very important immunosuppressive drug. More importantly, however, the induction of syngeneic GVHD by the administration of CsA provides a unique model system that may allow us to dissect further the fundamental processes of self-nonself discrimination.

The present review discusses the immunobiology of CsA-induced syngeneic GVHD with a particular emphasis on the effector mechanisms and on the disruption of central and peripheral processes that govern tolerance to self antigens. Although the salient features and mechanisms responsible for the induction syngeneic GVHD are known, many questions regarding this complex autoimmunological process remain unresolved. Nevertheless, the induction of autologous/syngeneic GVHD provides a significant antitumor effect after BMT. The application of this unique syndrome to clinical autologous BMT as antitumor immunotherapy will also be summarized.

II. INDUCTION OF SYNGENEIC GVHD

A. Initial Studies

The experimental induction of syngeneic GVHD after autologous or syngeneic BMT was first reported by Glazier et al. (8). Lethally irradiated rats reconstituted with syngeneic bone marrow and treated with CsA for 40 days develop a severe autoaggression syndrome 14 to 28 days after discontinuation of CsA treatment; non-CsA-treated syngeneic marrow recipients recover normally. The affected recipients with this autoaggressive disease exhibit erythroderma of the ears, dermatitis, and hair loss, classic clinical signs of GVHD. Histological evaluation reveals lesions characteristic of acute GVHD in the skin, tongue, and liver. Of particular interest is the presence of lymphocytic exocytosis, vacuolar changes in the basal layer, epidermal destruction, and dyskeratosis in the skin. The observed histological damage in this autoaggression syndrome is indistinguishable from the damage observed in GVHD after allogeneic BMT and included similar target organs (8,9). More recent studies show that following the onset of an acute syngeneic GVHD, there is a rapid progression to a chronic phase with complete alopecia, fibrosis, and scleroderma (9,14). Furthermore, the acute and chronic phases of syngeneic GVHD appear to be mediated by distinct autoreactive effector T cells, reflecting the histological damage observed (see below) (15). Of additional importance in this initial report is the observation that syngeneic GVHD could be induced in animals undergoing autologous marrow reconstitution after receiving total body irradiation, but with lead shielding of the tibia. The induction of syngeneic GVHD after autologous recovery rules out minor antigen differences due to genetic drift among syngeneic rats as the target antigens responsible for initiating this autoaggressive syndrome. Since GVHD after syngeneic BMT and CsA therapy and after allogeneic BMT are indistinguishable histologically, this single observation also reverses a landmark concept that histocompatibility differences are absolute requirements for the induction of GVHD, as postulated by Billingham (6). These observations suggest that the aberrant recognition of self antigens in syngeneic GVHD may also occur after allogeneic BMT. In fact, autoreactivity in chronic GVHD after allogeneic BMT can be documented (16,17).

B. Basic Requirements Necessary for the Induction of Syngeneic GVHD

Since the initial description of syngeneic GVHD, a number of studies clearly identify three important factors necessary for the induction of this autoaggression syndrome and provide some insight into this complex immunobiological process. First, syngeneic GVHD only occurs in syngeneic BMT recipients treated with CsA, indicating that this novel drug is an essential requirement. Second, irradiation or cytotoxic agents that ablate the lymphohematopoietic system also play an essential role. Cheney and Sprent (18) and Glazier et al. (9) reported that normal, nontransplanted animals treated with CsA generally do not develop this autoaggression syndrome, implicating a peripheral regulatory mechanism. The third essential requirement is an intact thymus. As shown by Sorokin et al. (19), syngeneic GVHD cannot be induced in thymectomized animals but requires the presence of an intact thymus.

It is important to note that recent studies question the role of irradiation in the induction of syngeneic GVHD. Shinozawa et al. (20) and Beschorner et al. (21) suggest that irradiation is not essential. Syngeneic GVHD can be induced if nonirradiated animals are treated with CsA for prolonged periods of time (>6 months) or if they are thymectomized at the end of the CsA treatment period (20,21). It appears that irradiation enhances the ability of CsA to induce this autoaggression syndrome by ablating the lymphohematopoietic system and by damaging the thymus. It follows that the peripheral lymphohematopoietic system can modify the induction of syngeneic GVHD. This premise is supported by recent investigations suggesting that the age of the animals is another critical requirement. Studies by Fischer and Hess in a rat model demonstrate that there is a correlation of age with the successful induction of syngeneic GVHD (22). Virtually a 100% incidence of syngeneic GVHD is observed if the animals are transplanted and treated with CsA prior to 6 weeks of age. Thereafter, the incidence of syngeneic GVHD decreases dramatically with the increasing age of the animals. Of particular importance in these studies is the finding that not only the age of the recipient is a significant variable but the age of the marrow donor has an even greater effect. Syngeneic GVHD can be consistently induced in older animals if the marrow is derived from animals under the age of 6 weeks, but not if the marrow donors are greater than 6 months of age. This autoimmune syndrome can be readily induced with marrow from older (6 months) animals, however, if the marrow is first depleted of mature T cells. Subsequently, the mature T cells in marrow from older animals were shown to have a powerful regulatory effect on the induction of syngeneic GVHD even when mixed with marrow from very young animals. These data support the hypothesis that mature peripheral T lymphocytes must be ablated by irradiation, since they exert a negative regulatory influence on the induction of syngeneic GVHD.

In summary, three essential requirements are necessary for the induction of syngeneic GVHD: (a) CsA treatment, (b) irradiation, and (c) an intact thymus. The requirements for irradiation to ablate the lymphohematopoietic system and an intact thymus, in fact, represent the peripheral and central lymphoid organs. Operationally, these observations suggest that the induction of syngeneic GVHD was at least two-tiered, requiring the elimination of the peripheral immune system and an active alteration of normal thymic function mediated by CsA treatment. The studies discussed below will show that CsA prevents the clonal deletion of autoreactive T cells in the thymus; in the absence of a peripheral autoregulatory mechanism (eliminated by irradiation), a permissive environment is provided for the activation and expansion of the autoreactive T cells and the subsequent generation of autoaggression.

III. EFFECTOR MECHANISMS IN SYNGENEIC GVHD

A. Target Antigens

Initial studies in the syngeneic GVHD model demonstrate that this autoaggression syndrome could be specifically transferred to secondary recipients with splenic T lymphocytes (9). These early studies, however, offer no indication of the complexity of the effector mechanisms, identification of the T-cell subsets involved, or the target antigens recognized in syngeneic GVHD. Because of the prominent effect of CsA on the reduction of major histocompatibility complex (MHC) class II antigen in the thymus, it seemed reasonable to assume that class II MHC determinants would be one of the primary target antigens in syngeneic GVHD, since developing T cells would fail to "learn" that these determinants are self (18,23,24). Although in retrospect this hypothesis is too simple, the experimental data supported this initial concept.

Initial studies by Hess et al. demonstrate that the induction of syngeneic GVHD is associated with the development of autoreactive $CD8^+$ cytotoxic T cells (24). These cells can be detected in the spleens of animals at the onset of syngeneic GVHD. Furthermore, the cytotoxic T cells associated with this autoaggression syndrome recognize a public determinant of MHC class II antigens, since, in addition to self, the effector cells are capable of lysing PHA blast cells from several different MHC disparate strains of rats. The lysis of the blast cells is effectively blocked by pretreating the target cells with monoclonal antibodies recognizing a public determinant on the MHC class II molecule. In contrast, anti-MHC class I–specific antibodies were ineffective. Additional blocking studies reveal that the RT1.B or I-A determinant is preferentially recognized by the cytolytic effector T cells in syngeneic GVHD, in contrast to minimal or no recognition of the RT1.D (I-E) determinant (25,29). Sorokin et al. also provided evidence that a $CD4^+$ autoreactive cell in a CsA-induced autoimmune model recognized self class II public MHC determinants (19).

The in vitro data clearly suggest that class II MHC determinants are the target antigens in syngeneic GVHD, and this is supported by initial in vivo studies attempting to block the development of syngeneic GVHD by treatment with monoclonal antibodies (25,29). Administration of antibody to the MHC class II determinant effectively delays or prevents the onset of syngeneic GVHD after adoptive transfer of effector cells. Furthermore, antibody to the RT1.B(I-A) subregion determinant was far superior at preventing development of syngeneic GVHD than treatment with antibodies to the RT1.D (I-E) antigen. These data parallel the in vitro studies showing that the effector cells in syngeneic GVHD predominantly recognize the RT1.B (I-A) antigen (25,29). On the other hand, administration of McAb to class I MHC determinants, also ineffective in vitro, fails to prevent the adoptive transfer of disease. Based on the observations that there is no alteration in the number of circulating T-cell subsets, it is likely that the antibodies to MHC class II determinants prevented recognition of these antigens in vivo. Similar results demonstrating the efficacy of treatment with McAb to MHC class II antigens were reported in several models of autoimmunity and in prolongation of xenogeneic islet transplants (26,27). In further support that MHC class II are the target antigens, recent studies in the mouse suggest that CsA induces an autoimmune syndrome primarily limited to the colon, which is due to MHC class II autoreactive T cells (28).

The apparent recognition of a public epitope by the effector cells from animals with syngeneic GVHD as defined in vitro, is rather perplexing. Studies utilizing $F_1 \rightarrow$ parent chimeras also provide evidence that a public determinant on the MHC class II antigen is recognized in vitro in syngeneic GVHD (29). Classically, GVHD does not develop in parental strain animals grafted with marrow from F_1 donors. Administration of CsA to $F_1 \rightarrow$ P chimeras, however, results in the induction of syngeneic GVHD. Effector T cells from $F_1 \rightarrow$ parent chimeras with syngeneic GVHD induced by CsA treatment after BMT transfer the disease into both parental strains. Thus, the effector cells recognized the class II MHC antigen on both parental strains. These data suggest that the thymic-dependent development and the specificity of the autoreactive T cells are not restricted by the MHC haplotype of the recipient thymus or the target tissue. A similar conclusion is provided by Babcock et al., who showed that development of syngeneic GVHD was dependent on the presence of a thymus but independent of its MHC haplotype (30). Thymectomized Lewis rats grafted with deoxyguanosine treated thymi from MHC-disparate DA-strain rats, develop syngeneic GVHD after syngeneic (Lewis donors) BMT and CsA treatment. Taken together, these data strongly support the concept that a MHC class II public determinant on the framework of the molecule is the target antigen in syngeneic GVHD. We cannot exclude, however, the recognition of a common minor antigenic peptide bound to class II molecules that mimics "public determinant" recognition in the $F_1 \rightarrow$ parent setting or the presentation of a highly conserved peptide fragment of MHC class II antigens, such as the invariant chain that can occupy the MHC class II binding site (31). Since CD8 and CD4 T cells primarily are associated with MHC class I and class II responses respectively, it is also possible that the recognition of class II molecules by $CD8^+$ autocytotoxic T cells rather than $CD4^+$ lymphocytes is promiscuous, since the appropriate accessory molecule is not present. Additional studies are needed to explore this issue.

B. Effector T-Cell Subsets

Although the demonstration that MHC class II specific autoreactive cytotoxic T cells appear with the onset of syngeneic GVHD could be a simple explanation of the pathogenesis of this autoaggression syndrome, recent studies suggest that syngeneic GVHD is more complex, requiring interaction between $CD8^+$ and $CD4^+$ autoreactive T cells (15). Furthermore, syngeneic GVHD can be separated into acute and chronic phases, each with distinct histology, suggesting two separate or interrelated immunological processes (14,32).

Initial histological evaluation reveals two separate phases of autoaggression. At the onset of syngeneic GVHD, the histology show changes primarily consistent with an acute response (dyskeratosis, epidermal lymphocyte infiltration), while later, these changes appear more chronic, with prominent fibrosis and dermal lymphocyte infiltration. The predominance of the $CD4^+$ T-helper-cell subset in the chronic GVHD phase is similar to the infiltrates associated with allogeneic chronic GVHD and with delayed-type hypersensitivity reactions (33,34). It is of interest that the histological damage observed also reflects differential infiltration of distinct T-lymphocyte subsets (14). At the onset of syngeneic GVHD, the majority of the infiltrating lymphocytes are the $CD8^+$ cytotoxic/suppressor T cells, which is consistent with the epithelial cell destruction observed histologically. During the chronic phase, however, the majority of the lymphocytes are $CD4^+$ T lymphocytes. The distinct immunobiological activities of the autoreactive $CD4^+$ and $CD8^+$ T-lymphocyte subsets were confirmed in adoptive transfer studies (15). Large numbers of $CD8^+$ T cells from animals with syngeneic GVHD only transfer a self-limited acute phase of the disease into secondary recipients that resolves within 2 weeks, whereas the $CD4^+$ subset by itself is ineffective. Progression of disease and development of chronic syngeneic GVHD, however, requires the addition of the $CD4^+$ T-helper-cell subset. Moreover, the onset of syngeneic GVHD correlates with the emergence of the $CD4^+$ T-cell subset in the peripheral blood (35,36). These data suggest that $CD4^+$ autoreactive T-helper cells play an essential role in amplifying the activity of the autoreactive $CD8^+$ cytolytic T cells and allowing the progression to the chronic phase. It appears likely that the autoreactive T-helper subset provides an amplification signal (i.e., IL-2) for the $CD8^+$ autocytoxic T cell, allowing subsequent clonal expansion and development of autoaggression. In fact, recent studies by Urdahl et al. in a murine system demonstrate that CsA treatment allows for the production of IL-2- producing autoreactive T-helper cells (38). On the other hand, it is important to note that in the rat model, addition of recombinant IL-2 does not amplify the $CD8^+$ but is effective at enhancing the adoptive transfer of syngeneic GVHD only if both $CD4^+$ and $CD8^+$ autoreactive T cells are present (15). These data suggest that an additional CD4-dependent factor is required to enhance autoaggression mediated by $CD8^+$ autoreactive T cells. Furthermore, cytokine production by the autoreactive T-helper-cell subset may also be responsible for the fibrosis observed in the chronic phase (16). Additional studies are required to identify the cytokines released to determine if the autoreactive $CD4^+$ T lymphocytes consist of both Th1 and Th2 type helper T cells, particularly since CsA can alter or modify Th1/Th2 responses (38). Similarly, it is unknown if amplification of the acute phase and the induction of the chronic phase are due to identical autoreactive T-helper populations with identical cytokine profiles. In this regard, recent studies by Fischer et al. suggest that there are two discrete T-helper populations defined by expression of the $V\beta$ 8.5 and $V\beta$ 10 T-cell receptor elements.

C. Limited T-Cell-Receptor V Region Repertoire of Syngeneic GVHD Autoreactive T Lymphocytes

The initial observation that set the stage for study of T-cell-receptor diversity in autoimmune disease was reported by Ben-Nunn et al., who demonstrated that irradiated autoreactive T-lymphocyte lines used as vaccines in naive animals confer protection or resistance to disease (40). The argument was raised that since the protection was specific, the diversity of the autoreactive T-cell receptor must be quite limited. Based on this assumption, several studies in a variety of autoimmune disorders suggest that the repertoire of autoreactive T cells may be quite limited, at least with respect to Vβ-region T-cell-receptor gene determinants (41–43). Apart from the obvious potential to control autoimmune disease by administration of V-region-specific antibodies, evaluation and identification of the genetic determinants of the autoreactive T-cell receptor in autoimmune models, such as syngeneic GVHD, will provide new insights into autoaggression, including the potential interaction with superantigens. In addition, identification of the autoreactive T-cell-receptor determinants will allow the opportunity to track the autoreactive T lymphocytes and determine potential interaction with peripheral regulatory mechanisms.

Recent studies in the Lewis rat evaluated the autoimmune T-cell receptor of T-cell clones from several models of autoimmunity, including experimental autoimmune encephalitis (EAE), experimental allergic neuritis (EAN), and adjuvant arthritis (AA) (44). Despite the fact that the clones are antigen-specific for each disease (antigen specificity conferred by the CD3 domain), there is an apparent restriction to the Vβ 8 family of T-cell receptor genes. Additionally, the autoreactive TcR in the Lewis rat recognizes the autoantigens in association with MHC class II determinants, the target antigen of syngeneic GVHD (44). Based on this evidence, initial studies assessed the role of Vβ 8^+ T cells in syngeneic GVHD. Severino et al. showed that CsA treatment following syngeneic BMT results in a marked increase in Vβ 8^+ T cells, which is primarily confined to the $CD8^+$ T-cell subset (45). Based on this study, Severino et al. suggest that a shift in the $CD4^+/CD8^+$ ratio of cells expressing the autoreactive Vβ 8 TcR may be an important factor in the breakdown of self-nonself recognition in the developing immune system. Since Vβ 8 T cells are not normally clonally deleted and are apparently preferentially confined to the $CD4^+$ T-cell subset, they postulate that, in the rat model of syngeneic GVHD, CsA primarily interferes with the thymic selection of $CD8^+$ T cells (45,46). Under normal circumstances, $CD8^+$ T cells expressing a T-cell receptor with a high affinity for class I MHC antigens are produced while clonally deleting the majority of $CD8^+$ T cells that have a T-cell receptor with a high affinity for class II MHC antigens (47).

Recent studies in our laboratory provide direct evidence that the Vβ 8.5/8.3 population is a major component of the autoreactive T-cell compartment in syngeneic GVHD, although a second population is also present (39). Adoptive transfer of syngeneic GVHD effector T cells in irradiated thymectomized secondary recipients reconstituted with T-cell-depleted marrow provides a selective environment (antigen-driven) for the preferential expansion of autoreactive T cells. Analysis of target tissues from these animals by the reverse transcriptase polymerase chain reaction using Vβ-specific oligonucleotide primers reveals T cells predominantly expressing the Vβ 8.5/8.3 and Vβ 10 TcR elements. More importantly, depletion of T cells from the effector population with a monoclonal antibody to the Vβ 8.5/8.3 determinant abrogates the ability to transfer syngeneic GVHD in this setting. Depletion of Vβ 10^+ T cells delays but does not prevent the adoptive transfer of syngeneic GVHD. Taken together, these results suggest that the repertoire of effector T cells appears to be limited and consists of cells expressing the Vβ 8.5/8.3 and the Vβ 10

TcR determinants. Fractionation of the autoreactive T-cell populations revealed two distinct helper T lymphocyte subsets expressing either Vβ 8.5 or Vβ 10 and the cytolytic CD8 population expressing the Vβ 8.5 T-cell receptor elements. Yet, not all Vβ 8.5^+ and Vβ 10^+ T cells are autoreactive; therefore, the autoaggressive T cells reside within a subset of cells expressing these determinants. Additionally, minor populations of cells expressing other V-region determinants also cannot be excluded. Similar observations were reported in a murine system demonstrating that IL-2–producing autoreactive T cells can be detected in the periphery after syngeneic BMT and CsA therapy (37). The autoreactive T-cell population in the periphery in this study was limited to a single Vβ determinant.

The identification of the autoreactive TcR determinants in syngeneic GVHD will provide unique insights into peripheral mechanisms of tolerance. In several studies, treatment of normal nonirradiated animals with CsA results in a marked increase of cells expressing the putative autoreactive T-cell receptor (29,37,49,50). Active autoaggression, however, was not observed, implying an active regulatory mechanism in the periphery (discussed below). The ability to mark autoreactive T cells that have potential to mediate syngeneic GVHD in a permissive environment will facilitate dissection of peripheral control mechanisms and identification of the mechanisms that mediate regulation of autoreactive T cells.

IV. FAILURE OF THYMIC-DEPENDENT CLONAL DELETION IN SYNGENEIC GVHD

Current evidence strongly indicates that the thymus plays a central role in the induction of syngeneic GVHD after CsA treatment. The primary effect of CsA in the induction of this autoaggressive syndrome is related to the ability of this immunosuppressive drug to alter thymic function and T-lymphocyte differentiation.

The importance of the thymus in syngeneic GVHD was first suggested by the observation of Glazier et al., that thymic shielding during irradiation prevents the development of autoaggression (9). The key observation was reported by Sorokin et al. (19). Syngeneic GVHD cannot be induced in rats if they were thymectomized prior to irradiation, bone marrow reconstitution, and CsA therapy. This autoaggression syndrome was induced in thymectomized rats, however, if thymic lobes were implanted prior to CsA therapy. The failure of a single cell suspension of thymocytes to replace the intact thymic lobe suggests that an intact cellular element within the thymus is essential for the successful induction of syngeneic GVHD. Additional studies by Sorokin et al. demonstrate that thymectomy is effective in preventing syngeneic GVHD only if performed prior to transplant. In contrast, thymectomy performed 2 weeks or later after syngeneic marrow transplant (CsA therapy was maintained for 6 weeks starting from the day of transplant) is ineffective at preventing the development of this autoaggressive syndrome. These data imply that the CsA-induced autoimmune cell population originates in the thymus and that these cells exit the thymus during the course of CsA treatment. The hypothesis that CsA treatment leads to the origin of the autoimmune cell population responsible for syngeneic GVHD is also supported by the observation of Beschorner et al. (50). Injection of thymocytes from irradiated, syngeneic bone marrow-reconstituted animals that are maintained on CsA into secondary irradiated recipients adoptively transfers of syngeneic GVHD into the secondary hosts. On the other hand, injection of thymocytes from non-CsA-treated animals fails to induce disease. These data, taken together, demonstrate the thymic origin of the cells responsible for the induction of syngeneic GVHD and the apparent role of CsA in allowing the generation of the autoreactive cells.

The mechanism whereby CsA allows for the generation of the cells that mediate syngeneic GVHD most likely is related to the effects of this novel immunosuppressive drug on the cellular architecture within the thymus. A number of studies demonstrate that CsA has remarkable effects on the structure of the thymus. Some of the first observations were made in normal (nonirradiated) animals (51,52). Treatment of both rats and mice with pharmacological doses of CsA results in the rapid ablation of the thymic medulla with a loss of medullary but not cortical epithelium. Recent studies, however, suggest that CsA treatment also selectively depletes thymic reticuloepithelial cells within the cortex (53). Furthermore, expression of MHC class II antigens is markedly reduced in the medulla, due mostly to the reduction of medullary epithelial cells (54). In contrast, MHC class II expression is virtually unchanged in the thymic cortex during CsA treatment. The changes observed after CsA treatment are rapidly reversible in nonirradiated animals but persist in the irradiated, bone- marrow-reconstituted recipient. Additional studies by Beschorner et al. indicate that there is an age-related variable on the effects of CsA on the thymus in rats receiving mediastinal irradiation (20,54). Pronounced changes of medullary ablation, reduction of a MHC class II antigen expression, and reduction of medullary epithelial cells including Hassall's corpuscles are observed in young animals (5 to 6 weeks of age). In contrast, treatment of older rats (48 to 60 weeks of age) that receive mediastinal irradiation and CsA treatment does not result in significant medullary involution. Although the Hassall's corpuscles are absent, fusiform epithelium, dendritic cells, and MHC class II antigen expression is not altered despite CsA treatment. The mechanism of resistance of the thymus from older animals to the effects of CsA remains unclear.

The above studies clearly demonstrate a marked effect of CsA on thymic architecture with elimination of thymocytes and epithelial cells in the medulla and a concomitant reduction of MHC class II antigen expression. On the other hand, CsA treatment does not appear to alter the thymic cortex significantly. These structural changes in the thymus induced by CsA reflect a significant change in the integrity of the thymic environment that governs T-cell differentiation and the clonal deletion of autoreactive lymphocytes. Cheney and Sprent and Hess et al. postulated that these thymic changes mediated by CsA, particularly the reduction or elimination of MHC class II antigen expression in the medulla, lead to a failure of T-cell differentiation and the clonal deletion of autoreactive T lymphocytes (18,24). Experimental evidence strongly supports this concept and suggests that CsA inhibits both positive and negative selection in the thymus.

Several recent studies clearly demonstrate that CsA alters T- lymphocyte differentiation as determined by monitoring expression of the α/β T-cell receptor and the CD4 and CD8 surface determinants that mark distinct T-cell functions restricted by class II and class I MHC antigens, respectively (21,36,48,54,55). Overall, CsA appears to induce a maturational arrest of T-cell development. There is a significant reduction in the number of thymocytes expressing the α/β T-cell receptor along with a virtual absence of CD4 single positive T cells and a marked (but not complete) reduction of CD8 single positive thymocytes. In contrast, the more immature thymocytes (CD4CD8 double negatives; CD4CD8 double positives) are significantly increased during CsA treatment. Additional studies suggest that immature or incompletely differentiated T cells are released prematurely during CsA treatment, since lymphocytes with early thymocyte differentiation antigens and coexpression of both CD4 and CD8 determinants can be detected in the peripheral circulation after CsA treatment (55,56). On the other hand, CsA does not appear to alter the development of γ/δ T cells, although this observation was recently disputed (48,57). The most informative series of experiments was reported by Jenkins et al., who studied the effect of CsA on clonal depletion in the thymus. In I-E$^+$ strains of mice, the majority of anti-I-E self-reactive T lymphocytes are deleted in the thymus. CsA treatment of these mice after syngeneic BMT results in the development of a significant number of single positive thymocytes with a high percentage (10 to 20%) of cells expressing a Vβ gene element associated with anti-I-E self reactivity. Only a very small number (0.6%) of single positive thymocytes were detected in the control non-CsA-treated animals. Similar studies were reported by Gao et al., showing that the autoreactive cells are released into the periphery (49). These data led to the conclusion that CsA interferes with the clonal deletion of autoreactive cells. It is thought that clonal deletion in the thymus occurs via apoptosis (or programmed cell death) after activation of T cells with receptors having high affinity for self MHC antigens (58). In this regard, recent studies show that CsA inhibits programmed cell death, presumably by inhibiting thymocyte activation via the T-cell receptor (59). Shi et al. demonstrate that CsA blocks anti-CD3 induced apoptosis in the thymus. Although this may likely explain the ability of CsA to inhibit clonal deletion, recent studies suggest that anti-CD3 triggering may not be a relevant model for negative selection. Anti-CD3 induced apoptosis does not occur in bcl-2 transgenic mice, despite the fact that thymocytes still undergo negative selection (60). Other factors may govern clonal deletion, including a requisite interaction with other cell-surface determinants. The mechanism of action of CsA in this process apparently may be more complex than just the inhibition of T-cell-receptor signaling. In this regard, recent studies in transgenic mice suggests that CsA inhibits positive selection of thymocytes. Urdahl et al. show that administration of CsA inhibited positive selection of cells transgenic for the T-cell receptor directed against the H-Y antigen and retarded negative selection (61). They also propose for a small subset of thymoctyes that CsA may convert a normally negatively selecting T-cell receptor signal to a positive selection signal, thus distorting clonal selection in the thymus.

Overall, these data strongly suggest that CsA interferes or alters normal intrathymic T-cell differentiation and abrogates normal clonal deletion mechanisms, as simplistically illustrated in Fig. 1. The precise mechanisms accounting for the inhibition of clonal deletion of autoreactive T cells remain elusive. Nevertheless, administration of CsA dramatically alters the thymic architecture in the medulla and inhibits both positive and negative selection processes. The production and export of autoreactive cells into a permissive environment (see below) results in systemic autoaggression.

Despite the attractive hypothesis that syngeneic GVHD is due to the inhibition of clonal deletion, several issues remain to be resolved. Without question, the abrogation of thymic-dependent clonal deletion by CsA gives rise to the effector cells of syngeneic GVHD. Yet, the production of autoreactive T cells alone is not sufficient to cause this autoaggression syndrome. T lymphocytes with an autoreactive T-cell

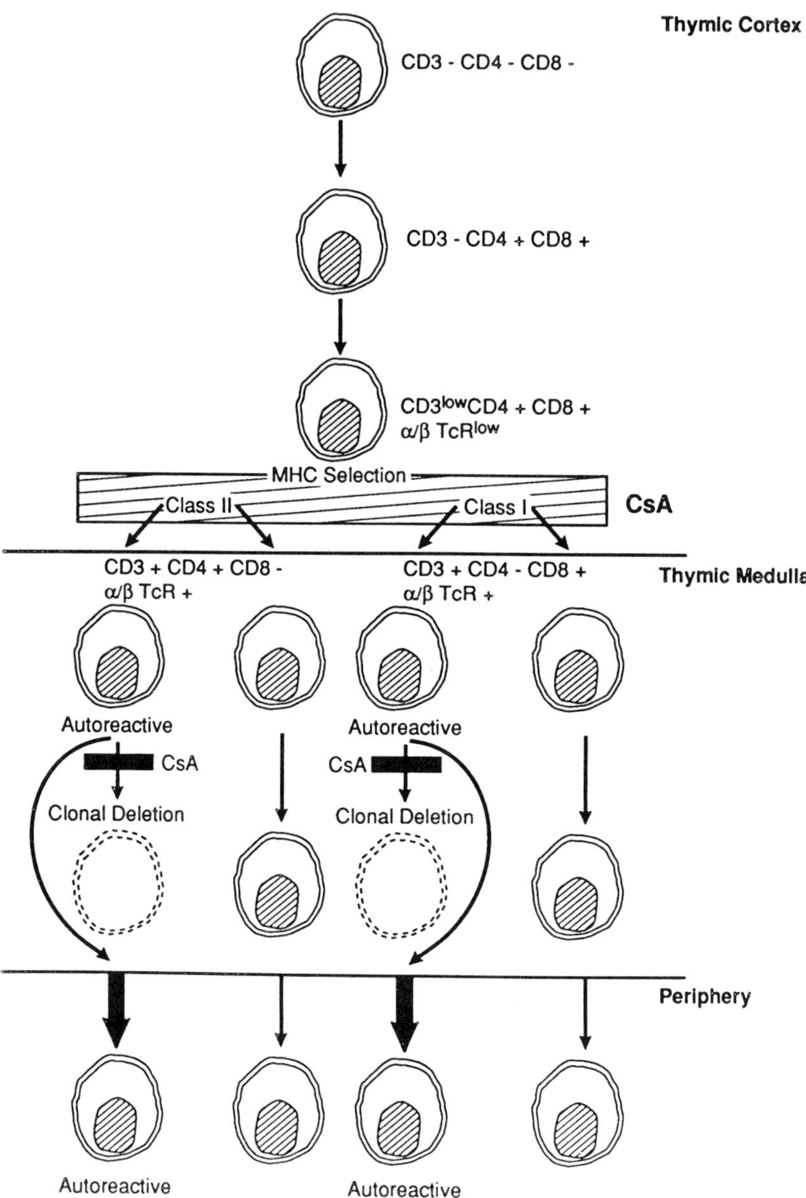

Figure 1 Effect of CsA on T lymphocyte differentiation and clonal deletion in the thymus.

receptor can be detected in the periphery of mice treated with CsA but without any evidence of autoaggressive disease (29,48,54). Similarly, autoreactive T cells can be detected in the peripheral lymphoid compartment of untreated mice, suggesting that, under normal conditions, clonal deletion is incomplete (62,63). Such findings imply the presence or absence (in syngeneic GVHD) of a peripheral regulatory mechanism controlling the expression of autoreactive T cells.

Other questions regarding the effect of CsA on the thymus also remain unanswered. For instance, the mechanism by which CsA prevents the maturation of T cells in the thymus is unknown. Inhibition of apoptosis by CsA cannot account for the marked reduction of thymocytes expressing the α/β T-cell receptor or for the maturational failure of CD4 and CD8 single positive T cells. Another distinct level of T-cell differentiation appears to be affected by CsA. Similarly, studies in the rat by Severino et al. suggest that CsA may alter the normal selection of MHC class I (CD8) and MHC class II (CD4) restricted T cells, leading to the production of $CD8^+$ T cells with MHC class II restricted T-cell receptors (45). Furthermore, the immunobiological mechanisms accounting for the elimination of epithelial and dendritic cells in the thymic medulla during CsA treatment remain undefined. The loss of specific architectural components of thymic medulla may alter T-cell differentiation at very distinct levels. In this regard, Beschorner et al. provide evidence that the dendritic cells in the thymus govern the development of peripheral regulatory mechanisms (64). Syngeneic GVHD develops if CsA treatment in nonirradiated rats is followed by thymectomy, whereas this autoaggression syndrome does not develop in the sham-thymectomized animals. This evidence also suggests that CsA treatment can inactivate established peripheral autoregulatory mechanisms (see below). Beschorner et al. propose that following CsA treatment, dendritic cells repopulate the thymus and allow the regeneration of regulatory T lymphocytes in the thymus (64). A similar concept suggesting that CsA acts on the thymus by preventing the development of regulatory cells was proposed by Sakaguchi and Sakaguchi (65). Thymectomy after CsA treatment of newborn mice accentuates the development of autoimmunity, a process that is inhibited by the infusion of splenic T cells from normal mice.

CsA remarkably affects many different aspects of thymic function and T-cell differentiation, permitting the production of autoreactive T cells while apparently inhibiting the generation of peripheral autoregulatory mechanisms. Are the divergent actions of CsA due to an effect on distinct cell populations within the thymus that control separate T-cell differentiation processes? Are these actions attributable to a single mechanism of action at the molecular level (i.e., inhibition of calcineurin) (66) or due to an effect on multiple enzyme systems? Certainly, our working knowledge of the effect of CsA on thymic function is quite rudimentary, and only intensive research will clarify this important issue.

V. ROLE OF PERIPHERAL REGULATORY MECHANISMS

The induction of syngeneic GVHD simply requires two elements; the production of autoreactive T cells and a permissive environment that allows the autoreactive T cells to mediate autoaggression. In normal animals, however, there is a peripheral autoregulatory mechanism that controls the expression of autoreactive T cells in syngeneic GVHD (67). A permissive environment can be achieved only after a T-lymphocyte-dependent peripheral mechanism is eliminated (by irradiation) or if the frequency of autoreactive T cells exceeds the capacity of the regulatory T lymphocytes. In fact, elimination of the peripheral autoregulatory mechanism is, perhaps, the single most important element necessary for the induction of syngeneic GVHD. Several studies utilized the experimental model of syngeneic GVHD to characterize this regulatory system, which appears to be important in the peripheral control of self nonself discrimination.

In some of the initial investigations, experimental evidence supported the presence of an autoregulatory system that modifies the action of the autoaggressive T cells mediating syngeneic GVHD. Studies by Glazier et al. demonstrate that syngeneic GVHD can be adoptively transferred only into irradiated secondary recipients (9). On the other hand, infusion of spleen cells from animals with active disease into normal animals is ineffective in transferring autoaggression, suggesting the presence of a resident regulatory system that modifies the activity of the effector cells. Other support for a regulatory system is provided by the studies of Cheney and Sprent, who show that CsA treatment of normal animals does not induce the syngeneic GVHD syndrome (18). Spleen cells from these animals, however, can adoptively transfer syngeneic GVHD when transplanted into irradiated secondary recipients reconstituted with normal bone marrow. The interpretation of these findings is that the effector cells were generated in the primary host treated with CsA but can mediate autoaggression only after removal of a radiation-sensitive regulatory component. The appearance of autoreactive T cells in the periphery of normal animals treated with CsA was confirmed by the detection of T cells with autoreactive T-cell receptors marked by specific Vβ-region determinants (described above). Since these initial reports, further evidence clearly documents the presence of peripheral autoregulatory cells that modulate the activity of syngeneic GVHD effector T cells.

The approach taken to document and characterize this autoregulatory system was the adoptive transfer of effector splenocytes from animals with active disease into secondary recipients that were differentially pretreated with radiation or cytotoxic drugs (67). The premise in these experiments is that radiation or chemotherapy (or both) perturbs the autoregulatory system, thus allowing for the successful adoptive transfer of syngeneic GVHD. Successful transfer of syngeneic GVHD only occurs if the secondary Lewis recipients receive total or upper body irradiation with 750R or treatment with 100 mg/kg of cyclophosphamide. In contrast, syngeneic GVHD cannot be transferred into secondary recipients either left untreated or prepared with low-dose total body irradiation (500R), lower body irradiation with 1050R, or treatment with busulfan. These results suggest that the autoregulatory system is sensitive to irradiation (750R) and cyclophosphamide but resistant to lower doses of irradiation (500R) and busulfan. It is important to note that syngeneic GVHD can be induced only if the radiation dose used in the preparative regimen exceeds 750R, suggesting that it is essential to eliminate the autoregulatory system in order to induce this autoaggression syndrome. Similarly, induction of autologous GVHD in humans (as antitumor immunotherapy) requires either total-body irradiation or cyclophosphamide in the preparative regimen, thereby compromising the peripheral regulatory compartment (68). Additionally, recent studies also suggest that the administration of CsA after syngeneic BMT prevents the regeneration of this autoregulatory system, thus, maintaining a permissive environment for the autoreactive T cells (69).

Direct support for a peripheral autoregulatory system is provided by the studies of Fischer et al. and Hess et al. (70,71). Adoptive transfer of splenic T lymphocytes from normal animals completely prevents the development of syngeneic GVHD in secondary recipients receiving autoimmune effector cells. The regulatory effect of the $CD5^+$, α/β TCR^+ T cells from normal animals, is critically dose-dependent, requiring a 2 : 1 ratio of normal T lymphocytes to syngeneic GVHD effector cells. It is of interest that in the initial studies, both $CD4^+$ and $CD8^+$ T cells from normal, unmodified animals were required to completely prevent the adoptive transfer of syngeneic GVHD. More recently, our results provide evidence that the autoregulatory system is in a resting state but undergoes upregulation in the presence of autoreactive T cells (71,72). Specific challenge or priming of normal animals with syngeneic GVHD effector cells results in a marked increase in the ability of the peripheral regulatory T-cell population to prevent the adoptive transfer of autoaggression. In addition, there is a maturation of the regulatory T-cell compartment, since after priming, the $CD4^+$ subset alone is capable of preventing the transfer of syngeneic GVHD. Although normal $CD8^+$ T cells are apparently required for the activation of the regulatory system, their precise role remains unclear.

Based on these observations, it is tempting to speculate that autoregulation is a dynamic process with active recognition of the syngeneic GVHD effector cells. A consequence of effector-cell recognition is the activation and clonal expansion of the autoregulatory T-cell compartment. Moreover, the primary autoregulatory activity resides within the $CD4^+$ T-cell subset after activation. Of interest is the finding that the $CD4^+$ T-cell subset appears to have regulatory activity in several different models, including peripheral infectious tolerance to allografts (73,74). The demonstration of regulatory activity occurs after challenge with antigen and immunosuppressive intervention. Challenge or priming of the regulatory system with antigen-reactive T cells may accelerate the activation of the regulatory compartment and obviate the need for immunosuppression. Such an approach with successful prevention of autoimmunity was recently described in an experimental allergic encephalomyelitis model (75).

The mechanism of peripheral regulation in syngeneic GVHD and in other CD4-dependent models remains unknown. Active regulation maybe mediated by secretion of modulatory cytokines that clonally inactivate the autoreactive T cells (76). Additionally, it is unclear if the autoregulatory T cells recognize antigen directly or if they recognize the autoreactive T cells, perhaps through an idiotype–anti-idiotype mechanism. Recent studies by Hess et al. in the rat model suggest that autoregulation of syngeneic GVHD requires a specific interaction of the α/β T-cell receptor on the autoregulatory cells with the MHC class II determinants on the autoreactive lymphocytes as illustrated in Fig. 2 (72). One possible explanation to account for the specificity observed in the priming response to the autoreactive T cells is that the T-cell receptor peptides are recognized in the context of class II MHC antigens. This hypothesis may have some merit in view of the results in the experimental allergic encephalomyelitis autoimmune model in which autoregulatory T cells recognized a $V\beta$ 8.2 peptide from the autoreactive lymphocytes (77).

On the other hand, CsA may also inhibit other mechanisms responsible for the peripheral control of autoreactivity including veto cells (78,79). Similarly, Vanier and Prud'homme showed that CsA prevents the induction of clonal anergy, findings that confirmed the original observations by Jenkins et al. (81,82). Inhibition of both peripheral regulatory mechanisms by CsA would lead to a permissive environment for expression of autoreactive T cells.

Although our understanding is incomplete, peripheral autoregulatory mechanisms are quite important in maintaining nonresponsiveness to self as documented in the syngeneic GVHD model. These mechanisms provide a safeguard to control autoreactive T cells that have escaped clonal deletion in the thymus. Current re-

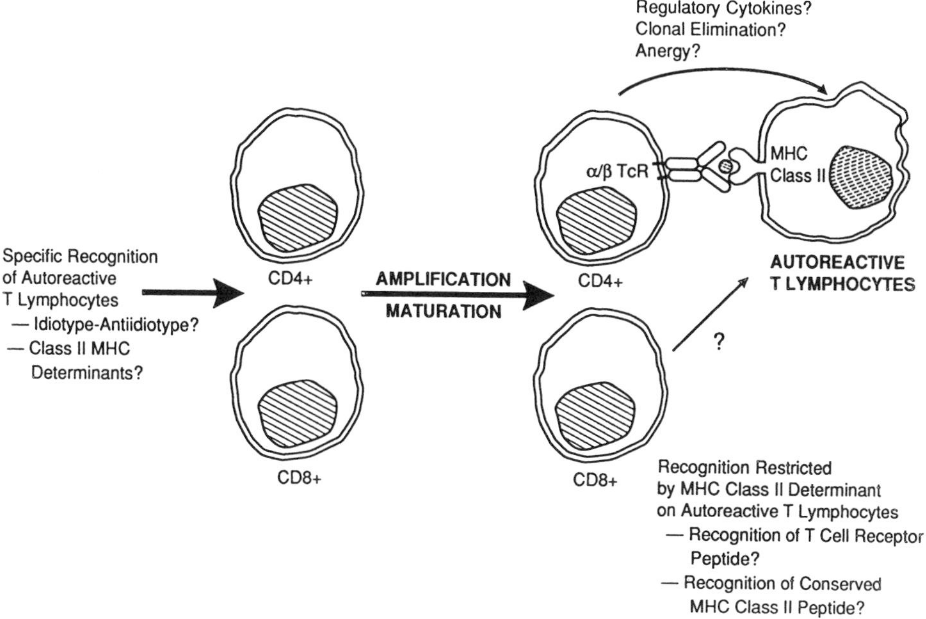

Figure 2 Possible mechanism of peripheral autoregulation in syngeneic GVHD.

search efforts in the syngeneic GVHD model should provide additional insights into the mechanisms of peripheral regulation.

VI. ANTITUMOR ACTIVITY OF SYNGENEIC/ AUTOLOGOUS GVHD

Several recent studies (summarized below) have attempted to assess whether this experimentally induced autoimmune syndrome could be mobilized to mediate a significant antitumor effect against tumor cells expressing the target antigen (MHC class II determinants) of syngeneic GVHD. This is particularly important, since one of the major limitations of autologous BMT as therapy for malignancy is the unacceptably high rate of tumor recurrence (84). In comparison, the rate of tumor recurrence after allogeneic BMT is significantly lower than the rate observed after autologous BMT, even though comparable preparative regimens are employed (84,85). The enhanced antitumor effect of allogeneic BMT is thought to be due to the occurrence of GVHD and suggests that tumor cells can be eliminated by immune mechanisms (86,87). Although autologous BMT avoids the morbidity and mortality associated with GVHD after allogeneic BMT, the graft-versus-tumor effect is absent. Certainly, the high rate of tumor recurrence in autologous BMT patients is, in large part, due to the lack of significant graft-versus-host disease. Based on the significant antitumor activity of GVHD, it seems likely that immune modulation should enhance the efficacy of autologous BMT in the treatment of malignancy. Immunological approaches for eradication of tumor in the autologous BMT setting should be particularly effective because they would be used at a time when there is minimal residual disease, thus limiting the number of tumor cells that need to be eliminated by the immune system.

The induction of syngeneic/autologous GVHD as antitumor therapy after autologous BMT is particularly attractive for several reasons. First, immune recognition of the tumor cells by the autoreactive T cells appears to be only dependent on expression of MHC class II determinants, as illustrated in Fig. 3. Comparatively, recognition of tumor cells by lymphocytes mediating allogeneic GVHD (recognizing minor histocompatibility antigens restricted by class I MHC determinants in transplants performed between MHC-matched siblings) requires that the tumor cells express not only the MHC class I antigen but also the relevant minor antigen. Based on these differences in target-cell recognition, it is conceivable that the antitumor effect of autologous/syngeneic GVHD may be equal to or greater than the antitumor activity observed with allogeneic GVHD. Second, expression of MHC class II antigens, the target antigen of autologous/syngeneic GVHD, can be upregulated by cytokines such as γ-interferon, thereby potentiating tumor targeting (Fig. 3). And third, administration of IL-2 could amplify the autoreactive T cells providing maximum tumor kill. Together, several different strategies can be utilized singly or in concert to enhance the antitumor effect of autologous/syngeneic GVHD after autologous BMT.

A. Animal Studies

Initial preclinical studies evaluated the antitumor effect of syngeneic GVHD in the rat model using the CRL 1662 myeloma derived from the Lou M strain of rat (88).

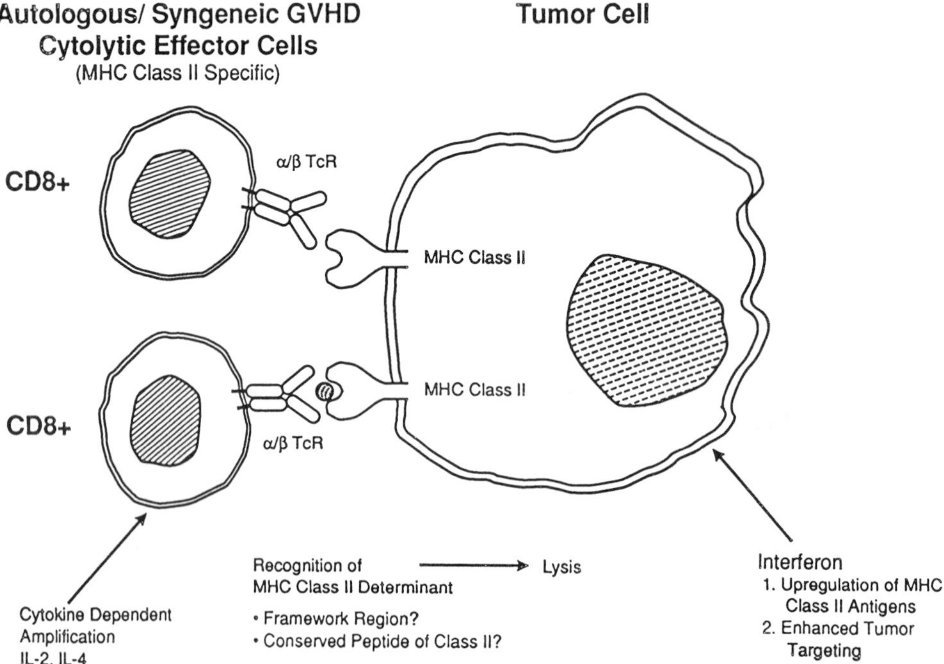

Figure 3 Tumor cell recognition by autoreactive T lymphocytes in autologous/syngeneic GVHD.

This tumor expresses MHC class II determinants and the expression of these antigens can be significantly enhanced by treatment with γ-interferon. Studies by Geller et al. demonstrate that $CD8^+$ splenic T cells from Lou M rats that developed syngeneic GVHD were able to lyse the myeloma cells in vitro (88). Lysis of the tumor cells was blocked by pretreating the tumor cells with antibodies to the MHC class II determinant but not by antibodies to MHC class I antigens. Furthermore, incubation of the tumor cells with γ- interferon not only increased the expression of MHC class II antigen but, more importantly, also increased their susceptibility to lysis by the effector lymphocytes from animals with syngeneic GVHD. These studies demonstrated that syngeneic GVHD could manifest significant antitumor activity in vitro and confirmed that the effector T cells recognized MHC class II antigens on the tumor cell.

Subsequent studies evaluated the antitumor activity of syngeneic GVHD in vivo and assessed if administration of the recombinant lymphokines, γ-interferon, or interleukin-2 (IL-2), could potentiate this effect (89,90). The results from these investigations indicate that syngeneic GVHD could mediate a significant antitumor effect achieving a 1–2 log tumor-cell kill. Additionally, administration of γ-interferon potentiated the antitumor effect of syngeneic GVHD, resulting in cure of 40% of the animals. Moreover, these animals are resistant to rechallenge with the tumor cells, suggesting that there is concomitant development of specific antitumor immunity. Treatment of the animals with γ-interferon augments (2- to 5-fold) MHC class II expression of the tumor cells in vivo. It seems likely that the increased expression of MHC class II antigens on the tumor cell results in the enhanced recognition of the tumor cells by the autoreactive effector lymphocytes. On the other hand, the use of high dose IL-2 treatment to amplify the effector mechanisms in syngeneic GVHD primarily exacerbates the autoaggression syndrome. Because of the potentiation of fatal autoaggression, the role of IL-2 in amplifying the antitumor activity cannot be accurately assessed. Lower doses of 15-10,000 units/day of IL-2 are more effective and appear to have an additive effect with administration of γ-interferon.

B. Clinical Studies

Encouraged by the results from the animals studies, clinical studies were initiated to assess the feasibility of inducing an autoimmune GVHD in autologous BMT patients and to evaluate whether there was any antitumor activity. Initially, five consecutive patients with either aggressive non-Hodgkins lymphoma or Hodgkin's disease in relapse and not responsive to conventional salvage therapy underwent autologous BMT and CsA treatment (91). CsA was started on the day of BMT and was continued for 28 days at 1 mg/kg per day. Histologically proven grade II GVHD of the skin developed in all five patients at a median of 11 days (range 9 to 13 days) after BMT, at the time of initial evidence of hematological recovery. The GVHD was confined to the skin (erythematous maculopapular rash affecting the face, ears, trunk, hands, and feet) with no evidence of extracutaneous involvement. The autologous GVHD resolved within 1 to 3 weeks either spontaneously or after a short course of corticosteriods. Moreover, cytolytic lymphocytes recognizing self and MHC- disparate lymphocytes could be detected during active disease, and the lysis was blocked by pretreating the target cells (self and unrelated) with monoclonal antibodies to class II MHC antigens. The autoreactive T cells could no longer be detected upon resolution of clinical autologous GVHD.

The findings in human autologous GVHD, for the most part, paralleled the results in the animal model. The CsA-induced autoaggression syndrome in humans was also associated with the development autocytotoxic T cells that recognize MHC class II determinants (91). The clinical results with the induction of GVHD with CsA treatment after autologous BMT have now been confirmed by several groups, including the detection of the MHC class II restricted autoreactive T-lymphocytes (92,93). Additionally, recent studies by Ruvolo et al. indicate that the appearance of the MHC class II autocytolytic T cells coincides with the onset of clinical autologous GVHD (94). These lytic T cells were primarily $CD8^+$ $CD4^-$ α/β TcR^+, although in a subgroup of patients, the lytic T cells expressed both CD8 and CD4 cell-surface accessory molecules. Also, it is of interest that the $V\beta$ T-cell receptor repertoire expressed by the infiltrating lymphocytes was limited, with a few common elements such as $V\beta$ 15 (94). Although these findings were unexpected in an outbred species such as the human, additional studies should define the importance of a restricted $V\beta$ T-cell receptor repertoire in autologous GVHD.

Despite similar effector mechanisms and histological lesions, there are a few differences between the induction of autologous/syngeneic GVHD in the human compared to the rat model. The major difference is that autologous GVHD develops in the patients while they are being treated with CsA. In the rat model, CsA must be discontinued, in most cases, prior to the onset of disease. This difference may be related to the higher doses of CsA administered to the animals, whereas lower doses in humans allow for the activation of the autoreactive T cells. The second difference is that a chronic phase of the disease develops in a majority of the animals. On the other hand, the development of a chronic phase in humans is rare. Since the development of the chronic phase is principally due to autoreactive $CD4^+$ T cells (15), it seems likely that the autoreactive T-helper cells may develop infrequently in humans, or they develop discordantly with the $CD8^+$ autoreactive T cells.

Encouraged by the fact that autologous GVHD could be induced in humans with similar effector mechanisms as defined in the animal model, several clinical trials were initiated to evaluate the antitumor activity of this experimentally induced autoaggression syndrome, especially since many lymphohematopoietic malignancies and solid tumors express MHC class II determinants (95–97). Included in these trials were a phase II study of high-grade non- Hodgkin's lymphoma in sensitive relapse (still responsive to salvage chemotherapy), a phase I study in acute myelogenous leukemia, and a phase I/II study in metastatic breast cancer. An additional phase I/II study in metastatic breast cancer was also started with the induction of autologous GVHD and the adjuvant administration of recombinant human γ-interferon. To date over 200 patients have been entered onto these clinical protocols. Although these clinical trials are ongoing, several important facts (as summarized in Table 1) have been established: (1) autologous GVHD was induced in over 70% of the patients; (2) this autoaggression syndrome was, in most cases, confined to the skin without any clinical evidence of internal organ disease (i.e., liver and gastrointestinal tract); (3) the appearance of autologous GVHD primarily occurred with the initial phases of engraftment while the patient was on CsA; (4) the autoimmune syndrome resolved spontaneously in most cases, although a small percentage of patients required a short course of corticosteroids; and (5) MHC class II–restricted autoreactive T cells could be detected that lysed not only pretransplant

Table 1 Characteristics of Clinical Autologous GVHD

Occurs in >70% of autologous BMT patients
Dose of CsA 1–2.0 mg/kg/day IV
Confined primarily to skin; generally no involvement of internal organs
Onset occurs with initial phases of engraftment; can occur 1–2 weeks after CsA withdrawal in a subset of patients
Lasts 1–3 weeks; resolves spontaneously, although a few patients require low-dose steroid treatment
INF-γ increases severity; has no effect on incidence
Associated with MHC class II autoreactive T cells; lysis of pretransplant lymphoblasts (PHA-transformed) and tumor cell lines

lymphocytes but also a number of tumor cell lines that expressed MHC class II determinants. Of further importance was the finding that administration of γ-interferon significantly increased the severity (greater incidence of grade II disease as defined by an erythematous rash covering >50% of the body) of the autologous GVHD. Subsequent studies revealed that γ-interferon administration resulted in upregulation of class II MHC antigens in the skin and probably accounted for the increased severity of the skin lesions (98).

More recently, a series of phase I pilot trials was initiated to maximize the induction of autologous GVHD in patients with metastatic breast cancer. Administration of granulocyte-colony stimulating factor (G-CSF) mobilized progenitor cells to the bone marrow graft plus CsA and γ-interferon treatment resulted in a significant increase in grade II autologous GVHD with a third of the patients requiring some corticosteroid therapy (99). This increase in the intensity of autologous GVHD was associated with an increase in the number of autoreactive cytolytic T cells and a rapid repopulation of the $CD4^+$ T-helper-cell compartment. The enhanced autocytolytic activity appears to be due to cytokine amplification provided by the proportional increase in helper T lymphocytes.

Ongoing analyses suggest that autologous GVHD does have a significant ántitumor activity. There is a significant increase in the event-free survival (62%) and decrease in the relapse rate (29%) of high-grade non-Hodgkin's lymphoma with autologous GVHD compared to recent historical controls (event-free survival, 40%; relapse rate, 50%) (95). Similarly, there is a marked early survival advantage for breast cancer patients who develop autologous GVHD compared with those who do not develop this autoaggression syndrome. Moreover, the antitumor effect appears to be enhanced by the administration of recombinant γ-interferon (98). Due to these encouraging results, several randomized trials with adjuvant administration of γ-interferon in a variety of lymphohematopoietic malignancies are now under way to confirm the antitumor effect of autologous GVHD in humans.

VII. SYNTHESIS AND CONCLUSIONS

The occurrence of syngeneic GVHD certainly challenges our previously held concepts that histocompatibility differences between donor and recipient are absolute requirements for the induction of GVHD. The induction of an autoaggression syndrome with CsA also underscores our rather incomplete understanding of how

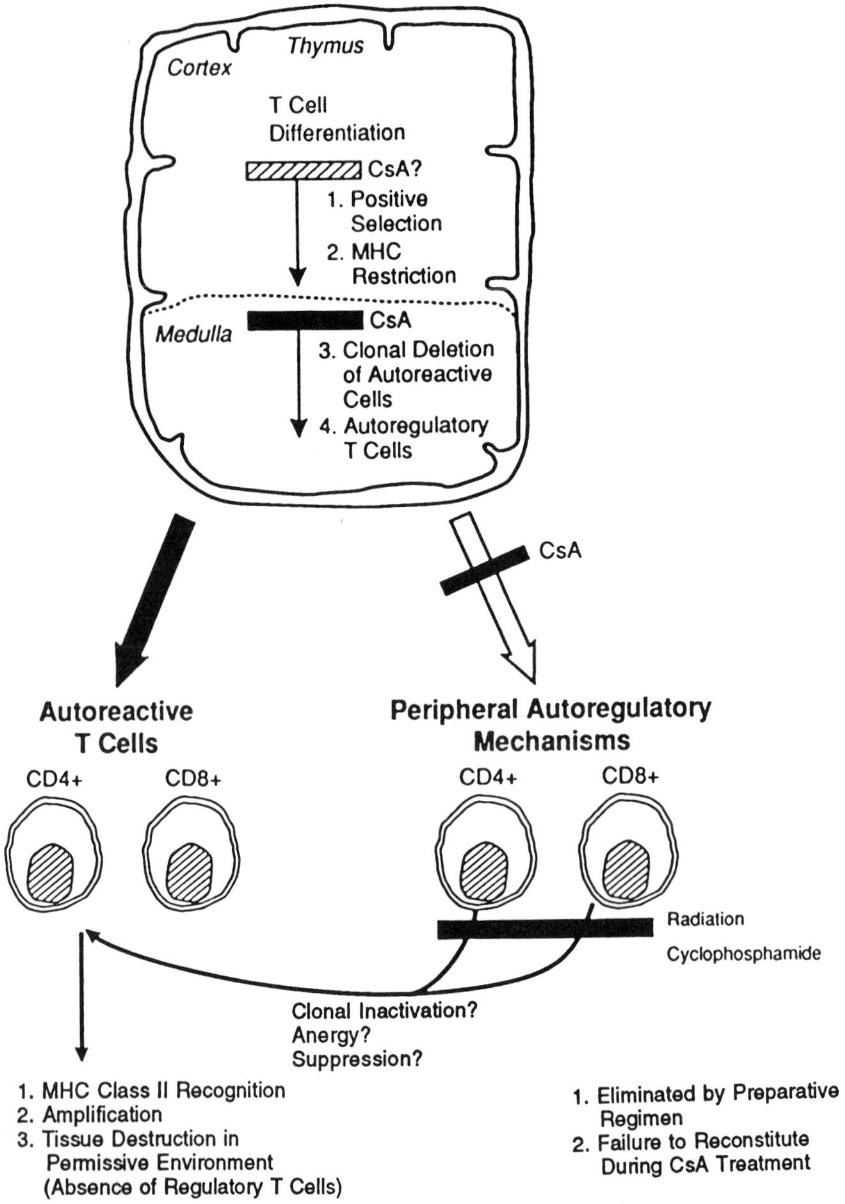

Figure 4 Autoreactive and autoregulatory immune mechanisms in autologous/syngeneic GVHD.

this novel immunosuppressive drug affects the complex immune system. A similar argument exists for FK 506, which can induce syngeneic GVHD (83). This finding is not surprising, since FK 506 and CsA have a common molecular mechanism of action (66).

This autoaggression syndrome, however, reflects a much more fundamental process in which the central and peripheral mechanisms governing nonresponsiveness to self are disrupted. This process is accentuated in the redeveloping immune system following autologous/syngeneic BMT. Perturbation of the developing immune system by interfering with clonal deletion mechanisms and the elimination of autoregulatory mechanisms alters the immunological homeostasis accounting for self–non-self discrimination leading to autoaggression, as simplistically illustrated in Fig. 4. Such a dysregulation of the immune system appears to be the cause of CsA-induced syngeneic GVHD. Although the precise mechanism of action of CsA remains to be elucidated, several important concepts that are important for the induction of syngeneic GVHD have been identified. They include (a) elimination of a peripheral autoregulatory mechanism by total body irradiation, (b) elimination or alteration of clonal deletion mechanisms in the thymus by CsA treatment, and (c) the failure to regenerate the autoregulatory system apparently due to the action of CsA. Elimination of peripheral autoregulatory mechanisms (i.e., by irradiation) provides a permissive environment for the autoreactive T cells emerging from the dyfunctional thymus compromised by CsA treatment. Thus, autoaggression can and does occur!

The ability of CsA to inhibit clonal deletion and induce autoaggression under certain experimental questions may also have far-reaching implications into its use as an immunosuppressive agent. Moreover, the induction of this syndrome may hold some promise as antitumor immunotherapy after autologous BMT. Although some of the mechanisms have been identified, many problems remain unresolved regarding syngeneic GVHD. Nevertheless, the induction of this autoimmune syndrome with CsA will provide unique insights into mechanisms of central and peripheral tolerance and provide a novel approach to treat certain neoplastic diseases.

ACKNOWLEDGMENTS

This work was supported by grants AI 24319, AI 33220, CA 54203, and CA 15396 from the National Institutes of Health.

REFERENCES

1. Santos GW, Hess AD, Vogelsang GB. Graft-versus-host disease. Immunol Rev 1985; 88:169.
2. Gluckman E, Devergie A, Sohier J, Sauret JH. Graft-versus-host disease in recipients of syngeneic bone marrow. Lancet 1980; 1:253.
3. Rappeport J, Reinherz E, Mihm M, et al. Acute graft-versus-host disease in recipients of bone marrow transplantation from identical twin donors. Lancet 1979; 2:717.
4. Thien SW, Goldman JM, Galton DG. Acute "graft-versus-host disease" after autografting for chronic granulocytic leukemia in transplantation. Ann Intern Med 1981; 94: 210.
5. Hood AF, Vogelsang GB, Black LP, et al. Acute graft-versus-host disease: Development following autologous and syngeneic bone marrow transplantation. Arch Dermatol 1987; 123:745.
6. Billingham RE. The biology of graft-versus-host reactions: Harvey Lect 1966–67; 62: 21.
7. Santos GW, Elfenbein GJ, Sharkis S, Tutschka PJ. Reconstitution of lymphohematopoietic function following allogeneic, syngeneic, and autologous marrow transplanta-

tion. In: Gelfand EW, Dorsch HM, eds. Advances in Pediatric Research: I. Biological Basis of Immunodeficiency. New York: Raven Press, 1979.
8. Glazier A, Tutschka PJ, Farmer ER, Santos GW. Graft-versus-host disease in cyclosporin: A treated rats after syngeneic and autologous bone marrow reconstitution. J Exp Med 1983; 158:1–8.
9. Glazier A, Tutschka PJ, Farmer ER. Studies on the immunobiology of syngeneic and autologous graft-versus-host disease in cyclosporine treated rats. Transplant Proc 1983; 15:3035.
10. Kahan BD. Cyclosporine. N Engl J Med 1989; 21:1725–1738.
11. Morris PJ. Cyclosporin A. Transplantation 1981; 349–354.
12. Borel JF. Pharmacology of cyclosporine: IV. Pharmacological properties in vivo. Pharmacol Rev 1989; 259–371.
13. Santos GW, Tutschka PJ, Brookmeyer R, et al. Cyclosporine plus methylprednisolone versus cyclophosphamide plus methylprednisolone as prophylaxis for graft-vs-host disease: A randomized double blind study in patients undergoing allogeneic marrow transplantation. Clin Transplant 1987; 1:21–28.
14. Beschorner WE, Shin CA, Fischer A, et al. Cyclosporine (CSA) induced pseudo-graft-vs host disease (CIPGVHD) in the early post CsA period. Transplant 1988; 46(suppl):112–117.
15. Hess AD, Fischer AC, Beschorner WE. Effector mechanisms in cyclosporine A induced syngeneic graft-vs-host disease: Role of $CD4^+$ and $CD8^+$ T lymphocyte subsets. J Immunol 1990; 140:526–533.
16. Parkman R. Clonal analysis of murine graft-versus-host disease: 1. Phenotypic and functional analysis of T lymphocyte clones. J Immunol 1985; 136:3542–3549.
17. Parkman R. Clonal analysis of graft-vs-host disease. In: Burakoft SJ, Deeg HJ, Ferrara J, Atkinson K, eds. Graft-vs-host Disease. New York: Marcel Dekker, 1990:51–60.
18. Cheney RT, Sprent J. Capacity of cyclosporine to induce autograft-versus-host disease and impair intrathymic T-cell differentiation. Transplant Proc 1985; 17:528–530.
19. Sorokin R, Kimura H, Schroder K, Wilson D. Cyclosporine-induced autoimmunity: Conditions for expressing disease, requirement for intact thymus, and potency estimates of autoimmune lymphocytes in drug-treated rats. J Exp Med 1986; 164:1615–1616.
20. Shinozawa T, Beschorner WE, Hess AD. Prolonged administration of cyclosporine and the thymus: Irreversible immunopathologic changes associated with autologous pseudo-graft-vs-host disease. Transplantation 1990; 50:106–111.
21. Beschorner WE, Ren H, Phillips J, et al. Recovery of thymic microenvironment after cyclosporine prevents syngeneic graft-vs-host disease. Transplantation 1991; 52:668–674.
22. Fischer AC, Hess AD. Age related factors in cyclosporine-induced syngeneic graft-vs-host disease: Regulatory role of marrow derived T lymphocytes. J Exp Med 1990; 172: 85–94.
23. Beschorner WE, DiGennaro KA, Hess AD, Santos GW. Cyclosporine A (CsA) and the thymus: Immunopathology and recovery. Cell Immunol 1988; 110:350–364.
24. Hess AD, Horwitz L, Beschorner WE, Santos GW. Development of graft-vs-host disease-like syndrome in cyclosporine-treated rats after syngeneic bone marrow transplantation: I. Development of cytotoxic T-lymphocytes with apparent polyclonal anti-Ia specificity, including autoreactivity. J Exp Med 1985; 161:718–730.
25. Hess AD, Horwitz LR, Laulis MK. Cyclosporine induced syngeneic graft-vs-host disease: Recognition of self MHC class II antigens in vivo. Transplant Proc 1993; 25:1218–1221.
26. Faustman D, Hauptfeld V, Lacy P, Davie J. Prolongation of murine islet allograft by pretreatment of islets with antibody directed to Ia determinants. Proc Natl Acad Sci USA 1981; 78:5156–5160.

27. Bryson JS, Carwood BE, Kaplan AM. Relationship of cyclosporine A-mediated inhibition of clonal delection and development of syngeneic graft-vs-host disease. J Immunol 1991; 147:391-397.
28. Kaufmann DS, Kong CD, Shizuru JA, et al. Use of anti-L3T4 and anti-Ia treatments for prolongation of neurogenic islet transplants. Transplantation 1988; 46:210-215.
29. Hess AD, Horwitz LR, Laulis MK. Cyclosporine induced syngeneic graft-vs-host disease: Prevention of autoaggression by treatment with monoclonal antibodies to T lymphocyte cell surface determinants and to MCH class II antigens. Clin Immunol Immunopathol 1993; 69:341.
30. Babock S, Niswender K, Wilson DB, Bellgrau D. Cyclosporine-induced autoimmunization in rats carrying thymus allografts. Transplantation 1990; 50:1278-1281.
31. Malcherek G, Gnau V, Jung G, et al. Supermotifs enable natural invariant chain-derived peptides to interact with many major histocompatibility complex class II molecules. J Exp Med 1995; 181:527.
32. Hess AD, Fischer AC. Immune mechanisms in cyclosporine- induced syngeneic graft-vs-host disease. Transplantation 1989; 48:895-900.
33. Beschorner WE, Tutschka PJ, Santos GW. Sequential Morphology of Graft-versus-host disease in the rat radiation chimera. Clin Immunol Immunopathol 1982; 22:203-224.
34. Korngold R, Sprent J. T-cell subsets in graft-vs-host disease: In: Burakoff SJ, Deeg HJ, Ferrara J, Atkison K, eds. Graft-vs-Host Disease. New York: Marcel Dekker, 1990:31-49.
35. Bos GM, Major GD, Van Breda-Vriesman PJ. Cyclosporin-A induces a selective, reversible suppression of T-helper lymphocyte regeneration after syngeneic bone marrow transplantation: Association with syngeneic graft-versus-host disease in rat. Clin Exp Immunol 1988; 74:443-448.
36. Fischer AC, Laulis MK, Horwitz L, Hess AD. Effect of cyclosporine on T lymphocyte development: Relationship to syngeneic graft-versus-host disease. Transplantation 1991; 51:252-259.
37. Urdahl KB, Pardoll DM, Jenkins MK. Self-reactive T cells are present in the peripheral lymphoid tissues of cyclosporin A-treated mice. Int Immunol 1992; 4:1341-1349.
38. Gajewski TF, Schell SR, Fitch FW. Evidence implicating utilization of different T-cell receptor associated signalling pathways by Th1 and Th2 clones. J Immunol 1990; 144: 4110-4120.
39. Fischer AC, Ruvolo P, Burt R, et al. Characterization of autoreactive T cell repertoire in cyclosporine-induced syngeneic graft-versus-host disease: A highly conserved repertoire mediates autoaggression. J Immunol, 1995; 154:3713-3725.
40. Ben-Nunn AH, Wekerle H, Cohen IR. Vaccination against autoimmune encephalomyelitis with a T lymphocyte line reactive against myelin basic protein. Nature 1981; 292: 60-63.
41. Acha-Orbea H, Mitchell DJ, Timmerman L, et al. Limited heterogeneity of T cell receptors from lymphocytes mediating autoimmune encephalomyelitis allows specific immune intervention. Cell 1988; 54:263-273.
42. Singer PA, Theofilopoulos AN. T cell receptor Vβ repertoire expression in murine models of SLE. Immunol Rev 1990; 118:102-127.
43. Gutierrez-Ramos JC, Andrew JL, Moreno Alboran I. Insights into autoimmunity; From classical models to current perspectives. Immunol Rev 1990; 118:73-101.
44. Heber-Katz E, Acha-Orbea H. The V-region hypothesis: Evidence from autoimmune encephalomyelitis. Immunol Today 1989; 19:64-67.
45. Severino ME, Laulis MK, Horwitz LR, Hess AD. Cyclosporine preferentially inhibits clonal deletion of CD8 positive T-cells with an MHC class II restricted autoreactive T-cell receptor. Transplantation 1993; 25:520-523.

46. Smith LR, Kono DH, Kammuller ME. Vβ repertoire in rats and implications for endogenous superantigens. Eur J Immunol 1992; 22:641–645.
47. von Boehmer H. The developmental biology of T lymphocytes. Annu Rev Immunol 1988; 6:309–376.
48. Jenkins MK, Schwartz RH, Pardoll DM. Effects of cyclosporin A on T cell development and clonal deletion. Science 1988; 241:1655–1658.
49. Gao EK, Lo D, Cheney R, Kanagawa O, Sprent J. Abnormal differentiation of thymocytes in mice treated with cyclosporin A. Nature 1988; 336:176–179.
50. Beschorner WE, Hess AD, Shinn CA, Santos GW. Transfer of cyclosporine-associated syngeneic graft-vs-host disease by thymocytes. Transplantation 1988; 45:209–215.
51. Ryffel B, Deysseroth R, Borel JF. Cyclosporin A: Effects on the mouse thymus. Agents Actions 1981; 11:373–381.
52. Beschorner WE, Namnoum JD, Hess AD, et al. Cyclosporin A and the thymus: Immunopathology. Am J Pathol 1987; 126:487–496.
53. Fabien NH, Auger C, Moreira A, et al. Effects of cyclosporin A on mouse thymus: Immunochemical and ultrastructural studies. Thymus 1992; 20:153–162.
54. Beschorner WE, Suresch DL, Shinozawa T, Hess AD. Influence of irradiation and age on the CsA induced thymic immunopathology. Transplant Proc 1988; 20(suppl 3): 1072–1078.
55. Hess AD, Vogelsang GB, Heyd J, Beschorner WE. Cyclosporine induced syngeneic graft-vs-host disease; Assessment of T cell differentiation. Transplant Proc 1987; 19: 2683–2686.
56. Zadeh HH, Goldschneider I. Demonstration of large-scale migration of cortical thymocytes to peripheral lymphoid tissues in cyclosporin A-treated rats. J Exp Med 1993; 178: 285.
57. Leclerq G, Plum J, Nandi D, et al. Intrathymic differentiation of V gamma 3T cells. J Exp Med 1993; 178:309–315.
58. Blue M-L, Daley JF, Levine H, et al. Class II major histocompatibility complex molecules regulate the development of the $T4^+T8$-inducer phenotype of cultured human thymocytes. Proc Natl Acad Sci USA 1985; 82:8178–8182.
59. Shi Y, Sahai BM, Green DR. Cyclosporin A inhibits activation-induced cell death in T-cell hybridomas and thymocytes. Nature 1989; 339:625–626.
60. Sentman CL, Shutter JR, Hockenberry D, et al. bc1-2 inhibits multiple forms of apoptosis but not negative selection in thymocytes. Cell 1991; 67:879–888.
61. Urdahl KB, Pardoll DM, Jenkins MK. Cyclosporin A inhibits positive selection and delays negative selection in γβ TcR transgenic mice. J Immunol 1994; 152:2853.
62. Siegel RM, Katsumata M, Komori S. Mechanisms of autoimmunity in the context of T-cell tolerance: Insights from natural and transgenic animal model systems. Immunol Rev 1990; 118:165–192.
63. Hammerling GJ, Schonrick G, Momburg F, et al. Non-deletional mechanisms of peripheral and central tolerance: Studies with transgenic mice with tissue-specific expression of a foreign MHC class I antigen. Immunol Rev 1991; 122:46–67.
64. Beschorner WE, Ren H, Phillips J, et al. Recovery of thymic microenvironment after cyclosporine prevents syngeneic graft-vs-host disease. Transplantation 1991; 52:668–674.
65. Sakaguchi S, Sakaguchi N. Organ-specific autoimmune diseases induced in mice by elimination of T-cell subsets: V. Neonatal administration of cyclosporin A causes autoimmune disease. J Immunol 1989; 142:471–480.
66. Schreiber SL, Crabtree GR. The mechanism of action of cyclosporin A and FK 506. Immunol Today 1992; 13:136–142.
67. Fischer AC, Beschorner WE, Hess AD. Requirements for the induction and adoptive

transfer of cyclosporine-induced syngeneic graft-vs-host disease. J Exp Med 1989; 169: 1031–1041.
68. Jones RJ, Hess AD, Mann RB, et al. Induction of graft-versus-host disease after autologous bone marrow transplantation. Lancet 1989; 1:754–757.
69. Fischer AC. Immunobiology of syngeneic graft-vs-host disease. PhD thesis. Baltimore: The Johns Hopkins University, 1991.
70. Fischer AC, Laulis MK, Horwitz L, et al. Host resistance to cyclosporine induced syngeneic graft-vs-host disease. J Immunol 1989; 143:827–832.
71. Hess AD, Fischer AC, Horwitz LR. Cyclosporine-induced autoimmunity: Critical role of autoregulation in the prevention of major histocompatibility class II-dependent autoaggression. Transplant Proc 1993; 25:2811–2813.
72. Hess AD, Fischer AC, Horwitz L, et al. Characterization of peripheral autoregulatory mechanisms that prevent development of cyclosporin-induced syngeneic graft-vs-host disease. J Immunol 1994; 153:400.
73. Qin S, Cobold SP, Pope, et al. "Infectious" transplantation tolerance. Science 1993; 259:974–977.
74. Pearce NW, Berger MF, Gurley KE, et al. Specific unresponsiveness in rats with prolonged cardiac allograft survival after treatment with cyclosporine. Transplantation 1993; 55:380–389.
75. Zhang J, Medaer R, Stinissen P. MHC-restricted depletion of human myelin basic protein-reactive T cells by T cell vaccination. Science 1993; 261:1451–1453.
76. Howard M, O'Garra A. Biological properties of interleukin 10. Immunol Today 1992; 13:198–200.
77. Offner H, Malotky MKH, Pope L, et al. Increased severity of experimental autoimmune encephalomyelitis in rats tolerized as adults but not neonatally to a protective TcR Vβ8 CDR2 idiotype. J Immunol 1995; 154:928.
78. Jenkins MK, Miller RA. Memory and anergy: Challenges to traditional models of T lymphocyte differentiation. FASEB J 1993; 6:2428–2433.
79. Mueller DL, Jenkins MK, Schwartz RH. Clonal expansions vs functional clonal inactivation. Annu Rev Immunol 1989; 7:445–481.
80. Hiruma K, Gress RE. Cyclosporin A and peripheral tolerance. J Immunol 1992; 149: 1539.
81. Vanier LE, Prud'homme GJ. Cyclosporin A markedly enhances superantigen-induced peripheral T-cell deletion and inhibits anergy induction. J Exp Med 1992; 176:37–46.
82. Jenkins MK, Pardoll DM, Mizuguchi J, et al. Molecular events in the induction of a nonresponsive state in interleukin 2-producing helper T lymphocyte clones. Proc Nat Acad Sci USA 1987; 84:5409–5414.
83. Cooper MH, Hartman GG, Starzl TE, et al. The induction of pseudo-graft-vs-host disease following a syngeneic bone marrow transplantation using FK 506. Transplant Proc 1991; 23:3234–3235.
84. Kersey JH, Weisdorf D, Nesbit ME, et al. Comparison of autologous and allogeneic bone marrow transplantation for treatment of high-risk refractory acute lymphoblastic leukemia. N Engl J Med 1987; 317:461.
85. Philip T, Armitage JO, Spitzer G, et al. High-dose therapy and autologous bone marrow transplantation after failure of conventional chemotherapy in adults with intermediate-grade non-Hodgkin's lymphoma. N Engl J Med 1987; 316:1493.
86. Horowitz MM, Gale RP, Sondel PM, et al. Graft-versus-leukemia reactions after bone marrow transplantation. Blood 1990; 75:555.
87. Weiden PL, Flournoy N, Thomas ED, et al. Antileukemic effect of graft-versus-host disease in human recipients of allogeneic marrow grafts. N Engl J Med 1979; 300:1068.
88. Geller RB, Esa AH, Beschorner We, et al. Successful in vitro graft-versus-tumor effect

against an Ia-bearing tumor using cyclosporine-induced syngeneic graft-versus-host disease in the rat. Blood 1989; 74:1165.

89. Hess AD, Noga SJ. Cyclosporine-induced syngeneic graft-versus-host disease: An immunotherapeutic approach after autologous bone marrow transplantation. Int J Cell Cloning 1992; 10(suppl 1):179.
90. Noga SJ, Horwitz L, Kim H, et al. γ-Interferon potentiates the anti-tumor effect of cyclosporine-induced autoimmunity. J Hematother 1992; 1:75.
91. Jones RJ, Vogelsang GB, Hess AD, et al. Induction of graft-versus-host disease after autologous bone marrow transplantation. Lancet 1989; 1:754.
92. Dale BM, Atkinson K, Kotasek D, et al. Cyclosporine-induced graft-versus-host disease in two patients receiving syngeneic bone marrow transplants. Transplant Proc 1989; 21: 3816.
93. Carella AM, Gaozza E, Piatti G. Induction of graft-versus-host disease (GVHD) after ABMT for high risk ALL in first CR and second chronic phase of chronic myeloid leukemia (abstr). Exp Hematol 1990; 18:684.
94. Ruvolo P, Bright EC, Kennedy MJ, et al. Cyclosporine-induced autologous graft-versus-host disease: Assessment of cytocytic effector mechanisms and the Vβ T cell receptor repertoire. Transplant Proc 1995; 27:1363–1365.
95. Jones RJ, Vogelsang GB, Ambinder RF, et al. Autologous marrow transplantation (ABMT) with cyclosporine (CsA)-induced autologous graft-versus-host disease (GVHD) for relapsed aggressive non-Hodgkin's lymphoma (NHL) (abstr). Blood 1991; 78:287a.
96. Yeager AM, Vogelsang GB, Jones RF, et al. Induction of cutaneous graft-versus-host disease by administration of cyclosporine to patients undergoing autologous bone marrow transplantation for acute myeloid leukemia. Blood, 1992; 79:3031.
97. Kennedy MJ, Beveridge R, Vogelsang GB, et al. Phase I study of cyclosporine (CsA) to induce graft-versus-host disease (GVHD) following high dose chemotherapy (HDC) with autologous marrow reinfusion (AMR) for metastatic breast cancer (MBC) (abstr). Am Soc Clin Oncol 1991; 10:43.
98. Kennedy MJ, Vogelsang GB, Jones RJ, et al. Phase I trial of interferon-gamma to potentiate cyclosporin A-induced graft-versus-host disease in women undergoing autologous bone marrow transplantation for breast cancer. J Clin Oncol 1994; 12:249.
99. Hess AD, Kennedy MJ, Bright EC, et al. Induction of autoimmune graft-vs-host disease after autologous bone marrow transplantation augmented with peripheral blood stem cells: Analysis of immune function (abstr). Blood 1994; 83(suppl 1):33.

21

Transfusion-Associated Graft-Versus-Host Disease

Kenneth C. Anderson
Dana-Farber Cancer Institute and Harvard Medical School
Boston, Massachusetts

I. INTRODUCTION

A. Comparison of Transfusion-Associated with Bone Marrow Transplant-Associated Graft-Versus-Host Disease

Graft-versus-host disease (GVHD) is a frequent complication of allogeneic bone marrow transplantation (ABMT), in which setting viable lymphocytes derived from donor bone marrow cannot be eliminated by an immunodeficient host. GVHD is mediated by donor T lymphocytes that recognize host HLA antigens as foreign and mount an immune response, which is manifested clinically by the development of fever, a characteristic cutaneous eruption, diarrhea, and liver function abnormalities (1) (Table 1). GVHD is less frequently encountered in the setting of solid-organ transplantation; in such cases, it is mediated by T lymphocytes that may be present in the transplanted organ (2–4). GVHD can also occur as a complication of transfusion of cellular blood components that contain donor T lymphocytes: multiple reports in the 1970s and 1980s served to establish transfusion-associated GVHD (TA-GVHD) as a distinct disease entity (5–10). In addition to the aforementioned clinical features, TA-GVHD is further characterized by marrow aplasia and pancytopenia. In contrast to GVHD that develops in the setting of ABMT, TA-GVHD is notoriously resistant to treatment with immunosuppressive therapies, including corticosteroids, cyclosporine, antithymocyte globulin, and ablative therapy followed by BMT. Clinical manifestations and death occur at 8 to 10 days and 3 to 4 weeks posttransfusion, respectively (11). The resistance to treatment and fatal outcome highlight the need for identification of patient groups at risk for TA-GVHD and use of methods for its prevention.

Table 1 Clinical and Pathological Comparison of Graft-Versus-Host Disease Associated with Bone Marrow Transplantation (BMTA-GVHD) and with Transfusions (TA-GVHD)

Manifestation	BMTA-GVHD	TA-GVHD
Skin rash	+[a]	+
GI involvement	+	+
Liver pathology	Obstructive	Hepatocellular
Liver tests		
Enzymes	±	Markedly increased
Alkaline phosphatase	Increased	−
Bilirubin	Increased	−
Bone marrow hypoplasia/aplasia	−	+
Pancytopenia	+[b]	+
Time of onset	20–100 days (gradual)	2–50 days (abrupt)
Response to therapy	60–70%	None
Mortality rate	10–15%	90–100%
Occurrence	50%	<1%

[a]+ present; ± mildly present; − absent.
[b]Predominantly thrombocytopenia.
Source: Ref. 12.

B. Epidemiology of TA-GVHD

All of the available epidemiological data on TA-GVHD are based upon reports of single patients or very small groups. A prospective study on the development of this disease has never been undertaken and would, in fact, be very difficult to perform. Estimates of the incidence and identification of patient groups at risk are therefore subject to the limitations of retrospective data analysis; foremost among these are the underreporting of cases and in many instances the absence of definitive diagnostic studies. At least two factors may contribute to the underreporting of cases of TA-GVHD: the diagnosis may not be considered, and it may be difficult or impossible to establish with certainty. Thus, while over 200 cases of presumed TA-GVHD have been reported or referenced in the Japanese and English literature, definitive diagnostic tests have been performed in only a minority of cases (11–15). The overall reported mortality is approximately 90%, although rare survivors have been documented (16,17). Two surveys of risk factors for the development of TA-GVHD have recently been completed in Japan, where TA-GVHD has commonly been reported. Takahashi and colleagues have analyzed 171 cases of TA-GVHD and found that risk factors included cardiovascular surgery, cancer, fresh and consanguineous blood transfusions, and being male (18). Ohto and Anderson have reviewed 122 cases of TA-GVHD in Japan and similarly found that TA-GVHD was most commonly noted in the setting of cardiovascular surgery, solid tumors, after transfusion of fresh blood, when donors were consanguineous, and when recipients were men (19).

C. Pathogenesis of TA-GVHD

The central issue in the pathogenesis of GVHD is the extent to which the recipient of a graft or transfusion is able to mount an immune response against donor T lymphocytes. The immune status of the host and the extent of HLA disparity between donor and recipient together determine the extent of any host-versus-graft reaction. Thus, Billingham has proposed three requirements for the development of GVHD: (a) differences in histocompatibility (HLA) antigens between the donor and the recipient; (b) the presence of immunocompetent cells in the graft; and (c) inability of the host to reject these immunocompetent cells (20). Since transfused cellular blood products are rarely tested for HLA antigens, the first of these requirements is almost always present in the circumstance of blood transfusion. As described above, TA-GVHD is mediated by viable T lymphocytes within nonirradiated transfused cellular blood components. Congenital or acquired immunodeficiency states provide the most common and obvious basis for an individual's failure to reject donor-derived cells, and TA-GVHD has been described in a wide variety of patients with apparent immune compromise (5). The naturally or iatrogenically immunosuppressed recipient has only a limited capacity to generate an effective host-versus-graft reaction, and greater HLA disparity confers increased probability that donor lymphocytes will attack host tissues.

Since immune cells in an immunocompetent host outnumber donor- derived T cells, the latter are effectively eliminated by virtue of a host-versus-graft reaction. However, if an immunocompetent individual heterozygous for a given HLA haplotype is transfused with even a small number of functional T lymphocytes from a donor who is homozygous for that HLA haplotype, the recipient's immune system may not recognize donor cells as foreign and therefore be incapable of eliminating them. In contrast, donor-derived T cells recognize those host HLA antigens that are encoded by the unshared haplotype as foreign, undergo clonal expansion, and establish TA-GVHD (21–23). The HLA relationship between such individuals is referred to as a "one-way HLA match," and the TA-GVHD expressed under these circumstances may be expected to occur regardless of the host's immune status, since the failure to eliminate donor-derived T lymphocytes is based on the sharing of HLA antigens with the donor rather than immune compromise within the recipient (Fig. 1) (24).

In both immunocompetent and immunodeficient hosts, TA-GVHD is characterized by inexorable proliferation of donor T lymphocytes and rapid elimination of all circulating host cellular blood elements, as described by Ito et al. (8). Moreover, a patient with chronic myelogenous leukemia who received a T-cell-depleted histocompatible BM allograft developed both graft rejection and GVHD; a variety of tests confirmed that cells in the patient's peripheral blood and BM were not derived from either the donor or the recipient (25). These cells were thought to represent a population of proliferating transfused cells that were alloreactive against both donor and host.

Recently, Lee and colleagues have applied a quantitative allele- specific polymerase chain reaction (PCR) to follow the fate of donor leukocytes after transfusion into humans and dogs (26). Their preliminary results demonstrate rapid clearance of cells on the first day, followed by a transient 1- to 2-log expansion after 4 to 6 days, presumably reflecting delayed clonal expansion of selected cells. Long-term donor-derived multilineage hematopoiesis has also recently been reported in a liver transplant recipient (27). The characteristics of the donor leukocytes surviving and proliferating in the recipient after transfusion, the mechanism for their subsequent elimination, and the role of HLA antigens in this process are all unknown, but such

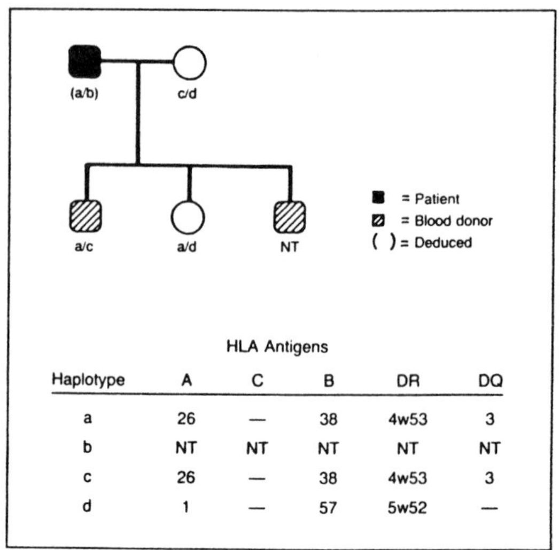

Haplotype	A	C	B	DR	DQ
a	26	—	38	4w53	3
b	NT	NT	NT	NT	NT
c	26	—	38	4w53	3
d	1	—	57	5w52	—

Figure 1 Results of HLA typing of Family 1. Squares indicate males, and circles females. NT denotes not tested.

studies are central to the understanding of TA-GVHD (28). The minimum number of donor lymphocytes required to mediate TA-GVHD is unclear, although the disease has been reported following transfusion of blood products expected to contain approximately 10^7 lymphocytes (29).

II. CLINICAL AND DIAGNOSTIC FEATURES OF TA-GVHD

A. Clinical Manifestations

The clinical manifestations of TA-GVHD are similar to those of GVHD in other settings and include fever, skin rash, watery or bloody diarrhea, elevated liver enzymes, and hyperbilirubinemia (Table 1). In addition, bone marrow failure, which manifests as pancytopenia, is a characteristic feature of the terminal phase of the disease and distinguishes it from GVHD occurring after BM or organ transplantation. The skin rash usually begins as an erythematous maculopapular eruption centrally, spreads to the extremities, and may progress to generalized erythroderma and bullous formation in severe cases. Similarly, diarrhea may be severe and elevation of liver function tests can be extreme, reflecting extensive hepatocellular damage. Additional manifestations may include anorexia, nausea, and vomiting. The majority of cases of TA-GVHD are rapidly fatal; time from onset of symptoms to death can be less than 1 week and rarely exceeds 3 to 4 weeks. Patients usually succumb to complications of bone marrow failure, primarily infection.

Since there are no pathognomonic features of GVHD, this syndrome is sometimes difficult to distinguish from viral infections or drug reactions (30). This assumes particular clinical importance in the transfusion-related disease, where the index of suspicion for this diagnosis may be low and a patient who has required blood product support may harbor significant comorbidity. Nonetheless, characteristic changes are demonstrable on skin biopsy, including degeneration of the epidermal basal cell layer with vacuolization; dermal-epithelial layer separation and bullae formation; mononuclear cell migration into and infiltration of the upper dermis; hyperkeratosis; and degenerative dyskeratosis (31,32). Liver biopsies reveal degeneration and eosinophilic necrosis of the small bile ducts, with intense periportal inflammation and mononuclear (lymphocytic) cell infiltration (33). Bone marrow aspirates may reveal lymphocytic infiltration, pancytopenia, and fibrosis.

B. Diagnostic Parameters

Although the clinical syndrome associated with TA-GVHD is dramatic and frequently fatal, the differential diagnosis is broad: a myriad of factors can result in the development of fevers, skin rashes, and liver function abnormalities. Certainly other etiologies, such as infection and drug reaction, are more commonly encountered in clinical practice and more likely to be investigated. Although histological findings in the skin and gastrointestinal tract may suggest the diagnosis of TA-GVHD, they are not pathognomonic; the only definitive diagnosis of TA-GVHD is the demonstration of donor-derived lymphocytes in the circulation and affected organs of the host in the appropriate clinical setting. This requires either careful HLA-typing or some other technique that reliably distinguishes between host and donor cells (34–36). However, since the disease involves rapid elimination of circulating host blood cells, samples adequate for HLA typing are frequently not available. Some workers have circumvented this problem by using PCR-based methods for HLA typing (34–36) or by deducing the patient's HLA type from those of surviving first-degree relatives (21). Cytogenetics have been employed in the event that donor and recipient have been of different gender or when the disease has followed transfusion of granulocytes donated by individuals with Philadelphia chromosome–positive chronic myeloid leukemia (37). Increasingly sophisticated techniques for confirming the diagnosis of TA-GVHD have included the detection of polymorphisms for restriction fragment lengths and human microsatellite markers (36). Even so, all too often the diagnosis is made postmortem.

III. CLINICAL SETTINGS IN WHICH TA-GVHD HAS BEEN REPORTED

A. Historical Perspective

In 1955, Shimoda reported the first Japanese case of "postoperative erythroderma," now considered to be the same disease as TA-GVHD (38). The syndrome was later described following transfusion in immunodeficient children in 1965 (39). Over the next 15 years, 38 cases of TA-GVHD were described in patients with severe combined immunodeficiency and Wiskott-Aldrich syndromes; in newborns with erythroblastosis fetalis; and in patients with hematological malignancies, including Hodgkin's disease and non-Hodgkin's lymphoma, acute lymphoblastic and myelocytic leukemia, and chronic lymphocytic leukemia (7). Although its true incidence remains unknown, TA-GVHD was estimated to occur in 0.1 to 1.0% of patients with hematological malignancies or lymphoproliferative diseases, and patients carrying the above diagnoses were felt to be at risk for TA-GVHD. In 1984 Weiden suggested that the risk of developing TA-GVHD be extended to patients with neuroblastoma who received high-dose therapy (40). In a 1987 review of 27 reported cases of TA-GVHD in patients with both hematological malignancies and solid tumors (neuroblastoma, rhabdomyosarcoma, and glioblastoma), Kessinger and colleagues noted that all affected patients had received cytotoxic chemotherapy and 13 had received prior radiation therapy (41). Cases of TA-GVHD have been documented in patients with Hodgkin's disease who were treated with either chemotherapy alone or with a combination of chemotherapy and ionizing radiation (42).

B. Reported Cases of TA-GVHD (Tables 2 to 4)

TA-GVHD continues to be reported, albeit rarely, in patients with malignancies. It was originally recognized in patients with solid tumors receiving intensive therapy for neuroblastoma (43,44). Of 34 patients with solid tumors (lung and germ-cell cancer) who were treated with high doses of chemotherapy and autologous BM infusions and subsequently received transfusions of nonirradiated blood cells, 4 also developed TA-GVHD (45,46). Case reports documenting TA-GVHD in patients with cervical, renal, esophageal, lung, bladder, and prostate carcinoma who did not receive aggressive chemotherapy indicate that a broader spectrum of patients with solid tumors may be at risk (21,37,39,47,48). Cases of TA-GVHD have also been documented in premature infants who received unirradiated blood products in the setting of hyaline- membrane disease or suspected sepsis and respiratory distress syndrome; these patients did not have congenital immunodeficiency syndromes or erythroblastosis fetalis (49,50).

It is interesting that there have been no reported cases of TA- GVHD in patients with AIDS. Perhaps some of the signs and symptoms (rashes, pancytopenia, liver function abnormalities) presently attributed to infections, drug reactions, and other coexistent medical conditions in patients with AIDS are related to TA-GVHD (30). Alternatively, qualitative aspects of the nature of the immune deficit in AIDS may not predispose patients to the development of TA-GVHD (51). In addition, the disease has also only rarely been reported in recipients of organ transplants or in patients on immunosuppressive medications. Although GVHD in organ transplant recipients has been attributed to passenger lymphocytes within the graft, molecular

Table 2 Transfusion Associated Graft-Versus-Host Disease in Patients with Congenital and Acquired Immunodeficiency Syndromes

Clinical Setting
Severe combined immunodeficiency syndrome
Thymic hypoplasia
Wiskott-Aldrich syndrome
Lenier's disease
5′ nucleotidase deficiency
Nonspecified immunodeficiency
Hemolytic disease of the fetus or newborn
Premature newborns
Neonatal alloimmune thrombocytopenia
Neonatal immunosuppressive medication

Table 3 Posttransfusion Graft-Versus-Host Disease in Patients with Malignancies

Clinical Setting
Hematologic
Hodgkin's disease
Non-Hodgkin's lymphoma
Acute Myelocytic leukemia
Acute Lymphocytic leukemia
Chronic Lymphocytic leukemia
Aplastic anemia
Solid tumors
Neuroblastoma
Lung carcinoma
Glioblastoma
Rhabdomyosarcoma
Cervical carcinoma
Esophageal carcinoma
Renal adenocarcinoma
Bladder carcinoma
Autologous bone marrow transplantation
Lung cancer
Germ cell tumor

techniques have recently been used to implicate transfused lymphocytes in a liver transplant recipient (4).

C. TA-GVHD in Immunocompetent Patients

TA-GVHD has been reported in individuals without obvious immunodeficiencies (18,19,52). In 1986 the syndrome was described following blood transfusion to a patient in Japan who had surgery for an aortic aneurysm and was not recognized to be immunodeficient (9). A survey of 340 Japanese hospitals documented "postoperative erythroderma," identical to TA-GVHD, in 96 of the 63,257 patients who

Table 4 Transfusion-Associated Graft-Versus-Host Disease in Immunocompetent Patients

Clinical Setting
Pregnancy
Cholecystectomy
Cardiac surgery
Vascular surgery
Gastrointestinal surgery
Abdominal surgery
Alpha thalassemia
Liver transplantation
Pancreosplenic transplantation

underwent cardiac surgery, with a mortality rate of 90% (53). Cases of TA-GVHD after cardiac surgery were subsequently reported from the United States and Israel (24,54). More recently, fatal GVHD has been reported in a number of HLA-heterozygous transfusion recipients who shared a haplotype with related or unrelated HLA-homozygous donors (15,21,24,55–58). Clinical settings in which TA-GVHD has been reported in immunocompetent hosts include pregnancy; cardiac, vascular, and abdominal surgeries; alpha thalassemia; rheumatoid arthritis; trauma; and short-term corticosteroid therapy (15,17–19,21,24,55–60).

Initial reports of TA-GVHD were limited to patients with either demonstrated or presumed immunodeficiency (7), which led to the belief that this was a prerequisite for the development of the disease. Indeed, immunodeficient patients constitute the largest group at risk for TA-GVHD within the United States. Since 1986, however, the syndrome has been reported among apparently immunocompetent individuals from Japan, Israel, Great Britain, Australia, and the United States (15,17–19,21,24,55–60). The clinical course and outcome in immunocompetent patients does not appear to be any different from that described above in immunocompromised transfusion recipients. A one-way HLA match, or significant sharing of HLA antigens between donor and recipient, may account not only for many of the cases of TA-GVHD in immunocompetent patients but also for at least some of the cases in immunocompromised patients. Based upon the likelihood of a one-way HLA match, certain groups are intrinsically at risk for the development of TA-GVHD: patients who receive blood products donated by close relatives and individuals from a population with limited genetic heterogeneity who receive blood products donated by other individuals within the same population (15,18,19).

Related-donor transfusions account for about half the cases of TA-GVHD reported in presumed immunocompetent patients (15). Kanter has employed a mathematical model to derive the risk of transfusion of blood from an HLA-homozygous donor to related HLA-heterozygous recipients who share that haplotype (61). Parents and children presented the greatest risk, but he concluded that some second-degree related donors presented a greater risk than siblings. More importantly, in this analysis there was no sharp cutoff of risk among the various classes of related donors. Indeed, transfusion from a grandson to his grandfather has now been implicated in causing GVHD (15). In a retrospective analysis of published cases of TA-GVHD in patients receiving chemotherapy for hematological or solid neoplasms, Charpentier and colleagues noted that 7 of 26 patients had received blood components donated by parents, children, or siblings and that a one-way HLA match was verified in 3 of these 7 cases (62). Other recent reports confirm that HLA-matched platelets may be implicated in TA-GVHD (63,64). These data support the view that HLA relatedness or haploidentity may account for a significant proportion of cases of TA-GVHD even in immunocompromised patients, and they underscore the notion that a one-way HLA match predisposes to the development of TA-GVHD regardless of the host's immune status.

The vast majority of reported cases of TA-GVHD occurring in patients who were presumed to be immunocompetent and who were transfused with blood products donated by an unrelated individual have been reported in Japan, where the population is relatively homogeneous (18,19). The application of a mathematical model to population data on HLA haplotypes in various countries has yielded useful estimates for the probability of transfusion of blood from HLA homozygotes to heterozygotes with a shared haplotype (65). These probability estimates range from 1/874 among the Japanese to 1/7174 among U.S. whites and 1/16,835 among the French. Interestingly, 6 of 8 Japanese cases involved the most common HLA haplotype in that country's population, A2-Bw52-C and two other cases involved an HLA haplotype that is represented in 5.8% of the Japanese population (55).

D. Patient Groups at Risk for Development of TA-GVHD (Table 5)

Clearly many, but not all, conditions or treatments that compromise immunity appear to predispose patients to the development of TA- GVHD. At the same time, immunocompetent individuals are not necessarily protected, particularly in the event of a one-way HLA match. The lack of reported GVHD after transfusion of unirradiated blood components to patients who are known to be immunodeficient, coupled with the development of this syndrome in patients without in vitro immune dysfunction, suggests that the risk factors predisposing to TA-GVHD are only partially defined. Blood transfusion itself may be immunosuppressive (66), and the argument can be made that almost every patient who requires transfusion of a blood product is potentially immunocompromised in some way that could facilitate the development of TA-GVHD. The low incidence of TA-GVHD in presumably immunocompetent patients may result from underrecognition of the syndrome, as discussed above, but likely also reflects effective defense against it in individuals with truly intact immune function (30,67).

IV. IMPLICATED BLOOD PRODUCTS

This syndrome has developed following exchange and intrauterine transfusions and after transfusion of whole blood, plasma, red blood cells, and platelets. Leukocytes

Table 5 Patient Groups at Risk for Developing TA-GVHD

A. Established risk
- Patients with:
  - Congenital immunodeficiencies
  - Hodgkin's disease
- Newborns with erythroblastosis fetalis
- Intrauterine transfusions
- Recipients of allogeneic bone marrow transplants
- Recipients of blood products donated by relatives
- Recipients of HLA-matched cellular transfusions

B. Probable risk
- Patients with:
  - Hematologic malignancies other than Hodgkin's disease
  - Solid tumors treated with cytotoxic agents
- Recipient-donor pairs from genetically homogeneous populations

C. No established risk
- Premature or term neonates
- Patients with acquired immunodeficiency syndrome (AIDS)
- Patients receiving immunosuppressive medications

harvested from normal donors and from donors with chronic myelocytic leukemia have also been transfused to patients with hematologic malignancies and been implicated in TA-GVHD. To date, transfusions of fresh frozen plasma, frozen deglycerolized red blood cells, or clotting factor concentrates have not definitively been implicated in causing TA-GVHD.

Transfusions of red cells or platelets account for the majority of cases of TA-GVHD, reflecting the higher frequency of transfusion of these components relative to other cellular blood products. The risk of developing TA-GVHD appears to be related to the presence of viable contaminating T lymphocytes rather than to any specific blood product. Many of these patients did receive transfusions of freshly donated—i.e., not stored—cellular blood products. Since fresh blood contains larger numbers of viable (and presumably competent) lymphocytes than blood that has been stored for a period prior to transfusion (68), it is not surprising that the use of unstored blood surfaces as a major risk factor for the development of TA-GVHD in univariate analysis (15). The practice of transfusing freshly donated blood is decreasing in Japan, where this was until recently a common clinical practice (69). However, it remains unclear whether the small numbers of lymphocytes that survive the storage process can mediate TA-GVHD in all susceptible patients; cases of TA-GVHD have occurred following transfusion of blood products that were stored for variable periods of time (68).

V. TREATMENT OF TA-GVHD

A. Therapy of Established TA-GVHD

Results on the treatment of TA-GVHD have been uniformly dismal, and failure at treatment accounts for the high mortality rate associated with the disease. Attempted immunosuppressive therapies have included glucocorticoids, antithymocyte globulin, cyclosporine, cyclophosphamide, and anti-T-cell monoclonal antibodies (52–57). Although some of these agents have been successful in the treatment of post-BMT GVHD, they have been ineffective for TA-GVHD. Resistance to treatment appears to reflect the pathophysiology rather than the common delays in diagnosis, since patients diagnosed early in the course of the disease fare no better than those diagnosed later. Rare responses to some of the commonly used agents have been reported (16,17), but it is difficult to extract meaningful guidelines for clinical practice. Since the disease has an immune basis, clinicians may consider a therapeutic trial of glucocorticoids, despite the low likelihood of efficacy. TA-GVHD is a serious and increasingly frequent disease for which new therapies are clearly needed.

B. Prevention of TA-GVHD

1. Gamma Irradiation

Since attempts at treatment of TA-GVHD have been unsuccessful, the primary emphasis has been on prevention. Prevention of TA-GVHD by gamma irradiation of blood was first described in mice in 1959 (70,71) and in humans 2 years later (72,73). As little as 500 cGy of gamma irradiation can abrogate the response of lymphocytes to allogeneic cells in a mixed lymphocyte culture, and 1500 cGy can reduce response to mitogen-induced stimulation by 90% (74). Button and colleagues have examined the function of blood components after irradiation doses of 500 to 20,000 cGy and demonstrated that doses up to 5000 cGy decreased mitogen stimulation by 98.5% without compromising the function of cells other than lymphocytes: specifically, irradiated red blood cells had no change in survival; granulocytes had normal in vitro bacterial killing capacity, chemotactic mobility, and superoxide production; and transfused irradiated platelets produced the expected increases in platelet counts and controlled hemostasis in thrombocytopenic patients (75). However, doses of 5000 cGy decreased the yield of platelets posttransfusion by one-third. At least two cases of GVHD after transfusion of irradiated blood components have been reported (25,76). Limiting dilution experiments suggest that the frequency of lymphocytes able to respond to mitogen is reduced by 5 to 6 logs by irradiation at 2500 to 3000 rads, compared to unirradiated controls (25,77,78). Based upon this and other similar studies, it has been recommended that 2500 cGy, be utilized to irradiate cellular blood components prior to transfusion (79); 97% of American Association of Blood Banks (AABB) institutions surveyed in 1989, when 1500 cGy was the minimum dose recommended, utilized doses of 1500 to 3500 cGy (80). Lowenthal and colleagues have observed a case of TA-GVHD in a recipient of irradiated cellular components and suggested that a dose of 3000 cGy may be more appropriate. Clearly the guidelines for irradiation may require reevaluation in the future, as more sensitive techniques become available for the detection of survival of transfused lymphocytes.

Several studies address the potential adverse consequences of irradiation followed by storage of blood products (81). Ramirez and colleagues irradiated red-cell concentrates at 3000 rads and noted a threefold elevation in potassium levels relative to controls (82). Rivet et al. confirmed that potassium levels increase with length of storage in both irradiated and nonirradiated red-cell concentrates, that the length of storage prior to irradiation does not significantly affect the potassium level, and that manual washing and reconstitution with fresh frozen plasma was effective in reducing the potassium levels of all red-cell concentrates (83). The total infusion load of potassium appears to be clinically insignificant in adults (84) but may be substantial in neonates (85,86); this has led to the recommendation that blood required for intrauterine, neonatal, or pediatric transfusion not be stored after irradiation or that irradiated red-cell concentrates used for neonatal transfusions be washed manually to reduce potassium levels (83). Most recent studies have documented decreases in ATP, increases in potassium, and increases in plasma hemoglobin after irradiation of red cells at 3000 to 3500 cGy and storage for 42 days (87,88). Red-cell survival has been reported to be decreased after transfusion of stored irradiated (68% survival) versus stored nonirradiated red cells (78% survival) (88). It has recently been shown that red cells can be irradiated, stored at 4°C for 6 days, and subsequently frozen with no increase in detectable damage as compared to controls that were not irradiated (89). Indeed, irradiated red cells can be frozen after being stored under various conditions and can still meet established guidelines requiring 75% recovery 24 hr after transfusion (90). Studies to date suggest that gamma irradiation of platelets with 2000 to 3000 cGy and subsequent storage for 5 days does not adversely affect in vitro platelet function or in vivo posttransfusion recovery and survival (91–94).

C. Current Practices and Guidelines for the Prevention of TA-GVHD

Attempts have recently been made to delineate blood component irradiation practices. Greenbaum surveyed 100 physicians selected at random from the membership directories of professional societies (14). Among 66 responders from 56 institutions, 30, 10, and 40.5% indicated that they provided irradiated blood products to all patients, potential or post-BMT patients, and selected patients, respectively. Blood component irradiation practice has also been examined in a survey of 2250 blood centers, hospital blood banks, or transfusion services that are institutional members of the American Association of Blood Banks: 12.3% of the institutions had on-site facilities for the irradiation of blood components; 952,516 of 9,397,516 (10.1%) components transfused in 1989 were irradiated; and 44 cases of TA-GVHD were identified (80). There was marked variability in blood component irradiation practice, even for patient groups in whom the risk of TA-GVHD is well defined. For example, 12, 19, and 32% of institutions did not provide irradiated components to recipients of allogeneic BMT, patients receiving autologous BMT, and those with congenital immunodeficiencies, respectively. Irradiated blood components were provided by 51.4, 34, 32, and 20% of institutions to patients with leukemias, Hodgkin's disease, non-Hodgkin's lymphomas, and solid tumors, respectively; and 24.5% of respondents provided irradiated blood products to patients with acquired immunodeficiency syndrome (AIDS), in spite of the fact that no cases of TA-GVHD have yet been noted in this setting.

The Transfusion Practices Committee of the AABB has delineated patient groups currently felt to be at risk for TA-GVHD and who should therefore receive only irradiated cellular blood components (80). Specifically, the risk of TA-GVHD is well defined in patients who have undergone BMT, in patients with congenital immunodeficiency syndromes, after intrauterine transfusion, in recipients of transfusions from first- or second- degree blood relatives, and in patients with Hodgkin's disease. In addition, many centers irradiate cellular blood products transfused into all patients with hematological malignancies or who have been treated with cytotoxic agents for neoplastic diseases. However, the risk of TA-GVHD remains under review in patients with hematological malignancies other than Hodgkin's disease, patients with solid tumors, premature newborns, and organ transplant recipients. Patients in whom no risks have yet been defined include term newborns and patients with AIDS.

Directed donations from immediate family members increase the likelihood of TA-GVHD because such donors share HLA antigens with recipients; homozygosity for HLA types is likely to be present not only among first-degree relatives but also among all related recipient-donor pairs (61). Irradiation of blood components from such directed donations may be utilized to avoid this complication, and the AABB has broadened its original recommendation, now suggesting that cellular blood components from all related donors be irradiated with at least 2500 cGy prior to transfusion (79).

In alloimmunized patients refractory to standard platelet transfusion therapy, the provision of HLA-matched platelets from donors sharing at least two antigens at the HLA-A and -B loci has been demonstrated to result in satisfactory platelet increments (95). However, the provision of platelets from donors sharing HLA antigens may predispose to TA-GVHD (62–64), and irradiation of transfused platelets under these circumstances may be prudent.

The recent cases of TA-GVHD reported after cardiac surgery in both Israel and Japan (18,19,23,24) occurred after transfusion of fresh whole blood, utilized due to the purported improved hemostatic effect of fresh whole blood versus platelet concentrates; however, there is no evidence that fresh blood is in fact more useful in this regard than stored blood (96,97). Moreover, there is no evidence that avoidance of the transfusion of fresh blood components can prevent GVHD. Indeed some components—i.e., platelets—must be used "fresh" or transfused after only 5 days of storage. At present, therefore, there is no reason to alter storage time between donation and transfusion of blood components due to concern for TA-GVHD.

The relatively low frequency of TA-GVHD in immunocompetent patients receiving blood donated by unrelated donors has thus far precluded the broad application of gamma irradiation to all transfused cellular blood products. Issues relating to cost, the logistics of irradiation in emergency and small clinic settings, and the exceedingly low risk of TA-GVHD in most cases have also been raised (98,99). However, this practice seems to be indicated within genetically homogenous populations, i.e., in the Japanese, when transfusion of unirradiated products from a nonblood relative homozygous for a given HLA haplotype to a recipient heterozygous for that haplotype can commonly occur.

VI. FUTURE DIRECTIONS

A. Leukodepletion of Cellular Blood Components to Prevent TA-GVHD

There are two potential alternatives to gamma irradiation for the prevention of TA-GVHD, but both are presently unproven. The first would involve depletion of lymphocytes from blood products prior to transfusion. Reductions in both the incidence and severity of GVHD postallogeneic BMT can be achieved if T cells are eliminated from the donor BM prior to grafting by a variety of techniques (100–104). Most currently utilized ex vivo methods are capable of removing >90% of T cells from donor marrow, with approximately 10^7 residual marrow T lymphocytes. Although these techniques abrogate GVHD in HLA-matched patients, almost every study reports at last some patients who develop GVHD, with more severe manifestations in HLA-mismatched patients. While it may not be either possible or practical to treat blood components in a similar fashion, techniques are presently available for the reduction of leukocytes from red cells: elimination of the buffy coat after centrifugation; direct or inverted dilution-centrifugation; washing; filtration; or freezing (105–107). Leukocytes can be removed from platelets by centrifugation or filtration or using current apheresis technology (106–108). These techniques may result in $<5 \times 10^6$ residual leukocytes (109–110) and have been developed primarily for the avoidance of febrile nonhemolytic transfusion reactions, alloimmunization, cytomegalovirus transmission, and immunomodulation. However, since the number and precise T-cell populations required to mediate TA-GVHD remain undefined, it is unknown whether depletion of leukocytes using these currently available techniques would decrease the risk of TA-GVHD. It is known that frozen deglycerolized blood contains less than 2% residual lymphocytes with intact proliferative ability (105), confirming that some immunocompetent T cells are present. Moreover, bedside filtration has been shown to be ineffective at prevention of HLA alloimmunization (111), suggesting that filtration as currently practiced may not be achieving expected leukodepletion. Indeed, TA-GVHD has been reported after transfusion of leukocyte-reduced (filtered) red cells in a patient with Hodgkin's disease (112). Although it remains important to determine whether leukocyte reduction can prevent TA-GVHD, it is critical to emphasize that at present even leukodepleted cellular components must be irradiated to avoid TA- GVHD.

B. Ultraviolet Irradiation of Blood Components to Prevent TA-GVHD

Second, a canine model has been used to demonstrate that ultraviolet (UV), rather than gamma, irradiation of transfused leukocytes can abrogate GVHD in recipient animals (113). Four dogs who received unirradiated leukocytes, two of three dogs given leukocytes irradiated with 20 mJ/cm^2 UV light (200–300 nm), and none of three dogs transfused with leukocytes irradiated to 1000 mJ/cm^2 developed GVHD. Preliminary studies in humans have utilized UV irradiation of blood components to minimize alloimmunization (114). Future studies will determine whether UV light can, in fact, avoid either alloimmunization or TA-GVHD in transfusion recipients without adverse effects on in vitro function or in vivo recovery of treated red cells and platelets.

Finally, van der Mast and colleagues have raised the provocative suggestion that host T cells may exert protective effects against the development of TA-GVHD, at least in immunocompetent patients (67). It remains to be seen whether such an effect can ever be harnessed therapeutically. Meanwhile, the practical emphasis remains on gamma irradiation, which has been shown to be effective not only in vitro in preventing lymphocyte reactivity, but also in vivo in decreasing the incidence of TA-GVHD when employed more generally within a given population (96).

REFERENCES

1. Ferrara JL, Deeg HJ. Graft-versus-host disease. N Engl J Med 1991; 324:667–674.
2. Burdick JF, Vogelsang GB, Smith WJ, et al. Severe graft-versus-host disease in a liver transplant recipient. N Engl J Med 1988; 318:689–691.
3. Collins RH, Anastasi J, Terstappen LWMM, et al. Brief report: Donor-derived long-term multilineage hematopoiesis in a liver-transplant recipient. N Engl J Med 1993; 328:762–765.
4. Wisecarver JL, Cattral MS, Langnas AN, et al. Transfusion-induced graft-versus-host disease after liver transplantation. Transplantation 1994; 58:269–271.
5. Hathaway WE, Fulginiti VA, Pierce CW, et al. Graft versus host reaction following a single blood transfusion. JAMA 1967; 201:1015–1020.
6. Dinsmore RE, Straus DJ, Pollack MS, et al. Fatal graft-versus-host disease following blood transfusion in Hodgkin's disease documented by HLA typing. Blood 1980; 55: 831–834.
7. Von Fliedner V, Higby DJ, Kim U. Graft versus host reaction following blood transfusion. Am J Med 1982; 72:951–956.
8. Ito K, Yoshida H, Yanagibashi K, et al. Change of HLA phenotype in postoperative erythroderma (letter). Lancet 1988; 2:413–414.

9. Sakakibara T, Juji T. Post-transfusion graft-versus-host disease after open heart surgery. Lancet 1986; 2:1099.
10. Sakakibara T, Ida T, Mannouji E, et al. Post-transfusion graft-versus-host disease following open heart surgery: Report of six cases. J Cardiovasc Surg 1989; 30:687-691.
11. Anderson KC. Clinical indications for blood component irradiation. In: Baldwin ML, Jeffries L, eds. Irradiation of Blood Components. Bethesda, MD: American Association of Blood Banks, 1992:31–49.
12. Brubaker DB. Transfusion-associated graft-versus-host disease. In Anderson KC, Ness PM, eds. Scientific Basis of Transfusion Medicine: Implications for Clinical Practice. Philadelphia: Saunders, 1994:544–580.
13. Anderson KC, Weinstein HJ. Transfusion-associated graft-versus-host disease. N Engl J Med 1990; 323:315–321.
14. Greenbaum BH. Transfusion associated graft versus host disease: Historical perspectives, incidence, and current use of irradiated blood products. J Clin Oncol 1991; 9: 1889-1902.
15. Petz LD, Calhoun L, Yam P, et al. Transfusion-associated graft-versus-host disease in immunocompetent patients: Report of a fatal case associated with transfusion of blood from a second- degree relative, and a survey of predisposing factors. Transfusion 1993; 33:742–750.
16. Cohen D, Weinstein H, Mihm M, Yankee R. Nonfatal graft-versus-host disease occurring after transfusion with leukocytes and platelets obtained from normal donors. Blood 1979; 53:1053–1059.
17. Prince M, Pedersen JS, Szer J, et al. Transfusion associated graft-versus-host disease after cardiac surgery: Response to antithymocyte globulin and corticosteroid therapy. Aust NZ J Med 1991; 21:43–46.
18. Takahashi K, Juji T, Miyamoto M, et al. Analysis of risk factors for post-transfusion graft-versus-host disease in Japan. Lancet 1994; 1:700–702.
19. Ohto H, Anderson KC. Survey of transfusion-associated graft-versus-host disease in immunocompetent recipients. Trans Med Rev 1996; X:31–43.
20. Billinghan RE. The biology of graft-versus-host reactions. Harvey Lect 1967; 62:21-78.
21. Shivdasani RA, Haluska FG, Dock NL, et al. Graft-versus-host disease associated with transfusion of blood from unrelated HLA-homozygous donors. N Engl J Med 1993; 328:766–770.
22. Shivdasani RA, Anderson KC. HLA homozygosity and shared HLA haplotypes in the development of transfusion-associated graft-versus-host disease. Leuk Lymph 1994; 15:227–234.
23. Takahashi K, Juji T, Miyazaki H. Post-transfusion graft-versus-host disease occurring in non-immunocompromised patients in Japan. Trans Sci 1991; 12:281–289.
24. Thaler M, Shamiss A, Orgad S, et al. The role of blood from HLA-homozygous donors in fatal transfusion-associated graft-versus-host disease after open heart surgery. N Engl J Med 1989; 321:25–28.
25. Drobyski W, Thibodeau S, Truitt RL, et al. Third party mediated graft rejection and graft-versus-host disease after T cell depleted bone marrow transplantation, as demonstrated by hypervariable DNA probes and HLA-DR polymorphism. Blood 1989; 74:2285–2294.
26. Lee TH, Donegan E, Slichter S, Busch MP. In vivo proliferation of donor leukocytes following allogeneic transfusions of immunocompetent recipients (abstr). Transfusion 33(suppl):51S, 1993.
27. Collins RH, Cooper B, Nikaein A, et al. Graft-versus- host disease in a liver transplant recipient. Ann Intern Med 1992; 116:391–392.

28. Dzik W. Mononuclear cell microchimerism and the immunomodulatory effect of transfusion. Transfusion 1994; 34:1007–1012.
29. Rubinstein A, Radl J, Cottier H, et al. Unusual combined immunodeficiency syndrome exhibiting kappa-IgD paraproteinemia, residual gut immunity and graft-versus-host reaction after plasma infusion. Acta Paediatr Scand 1973; 62:365.
30. Shivdasani RA, Anderson KC. Transfusion-associated graft-versus-host disease: Scratching the surface. Transfusion 1993; 33:696–697.
31. DeDobbeleer GD, Ledoux-Corbusier MH, Achten GA. Graft versus host reaction: An ultrastructural study. Arch Dermatol 1975; 111:1597–1602.
32. Sale GE, Lerner KG, Barker EA, et al. The skin biopsy in the diagnosis of acute graft versus host disease in man. Am J Pathol 1977; 89:621–635.
33. Sale GE, Storb R, Kolb H. Histopathology of hepatic acute graft versus host disease in the dog. Transplantation 1978; 26:102–110.
34. Kunstmann E, Bocker T, Roewer L, et al. Diagnosis of transfusion-associated graft-versus-host disease by genetic fingerprinting and polymerase chain reaction. Transfusion 1992; 32:766–770.
35. Hayakawa S, Chishima F, Sakata H, et al. A rapid molecular diagnosis of posttransfusion graft-versus-host disease by polymerase chain reaction. Transfusion 1993; 33:413–417.
36. Wang L, Juji T, Tokunaga K, et al. Brief report: Polymorphic microsatellite markers for the diagnosis of graft-versus-host disease. N Engl J Med 1994; 330:398–401.
37. Matsushita M, Shibata Y, Fuse K, et al. Sex chromatin analysis of lymphocytes invading host organs in transfusion-associated graft-versus-host disease. Virchows Arch B Cell Pathol 1988; 55:237–239.
38. Shimoda T. The case report of post-operative erythroderma. Geka 1955; 17:487.
39. Hathaway WE, Githens JH, Blackburn WR, et al. Aplastic anemia, histiocytosis, and erythroderma in immunologically deficient children. N Engl J Med 1965; 273:953–958.
40. Weiden P. Graft-vs-host disease following transfusion. Arch Intern Med 1984; 144: 1557–1558.
41. Kessinger A, Armitage JO, Klassen LW, et al. Graft versus host disease following transfusion of normal blood products to patients with malignancies. J Surg Oncol 1987; 36:206–209.
42. Ekert H, Waters KD, Smith PJ, et al. Treatment with MOPP or ChlVPP chemotherapy only for all stages of childhood Hodgkin's disease. J Clin Oncol 1988; 6:1845–1850.
43. Woods WG, Lubin BH. Fatal graft-versus-host disease following a blood transfusion in a child with neuroblastoma. Pediatrics 1981; 67:217–221.
44. Kennedy JS, Ricketts RR. Fatal graft versus host disease in a child with neuroblastoma following a blood transfusion. J Pediatr Surg 1986; 21:1108–1109.
45. Postmus PE, Mulder NH, Elema JD. Graft versus host disease after transfusion of non-irradiated blood cells in patients having received autologous bone marrow. Eur J Cancer Clin Oncol 1988; 24:889–894.
46. Mulder NH, Elema JD, Postmus PE. Transfusion associated graft-versus-host disease in autologous bone marrow transplantation. Lancet 1989; 1:735–736.
47. Capon SM, DePond WD, Tynan DB, et al. Transfusion-associated graft-versus-host disease in an immunocompetent patient. Ann Intern Med 1991; 114:1025–1026.
48. Saito M, Takamatsu H, Nakao S, et al. Transfusion-associated graft-versus-host disease after surgery for bladder cancer (letter). Blood 1993; 82:326–327.
49. Sanders M, Graeber J, Zehnbauer B, et al. Post transplant graft-versus-host disease in a premature infant without known risk factors (abstr). Blood 1988; 72(suppl 1):384a.
50. Berger RS, Dixon SL. Fulminant transfusion-associated graft-versus-host disease in a premature infant. J Am Acad Derm 1989; 20:945–950.

51. Ammann AJ. Hypothesis: Absence of graft-versus-host disease in AIDS is a consequence of HIV-1 infection of $CD4^+$ T cells. J AIDS 1993; 6:1224–1227.
52. Vogelsang GB. Transfusion-associated graft-versus-host disease in nonimmunocompromised hosts. Transfusion 1990; 30:101–103.
53. Juji T, Takahashi K, Shibata Y, et al. Post-transfusion graft-versus-host disease in immunocompetent patients after cardiac surgery (letter). N Engl J Med 1989; 321:56.
54. Arsura EL, Bertelle A, Minkowtiz S, et al. Transfusion-associated graft-versus-host disease in a presumed immunocompetent patient. Arch Intern Med 1988; 148:1941–1944.
55. Otsuka S, Kunieda K, Kitamura F, et al. The critical role of blood from HLA-homozygous donors in fatal transfusion-associated graft-versus-host disease in immunocompetent patients. Transfusion 1991; 31:260–264.
56. Otsuka S, Kunieda K, Hirose M, et al. Fatal erythroderma (suspected graft-versus-host disease) after cholecystectomy. Transfusion 1989; 29:544–548.
57. O'Connor NTJ, Mackintosh P. Transfusion associated graft versus host disease in an immunocompetent patient. J Clin Pathol 1992; 45:621–622.
58. Kobayashi H, Kitano K, Kishi E, et al. Transfusion-associated graft-versus-host disease in an immunocompetent patient following accidental injury. Am J Hematol 1993; 43:51–53.
59. Sheehan T, McLaren KM, Brettle R, Parker AC. Transfusion-induced graft versus host disease in pregnancy. Clin Lab Haematol 1987; 9:205–207.
60. Bell C. Fatal transfusion-associated graft-versus-host disease caused by blood from an unrelated donor in an immunocompetent patient (letter). Transfusion 1993; 33:785–786.
61. Kanter MH. Transfusion-associated graft-versus-host disease: Do transfusions from second-degree relatives pose a greater risk than those from first-degree relatives? Transfusion 1992; 32:323–327.
62. Charpentier F, Bracq C, Bonin P, et al. HLA-matched blood products and post-transfusion graft-versus-host disease (letter). Transfusion 1990; 30:850.
63. Grishaber JE, Birney SM, Strauss RG. Potential for transfusion-associated graft-versus-host disease due to apheresis platelets matched for HLA class I antigens. Transfusion 1993; 33:910–914.
64. Benson K, Marks AR, Marshall J, Goldstein JD. Fatal graft-versus-host disease associated with HLA-matched, HLA-homozygous platelet transfusions from unrelated donors. Transfusion 1994; 34:432–437.
65. Ohto H, Yasuda H, Noguchi M, Abe R. Risk of transfusion-associated graft-versus-host disease as a result of directed donations from relatives (letter). Transfusion 1992; 32:691–693.
66. Perkins HA. Transfusion-induced immunologic unresponsiveness. Trans Med Rev 1988; 2:196–203.
67. van der Mast BJ, Hornstra N, Ruigrok MB, et al. Transfusion-associated graft-versus-host disease in immunocompetent patients: A self-protective mechanism. Lancet 1994; 343:753–757.
68. Suzuki K, Akiyama H, Takamoto S, et al. Transfusion-associated graft-versus-host disease in a presumably immunocompetent patient after transfusion of stored packed red cells. Transfusion 1992; 32:358–360.
69. Hato T, Yasukawa M, Takeuchi N. Decrease in transfusion-associated graft-versus-host disease. Transfusion 1994; 34:45.
70. Goodman JW, Congdon CC. The killing effect of blood-bone marrow mixtures given to irradiated mice. Radiation Res 1960; 12:439–440.
71. Cole LJ, Garver RM. Abrogation by injected mouse blood of the protective effect of foreign bone marrow in lethally x- irradiated mice. Nature 1959; 184:1815–1816.

72. Thomas ED, Herman EC Jr, Greenough WB III, et al. Irradiation and marrow infusion in leukemia. Arch Intern Med 1961; 107:829–845.
73. Sprent J, Anderson RE, Miller JFAP. Radiosensitivity of T and B lymphocytes: II. Effect of radiation on response of T cells to alloantigens. Eur J Immunol 1974; 4:204–210.
74. Valerius NH, Johansen KS, Nielson OS, et al. Effect of in vitro x-irradiation on lymphocyte and granulocyte function. Scand J Hematol 1981; 27:9–18.
75. Button LN, DeWolf WC, Newburger PE, et al. The effects of irradiation on blood components. Transfusion 1981; 21:419–426.
76. Lowenthal RM, Challis DR, Griffiths AE, et al. Transfusion-associated graft-versus-host disease: Report of a case following administration of irradiated blood. Transfusion 1993; 33:524–529.
77. Rosen NR, Weidner JG, Boldt HD, Rosen DS. Prevention of transfusion-associated graft-versus-host disease: Selection of an adequate dose of gamma radiation. Transfusion 1993; 33:125–127.
78. Pelszynski MM, Moroff G, Luban NLC, et al. Effect of γ irradiation of red blood cell units on T-cell inactivation as assessed by limiting dilution analysis: Implications for prevention transfusion-associated graft-versus-host disease. Blood 1994; 83:1683–1689.
79. Klein H, ed. Standards for Blood Banks and Transfusion Services. 16th ed. Bethesda, MD: American Association of Blood Banks, 1994:33.
80. Anderson KC, Goodnough LT, Sayers M, et al. Variation in blood component irradiation practice: Implications for prevention of transfusion-associated graft-versus-host disease. Blood 1991; 77:2096–2102.
81. Moroff G, Luban NLC. The influence of gamma irradiation on red cell and platelet properties. Transfus Sci 1994; 15:141–148.
82. Ramirez AM, Woodfield DG, Scott R, McLachlan J. High potassium levels in stored irradiated blood (letter). Transfusion 1987; 27:444–445.
83. Rivet C, Baxter A, Rock G. Potassium levels in irradiated blood (letter). Transfusion 1989; 29:185.
84. Ferguson DJ. Potassium levels in irradiated blood (letter). Transfusion 1989; 29:749.
85. Rock G, Shear JM. Potassium levels in irradiated blood (letter). Transfusion 1989; 29:749.
86. Bernard DR, Chapman RG, Simmons MA, et al. Blood for use in exchange transfusions in the newborn. Transfusion 1980; 20:401–408.
87. Hillyer CD, Tiegerman KO, Berkman EM. Evaluation of the red cell storage lesion after irradiation in filtered packed red cell units. Transfusion 1991; 31:497–499.
88. Davey RJ, McCoy NC, Yu M, et al. The effect of prestorage irradiation on posttransfusion red cell survival. Transfusion 1992; 32:525–528.
89. Suda BA, Leitman SF, Davey RJ. Characteristics of red cells irradiated and subsequently frozen for long-term storage. Transfusion 1993; 33:389–392.
90. Miraglia CC, Anderson G, Mintz PD. Effect of freezing on the in vivo recovery of irradiated red cells. Transfusion 1994; 34:775–778.
91. Rock G, Adams GA, Labow RS. The effects of irradiation on platelet function. Transfusion 1988; 28:451–455.
92. Read EJ, Kodis C, Carter CS, Leitman SF. Viability of platelets following storage in the irradiated state. Transfusion 1988; 28:446–450.
93. Duguid JKM, Carr R, Jenkins JA, et al. Clinical evaluation of the effects of storage time and irradiation on transfused platelets. Vox Sang 1991; 60:151–154.
94. Sweeney JD, Holme S, Moroff G. Storage of apheresis platelets after gamma radiation. Transfusion 1994; 34:779–783.
95. Yankee RA, Grumet FC, Rogentine GN. Platelet transfusion therapy: The selection of

compatible platelet donors for refractory patients by lymphocyte HL-A typing. N Engl J Med 1969; 281:1208–1212.
96. Mohr R, Martinowitz Y, Lavee J, et al. The hemostatic effect of transfusing fresh whole blood versus platelet concentrates after cardiac operations. J Thorac Cardiovasc Surg 1988; 96:530–534.
97. Wasser MN, Houblers JG, D'Amaro J, et al. The effect of fresh versus stored blood on post-operative bleeding after coronary bypass surgery: A prospective randomized study. Br J Haematol 1989; 72:81–84.
98. Lind SE. Has the case for irradiating blood products been made? Am J Med 1985; 78: 543–544.
99. Perkins HA. Should all blood from related donors be irradiated? Transfusion 1992; 32:302–303.
100. Korngold R, Sprent J. T cell subsets and graft-versus-host disease. Transplantation 1987; 44:335–339.
101. Filipovich AH, Vallera DA, Youle RJ, et al. Graft-versus-host disease prevention in allogeneic bone marrow transplantation from histocompatible siblings: A pilot study using immunotoxins for T cell depletion of donor bone marrow. Transplantation 1987; 44:62–69.
102. Anderson KC, Nadler LM, Takvorian T, et al. Monoclonal antibodies: their use in bone marrow transplantation. In: Brown E, ed. Progress in Hematology. Orlando, FL. Grune & Stratton, 1987:137–181.
103. Reisner Y, Kapoor N, Kirkpatrick D, et al. Transplantation for acute leukaemia with HLA-A and B nonidentical parental marrow cells fractionated with soybean agglutinin and sheep red blood cells. Lancet 1981; 2:327–331.
104. de Witte T, Hoogengout J, de Pauw B, et al. Depletion of donor lymphocytes by counterflow centrifugation successfully prevents acute graft-versus-host disease in matched allogeneic marrow transplantation. Blood 1988; 5:1302–1308.
105. Crowley JP, Skrabut EM, Valeri CR. Immunocompetent lymphocytes in previously frozen washed red cells. Vox Sang 1974; 26:513–157.
106. Lane TA, Anderson KC, Goodnough LT, et al. Leukocyte reduction in blood component therapy. Ann Intern Med 1992; 177:151–162.
107. Bordin JO, Heddle NM, Blajchman MA. Biologic effects of leukocytes present in transfused cellular blood products. Blood 1994; 84:1703–1721.
108. Dzieckowski JS, Barrett BB, Nester D, et al. Characterization of reactions after exclusive transfusion of white cell-reduced cellular blood components. Transfusion 1995; 35:20–25.
109. Lee TH, Stromberg RR, Heitman J, Tran K, Busch MP. Quantitation of residual white cells in filtered blood components by polymerase chain reaction amplification of HLA DQ-ADNA. Transfusion 1994; 34:986–994.
110. Kao KJ, Michel M, Braine HG, et al. White cell reduction in platelet concentrates and packed red cells by filtration: A multicenter clinical trial. Transfusion 1995; 35:13–19.
111. Williamson LM, Wimperis JZ, Williamson P, et al. Bedside filtration of blood products in the prevention of HLA alloimmunization: A prospective randomized study. Blood 1994; 83:3028–3035.
112. Akahoshi M, Takanashi M, Masuda M, et al. A case of transfusion-associated graft-versus-host disease not prevented by white cell-reduction filters. Transfusion 1992; 32: 169–172.
113. Deeg HJ, Graham TC, Gerhard-Miller L, et al. Prevention of transfusion-induced graft-versus-host disease in dogs by ultraviolet irradiation. Blood 1989; 74:2592–2595.
114. Brand A, Claas FHJ, van Rood JJ. UV-irradiated platelets: Ready to use? Transfusion 1989; 29:377–378.

22

Role of Histocompatibility Antigens in the Development of Graft-Versus-Host Disease

Patrick G. Beatty

University of Utah Health Sciences Center
Salt Lake City, Utah

I. INTRODUCTION

For the last several decades, progress in the science of immunogenetics has been directly linked with increasing success in clinical marrow transplantation. In the late 1930s, Gorer (1) demonstrated that control of the rejection of tumors by inbred mice could be traced to specific genetic loci. These observations were elaborated upon in the 1940s by Snell (2), who systematically explored a similar model and was able to demonstrate a large number of codominant, independently segregating loci that were capable of eliciting alloreactivity.

The possible relevance of these observations to transplantation was demonstrated in 1951 by Lorenz (3), who showed that mice and guinea pigs could be rescued from lethal radiation doses by infusion of autologous or syngeneic marrow. This finding led to futile attempts in about 200 humans between 1951 and 1967 to perform allogeneic bone marrow transplants for various diseases (4). None of these patients survived with documentation of stable engraftment, at least in part due to unavailability of histocompatibility testing.

A key breakthrough in histocompatibility testing was initiated in 1954, when Dausset (5) demonstrated that luekoagglutinins were capable of demonstrating segregating polymorphic systems of histocompatibility. It was realized that these loci might be analogous to those demonstrated by Snell and Gore in mice and hence could be of critical importance in transplantation. Over the next several years, such antisera were collected and systematically analyzed (6,7). These efforts culminated in the First International Histocompatibility Workshop in 1964, where several different tissue typing technologies were compared, and in 1965, when the techniques and nomenclature were standardized (8). Over the next three decades, periodic international workshops led to a dramatic expansion in the knowledge of histocompatibility testing to the point that we can now define at the DNA sequence level virtually all known alleles of all loci within the major histocompatibility complex (9).

The convergence of these lines of scientific investigation led to the dawn of the modern era of marrow transplantation, which commenced in the late 1960s when three allogeneic marrow transplants were performed in children with otherwise fatal inborn defects in their immune systems (10–12). All three patients and their families were tested with the state-of-the-art histocompatibility technology of that time and were found to have HLA-identical siblings. As of 1993, some 25 years later, all three of these initial patients remain alive and engrafted (13). In the early 1970s, clinical oncology investigators hypothesized that if inborn immunodeficiencies could be corrected by marrow transplant, it might be possible to correct iatrogenic marrow ablation included by high-dose chemoradiotherapy given to cure patients of their underlying malignancies (14–16). From the immunogenetic perspective, the challenge was to develop technology allowing discrimination of all possible HLA alleles, to define the relative importance of incompatibility at different loci, and to ascertain whether there might be other loci outside the HLA region that might be of importance in the outcome of marrow transplantation.

II. HISTOCOMPATIBILITY SYSTEMS OF RELEVANCE TO MARROW TRANSPLANTATION

First in experimental animals and later in humans, it was recognized that the most important antigens for alloreactivity were encoded on a small portion of a single chromosome inherited in a codominant fashion by an individual from his or her parents. In humans, this region is on the short arm of chromosome 6. Within this region, a large number of loci have been identified (Table 1). Many loci have no apparent relevance to histocompatibility; some loci appear to be expressed on a limited distribution of tissues and/or at low levels; others are pseudogenes, that is, not transcribable; and others appear to be widely expressed at high levels. The most carefully studied loci, and those thought to be most important to clinical transplantation, include the HLA-A locus (50 recognized alleles), HLA-B locus (107 alleles), and the HLA-DRB1 locus (106 alleles) (17). Also in close proximity but of less certain importance, are the HLA-C, -DRB3, -DRB4, -DRB5, -DRB6, and the -DRB7 loci. Recent data suggest that nonidentity for the alleles of the HLA-C locus may increase the risk of nonengraftment, especially in patients with chronic myelogenous leukemia (E. Petersdorf, personal communication). Of

Table 1 HLA Loci and Number of Alleles[a]

Class I				
A	B	C	E	G
50	107	34	4	4

Class II											
DRA	DRB1	DRB3	DRB4	DRB5	DRB7	DQA1	DQB1	DPA1	DPB1	DMA	DMB
2	106	4	5	5	2	15	2	8	59	4	4

[a]Number of possible haplotypes: 3.6345×10^{17}; number of possible phenotypes: 1.351×10^{31}.

greater complexity are the DQ and DP regions, where the DQA1 or DPA1 genes products can affiliate as a heterodimer with the DQB1 or DPB1 gene products, respectively; thus an even greater polymorphism is possible. The potential polymorphism given so many loci, and the very large number of alleles at each locus, would seemingly render it theoretically impossible for any two random individuals to be truly histocompatible. However, in considering searching for an HLA-matched donor within a family, the genetics of HLA allows the problem to simplify. These HLA loci are all encoded on a short portion of a single chromosome, hence they are usually inherited en bloc, implying that any given pair of siblings would have a 1 in 4 chance of inheriting the same two HLA haplotypes and would therefore be genetically identical for their histocompatibility alleles.

In considering the possibility of finding HLA-matched unrelated donors for a patient, the issues become much more complex. It becomes critically important to be able to define all the relevant alleles, to have some understanding of their relative frequency—and most important—to understand which loci are of the greatest importance to allogeneic complications so that the clinician can prioritize amongst potential donors, none of whom may be fully matched with the patient.

By definition, the antigens so far discussed are all encoded on one short portion of one chromosome. It is clear from a cursory examination of the clinical data that despite genotypic matching for all of HLA, as would be obtained in matched sibling transplantation, the incidence of graft-versus-host disease, including fatal graft-versus-host disease, can be 10 to 50%, depending upon the selected mode of immunosuppression (18). These clinical observations led to the postulate that there must exist other loci of major clinical relevance outside of the major histocompatibility complex (19). From limited human data and more extensive murine data, it appears that there are a large number of such loci, with different degrees of clinical importance and different degrees of polymorphism. The study of these antigens has been impeded by the complicated biology of their presentation to the immune system (20). These antigens can only be recognized by the immune system when they are presented within the binding groove of an HLA molecule. Each individual T cell must therefore concordantly recognize both a specific minor antigen and the one specific HLA allele that binds it. Furthermore, these T cells can usually be generated only via in vivo stimulation, such as that obtained in an allogeneic marrow transplant. This complex biology and cumbersome method of obtaining necessary testing reagents has made it impossible to develop an easy means of determining the compatibility of patient and prospective donors. However, their importance of such compatibility cannot be minimized, particularly in unrelated transplantation. In HLA-identical sibling transplants, one can assume that there will be some degree of chance matching due to inheritance; in unrelated donor transplants, however, it must be presumed that any matching will be strictly random (21).

III. CLINICAL HISTOCOMPATIBILITY TESTING TECHNOLOGY

As noted above, the first available reagents for histocompatibility testing were antibodies that were reactive with white blood cells, most commonly obtained from women who had been pregnant. Serum obtained from most women reacts with a very high proportion of test cells, thus making it difficult to identify reagents that might be informative for individual alleles. This apparent propensity of women to make antibodies that can recognize many different alleles is, of course, in part due to the codominant expression of two alleles per each of the several histocompatibility loci. Thus, much of the early history of histocompatibility testing was focused upon identifying those very rare alloantisera that recognized a single epitope on a single allele. As a result, many histocompatibility laboratories set up extensive screening programs in which female blood donors were asked if they had previously been pregnant and if they would be willing to have their blood tested for antibodies. Whenever a potentially interesting antibody was found among many of the hundreds of samples tested, these women would be reapproached and asked if they would donate about 300 mL of plasma. Given the scarcity of reagents, it was critical that technology be developed to allow utilization of the smallest possible amount of serum. Histocompatibility workshops allowed one-to-one comparison of these scarce reagents as well as further characterization of new alleles and location of variants of previously described alleles. In the 1970s, the technology to make mouse monoclonal antibodies became available, thus allowing development of reagents that were truly specific for a single epitope. However, the goal of developing a full panel of such reagents specific for human antigens was not attainable, as the mouse antibody repertoire was apparently incapable of recognizing all human alleles.

Simultaneous with the development of serological reagents, the observation was made that if lymphocytes from two unrelated individuals were mixed, in the vast majority of cases these cells would begin dividing. It was possible to measure the rate of cellular division by determining incorporation into the cell's DNA of such agents as tritiated thymidine. Dupont et al., using methodology similar to that employed by their colleague serologists, were able to define alleles recognizable by such cellular reagents (22). Eventually, it proved possible to cross- correlate the epitopes and alleles recognized by cellular reagents with epitopes and alleles recognized by serological reagents.

In the early 1980s, technology evolved making it possible to isolate and define the proteins encoded by the histocompatibility genes. Methodology such as one- or two-dimensional isoelectric focusing made it possible to distinguish the protein products of various alleles after they had been labeled on the cell surface. This technology was quite cumbersome and required a significant amount of protein for adequate testing (23).

Most recently, technology based on DNA sequencing has evolved and become widely available, so that virtually all HLA-DRB1, DQA1, DQB1, DPA1, and DPB1 alleles can be unambiguously defined (9). Furthermore, it is likely that within the next few years it will be possible to do likewise for the class I alleles. This advancement has provided a cost-effective means of determining the complete genotype of all tested loci. Indeed, the robustness of this technology has made it possible to eliminate the cellular typing technology and is rapidly displacing serological technology.

IV. CLINICAL RESULTS

As outlined above, the science of histocompatibility testing has provided the clinician with an overwhelming compendium of loci and alleles. Only large, well-designed clinical trials can hope to determine which loci are of premiere importance in outcome and which may be safely disregarded. There are two categories of transplantation that might provide information in this respect: transplants from HLA mismatched relatives and transplants from unrelated donors.

The Seattle Transplant Team has published a series of analyses of patients who received HLA partially incompatible grafts from close relatives (24,25). In all cases, the patient and donor shared one HLA haplotype by inheritance but variably differed for the alleles encoded on the nonshared HLA haplotype. In the early studies, HLA class I alleles were defined by serological methods, with the emphasis being placed on HLA-A and -B. With respect to HLA class II, the emphasis was placed on HLA-DR as defined by serology, which was then subcategorized into HLA-D phenotypes using homozygous typing cells. More recent methodology has included DNA-based typing for HLA-DRB1, with recently collected data on HLA-C, DQ, and DP. The first major analysis, published in 1985, compared results of 105 HLA-mismatched transplants to a contemporaneous cohort of 728 patients receiving HLA-matched transplants from their siblings. All patients received similar graft-versus-host disease (GVHD) prophylaxis and had similar diagnoses. Increasing disparity (considering HLA-A, -B, and -DR) led to increasing risk of acute GVHD. However, there were patients who, despite mismatch for one or more HLA loci, did not develop significant GVHD, whereas some patients who received HLA genotypically identical grafts did develop significant GVHD. This shows that, on the one hand, the engrafting immune system is capable of becoming tolerant to the mismatched HLA alleles, while, on the other hand, HLA antigens do not represent the complete immunogenetic picture. Rather, minor histocompatibility antigens can clearly play a significant role. The study also noted that patients who received mismatched transplants tended to develop their GVHD several days earlier than did patients who received HLA-matched transplants, a phenomenon sometimes referred to "hyperacute" GVHD. This often represents a significant clinical problem, as these patients may still be recovering from toxicity induced by the chemoradiotherapy preparative regimen, thus making it difficult to deliver adequate prophylactic doses of immunosuppressive agents capable of controlling the rapidly developing GVHD. This original study included only patients who received methotrexate for GVHD prophylaxis. Based on observations in HLA-matched siblings that a combination of methotrexate and cyclosporine was superior to either drug alone (26), HLA-mismatched transplants in Seattle subsequent to 1985 were treated prophylactically with this combination. This led to a decrease in the incidence of severe GVHD although the hierarchical increase in risk was still observed. Thus far, analyses of which loci might be most important in the risk of developing GVHD have been inconclusive. In patients who received only methotrexate for GVHD, there was no differential impact of mismatching for A, B, or D loci. However, when a combination of methotrexate and cyclosporine was utilized, it appeared that a D-locus mismatch could lead to an increased risk compared to mismatches for the A and B loci. One might hypothesize that incompatibility for a particular locus might be best controlled by a particular prophylactic immunosuppressive regimen, but incompatibility for another locus might be better controlled by another.

If one analyzes these HLA-mismatched transplants not only with respect to risk for GVHD, but also with respect to survival, mismatch for one HLA locus does not substantially change the probability of survival, but mismatch for two or three loci does affect survival rates. This is a critical issue, since if it were possible to routinely accept two- and three-antigen-mismatch related donors, the probability of finding a donor within the family would reach nearly 100%. Over the past decade, there have been numerous attempts to develop means of allowing such incompatible transplants. These include different methods of T-cell depletion, both in vivo and in vitro, and new means of immunosuppression, but none have yet become established (27).

Particularly as it became clear that the use of highly HLA- mismatched donors was not going to be clinically feasible soon, and as the science of histocompatibility testing reached the point at which it was possible to define all alleles unambiguously, several teams began investigating the feasibility and clinical efficacy of transplantation for HLA-match unrelated volunteer donors. Given the extreme polymorphism of HLA (28), it was difficult to find suitable matches for most patients during these early clinical trials. However, the initial data (29,30) showed that it was possible to carry out successful transplants. In 1986 this led to the establishment of the National Marrow Donor Program, whose objective was to recruit sufficient numbers of HLA-matched unrelated donors to provide acceptable matches for most patients (31). As data accumulated, it became apparent that even if a patient and the unrelated donor were HLA-matched, the incidence of GVHD was substantially higher than that which would be expected had the patients received transplants from HLA-matched siblings (32–34). In a study of 112 transplants from one-antigen-mismatched unrelated donors, the Seattle team showed that this degree of incompatibility raised the risk of grade III GVHD from 36 to 51%, compared to patients receiving marrow from HLA-matched unrelated donors (35). Thus, with respect to the risk of acute GVHD, one can equate an HLA-matched unrelated donor to a one-antigen-mismatched related donor and a one-antigen-mismatched unrelated donor to a two-antigen-mismatched related donor. Clearly, the problem of HLA incompatibility has not yet been solved and will require further research.

V. CONCLUSIONS

The evolution of the field of histocompatibility testing over the past four decades initially allowed clinicians to reliably identify HLA-matched siblings, then closely HLA-matched relatives and, most recently, HLA-matched unrelated donors. With the advent of DNA-based typing technology, it has become possible to precisely characterize all HLA differences between patient and donor, thus allowing clinicians to embark on the task of clarifying which loci are of the most importance. Thus, the relevant question for a given patient is less "Is there a donor available?" but rather "Which donor is most appropriate?"

REFERENCES

1. Gorer PA. The genetic and antigenic basis of tumor transplantation. J Pathol 1937; 44: 691–697.
2. Snell GD. The genetics of transplantation. J Natl Cancer Inst 1953; 14:691–700.
3. Lorenz E, Uphoff D, Reid TR, Shelton E. Modification of irradiation injury in mice and guinea pigs by bone marrow injections. J Natl Cancer Inst 1951; 12:197–201.
4. Bortin MM. A compendium of reported human bone marrow transplants. Transplantation 1970; 9:571–587.
5. Dausset J, Nenna A, Brecy H. Leuco-agglutinins: V. Leuco-agglutininis in chronic

idiopathic or symptomatic pancytopenia and in paroxysmal nocturnal hemoglobinuria. Blood 1954; 9:696–720.
6. Payne R, Rolfs MR. Fetomaternal leukocyte incompatibility. J Clin Invest 1958; 37: 1756–1763.
7. van Rood JJ, Eernisse JG, van Leeuwen A. Leukocyte antibodies in sera from pregnant women. Nature 1958; 181:1735–1736.
8. Halner H, Cleton FJ, Eernisse JF (eds). Histocompatibility Testing, 1965. Copenhagen: Munksgaard, 1965.
9. Begovich AB, Erlich HA. HLA typing for bone marrow transplantation: New polymerase chain reaction-based methods. JAMA 1995; 273:586–591.
10. Good RA, Gatti A, Hong R, Meuwissen HJ. Successful marrow transplantation for correction of immunological deficit in lymphopenic agammaglobulinemia and treatment of immunologically induced pancytopenia. Exp Hematol 1969; 19:4–10.
11. Bach FH, Albertini RJ, Anderson JL, et al. Bone marrow transplantation in a patient with Wiskott-Aldrich syndrome. Lancet 1968; 2:1364–1366.
12. de Koning J, van Bekkum DW, Dicke KA, et al. Transplantation of bone marrow cells and fetal thymus in an infant with lymphopenic immunological deficiency. Lancet 1969; 1:1223–1227.
13. Bortin MM, Bach FH, van Bekkum DW, et al. 25th anniversary of the first successful allogeneic bone marrow transplants. Bone Marrow Transplant 1994; 14:211–212.
14. Thomas ED, Lochte HL Jr, Lu WC, Ferrebee JW. Intravenous infusion of bone marrow in patients receiving radiation and chemotherapy. N Engl J Med 1957; 257:491–496.
15. Mathe G, Amiel JL, Schwarzenberg L, et al. Greffe de moelle osseuse allogenique chez l'homme prouvee par six marquerurs antigeniques apres conditionnement du receveur et du donneur par le serum antilymphocytaire. Rev Franc Etudes Clin et Biol 1968; 13: 1025–1027.
16. Thomas ED, Storb R, Clift RA, et al. Bone marrow transplantation. N Engl J Med 1975; 292:832–843, 895–902.
17. Bodmer JG, Marsh SGE, Albert ED, et al. Nomenclature for factors of the HLA system, 1994. Hum Immunol 1994; 41:1–20.
18. Beatty PG. The immunogenetics of bone marrow transplantation. Transfus Med Rev 1994; 8:45–58.
19. de Bueger M, Goulmy E. Human minor histocompatibility antigens. Transplant Immunol 1993; 1:28–38.
20. Beatty PG. Minor histocompatibility antigens. Exp Hematol 1993; 21:1514–1516.
21. Martin PJ. Increased disparity for minor histocompatibility antigens as a potential cause of increased GVHD risk in marrow transplantation from unrelated donors compared with related donors. Bone Marrow Transplant 1991; 8:217–223.
22. Dupont B, Braun DW, Yunis EF, Carpenter CB. HLA-D by cellular typing, in Teraski P (ed): Histocompatibility Testing 1980. Los Angeles, CA: UCLA Press, 1980:229.
23. Beatty PG, Mickelson EM, Petersdorf EW, et al. Histocompatibility 1991. Transfusion 1991; 31:847–856.
24. Beatty PG, Clift RA, Mickelson EM, et al. Marrow transplantation from related donors other than HLA-identical siblings. N Engl J Med 1985; 313:765–771.
25. Anasetti C, Amos D, Beatty PG, et al. Effect of HLA compatibility on engraftment of bone marrow transplants in patients with leukemia or lymphoma. N Engl J Med 1989; 320:197–204.
26. Storb R, Deeg HJ, Fischer L, et al. Cyclosporine vs methotrexate for graft-vs.-host disease prevention in patients given marrow grafts for leukemia: Long term follow-up of three controlled trials. Blood 1988; 71:293–298.
27. Aversa F, Tabilio A, Ternzi A, et al. Successful engraftment of T-cell-depleted haploidentical "three-Loci" incompatible transplants in leukemia patients by addition of

recombinant human granulocyte colony-stimulating factor-mobilized peripheral blood progenitor cells to bone marrow infusion. Blood 1994; 84:3948–3955.
28. Beatty PG, Dahlberg S, Mickelson EM, et al. Probability of finding HLA-matched unrelated marrow donors. Transplantation 1988; 45:714–718.
29. Hansen JA, Clift RA, Thomas ED, et al. Transplantation of marrow from an unrelated donor to a patient with acute leukemia. N Engl J Med 1980; 303:565–567.
30. Gingrich RD, Ginder GD, Goeken NE, et al. Allogeneic marrow grafting with partially mismatched, unrelated marrow donors. Blood 1988; 71:1375–1381.
31. Champlin R, Coppo P, Howe C. National Marrow Donor Program: Progress and challenges. Bone Marrow Transplant 1993; 33:567–577.
32. Beatty PG, Hansen JA, Longton GM, et al. Marrow transplantation from HLA-matched unrelated donors for treatment of hematologic malignancies. Transplantation 1991; 51:443–447.
33. Ash RC, Casper JT, Chitambar CR, et al. Successful allogeneic transplantation of T-cell-depleted bone marrow from closely HLA-matched unrelated donors. N Engl J Med 1990; 322:485–494.
34. Kernan NA, Bartsch G, Ash RC, et al. Analysis of 462 transplantations from unrelated donors facilitated by the National Marrow Donor Program. N Engl J Med 1993; 328: 593–602.
35. Beatty PG, Anasetti C, Hansen JA, et al. Marrow transplantation from unrelated donors for treatment of hematologic malignancies: Effect of mismatching for one HLA locus. Blood 1993; 81:249–253.

23

T-Cell Depletion for GVHD Prevention in Humans

Paul J. Martin
Fred Hutchinson Cancer Research Center and University of Washington
Seattle, Washington

Nancy A. Kernan
Memorial Sloan-Kettering Cancer Center
New York, New York

I. INTRODUCTION

The ability to prevent graft-versus-host disease (GVHD) by removing T cells from donor marrow has been demonstrated in numerous experimental models. Impetus for testing this approach for preventing GVHD in clinical trials came from the development of a variety of methods for selective depletion of T cells in human marrow. Data from animal models indicated that the need for posttransplant immunosuppression could be entirely circumvented by T-cell depletion (reviewed in Chap. 00). This led to the anticipation that the risks of mucositis, delayed engraftment, renal impairment, infections, and other complications could be diminished by avoiding the necessity of GVHD prophylaxis with methotrexate, cyclosporine, antithymocyte globulin, prednisone, or cyclophosphamide. It was hoped that more effective GVHD prevention would lead to improved survival.

Initially, there was little information from animal experiments to indicate that T-cell depletion could lead to complications. Early enthusiasm for this approach in humans was reflected by widespread testing in many centers. More than 800 T-cell-depleted marrow transplants were carried out worldwide during the 6-year period between 1981, when the initial reports were published, and the end of 1986 (1). Data from these studies confirmed the expectation of decreased incidence and severity of GVHD but led to recognition of the problems of increased graft failure and leukemic relapse and delayed immune reconstitution. This recognition indicated the need for greater understanding of the immunobiology of marrow transplantation, particularly in terms of the relationship between engraftment, GVHD, and immunological control of malignant cells.

During the past 5 years, some progress has been made in elucidating the complex interplay between engraftment, GVHD, immune reconstitution, and graft-versus-leukemia (GVL) effects. Much of this understanding has come from laboratory studies prompted by unexpected findings in the initial clinical trials of T-cell depletion. This chapter will summarize the overall clinical results of T-cell depletion, providing a broad perspective without attempting a comprehensive review. Discussion will include laboratory studies that have addressed the mechanisms involved in the complications now recognized to be caused by T-cell depletion. The understanding of marrow transplant immunobiology gained from such studies could make it possible for T-cell depletion to emerge as a safe, effective, and widely applicable method for preventing GVHD in humans.

II. METHODS OF T-CELL DEPLETION

Marrow aspirated for human transplantation typically contains on the order of 10^{10} nucleated cells (2), of which approximately 10% or 10^9 represent mature T cells, depending on the amount of blood coaspirated with marrow. Marrow obtained directly from cadaveric vertebral bodies contains 4- to 5-fold fewer T cells (3). Patients transplanted with unmodified marrow generally receive on the order of 10^7 T cells/kg recipient body weight. Initially it was not known how much depletion of T cells would be required in order to prevent GVHD in humans, and efforts were therefore made to develop methods that could achieve a maximum degree of depletion without damage to hematopoietic progenitors.

Both physical methods and antibody-based methods have been used for depletion of T cells in human marrow. Highly efficient removal of T cells and enrichment of hematopoietic progenitors in human marrow can be achieved by differential agglutination with soybean lectin followed by rosetting with sheep erythrocytes (4–7). Counterflow centrifugal elutriation (8–11) and density gradient fractionation (12) exploit physical differences to separate T cells and hematopoietic stem cells. Anti T-cell antibodies have been employed alone (13–15), together with homologous or heterologous complement (16–27), as immunotoxins (28–33), or with immunomagnetic beads (34,35). A variety of antibodies and combinations of antibodies have been used in different clinical trials. The most extensive experience worldwide has been with the rat IgM monoclonal antibody Campath-1 (36–37), which recognizes CDw52, a heterogeneous 23- to 30-kDa glycoprotein expressed by all lymphocytes and monocytes (38,39). Other trials have employed antibodies that recognize antigens with a more restricted pattern of expression specific for T cells. (See Ref. 1 for summary and Refs. 40 to 42 for descriptions of T-cell antigens.) These include CD2, which represents the E-rosette receptor; CD3, which is noncovalently associated with the antigen receptor of T cells; CD5, which represents the human equivalent of murine Lyt-1 (also expressed by a small subpopulation of B lymphocytes); CD6 (a 120-kDa molecule of undefined function); and CD7 (a 41-kDa molecule of undefined function). Antibodies against T-cell subset antigens such as CD4, CD8, and CD28 have also been tested either alone (26,43) or as components of mixtures. With sufficient preclinical development and testing, most physical methods and antibody-based methods are capable of at least 2 $\log_{10}$ (99%) depletion of T cells (44).

Evaluation of various marrow treatment methods has required the development of suitable assays for enumerating residual T cells (45–50). E-rosetting assays can be very sensitive, but many CD2-specific antibodies interfere with rosette formation. Mitogen-stimulated proliferation measured as ^{3}H-thymidine incorporation lacks sensitivity because of the high background proliferation of marrow cells (51). Under optimal conditions, indirect immunofluorescence and flow cytometry can reliably detect T cells at levels of approximately 0.1% after complement-mediated lysis (46), but this method does not provide information about the functional competence of residual cells. Direct immunofluorescence and flow cytometry can reliably detect T cells at levels less than 0.01% after depletion by physical methods. Mitogen stimulation and short-term culture of treated marrow can improve the sensitivity of immunofluorescent methods and provide a semiquantitative measure of the number of residual T cells (46). Limiting dilution analysis represents the assay method best able to provide a highly sensitive and quantitative assessment of functional T cells remaining after marrow treatment. Limiting dilution assays to enumerate cells capable of proliferating in response to PHA and IL-2 (46–48) or Con A and IL-2 (49) have been described by several investigators. More recently, assays for cells capable of producing IL-2 in response to PHA or ConA and assays for cells capable of developing cytotoxic activity have also been described (49–50). With cell-surface phenotyping included as a readout, limiting dilution assays can be adapted to assess the results of T-cell subset depletion.

In vitro assays do not provide insight regarding the clinical utility of various methods, nor do they indicate which cell surface antigen(s) would serve as the best target(s) for T-cell depletion. Too little is known about the effects of different T-cell subtypes to predict optimal depletion strategies based solely on in vitro depletion data. Nonetheless, the interpretation of clinical outcome always requires enumeration and functional assessment of T cells remaining in treated marrows.

III. EFFECTS ON GVHD

Initially it was reported that treatment of marrow with a murine IgG2a anti-CD3 antibody alone was sufficient to prevent GVHD (13), but this finding was not confirmed in subsequent studies (14,15). Thus it appeared that in vivo mechanisms such as complement-mediated lysis, antibody-dependent cell-mediated cytotoxicity, and reticuloendothelial clearance were inadequate to eliminate the antibody-coated T cells in marrow transplant recipients. In vitro testing has indicated that most murine and T-cell antibodies do not lyse human T cells with human serum as a source of complement. Certain rat antibodies such as Campath-1, however, show highly efficient complement-mediated lysis in the presence of human serum (52). Variation in ability to mediate complement-dependent lysis reflects not only the species- and isotype-specific interactions between antibody and human complement components (53,54) but also other factors such as the cell surface density of antigen expression and the valency of antibody binding (55).

Retrospective data collected by the International Bone Marrow Transplant Registry (IBMTR) have confirmed the results of many previous studies indicating that T-cell depletion is associated with a decreased risk of clinically significant (grades II–IV) acute GVHD after marrow transplantation from an HLA-identical sibling (relative risk = 0.45) (56). With in vitro procedures that assure removal or destruction of T cells before infusion of marrow into the recipient, the number of viable T cells remaining in the graft can be estimated. In clinical studies where 2 $\log_{10}$ depletion of T cells was achieved by in vitro marrow treatment, there was approximately a 10% incidence of grades II–IV acute GVHD among durably engrafted patients transplanted with HLA-identical marrow when no posttransplant immunosuppression was administered (12,33,57,58). This contrasts with a GVHD incidence of at least 80% when posttransplant immunosuppression is omitted in patients given marrow without T-cell depletion (59). Thus it appears that as many as 1.0×10^5 HLA-identical donor T cells/kg recipient body weight can generally be tolerated with a minimal risk of acute GVHD in patients given no posttransplant immunosuppression. Studies in which only 1 $\log_{10}$ depletion of T cells was achieved showed correspondingly higher rates of acute GVHD (12). In some studies, clinically significant acute GVHD was not seen in patients who received HLA-identical marrow containing less than 1.0×10^5 cells/kg (60,61), but other investigators have reported acute GVHD in patients receiving as few as 4×10^3 T cells/kg (62). Technical differences between assays for enumerating residual viable T cells remaining in the marrow after treatment and additional in vivo elimination of T cells with certain treatment methods may account for some of the variation in estimates of the number of T cells required to cause GVHD.

The extent of T-cell depletion required to prevent GVHD probably depends on multiple factors already known to affect the risk of GVHD in patients transplanted with unmodified marrow (63). These include recipient age, parity of the donor, the underlying diagnosis and preparative regimen, the amount of posttransplant immunosuppression, and the type of reverse isolation and antimicrobial prophylaxis. HLA genetic disparity between the donor and recipient probably represents the single factor having greatest influence on GVHD risk (64). Attempts to employ T-cell depletion for HLA-mismatched marrow transplantation without posttransplant immunosuppression in patients with diseases other than congenital immunodeficiency have been discouraging, since either acute GVHD or graft rejection has been encountered in as many as 50% of the patients (6). To some extent, these results may reflect the greater degree of T-cell depletion required to prevent GVHD in the setting of HLA disparity. With a sufficient degree of depletion (3.0 to 3.5 logs), the incidence of clinically significant acute GVHD in HLA-haploidentical recipients can be reduced to 10% or less (65).

There is relatively little published information concerning the effects of T-cell depletion on chronic GVHD. Data from the IBMTR have indicated that T-cell depletion is associated with a decreased risk of chronic GVHD after marrow transplantation from an HLA-identical sibling (relative risk = 0.56) (56). The incidence of chronic GVHD in some studies of T-cell depletion was reported to be as low as 0 to 5% (57,58,66), substantially lower than the 40 to 50% incidence usually seen with conventional marrow transplantation from HLA-identical donors (67). These findings are noteworthy because conventional posttransplant immunosuppressive regimens have had little impact on chronic GVHD (68–70).

IV. GRAFT FAILURE

In virtually all clinical studies, the use of T-cell-depleted marrow for allogeneic transplantation has been complicated by an increased incidence of graft failure (6,11,12,19,20,22–26,29–31,36,37,57,65,71–74). At least three patterns of graft failure have been recognized: (a) failure of initial engraftment, (b) prompt initial engraftment followed by the subsequent development of pancytopenia and marrow aplasia, and (c) late graft failure associated with autologous reconstitution. The incidence of graft failure has varied widely among different centers and in different patient populations. For patients with HLA-identical related donors, the incidence has ranged from less than 5% (11,57) to more than 60% (62,75). At least five factors could contribute to this variation: patient selection, the pretransplant and posttransplant immunosuppressive regimens, the method and extent of T-cell depletion, and the small size of most studies. Overall, T-cell depletion has been associated with a nearly 10-fold increased risk of graft failure after transplantation from an HLA-identical sibling (56). When results from different studies are pooled, it appears that graft failure occurs in approximately 10% of patients transplanted with T-cell-depleted HLA-identical sibling marrow (56) and in approximately 30% of those transplanted with HLA-mismatched marrow from a related donor (76).

In some studies, risk factors associated with graft failure have been identified by retrospective analysis. At least four retrospective studies showed an inverse relationship between the risk of graft failure and the amount of pretransplant cytoreduction and immunosuppression achieved by increased total-body irradiation (TBI) (62,75,77,78). These observations were confirmed in a retrospective multicenter analysis of T-cell depletion (56), although a randomized prospective trial indicated no benefit of adding 6 Gy total lymphoid irradiation to a conditioning regimen of cyclophosphamide and 10 Gy single-exposure TBI (79). In the multicenter analysis, patient age greater than 20 years, sex disparity between the donor and recipient, and the omission of posttransplant immunosuppression were factors associated with an increased risk of graft failure (56). It is possible that posttransplant immunosuppression was administered preferentially to patients transplanted with grafts that contained larger numbers of T cells, but low T-cell dose per se was not associated with an increased risk of graft failure among patients for whom the relevant information was available. The inverse relationship between TBI exposure and risk of graft failure indicated that host factors can contribute to graft failure in at least some patients. These observations suggested the hypothesis that host T cells surviving the conditioning regimen could cause rejection and that agents such as methotrexate or cyclosporine could suppress the activity of these host T cells.

Data supporting this hypothesis have come from careful in vitro studies of lymphoid cells in patients with graft failure. Host lymphocytes with antidonor cytotoxic activity have been identified in the blood of patients with graft failure after T-cell-depleted HLA-mismatched marrow transplantation (80–89). In some cases, it was possible to show that these cells had specificity for donor HLA antigens, indicating that the effectors were T lymphocytes. In general, however, it has not been possible to detect direct antidonor cytotoxic activity in lymphocytes from patients with graft failure after T-cell-depleted HLA-identical marrow transplantation (85). As a different approach, hematopoietic progenitors have been tested as targets for cytotoxic activity or suppression. One group found that cells from patients with graft failure before day 29 showed specific suppression of HLA-identical donor granulocyte-macrophage colony-forming units (CFU-GM) but not burst-forming units–erythroid (BFU-E) (85). Cells from patients with graft failure at later time points did not show this suppression. Another group reported nonspecific suppression of CFU-GM but, again, not BFU-E (81). Similar results were seen when culture supernates from patient cells were tested. The inconsistency of results might reflect technical differences in the assay systems or might indicate the involvement of multiple mechanisms contributing to graft failure. Interpretations must be made with caution, since in vitro results do not necessarily reflect causal mechanisms of graft failure in vivo.

Other clinical observations in trials of T-cell depletion may offer some insight regarding causes of graft failure. Many studies have noted a high incidence of mixed lymphoid and mixed hematopoietic chimerism in patients transplanted with T-cell-depleted marrow compared to similar patients transplanted with unmodified marrow (20,62,75,78,91–104). In keeping with these observations, it has been possible to recover viable host cells after administration of the conditioning regimen but before infusion of the marrow (105,106). In general, the proportion of persisting host lymphoid cells was much higher than the proportion of host myeloid cells. The host lymphoid cells persisted in some patients for more than a year after transplantation. It was noteworthy that some of the patients with persisting mixed lymphoid chimerism had fully functional donor hematopoietic grafts, indicating no strict relationship between mixed lymphoid chimerism and the risk of graft failure (62,97). The association between T-cell depletion and mixed chimerism suggests that donor T cells help to eliminate host lymphoid and hematopoietic cells that survive the conditioning regimen.

The role of donor T cells in preventing graft rejection has been investigated in murine marrow transplant models. In mice, marrow graft rejection can be caused by both CD4 cells and CD8 cells and also by natural killer (NK) cells of the host (107–112). Under certain circumstances, the absence of T cells in the graft can cause an increased susceptibility to rejection by either NK cells or T cells of the host (110,113–116). In such circumstances, the addition of certain cell populations to the graft can prevent rejection (110,115,116). The observations with murine marrow transplant models have indicated that donor lymphoid cells can prevent rejection or promote allogeneic engraftment by at least three different mechanisms not yet fully characterized but probably differing in potency and importance, depending to a great extent on the types of genetic disparity between the donor and recipient. The most potent mechanism may involve the ability of donor T cells or lymphoid activated killer (LAK) cells to recognize and eliminate or inactivate host lymphoid populations containing the effectors responsible for causing rejection (110,117). Direct recognition of host cells by donor cells is not strictly necessary, however, for donor lymphoid cells to be able to prevent rejection. T cells from donors tolerant of host alloantigens can prevent rejection (14,116,118–123), although larger numbers of cells from tolerant donors were needed compared to cells from nontolerant donors (116), suggesting that the cells from tolerant donors were less potent than the cells from nontolerant donors.

The ability of tolerant cells to prevent rejection may involve passive or reverse recognition of donor T cells by host T cells, resulting in "veto" inactivation of the host T cells involved in rejection (124,125). In order to prevent rejection, the cells with veto activity must express the antigens that are involved in causing rejection (126,127). Some experiments have suggested, however, that rejection can be prevented by cells that neither recognize the recipient nor express any antigens involved in causing rejection (121). Therefore, the veto hypothesis cannot fully explain the ability of tolerant T cells to prevent allogeneic marrow graft rejection in mice. Other data have suggested that CD8 cells (128) and LAK cells (129) may produce cytokines that promote donor hematopoiesis in allogeneic recipients, but the cytokines involved in these effects have not been identified.

The crucial question emerging from murine marrow transplant models is whether it might be possible to identify a donor cell population capable of preventing rejection without causing GVHD. Several candidate phenotypes have been identified (122,123,130), and clinical trials to test the relevance of these findings in human marrow transplantation are likely to be forthcoming in the future. At present, the use of more intensive pretransplant immunosuppression (27,33,131–137), larger numbers of stem cells in the graft (138), and less complete removal of T cells (57,66,132,137–141) or T-cell subset depletion (43) represent the empirical approaches under most active investigation as possible ways of avoiding graft failure. Attempts to employ more intensive pretransplant immunosuppression generally cause increased toxicity, which may offset any possible benefits (22). The use of monoclonal antibodies for this purpose may offer an attractive alternative to increased doses of chemotherapy or irradiation (37,135,142–145), although this approach has not been uniformly successful (146,147). Attempts to obtain larger amounts of marrow may increase the risk of complications for the donor and may disproportionately increase the number of T cells, due to the blood coaspirated with the marrow, although this difficulty can be circumvented by the use of stem cells mobilized into the peripheral blood by administration of hematopoietic growth factors (136). Less complete removal of T cells requires the adjunctive use of posttransplant immunosuppression, thus negating one of the major benefits potentially to be gained by T-cell depletion. Various combinations of these approaches can decrease the risk of graft failure to approximately 2 to 3% with HLA-identical sibling donors (57) and to 5 to 10% with unrelated donors (132). The use of lymphokines to promote growth of donor hematopoietic stem cells in vitro before transplantation or in vivo after transplantation is also being explored as a method for avoiding graft failure. These studies follow from the concept that factors elaborated by T cells are directly or indirectly responsible for sustaining hematopoietic function after marrow transplantation and that graft failure after T-cell depletion is caused by deficiency of one or more lymphokines (148). At present, there are no published data indicating that this approach used by itself can prevent rejection (149).

V. LEUKEMIC RELAPSE

Data suggesting an increased incidence of leukemic relapse in patients transplanted with T-cell-depleted marrow were first reported in a prospective randomized study of patients with acute leukemia in remission or chronic myelogenous leukemia (CML) in various phases, but the trend in this study was not statistically significant (24). More convincing evidence came from retrospective studies that found an increased relapse rate in patients transplanted with T-cell-depleted marrow during the first chronic phase of CML compared to similar historical patients transplanted with unmodified marrow (36,150,151).

Many retrospective multivariate analyses have confirmed an increased relapse hazard associated with T-cell depletion in CML patients transplanted with marrow from HLA-identical sibling donors (56,152–158). The relative risk of relapse after transplantation during chronic phase has been estimated at approximately five- to sixfold higher in recipients of T-cell-depleted marrow compared to recipients of unmodified marrow (56,152), and the corresponding relative risk after transplantation during accelerated phase was estimated at 2.65 (56). One study estimated the relative risk of relapse at 18 for patients transplanted during accelerated phase (153). Separate analyses of patients with and without clinically evident acute or chronic GVHD confirmed an increased risk of relapse associated with T-cell depletion in all subgroups (152,154). Thus, decreased GVHD produced by T-cell depletion could not in itself entirely account for the increased relapse risk. Retrospective studies of chronic-phase CML have suggested an association between T-cell depletion and decreased relapse-free survival, but the results did not reach statistical significance despite the marked impact of T-cell depletion on relapse risk (56).

Mechanisms for the association between T-cell depletion and relapse in CML patients could well be identical to those responsible for the increased mixed hematopoeitic chimerism seen after T-cell depletion (20,62,75,78,91–104), since in CML, hematopoiesis originates from a clonal population of pluripotent stem cells that have largely replaced their normal counterparts (159). No relationship between unmanipulated marrow cell dose and relapse rate has been found (56), arguing against the idea that the increased relapse (and increased mixed hematopoietic chimerism) associated with T-cell depletion might be related to a small number of stem cells in the graft (36). Overall, the data best fit the hypothesis that donor T cells help to eliminate residual malignant and normal host hematopoietic stem cells and that overt GVHD is not necessary for this effect.

In HLA-identical marrow transplantation, T-cell depletion increases the risk of relapse not only in patients with CML but also in patients with acute leukemia (56,154). In some studies, this biological effect might not be detectable either because of inadequate statistical power or because an intensified conditioning regimen used to avoid rejection may overcome a small increment in relapse risk caused by T-cell depletion. Moreover, the risk of leukemic relapse appears to be influenced by the method of T-cell depletion (56) and by the posttransplant immunosuppressive regimen (68). Nevertheless, retrospective data collected by the IBMTR have indicated that T-cell depletion was associated with a 1.7 to 2.0-fold increased risk of recurrence in patients with acute lymphoblastic leukemia (ALL) in any phase of the disease and in patients with acute myelogenous leukemia (AML) in first remission or in relapse at the time of transplant. The risk of relapse was not detectably increased in patients with CML in blast crisis at the time of transplant, possibly reflecting the high risk of recurrence in patients with this disease even without T-cell depletion. Patients with AML in second or subsequent remission at the time of transplant were the only group in which T-cell depletion could have been associated with a decreased risk of recurrence, but this trend was not statistically significant. The combined results for patients with chronic-phase CML or acute leukemia in remission demonstrated that T-cell depletion was associated with decreased relapse-free survival after transplantation (56). The overall results for patients with blast-phase CML or acute leukemia in relapse showed a similar decrease in relapse-free survival associated with T-cell depletion. A similar trend was evident in patients with ALL in second or subsequent remission but not in patients with AML in second or subsequent remission.

To some extent, the increased risk of relapse associated with T-cell depletion in patients with acute leukemia could result from the decreased risk of GVHD in this population, since overt GVHD per se seems to account for at least part of the GVL effect (154). Thus inflammatory mediators such as interferon-γ released by activated effectors during GVHD could have a bystander cytotoxic effect on susceptible leukemic progenitors. Alternatively, activated effectors could have a direct cytotoxic effect on leukemic progenitors. In retrospective studies, the risk of recurrence after transplantation for AML in first remission appeared to be higher with syngeneic twin donors than with allogeneic donors in patients who had no GVHD (154). For this malignancy, as with CML, allogeneic T cells may be able to mediate some degree of graft-versus-leukemia (GVL) activity without causing overt GVHD.

For patients with a related donor other than an HLA-identical sibling, the available evidence does not indicate an association between T-cell depletion and an increased risk of recurrent malignancy after transplantation (76), but the statistical power in this study was low. The absence of an increased relapse risk associated with T-cell depletion could be explained by the higher baseline risk of GVHD in this setting compared to transplantation from an HLA-identical sibling or by the antileukemic effects of more intensive conditioning regimens or less complete removal of T cells employed to avoid graft rejection.

Conflicting evidence has been reported for the association between T-cell depletion and recurrent malignancy after unrelated marrow transplantation. Two early retrospective studies did not detect any such association (160,161), but a preliminary report of more recent data has suggested that T-cell depletion was associated with an increased risk of recurrent malignancy after unrelated marrow transplantation in patients with CML (162). The earlier studies suggested that T-cell depletion might be associated with improved relapse-free survival after unrelated marrow transplantation, but the more recent retrospective study showed a statistically significant decrease in relapse-free survival in patients with CML, similar to the previously reported finding in patients with HLA-identical sibling donors.

The role of donor lymphoid cells in controlling minimal residual malignancy has been investigated in murine marrow transplant models (see Chap. 00). These studies have demonstrated that several different types of cells may be able to mediate antileukemic effects in marrow transplant recipients. The relative importance of different cell types and mechanisms may depend not only on the type of genetic disparity between the donor and recipient but also on the type of malignancy involved. Many of these studies have focused on the question of whether it might be possible to preserve GVL effects while decreasing the risk of GVHD, and with certain models, such discrimination between GVL activity and GVHD has been possible.

Clinical trials during the past 5 years have used more intensive conditioning regimens (27,33,131–136) and less complete removal of T cells (57,66,132,137–141) or T-cell subset depletion (43) in order to decrease the risk of recurrent malignancy after T-cell-depleted marrow transplantation. More recently, studies have been initiated to test cytokine administration (163,164) or delayed infusion of T cells (165–168) as methods for decreasing the risk of leukemic relapse. Given the probable diversity of antileukemic effects, full evaluation of these approaches will require separate studies with different malignancies and lengthy follow-up in order to assess results.

IV. IMMUNOLOGICAL RECONSTITUTION

Transplantation of syngeneic, autologous, or allogeneic marrow is followed by a period of immunodeficiency frequently complicated by serious, life-threatening infections. It is well documented that GVHD and its treatment can further delay or inhibit immune recovery (169,170). On the other hand, it is unknown to what extent initial immune reconstitution depends on mature T cells in the graft, particularly in older individuals with impaired thymic function. Studies with murine marrow transplant models have shown that posttransplant T-cell regeneration in recipients lacking thymic function occurs by expansion of peripheral T cells in the graft (171). These regenerated T cells had a diverse T-cell-receptor repertoire and a cell surface phenotype consistent with derivation from memory T cells. In recipients with a functional thymus, expansion of memory T cells was downregulated, and posttransplant T cell regeneration occurred by the differentiation of prethymic progenitors and expansion of thymic emigrants with cell surface markers indicating a "naive" phenotype.

The tempo of reconstitution following allogeneic unmodified marrow transplantation has been well documented by in vitro studies (172–174), thereby providing a baseline for comparisons with T-cell-depleted transplantation. At the initiation of clinical trials, it was unclear how depletion of mature T cells from allogeneic donor marrow would affect the duration of immunodeficiency after transplantation. It is now known that T-cell depletion can cause delayed immune reconstitution whether recipients received marrow depleted of T cells by treatment with monoclonal antibodies plus complement (175–182) or by soybean lectin agglutination and E-rosetting (183–185).

Immune recovery has been compared concurrently in recipients of HLA-identical marrow depleted of T cells by soybean lectin agglutination and E-rosetting and in recipients of unmodified marrow (183). In this study and in other reports (175,177,182,186), NK cells were the first lymphoid subset to recover in all recipients irrespective of the type of transplant, with initial recovery occurring between 2 and 3 weeks after transplantation. Phenotypic analysis of blood leukocytes indicated that the total number of lymphocytes was slightly higher in conventional marrow recipients during the first month. Thereafter, patients with chronic GVHD had a lymphocytosis, while recipients of T-cell-depleted marrow remained normal, consistent with the absence of chronic GVHD. Lymphocytes predominantly had a $CD3^+$, $CD8^+$ phenotype, with the number of $CD4^+$ cells remaining well below normal in both groups of patients throughout the first 6 months. The number of $CD4^+$ cells began to increase at 7 to 9 months posttransplant in recipients of unmodified marrow and at 10 to 12 months in recipients of T-cell-depleted marrow. T-cell function measured by proliferative response to phytohemagglutinin recovered to the normal range at 4 to 6 months after conventional transplantation and at 10 to 12 months after T cell-depleted transplantation.

In this study (183) as well as in other reports (175,180,184,187–189), the number of circulating B lymphocytes recovered to the normal range by the second month and exceeded normal levels after 7 months. Similarly, responses to *Staphylococcus aureus* (SAC) were normal in both groups of patients by 2 to 3 months posttransplant. In fact, by 4 months, the responses were higher than normal and remained elevated for at least 18 months. In vitro assays showed that normal levels of IgM production were achieved in both groups of patients by 4 to 6 months posttransplant. In contrast, the time to achieve normal IgG production differed in the two groups of patients. Recipients of conventional grafts reached normal production at 7 to 9 months, while recipients of T-cell-depleted grafts did not recover until 13 to 15 months.

Further evidence for T-cell functional impairment has come from limiting dilution assays that enumerated precursors for helper, cytotoxic, and proliferative T lymphocytes (190). During the first 180 days, precursor frequencies for cytotoxic and proliferating T cells were lower in patients transplanted with T-cell-depleted marrow than in patients transplanted with unmodified marrow. After the first 6 months, the precursor frequencies for these cells were similar in the two groups but still well below normal values. T-cell depletion did not have a statistically significant effect on the precursor frequency for helper T cells, but only limited data were available. Other factors such as age and GVHD did not detectably affect the results.

Despite the in vitro observations described above, there is little reported evidence to suggest an increased risk of infectious complications in durably engrafted recipients of T-cell-depleted marrow. Three groups, however, have suggested that the incidence of Epstein-Barr virus–associated lymphoproliferative syndromes (EBV-LPS) may be increased in recipients of T-cell-depleted marrow (33,191–193). In two studies, the occurrence of EBV-LPS appeared to be associated with T-cell depletion of marrow from HLA-mismatched donors (33,191). In the other study, the EBV-LPS occurred in recipients of T-cell-depleted HLA-identical marrow (192). By multivariate proportional hazards analysis, the relative risk for EBV-LPS was estimated to be sevenfold greater in recipients of HLA-identical T-cell-depleted marrow compared to recipients of unmodified marrow (192). EBV-specific cytotoxic T lymphocytes represent the primary mechanism for controlling the proliferation of EBV-infected B lymphocytes (194). Thus the increased incidence of EBV-LPS after T-cell-depleted transplantation may correspond with the impaired reconstitution of cytotoxic precursors observed during the first 6 months (190). Evidence in support of this hypothesis has come from the finding that EBV-LPS can resolve after infusion of unirradiated donor leukocytes (195).

VII. CONCLUSIONS

Clinical trials evaluating T-cell depletion of donor marrow have clearly indicated both the benefits and the drawbacks of this method for preventing GVHD. Insights concerning mechanisms for the detrimental effects associated with this procedure are beginning to emerge, and new approaches to solve the problems of increased graft failure, leukemic relapse, and delayed immune reconstitution are being explored. Although most trials have employed methods aimed at global T-cell depletion, it should be recognized that GVHD is initiated by the relatively small subset of cells that are specifically alloreactive against host histocompatibility antigens. The extent to which these same cells are necessary for engraftment and antileukemic activity in humans remains unknown. If separate populations are responsible for these different functional activities, then methods for depleting the subset(s) specifically involved in causing GVHD may solve many of the problems associated with currently used methods of T-cell depletion. On the other hand, if a single subset is responsible for all three effects, then alternative methods must be developed for assuring adequate engraftment and eliminating residual malignant cells if T-cell depletion of donor marrow is used to prevent GVHD.

ACKNOWLEDGMENT

The authors' investigations were supported by U.S. Public Health Service grants CA18029, CA29548, CA22507, CA23766, CA08748, and AI27951, awarded by the

Department of Health and Human Services, National Institutes of Health. We gratefully thank Alison Sell for assistance in preparation of the manuscript.

REFERENCES

1. Gale RP. T cells, bone marrow transplantation and immunotherapy: Use of monoclonal antibodies. Ann Intern Med 1987; 106:257–274.
2. Thomas ED, Storb R. Technique for human marrow grafting. Blood 1970; 46:507–515.
3. Lucas PJ, Quinones RR, Moses RD, et al. Alternative donor sources in HLA-mismatched marrow transplantation: T cell depletion of surgically resected cadaveric marrow. Bone Marrow Transplant 1988; 3:211–220.
4. Reisner Y, Kapoor N, Kirkpatrick D, et al. Transplantation for acute leukaemia with HLA-A and B nonidentical parental marrow cells fractionated with soybean agglutinin and sheep red blood cells. Lancet 1981; 2:327–331.
5. Reisner Y, Kapoor N, Kirkpatrick D, et al. Transplantation for severe combined immunodeficiency with HLA-A, B, D, DR incompatible parental marrow cells fractionated by soybean agglutinin and sheep red cells. Blood 1983; 61:341–348.
6. O'Reilly RJ, Collins NH, Kerman NA, et al. Transplantation of marrow depleted of T cells by soybean lectin agglutination and E-rosette depletion: Major histocompatibility complex-related graft resistance in leukemic transplant patients. Transplant Proc 1985; 17:455–459.
7. Matthay KK, Wara DW, Ammann AJ, et al. Mismatched bone marrow transplantation using soybean agglutinin processed T-cell depleted marrow. In: Gale RP, Champlin RE, eds. Progress in Bone Marrow Transplantation. New York: Liss, 1987:343–351.
8. DeWitte T, Raymakers R, Plas A, et al. Bone marrow repopulation capacity after transplantation of lymphocyte-depleted allogeneic bone marrow using counterflow centrifugation. Transplantation 1984; 37:151–155.
9. DeWitte T, Hoogenhout J, DePauw B, et al. Depletion of donor lymphocytes by counterflow centrifugation successfully prevents acute graft-versus-host disease in matched allogeneic marrow transplantation. Blood 1986; 67:1302–1308.
10. Noga SJ, Donnenberg AD, Schwartz CL, et al. Development of a simplified counterflow centrifugation elutriation procedure for depletion of lymphocytes from human bone marrow. Transplantation 1986; 41:220–229.
11. Wagner JE, Donnenberg AD, Noga SJ, et al. Lymphocyte depletion of donor marrow by counterflow centrifugal elutriation: Results of a phase I clinical trial. Blood 1988; 72:1168–1176.
12. Lowenberg B, Wagemaker E, van Bekkum DW, et al. Graft-versus-host disease following transplantation of "one log" versus "two log" T-lymphocyte depleted bone marrow from HLA-identical donors. Bone Marrow Transplant 1986; 1:133–140.
13. Prentice HG, Blacklock HA, Janossy G, et al. Use of anti-T cell monoclonal antibody OKT3 to prevent acute graft-versus-host disease in allogeneic bone-marrow transplantation for acute leukaemia. Lancet 1982; 1:700–703.
14. Filipovich AH, McGlave PB, Ransay NKC, et al. Pretreatment of donor bone marrow with monoclonal antibody OKT3 for prevention of acute graft-versus-host disease in allogeneic histocompatible bone-marrow transplantation. Lancet 1982; 1:1266–1269.
15. Martin PJ, Hansen JA, Thomas ED. Preincubation of donor bone marrow cells with a combination of murine monoclonal anti-T-cell antibodies without complement does not prevent graft-versus-host disease after allogeneic marrow transplantation. J Clin Immunol 1984; 4:18–22.

16. Reinherz EL, Geha R, Rappeport JM, et al. Reconstitution after transplantation with T-lymphocyte-depleted HLA haplotype-mismatched bone marrow for severe combined immunodeficiency. Proc Natl Acad Sci USA 1982; 79:6047–6051.
17. Gilmore MJML, Prentice HG, Price-Jones E, et al. Allogeneic bone marrow transplantation: The monitoring of granulcoyte macrophage colonies following the collection of bone marrow mononuclear cells and after the subsequent in-vitro cytolysis of OKT3 lymphocytes. Br J Haematol 1983; 55:587–593.
18. Prentice HG, Janossy G, Price-Jones L, et al. Depletion of T lymphocytes in donor marrow prevents significant graft-versus-host disease in matched allogeneic leukaemic marrow transplant recipients. Lancet 1984; 1:472–475.
19. Waldmann H, Hale G, Cividalli G, et al. Elimination of graft-versus-host disease by in vitro depletion of alloreactive lymphocytes with a monoclonal rat anti-human lymphocyte antibody (Campath-1). Lancet 1984; 2:483–486.
20. Martin PJ, Hansen JA, Buckner CD, et al. Effects of in vitro depletion of T cells in HLA-identical allogeneic marrow grafts. Blood 1985; 66:664–672.
21. Herve P, Flesch M, Cahn JY, et al. Removal of marrow T cells with OKT3-OKT11 monoclonal antibodies and complement to prevent graft-versus-host disease. Transplantation 1985; 39:138–143.
22. Sondel PM, Bozdech MJ, Trigg ME, et al. Additional immunosuppression allows engraftment following HLA-mismatched T cell-depleted bone marrow transplantation for leukemia. Transplant Proc 1985; 17:460–461.
23. Trigg ME, Billing R, Sondel PM, et al. Clinical trial depleting T lymphocytes from donor marrow for matched and mismatched allogeneic bone marrow transplant. Cancer Treat Rep 1985; 69:377–386.
24. Mitsuyasu RT, Champlin RE, Gale RP, et al. Treatment of donor bone marrow with monoclonal anti-T cell antibody and complement for the prevention of graft-versus-host disease: A prospective, randomized, double-blind trial. Ann Intern Med 1986; 105:20–26.
25. Maraninchi D, Blaise D, Rio B, et al. Impact of T-cell depletion on outcome of allogeneic bone marrow transplantation for standard-risk leukaemias. Lancet 1987; 2: 175–178.
26. Maraninchi D, Mawas C, Guyotat D, et al. Selective depletion of marrow-T cytotoxic lymphocytes (CD8) in the prevention of graft-versus-host disease after allogeneic bone-marrow transplantation. Transplant Int 1988; 1:91–94.
27. Cahn JY, Herve P, Flesch M, et al. Marrow transplantation from HLA non-identical family donors for the treatment of leukaemia: A pilot study of 15 patients using additional immunosuppression and T-cell depletion. Br J Haematol 1988; 69:345–349.
28. Filipovich AH, Youle RJ, Neville DM, et al. Ex-vivo treatment of donor bone marrow with anti-T-cell immunotoxins for prevention of graft-versus-host disease. Lancet 1984; 1:469–472.
29. Filipovich AH, Vallera DA, Youle RJ, et al. Graft-versus-host disease prevention in allogeneic bone marrow transplantation from histocompatible siblings. Transplantation 1987; 44:62–69.
30. Martin PJ, Hansen JA, Torok-Storb B, et al. Effects of treating marrow with a CD3-specific immunotoxin for prevention of acute graft-versus-host disease. Bone Marrow Transplant 1988; 3:437–444.
31. Laurent G, Maraninchi D, Gluckman E, et al. Donor bone marrow treatment with T101 Fab fragment-ricin A-chain immunotoxin prevents graft-versus-host disease. Bone Marrow Transplant 1989; 4:367–371.
32. Filipovich AH, Vallera D, McGlave P, et al. T cell depletion with anti-CD5 immunotoxin in histocompatible bone marrow transplantation. Transplantation 1990; 50:410–415.

33. Antin JH, Bierer BE, Smith BR, et al. Selective depletion of bone marrow T lymphocytes with anti-CD5 monoclonal antibodies: Effective prophylaxis for graft-versus-host disease in patients with hematologic malignancies. Blood 1991; 78:2139–2149.
34. Vartdal F, Albrechtsen D, Ringden O, et al. Immunomagnetic treatment of bone marrow allografts. Bone Marrow Transplant 1987; 2(suppl 2):94–98.
35. Knobloch C, Spadinger U, Rueber E, Friedrich W. T cell depletion from human bone marrow using magnetic beads. Bone Marrow Transplant 1990; 6:21–24.
36. Hale G, Cobbold S, Waldmann H. T cell depletion with Campath-1 in allogeneic bone marrow transplantation. Transplantation 1988; 45:753–759.
37. Hale G, Waldmann H, for Campath users. Control of graft-versus-host disease and graft rejection by T cell depletion of donor and recipient with Campath-1 antibodies: Results of matched sibling transplants for malignant diseases. Bone Marrow Transplant 1994; 13:597–611.
38. Cobbold S, Hale G, Waldmann H. Non-lineage, LFA-1 family, and leucocyte common antigens: New and previously defined clusters. In: McMichael AJ, ed. Leucocyte Typing III: White Cell Differentiation Antigens. Oxford, England: Oxford University Press, 1987:788–803.
39. Hale G, Xia M-Q, Tight HP, et al. The Campath-1 antigens (CDw52). Tissue Antigens 1990; 35:118–127.
40. Bernard A, Boumsell L, Hill C. Joint report of the First International Workshop on Human Leucocyte Differentiation Antigens by the investigators of the participating laboratories. In: Bernard A, Boumsell L, Dausset J, et al., eds. Leucocyte Typing. New York: Springer-Verlag, 1984:9–142.
41. Haynes BF. Summary of T cell studies performed during the Second International Workshop and Conference on Human Leukocyte Differentiation Antigens. In: Reinherz E, Haynes BF, Nadler LM, Bernstein ID, eds. Leukocyte Typing II, vol 1. New York: Springer-Verlag, 1986:3–30.
42. McMichael AJ, Gotch FM. T-cell antigens: New and previously defined clusters. In: McMichael AJ, ed. Leucocyte Typing III, White Cell Differentiation Antigens. Oxford, England: Oxford University Press, 1987:31–62.
43. Champlin R, Ho W, Gajewski J, et al. Selective depletion of $CD8^+$ T lymphocytes for prevention of graft-versus-host disease after allogeneic bone marrow transplantation. Blood 1990; 76:418–423.
44. Frame JN, Collins NH, Cartagena T, et al. T cell depletion of human bone marrow: comparison of Campath-1 plus complement, anti-T cell ricin A chain immunotoxin, and soybean agglutinin alone or in combination with sheep erythrocytes or immunomagnetic beads. Transplantation 1989; 47:984–988.
45. Knott LJ, Levinsky RJ, Newland A, et al. Bone marrow T-cell colony-forming cells: Studies of their origin and use in monitoring T cell-depleted bone marrow grafts. Clin Exp Immunol 1985; 62:561–569.
46. Martin PJ, Hansen JA. Quantitative assays for detection of residual T cells in T-depleted human marrow. Blood 1985; 65:1134–1140.
47. Kernan NA, Flomenberg N, Collins NH, et al. Quantitation of T lymphocytes in human bone marrow by a limiting dilution assay. Transplantation 1985; 40:317–322.
48. Rohatiner A, Gelber R, Schlossman SF, Ritz J. Depletion of T cells from human bone marrow using monoclonal antibodies and rabbit complement. Transplantation 1986; 42:73–80.
49. Rozans MK, Smith BR, Emerson S, et al. Functional assessment of T cell depletion from bone marrow prior to therapeutic transplantation using limiting dilution culture methods. Transplantation 1986; 42:380–387.
50. Irle C, Kaestli M, Aapro M, et al. Quantity and nature of residual bone marrow T cells after treatment of the marrow with Campath-1. Exp Hematol 1987; 15:163–170.

51. Sharp TG, Sachs DH, Fauci AS, et al. T cell depletion of human bone marrow using monoclonal antibody and complement-mediated lysis. Transplantation 1983; 35:112–120.
52. Hale G, Bright S, Chumbley G, et al. Removal of T cells from bone marrow for transplantation: A monoclonal antilymphocyte anti-antibody that fixes human complement. Blood 1983; 62:873–882.
53. Cobbold SP, Thierfelder S, Waldmann H. Immunosuppression with monoclonal antibodies: A model to determine the rules for effective serotherapy. Mol Biol Med 1984; 1:285–304.
54. Kummer U, Thierfelder S, Hoffman-Fezer G, Schuh, R. In vivo immunosuppression by pan-T cell antibodies relates to their isotype and to their Clq uptake. J Immunol 1987; 138:4069–4074.
55. Cobbold SP, Waldmann H. Therapeutic potential of monovalent monoclonal antibodies. Nature 1984; 308:460–462.
56. Marmont AM, Horowitz MM, Gale RP, et al. T-cell depletion of HLA-identical transplants in leukemia. Blood 1991; 78:2120–2130.
57. Soiffer RJ, Murray C, Mauch P, et al. Prevention of graft-versus-host disease by selective depletion of CD6-positive T lymphocytes from donor bone marrow. J Clin Oncol 1992; 10:1191–1200.
58. Young JW, Papadopoulos EB, Cunningham I, et al. T-cell-depleted allogeneic bone marrow transplantation in adults with acute nonlymphocytic leukemia in first remission. Blood 1992; 79:3380–3387.
59. Sullivan KM, Deeg JH, Sanders J, et al. Hyperacute graft-versus-host disease in patients not given immunosuppression after allogeneic marrow transplantation. Blood 1986; 67:1172–1175.
60. Kernan NA, Collins NH, Juliano L, et al. Clonable T lymphocytes in T cell-depleted bone marrow transplants correlate with development of graft-versus-host disease. Blood 1986; 68:770–773.
61. Atkinson K, Farrelly H, Cooley M, et al. Human marrow T cell dose correlates with severity of subsequent acute graft-versus-host disease. Bone Marrow Transplant 1987; 2:51–57.
62. Martin PJ, Hansen JA, Torok-Storb B, et al. Graft failure in patients receiving T cell-depleted HLA-identical allogeneic marrow transplants. Bone Marrow Transplant 1988; 3:445–456.
63. Gale RP, Bortin MM, van Bekkum DW, et al. Risk factors for acute graft-versus-host disease. Br J Haematol 1987; 67:397–406.
64. Beatty PG, Clift RA, Mickelson EM, et al. Marrow transplantation from related donors other than HLA-identical siblings. N Engl J Med 1985; 313:765–771.
65. O'Reilly RJ, Keever CA, Small TN, Brochstein J. The use of HLA-non-identical T-cell depleted marrow transplants for correction of severe combined immunodeficiency disease. Immunodef Rev 1989; 1:273–309.
66. Wagner JE, Santos GW, Noga SJ, et al. Bone marrow graft engineering by counterflow centrifugal elutriation: Results of a phase I-II clinical trial. Blood 1990; 75:1370–1377.
67. Atkinson K, Horowitz MM, Gale RP, et al. Risk factors for chronic graft-versus-host disease after HLA-identical sibling bone marrow transplantation. Blood 1990; 75: 2459–2464.
68. Storb R, Deeg J, Pepe M, Appelbaum FR, et al. Methotrexate and cyclosporine versus cyclosporine alone for prophylaxis of graft-versus-host disease in patients given HLA-identical marrow grafts for leukemia: Long term follow-up of a controlled trial. Blood 1989; 73:1729–1734.
69. Storb R, Deeg HG, Pepe M, et al. Graft-versus-host disease prevention by methotrex-

ate combined with cyclosporine compared to methotrexate alone in patients given marrow grafts for severe aplastic anemia: Long term follow-up of a controlled trial. Br J Haematol 1989; 72:567–572.

70. Sullivan KM, Storb R, Witherspoon RP, et al. Deletion of immunosuppressive prophylaxis after marrow transplantation increases hyperacute graft-versus-host disease but does not influence chronic graft-versus-host disease or relapse in patients with advanced leukemia. Clin Transplant 1989; 3:5–11.
71. Herve P, Cahn JG, Flesch M, et al. Successful graft-versus-host disease prevention without graft failure in 32 HLA-identical allogeneic bone marrow transplantations with marrow depleted of T cells by monoclonal antibodies and complement. Blood 1987; 69:388–393.
72. Kernan NA, Bordignon C, Heller G, et al. Graft failure following T cell depleted HLA-identical marrow transplants for leukemia: Analysis of risk factors and results of secondary transplants. Blood 1989; 74:2227–2236.
73. Champlin RE, Horowitz MM, van Bekkum DW, et al. Graft failure following bone marrow transplantation for severe aplastic anemia: risk factors and treatment results. Blood 1989; 73:606–613.
74. Delain M, Cahn JY, Racadot E, et al. Graft failure after T cell depleted HLA identical allogeneic bone marrow transplantation: risk factors in leukemic patients. Leuk Lymph 1993; 11:359–368.
75. Patterson J, Prentice HG, Brenner MK, et al. Graft rejection following HLA matched T-lymphocyte depleted bone marrow transplantation. Br J Haematol 1986; 63:221–230.
76. Ash RC, Horowitz MM, Gale RP, et al. Bone marrow transplantation from related donors other than HLA-identical siblings: effect of T cell depletion. Bone Marrow Transplant 1991; 7:443–452.
77. Guyotat D, Dutou L, Erhsam A, et al. Graft rejection after T cell-depleted marrow transplantation: Role of fractionated irradiation. Br J Haematol 1987; 65:499–507.
78. Burnett AK, Hann IM, Robertson AG, et al. Prevention of graft-versus-host disease by ex vivo T cell depletion: Reduction in graft failure with augmented total body irradiation. Leukemia 1988; 2:300–303.
79. Ganem G, Kuentz M, Beaujean F, et al. Additional total-lymphoid irradiation in preventing graft failure of T-cell depleted bone marrow transplantation from HLA-identical siblings. Transplantation 1987; 45:244–248.
80. Sondel PM, Hank JA, Trigg ME, et al. Transplantation of HLA-haploidentical T cell-depleted marrow for leukemia: Autologous marrow recovery with specific immune sensitization to donor antigens. Exp Hematol 1986; 14:278–286.
81. Bunjes D, Heit W, Arnold R, et al. Evidence for the involvement of host-derived OKT8-positive T cells in the rejection of T-depleted, HLA-identical bone marrow grafts. Transplantation 1987; 43:501–505.
82. Kernan NA, Flomenberg N, Dupont B, O'Reilly RJ. Graft rejection in recipients of T-cell depleted HLA-nonidentical marrow transplants for leukemia. Transplantation 1987; 43:842–847.
83. Bierer BE, Emerson SG, Antin J, et al. Regulation of cytotoxic T lymphocyte-mediated graft rejection following bone marrow transplantation. Transplantation 1988; 46:835–839.
84. Bosserman LD, Murray C, Takvorian T, et al. Mechanism of graft failure in HLA-matched and HLA-mismatched bone marrow transplant recipients. Bone Marrow Transplant 1989; 4:239–245.
85. Bordignon C, Keever CA, Small TN, et al. Graft failure after T-cell-depleted human leukocyte antigen identical marrow transplants for leukemia: II. In vitro analyses of host effector mechanisms. Blood 1989; 74:2237–2243.

86. Voogt PJ, Fibbe WE, Marijt WA, et al. Rejection of bone marrow graft by recipient-derived cytotoxic T lymphocytes against minor histocompatibility antigens. Lancet 1990; 335:131–134.
87. Bunjes D, Theobald M, Wiesneth M, et al. Graft rejection by a population of primed CDw52-host T cells after in vivo/ex vivo T-depleted bone marrow transplantation. Bone Marrow Transplant 1993; 12:209–215.
88. Fleischhauer K, Kernan NA, O'Reilly RJ, et al. Bone marrow allograft rejection by host-derived allocytotoxic T lymphocytes recognizing a single amino acid at position 156 of the HLA-B44 class I antigen. N Engl J Med 1990; 323:1818–1822.
89. Donohue J, Homge M, Kernan NA. Characterization of cells emerging at the time of graft failure after bone marrow transplantation from an unrelated marrow donor. Blood 1993; 82:1023–1029.
90. Walker H, Singer CRJ, Patterson J, et al. The significance of host hematopoietic cells detected by cytogenetic analysis of bone marrow from recipients of bone marrow transplants. Br J Haematol 1986; 62:385–391.
91. Bretagne S, Vidaud M, Kuentz M, et al. Mixed blood chimerism in T cell-depleted bone marrow recipients: Evaluation using DNA polymorphisms. Blood 1987; 70:1692–1695.
92. Lawler SD, Harris H, Millar J, Barrett-Powles RL. Cytogenetic follow-up studies of recipients of T-cell depleted allogeneic bone marrow. Br J Haematol 1987; 65:143–150.
93. Korver K, Delange GG, Van den Bergh RL, et al. Lymphoid chimerism after allogeneic bone marrow transplantation. Transplantation 1987; 44:643–650.
94. Bertheas MF, Maraninchi D, Lafage M, et al. Partial chimerism after T-cell depleted allogeneic bone marrow transplantation in leukemic HLA-matched patients: A cytogenetic documentation. Blood 1988; 72:89–93.
95. Schouten HC, Sizoo W, vant Veer MB, et al. Incomplete chimerism in erythroid, myeloid and B lymphocyte lineage after T cell-depleted allogeneic bone marrow transplantation. Bone Marrow Transplant 1988; 3:407–412.
96. Offit K, Burns JP, Cunningham I, et al. Cytogenetic analysis of chimerism and leukemia relapse in chronic myelogenous leukemia patients following T cell depleted bone marrow transplantation. Blood 1990; 75:1346–1355.
97. Roy DC, Tantravahi R, Murray C, et al. Natural history of mixed chimerism after bone marrow transplantation with CD6-depleted allogeneic marrow: A stable equilibrium. Blood 1990; 75:296–304.
98. Lawler M, Humphries P, McCann SR. Evaluation of mixed chimerism by in vitro amplification of dinucleotide repeat sequences using the polymerase chain reaction. Blood 1991; 77:2504–2514.
99. Roux E, Helg C, Chapuis B, et al. Evolution of mixed chimerism after allogeneic bone marrow transplantation as determined on granulocytes and mononuclear cells by the polymerase chain reaction. Blood 1992; 79:2775–2783.
100. Mackinnon S, Barnett L, Bourhis JH, et al. Myeloid and lymphoid chimerism after T-cell-depleted bone marrow transplantation: Evaluation of conditioning regimens using the polymerase chain reaction to amplify human minisatellite regions of genomic DNA. Blood 1992; 80:3235–3241.
101. Schattenberg A, De Witte T, Salden M, et al. Mixed hematopoietic chimerism after allogeneic transplantation with lymphocyte-depleted bone marrow is not associated with a higher incidence of relapse. Blood 1989; 73:1367–1372.
102. Roux E, Abdi K, Speiser D, et al. Characterization of mixed chimerism in patients with chronic myeloid leukemia transplanted with T-cell-depleted bone marrow: Involvement of different hematologic lineages before and after relapse. Blood 1993; 81:243–248.
103. Mackinnon S, Barnett L, Heller G, O'Reilly RJ. Minimal residual disease is more

common in patients who have mixed T-cell chimerism after bone marrow transplantation for chronic myelogenous leukemia. Blood 1994; 83:3409–3416.

104. van Leeuwen JE, van Tol MJ, Joosten AM, et al. Persistence of host-type hematopoiesis after allogeneic bone marrow transplantation for leukemia is significantly related to the recipient's age and/or the conditioning regimen, but it is not associated with an increased risk of relapse. Blood 1994; 83:3059–3067.
105. Butturini A, Seger RC, Gale RP. Recipient immune-competent T-lymphocytes can survive intensive conditioning for bone marrow transplantation. Blood 1986; 68:948–956.
106. Kedar E, Or R, Naparstek E, et al. Preliminary characterization of functional residual host-type T lymphocytes following conditioning for allogeneic HLA-matched bone marrow transplantation (BMT). Bone Marrow Transplant 1988; 3:129–140.
107. Cobbold SP, Martin G, Qin S, Waldmann H. Monoclonal antibodies to promote marrow engraftment and tissue graft tolerance. Nature (Lond) 1986; 323:164–166.
108. Murphy WJ, Kumar V, Bennett M. Acute rejection of murine bone marrow allografts by natural killer cells and T cells. Differences in kinetics and target antigens recognized. J Exp Med 1987; 166:1499–1509.
109. Nakamura H, Gress RE. Graft rejection by cytolytic T cells. Transplantation 1990; 49: 453–458.
110. Martin PJ. Donor CD8 cells prevent allogeneic marrow graft rejection in mice: Potential implications for marrow transplantation in humans. J Exp Med 1993; 178:703–712.
111. Vallera DA, Taylor PA, Sprent J, Blazar BR. The role of host T cell subsets in bone marrow rejection directed to isolated major histocompatibility complex class I versus class II differences of bm1 and bm12 mutant mice. Transplantation 1994; 57:249–256.
112. Bennett M. Biology and genetics of hybrid resistance. Adv Immunol 1987; 41:333–445.
113. Chester CH, Sykes M, Sachs DH. The recovery of resistance to alloengraftment following lethal irradiation and administration of T cell-depleted syngeneic bone marrow. Bone Marrow Transplant 1989; 4:195–200.
114. Pierce GE, Watts LM. Effects of Thy-1^+ cell depletion on the capacity of donor lymphoid cells to induce tolerance across an entire MHC disparity in sublethally irradiated adult hosts. Transplantation 1989; 48:289–296.
115. Murphy WJ, Kumar V, Cope JC, Bennett M. An absence of T cells in murine bone marrow allografts leads to an increased susceptibility to rejection by natural killer cells and T cells. J Immunol 1990; 144:3305–3311.
116. Lapidot T, Lubin I, Terenzi A, et al. Enhancement of bone marrow allografts from nude mice into mismatched recipients by T cells void of graft-versus-host activity. Proc Natl Acad Sci USA 1990; 87:4595–4599.
117. Murphy WJ, Bennett M, Kumar V, Longo DL. Donor-type activated natural killer cells promote marrow engraftment and B cell development during allogeneic bone marrow transplantation. J Immunol 1992; 148:2953–2960.
118. Pierce GE. Allogeneic versus semiallogeneic F1 bone marrow transplantation into sub-lethally irradiated MHC-disparate hosts: Effects on mixed lymphoid chimerism, skin graft tolerance, host survival, and alloreactivity. Transplantation 1990; 49:138–144.
119. Pierce GE, Steers JL. Thy 1^+ donor cells that promote allograft tolerance in sublethally irradiated MHC-disparate hosts. Transplantation 1991; 52:526–530.
120. Navarro J, Touraine J-L. Promotion of fetal liver engraftment by T cells in a murine semiallogeneic model without graft-versus-host reaction. Transplantation 1989; 47: 871–876.
121. Faktorowich Y, Lapidot T, Lubin I, Reisner Y. Enhancement of BM allografting from C57BL/6 'nude' mice into C3H/HeJ recipients by tolerized T cells from (C57BL/6 →

C3H/HeJ) and (C3H/HeJ → C57BL/6) chimeras. Bone Marrow Transplant 1993; 12:15–20.
122. Sykes M, Sheard M, Sachs DH. Effects of T cell depletion in radiation bone marrow chimeras: I. Evidence for a donor cell population which increases allogeneic chimerism but which lacks the potential to produce GVHD. J Immunol 1988; 141:2282–2288.
123. Sykes M, Chester CH, Sundt TM, et al. Effects of T cell depletion in radiation bone marrow chimeras: III. Characterization of allogeneic bone marrow cell populations that increase allogeneic chimerism independently of graft-vs-host disease in mixed marrow recipients. J Immunol 1989; 143:3503–3511.
124. Azuma E, Kaplan J. Role of lymphokine-activated killer cells as mediators of veto and natural suppression. J Immunol 1988; 141:2601–2606.
125. Nakamura H, Gress RE. Interleukin 2 enhancement of veto suppressor cell function in T-cell-depleted bone marrow in vitro and in vivo. Transplantation 1990; 49:931–937.
126. Fink PJ. Veto cells. Ann Rev Immunol 1988; 6:115–137.
127. Rammensee HG. Veto function in vitro and in vivo. Int Rev Immunol 1989; 4:175–191.
128. Lapidot T, Faktorowich Y, Lubin I, Reisner Y. Enhancement of T cell-depleted bone marrow allografts in the absence of graft-versus-host disease is mediated by $CD8^+CD4^-$ and not by $CD8^-CD4^+$ thymocytes. Blood 1992; 80:2406–2411.
129. Murphy WJ, Keller JR, Harrison CL, et al. Interleukin-1 activated natural killer cells can support hematopoiesis in vitro and promote marrow engraftment in vivo. Blood 1992; 80:670–677.
130. Kaufman CL, Colson YL, Wren SM, et al. Phenotypic characterization of a novel bone marrow-derived cell that facilitates engraftment of allogeneic bone marrow stem cells. Blood 1994; 84:2436–2446.
131. Trigg ME, Gingrich R, Goeken N, et al. Low rejection rate when using unrelated or haploidentical donors for children with leukemia undergoing marrow transplantation. Bone Marrow Transplant 1989; 89:431–437.
132. Ash RC, Casper JT, Chitambar CR, et al. Successful allogeneic transplantation of T-cell depleted bone marrow from closely HLA-matched unrelated donors. N Engl J Med 1990; 322:485–494.
133. Aversa F, Pelicci PG, Terenzi A, et al. Results of T-depleted BMT in chronic myelogenous leukaemia after a conditioning regimen that included thiotepa. Bone Marrow Transplant 1991; 7(suppl 2):24.
134. Soiffer RJ, Mauch P, Tarbell NJ, et al. Total lymphoid irradiation to prevent graft rejection in recipients of HLA non-identical T cell-depleted allogeneic marrow. Bone Marrow Transplant 1991; 7:23–33.
135. Or R, Mehta J, Kapelushnik J, Aker M, et al. Total lymphoid irradiation, antilymphocyte globulin and Campath 1-G for immunosuppression prior to bone marrow transplantation for aplastic anemia after repeated graft rejection. Bone Marrow Transplant 1994; 13:97–99.
136. Aversa F, Tabilio A, Terenzi A, et al. Successful engraftment of T-cell-depleted haploidentical "three-loci" incompatible transplants in leukemia patients by addition of recombinant human granulocyte colony-stimulating factor-mobilized peripheral blood progenitor cells to bone marrow inoculum. Blood 1994; 84:3948–3955.
137. Drobyski WR, Ash RC, Casper JT, et al. Effect of T-cell depletion as graft-versus-host disease prophylaxis on engraftment, relapse, and disease-free survival in unrelated marrow transplantation for chronic myelogenous leukemia. Blood 1994; 83:1980–1987.
138. Verdonck LF, de Gast GC, van Heugten HG, Dekker AW. A fixed low number of T-cells in HLA-identical allogeneic bone marrow transplantation. Blood 1990; 75:776–780.

139. Potter MN, Pamphilon DH, Cornish JM, Oakhill A. Graft-versus-host disease in children receiving HLA-identical allogeneic bone marrow transplants with a low adjusted T-lymphocyte dose. Bone Marrow Transplant 1991; 8:357–361.
140. Quinones RR, Gutierrez RH, Dinndorf PA, et al. Extended-cycle elutriation to adjust T-cell content in HLA-disparate bone marrow transplantation. Blood 1993; 82:307–317.
141. Verdonck LF, Dekker AW, de Gast GC, et al. Allogeneic bone marrow transplantation with a fixed low number of T-cells in the marrow graft. Blood 1994; 83:3090–3096.
142. Fischer A, Blanche S, Veber F, et al. Prevention of graft failure by an anti-HLFA-1 monoclonal antibody in HLA-mismatched bone marrow transplantation. Lancet 1986; 2:1058–1061.
143. Theobald M, Hoffmann T, Bunjes D, Heit W. Comparative analysis of in vivo T cell depletion with radiotherapy, combination chemotherapy, and the monoclonal antibody Campath-1G, using limiting dilution methodology. Transplantation 1990; 49: 553–559.
144. Fischer A, Friedrich W, Fasth A, et al. Reduction of graft failure by a monoclonal antibody (anti-LFA-1 CD11a) after HLA nonidentical bone marrow transplantation in children with immunodeficiencies, osteopetrosis, and Fanconi's anemia: A European group for immunodeficiency/European group for bone marrow transplantation report. Blood 1991; 77:249–256.
145. Willemze R, Richel DJ, Falkenburg JHF, et al. In vivo use of Campath-1G to prevent graft-versus-host disease and graft rejection after bone marrow transplantation. Bone Marrow Transplant 1992; 9:255–261.
146. Baume D, Kuentz M, Pico JL, et al. Failure of a CD18/anti-LFA1 monoclonal antibody infusion to prevent graft rejection in leukemic patients receiving T-depleted allogeneic bone marrow transplantation. Transplantation 1989; 47:472–474.
147. Maraninchi D, Mawas C, Stoppa AM, et al. Anti LFA1 monoclonal antibody for the prevention of graft rejection after T cell-depleted HLA-matched bone marrow transplantation for leukemia in adults. Bone Marrow Transplant 1989; 4:147–150.
148. Mangan KF, Mullaney MT, Barrientos TD, Kernan NA. Serum interleukin-2 levels following autologous or allogeneic bone marrow transplantation: Effects of T-cell depletion, blood stem cell infusion, and hematopoietic growth factor treatment. Blood 1993; 81:1915–1922.
149. DeWitte T, Gratwohl A, Van Der Lely N, et al. Recombinant human granulocyte-macrophage colony-stimulating factor accelerates neutrophil and monocyte recovery after allogeneic T-cell-depleted bone marrow transplantation. Blood 1992; 79:1359–1365.
150. Apperley JF, Jones L, Hale G, et al. Bone marrow transplantation for patients with chronic myeloid leukaemia: T cell depletion with Campath-1 reduces the incidence of graft-versus-host disease but may increase the risk of leukaemic relapse. Bone Marrow Transplant 1986; 1:53–66.
151. Papa G, Arcese W, Mauro FR, et al. Standard conditioning regimen and T-depleted donor bone marrow for transplantation in chronic myeloid leukaemia. Leuk Res 1986; 10:1469–1475.
152. Goldman JM, Gale RP, Horowitz MM, et al. Bone marrow transplantation for chronic myelogenous leukemia in chronic phase: Increased risk for relapse associated with T-cell depletion. Ann Intern Med 1988; 108:806–814.
153. Martin PJ, Clift RA, Risher LD, et al. HLA-identical marrow transplantation during accelerated-phase chronic myelogenous leukemia: Analysis of survival and remission duration. Blood 1988; 72:1978–1984.
154. Horowitz MM, Gale RP, Sondel PM, et al. Graft-versus-leukemia reactions after bone marrow transplantation. Blood 1990; 75:555–562.

155. Devergie A, Reiffers J, Vernant JP, et al. Long-term follow-up after bone marrow transplantation for chronic myelogenous leukemia: Factors associated with relapse. Bone Marrow Transplant 1990; 5:379–386.
156. Marks DI, Hughes TP, Szydlo R, et al. HLA-identical sibling donor bone marrow transplantation for chronic myeloid leukaemia in first choice phase: Influence of GVHD prophylaxis on outcome. Br J Haematol 1992; 81:383–390.
157. Wagner JE, Zahurak M, Piantadosi S, et al. Bone marrow transplantation of chronic myelogenous leukemia in chronic phase: Evaluation of risks and benefits. J Clin Oncol 1992; 10:779–789.
158. Gratwohl A, Hermans J, Niederwieser D, et al. Bone marrow transplantation for chronic myeloid leukemia: long-term results: Chronic Leukemia Working Party of the European Group for Bone Marrow Transplantation. Bone Marrow Transplant 1993; 12:509–516.
159. Fialkow PJ, Jacobson RJ, Papayannopoulou T. Chronic myelocytic leukemia: Clonal origin in a stem cell common to the granulocyte, erythrocyte, platelet and monocyte/macrophage. Am J Med 1977; 63:125–130.
160. Kernan NA, Bartsch G, Ash RC, et al. Analysis of 462 transplantations from unrelated donors facilitated by the National Marrow Donor Program. N Engl J Med 1993; 328: 593–602.
161. McGlave P, Bartsch G, Anasetti C, et al. Unrelated donor marrow transplantation therapy for chronic myelogenous leukemia: Initial experience of the National Marrow Donor Program. Blood 1993; 81:543–550.
162. Devergie A, Labopin M, Apperley J, et al. European results of 537 matched unrelated donor (MUD) transplants for chronic myeloid leukemia (CML). Blood 1994; 84:537a.
163. Soiffer RJ, Murray C, Cochran K, et al. Clinical and immunologic effects of prolonged infusion of low-dose recombinant interleukin-2 after autologous and T-cell depleted allogeneic bone marrow transplantation. Blood 1992; 79:517–526.
164. Soiffer RJ, Murray C, Gonin R, Ritz J. Effect of low-dose interleukin-2 on disease relapse after T-cell-depleted allogeneic bone marrow transplantation. Blood 1994; 84: 964–971.
165. Kolb HJ, Mittermuller J, Clemm C, et al. Donor leukocyte transfusions for treatment of recurrent chronic myelogenous leukemia in marrow transplant patients. Blood 1990; 76:2462–2465.
166. Cullis JO, Jiang YZ, Schwarer AP, et al. Donor leukocyte infusions for chronic myeloid leukemia in relapse after allogeneic bone marrow transplantation. Blood 1992; 79:1379–1381.
167. Drobyski WR, Roth MS, Thibodeau SN, Gottschall JL. Molecular remission occurring after donor leukocyte infusions for the treatment of relapsed chronic myelogenous leukemia after allogeneic bone marrow transplantation. Bone Marrow Transplant 1992; 10:301–304.
168. Porter DL, Both MS, McGarigle C, et al. Induction of graft-versus-host disease as immunotherapy for relapsed chronic myeloid leukemia. N Engl J Med 1994; 330:100–106.
169. Noel DR, Witherspoon RP, Storb R, et al. Does graft-versus-host disease influence the tempo of immunologic recovery after allogeneic human bone marrow transplantation? An observation on 56 long-term survivors. Blood 1978; 51:1087–1105.
170. Paulin T, Ringden O, Nilsson R, et al. Variables predicting bacterial and fungal infections after allogeneic marrow engraftment. Transplantation 1987; 43:393–398.
171. Mackall CL, Granger L, Sheard MA, et al. T-cell regeneration after bone marrow transplantation: Differential CD45 isoform expression on thymic-derived versus thymic-independent progeny. Blood 1993; 82:2585–2594.
172. Witherspoon RP, Lum LG, Storb R. Immunologic reconstitution after human marrow grafting. Semin Hematol 1984; 21:2–10.

173. Welte K, Ciobanu N, Moore MAS, et al. Defective interleukin-2 production in patients after bone marrow transplantation and in vitro restoration of defective T lymphocyte proliferation by highly purified interleukin-2. Blood 1984; 64:380–385.
174. Lum LG. The kinetics of immune reconstitution after human marrow transplantation. Blood 1987; 69:369–380.
175. Ault KA, Antin JH, Ginsburg D, et al. Phenotype of recovering lymphoid cell populations after marrow transplantation. 1985; 161:1483–1502.
176. Janossy G, Prentice HG, Grob JP, et al. T lymphocyte regeneration after transplantation of T cell depleted allogeneic bone marrow. Clin Exp Immunol 1986; 63:577–586.
177. Rooney CM, Wimperis JZ, Brenner MK, et al. Natural killer cell activity following T-cell depleted allogeneic bone marrow transplantation. Br J Haematol 1986; 62:413–420.
178. Wimperis JZ, Prentice HG, Karayiannis P, et al. Transfer of a functioning humoral immune system in transplantation of T-lymphocyte depleted bone marrow. Lancet 1986; 1:339–343.
179. Parreira A, Smith J, Hows JM, et al. Immunological reconstitution after bone marrow transplant with Campath-1 treated bone marrow. Clin Exp Immunol 1987; 67:142–150.
180. Wimperis JZ, Brenner MK, Prentice HG, et al. B cell development and regulation after T cell-depleted marrow transplantation. J Immunol 1987; 138:2445–2350.
181. de Gast GC, Gratama JW, Verdonck LF, et al. The influence of T cell depletion on recovery of T cell proliferation to herpes viruses and Candida after allogeneic bone marrow transplantation. Transplantation 1989; 48:111–115.
182. Drobyski WR, Piaskowski V, Ash RC, et al. Preservation of lymphokine-activated killer activity following T cell depletion of human bone marrow. Transplantation 1990; 50:625–632.
183. Keever CA, Small TN, Flomenberg N, et al. Immune reconstitution following bone marrow transplantation: Comparison of recipients of T cell depleted marrow with recipients of conventional marrow grafts. Blood 1989; 73:1340–1350.
184. Small TN, Keever CA, Weiner-Fedus S, et al. B-cell differentiation following autologous, conventional, or T-cell depleted bone marrow transplantation: A recapitulation of normal B-cell ontogeny. Blood 1990; 76:1647–1656.
185. Welte K, Keever CA, Levick J, et al. Interleukin-2 production and response to interleukin-2 by peripheral blood mononuclear cells from patients after bone marrow transplantation: II. Patients receiving soybean lectin-separated and T cell-depleted bone marrow. Blood 1987; 70:1595–1603.
186. Soiffer RJ, Bosserman L, Murray C, et al. Reconstitution of T-cell function after CD6-depleted allogeneic bone marrow transplantation. Blood 1990; 75:2076–2084.
187. Brenner MK, Wimperis JZ, Reittie JE, et al. Recovery of immunoglobulin isotypes following T cell depleted allogeneic bone marrow transplantation. Br J Haematol 1986; 64:125–132.
188. Brenner MK, Reittie JE, Grob J-P, et al. The contribution of large granular lymphocytes to B cell activation and differentiation after T-cell-depleted allogeneic bone marrow transplantation. Transplantation 1986; 42:257–261.
189. Antin JH, Ault KA, Rappeport JM, Smith BR. B lymphocyte reconstitution after human bone marrow transplantation: Leu-1 antigen defines a distinct population of B lymphocytes. J Clin Invest 1987; 80:325–332.
190. Daley JP, Rozans MK, Smith BR, et al. Retarded recovery of functional T cell frequencies in T cell-depleted bone marrow transplant recipients. Blood 1987; 70:960–964.
191. Shapiro RS, McClain K, Frizzera G, et al. Epstein-Barr virus associated B cell lympho-

proliferative disorders following bone marrow transplantation. Blood 1988; 71:1234–1243.

192. Zutter MJ, Martin PJ, Sale GE, et al. Epstein-Barr virus lymphoproliferation after bone marrow transplantation. Blood 1988; 72:520–529.
193. Witherspoon RP, Fisher LD, Schoch G, et al. Secondary cancers after bone marrow transplantation for leukemia or aplastic anemia. N Engl J Med 1989; 321:784–789.
194. Rickinson AB. Cellular immunological responses to the virus infection. In: Epstein MA, Achong BG, eds. the Epstein-Barr Virus: Recent Advances. New York: Wiley, 1986:75–126.
195. Papadopoulos EB, Ladanyi M, Emanuel D, et al. Infusions of donor leukocytes to treat Epstein-Barr virus-associated lymphoproliferative disorders after allogeneic bone marrow transplantation. N Engl J Med 1994; 330:1185–1191.

24

In Vivo Prevention and Treatment of GVHD

Nelson J. Chao
Stanford University Medical Center
Stanford, California

H. Joachim Deeg
Fred Hutchinson Cancer Research Center and University of Washington
Seattle, Washington

I. HISTORICAL PERSPECTIVE

The early experience with "secondary disease" or graft-versus-host disease (GVHD) has been well summarized by van Bekkum and Vries (1). In the same year, Billingham outlined the basic requirements for GVH reaction and the development of the clinical picture of GVHD as follows (2):

1. The graft must contain immunogically competent cells.
2. The host must possess relevant tissue antigens that are lacking in the donor, so that the host appears foreign and therefore is capable of activating donor cells.
3. The host must be incapable of mounting an effective immunological reaction against donor cells, at least for sufficient time for the latter to manifest its immunological capabilities—i.e., the graft must have some security of tenure.

These criteria immediately suggest where intervention aimed at preventing GVHD should be possible. However, since "security of tenure" or sustained engraftment is the very purpose of transplantation, it is generally not advisable to intervene at the level of engraftment. This leaves the option of selecting histocompatible donor and controlling the functions of immunocompetent donor cells.

As early as the 1960s, different methods were employed to prevent GVHD. One approach was the use of amethopterin, a folate antagonist that reduced the incidence of secondary disease in murine models (3). These studies led to the use of a related drug, methotrexate, for the prophylaxis of GVHD in animal models and eventually following human BMT. Cosgrove et al. showed that in vitro exposure of B6 spleen cells to a (B6 × 101) F1 liver homogenate at 10°C for about 10 hr before transplantation into (B6 × 101) F1 recipients reduced the capacity of these cells to cause secondary disease (4). Mathe et al. suggested that maintaining suspensions of lymphoid or myeloid cells in Tyrode's solution or autologous serum at 37°C for 1 to 2 hr profoundly depressed the immunologic activity (5). A similar rationale underlies more recent studies on inactivation of alloreactive lymphocytes by ultraviolet (UV) light (6). A more radical approach is that of completely eliminating donor lymphocytes from the marrow inoculum (see Chap. 23) by physicochemical means or by poly- or monoclonal antibodies as advanced by Euler et al., Kolb et al., and Korngold and Sprent (7–9).

Haller showed in neonatal B6 mice that splenectomy within a few hours of intravenous injection of CBA donor spleen cells reduced the mortality from runt disease by half (10). No protective effect was seen if the spleen was removed prior to inoculation of donor cells. An observation supporting this hypothesis pursued more recently in elegant experiments by Korngold and Sprent, is that, in intact animals, immunologically competent alloreactive cells settle at least transiently in the host spleen from which a variety of antihost responses are initiated. It is these events in and against primary and secondary lymphoid organs (thymus, spleen, lymph nodes, etc.), which compromise the host posttransplant. The host is highly susceptible to infectious complications for extended periods of time (11,12). These issues are discussed in detail elsewhere in this volume. It is important to emphasize, however, that treatment of GVHD generally consists of immunosuppressive therapy, contributing further to the host's lack of immunocompetence. Therefore, not surprisingly, infection is a frequent and serious complication of GVHD, often responsible for a fatal outcome.

II. PROPHYLAXIS OF ACUTE GVHD

Clinically significant acute GVHD occurs in 10 to 50% of patients who receive an allogeneic bone marrow graft from an HLA genotypically identical sibling, even if intensive prophylaxis with immunosuppressive agents such as methotrexate, cyclosporine, corticosteroids or antithymocyte globulin are used. Without postgrafting prophylaxis, the incidence of acute GVHD was 100% in some trials (13). Mild GVHD (grade I, limited skin involvement only) often is self-limited and generally is not of clinical consequence but may predict a higher incidence of chronic GVHD compared to patients who never had any acute GVHD. Development of moderate (grade II) or severe (grades III or IV) acute GVHD after marrow transplantation is associated with a significant decrease in the probability of survival. The mainstay of prophylaxis remains in vivo administration of pharmacological combinations of drugs which, individually, have been shown to affect GVHD. Prevention of GVHD has generally been measured and equated as the prevention of significant GVHD—that is, grade II or greater. Thus, the studies discussed will refer to prevention of grades II–IV acute GVHD in recipients of matched related bone marrow grafts. The approach to HLA-nonidentical and unrelated BMT will be addressed separately.

A. In Vivo Manipulation

1. Omission of Prophylaxis

Prevention is the most important aspect of the approach to GVHD, and allogeneic transplant recipients not given GVHD prophylaxis are expected to develop GVHD. Nonetheless, three small trials of allogeneic BMT without GVHD prophylaxis have been conducted with the rationale that the development of GVHD may also confer a graft-versus-leukemia (GVL) effect (13–15). There were no differences in the overall survival or in the incidence of GVHD (although there may have been a difference in the severity of chronic GVHD). The current consensus is that the potential gain of omission of GVHD prophylaxis (for the GVL effect) is not convincing and that all patients should be given some form of GVHD prophylaxis.

2. Methotrexate and Cyclophosphamide

The initial studies used a single drug for prophylaxis of GVHD based on the observation with aminopterin in murine and canine BMT models (3,16). In dogs, the use of methotrexate resulted in a greater than 90% disease-free survival following BMT from a DLA-identical littermate, compared to a 55% incidence of acute GVHD and a survival probability of only 45% in dogs not receiving post-transplant prophylaxis (16). In 1966, Santos and Owens demonstrated that cyclophosphamide was useful for the prevention and treatment of GVHD in rats (17). Additional single agents, including cytosine arabinoside, 6-mercaptopurine, L-asparaginase, and others were tested in experimental models but did not offer any advantage compared to either methotrexate or cyclophosphamide (18). Accordingly, clinical trials involved either methotrexate or, less frequently, cyclophosphamide. With either one of these agents, GVHD occurred in up to 55 to 70% of patients transplanted from an HLA genotypically identical sibling donor (19,20). The major disadvantages of both agents are myelosuppression and mucositis. Nevertheless, until the introduction of cyclosporine, these two drugs served as the mainstay of therapy. Cyclophosphamide is not used any longer. Methotrexate as a single agent continues to be given to patients considered at high risk for recurrence of the underlying disease, since there is evidence that leukemic recurrence may be less frequent with the use of methotrexate alone rather than the combination of cyclosporine and methotrexate (21,22).

3. Cyclosporine

Cyclosporine A was introduced in the late 1970s. Its mechanism of action involves binding to cyclophilin, interference with the function of calcineurin, and, as a result, prevention of interleukin-2 (IL-2) gene expression and activation of T lymphocytes, as described by Bierer et al. (23). Studies in rats demonstrated that cyclosporine was a potent agent to prevent GVHD (24). Studies in dogs yielded results similar to those obtained with methotrexate in DLA-identical littermate transplants but failed to show tolerance induction with DLA nonidentical transplants (25). Early clinical trials suggested that cyclosporine was useful in reducing the incidence of GVHD and improving survival (26,27). However, follow-up of controlled studies showed that although cyclosporine was a useful agent, it was not superior to either methotrexate or cyclophosphamide (19,28,29). In one study of 75 patients, 33% of those on cyclosporine and 56% on methotrexate developed acute GVHD of grades II to IV ($p = 0.07$). A recent update of three studies (179 patients) comparing cyclosporine and methotrexate, with follow-up ranging from 8 to 11 years, indicated that patients with advanced disease receiving cyclosporine tended to have higher relapse rates, although the difference did not reach statistical significance (21).

Other teams have used a prolonged course of cyclosporine (12 months, followed by gradual tapering) and instituted early treatment of acute GVHD with high-dose corticosteroids (28). In 45 patients, acute GVHD was treated at the first clear sign of the disease with methylprednisolone at 10 to 20 mg/kg/day divided into four doses. This regimen proved to be quite efficacious for the prevention of severe GVHD. The incidence of severe acute GVHD was 5% and, of chronic GVHD, 9%.

4. Cyclosporine and Methotrexate

These results with cyclosporine alone, while encouraging, were not satisfactory. This led to the development of a regimen combining cyclosporine and methotrexate. Studies in dogs that received DLA-nonidentical marrow from an unrelated donor and were given a short course of methotrexate (days 1, 3, 6, and 11) and a 100-day course of cyclosporine showed approximately 35% survival. These results were clearly superior to the 10% seen with single agents, although chronic GVHD was not prevented (25). Among dogs given the same regimen and transplanted with DLA-haploidentical marrow from littermates, GVHD was almost completely prevented and 75% survived (29).

In several clinical trials, there was a survival advantage for patients who received the combination of cyclosporine and methotrexate compared to either one of those drugs utilized alone (30,31). A retrospective study of 595 patients with aplastic anemia receiving allogeneic bone marrow transplants analyzed the effect of three GVHD regimens: methotrexate, cyclosporine, and the combination of methotrexate plus cyclosporine (32). Due to a lower incidence of interstitial pneumonia and chronic GVHD, patients who received cyclosporine alone or combined with methotrexate had a significantly higher probability of 5-year survival (69%) than did patients receiving methotrexate only (56%).

Two prospective randomized trials in patients with leukemia or aplastic anemia, demonstrated that the combination of cyclosporine and methotrexate was superior to either drug alone in preventing GVHD (33,34). Among 93 patients with acute myelogenous leukemia in first complete remission or chronic myelogenous leukemia in chronic phase randomized to receive cyclosporine plus methotrexate, 33% developed acute GVHD compared to 54% among patients receiving cyclosporine alone (34). Another trial compared the combination of cyclosporine plus methotrexate to methotrexate alone in patients with leukemia and aplastic anemia (33). With the combination, 18% of patients developed grades II to IV acute GVHD, compared to 52% among patients receiving methotrexate alone. The long-term follow-up results of these trials have been reported (21,35–37). There was a trend toward improved event-free survival in the subgroup of patients with chronic myelogenous leukemia treated with the drug combination, but the early survival benefit was offset by an increase in the relapse rate. There was no effect on the rate of development of chronic GVHD, and the incidence of chronic GVHD was not reduced by the methotrexate-plus-cyclosporine combination. Among patients with aplastic anemia, however, long-term disease-free survival was improved due to a significant decrease in the incidence and severity of acute GVHD (37). A three-way comparison of T-cell depletion versus cyclosporine alone and the combination of cyclosporine plus methotrexate was recently carried out in 140 consecutive patients with chronic myelogenous leukemia (38). The combination of cyclosporine and methotrexate was associated with the best disease-free survival. Accordingly, the combination of cyclosporine and methotrexate is currently the most widely utilized regimen for GVHD prophylaxis. Table 1 details the regimen.

Various modifications of this regimen (known as the Seattle regimen) have been investigated, but none in a prospective randomized fashion. One study used

Table 1 Cyclosporine/Methotrexate Prophylaxis Regimen[a]

Day	Cyclosporine	Methotrexate
−2	5.0 mg/kg IV daily	—
+1	"	15 mg/m^2 IV single dose[b]
+3	"	10 mg/m^2 IV single dose
+4	3.0 mg/kg IV daily	—
+6	"	10 mg/m^2 IV single dose
+11	"	10 mg/m^2 IV single dose
+15	3.75 mg/kg IV daily	
+36	5 mg/kg PO bid	
+84	4 mg/kg PO bid	
+98	3 mg/kg PO bid	
+120	2 mg/kg PO bid	
+180	off	

[a]Note that cyclosporine is given on a daily basis while only four total doses of methotrexate are administered.
[b]Some investigators recommend a dose of 10 mg/m^2 even on day 1 (41).

continuous intravenous infusion of cyclosporine until day +45 (rather than switching to oral administration) combined with a short course of methotrexate. This regimen was well tolerated and resulted in a 16% incidence of acute GVHD and 13% de novo chronic GVHD (39). In a recent pilot study, 19 patients received cyclosporine at a 50% decreased dose for the first 2 weeks in an attempt to decrease toxicity (40). As compared to a matched cohort receiving standard-dose cyclosporine, there was no difference in the incidence of acute GVHD (42% versus 51% in the standard-dose group). However, patients receiving the "low-dose" prophylaxis appeared to have less hepatotoxicity and the doses of methotrexate and cyclosporine administered were closer to the intended doses, an observation quite similar to those from another trial in which the methotrexate dose was reduced (41).

Determination of cyclosporine blood levels and correlation with dose and clinical events, using as many as four different assay methods, has remained a problem. Even within the same institution, one study found a correlation of cyclosporine levels and GVHD prevention (42), whereas a follow-up study did not (43).

5. Prednisone

Prednisone, while considered standard for the therapy of acute GVHD, has been used less commonly for prophylactic purposes. However, interesting data in regards to its use in combination with cyclosporine, methotrexate, or cyclophosphamide for prophylaxis of acute GVHD have been presented (20,44–49). In 1976, the City of Hope investigators performed a prospective randomized study comparing methotrexate plus prednisone versus cyclosporine plus prednisone. Grades II to IV acute GVHD were reduced from 47 to 28% with the cyclosporine-plus-prednisone combination (45). In 1986, the combination of cyclosporine plus prednisone was modified by increasing the dose of prednisone and starting it on day +7, as described by the team at Ohio State University, rather than on day +15 (48). This modification resulted in a reduction of the incidence of grades II to IV acute GVHD to 12% (S. Forman, personal communication).

Methotrexate in combination with cyclosporine (see above) had been found to offer effective prophylaxis for many patients; thus, the addition of methotrexate to a regimen of cyclosporine and prednisone might further improve the outcome (Table 2). The rationale for using only three doses of methotrexate, as previously suggested by Deeg et al. (41), was twofold: first, many patients never receive the prescribed fourth dose of methotrexate, due to cumulative toxicity, and second, there was concern with the potential added toxicity of this GVHD regimen to the preparatory regimen containing high doses of etoposide. All patients were in first complete remission of acute leukemia or chronic-phase of chronic myelogenous leukemia and conditioned with fractionated total body irradiation and etoposide. There was a significantly lower incidence of grades II to IV acute GVHD (9%) with the three-drug regimen compared to the two drug regimen of cyclosporine and prednisone (23%, $p = 0.02$). Although the lower incidence of acute GVHD did not result in a higher relapse rate, disease-free survival at 3 years was comparable (64% for the triple-drug regimen versus 59% for the two-drug combination, $p = 0.57$) (46). The Seattle team also conducted a study using a regimen of cyclosporine and

Table 2 Cyclosporine/Methotrexate/Prednisone Prophylaxis Regimen[a]

Day	Cyclosporine	Prednisone	Methotrexate
−2	5.0 mg/kg IV daily	—	
+1	"	—	15 mg/m^2 IV single[b]
dose			
+3	"	—	10 mg/m^2 IV single
dose			
+4	3.0 mg/kg IV daily	—	
+6	"	—	10 mg/m^2 IV single
dose			
+7	"	0.5 mg/kg IV daily	
	"	"	
+15	3.75 mg/kg IV daily	1.0 mg/kg IV daily	
	"	"	
+29	"	0.8 mg/kg PO daily	
+36	5 mg/kg PO bid	"	
+43	"	0.5 mg/kg PO daily	
	"	"	
+57	"	0.2 mg/kg PO daily	
+84	4 mg/kg PO bid	"	
	"	"	
+98	3 mg/kg PO bid	"	
	"	"	
+120	2 mg/kg PO bid	0.1 mg/kg PO daily	
	"	"	
+180	off	off	

[a]Note that cyclosporine is given on a daily basis while only three total doses of methotrexate are administered.

[b]Some investigators recommend a dose of 10 mg/m^2 even on day 1 (41).

methotrexate (four doses) plus prednisone, starting on day 1 (50). Interestingly, this study yielded an increased incidence of acute GVHD, albeit a lower probability of leukemic relapse. Presumably this was related to a negative interaction between prednisone and methotrexate. If prednisone was delayed until day 15, the incidence of GVHD returned to the level seen with cyclosporine plus methotrexate. Thus, initiating prednisone on day 7 may be the optimum timing. Another study also did not find a difference with the addition of prednisone (51), while preliminary data from a fourth study (52) showed a highly significant difference in acute GVHD incidence between patients given cyclosporine plus methotrexate and patients given cyclosporine, methotrexate, and prednisolone (22/48 versus 6/50 respectively; $p < 0.00001$).

One concern in using combination regimens is additional toxicity. A marked increase in hepatotoxicity was observed in patients who received cyclosporine and methotrexate following a preparative regimen consisting of busulfan and cyclophosphamide (54). Venoocclusive disease (VOD) occurred in 70% of patients and contributed to death in 25% compared to 18 and 4.5%, respectively, in patients who received cyclosporine and prednisone.

6. Antibodies

Antithymocyte globulin (ATG) has also been utilized for the prevention of GVHD. The compelling rationale is that GVHD is triggered by donor T lymphocytes. In two studies, the addition of ATG to methotrexate failed to decrease the incidence of GVHD (55,56). However, when ATG was combined with methotrexate and prednisone, there was a decrease of acute GVHD from 48 to 21% (44). Unfortunately there was no difference in survival.

More recently, numerous monoclonal antibodies have been used, since the binding of IL-2 to its receptor is an essential requirement for T-cell proliferation. The use of murine monoclonal antibodies that bind to the IL-2 receptor light chain and block IL-2 binding can be expected to block alloreactivity and thereby interfere with GVHD (57,58). These IL-2 receptor-specific monoclonal antibodies may also allow selective targeting and destruction of activated T cells. In one study, a murine monoclonal IgG1 antibody (2A3) specific for the 55-kDa chain of the human IL-2 receptor was used in addition to cyclosporine and methotrexate. While there was no appreciable toxicity, efficacy was also limited, since 70% of patients developed grades II to IV acute GVHD. These results suggested that administration of this particular antibody suppressed or delayed the activation of alloantigen-specific T cells but did not result in the elimination of these cells and therefore, did not have a significant impact in the prophylaxis of GVHD, although it should be noted that these patients had received BMT from HLA nonidentical donors. A refined approach to the use of IL-2-receptor antibodies involves molecular engineering such that only the complementary determining regions remain of murine original, whereas the remainder of the molecule is replaced by human sequences. This should be accompanied by high efficiency and low immunogenecity. One such antibody, humanized anti-Tac (HAT), has been used on a limited scale for the prophylaxis of acute GVHD, but failed in a randomized perspective trial in matched unrelated donor BMT (59).

Other antibodies—e.g., anti-CD5 conjugated to ricin A chain (A9B10)—have been used, generally in conjunction with partial in vitro T-cell depletion, in patients receiving transplants from donors other than HLA-identical siblings (60). Monoclonal antibodies targeting various adhesion molecules have been tested in murine models (61–64) and have seen only limited clinical application (65).

7. Intravenous Immunoglobulins (IVIg)

Following marrow transplantation, serum Ig levels often decrease dramatically. With posttransplant recovery, IgG and IgM return to normal within 3 to 4 months, while serum IgA levels may remain low for up to 2 years. Other studies have reported subclass deficiencies of IgG2 and IgG4 even though total serum IgG levels were normal (66,67). Initial studies of intravenous immunoglobulins (IVIg) following BMT were carried out with the aim of achieving a reduction in the incidence and severity of cytomegalovirus (CMV) and other infections. Tutschka and colleagues and, in a large randomized study, Sullivan et al. noticed that there was a reduced incidence of gram-negative septicemia and local infections in patients receiving IVIg but also a reduced incidence of acute GVHD in patients aged 20 years and older (69,70).

8. Newer Agents

FK506, a macrolide molecule, has been found to be as effective as cyclosporine for the prevention of rejection of cell or organ allografts (71). FK506 has been utilized extensively in animal models. In a comparison between FK506 and cyclosporine, FK506 appeared to be more effective (on a weight basis), but there was delayed appearance of GVHD after discontinuation of treatment (72). However, small doses of maintenance FK506 every other day suppressed GVHD once the induction period was completed. FK506 can also reverse established GVHD in an experimental model (73) as well as ameliorate chronic GVHD in humans (74). Several clinical trials on GVHD prevention by FK506, either alone or combined with methotrexate or prednisone, are under way. Single and multi-instution pilot trials (Ref. 75 and Nash et al., personal communication) suggest that FK506 is efficacious for GVHD prophylaxis, possibly at a level similar to that of cyclosporine.

A second approach using FK506, similar to a previous study using cyclosporine, is donor pretreatment with FK506 (76). This appears to prevent acute GVHD after allogeneic BMT (77). A study using FK506 for donor treatment only, as well as in combination with recipient treatment, was performed. A single dose of FK506 given to the allogeneic bone marrow donor can significantly prolong the mean GVHD-free interval after allogeneic BMT. The results were clearly better when combined with a recipient course of FK506. Explanations for efficacy of donor pretreatment may be related to drug carryover versus a direct effect on the donor cells prior to BMT.

Rapamycin is a macrolide similar to FK-506 and acts as reciprocal antagonists on T cells (78,79). In contrast to FK-506, however, its acts further downstream in the T-cell activation pathway. Rapamycin has been used successfully to suppress both host-versus-graft (HVG) and GVH disease in MHC-mismatched rats (80) and murine transplants (81). The use of rapamycin also resulted in significant suppression in both HVG and GVH versus-host reaction (GVHR) after small bowel transplantation in rats.

Trimetrexate is a 2,4-diaminoquinazoline folate analog synthesized in the early 1970s as an antimalarial agent. Like methotrexate, trimetrexate is a potent inhibitor of the enzyme dihydrofolate reductase. Unlike methotrexate, trimetrexate is not excreted in the urine but rather is metabolized by the liver, which may offer an advantage in patients with compromised renal function. In a canine study of one DLA haplotype, mismatched littermate transplant results with a combination of trimetrexate and cyclosporine (82) were almost equivalent to results achieved with the combination of methotrexate and cyclosporine (29), suggesting that the substitution of methotrexate by trimetrexate can be made. In a phase I study in humans, trimetrexate was well tolerated at doses of 120 to 200 mg/m^2 as a single dose and pilot trials in marrow transplantation are encouraging (Doney, et al., personal communication).

Studies in a murine model show that UVB irradiation of lymphohematopoietic cells results in the prevention of GVHD (82–84). UVB exposure preferentially inhibits lymphocyte function while preserving hematopoietic precursors. Mice treated with UVB-exposed spleen and marrow cells showed donor-specific tolerance of skin grafts. The mechanism of UVB is not clear. However, UVB modifies class II antigen expression and interferes with transmembrane signaling (85,86). Suppressor T cells can be found in the spleen of UV-irradiated antigen-sensitized mice. This suggests that antigen-specific suppressor T cells are present in the spleens of UV-irradiated alloantigen-sensitized mice, which suppresses the immune response against such alloantigens. UV irradiation also modifies cytokine expression (e.g., IL-1, IL-2, IL-4 and others) and interferes with antigen presentation. There is also evidence of an increased production of *cis*-urocanic acid, which by itself is immunosuppressive (87).

Since antigen-activated T (and B) cells depend on purine de novo synthesis whereas most other cells can utilize the salvage pathway, inhibition of purine synthesis may also be an attractive approach. A study to evaluate the possibility of using 2-deoxy-chloroadenosine (2-CdA) for the prophylaxis and treatment of GVHD would be of interest. However, caution is indicated, since not all species have the necessary target enzyme.

Mycophenolate mofetil, also known as RS-61443, an ester product of mycophenolic acid that inhibits de novo synthesis of guanine nucleotides (88) was found useful in preventing GVHD after allogeneic rat small bowel transplants. Long-term tolerance against GVHD after discontinuation of therapy was established (89). Similar observations have been made with mizorbine (90). Neuraminidase pretreatment of donor lymphocytes decreased the incidence of acute GVHD without a compromise in engraftment or adverse effect on T- or B-cell function following adoptive transfer experiments (91). Although the exact mechanism by which this treatment prevents GVHD is unknown, the data suggest that it does provide such protection.

Deoxyspergualin, a derivative of spergualin, was isolated from *Bacillus laterosporus* and abolishes the activity of cytotoxic T lymphocytes, not only at the induction stage but also at further stages of cell maturation (92). Deoxyspergualin inhibits alloreactive cytotoxic activity in GVHD (93). Various experiments demonstrate that bone marrow and spleen cells from deoxyspergualin-treated survivors lack the ability to induce lethal GVHD (94). These results suggest that the survivors have immunological unresponsiveness. Deoxyspergualin has also been combined with methotrexate, and this combination appears to be even more effective than using either alone (95).

Many of these newer agents hold some promise in the preclinical trials to proceed to clinical trials. However, more effective GVHD prophylaxis will depend on a more selective inhibition of T-cell activation and the control of the cytokine cascade that occurs following T-cell activation. As the immunological events associated with GVHD become clearer, such selective inhibition may be more appropriately designed.

9. Other Methods

Gnotobiosis is effective in preventing GVHD in murine models (96). Clinically protective environment and suppression of gastroinestinal flora have met with some success in preventing infection (97–99). A beneficial effect on GVHD prevention has been observed only in patients with severe aplastic anemia (100,101). A major problem is compliance and failure to actually achieve gnotobiosis. In mice, gnotobiosis is achieved by delivering newborn fetuses into a sterile environment prior to any oral intake and, therefore, prior to colonization of intestinal flora. Such a situation is probably never achieved in human patients. Once intestinal flora has been established, there is likely to be continued competition of various organisms.

Another method to prevent GVHD that follows the reasoning of gnotobiosis is to decrease gram-negative bacteria using antibodies. One hypothesis for the efficacy of gnotobiosis is that bacterial endotoxin can activate monocytes and macrophages to release IL-1, tumor necrosis factor alpha (TNF-α), and gamma interferon (γ-IFN), all of which can lead to or enhance T-cell proliferation and result in tissue damage. Endotoxin is a lipopolysaccharide that may enter the bloodstream, especially if the GI tract is denuded from the high-dose therapy prior to transplantation or from methotrexate used in the prophylaxis of GVHD. It has recently been suggested that the use of immunoglobulin enriched for IgM (pentaglobulin), which contains antibodies that are active against intestinal organisms (102), may result in decontamination and a beneficial effect on GVHD.

In summary, the standard approach is to prevent the occurrence of acute GVHD. The target for most of the drugs is the GVHD effector T cells. The most commonly utilized regimen is that of cyclosporine and four doses of methotrexate, as developed by the BMT group in Seattle. The combination of cyclosporine, methotrexate (three doses), and methylprednisolone (starting on day +7) also shows excellent activity in the prevention of grades II to IV acute GVHD. Other approaches for the prevention of GVHD, some of which are in ongoing clinical or just beginning clinical trials, include new immunosuppressants such as FK506 and possibly rapamycin. Alternatively, immunosuppressive regimens have combined monoclonal antibodies with standard drug prophylaxis. Finally, as the afferent and efferent pathways leading to GVHD are elucidated, more specific targeting of the selected cytokines involved may lead to more effective approaches.

III. TREATMENT OF ACUTE GVHD

Since the development of GVHD generally has a negative effect on survival, the basic goal is to *prevent* GVHD. As discussed above, this goal is not always achieved and therapy is required. Therapy should be aggressive, since the completeness of response correlates directly with survival. Many agents have been used for therapy. Glucocorticoids have remained the standard.

A. Glucocorticoids

Despite aggressive use of immunosuppressant prophylaxis, 10 to 50% of the patients will still develop significant acute GVHD (grades II to IV). First-line therapy consists of glucocorticoids (steroids). The mechanism of action of glucocorticoids is presumably related to its lympholytic effects. All therapies aimed at treatment of acute GVHD have been measured against steroids, and "second-line" therapy has generally been administered only for "steroid resistant" disease. Although responses occur, recrudescence is frequent with dose reduction, and almost all of the long-term survivors developed chronic GVHD, with considerable morbidity and mortality from secondary opportunistic infection or interstitial pneumonitis (103–105). Higher doses of steroids may increase the response rate, and while patients with mild to moderate GVHD often show excellent responses, this response is not associated with improved survival. Patients with severe GVHD often do poorly.

Several analyses of GVHD therapy have recently been presented (106,107). Among 469 patients receiving allogeneic BMT in Minneapolis, 179 (42%) developed grade II or greater acute GVHD. Seventy two patients (41%) achieved complete and continued resolution of acute GVHD after a median of 21 days of therapy. While most of these responders primarily received corticosteroids, other immunosuppressive therapies—including cyclosporine A, anti-T-cell immunotoxin, or antilymphocyte globulin—were also used. Patients not responding to the initial immunosuppressive agent received high-dose methylprednisolone, ATG with steroids, or other therapies. Only 7 of those 61 patients eventually attained a complete continued remission. The overall incidence of chronic GVHD among patients who developed acute GVHD was 70%. More favorable responses to therapy occurred in patients without liver or skin involvement, patients with acute lymphoblastic leukemia, and donor/recipient pairs other than male patients with female donors. Most of these patients had received GVHD prophylaxis with methotrexate either alone or in conjunction with ATG and prednisone or in vitro T-cell depletion.

Martin and colleagues analysed results in 740 patients with grades II to IV GVHD (108). Initial therapy was with steroids in 532 patients, cyclosporine in 170, ATG in 156, and monoclonal antibody in 3. Improvement was seen in the skin in 43%; liver, 35%; and intestinal tract, 50%—for an overall complete response of 18% and another partial response of 26%. GVHD prophylaxis with the combination of methotrexate and cyclosporine and treatment with glucocorticoids or cyclosporine represented favorable risk factors. Unfavorable factors were transplant from an HLA nonidentical donor, liver complications other than GHVD, and early-onset GVHD. A subsequent analysis comprised 427 patients who had failed initial therapy (107). Most of the patients had a skin rash (75%), with liver dysfunction the second most common manifestation (59%) and gastrointestinal complications the third in 53% of the patients. Secondary treatment consisted of glucocorticoids in 249 patients, cyclosporine in 80, ATG in 214, or monoclonal antibody in 19. Most patients received single-agent treatments; however, 37 received a combination of these agents. Improvement or resolution of GVHD in the respective organs was seen in 45% of the patients with skin disease, 25% of the patients with liver disease, and 35% of the patients with gut disease. Forty percent of the patients showed some response. The highest complete response rate was seen when GVHD recurred during the taper phase of primary glucocorticoid treatment. Increasing the dose of glucocorticoids seemed to allow for a second complete response. Severe dysfunction of the liver, gut, or skin at the beginning of treatment was associated with lower incidence of response and lack of improvement in outcome. Although increasing the dose of glucocorticoids appeared to represent the most effective therapy or strategy when GVHD recurred during the taper phase or primary treatment, less than half the patients showed a durable improvement. These results suggest that the potential efficacy of immunosuppressive agents can be assessed meaningfully in patients who have not responded adequately to primary treatment and that more effective treatments are needed.

B. Antithymocyte Globulin (ATG)

Only few therapeutic studies using ATG have been reported. In initial studies in Seattle, ATG was used as a single agent and 30 to 50% of patient responded; results were inferior to those with steroids but not significantly so (109,110). Another study investigated the usefulness of a combination of ATG and cyclosporine (111); some patients also received methylprednisolone. Interestingly, while survival was low in patients receiving the triple immunosuppression of cyclosporine, ATG, and methylprednisolone, mostly due to infectious complications, approximately 60% given ATG plus cyclosporine responded. All these patients had received methotrexate for prophylaxis, and this regimen is not truly applicable to patients already on cyclosporine.

C. Monoclonal Antibodies

Since treatment with monoclonal antibody OKT3, specific for the CD3 complex, can reverse or cure rejection of human renal allografts, its use was attractive for the treatment of GVHD. A pilot trial in 8 allogeneic recipients with grades II or IV acute GVHD showed responses in 6 patients, especially those with minimal disease (112). In a second study of 10 patients with grades III to IV acute GVHD who were resistant to cyclosporine and methylprednisolone, OKT3 induced complete responses in 5 and partial responses in 4 patients. However, acute GVHD recurred frequently (113). Since these anti-CD3 antibodies were mitogenic, T-cell activation might have been dose-limiting.

A different approach was utilized in a phase I/II study with an anti-CD3 antibody called BC3, that cannot cross-link CD3 with Fc receptors on accessory cells and therefore cannot induce T-cell proliferation (114). A total of 17 patients were enrolled into this study, and 5 patients achieved a complete resolution of GVHD; 8 patients had partial improvement, 2 had no change, and 2 had progression. Of the 13 patients, 8 had sustained responses. The mechanism of action of this antibody appears to be related to some form of immunosuppression through modulation of T-cell function. Unfortunately, the use of OKT3 or other anti-CD3 monoclonal antibodies in several patients has resulted in a lymphoproliferative syndrome (frequently a fatal complication) due to proliferation of polyclonal B cells infected with the Epstein-Barr virus. In another trial by the Seattle team, four different IgG2a anti-T-cell monoclonal antibodies designated 9.6, 35.1, 10.2, and 12.1 were given to 15 patients (115). Of 10 patients, 6 had at least partial improvement in one organ system involved.

Another approach has been the use of anti-IL-2 receptor monoclonal antibody to treat patients with steroid-resistant grades II to IV acute GVHD (116,117). In a multicenter pilot trial, patients with severe GVHD refractory to conventional therapy received an anti-IL-2 receptor monoclonal antibody. Unfortunately, no complete responses were observed; however, 8 of 19 patients achieved a good partial response (117). Gut lesions responded best, followed by skin and then liver. GVHD recurred when treatment was discontinued. Another anti-IL-2 receptor monoclonal antibody (B-B10) for the treatment of acute GVHD showed promising results (118). In a multicenter pilot study, 32 patients who experienced steroid-resistant acute GVHD were treated with this anti IL-2 receptor monoclonal antibody. A full response of organ involvement was achieved in 22 patients (68.7%). Unfortunately, this study did not state whether these responses were durable. A follow-up study of 58 patients reported that 26 (44.8%) were alive between 240 and 900 days after GVHD treatment with B-B10 (119). Although the response rate was gratifying, the GVHD recurrence rate remained high at 41%. However, there was a significant survival advantage for those who responded to treatment with B-B10.

Monoclonal antibody against TNF-α is another potential method for the treatment of severe acute GVHD. A monoclonal anti-TNF-α, termed B-C7, has been used to treat patients suffering from grades III to IV acute GVHD. Eighteen patients responded, 21% with a complete response and 61% with improvement. Only 22% of the patients were alive following treatment (114). This pilot study suggests that a monoclonal anti-TNF-α antibody may be of benefit for some patients with severe refractory acute GVHD but is ineffective in preventing GVHD recurrence in the majority of the patients.

Another approach has been to use Xomazyme (anti-CD5 conjugated to ricin A chain) (121). Thirty-four patients with moderate to severe steroid-resistant acute GVHD were treated with Xomazyme. Of these patients, 72% responded in at least one organ and another 16% had stable disease. However, GVHD recurrence was frequent. Major difficulties with using murine monoclonal antibody included febrile reactions, fluctuation in blood counts, and flulike symptoms, including fever, tremors, lethargy, anorexia, myalgias, and arthralgias.

In summary, for patients who "break through" the prophylactic regimen, steroids are the first-line therapy. For those who fail high doses of steroids, various approaches are possible, including ATG and monoclonal antibodies. Unfortunately, although responses are seen to such attempts, none of these agents have resulted in a large number of reproducible and sustained responses. The recent advances in understanding the cytokine cascade that leads to acute GVHD may allow for more specific targeting of therapies and to a higher response rate.

IV. Chronic GVHD

A. Introduction

Graft-versus-host disease has historically been divided into acute and chronic phases. Acute GVHD occurs within the first 100 days and chronic GVHD was defined as GVHD occurring after the first 100 days following allogeneic BMT. Acute GVHD generally occurs within 30 to 40 days of BMT, and it is clear now that cases of chronic GVHD, both by clinical and histological criteria, can occur as early as 50 days posttransplant (124). Chronic GVHD is the single major determinant of long-term outcome and quality of life following BMT. The morbidity and mortality associated with chronic GVHD remains a serious problem.

Chronic GVHD involves target tissues which are often different from sites affected by acute GVHD. Moreover, acute and chronic GVHD differ histologically. Chronic GVHD appears to present more as an autoimmune phenomenon, including autoantibody formation. Aspects of chronic GVHD may mimic systemic lupus erythematosus, scleroderma, progressive systemic sclerosis, lichen planus, sicca syndrome, eosinophilic fasciitis, rheumatoid arthritis, and primary biliary sclerosis (125). None of these collagen vascular diseases, however, explain the entire spectrum observed with chronic GVHD. Renal and CNS involvement are rarely seen in chronic GVHD. Chronic GVHD can be classified as limited or extensive, depending on the clinical presentation in patients. Chronic GVHD has further been categorized as "progressive," i.e., evolving directly out of acute GVHD; "quiescent" if acute GVHD had at least transiently responded to therapy; and "de novo" in patients who never showed signs of acute GVHD (126).

Chronic GVHD is associated with marked immunodeficiency, and treatment of chronic GVHD, usually involving the use of more immunosuppressive agents, results in increased immunosuppression. The recovery of immune function is delayed in comparison to patients without GVHD. These patients remain immunodeficient as long as the disease is active (127). T- and B-lymphocyte control remains dysregulated (128). With prolonged observation, recurrent infectious processes may occur in up to 100% of these patients. These infectious complications largely account for morbidity and mortality associated with chronic GVHD.

Chronic GVHD occurs in approximately 50% of long-term survivors of HLA-identical sibling transplants (129). There appears to be moderate to high concordance for the diagnosis, grading, and treatment of chronic GVHD. However, major disagreements were observed in the diagnosis of uncommon manifestations of chronic GVHD, interpretation of symptoms which occur less than 2 months after transplantation, interpretation of persistent stable symptoms, and deciding whether to treat chronic GVHD limited to skin. One interesting observation was that time of onset is an important clinical feature for some but not all transplanters in establishing diagnosis of chronic GVHD. Consistency in grading the severity of the symptoms may be improved by using, for example, the Karnofsky performance status to differentiate between limited versus extensive chronic GVHD.

Patients who have limited disease have a favorable prognosis even without therapy. Patients with extensive, particularly multiorgan disease have an unfavorable natural history. Approximately 50% of patients will develop chronic GVHD at some point after the first 100 days.

B. Prevention of Chronic GVHD

The best prophylaxis of chronic GVHD is effective prevention of acute GVHD. Only 15 to 20% of patients without acute GVHD will develop "de novo" chronic GVHD, compared to 40 to 100% of those who suffer from acute GVHD (130). Thus several attempts have been made to include additional preventive measures in the early posttransplant period. Many of such attempts have been aimed at establishing T-cell tolerance.

Thymus tissue implants, thymic endothelial cells obtained from third party (usually pediatric) donors sharing one HLA-A and B locus with the recipient, thymosin fraction 5, and thymopentin administration to recipients of HLA-identical sibling BMT have been used in order to prevent chronic GVHD and to accelerate immunological reconstitution (126). However, the clinical courses of these patients were not different compared to concurrent or historical controls. Trials using prolonged administration of glucocorticoids have also been unsuccessful (132,133). Several European groups have suggested that an extended regimen of cyclosporine covering 12 to 24 months may be beneficial (134), and a randomized prospective trial addressing this question is currently under way [KM Sullivan, personal communication].

C. Therapy of Chronic GVHD

1. Prednisone and Cyclosporine

Sullivan and colleagues at Seattle have utilized "day 100 screening studies" to demonstrate that a positive skin biopsy and a history of prior acute GVHD independently predicted subsequent development of chronic GVHD. The study was designed to treat patients with subclinical GVHD—i.e., patients who were asymptomatic with a positive random skin or oral biopsy (or both) showing histological evidence of chronic GVHD. Patients were randomized to prednisone plus placebo versus prednisone plus azathioprine. Early treatment with prednisone alone in standard risk chronic GVHD patients was superior to treatment with a combination of prednisone and azathioprine (135). However, in high-risk patients with persistent thrombocytopenia, prednisone alone resulted in only 26% long-term survival. Survival can be improved and transplant-related mortality reduced in patients with high-risk chronic GVHD by treatment with an alternating-day regimen of cyclosporine and prednisone (136). The 5-year actuarial survival increased from 26% with prednisone alone in the earlier study to 51% in the subsequent study. A randomized study in standard-risk patients with platelet counts $>100{,}000/\mu L$ has compared the effect of prednisone alone versus cyclosporine and prednisone. Patients with high-risk chronic GVHD were randomized to receive either cyclosporine alone or the cyclosporine and prednisone combination. Among standard-risk patients, 33% given prednisone had complete responses compared to 46% with prednisone/cyclosporine ($p = 0.032$). Among high-risk patients, 18% had complete responses to cyclosporine compared to 33% with cyclosporine/prednisone ($p = 0.031$). Progressive onset of GVHD and elevated bilirubin were associated with an increased risk of failure in both groups.

2. Thalidomide

Thalidomide (*N*-phthalidoglutarimide) was introduced as a sleeping pill and showed activity and absence of acute toxicity or side effects. Unfortunately, with long-term use, neurotoxicity became evident and the confirmed teratogenic activity led to the withdrawal of thalidomide from the market. Its immunosuppressive activity, however, has been clearly documented (137). It was first noted that patients with leprosy who received thalidomide as a sedative experience relief of their symptoms of leprosy (138). Thalidomide has found a place in the therapy of primary mucocutaneous disorders, including lepromatous leprosy, apthous stomatitis, and discoid lupus erythematosus (139). Because of the severe teratogenic effects, thalidomide's immunosuppressive properties have not been fully explored. Investigators at Johns

Hopkins University reported on the use of thalidomide in the treatment of acute GVHD in a rat model of BMT, and subsequent studies confirmed its value in chronic GVHD (140,141). In a clinical study at Johns Hopkins University, 44 patients with GVHD were treated and an overall response rate of 64% was observed (142). Survival was 76% among the patients receiving salvage therapy for refractory GVHD and 48% among those with high-risk GVHD. These studies suggested that thalidomide was effective in treating established chronic GVHD. Another phase I–II trial with thalidomide in patients with chronic GVHD who had failed prednisone therapy confirmed these data. Eighty patients were treated at the City of Hope National Medical Center and Stanford University, and overall responses were seen in 16 of 80 patients (20%) (174). In this trial, the adverse effects experienced were significant and several patients had the thalidomide discontinued due to these side effects.

3. Psoralen plus Ultraviolet Irradiation (PUVA)

Ultraviolet irradiation of methoxypsoralen-sensitized patients (PUVA) has been used widely for the treatment of dermatologic disorders (6,143–145). Experimental models have revealed a profound immunosuppressive effect of PUVA (144). The proposed mechanism of PUVA is inhibition of DNA transcription and mitosis. Upon activation with ultraviolet A light, photoexcited psoralen covalently binds to one or both strands of DNA. The psoralen forms monoadducts or bifunctional adducts with intrastrand linkage between opposite DNA strands and therefore damages DNA. Psoralen can also damage mitochondria and thereby affects cell function. During PUVA treatment, the circulating lymphocytes are exposed to 1 to 5% of the skin surface dose of UVA. This results in a decrease in the number and function of circulating lymphocytes. There is a decrease in T-cell proliferation, mitogen responses, and NK activity (147). There is evidence for UV-resistant antigen-presenting cells that activate suppressor pathways (148). Ultraviolet radiation also has an effect on cytokine production, specifically on IL-1 and IL-2; however, these observations have been made either in vitro or in patients with psoriasis (149). The results in patients after BMT may be different. A recent review of PUVA for the treatment of GVHD reported that 3 of 11 patients achieved a complete remission of chronic GVHD (150). A 60% response rate has been observed by others (151,152). The efficacy of PUVA may be limited by skin complications of chronic GVHD. Perhaps use of this modality earlier in the course of chronic GVHD may be more effective. There are data that ultraviolet irradiation may modulate MHC-alloreactive cytotoxic T-cell precursors that are involved in the onset of GVHD (153). Also, the rather shallow depth penetration of UVA may limit the application of PUVA in patients with liver or intestinal GVHD. Use of methoxypsoralen with extracorporeal photopheresis has also been attempted. The results in a limited number of patients treated so far at one institution (NJC) suggest only a transient improvement.

4. Specific Therapies

Since chronic GVHD affecting the liver is a cholestatic disease associated with jaundice and elevation of alkaline phosphatase similar to primary biliary cirrhosis, a trial was carried out to evaluate the effect of ursodeoxycholic acid treatment (154). Ursodeoxycholic acid is a relatively nontoxic hydrophilic bile acid with a striking choleresis effect. Patients with chronic GVHD on this drug improved with a 33% decrease in the bilirubin level compared to baseline ($p < 0.005$), 32% decrease in alkaline phosphatase ($p < 0.038$), and a 37% decrease in AST ($p < 0.007$). The levels of these serum tests rose again after discontinuation of the drug. One possibility for the mechanism of action is that ursodeoxycholic acid simply replaces the more hydrophobic detergent and toxic bile acids. A more intriguing possibility could be an effect on the immune system suggested by the disappearance of aberrant expression of HLA class I antigens on hepatocytes after ursodeoxycholic acid treatment of primary biliary cirrhosis (155).

As mentioned previously, infectious complications are a common occurrence due to the impaired immune system, especially in patients with chronic GVHD. The most common pathogens are those found in the upper airways, including *Streptococcus* and *Haemophilus* species (156,157). Patients who have recurrent pulmonary infections have been placed on rotating antibiotics (one antibiotic per week) for 3 weeks with one week off (NJC). Prophylaxis for *Pneumocystis carinii* with trimethoprim-sulfamethoxazole is instituted and continued for as long as patients are on corticosteroids. Patients who are unable to tolerate trimethoprim-sulfamethoxazole can receive nebulized pentamidine. Hypogammaglobulinemia is also found in patients who develop chronic GVHD (158). Use of intravenous immunoglobulins may be of help in preventing recurrent infections. Such prophylactic approaches are important as part of the continued supportive care of such patients.

In summary, chronic GVHD is a critical determinant of long-term outcome and quality of life following BMT. The best method to prevent chronic GVHD is to prevent acute GVHD. For those patients who develop extensive chronic GVHD, newer immunosuppressive regimens are clearly needed. Since chronic GVHD in of itself causes immunosuppression, intensive supportive care such as antibiotic prophylaxis, intravenous immunoglobulins (if the patient is hypogammaglobulinenic), and nutritional support is of paramount importance. The usual course if such patients can be supported is that the disease will "burn out" (i.e. tolerance occurs) and the patient improves.

V. Unrelated Donor BMT

The reported incidence of acute GVHD for patients who receive matched unrelated donor transplantation is high and ranges from 53% following T-cell-depleted bone marrow to as high as 80% with drug prophylaxis (159–162). Various groups have reported grades III to IV acute GVHD as high as 54% as well as extensive chronic GVHD at 52%. Analysis of 462 transplants from unrelated donors from the National Marrow Donor Program revealed that the probability of having grades II to IV acute GVHD was 64%, whereas 47% had severe grade III to IV acute GVHD (162). In that study, the probability of limited or extensive chronic GVHD 1 year after transplantation was 55%. Another report using T-cell depletion for GVHD prophylaxis suggested that the actuarial probability of developing grades II to IV GVHD was 40% and of developing grade III to IV acute GVHD was only 8.3% (161). Moreover, in this trial, there was no difference in the incidence of grade II to IV acute GVHD between patients receiving matched or mismatched unrelated marrow grafts. Even more surprising, there was only one cytogenetic relapse in this cohort of patients with chronic myelocytic leukemia. Two recent reviews suggest that in spite of the high incidence of acute GVHD and higher morbidity and mortality, the overall outcome of unrelated donor BMT parallels that achieved with autologous BMT or HLA-matched sibling donors (163,164). These results suggest that continued use of matched unrelated donors is justified.

One of the interesting observations has been a suggestion that the role of HLA-DPB1 disparity may be related to the higher incidence of acute GVHD. One study suggested that there was a significant contribution of the HLA-DP antigen mismatches to the incidence of severe GVHD (165). However, a follow-up study did not corroborate that disparity of DPB1 influences the risk of acute GVHD (166).

Treatment for acute GVHD following unrelated donor marrow transplantation suggests that more aggressive therapies are warranted in these patients (122). Standard treatment with prednisone and ATG appears to be ineffective. In comparing with histocompatible sibling BMT, the Minnesota group reported that therapy for acute GVHD is associated with a 41% complete and continuing response rate (106). But of the 42 patients who underwent treatment with prednisone and ATG, only 9 achieved a complete and continuous response of acute GVHD by day +100 (21%). This increase in GVHD following unrelated donor BMT is due to the greater histocompatibility differences between the donor and recipient.

There is some suggestion that acute GVHD following a matched unrelated donor transplantation may respond to very high doses of methylprednisolone. In one small series of eight patients, high dose methylprednisolone, 5 mg/kg/day for four days, and dose escalation to 10 mg/kg/day for nonresponders as initial therapy for acute GVHD was associated with a response in a majority of the patients (123). Unfortunately, high-dose methylprednisolone was associated with severe, life-threatening infectious complications. Currently, there is not one standard prophylactic regimen for patients receiving unrelated donor BMT. Various groups are interested in exploring the combination of T-cell depletion and chemoprophylaxis. There is no doubt that an unrelated donor BMT presents a unique set of problems that are difficult to prevent or control.

VI. Autologous GVHD

GVHD occurs due to histocompatibility differences between the donor and recipient. Occasionally, this does not seem to be necessary. Several reports suggested that recognition of autoantigens occurs, and a syndrome similar to acute GVHD has been described in recipients of syngeneic or autologous BMT (167–170). In an experimental rat model of GVHD, there are data suggesting that autoreactive T cells that recognize Ia (major histocompatibility class II molecules) can be found (171). Moreover, this autologous GVHD can be enhanced by the early and transient administration of cyclosporine. When the cyclosporine is withdrawn, acute GVHD is induced. This auto-GVHD may be associated with thymic damage, presumably from the preparatory regimen or from cyclosporine, which allows the development of autoreactive T cells (172). Such a GVHD syndrome has been reported in patients after syngeneic and autologous BMT. The usual manifestation is that of a mild skin rash, which promptly resolves either without therapy or with methylprednisolone. Rarely, other organ involvement with GVHD has been described (173).

One difficulty with the description of autologous GVHD is the establishment of a definitive histological diagnosis, since the skin biopsy is generally done shortly after high doses of radiation or drugs (or both). The damage observed histologically may be indistinguishable. However, the data obtained in experimental models do indicate that a GVHD syndrome may develop in the absence of histocompatibility barriers.

ACKNOWLEDGMENTS

NJC is supported by grant CA 49605 and an American Cancer Society Junior Faculty Research Award (JFRA 446). HJD is supported by grants CA 18029, CA 15704, CA 18221, and HL 36444 and a grant from the National Marrow Donor Program/Baxter Health Care Division.

REFERENCES

1. Van Bekkum DW, De Vries MJ. Radiation Chimaeras. New York: Academic Press, 1967.
2. Billingham R. The biology of graft-versus-host reaction. Harvey Lect 1966:21.
3. Uphoff D. Alteration of homograft reaction by a-methopterin in lethally irradiated mice treated with homologous marrow. Proc Soc Exp Biol Med 1958; 99:651.
4. Cosgrove GE, Upton AC, Popp RA, Congdon CC. Inhibition of foreign spleen reaction by inactivation of donor cells with recipient antigens. Proc Soc Exp Biol Med 1959; 102:525.
5. Mathe G, Amiel JL, Schwarzenberg M, et al. Conditioning of immunologically competent cells by incubation at 37 degrees C. Ann NY Acad Sci 1966; 129:355.
6. Deeg H. Ultraviolet irradiation in transplantation biology: Manipulation of immunity and immunogenicity. Transplantation 1988; 45:845.
7. Rodt HV, Eulitz M, Thierfelder S. Suppression of acute secondary disease by heterologous anti-brain serum. Blut 1972; 25:385.
8. Kolb HJ, Scholz S, Rieder I, et al. Antilymphocytic antibodies and marrow transplantation: VI. Graft-versus-host tolerance in DLA-incompatible dogs after in vitro treatment of bone marrow with absorbed antithymocyte globulin. Transplantation 1979; 27:242.
9. Korngold R, Sprent J. T cell subsets and graft-versus-host disease. Transplantation 1987; 44:335.
10. Haller J. The effect of neonatal splenectomy on mortality from runt disease in mice. Transplantation 1964; 2:287.
11. Lum LG. The kinetics of immune reconstitution after human marrow transplantation. Blood 1987; 69:369.
12. Bowden RA. Infections in patients with graft-vs.-host disease. In: Burakoff SJ, Deeg HJ, Ferrara J and Atkinson K, eds. Graft-vs.-Host-Disease: Immunology, Pathophysiology and Treatment. New York: Marcel Dekker, 1990:525.
13. Sullivan K, Deeg HJ, Sanders A, et al. Hyperacute graft-v-host disease in patients not given immunosuppression after allogeneic marrow transplantation. Blood 1986; 67: 1172.
14. Lazarus H, Coccia PF, Herzig RH, et al. Incidence of acute graft-versus-host disease with and without methotrexate prophylaxis in allogeneic bone marrow transplantation. Blood 1984; 64:215.
15. Elfenbein G, Goedect T, Graham-Pole J, et al. Is prophylaxis against acute graft-versus-host disease necessary if treatment is effective and survival is not impaired? Proc Am Soc Clin Oncol 1986; 5:643.
16. Storb R, Epstein RB, Graham TC, Thomas ED. Methotrexate regimens for control of

graft-versus-host disease in dogs with allogeneic marrow grafts. Transplantation 1970; 9:240.

17. Santos G, Owens AH. Production of graft-versus-host disease in the rat and its treatment with cytotoxic agents. Nature 1966; 210:139.
18. Storb R, Appelbaum F, Kolb HJ, et al. Prevention of graft-versus-host disease by immunosuppressive agents after transplantation of DLA-nonidentical canine marrow. Bone Marrow Transplant 1986; 1:167.
19. Storb R, Deeg HJ, Fisher L, et al. Cyclosporine v methotrexate for graft-v-host disease prevention in patients given marrow grafts for leukemia: Long-term follow-up of three controlled trials. Blood 1988; 71:293.
20. Santos G, Tutschka PJ, Brookmeyer R, et al. Cyclosporine plus methylprednisolone versus cyclophosphamide plus methylprednisolone as prophylaxis for graft-versus-host disease: A randomized double-blind study in patients undergoing allogeneic marrow transplantation. Clin Transplant 1987; 1:21.
21. Storb R, Deeg HJ, Pepe M, et al. Long-term follow-up of three controlled trials comparing cyclosporine versus methotrexate for graft-versus-host disease prevention in patients given marrow grafts for leukemia. Blood 1992; 79:3091.
22. Backman L, Ringden O, Tollemar J, Lonnqvist B. An increased risk of relapse in cyclosporin-treated compared with methotrexate-treated patients: Long-term follow-up of a randomized trial. Bone Marrow Transplant 1988; 3:463.
23. Bierer BE, Fruman D, Hollander G, et al. Cyclosporin A and FK506: Molecular mechanisms of immunosuppression and probes for transplantation biology. Curr Opin Immunol 1993; 5:763.
24. Tutschka P, Beschorner WE, Allison AC, et al. Use of cyclosporin A in allogeneic bone marrow transplantation in rats. Nature 1979; 280:148.
25. Deeg H, Storb R, Weiden PL, et al. Cyclosporin A and methotrexate in canine marrow transplantation: Engraftment, graft-versus-host disease, and induction of tolerance. Transplantation 1982; 34:30.
26. Tutschka P, Beschorner WE, Hess AD, Santos GW. Cyclosporine A to prevent graft-versus-host disease: A pilot study in 22 patients receiving allogeneic marrow transplant. Blood 1983; 61:318.
27. Powles R, Clink HM, Spence D, et al. Cyclosporin A to prevent graft-versus-host disease in man after allogeneic bone marrow transplantation. Lancet 1980; 1:327.
28. Santos G, Brookmeyer R, Saral R, Tutschka PJ. Cyclosporine (CsA) versus cyclophosphamide (CY): Prevention of graft-versus-host disease (GVHD). Exp Hematol 1985; 13:427.
29. Deeg HJ, Storb R, Appelbaum FR, et al. Combined immunosuppression with cyclosporine and methotrexate in dogs given bone marrow grafts from DLA haploidentical littermates. Transplantation 1984; 37:62.
30. Ringden O, Klaesson S, Sundberg B, et al. Decreased incidence of graft-versus-host disease and improved survival with methotrexate combined with cyclosporin compared with monotherapy in recipients of bone marrow from donors other than HLA identical siblings. Bone Marrow Transplant 1992; 9:19.
31. Mrsic M, Labar B, Boganic V, et al. Combination of cyclosporin and methotrexate for prophylaxis of acute graft-versus-host disease after allogeneic bone marrow transplantation for leukemia. Bone Marrow Transplant 1990; 6:137.
32. Gluckman E, Horowitz MM, Champlin RE, et al. Bone marrow transplantation for severe aplastic anemia: Influence of conditioning and graft-versus-host disease prophylaxis regimens on outcome. Blood 1992; 79:269.
33. Storb R, Deeg HJ, Farewell V, et al. Marrow transplantation for severe aplastic anemia: Methotrexate alone compared with a combination of methotrexate and cyclosporine for prevention of acute graft-versus-host disease. Blood 1986; 68:119.

34. Storb R, Deeg HJ, Whitehead J, et al. Methotrexate and cyclosporine compared with cyclosporine alone for prophylaxis of acute graft-versus-host disease after marrow transplantation for leukemia. N Engl J Med 1986; 314:729.
35. Storb R, Deeg HJ, Whitehead J, et al. Marrow transplantation for leukemia and aplastic anemia: Two controlled trials of a combination of methotrexate and cyclosporine v cyclosporine alone or methotrexate alone for prophylaxis of acute graft-v-host disease. Transplant Proc 1987; 19:2608.
36. Storb R, Deeg HJ, Pepe M, et al. Methotrexate and cyclosporine versus cyclosporine alone for prophylaxis of graft-versus-host disease in patients given HLA-identical marrow grafts for leukemia: Long-term follow-up of a controlled trial. Blood 1989; 73:1729.
37. Storb R, Leisenring W, Deeg HJ, et al. Long-term follow-up of a randomized trial of graft-versus-host disease prevention by methotrexate/cyclosporine versus methotrexate alone in patients given marrow grafts for severe aplastic anemia (letter). Blood 1994; 83:2749–2750.
38. Marks D, Hughes TP, Szydlo R, et al. HLA-identical sibling donor bone marrow transplantation for chronic myeloid leukemia in first chronic phase: Influence of GVHD prophylaxis on outcome. Br J Haematol 1992; 81:383.
39. Beelen D, Quabeck K, Kaiser B, et al. Six weeks of continuous intravenous cyclosporine and short-course methotrexate as prophylaxis for acute graft-versus-host disease after allogeneic bone marrow transplantation. Transplantation 1990; 50:421.
40. Stockschlaeder M, Storb R, Pepe M, et al. A pilot study of low-dose cyclosporin for graft-versus-host prophylaxis in marrow transplantation. Br J Haematol 1992; 80:49.
41. Deeg HJ, Cahill R, Spitzer TR, et al. Conditioning-related toxicity and acute graft-versus-host disease in patients given methotrexate/cyclosporine prophylaxis. Bone Marrow Transplant 1991; 7:193.
42. Yee GC, Self SG, McGuire TR, et al. Serum cyclosporine concentration and risk of acute graft-versus-host disease after allogeneic marrow transplantation. N Engl J Med 1988; 319:65.
43. Nash R, Pepe MS, Storb R, et al. Acute graft-versus-host disease: Analysis of risk factors after allogeneic marrow transplantation and prophylaxis with cyclosporine and methotrexate. Blood 1992; 80:1838.
44. Ramsay N, Kersey J, Robison LL, et al. A randomized study of the prevention of acute graft-versus-host disease. N Engl J Med 1982; 306:392.
45. Forman S, Blume KG, Krance RA, et al. A prospective randomized study of acute graft-v-host disease in 107 patients with leukemia: Methotrexate/prednisone v cyclosporin a/prednisone. Transplant Proc 1987; 19:2605.
46. Chao NJ, Schmidt GM, Niland JC, et al. Cyclosporine, methotrexate, and prednisone compared with cyclosporine and prednisone for prophylaxis of acute graft-versus-host disease. N Engl J Med 1993; 329:1225.
47. Martin P, Schoch G, Fisher L, et al. A retrospective analysis of therapy for acute graft-versus-host disease: Secondary treatment. Blood 1991; 77:1821.
48. Tutschka P, Copelan EA, Klein JP. Bone marrow transplantation for leukemia following a new busulfan and cyclophosphamide regimen. Blood 1987; 70:1382.
49. Yau J, LeMaistre CF, Zagars GK, et al. Methylprednisone, cyclosporine and methotrexate for prophylaxis for acute graft-versus-host disease. Bone Marrow Transplant 1990; 5:269.
50. Storb R, Pepe M, Anasetti C, et al. What role for prednisone in prevention of acute graft-versus-host disease in patients undergoing marrow transplants? Blood 1990; 76:1037.
51. Atkinson K, Biggs J, Concannon A, et al. A prospective randomised trial of cyclosporin and methotrexate versus cyclosporin, methotrexate and prednisolone for

prevention of graft-versus-host disease after HLA-identical sibling marrow transplantation for haematological malignancy. Aust NZ J Med 1991; 21:850.

52. Ruutu T, Volin L, Elonen E, et al. Triple prophylaxis with cyclosporine A (CsA), methotrexate (METHOTREXATE), and methylprednisolone (MP): More effective prevention of acute GVHD than with CsA + METHOTREXATE. Bone Marrow Transplantation, 20th Annual Meeting of the EBMT, Harrogate, UK, 1994:183.
53. Biggs J, Szer J, Crilley P, et al. Treatment of chronic myeloid leukemia with allogeneic bone marrow transplantation after preparation with BuCy2. Blood 1992; 80:1352.
54. Essell J, Thompson JM, Harman GS. Marked increase in veno-occlusive disease of the liver associated with methotrexate use for graft-versus-host disease prophylaxis in patients receiving busulfan/cyclophosphamide. Blood 1992; 79:2784.
55. Weiden P, Doney K, Storb R, Thomas ED. Anti-human thymocyte globulin prophylaxis of acute graft-versus-host disease: A randomized trial in patients with leukemia treated with HLA-identical sibling matched grafts. Transplantation 1979; 27:227.
56. Doney K, Weiden PL, Storb R, Thomas ED. Failure of early administration of antithymocyte globulin to lessen graft-versus-host disease in human allogeneic marrow transplant recipients. Transplantation 1981; 31:141.
57. Anasetti C, Martin PJ, Storb R, et al. Prophylaxis of graft-versus-host disease by administration of the murine anti-IL-2 receptor antibody 2A3. Bone Marrow Transplant 1991; 7:375.
58. Blaise D, Olive D, Hirn M, et al. Prevention of acute GVHD by in vivo use of anti-interleukin-2 receptor monoclonal antibody (33b3.1): A feasibility trial in 15 patients. Bone Marrow Transplant 1991; 8:105.
59. Anasetti C, Lin A, Nademanee A, et al. A Phase II/III randomized, double-blind, placebo-controlled multicenter trial of humanized anti-TAC for prevention of acute graft-versus-host disease (GVHD) in recipients of marrow transplants from unrelated donors. Blood 1995; 86:621a.
60. Henslee-Downey PJ. Choosing an alternative bone marrow donor among available family members. Am J Pediatr Hematol Oncol 1993; 15:150.
61. Davignon D, Martz E, Reynolds T, et al. Monoclonal antibody to a novel lymphocyte function-associated (LFA-1): Mechanisms of blockade of T lymphocyte-mediated killing and effects on other T and B lymphocyte functions. J Immunol 1981; 127:590.
62. Krensky A, Sanchez-Madrid F, Robbins E, et al. The functional significance, distribution, and structure of LFA-1, LFA-2, and LFA-3: Cell surface antigens associated with CTL-target interactions. J Immunol 1983; 131:611.
63. Harning R, Pelletier J, Lubbe K, et al. Reduction in the severity of graft-versus-host disease and increased survival in allogeneic mice by treatment with monoclonal antibodies to cell adhesion antigens LFA-1a and MALA-2. Transplantation 1991; 52:842.
64. Schlegel P, Vaysburg M, Butcher E, et al. Selective inhibition of T cell costimulation mediated by VCAM-1 prevents murine graft-versus-host disease. J Immunol 1995; 155:3856.
65. Fischer A, Veber F, Friedrich W, et al. Reduction of graft failure by a monoclonal antibody (anti-LFA-1 CD11a) after HLA nonidentical bone marrow transplantation in children with immunodeficencies, osteopetrosis, and Fanconi's anemia: A European Group for Immunodeficiency/European Group for Bone Marrow Transplantation report. Blood 1991; 77:249.
66. Sheridan J, Tutschka PJ, Sedmak DD, et al. Immunoglobulin G subclass deficiency and pneumococcal infection after allogeneic bone marrow transplantation. Blood 1990; 75:1583.
67. Lum LG, Seigneuret MC, Orcutt-Thordason N, et al. The regulation of immunoglobulin synthesis after HLA-identical bone marrow transplantation II. Differential rates of

maturation of distinct functional groups within lymphoid subpopulation in patients after human marrow grafting. Blood 1985; 65:1422.
68. Aucouturier P, Barra A, Intrator L, et al. Long lasting IgG subclass and antibacterial polysaccharide antibody deficiency after allogeneic bone marrow transplantation. Blood 1987; 70:779.
69. Copelan EA, Bechtel T, Avalos BR, et al. Alternate applications of immunoglobulin following bone marrow transplantation. Semin Hematol 1992; 29:96.
70. Sullivan K, Kopecky KJ, Jocom J, et al. Immunomodulatory and antimicrobial efficacy of intravenous immunoglobulin in bone marrow transplantation. N Engl J Med 1990; 323:705.
71. Thomson A. FK-506 enters the clinic. Immunol Today, 1990; 11:35.
72. Markus P, Cai X, Ming W, et al. Prevention of graft-versus-host disease following allogeneic bone marrow transplantation in rate using FK506. Transplantation 1991; 52:590.
73. Markus P, Cai X, Ming W, et al. FK 506 reverses acute graft-versus-host disease following allogeneic bone marrow transplantation in rats. Surgery 1991; 110:357.
74. Fung J, Todo S, Tzakis AG, et al. Current status of FK 506 in liver transplantation. Transplant Proc 1991; 23:1902.
75. Fay JW, Wingard JR, Antin JH, et al. FK506 (Tacrolimus) monotherapy for prevention of graft-versus-host disease after histocompatible sibling allogeneic bone marrow transplantation. Blood 1996; 87:3514.
76. Jacobs P. Cyclosporin A pretreatment of both donor and recipient undergoing allogeneic bone marrow transplantation. Scand J Haematol 1985; 35:386.
77. Cooper M, Markus PM, Cai X, et al. Prolonged prevention of acute graft-versus-host disease after allogeneic bone marrow transplantation by donor pretreatment using FK 506. Transplant Proc 1991; 23:3238.
78. Dumont F, Melino MR, Staruch MJ, et al. The immunosuppressive macrolides FK-506 and rapamycin act as reciprocal antagonists in murine T cells. J Immunol 1990; 144: 1418.
79. Dumont F, Staruch MJ, Koprak SL, et al. Distinct mechanisms of suppression of murine T cell activation by the related macrolides FK-506 and rapamycin. J Immunol 1990; 144:251.
80. Fabian M, Denning SM, Bollinger RR. Rapamycin suppression of host-versus-graft and graft-versus-host disease in MHC-mismatched rats. Transplant Proc 1992; 24: 1174.
81. Mollison KW, Thomas VA, Fey TA, et al. Comparison of FK-506, rapamycin, ascomycin, and cyclosporine in mouse models of host-versus-graft disease and heterotopic heart disease. Ann NY Acad Sci 1993; 685:55.
82. Appelbaum F, Raff RF, Storb R, et al. Use of trimetrexate for the prevention of graft-versus-host disease. Bone Marrow Transplant 1989; 4:421.
83. Pamphilon DH, Alaqdy AA, Godwin V, et al. Studies of allogeneic bone marrow and spleen cell transplantation in a murine model using ultraviolet-B light. Blood 1991; 77: 2072.
84. Okamoto H, Horio T, Meader M. Alteration of lymphocyte functions by 8 methoxypsoralen and long wave ultraviolet radiation: II. The effect of in vivo PUVA on IL-2 production. J Invest Dermatol 1987; 89:24.
85. Deeg H, Sigaroudinia M. Ultraviolet B-induced loss of HLA class II antigen expression on lymphocytes is dose, time, and locus dependent. Exp Hematol 1990; 18:916.
86. Spielberg H, June CH, Blair OC, et al. Ultraviolet-irradiation of lymphocytes triggers increase in intracellular CA^{2+} and prevents lectin-stimulated CA^{2+} mobilization: Evidence for UV and nifedipine sensitive calcium channels. Exp Hematol 1991; 19:742.

87. Gruner S, Oesterwitz H, Stoppe H, et al. Cis-urocanic acid as a mediator of ultraviolet-light-induced immunosuppression. Semin Hematol 1992; 29:102.
88. Allison A, Almquist SJ, Muller CD, Eugui EM. In vitro immunosuppressive effects of mycophenolic acid and an ester pro-drug RS-61443. Transplant Proc 1991; 23:10.
89. Sonnino R. RS-61443 prevents graft-versus-host disease but not rejection in allogeneic rat small bowel transplants. Transplant Proc 1992; 24:1190.
90. Dayton JS, Turka LA, Thompson CB, et al. Comparison of the effects of mizoribine with those of azathioprine, 6-mercaptopurine, and mycophenolic acid on T lymphocyte proliferation and purine ribonucleotide metabolism. Mol Pharmacol 1992; 41: 671.
91. Stacey N, Cox J, Loblay R, Crosbie J. Neuraminidase pretreatment of donor lymphocytes and graft-versus-host disease. Int Soc Exp Hematol 1989; 17:273.
92. Takeuchi T, Iinuma H, Kunimoto S, et al. A new antitumor antibiotic spergualin: Isolation and antitumor activity. J Antibiot 1981; 34:1619.
93. Nemoto K, Hayashi M, Abe F, et al. Inhibition by deoxyspergualin of allo-reactive cytotoxic activity in graft-versus-host disease. Transplant Proc 1989; 21:3028.
94. Nemoto K, Sugawara Y, Mae T, et al. Immunological unresponsiveness by deoxyspergualin therapy in mice undergoing lethal graft-vs-host disease, and successful adoptive transfer of unresponsiveness. Transplant Proc 1991; 23:862.
95. Nemoto K, Hayshi M, Ito J, et al. Deoxyspergualin in lethal murine graft-versus-host disease. Transplantation 1991; 51:712.
96. Jones JM, Wilson R, Baelmaer PM. Mortality and gross pathology of secondary disease in germfree mouse radiation chimeras. Radiat Res 1971; 45:577.
97. Buckner C, Clift RA, Sanders JE, et al. Protective environment for marrow transplant recipients: A prospective study. Ann Intern Med 1978; 89:893.
98. Levine A, Siegel SE, Schreiber AD, et al. Protected environments and prophylactic antibiotics: A prospective controlled study on their utility in the therapy of acute leukemia. N Engl J Med 1973; 288:477.
99. Schimpff S, Greene WH, Young VM, et al. Infection prevention in acute nonlymphoblastic leukemia: Laminar air flow reverse isolation with oral, non-absorbable antibiotic prophylaxis. Ann Intern Med 1975; 82:351.
100. Storb R, Hansen JA, Prentice RL, et al. Graft-versus-host disease and survival in patients with aplastic anemia treated by marrow grafts from HLA-identical siblings. Beneficial effect of a protective environment. N Engl J Med 1983; 308:302.
101. Vossen J, Heidt PJ, van den Berg H, et al. Prevention of infection and graft-versus-host disease by suppression of intestinal microflora in children treated with allogeneic bone marrow transplantation. Eur J Clin Micro Inf 1990; 9:14.
102. Klingemann H, Barnett MJ, Reece DE, et al. Use of an immunoglobulin preparation enriched for IgM (pentaglobin) for the treatment of acute graft-versus-host disease. Bone Marrow Transplant 1990; 6:199.
103. Bagacilupo A, van Lint MT, Frassoni F, et al. High dose bolus methylprednisolone for the treatment of acute graft-versus-host disease. Blut 1983; 46:125.
104. Kanojia M, Anagnostou AA, Zander AR, et al. High dose methylprednisolone treatment for acute graft-versus-host disease after bone marrow transplantation in adults. Transplantation 1984; 37:246.
105. Neudorf S, Filipovich A, Ramsay N, Kersey J. Prevention and treatment of acute graft-versus-host disease. Semin Hematol 1984; 21:91.
106. Weisdorf D, Haake R, Blazar, et al. Treatment of moderate/severe acute graft-versus-host disease after allogeneic bone marrow transplantation: An analysis of clinical risk factors and outcome. Blood 1990; 75:1024.
107. Martin PJ, Schoch G, Fisher L, et al. A retrospective analysis of therapy for acute graft-versus-host disease: Initial treatment. Blood 1990; 76:1464.

108. Martin P, Schoch G, Fisher L, et al. A retrospective analysis of therapy for acute graft-versus-host disease: Secondary treatment. Blood 1991; 77:1821.
109. Storb R, Gluckman RE, Thomas ED, et al. Treatment of established human graft-versus-host disease by antithymocyte globulin. Blood 1974; 44:57.
110. Doney K, Weiden PL, Storb R, Thomas ED. Treatment of graft-versus-host disease in human allogeneic marrow graft recipients: A randomized trial comparing antithymocyte globulin and corticosteroids. Am J Hematol 1981; 11:1.
111. Deeg H, Loughran TP Jr, Storb R, et al. Treatment of human acute graft-versus-host disease with anti-thymocyte globulin and cyclosporine with or without methylprednisolone. Transplantation 1985; 401:162.
112. Gratama J, Jansen J, Lopovich RA, et al. Treatment of acute graft-versus-host disease with monoclonal antibody OKT3. Transplantation 1984, 38:469.
113. Gluckman E, Devergie A, Varin F, et al. Treatment of steroid resistant severe acute graft-versus-host disease with a monoclonal pan T OKT3 antibody. Exp Hematol 1984; 12:66.
114. Anasetti C, Martin PJ, Storb R, et al. Treatment of acute graft-versus-host disease with a nonmitogenic anti-CD3 monoclonal antibody. Transplantation 1992; 54:844.
115. Martin P, Remlinger K, Hansen JA, et al. Murine monoclonal anti-T cell antibodies for treatment of refractory acute graft-versus-host disease. Transplant Proc 1984; 16: 1494.
116. Herve P, Wijdenes J, Bergerat JP, et al. Treatment of corticosteroid resistant acute graft-versus-host disease by in vivo administration of anti-interleukin-2 receptor monoclonal antibody (B-B10). Blood 1990; 75:1017.
117. Herve P, Flesch M, Tiberghien P, et al. Phase I-II trail of a monoclonal anti-tumor necrosis factor α antibody for the treatment of refractory severe acute graft-versus-host disease. Blood 1992; 79:3362.
118. Wijdenes J, Beliard R, Muot S, et al. A semi-pharmaceutical approach for the preparation of an anti-IL2 receptor monoclonal antibody in the treatment of acute GvHD in a multicentric study. Develop Biol Stand 1990; 71:103.
119. Herve P, Bordigoni P, Cahn JY, et al. Use of monoclonal antibodies in vivo as a therapeutic strategy for acute GvHD in matched and mismatched bone marrow transplantation. Transpl Proc 1991; 23:1692.
120. Herve P. Perspectives in the prevention and treatment of acute graft versus host disease. Bone Marrow Transplant 1991; 7(suppl):117.
121. Byers V, Henslee PJ, Kernan NA, et al. Use of anti-pan T-lymphocyte ricin A chain immunotoxin in steroid-resistant acute graft-versus-host disease. Blood 1990; 75: 1426.
122. Roy J, McGlave PB, Filipovich AH, et al. Acute graft-versus-host disease following unrelated donor marrow transplantation: Failure of conventional therapy. Bone Marrow Transplant 1992; 10:77.
123. Oblon D, Felker D, Coyle K, Myers L. High-dose methylprednisolone therapy for acute graft-versus-host disease associated with matched unrelated donor bone marrow transplantation. Bone Marrow Transplant 1992; 10:355.
124. Atkinson K, Horowitz M, Gale RP, et al. Consensus among bone marrow transplanters for diagnosis, grading and treatment of chronic graft-versus-host disease. Bone Marrow Transplant 1989, 4:247.
125. Shulman HM. Pathology of chronic graft-vs.-host disease. In: Burakoff SJ, Deeg HJ, Ferrara J and Atkinson K, eds. Graft-vs-Host Disease: Immunology, Pathophysiology and Treatment. New York: Marcel Dekker, 1990.
126. Sullivan KM, McDonald GB, Shulman HM, et al. Chronic graft-versus-host disease in 52 patients: Adverse natural course and successful treatment with combination immunosuppression. Blood 1981; 57:267.

127. Sullivan K. Acute and chronic graft-versus-host disease. Int J Cell Cloning 1986; 4(suppl 1):42.
128. Lum L, Orcutt-Thordarson N, Seigneuret MC, Storb R. The regulation of Ig synthesis after marrow transplantation: IV. T4 and T8 subset function in patients with chronic graft-versus-host disease. J Immunol 1982; 129:113.
129. Atkinson K, Horowitz MM, Gale RP, et al. Consensus among bone marrow transplanters for diagnosis, grading and treatment of chronic graft-versus-host disease. Bone Marrow Transplant 1989; 4:247.
130. Storb R, Clift RA, Prentice RL, et al. Predictive factors in chronic graft-versus-host disease in patients with aplastic anemia treated by marrow transplantation from HLA-identical siblings. Ann Intern Med 1983; 98:461.
131. Witherspoon R, Sullivan KM, Lum LG, et al. Use of thymic grafts or thymic factors to augment immunologic recovery after bone marrow transplantation: Brief report with 2 to 12 years' follow-up. Bone Marrow Transplant 1988; 3:425.
132. Blume KG, Beutler E, Bross KJ, et al. Bone-marrow ablation and allogeneic marrow transplantation in acute leukemia. N Engl J Med 1980; 302:1041.
133. Ringden O, Persson U, Gunnar S, et al. Early diagnosis and treatment of acute human graft-versus-host disease. Transplant Proc 1983; 15:1490.
134. Gratwohl A. Cyclosporin A in allogeneic bone marrow transplantation for leukemia: Basel experience 1979 to 1984. Tokai J Exp Clin Med 1985; 10:127.
135. Sullivan K, Witherspoon RP, Storb R, et al. Prednisone and azathioprine compared to prednisone and placebo for treatment of chronic graft-v-host disease: Prognostic influence of prolonged thrombocytopenia after allogeneic marrow transplantation. Blood 1988; 72:546.
136. Sullivan K, Witherspoon RP, Storb R, et al. Alternating-day cyclosporine and prednisone for treatment of high-risk chronic graft-v-host disease. Blood 1988; 72:555.
137. Fields E, Gibbs JE, Tucker DF, Hellman K. Effect of thalidomide on the graft versus host reaction. Nature 1966; 211:1308.
138. Sheskin J. Thalidomide in the treatment of lepra reactions. Clin Pharmacol 1968; 6: 303.
139. Barnhill R, McDougall AC. Thalidomide: Use and possible mode of action in reactional lepromatous leprosy and in various other conditions. J Am Acad Dermatol 1982; 7:317.
140. Vogelsang G, Wells MC, Santos GW, et al. Combination low-dose thalidomide and cyclosporine prophylaxis for acute graft-versus-host disease in a rat mismatched model. Transplant Proc 1988; 20(2 suppl 2):226.
141. Heney D, Bailey CC, Lewis IJ. Thalidomide in the treatment of graft-versus-host disease. Biomed Pharmacother 1990; 44:199.
142. Vogelsang G, Farmer ER, Hess AD, et al. Thalidomide for the treatment of chronic graft-versus-host disease. N Engl J Med 1992; 326:105.
143. Hymes S, Morison WL, Farmer ER, et al. Methoxypsoralen and ultraviolet A radiation in treatment of chronic cutaneous graft-versus-host reaction. Acad Dermatol 1985; 12:30.
144. Atkinson K, Weller P, Ryman W, et al. PUVA therapy for drug-resistant graft-versus-host disease. Bone Marrow Transplant 1990; 1:227.
145. Eppinger T, Ehninger G, Steinert M, et al. 8-methoxypsoralen and ultraviolet A therapy for cutaneous manifestations of graft-versus-host disease. Transplantation 1990; 50:807.
146. Kripke M. Immunological unresponsiveness induced by ultraviolet radiation. Immunol Rev 1984; 80:87.
147. Bredberg A, Forsgren A. Effects of in vitro PUVA on human leukocyte function. Br J Dermatol 1984; 111:159.

148. Granstein R, Lowy A, Greene M. Epidermal antigen presenting cells in activation of suppression: Identification of a new functional type of ultraviolet radiation resistant epidermal cell. J Immunol 1985; 132:563.
149. Okamoto H, Horio T, Meader M. Alteration of lymphocyte functions by 8 methoxypsoralen and long wave ultraviolet radiation: II. The effect of in vivo PUVA on IL-2 production. J Invest Dermatol 1987; 89:24.
150. Kapoor N, Pelligrini AE, Copelan EA, et al. Psoralen plus ultraviolet A (PUVA) in the treatment of chronic graft versus host disease: Preliminary experience in standard treatment resistant patients. Semin Hematol 1992; 29:108.
151. Deeg HJ, Storb R, Erickson K, et al. Photoinactivation of lymphohemopoietic cells: Studies in transfusion medicine and bone marrow transplantation. Blood Cells 1992; 18:151.
152. Erickson KW, Sullivan KM, Deeg HJ, et al. Psoralen and ultraviolet A irradiation (PUVA) as salvage therapy for refractory cutaneous acute graft-versus-host disease following allogeneic marrow transplantation: Long-term efficacy and safety. Blood. In press.
153. van Prooijen H, Aarts-Riemens MI, Grijzenhout MA, van Weelden H. Ultraviolet irradiation modulates MHC-alloreactive cytotoxic T-cell precursors involved in the onset of graft-versus-host disease. Br J Haematol 1992; 81:73.
154. Freid R, Murakami CS, Willson RA, et al. Chronic graft-vs-host disease of the liver: Another indication of ursodeoxycholic acid. Ann Intern Med 1992; 116:233.
155. Eslinger S. Hepatology elsewhere. Hepatology 1992; 16:1305.
156. Atkinson K, Farewell V, Storb R, et al. Analysis of late infections after human bone marrow transplantation: Role of genotypic nonidentity between marrow donor and recipient and of nonspecific suppressor cells in patients with chronic graft-versus-host disease. Blood 1982; 60:714.
157. Winston DJ, Schiffman G, Wand DC, et al. Pneumococcal infections after human bone marrow transplantation. Ann Intern Med 1979; 91:835.
158. Sullivan KM, Mori M, Sanders J, et al. Late complications of allogeneic and autologous bone marrow transplantation. Bone Marrow Transplant 1992; 10(suppl 1):127.
159. Beatty PG, Hansen JA, Longton GM, et al. Marrow transplantation from HLA-matched unrelated donors for treatment of hematologic malignancies. Transplantation 1991; 51:443.
160. McGlave PB, Beatty T, Ash R, Hows JM. Therapy for chronic myelogenous leukemia with unrelated donor bone marrow transplantation: Results in 102 cases. Blood 1990; 75:1728.
161. Drobyski WR, Ash RC, Casper JT, et al. Effect of T-cell depletion as graft-versus-host disease prophylaxis on engraftment, relapse, and disease-free survival in unrelated marrow transplantation for chronic myelogenous leukemia. Blood 1994; 83:1980.
162. Kernan NA, Bartsch G, Ash RC, et al. Analysis of 462 transplantations from unrelated donors facilitated by the National Marrow Donor Program. N Engl J Med 1993; 328: 593.
163. Kato Y, Mitsuishi Y, Cecka M, et al. HLA-DP incompatibilities and severe graft-versus-host disease in unrelated bone marrow transplants. Transplantation 1991; 52:374.
164. Petersdorf EW, Smith AG, Mickelson EM, et al. The role of HLA-DPB1 disparity in the development of acute graft-versus-host disease following unrelated donor marrow transplantation. Blood 1993; 81:1923.
165. Busca A, Anasetti C, Anderson G, et al. Unrelated donor or autologous marrow transplantation for treatment of acute leukemia. Blood 1994; 83:3077.
166. Marks DI, Cullis JO, Ward KN, et al. Allogeneic bone marrow transplantation for chronic myeloid leukemia using sibling and volunteer unrelated donors. Ann Intern Med 1993; 119:207.

167. Hood AF, Vogelsang GB, Black LP, et al. Acute graft-versus-host disease: Development following autologous and syngeneic bone marrow transplantation. Arch Dermatol 1987; 123:745.
168. Santos GW. Syngeneic or autologous graft-versus-host disease. Int J Cell Cloning 1989; 7:92.
169. Rappeport JM, Mihm M, Reinherz EL, et al. Acute graft-vs-host disease in recipients of bone marrow transplants from identical twin donors. Lancet 1979; 2:712.
170. Gluckman E, Devergie A, Sohier J, Saurat JH. Graft-versus-host disease in recipients of syngeneic bone marrow. Lancet 1980; 1:253.
171. Hess AD, Horwitz L, Beschorner WE, Santos GW. Development of graft-vs-host disease-like syndrome in cyclosporine treated rats after syngeneic bone marrow transplantation: I. Development of cytotoxic T lymphocytes with apparent polyclonal anti-Ia specificity, including autoreactivity. J Exp Med 1985; 161:718.
172. Shinozawa T, Beschorner WE, Hess AD. The thymus and prolonged administration of cyclosporine. Transplantation 1990; 50:106.
173. Einsele H, Ehninger G, Schneider EM, et al. High frequency of graft-versus-host-like syndromes following syngeneic bone marrow transplantation. Transplantation 1988; 45:579.
174. Parker P, Chao NJ, Snyder DS, et al. Thalidomide therapy for chronic graft-versus-host disease. Blood 1995; 86:3604.

25

Antagonists of Inflammatory Cytokines: Prophylactic and Therapeutic Applications

Ernst Holler
Klinikum Grosshadern der Universitat
Munich, Germany

James L. M. Ferrara
Dana-Farber Cancer Institute, Children's Hospital, and Harvard Medical School
Boston, Massachusetts

I. RATIONALE FOR THE USE OF INFLAMMATORY CYTOKINE ANTAGONISTS IN ALLOGENEIC BMT

A. Inflammatory Cytokines in GVHD: TNFα and IL-1

The proteins tumor necrosis factor alpha (TNFα) and interleukin-1 (IL-1) are secreted during inflammatory processes of natural or "innate" immunity to infectious microbes of other foreign proteins, and are therefore prime examples of inflammatory cytokines. Because IL-1 and TNFα are produced by activated mononuclear cells, they are sometimes called monokines. The cellular sources of TNFα and IL-1 are not always mononuclear cells, however; in fact, numerous cell types are known to produce them. These proteins are often produced during processes of acquired immunity, thus enhancing natural immunity, and may have synergistic, pleiotropic, and occasionally redundant effects on target cells; thus they are able to activate lymphocytes as well as perform certain effector functions.

TNFα was originally described as a protein produced after activation of macrophages following lipopolysaccharide (LPS) stimulation and which induced hemorrhagic necrosis of transplantable murine sarcomas (1). Subsequently, TNFα became a major focus of interest as a central proinflammatory cytokine capable of mediating the deleterious effects of severe infectious complications such as septic shock (2,3). This protein is pivotal in inflammatory responses that result in a wide variety of systemic effects, including fever, acute-phase actions, hematopoietic growth factor production, the activation of endothelial cells, and the destruction of epithelial cells and keratinocytes (4–6). These direct effects of TNFα are accompanied by increased expression of a variety of molecules critical to immune responses, such as intercellular adhesion molecules (ICAMs) and HLA class I antigens on epithelial and endothelial cells (6,7). Furthermore, a costimulatory role for TNFα in activation of cytotoxic T cells has recently been reported (8).

IL-1 shares multiple proinflammatory properties with TNFα (2), making both cytokine candidates for involvement in the pathophysiology of bone marrow transplantation (BMT)-related complications (see Chap. 7). IL-1 is a polypeptide with two isoforms, IL-1α and IL-1β. IL-1 was first described as "endogenous pyrogen" and was later shown to be a lymphocyte-stimulating factor. Endotoxin is the most important known stimulus for IL-1 production, and approximately five molecules per lymphocyte is sufficient to stimulate IL-1 mRNA transcription. Recent studies suggest that cells undergoing apoptosis or programmed cell death produce IL-1 more efficiently (9) and IL-1 appears to be important in the regulation of apoptosis. Overexpression of IL-1 converting enzyme (ICE) induces apoptosis in cell lines (10) and ICE-deficient mice are resistant to apoptosis through the Fas pathway (11,12). IL-1 and TNFα appear to be linked in this pathway because the Fas antigen (CD95) is a cell-surface protein with high homology to the TNFα receptor (13,14).

A third member of the IL-1 family, interleukin-1 receptor antagonist (IL-1ra), is an important, specific inhibitor of IL-1 activity. IL-1ra was isolated from human mononuclear cells and its cDNA was sequenced in 1990 (15). IL-1ra is a 17-kDa popypeptide (with a glycosylated form of 25 kDa) that has a 26% homology to IL-1β and a 19% homology to IL-1α. IL-1ra, which contains a leader sequence and a signal peptide, is secreted from cells and acts as a pure antagonist with no agonist activity (16). The biological activity of IL-1 is therefore extremely tightly regulated, with the same cell producing both agonists and antagonists. Purified IL-1ra competes with both IL-1α and IL-1β to bind IL-1 receptors with approximately the same affinity as either isoform. IL-1ra blocks IL-1 activity both in vitro and in vivo, including thymocyte proliferation, endothelial and neutrophil adhesion, and cytokine synthesis, but 100-fold excesses of IL-1ra are required to produce such inhibition in vitro (17,18). In addition to the secreted form of IL-1ra, an intracellular form (icIL-1ra) is known to exist in keratinocytes and epithelial cells; the function of this molecule is not yet completely understood (19). Immunoglobulins are known to induce the production of IL-1ra (20), and thus the therapeutic consequences of intravenous immunoglobulin (IVIg), which is known to reduce the incidence of GVHD, may involve the regulatory effect of Ig on networks of inflammatory cytokines.

Endotoxin is a principal inducer of inflammatory cytokines, and stimulation of TNFα and IL-1 by endotoxin is the most likely explanation for the well-known role of bacterial microflora in development of GVHD (see Chap. 18). Sensitivity to endotoxin and its ability to trigger release of TNFα are greatly enhanced in mice with graft-versus-host disease (GVHD), and this priming is predominantly due to the costimulatory role of IFNγ (21). The induction of IFNγ in the setting of BMT is the result of activation of donor Th1 cells, which occurs subsequent to the T-cell recognition of alloantigens (see Chap. 7). A second mechanism of IFNγ induction involves viral infections such as cytomegalovirus (22,23), a pathway of great potential significance in the context of BMT. Reproducible increases of IFNγ serum levels have also been noted during pretransplant conditioning by Niederwieser et al. (22).

There is increasing evidence for induction of inflammatory cytokines by cytotoxic drugs and ionizing irradiation. Induction of TNFα mRNA by irradiation has been demonstrated in cultures of human sarcoma cells (24) and in myeloid cell lines as well as in normal monocytes/macrophages (25,26). In these systems, doses as low as 2 Gy induced TNFα mRNA after 1hr and reached a maximum after 3 hr. Clinically, increases of serum TNFα and soluble TNF-receptor p55 (sTNF-R p55) have been observed following total-body irradiation (TBI) with fractions of 4 Gy in patients prepared for allogeneic BMT (27). Both TNFα and interleukin 6 (IL-6) are released after a single TBI dose of 10 Gy (28). In an experimental SCID model, pretransplant conditioning induced systemic TNFα within 4 hr of TBI. IL-1α levels increased slightly later, peaking at 72 hr (29). Systemic cytokine release was accompanied by increased expression of TNFα, and subsequently, IL-6 in colonic tissue. These results have been independently confirmed in other experimental models (see below), where IL-1α mRNA was induced 100-fold in the spleens of mice 1 week after they received either syngeneic or allogeneic BMT; IL-1α production then returned to normal in syngeneic (but not allogeneic) BMT recipients (30). Though experimental data are sparse regarding cytokine induction by cytotoxic drugs used for pretransplant conditioning, significant increases seem likely. Xun et al. detected only minimal amounts of systemic and tissue expression of TNFα and IL-1α in mice conditioned by busulfan/cyclophosphamide regimens (29), but large increases in TNFα serum levels have been seen in patients receiving CVB (cyclophosphamide, etoposide, BCNU) prior to autologous BMT, suggesting that at least this combination can cause TNFα release (see below). Cyclophosphamide is also known to trigger TNFα release from normal mononuclear cells in vitro (27).

Parallel to the heterogeneity of mechanisms resulting in the release of inflammatory cytokines, a vast number of cellular sources may be involved in this process. Donor monocytes and, to a lesser extent, CD4$^+$ cells, can produce TNFα. Host macrophages are also candidate sources of TNFα (31). Organs such as the lung and the liver (with significant populations of alveolar macrophages and Kupffer cells, respectively) are likely to be important producers of systemic cytokines. The concept of macrophage-derived cytokines might also help to explain the causal relationship between pretransplant risk factors and posttransplant complications, because macrophages have a half-life of about 2–3 months and are only slowly replaced by donor monocytes (32,33). In patients with chronic myeloid leukemia (CML), tissue macrophages are *bcr-abl* positive, and if allogeneic T cells recognize this foreign peptide, targeted host macrophages may be a source of cytokine dysregulation throughout the period of acute GVHD. Additional cells capable of TNFα production are NK cells and keratinocytes (34). Mast cells have also recently been recognized as potent reservoirs of preformed TNFα, which can be released rapidly during the process of degranulation; these cells are thus ideal candidates for initiation of an inflammatory cascade without prior de novo synthesis of cytokines (35,36).

B. Experimental Evidence for Pathophysiological Involvement of Inflammatory Cytokines in Allogeneic BMT

Mixed lymphocyte cultures (MLC) are thought to represent in vitro models of host-versus-graft and graft-versus-host reactions, but MLC reactivity does not generally correlate with the incidence and severity of GVHD (J. Hansen, personal communication). Nevertheless, in many centers MLCs are used in the selection of suitable donors in allogeneic BMT. MLCs from HLA-nonidentical donors produce significant amounts of TNFα, which occurs subsequent to production of IL-2 and

IFNγ (37). Antibodies that neutralize IFNγ also inhibit TNFα secretion, clearly reflecting the hypothesized cascade of sequential T-cell and monocyte activation in acute GVHD (21,38,39). In a study of HLA-disparate MLCs, Dickinson et al. used MLC supernatants to induce GVHD histology in skin explant assays (37). In these experiments, histological severity of GVHD was significantly associated with the amount of TNFα and IFNγ released to the supernatants; in addition, skin pathology could be prevented by addition of polyclonal or monoclonal antibodies neutralizing TFNα (40) or both TFNα and IFNγ (37). Thus, in a simplified model of GVHD in vitro, TNFα is not merely an index of cellular activation but is also a direct mediator of target organ pathology.

Convincing data regarding a direct pathophysiological role of TNFα were first presented by Piguet et al. in 1987 (41). In a P → F1 model of MHC-incompatible BMT, lethally irradiated mice were injected with bone marrow and lymph node T cells. The observed skin and gut lesions of acute GVHD as well as weight loss (a systemic indicator of GVHD) were significantly prevented by weekly administration (day +7 to day +35) of a polyclonal antibody that neutralized TNFα (41,42). Since that time, several investigators have confirmed Piguet's observations, and application of TNFα antibodies starting either before BMT or from day +7 have reduced the mortality from GVHD and its associated signs, including immunosuppression and mast cell degranulation (36,43–45).

In most of these experimental studies, antibodies neutralizing TNFα were less effective than T-cell depletion of the bone marrow in preventing GVHD, suggesting that TNFα release may occur as a consequence of donor T-cell activation (36,41,43–45). In one study, the protective effects of TNF antibodies seems to be restricted to acute GVHD induced by $CD4^+$ T cells and were not observed in a $CD8^+$-dependent model of GVHD (36). The predominance of TNFα-related lesions in CD4-induced GVHD is consistent with IFNγ-mediated activation of monocytes/macrophages; however, administration of anti-IFNγ antibodies during GVHD induction showed variable results and occasionally intensified the severity of GVHD in some studies (45; P. F. Piguet, unpublished observations). The role of IFNγ in GVHD is therefore quite complex, and interference with its immunoregulatory role in the context of a Th1/Th2 balance might have unpredictable consequences.

Murine studies have occasionally shown conflicting results with regard to the importance of systemic release of TNFα in GVHD (46). This confusion may be related to the type of immunoassays used in these studies (see below). Recent introduction of PCR techniques and immunohistology have allowed analysis of cytokine protein and gene expression in various organs of acute GVHD. In such studies, increased TNFα protein and mRNA expression have been reported for spleen, gut, and skin in the early period of acute GVHD; in several studies, expression of TFNα was less pronounced than the expression of IL-1 or IFNγ, demonstrating that TNFα is but one important cytokine among several that are dysregulated (47,48).

Convincing data regarding a direct role for IL-1 in GVHD were published by Abhyankar et al. in 1993 (30). Using a well-described mouse model of GVHD to minor histocompatibility antigens in a BMT model, mRNA for IL-1, IL-2, and TNFα were evaluated after transplant by a semiquantitative RT-PCR technique. In the spleen, IL-1α levels were increased almost two orders of magnitude the first week after transplant in both syngeneic and allogeneic BMT recipients (Fig. 1).

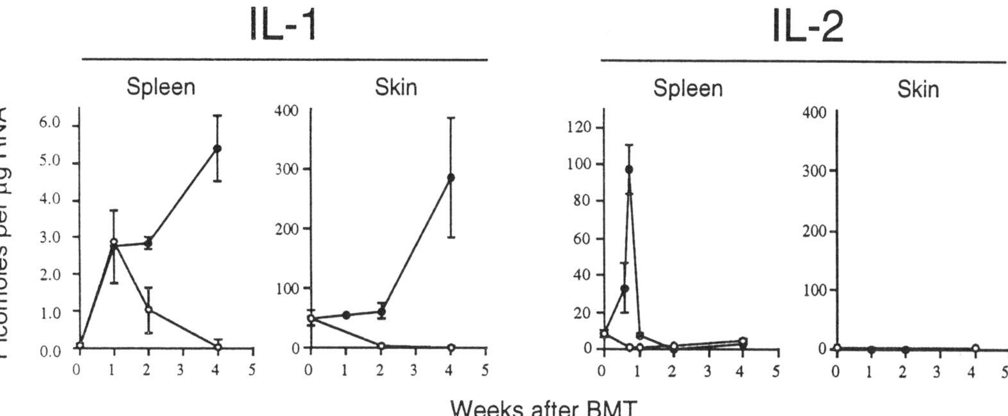

Figure 1 Kinetics of IL-2 mRNA transcript levels during the first month after transplant. Syngeneic B10.BR (○) and allogeneic CBA (●) mice were transplanted with B10.BR bone marrow and splenic T cells (as described in 30); epidermis and spleen were harvested and quantitative PCR was performed at the times indicated (as described in 30), $n = 2$–6 animals/group. Data are presented as mean ± SE. (Reprinted from Ref. 30.)

After that time, IL-1α mRNA decreased in animals without GVHD, but it continued to increase in animals with GVHD. IL-1α mRNA was also markedly elevated in the skin of animals with GVHD, but not in syngeneic controls. A large increase in IL-2 mRNA was observed only in recipients of allogenic BMT during the first week after transplant in the spleen, which is the first site where donor T cells recognize host alloantigens. One month after transplant, when GVHD was clinically apparent, IL-1α mRNA levels were 600-fold higher in the skin of animals with GVHD, where TNFα levels in the skin were only sixfold higher, although this latter difference was significant.

A causal relationship between IL-1 and the development of GVHD was established by injection of IL-1ra into transplanted mice. Surviving animals eventually developed skin disease consistent with GVHD. Administration of IL-1ra from either day 0–10 or from day 10–20 after transplant reduced the mortality of GVHD from approximately 80% to 20% (Fig. 2). Thus, IL-1 appears to be a critical effector molecule in this experimental model of acute GVHD, and its dysregulation occurs with completely different kinetics from that observed for IL-2.

The observation of systemic inflammatory cytokine release during pretransplant conditioning and its correlation with poor outcome following BMT in clinical studies (see below) suggest that release of inflammatory cytokines before the transplant might increase activation of donor T cells, perhaps by upregulating HLA and adhesion molecules on epithelial and endothelial targets (6,7). To explore the pathophysiological relevance of this pathway in an experimental model, a P → F1 mouse system comparable to the design reported by Piguet was investigated, giving only two injections of a polyclonal neutralizing TNFα antibody prior to irradiation and BMT. Using a low dose of donor T cells for induction of GVHD, this approach was as effective in prevention of mortality and weight loss as multiple injections of TNFα antibodies from day +7 to day +35 after BMT (44). In contrast, daily

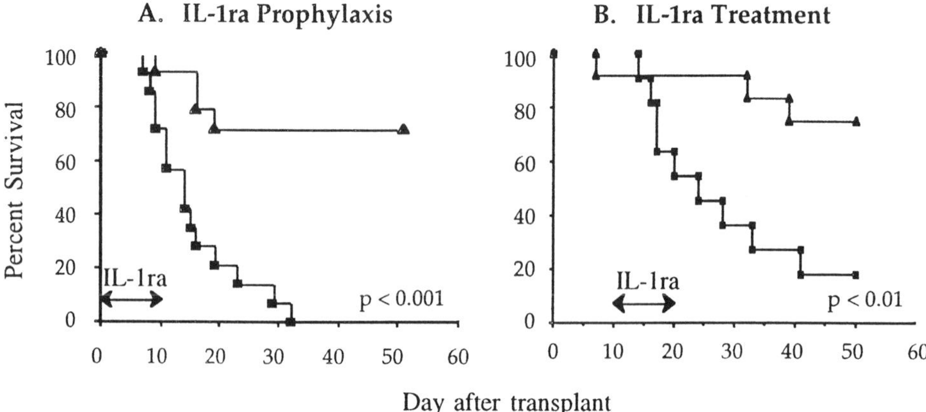

Figure 2 Survival of CBA mice transplanted with B10.BR bone marrow and splenic T cells and injected with saline (■, *n* eq 11) or IL-1ra (▲, $n = 12$) from day 10 to day 20 after transplant. Transplants were performed as described in Ref. 30. Mice were injected intraperitoneally twice a day with 75 μg of purified, recombinant human IL-1ra in 0.2 ml saline or saline alone. Mice surviving to day 60 did not show clinical evidence of GVHD such as weight loss or hunched posture. Results are combined from two separate experiments.(Reprinted from Ref. 30.)

injections of pentoxifylline (PTX), an alternative TNF antagonist, failed to protect mice from GVHD.

The role of conditioning-related release of TNFα in the induction of GVHD was elegantly confirmed in a study by Xun and his colleagues (29). In this study, lethal, acute GVHD was prevented by prolonging the interval between TBI and BMT for at least 4 days, i.e., to a time when conditioning-related TNFα levels had declined. Injection of soluble rhuTNFR : Fc, an engineered TNFα-antagonist made by linking two soluble TNF receptors (p80) with the Fc portion of human IgG1, resulted in a comparable protection from GVHD without any interval between TBI and BMT. However, neither of these approaches completely eliminated acute GVHD, nor did the use of a less aggressive conditioning regimen with busulfan and cyclophosphamide.

The importance of timing between the conditioning regimen and the injection of donor cells has been confirmed by several independent laboratories, including an analysis of a murine model of GVHD using cyclophosphamide alone (49). The role of pretransplant conditioning, especially ionizing irradiation, in the induction of GVHD is also supported by the clinical observation of intensified GVHD lesions in irradiated areas (50). This mechanism has been confirmed by experimental studies where GVHD histology occurred primarily in murine skin that had been irradiated and transplanted prior to the induction of GVHD in the recipients (51).

Chronic GVHD has been observed in experimental models where acute GVHD is prevented with anti-TNFα, suggesting that early release of TNFα and conditioning-related tissue damage accelerate and amplify acute GVHD but are not relevant to the induction of chronic GVHD. This dichotomy implies that prophylactic neutralization of inflammatory cytokines will not be able to induce tolerance to host antigens, a fact that might be advantageous with respect to the preservation of GVL effects. So far, only one study has documented TNFα expression in a murine model of chronic GVHD (47). In this report, TNFα mRNA expression was not increased, IFNγ was suppressed, and IL-4 was overexpressed in splenocytes, suggesting a shift toward a Th2 profile in chronic GVHD. These results suggest that the proinflammatory cascade involving IFNγ and TNFα does not operate during the pathophysiology of chronic GVHD, but further documentation is required.

C. Clinical Evidence for Involvement of Inflammatory Cytokines in Acute GVHD

In clinical allogeneic BMT, the first analyses of TNFα levels have focused on the postransplant period. Discrepancies reported in the first studies are probably explained by the heterogeneity of assays and the short half-life of systemic cytokine levels (52–56). Results of cytokine serum or plasma assays strongly depend on the type of assays employed, because these fluids contain not only bioactive cytokine but also large amounts of soluble TNF receptors (p55 and p75) that bind TNFα and circulate as receptor-ligand complexes. TNFα bound to its receptor is unlikely to be detected in bioassays, and detection of complexed TNFα in immunoassays depends on the epitope specificity of antibodies used (57). Standardization of TNFα-TNFR interactions is missing in most current assays and therefore accurate comparison of analyses is problematic.

A review of all the published data on systemic TNFα levels during the first 3 months following BMT clearly demonstrates that TNFα serum levels are increased not only in patients developing acute GVHD, but also in those experiencing acute endothelial complications such as venooclusive disease (VOD) or capillary leakage syndrome (55,58,59). This association of elevated TNF level with a variety of pathological conditions, as well as its wide range of normal values, has so far precluded its use as an independent diagnostic parameter for acute GVHD. We have shown that a close correlation exists between acute GVHD and elevated sTNFR p55 levels (60) (Table 1). The shedding of soluble receptors subsequent to induction of TNFα has been reported for a variety of clinical conditions; in the future, soluble TNF receptor (sTNFR) levels might prove to be a more suitable and sensitive approach for clinical monitoring, because soluble receptors are more stable than native cytokines and circulate in normal individuals with significant (nanogram) levels, which may facilitate the detection of minor shifts in their concentrations.

A second and more precise approach to predictive assays for GVHD may be the analysis of cytokine production by peripheral blood mononuclear cells (PBMC). In studies performed in Munich, monitoring of spontaneous and LPS-induced secretion of TNFα in PMBC cultures obtained after engraftment revealed a significant increase in patients who developed GVHD (and other complications) compared to patients with uneventful courses. Quantitative data can be obtained by evaluation of cytokine expression using either immunodetection of intracytoplasmatic cytokine protein (56) or PCR analysis of cytokine mRNA (30,59). Such techniques have shown increased expression of both TNFα and IL-1 in patients with GVHD. Rowbottom and colleagues performed PCR in postmortem specimens and showed significant expression of TNFα mRNA in skin biopsies in 3/5 patients with GVHD, but in no patient without GVHD (61). Similar induction of TNFα mRNA was

Table 1 Maximal Release of TNFα and Soluble TNF Receptor p55 (sTNFR p55) in Sequential Serum Samples Obtained Between Day 0 and Day +100 Following BMT (mean ± SEM, pg/ml)

BMT type	Autologous	Allogeneic			
Complication	—	a GVHD grade 0–I	aGVHD grade II	aGVHD grade III/IV	VOD/ capillary leak
TNFα (cryo)	30 (46) $n = 4$	50 (11) $n = 21$	97 (36) $n = 8$	326 (152) $n = 17$	726 (360) $n = 6$
TNFα (fresh)	111 (28) $n = 14$	181 (48) $n = 13$	365 (80) $n = 11$	477 (103) $n = 14$	554 (161) $n = 13$
sTNFR p55	5500 (1800) $n = 5$	4100 (1200) $n = 9$	8500 (2400) $n = 12$	14,300 (5,700) $n = 11$	26,400 (10,800) $n = 6$

TNFα was determined by ELISA either in cryopreserved (cryo) or in fresh (fresh) serum samples; sTNFR p55 was determined by IRMA using cryopreserved samples. Patients were grouped according to the type of BMT and occurrence or absence of complications. Maximal levels between groups were compared by Wilcoxon tests; both TNFα and sTNFR were significantly elevated in patients with GVHD grade II ($p < 0.01$). TNFα levels in frozen control samples ($n = 20$) were 28 ± 36 pg/ml, sTNFR p55 levels 3000 ± 300 pg/ml. TNFα levels in fresh control samples ($n = 30$) were 48 ± 20 pg/ml.

observed in lymph nodes or spleen of 7/10 patients with GVHD. Interestingly, in three patients there was absent TNFα mRNA production but high expression of IL-4 mRNA, indicating a reciprocal expression of these cytokines. This reciprocity may have important consequences in terms of the type of GVHD that is manifest, i.e., acute versus chronic (see below). Furthermore, TNFβ, the isoform of TNF produced by T cells, appeared to be increased in skin and lymphoid organs of patients with GVHD. In contrast, TNFβ was not detected in more than 400 serum samples obtained following BMT in Munich, and strong suppression of T-cell TNFβ release in PBMNC was seen throughout the period of acute GVHD (62). These contradictory findings may be due to a more localized proinflammatory action of TNFβ, and they illustrate the potential pitfalls of using PBMC as indicators of GVHD effector cell populations. It should be noted that PBMC analysis presumes that peripheral circulating cells are relevant to the pathophysiology of acute GVHD; other critical cell poluations, such as tissue macrophages or endothelial cells, may be major producers of relevant cytokines but may be inaccessible to analysis. Detailed correlations of serum or PBMC cytokine levels with tissue cytokine expression are therefore needed.

One of the most important findings in studies regarding the systemic release of TNFα is the strong correlation between the time of first elevated levels of TNFα and the occurrence of transplant-related complications (TRC) (63). In an update of studies in Munich, 222 patients receiving either allogeneic related donor ($n = 161$), unrelated donor ($n = 34$), or autologous BMT ($n = 35$) have been analyzed for daily serum TNFα levels starting from admission until day +10 after BMT. As shown in Fig. 3 and Table 2, patients receiving HLA-identical sibling donor BMT

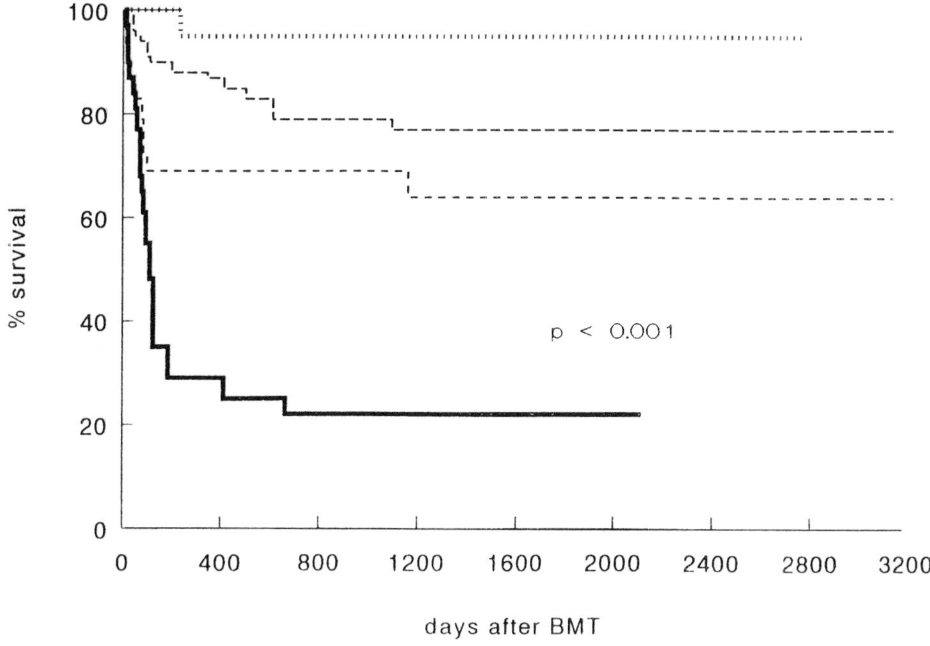

Figure 3 Actuarial survival of patients receiving allogeneic family member donor BMT. Patients were grouped according to the first observation of pathological TNFα serum levels: chronic release at the time of admission (| | |, $n = 24$), de novo release during conditioning (–, $n = 31$), de novo release in the first 10 days following BMT (--, $n = 29$), de novo release after day +10 or not observed (---, $n = 77$). Deaths from relapses were censored and are described in Table 3. Survival was significantly worse in patients with acute TNFα release during pretransplant conditioning ($p < 0.005$ as compared to group d+1 to +10, $p < 0.001$ as compared to others).

are divided into four subgroups: (1) patients with increased TNFα serum levels prior to treatment and without any clinical symptoms of "chronic" cytokine release [as previously described (64)]; (2) patients with low levels prior to chemotherapy and an acute increase during pretransplant conditioning; (3) patients with acute release observed between day +1 and day +10 following BMT; and (4) patients without any pathological TNFα serum levels prior to day +10 after BMT. Patients with de novo release of TNFα (group 2) have an extremely poor prognosis owing to occurrence of severe TRC (including acute GVHD). Their outcome is significantly worse than that of patients with TNFα release between day +1 and +10 ($p <$ 0.005, log rank) and all other subgroups ($p < 0.0001$), strongly supporting a pivotal role for host-associated cytokine release in induction of acute GVHD and related complications. We have now extended our observations to unrelated donor BMT (Fig. 4); even in this small subgroup, outcome is significantly worse when release of TNFα occurs during pretransplant conditioning, indicating that host-derived cytokine release is important to the induction of GVHD even when the histocompatibility differences between donor and recipient are increased.

A still puzzling observation is the extremely low incidence of TRC in patients

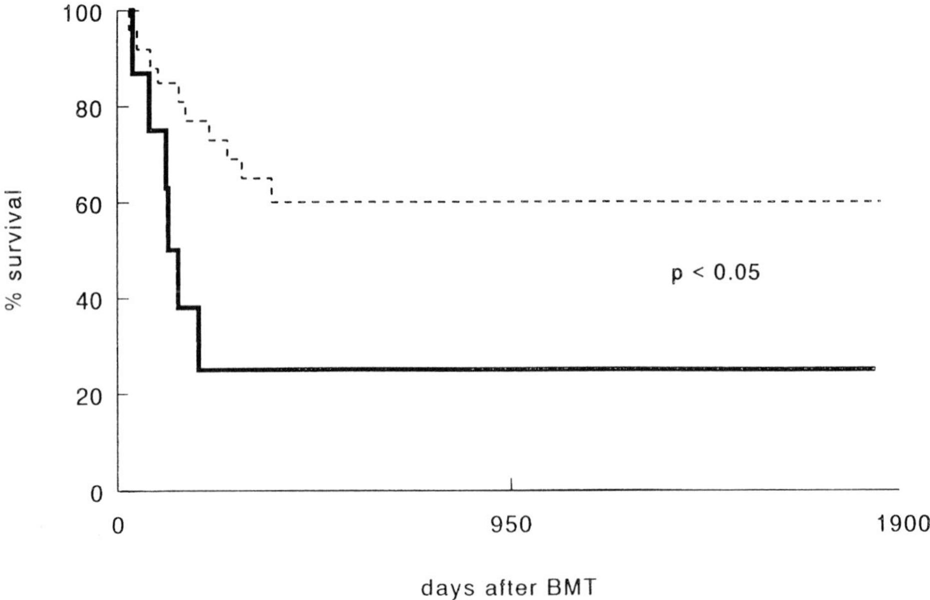

Figure 4 Actuarial survival of patients receiving allogeneic BMT from unrelated donors. Deaths due to relapses were censored and occurred in four patients with TNFα release after BMT. Patients were grouped according to the time of first pathological release of serum TNFα: during conditioning (—, $n = 8$), after BMT; release after BMT or not observed (— —, $n = 26$). Differences between both groups are significant with $p < 0.05$ (log rank test).

Table 2 Actuarial Distribution of Complications in Patients Receiving Allogeneic Related Donor BMT and Grouped Acccording to the Time of First Pathological Systemic Release of TNFα

	Time of first pathological release of TNFα (>100 pg/ml)			
Actuarial outcome	Chronic release ($n = 24$)	During conditioning ($n = 31$)	Day +1 → +10 ($n = 29$)	≥day +10 ($n = 77$)
Died of TRC	1	24	10	16
Died of relapse	5	2	3	11
Survived	18	5	16	49
after aGVHD	2 (11%)	4 (80%)	9 (56%)	16 (33%)
without GVHD	16 (89%)	1 (20%)	7 (44%)	33 (67%)
Median follow-up (months) for survivors	55 (7–93)	60 (44–70)	70 (6–104)	39 (6–105)

Actuarial complication-free survival is shown in Fig. 1.

with "chronic" release of TNFα (Table 2). Increased serum levels of these patients correlate with increased spontaneous production of TNFα by PBMC in culture. Unique features of this subgroup are its low incidence of GVHD and the absence of disease correlations to stage, age, or previous infectious complications, implying existence of some intrinsic or even genetically fixed mechanisms responsible for the increased production of TNFα. Analyses of polymorphisms within the TNFα gene are presently being performed to investigate this hypothesis. In thalassemia patients, a subgroup with high TNFα levels prior to BMT has also been observed; although there was some correlation of TNFα level with liver fibrosis, there is a stronger association with HLA-DQw1, suggesting a mechanism of genetically fixed cytokine dysregulation (65). In spite of the small numbers of patients with spontaneous TNFα release, further evaluation of this group may lead to important insights regarding mechanisms of cytokine-mediated damage. For example, chronic TNFα secretion may lead to desensitization of TNF, or other cytokines, such as IL-10, may be simultaneously induced in this network that have protective effects. Recently, Tan and colleagues have identified a novel factor produced by Th1 T-cell clones that protects nonobese diabetic mice (NOD) from the development of diabetes (66). In addition, polymorphisms of the TNFα gene and promoter region have been found to correlate with increased TNFα production in heart transplant recipients (67). Further insights into regulation of cytokine networks and their impact on disease could lead to therapeutic interventions and provide an alternative approach to the prevention of TRC in the future.

Correlation of conditioning-related release of TNFα and BMT outcome has now been confirmed in experiments from several laboratories (29,49) and has been observed in a Swedish clinical study (68). Although the murine models have shown an almost exclusive role for TBI in the induction of excess TNFα, comparison of conditioning regimens in patients in Munich has not yet shown a significantly higher incidence of TNFα release in those receiving total body irradiation and cyclophosphamide (TBICY) regimens (23% have increased TNFα release during conditioning, 24% between day +1 and day +10) compared to busulfan and cyclophosphamide (BUSCY) regimens (16% have increased TNFα release during conditioning, 15% between day +1 and +10). These data suggest that some cytokine is released during non-TBI-containing regimens, but a more detailed analysis is needed. Recently, we were able to clarify one aspect of this issue by analyzing circadian kinetics of TNF–anti-TNF complexes in patients receiving anti-TNFα monoclonal antibody throughout conditioning (69). In these patients, the binding of TNFα to circulating antibody facilitated detection of TNFα production during both TBICY and BUSCY conditioning regiments. In TBICY-treated patients, every single dose of TBI (as well as every dose of CY) was followed by an increase of TNF–anti-TNF complexes in patients receiving anti-TNFα monoclonal antibody throughout conditioning (69). In BUSCY-treated patients, only CY induced significant peaks of cytokine. In contrast, oral administration of BUS had no effect on levels of these complexes. These data clearly indicated TNFα is induced by both TBI and CY in vivo, confirming that cytokine release is not restricted to TBI in humans. As already discussed, the concept of chemotherapy-induced cytokine release is further supported by analysis of patients receiving autologous BMT following cyclophosphomide, etoposide, and bleomycin (CVB)-conditioning, where 8/35 patients showed significant release of TNFα during the course of conditioning. Even in autologous BMT, transplant-related mortality (mainly due to pulmonary complications) was increased with early TNFα secretion (37.5% vs. 7.4%).

In our previous studies, clinical risk factors predisposing to acute release of TNFα during the course of conditioning were identified (70). Increases of TNFα serum levels were significantly ($p < 0.001$) correlated with a diagnosis of CML or myelodysplastic syndrome. Fever or skin exanthems during conditioning were strongly associated ($p < 0.001$) with TNFα release; in addition, failure of gastrointestinal decontamination, as indicated by the presence of pathological stool specimens on the day of BMT, was also associated with acute release of TNFα ($p < 0.05$). Interestingly, these risk factors correspond to the three major mechanisms postulated in host-associated cytokine dysregulation: pretransplant conditioning itself, underlying disease, and translocation of bacteria from a damaged intestinal mucosa.

II. CLINICAL STUDIES WITH ANTAGONISTS OF INFLAMMATORY CYTOKINES

A. Corticosteroids

When discussing the use of specific cytokine antagonists for treatment and prevention of acute GVHD, it should be remembered that corticosteroids, which are still the first-line treatment of choice of acute GVHD, exhibit potent and broad cytokine antagonism. There is increasing evidence that corticosteroids act via suppression of cytokine gene activation rather than by cytotoxicity (71). In our studies on treatment of acute GVHD, both TNFα and sTNFR p55 serum levels as well as PBMC production of TNFα significantly decreased 48–72 hr after initiation of first-line treatment of GVHD with 5 mg/kg prednisolone (72). In patients with progressive GVHD, TNFα levels started to rise again as soon as corticosteroids were tapered to 2 mg/kg, indicating that the threshold for suppression of TNFα release might be higher than expected. Owing to their broad suppression of cytokine production, the use of corticosteroids must be considered in clinical trials that examine the effects of specific cytokine antagonists. In addition, some of the well-known effects and side effects of corticosteroid treatment, especially the increase in infectious complications and existence of thresholds pertaining to control of GVHD, should be anticipated for other cytokine antagonists. Finally, the optimal dosages for corticosteroids as they relate to the suppression of inflammatory cytokines still need to be defined.

B. Anti-TNFα Monoclonal Antibodies

Two differnt monoclonal antibodies (MAb) that neutralize human TNFα have been tested in clinical trials. Both studies were performed in BMT patients with acute GVHD that was resistant to corticosteroids and to at least one additional experimental treatment (either monoclonal or polyclonal antibodies directed against T cells or the IL-2-receptor). In a French trial (73), BC7, a complete murine IgG1 MAb, was given to 19 patients with grade III or IV acute GVHD over 8–12 days in addition to baseline immunosuppression that included cyclosporin and corticosteroids. Eight patients achieved a very good partial response (42.1%) and an additional six patients had a partial response (31.5%), while five patients (26.3%) had no response.

Skin (61%) and gut (72%) lesions responded better than liver lesions (38.5%). In 9/11 evaluable responding patients, acute GVHD recurred after cessation of BC7 treatment; two patients became long-term survivors.

A second trial in five patients with advanced acute GVHD used MAb 195F, a F(ab) '2 fragment of a murine IgG3 antibody with a high capacity for neutralization of human TNFα (74). Again, symptoms of GVHD improved quite rapidly in four of these five patients with a skin response in 4/4 and a liver and gut response in 3/4 (70). As observed in the earlier study, signs of GVHD recurred after cessation of treatment and in parallel with the decline in anti-TNFα activity in the serum of three of four responding patients. One patient became a long-term survivor. In both studies, administration of anti-TNFα MAbs was safe and did not result in an increased incidence of infections or hematopoietic side effects. These clinical studies were the first to demonstrate that TNFα is not only associated with acute GVHD, but is also an effector molecule, at least in skin and gut lesions. These studies also clearly indicated that established GVHD will not resolve with short-term treatment of anti-TNFα alone, given the rapid recurrence of GVHD symptoms in the majority of patients.

We investigated combined treatment of refractory acute GVHD using a 7-day course of daily injections of MAb 195F and OKT3 ($n = 7$), OKT3 and PTX (in a daily continuous infusion ($n = 7$), or OKT3 and high-dose corticosteroids ($n = 8$). Combination of OKT3 with MAb 195F not only resulted in improvement of acute responses and intermediate survival but also proved to be very effective with regard to prevention of the cytokine relase syndrome associated with the first dose of OKT3 (Table 3). Alternative approaches, such as combining anti-TNFα MAb BC7 with anti-CD2 MAb followed by maintenance treatment with anti-IL-2 receptor MAb, are currently underway in other centers.

In an earlier attempt to use TNFα antagonists in earlier period of acute GVHD, a multicenter phase II trial was initiated combining a 7-day course of MAb 195F with high-dose corticosteroids for primary treatment of acute GVHD. In an interim analysis of 33 patients treated thus far in our center, the response rate at day +30 was 75% in 12 patients following HLA-identical sibling donor BMT but only 36% in 11 patients following unrelated donor BMT, indicating that neutralization of TNFα may not be sufficient to treat the more intense forms of acute GVHD. Though the final analysis is pending, we have not observed an increase in infectious

Table 3 Combined Treatment of Refractory Acute GVHD with OKT3 (5 mg/day) and TNF Antagonists (7-day course)

Treatment regimen	Fever >39°C after 1st dose of OKT3	Dyspnea after 1st dose of OKT3	CR/PR of acute GVHD at day +14	4-month survival
OKT3 + Pred.	8/8	6/8	5/8	3/8
OKT3 + PTX	4/7	2/7	6/7	3/7
OKT3 + MAb195	2/7	1/7	6/7	4/7

Pred. = prednisolone 4 mg/kg/day; PTX = pentoxifylline (2100 mg/day) + low-dose prednisolone (<3 mg/kg); MAb195 = monoclonal antibody 195F, which neutralizes TNFα (d1–3:3 × 1 mg/kg, d4–7: 1 × 1 mg/kg) + low-dose prednisolone (<3 mg/kg).

complications and no interference with hematopietic recovery, because GVHD occurred in the majority of the patients prior to marrow engraftment.

C. IL-1ra

In a Boston trial of IL-1ra for patients with steroid-resistant GHVD, IL-1ra was administered as 24 hr continuous infusions for 7 days and in four separate doses (75). Seventeen patients were treated with escalating doses of IL-1ra. Twelve of 17 patients (71%) had received allogeneic marrow grafts from matched (either five or six antigens) unrelated donors, and five of 17 (29%) received marrow from HLA-identical siblings. Four patients died of accelerated GVHD before completing the course of IL-1ra but were analyzed for response; only one patient, with *Candida albicans* hepatitis and sepsis, had a liver that was inevaluable. The majority of patients had received cyclosporine and methotrexate as GVHD prophylaxis; matched unrelated donor (MUD) BMT recipients also received methylprednisolone 3 mg/kg/day beginning on day 7 after BMT. All patients with acute GVHD received methylprednisolone at 3 mg/kg/day for a minimum of 3 days before being considered resistant to steroids. Table 4 summarizes the response to IL-1ra infusion. Improvements in intestinal GVHD by at least one stage occurred in nine of 11 (92%) of evaluable patients. Complete resolution of diarrhea occurred in six of 11 (55%) of the entire group, and a reduction in the severity of gut GVHD to stage 0 or 1 occurred in eight of 11 patients (73%). Acute GVHD of the skin was improved in eight of 14 patients (57%), with complete resolution of the rash observed in three of those cases (21%). Liver responses were the most difficult to evaluate. Most patients were thrombocytopenic at the commencement of the trial and therefore liver biopsies were not performed; diagnosis of liver GVHD is based solely on clinical and laboratory findings. Improvement or resolution of GVHD occurred in only two of 11 (18%) patients. Overall reduction of acute GVHD by at least one grade was observed in 10 of 16 patients (63%). The only toxicity attributable to IL-1ra was a reversible transaminase evaluation in two patients. In this study, it thus appeared that IL-1ra was safe and had demonstrable efficacy even in acute GVHD that had failed to respond to conventional treatment. Two patients had good initial responses but acute GVHD flared upon discontinuation of the infusion and neither patient responded to a second course of IL-1ra. In addition, five of seven patients who were at risk for relapse of their acute GVHD did so after cessation of the IL-1ra. Five patients, all of whom received marrow from unrelated donors, had severe "hyperacute" GVHD occurring within 2 weeks of marrow infusion, and died of GVHD despite therapy.

Serum peripheral blood samples obtained at the beginning and end of IL-1ra treatment were available for 10 patients, and cytokine IL-1β and TNFα mRNA levels were measured using the same quantitative PCR technique developed for the mouse models (see above). Clinical data were generally consistent with observations in the murine GVHD experiments. IL-2 mRNA was below the level of detection in all samples, whereas IL-1β mRNA ranged between 1.0 and 45 pg/mg total cellular mRNA; TNFα ranged between 0.04 and 50 pg/mg. The absolute amount of cytokine mRNA at the beginning of treatment did not correlate with the severity of GVHD. When comparisons of cytokine mRNA were made at the end and at the beginning of treatment (Fig. 5), those responding to IL-1ra had approximately half

Table 4 IL-1ra Treatment for Steroid-Resistant GVHD

Age	GVHD proph.	GVHD therapy	IL → 1ra dose (mg/kg)	GVHD stage Skin	Gut	Liver	Overall grade
40	CSA/PRED	Cyc., Pred.	3200	0 → 0	4 → 1	NE	2 → 1
41	None	Cyc., MePr	1600	2 → 0	4 → 0	3 → 3	3 → 2
47	3	MePr	3200	3 → 4	NE	3 → 4	3 → 4
37	1	MePr	800	0 → 0	4 → 0	0 → 0	3 → 0
4	1	MePr	6	3 → 3	3 → 0	0 → 0	3 → 2
3	1	MePr	6	3 → 4	3 → 2	2 → 3	3 → 4
34	1	MePr	400	3 → 0	0 → 0	3 → 0	3 → 0
33	1	MePr	800	4 → 2	0 → 0	2 → NE	2 → 1
39	1	MePr	800	2 → 1	0 → 0	2 → 1	2 → 1
31	2	MePr	1600	3 → 3	2 → 0	3 → 4	4 → 4
34	2	MePr	1600	3 → 1	1 → 0	0 → 3	2 → 2
42	2	MePr	1600	3 → 4	4 → 4	2 → 3	4 → 4
20	3	MePr	3200	1 → 2	1 → 1	1 → 4	2 → 3
40	3	MePr	3200	0 → 0	3 → 1	1 → NE	2 → 1
50	4	MePr	3200	3 → 2	0 → NE	2 → NE	2 → NE
29	3	MePr	3200	4 → 1	0 → 0	0 → 1	3 → 1
5	3	MePr	12	2 → 0	4 → 0	2 → 3	3 → 2
			Response (%)	8/14 (57%)	9/11 (82%)	2/11 (18%)	10/16 (63%)

Median age (range): 34 years (3–50). Median time to IL-1ra (range): 33 days (8–128).
MePr = methylprednisolone; CSA/PRED = cyclosporine/prednisone; Cyc. = cyclosporine; Pred. = prednisone; NE = unevaluable.
Prophylactic regimens used: (1) = cyclosporine 1.5 mg/kg twice a day, methorexate 10 mg/m^2 days 1, 8, 15, 22, and 28; (2) = cyclosporine 1.5 mg/kg twice a day, methotrexate 10 mg/m^2 days 1, 8, 15, 22, and 28, plus methylprednisolone 3 mg/kg/day beginning on day 7; (3) = cyclosporine 1.5 mg/kg twice a day, methotrexate 15 mg/m^2 on day 1, and then 10 mg/m^{2}on days 3, 6, and 11, plus methylprednisolone 3 mg/kg/day beginning on day 7; (4) = cyclosporine 1.5 mg/kg twice a day, methotrexate 15 mg/m^2 on day 1, and then 10 mg/m^2 on days 3, 6, and 11.

of the IL-1β message present at the initiation of treatment, whereas those who did not respond had more than twice the amount of IL-1β mRNA. A more profound difference was seen with respect to TNFα, where at the end of 7 days responders had only 80% of pretreatment levels and nonresponders had nearly 16 times pretreatment levels (p = 0.001, matched pair t-test). Thus in those cases where IL-1ra had clinical efficacy the production of both these inflammatory cytokines was reduced. Univariate and multivariate analysis showed that only the change in TNFα mRNA between the start and conclusion of therapy was significantly associated with response in this small cohort.

In summary, the studies performed so far using specific cytokine inhibitors to neutralize IL-1 or TNFα for treatment of acute GVHD confirm their role as effector molecules, but suggest that selective interference with either cytokine alone is unable to reverse severe acute GVHD for any length of time. Thus, in established acute GVHD, cytokine antagonists might serve as temporary "bridging" treatments, providing time for additional strategies to limit tissue damage.

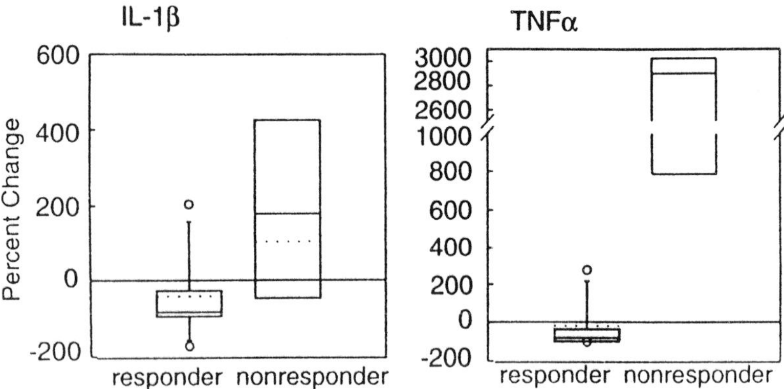

Figure 5 Box and whisker plot of the percent change in mRNA levels between the start and completion of IL-1ra therapy. (.....) Average percent change; (○) individual values that are beyond the 10th or 90th percentiles. Peripheral blood mononuclear cells were obtained by separation of heparinized whole blood on Ficoll-Hypaque, and total cellular RNA was extracted using RNAzol (Biotecx, Houston, TX) and reverse-transcribed into cDNA. IL-1β and TNFα levels were quantified using a polymerase chain reaction as previously described. (Adapted from Ref. 75.)

D. Phase I/II Trial of Prophylactic Neutralization of TNFα in the Course of Pretransplant Conditioning

Based on the above studies on systemic TNFα in GVHD and the beneficial effects of early neutralization of TNFα in murine models, a phase I/II trial of MAb 195F was started in 1991. The MAb was given throughout the period of pretransplant conditioning in addition to standard immunosuppression with cyclosporine and methotrexate. This study included high-risk patients receiving related donor BMT defined by an age above 40 years and a diagnosis of CML or myelodysplastic syndrome. Treatment was started prior to the first dose of TBI or cytotoxic drugs and stopped at midnight at the day before BMT. Three doses of MAb were tested; while the low dose proved inefficient with regard to prevention of GVHD, the high-dose group was stopped owing to observation of two late graft failures occurring more than 3 months after BMT without complete prevention of GVHD (for details see 69). Because beneficial effects were seen in the first four patients receiving the intermediate dose (1.0 mg/kg/day), this dose was chosen according to the study protocol for evaluation in an additional 10 patients. Results of this study group were compared with those of a historical control group of patients marked for age and disease. The study group and historical controls were not balanced with regard to the conditioning regimens used (TBICY vs. BUSCY), and a recent study from Seattle suggested a reduced incidence of acute GVHD in patients receiving BUSCY (76). Results of the MAb 195F prophylaxis study were therefore analyzed separately for patients receiving TBICY and BUSCY regimens (Table 5). With regard to toxicity, patients receiving MAb 195F prophylaxis showed no increase of infectious complications during the first 100 days following BMT and no delay of hematopoietic engraftment. Donor engraftment, as detected by isoenzyme typing and cytogenetic analysis of bone marrow in CML patients, was complete at day

Table 5 Summary of the Results of the Phase II Trial Using the anti-TNFα MAb195F (3 × 1 mg/kg) During Pretransplant Conditioning as an Additive Prophylaxis

	Overall incidence of GVHD grade II		Median time to onset of GVHD II (days)		Overall incidence of GVHD grade III/IV	
	TBI	BUS	TBI	BUS	TBI	BUS
Anti-TNF-alpha	2/3	5/11	26	50	0/3	2/11
Historical control	9/9	7/9	14	35	6/9	4/9

Patients were separately analyzed according to the type of pretransplant conditioning. TBI = total body irradiation (3 × 4 Gy/day) followed by cyclophosphamide; BUS = oral busulfan (4 × 4 mg/kg/day) followed by cyclophosphamide. The overall incidence of GVHD grade II observed until day 100 was not statistically different between groups; onset of aGVHD was delayed ($p < 0.05$ for TBI, < 0.10 for BUS) in anti-TNFα-treated patients. This trended toward reduced incidence of severe GVHD (grade III/IV) in patients receiving TNFα during TBI conditioning ($p < .10$).

+30 in 17/18 patients of the historical control and in 12/14 patients receiving MAb 195F prophylaxis. In addition, the onset of acute GVHD was delayed in the study group, with a trend toward reduction in overall GVHD incidence (Fig. 6). Importantly, there was a reduction of severe GVHD (grade III/IV) and a 4-month survival rate of 79% in the MAb 195F groups versus 67% in the historical control group. These phase II data demonstrate that neutralization of TNFα in the period of pretransplant conditioning can be safely applied in the setting of human allogeneic BMT, and potential benefits await confirmation in a randomized trial, which is currently underway.

E. Pentoxifylline as a Pharmacological TNF Antagonist

Pentoxifylline (PTX), a well-established drug formerly used for its feasible rheological effects in patients with arteriosclerosis, has recently generated considerable interest for its suppression of TNFα transcription via its phosphodiesterase inhibitor activity. This effect could be clearly demonstrated in animals and human volunteers receiving LPS injections as well as in several studies on prevention of the cytokine release syndrome following the first dose of anti-CD3 MAbs (for review see 63). Based on these effects and on the first reports on favorable effects of PTX in patients with amphotericin nephrotoxicity in the setting of BMT, a phase I/II study with oral PTX given for the whole period of allogeneic BMT was performed by Bianco et al. (77) and suggested reduction of regimen-related toxicity as well as of acute GVHD when compared with historical controls. Since that report, several studies (78–80) were unable to repeat these beneficial observations. These negative results in subsequent trials are confusing, as TNF-suppressing activities of PTX have been clearly documented in a variety of experimental conditions. However, TNFα levels were not evaluated in these trials. The most likely explanation for the negative results observed in randomized PTX trials is that clinically achievable PTX levels are too low to suppress TNFα release; this effect has been directly documented in a recent small study where patients receiving PTX prophylaxis and suffering from

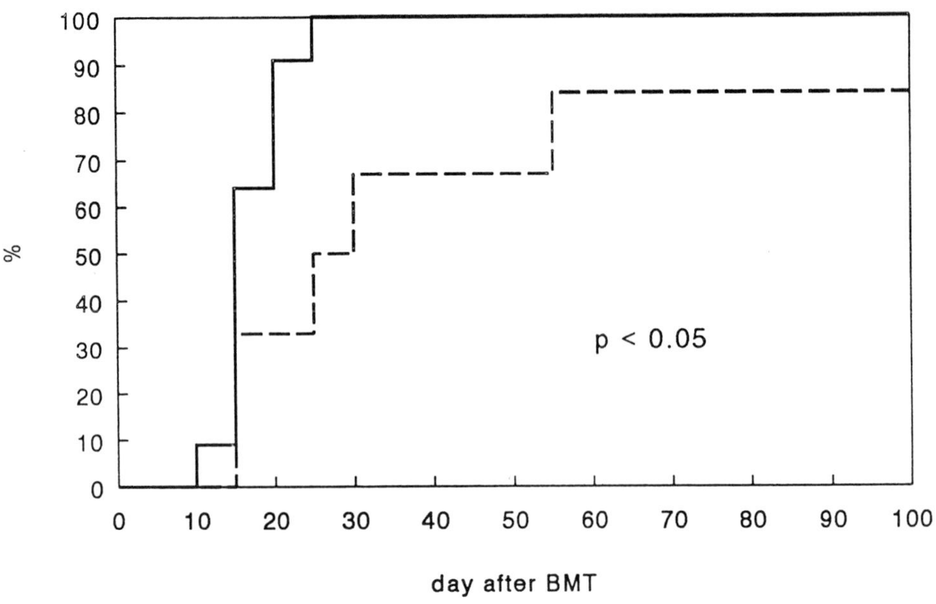

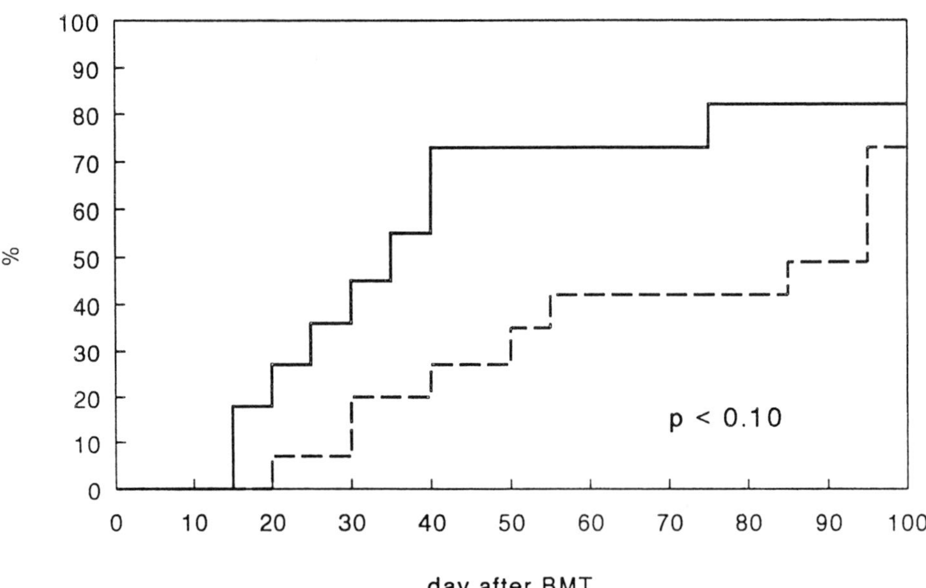

Figure 6 Cumulative incidence of acute GVHD (≥grade II) in patients receiving prophylactic anti-TNFα MAb as compared to historical controls (see Table 5). (A) Patients receiving conditioning regimen of total body irradiation (TBI, fractions of 4 Gy on three consecutive days) followed by cyclophosphamide (CY, 60 mg/kg for 2 days or 50 mg/kg for 4 consecutive days). Control, $n = 11$ (–); anti-TNF, $n = 6$ (---); $p < 0.05$. (B) Patients receiving oral busulfan (BUS) (4 mg/kg/day on 4 consecutive days) followed by CY. Control, $n = 11$ (–); anti-TNF, $n = 15$ (---); $p < 0.10$.

acute GVHD nevertheless demonstrated significant levels of TNFα in their serum (81). It is also possible that PTX has other deleterious effects that counterbalance the beneficial reduction in TNFα secretion. Investigation of new phosphodiesterase inhibitors or related drugs that inhibit transcription of TNFα still seems an attractive approach for prevention of TNFα release in the setting of allogeneic BMT and deserves more detailed analysis of bioavailability and efficacy with respect to experimental and clinical endpoints.

III. SYNOPSIS AND CRITICAL OUTLOOK

A. Major Concerns and Unresolved Issues in the Use of Inflammatory Cytokine Antagonists

Though the data discussed up to now demonstrate a substantial role of IL-1 and TNFα as a critical mediator involved in induction as well as in the effector phase of acute GVHD, a variety of issues still require examination. A major concern is still the lack of information regarding the various phases of cytokine-mediated effects. So far, both TNFα and IL-1 have been identified as critical mediators released in the host phase as well as in the effector phase of acute GVHD. Both mediators may need to be neutralized to achieve an optimal effect. In that case, broader cytokine antagonists would be preferable, and it might be difficult to prove superiority of any single antagonist as compared to corticosteroids.

Involvement of inflammatory cytokines in various phases of BMT suggests that prolonged neutralization is needed to optimize protection from cytokine-mediated damage. Chronic administration of potent antagonists, such as MAbs, raises concerns regarding interference with antimicrobial defense. Neutralization of TNFα in models of chronic bacterial infection such as peritonitis has been reported to increase morality (82), presumably due to the need for TNFα in focusing the inflammatory response and subsequently preventing bacterial spread and diffuse inflammation. A similar mechanism may pertain to the containment of viral infections, stressing the need to define optimal windows for neutralizations of TNFα in immunocompromised BMT patients.

The exact role of inflammatory cytokines in mediating the cytotoxic effects of irradiation or cytotoxic drugs is still poorly defined. There is some evidence that TNFα augments tumor cell cytotoxicity of drugs like etoposide or cisplatin, and TNFα has been demonstrated to suppress growth of normal as well as malignant hematopoietic progenitors (83). Thus neutralization of TNF α might interfere with eradication of leukemic cells during pretransplant conditioning. Graft-versus-leukemia (GVL) effects are the major therapeutic principle of allogeneic BMT (see Truitt chap. 14). Because both the IL-1 and TNFα are produced by all cellular components postulated to be involved in GVL (84,85), their neutralization might diminish GVL as well.

Finally, the optimal approach to neutralization of inflammatory cytokines is an important topic. In experimental studies, both neutralizing antibodies and recombinant soluble TNF receptors have proved effective in reducing GVHD. In a direct comparison of anti-TNF-MAbs and soluble TNF receptors in various T-cell-mediated immunopathological conditions, Piguet and Grau postulated superiority of MAbs in diseases characterized by systemic release of TNFα (86); however, further studies comparing the existing antagonists, pharmacological agents, and new drugs in development are needed to clarify this question. For evaluation of the pathophysiological role of cytokines in allogeneic BMT, the specific agent used for neutralization seems to be of minor relevance as long as efficacious neutralization of release or production is assured.

B. Potential Advantages of Inflammatory Cytokine Antagonists

Neutralization of inflammatory cytokines as an alternative approach to prevent or treat early GVHD should be considered in the context of effective GVHD prevention by T-cell depletion. The problem of an increased relapse rate observed after T-cell depletion might be approached by subsequent reinfusion of donor T cells in a period when patients have recovered from conditioning-related damage, as suggested by Waldmann et al. (87). However, the period when the presence of donor T cells is required to control residual disease is still poorly defined. Recent work in murine GVL models suggests that there is a limited window of time in which T cells are required to produce an antitumor effect (see Truitt chap. 14). Reducing nonspecific inflammation induced by pretransplant conditioning but preserving donor T-cell maturation in an early posttransplant period as is achieved by prophylactic neutralization of cytokines might prove an attractive alternative approach to temporal dissociation of GVHD and GVL effects. Such an approach appears to be supported by murine studies (29) as well as by results of our phase I/II trial on prophylactic neutralization of TNFα, because the incidence and severity of acute GVHD are reduced without modulation of chronic GVHD.

A second and as yet poorly analyzed issue is the pathophysiological role of cytokines in other acute transplant-related complications that contribute to early mortality following BMT. There is clinical evidence that systemic release of TNFα is associated with the occurrence of VOD (70,88). A possible contribution of liver macrophages, i.e. Kupffer cells, to pathophysiology of VOD seems likely because they are the largest macrophage compartment of the body and the first macrophages in the line of defense against endotoxin and other microbial products translocated from a damaged gastrointestinal mucosa. Prostaglandins have been reported to interfere with Kupffer cell activation and cytokine production, which may explain the beneficial effects of prophylactic PGE_2 infusion on occurrence and severity of VOD (89). Such effects may be partially explained by local cytokine production, although we have been unable to observe modulation of TNFα levels in patients receiving PGE_2 prophylaxis (E. Holler, unpublished data). Similar pathways of cytokine-mediated pathophysiology appear to underlie interstitial pneumonitis or idiopathic pneumonia syndrome (see Chap. 15) and late pulmonary complications such as fibrosis. Piguet et al. have reported a necrotizing alveolits associated with experimental GVHD, which is characterized by massive expression of TNFα mRNA within the lung (90) and which is reversed by anti-TNFα mAbs. In a more recent study, neutralizing anti-TNFα antibodies strongly suppressed development of CMV-mediated pneumonitis (23). In addition, radiation-induced damage of the lung, which contributes significantly to pulmonary complications in clinical BMT, is characterized by enhanced expression of fibrogenic cytokines such as TGFβ (91), which in turn is strongly induced by TNFα. Thus, further investigation on the use of TNF antagonists for prevention or even early treatment of interstitial pneumonitis is clearly justified.

Analysis of inflammatory cytokine production and release has provided novel insights into the complex patterns of immunoregulatory mechanisms involved in the pathophysiology of acute GVHD. The identification of a subgroup of patients that seems to be protected by an altered pattern of high spontaneous TNFα release prior to conditioning is a strong argument that future patients can be stratified for their risk of developing TRC after BMT based on a detailed analysis of individual cytokine regulation, which includes proinflammatory as well as antagonistic cytokines. Thus, with improving knowledge of cytokine dysregulation in the various phases of BMT, blockade of inflammatory cytokines may emerge as a beneficial approach to the prevention and treatment of transplant-related complications.

ACKNOWLEDGMENTS

This work was supported by grants from the Deutsche Forschungs Gemeinschaft (DFG Grant Ho 1142) and NIH Grants CA4952, AI30018, and HL55162.

REFERENCES

1. Carswell EA, Old LJ, Kassel RL, Green S, Fiore N, Williamson B. An endotoxin induced serum factor that causes necrosis of tumors. Proc Natl Acad Sci USA 1975; 72: 3666–3670.
2. Fiers W. Tumor necrosis factor – Characterization at the molecular, cellular and in vivo level. FEBS 1991; 285:199–212.
3. Tracey KJ, Vlassara H, Cerami A. Cachectin/tumour necrosis factor. Lancet 1989; 1122–1126.
4. Deem RL, Shanahan F, Targan SR. Triggered human mucosal T cells release tumour necrosis factor alpha and interferon gamma which kill human colonic epithelial cells. Clin Exp Immunol 1991; 83:79–84.
5. Symington FW. Lymhotoxin, tumor necrosis factor and gamma interferon are cytostatic for normal human keratinocytes. J Invest Dermatol 1989; 92:798–804.
6. Pober JS. Effects of tumour necrosis factor and related cytokines on vascular endothelial cells. In:Tumour Necrosis Factor and Related Cytotoxins. Chichester, Sussex: Wiley, 1987:170–184.
7. Johnson DR, Pober JS. Tumor necrosis factor regulation of major histocompatibility complex gene expression. Immunol Res 1991; 10:141–155.
8. Robinet E, Branellec D, Termijtelen AM, Blay JY, Gay F, Chouaib S. Evidence for tumor necrosis factor alpha involvement in the optimal induction of class I allospecific cytotoxic T cells. J Immunol 1990; 144:4555–4561.
9. Hogquist KA, Nett MA, Unanue ER, Chaplin DD. Interleukin-1 is processed and released during apoptosis. Proc Natl Acad Sci USA 1991; 88:8485–8489.
10. Yuan J, S. S, S. L, et al. The *C. elegans* cell death gene *ced*-3 encodes a protein similar to mammalian interleukin-1 beta converting enzyme. Cell 1993; 75:641–652.
11. Kuida K, Lippke JA, Ku G, Harding MW, Livingston DJ, Su MS-S, Flavell RA. Altered cytokine export and apoptosis in mice deficient in interleukin-1β converting enzyme. Science 1995; 268:2000–2003.
12. Miura M, Zhu H, Rotello R, et al. Induction of apoptosis in fibroblasts by IL-1 beta converting enzyme, a mammalian homolog of the *C. elegans* cell death gene *ced*-3. Cell 1993; 75:653–660.
13. Itoh N, Yonehara S, Ishii A, et al. The poypeptide encoded by the cDNA for human cell surface antigen Fas can mediate apoptosis. Cell 1991; 66:233–243.

14. Ju ST, Panka, DJ, Cui H, et al. Fas (CD95)/FasL interactions required for programmed cell death after T-cell activation. Nature 1995; 373:444–448.
15. Eisenberg SP, Evans RJ, Arend WP, Verderberr E, Brewer MT, Hannum CH, Thompson RC. Primary structure and functional expression from complementary DNA of a human interleukin-1 receptor antagonist. Nature 1990; 343:341.
16. Arend WP. Interleukin-1 receptor antagonist. Adv Immunol 1993; 54:167–227.
17. Granowitz EV, Clark BD, Mancilla J, et al. Interleukin-1 receptor antagonist competitively inhibits the binding of interleukin-1 to the type II interleukin-1 receptor. J Biol Chem 1991; 266:14147–14150.
18. Arend WP, Welgus HG, Thompson RC, Eisenberg SP. Biological properties of recombinant human monocyte-derived interleukin-1 receptor antagonist. J Clin Invest 1990; 85:1694–1697.
19. Haskill S, Martin G, Van Le L, Morris J, Peace A, Bigler CF, Jaffe GJ, Hammerberg C, Sporn SA, Fong S, Arend WP, Raph P. cDNA cloning of an intracellular form of the human interleukin-1 receptor antagonist associated with epithelium. Proc Natl Acad Sci USA 1990; 88:3681–3685.
20. Aukrust P, Froland S, Liabakk NB, Muller F, Nordoy I, Haug C, Espevik T. Release of cytokines, soluble cytokine receptors, and interleukin-1 receptor antagonist after intravenous immunoglobulin administration in vivo. Blood 1994; 84:2136–2143.
21. Nestel FP, Price KS, Seemayer TA, Lapp WS. Macrophage priming and lipolysaccharide-triggered release of tumor necrosis factor alpha during graft-versus-host disease. J Exp Med 1992; 175:405–413.
22. Niederwieser D, Herold M, Woloszczuk W, Aulitsky W, Meister B, Tilg H, Gastl G, Bowden R, Huber C. Endogenous IFN-gamma during human bone marrow transplantation. Transplantation 1990; 50:620–625.
23. Haagmans BL, Stals FS, van der Meide PH, Bruggeman CA, Horzinek MC, Schijns VEC. Tumor necrosis factor alpha promotes replication and pathogenicity of rat cytomegalovirus. J Virol 1994; 68:2297–2304.
24. Hallahan DE, Spriggs DR, Beckett MA, Kufe DW, Weichselbaum RR. Increased tumor necrosis factor alpha mRNA after cellular exposure to ionizing radiation. Proc Natl Acad Sci USA 1989; 86:10104–10107.
25. Sherman ML, Datta R, Hallahan D, Weichselbaum RR, Kufe DW. Regulation of tumor necrosis factor gene expression in human myeloid leukemia cells and peripheral blood monocytes. J Clin Invest 1991; 87:1794–1797.
26. Iwamoto KS, McBride WH. Production of 13-hydroxyoctadecadienoic acid and tumor necrosis factor alpha by murine peritoneal macrophages in response to irradiation. Radiat Res 1994; 139:103–108.
27. Hoffmann B, Hintermeier-Knabe R, Holler E, Kempeni J, Brockhaus M, Kolb HJ, Wilmanns W. Evidence for induction of TNFalpha by irradiation and cytotoxic therapy preceding bone marrow transplantation—in vivo and in vitro studies. Netw 1992; 3:257 (abstract).
28. Girinsky TA, Pallardy M, Comoy E, Benassi T, Roger R, Ganem G, Cosset JM, Socie G, Magdelenat H. Peripheral blood corticotropin-releasing factor, adrenocorticotropic hormone and cytokine (interleukin beta, interleukin 6, tumor necrosis factor alpha) levels after high- and low dose total-body irradiation in humans. Radiat Res 1994; 139: 360–363.
29. Xun CQ, Thompson JS, Jennings CD, Brown SA, Widmer MB. Effect of total body irradiation, busulfan-cyclophosphamide, or cyclophosphamide conditioning on inflammatory cytokine release and development of acute and chronic graft-versus-host disease in H-2-incompatible transplanted SCID mice. Blood 1994; 83:2360–2367.
30. Abhyankar S, Gilliland DG, Ferrara JLM. Interleukin 1 is a critical effector molecule

during cytokine dysregulation in graft-versus-host disease to minor histocompatibility antigens. Transplantation 1993; 56:1518–1523.
31. Brugger W, Reinhardt D, Galanos C, Andreesen R. Inhibition of in vitro differentiation of human monocytes to macrophages by lipopolysaccharides (LPS): Phenotypic and functional analysis. Intern Immunol 1991; 3:221–227.
32. Thomas ED, Ramberg RE, Sale GE, Sparkes RS, Golde DW. Direct evidence for a bone marrow origin of the alveolar macrophage in man. Science 1976; 192:1016–1018.
33. Perreault C, Pelletier M, Belanger R, Boileau J, Bonny Y, David M, Gyger M, Landry D, Montplaisir S. Persistence of host Langerhans cells following allogeneic bond marrow transplantation: Possible relationship with acute graft-versus-host disease. Br J Haematol 1985; 60:253–260.
34. Barker JNWN, Mitra RS, Griffiths CEM, Dixit VM, Nickoloff BJ. Kerationocytes as initiators of inflammation. Lancet 1991; 337:211–214.
35. Walsh LJ, Trinchieri G, Waldorf HA, Whitaker D, Murphy GF. Human dermal mast cells contain and release tumor necrosis factor alpha which induces endothelial leukocyte adhesion molecule 1. Proc Natl Acad Sci USA 1991; 88:4420–4424.
36. Murphy GF, Sueki H, Teuscher C, Whitaker D, Korngold R. Role of mast cells in early epithelial target cell injury in experimental acute graft-versus-host disease. J Invest Dermatol 1994; 102:451–461.
37. Dickinson AM, Sviland L, Dunn J, Carey P, Proctor SJ. Demonstration of direct involvement of cytokines in graft-versus-host reactions using an in vitro skin explant model. Bone Marrow Transplant 1991; 7:209–216.
38. Antin JH, Ferrara JLM. Cytokine dysregulation and acute graft-versus-host disease. Blood 1992; 80:2964–2968.
39. Danzer SG, Kirchner H, Rink L. Cytokine interactions in human mixed lymphocyte culture. Transplanation 1994; 57:1638–1642.
40. Dickinson AM, Sviland L, Jackson G, Dunn J, Stephens S, Proctor SJ. Monoclonal anti-TNF-alpha supresses graft-vs host disease reactions in an vitro human skin model. Cytokine 1994; 6:141–146.
41. Piguet PF, Grau GE, Allet B, Vassalli PJ. Tumor necrosis factor/cachectin is an effector of skin and gut lesions of the acute phase of graft-versus-host disease. J Exp Med 1987; 166:1280–1289.
42. Piguet PF, Grau GE, Vassalli P. Tumor necrosis factor and immunopathology. Immunol Res 1991; 10:122–140.
43. Shalaby MR, Fendly B, Sheehan KC, Schreiber RD, Ammann AJ. Prevention of the graft-vs-host reaction in newborn mice by antibodies to tumor necrosis factor-alpha. Transplantation 1989; 47:1057–1061.
44. Holler E, Thierfelder S, Behrends U, Daum L, Hintermeier-Knabe R, Kolb HJ, Kempeni J, Wilmanns W. Anti-TNF-alpha and pentoxifylline for prophylaxis of a GVHD in murine allogeneic bone marrow transplantation. Oncologie 1992; 15:31–35.
45. Wall DA, Sheehan KCF. The role of tumor necrosis factor and interferon gamma in graft-versus-host disease and related immunodeficiency. Transplantation 1994; 57:273–279.
46. Cohen J. Cytokines as mediators of graft-versus-host disease. Bone Marrow Transplant 1988; 3:193–197.
47. Allen RD, Staley TA, Sidman CL. Differential cytokine expression acute and chronic murine graft-versus-host disease. Eur J Immunol 1993; 23:333–337.
48. Ferrara JLM, Abhyankar S, Gilliland DG. Cytokine storm of graft-versus-host disease: A critical effector role for interleukin-1. Transplant Proc 1993; 25:1216–1217.
49. Lehnert S, W. B. R. Amplification of the graft-versus-host reaction by cylophosphamide: Dependence on timing of drug administration. Bone Marrow Transplant 1994; 13:473–477.

50. Zwaan FE, Janson J, Noordijk EM. Graft-versus host disease limited to area of irradiated skin. Lancet 1980; 1:1081–1082.
51. Desbarats J, Seemayer TA, Lapp WS. Irradiation of the skin and systemic graft-versus-host disease synergize to produce cutaneous lesions. Am J Pathol 1994; 144:883–888.
52. Irle C, Salamin AF, Bacigalupo A, Chapuis B, Gratwohl A, Hows J, Piguet PF, Grau GE. Serum TNF levels during graft versus host disease after bone marrow transplantation. Bone Marrow Transplant 1988; 3:127 (abstract).
53. Robinet E, Ibrahim A, Truneh A, Ostronoff M, Mishal Z, Zambon E, Gay F, Hayat M, Pico J-L, Chouaib S. Serum levels and receptor expression of tumor necrosis factor-alpha following human allogeneic and autologous bone marrow transplantation. Transplantation 1992; 53:574–579.
54. Symington FW, Pepe MS, Chen A, Deliganis A. Serum tumor necrosis factor alpha associated with acute graft-versus-host disease in humans. Transplantation 1990; 50: 518–521.
55. Holler E, Kolb HJ, Moller A, Kempeni J, Lisenfeld S, Pechumer H, Lehmacher W, Ruckdeschel G, Gleixner B, Riedner C, Ledderose G, Brehm G, Mittermuller J, Wilmanns W. Increased serum levels of tumor necrosis factor alpha precede major complications of bone marrow transplanation. Blood 1990; 75:1011–1016.
56. Rowbottom AW, Riches PG, Downie C, Hobbs JR. Monitoring cytokine production in peripheral blood during acute graft-versus-host disease following allogeneic bone marrow transplantation. Bone Marrow Transplant 1993; 12:635–641.
57. Engelberts I, Stephens S, Francot GJM, Van der Linden CJ, Buurman WA. Evidence for different effects of soluble TNF-receptors on various TNF measurements in human biological fluids. Lancet 1991; 338:515–516.
58. Tanaka J, Imamura M, Kasai M, Masauzi N, Watanabe M, Matsuura A, Morii K, Kiyama Y, Naohara T, Higa T, Honke K, Gasa S, Sakurada K, Miyazaki T. Rapid analysis of tumor necrosis factor-alpha mRNA expression during venooclusive disease of the liver after allogeneic bone marrow transplantation. Transplantation 1993; 55: 430–432.
59. Tanaka J, Imamura M, Kasai M, Masauzi N, Matsuura A, Ohizumi H, Morik Y, Naohara T, Saitho M, Higa T, Honke K, Gasa S, Sakurada K, Miyazaki T. Cytokine gene expression in peripheral blood mononuclear cells during graft-versus-host disease after allogeneic bone marrow transplantation. Br J Haematol 1993; 85:558–565.
60. Holler E, Kolb HJ, Hintermeier-Knabe R, Mittermuller J, Thierfelder S, Behrends U, Hultner L, Kempeni J, Kaul M, Silmanns W. Involvement in cytokines in graft-versus-host disease and graft-versus-leukemia activity. In: Bergmann L, Mitrou PS, eds. Cytokines in Cancer Therapy. Basel; Karger, 1994:318–329.
61. Rowbottom AW, Norton J, Riches PG, Hobbs JR, Powles RL, Sloane JP. Cytokine gene expression in skin and lymphoid organs in graft versus host disease. J Clin Pathol 1993; 46:341–345.
62. Remberger M, Ringden O, Marhlin L. TNF alpha levels during bone marrow transplantation (BMT) conditioning are increased in patients who develop GVHD and decreased in patients who relapse. In: 1st Intern. Symposium on Cytokines in Bone Marrow Transplantation. New Zealand: Christchurch, 1993.
63. Holler E, Kolb HJ, Hintermeier-Knabe R, Mittermuller J, Thierfelde S, Kaul M, Wilmanns W. The role of tumor necrosis factor alpha in acute graft-versus-host disease and complications following allogeneic bone marrow transplantation. Transplant Proc 1993; 25:1234–1236.
64. Holler E, Hintermeier-Knabe R, Kolb HJ, Kempeni J, Moller A, Liesenfeld S, Daum L, Wilmanns W. Low incidence of transplant related complications in patients with chronic release of TNFalpha before admission to bone marrow transplantation—A clinical correlate of cytokine desensitization? Pathobiology 1991; 59:171–175.

65. Meliconi R, Uguccioni M, Lalli E, Nesci S, Delfini C, Paradisi O, Lucarrelli G, Gasbarrini G, Facchini A. Increased serum concentrations of tumour necrosis factor in beta-thalassaemia: Effect of bone marrow transplantation. J Clin Pathol 1992; 45:61–65.
66. Akhtar I, Gold JP, Pan LY, Ferrara JLM, Yang XD, Kim JI, Tan KN. $CD4^{+}\beta$ islet cell-reactive T cell clones that suppress autoimmune diabetes in nonobese diabetic mice. J Exp Med 1995; 182:87–97.
67. Turner DM, Grant SCD, Lamb WR, Brenchley PEC, Dyer PA, Sinnott PJ, Hutchinson IV. A genetic marker of high TNF-α production in heart transplant recipients. Transplantation 1995; 60:1113–1117.
68. Remberger M, Ringden O, Markling L. TNFα levels are increased during bone marrow transplantation conditioning in patients who develop acute GVHD. Bone Marrow Transplant 1995; 15:99–104.
69. Holler E, Kolb HJ, Mittermüller J, Kaul M, Ledderose G, Duell T, Seeber B, Schleuning M, Hintermeier-Knabe R, Ertl B, Kempeni J, Wilmanns W. Modulation of acute graft-versus-host disease after allogeneic bone marrow transplantation by tumor necrosis factor α (TNFα) release in the course of pretransplant conditioning: Role of conditioning regimens and prophylactic application of a monoclonal antibody neutralizing human TNFα (MAK 195F). Blood 1995; 86:890–899.
70. Holler E, Kolb HJ, Hintermeier-Knabe R, Kempeni J, Moller A, Wilmanns W. Systemic release of tumor necrosis factor alpha in human allogeneic bone marrow transplantation: Clinical risk factors, prognostic significance and therapeutic approaches. In: Link, Freund, Schmidt, Welte, eds. Cytokines in Hempoiesis, Oncology and AIDS II. Berlin-Heidelberg: Springer, 1992:435–442.
71. Almawi WY, Lipman ML, Stevens AC, Zanker B, Hadro ET, Strom TB. Abrogation of glucocorticosteroid-mediated inhibition of T cell proliferation by the synergistic action of IL-1, IL-6 and IFNgamma. J Immunol 1991; 146:3523–3527.
72. Holler E, Kolb HJ, Wilmanns W. Treatment of GVHD-TNF-antibodies and related antagonists. Bone Marrow Transplant 1993; 12 Suppl 3:29–31.
73. Herve P, Flesch M, Tiberghien P, Wijdenes J, Racadot E, Bordigoni P, Plouvier E, Stephan JL, Bourdeau H, Holler E, Lioure B, Roche C, Vilmer E, Demeocq F, Kuentz M, Cahn YJ. Phase I–II trial of a monoclonal anti-tumor necrosis factor alpha antibody for the treatment of refractory severe acute graft-versus-host disease. Blood 1992; 79: 3362–3368.
74. Möller A, Emling F, Blohm D, Schlick E, Schollmeier K. Monoclonal antibodies to human tumor necrosis factor alpha: In vitro and in vivo application. Cytokine 1990; 2: 162–169.
75. Antin JH, Weinstein HJ, Guinan EC, McCarthy P, Bierer BE, Gilliland DG, Parsons SK, Ballen KK, Rimm IJ, Falzarano G, Bloedow DC, Abate L, Lebsack M, Burakoff SJ, Ferrara JLM. Recombinant human interleukin-1 receptor antagonist in the treatment of steroid-resistant graft-versus-host disease. Blood 1994; 84:1342–1348.
76. Clift RA, Buckner CD, Thomas WI, Bensinger WI, Bowden R, Bryant E, Deeg HJ, Doney KC, Fisher LD, Hansen JA, Martin P, McDonald GB, Sanders JE, Schoch G, Singer J, Storb R, Sullivan KM, Witherspoon RP, Appelbaum FR. Marrow transplantation for chronic myeloid leukemia: A randomized study comparing cyclophosphamide and total body irradiation with busulfan and cyclophosphamide. Blood 1994; 84:2036–2043.
77. Bianco JJ, Appelbaum FR, Guiffre A, et al. Phase I–II trial of pentoxifylline for the prevention of transplant-related toxicities following bond marrow transplantation. Blood 1991; 78:1205–1211.
78. Clift RA, Bianco JA, Appelbaum FR, Buckner CD, Singer JW, Bakke L, Bensinger WI, Bowden RA, McDonald GB, Schubert M, Shields AF, Slattery JT, Storb R, Fisher LD, Mori M, Thomas ED, Hansen JA. A randomized controlled trial of

pentoxifylline for the prevention of regimen-related toxicities in patients undergoing allogeneic bone marrow transplantation. Blood 1993; 82:2025–2030.

79. Attal M, Huguet F, Rubie H, Charlet J-P, Schlaifer D, Huynh A, Laurent G, Pris J. Prevention of regimen-related toxicities after bone marrow transplantation by pentoxifylline: A prospective, randomized trial. Blood 1993; 82:732–736.

80. Kahls P, Lechner K, Stockschlader M, Kruger W, Peters S, Zander A. Pentoxifylline did not prevent transplant-related toxicity in 31 consecutive allogeneic bone marrow transplant recipients. Blood 1992; 80:2683 (letter).

81. Malich U, Tischler HJ, Petersen D, Freund M, Lux E, Link H. Pentoxifylline and levels of tumor necrosis factor alpha after bone marrow transplantation. In Garmisch-PartenKirchen, ed. 19th Annual Meeting of the EBMT. Munich: MMV-Verlag, 1993: 807 (abstract).

82. Echtenacher B, Falk W, Maennel DN, Krammer PH. Requirement of endogenous tumor necrosis factor/cachectin for recovery from experimental peritonitis. J Immunol 1990; 145:3762–3766.

83. Wisniewski D, Strife A, Atzpodien J, Clarkson BD. Effects of recombinant human tumor necrosis factor on highly enriched progenitor cell populations from normal human bone marrow and peripheral blood and bone marrow from patients with chronic myeloid leukemia. Cancer Res 1987; 47:4788–4794.

84. Kohn FR, Phillips GL, Klingemann H-G. Regulation of tumor necrosis factor-alpha production and gene expression in monocytes. Bone Marrow Transplant 1992; 9:369–376.

85. Bruserud O, Hamann W, Patel S, Ehninger G, H. S, Pawelec G. γ and α secretion by CD4$^+$ and CD8$^+$ TCR$\alpha\beta$+ T-cell clones derived early after allogeneic bone marrow transplantation. Eur J Haematol 1993; 51:73–79.

86. Piguet PF, Grau GE. TNF and IL-1 antagonists in immunopathological reactions. Eur Cytokine Network 1992; 3:126 (abstract).

87. Waldmann H, Cobbold S, Hale G. What can be done to prevent graft versus host disease? Curr Opin Immunol 1994; 6:777–783.

88. Bearman SI. The syndrome of hepatic veno-occlusive disease after marrow transplantation. Blood 1995; 85:3005–3020.

89. Gluckman E, Jolivet I, Scrobohaci ML, Devergie A, Traineau R, Bourdeau-Esperou H, Lehn P, Faure P, Drouet L. Use of prostaglandin E1 for prevention of liver veno-occlusive disease in leukemic patients treated with allogeneic bone marrow transplantation. Br J Haematol 1990; 74:277–281.

90. Piguet PF, Grau GE, Collart MA, Vassalli P, Kapanci Y. Pneumopathies of the graft-versus-host reaction: Alveolitis associated with an increased level of tumor necrosis factor MRNA and chronic interstitial pneumonities. Lab Invest 1989; 61:37–45.

91. Rubin P, Finkelstein J, Shapiro D. Molecular biology mechanisms in the radiation induction of pulmonary injury syndromes: Interrelationship between the alveolar macrophage and the septal fibroblast. Int J Radiat Oncol Biol Phys 1992; 24:93–101.

26

The Role of Interleukin-10 in Transplantation and GVHD

Maria-Grazia Roncarolo
DNAX Research Institute of Molecular and Cellular Biology
Palo Alto, California

I. INTRODUCTION

Despite significant progress in the past 20 years, acute and chronic graft-versus-host disease (GVHD) remains the principal complication after allogeneic bone marrow transplantation and is still a major obstacle to reaching long-term engraftment and disease-free survival in transplanted patients (for review, see Ref. 1). GVHD is due to activation of alloreactive T cells of donor origin, which recognize alloantigens expressed on host antigen-presenting cells (APC). After contact with antigen on APC, activated T cells profilerate extensively and release various cytokines. This initial immune response leads to a cascade of events, including upregulation of adhesion and costimulatory molecules, migration and dissemination of T cells throughout the body, recruitment of other effector cells, and activation of macrophages that release proinflammatory cytokines and cause tissue damage (for reviews, see Refs. 2 and 3). These complications are more serious in patients receiving chemotherapy and irradiation prior to the transplant, which also result in inflammation and tissue damage (for review, see Ref. 4). Therefore, two major mechanisms play a key role in the pathogenesis of GVHD: the activation of the alloreactive T cells and the inflammation elicited by both irradiation and the chain of events that constitutes a graft-versus-host reaction (GVHR). The relative contribution of these two events to the clinical manifestations of the disease remains to be determined.

Several therapeutic approaches have been explored to prevent or overcome T-cell activation and inflammation. One strategy is based on purging the donor marrow inoculum of mature T cells by ex vivo T-cell depletion or by in vivo administration of T-cell–depleting antibodies. Although a significant reduction in the incidence of GVHD was achieved with T-cell depletion, the rate of allograft failure and tumor relapse increased substantially, indicating that the donor-derived T cells also had a beneficial role in promoting engraftment and mediating anti-tumor effects (5,6). Another strategy currently employed in several clinical protocols is the use of nonspecific immunosuppressive drugs, mainly cyclosporin A (CsA) and FK506. Although these drugs have been used successfully to prevent and treat GVHD, they have unwanted side effects, such as infectious complications, nephrotoxicity, and hepatotoxicity. In addition, treatment with these drugs often fails to induce permanent tolerance of the allograft (7,8).

Recently, much attention has been focused on the induction of tolerance, either in the thymus or in the periphery, by blocking the costimulatory signals required for optimal T-cell activation. Clinical trials using monoclonal antibodies or soluble antagonists directed against adhesion and costimulatory molecules are in progress (9,10). Whether this approach in humans will result in host-specific tolerance, with long-term deletion or inactivation of host-specific T cells without affecting normal immune responses, remains to be established.

A large body of evidence supports the notion that cytokine dysregulation plays a critical role in the events leading to GVHD (4,11). In particular, interleukin-2 (IL-2) and interferon-gamma (IFN-γ) produced by the donor-derived T cells are involved in the initial amplification of allogeneic responses, whereas IL-1, IL-6, tumor necrosis factor alpha (TNF-α), and chemokines, produced by the host APC, significantly contribute to the strong inflammatory responses characteristic of this disease. Therefore, modulation of the production and biological effects of certain cytokines may represent a logical target to achieve immunosuppression. Furthermore, to prevent GVHD, therapy with cytokines or cytokine antagonists or with neutralizing antibodies to either cytokines or cytokine receptors may have fewer side effects than other therapeutic interventions currently available. The use of either IL-1α receptor antagonist, anti-IL-2α receptor mAb, or anti-TNF-α mAb has shown promising results in both the prophylaxis and treatment of GVHD (reviewed elsewhere in this book and in Refs. 12–14).

The cytokine IL-10 is a potent immunosuppressant. IL-10 was initially described as cytokine synthesis inhibitory factor (CSIF), a product of mouse T-helper 2 (Th2) cell clones, which inhibited cytokine synthesis and effector functions of mouse T-helper 1 (Th1) cell clones (15). This novel activity was the basis for the isolation of cDNA clones coding for both murine IL-10 (mIL-10) and human IL-10 (hIL-10). Like all other cytokines, mIL-10 and hIL-10 are pleiotropic in function. Among other activities, IL-10 inhibits T-cell activation and proliferation and has strong anti-inflammatory effects (for reviews, see Refs. 16–19). These biological properties of IL-10 suggest that this cytokine may be useful in the prophylaxis and treatment of GVHD. In this chapter, current knowledge of the structural and biological properties of IL-10 is discussed. Special emphasis is given to the potential role of IL-10 in transplantation.

II. STRUCTURAL PROPERTIES OF IL-10 AND ITS RECEPTOR

Mouse IL-10 and hIL-10 cDNAs were cloned from a mouse Th2 cell line stimulated with concanavalin A and from an activated tetanus toxin-specific human T-cell clone, respectively (20,21). hIL-10 is active on both mouse and human cells, but mIL-10 is not active on human cells. The mIL-10 and hIL-10 cDNA clones exhibit a high degree of nucleotide sequence homology (>80%). Both encode very similar (73% identical) polypeptides composed of 178 amino acids. Recombinant hIL-10 is a nonglycosylated 18-kDa polypeptide, but mIL-10 is N-glycosylated at a site near its N terminus. Glycosylation is heterogeneous, resulting in a mixture of 17-, 19-, and 21-kDa glycoproteins. mIL-10 and hIL-10 appear to be expressed as acid-sensitive noncovalent homodimers. Whether the monomeric cytokine is biologically active has not been established. Both cytokines contain two intrachain disulfide bonds. Reduction of these disulfide bonds abolishes the cytokine's activities (22).

The IL-10 genes in mouse and humans are located on chromosome 1. The murine IL-10 gene is encoded by five exons spanning ~5.5 kb of genomic DNA, and the human IL-10 gene has a similar structure (22,23).

Both Epstein-Barr virus (EBV) and equine herpesvirus type 2 (EHV2) genomes contain viral homologs of IL-10. EBV, which transforms human B lymphocytes, carries a gene, BCRF1, that is 84% homologous at the protein level to hIL-10 and is called viral IL-10 (vIL-10). Most of the divergence between hIL-10 and vIL-10 is found in the N-terminal 20 amino acids of the mature proteins. Recombinant vIL-10 is a 17-kDa nonglycosylated polypeptide that shares some but not all of the known activities of IL-10, although its specific activity is 3 to 10-fold lower than that of the cellular cytokine (22).

The biological effects of IL-10 are mediated by interaction with its cell surface receptor. Recently, both mouse and human receptors for IL-10 (mIL-10R, hIL-10R) were identified and characterized (22,24,25). The mIL-10R cDNA was isolated by expression cloning from a cDNA library established from mouse mast cell and macrophage cell lines. The hIL-10R cDNA was cloned from a library obtained from a Burkitt's lymphoma cell line. The hIL-10R exhibits 70% DNA sequence homology with the mIL-10R cDNA. hIL-10 binds to both mIL-10R and hIL-10R expressed in heterologous cells, whereas mIL-10 binds only to mIL-10R, as expected from the species specificity of mIL-10. Murine IL-10R and hIL-10R bind hIL-10, with a kDa of ~70 pM and 200 to 250 pM, respectively. mIL-10R mRNA was detected in a number of hematopoietic tissues and cell lines, including cells known to respond to mIL-10 (B cells, thymocytes, mast cells, and macrophage cell lines). Similarly, hIL-10R mRNA was found mainly in human hematopoietic cells and cell lines. Activation by anti-CD3 mAb and phorbol ester of different subsets of human T-cell clones, including $CD8^+$ T-cell clones, and Th0, Th1, and Th2 $CD4^+$ clones, resulted in downregulation of hIL-10R mRNA detected in the cells. This decrease in hIL-10R mRNA ranged from 2- to 10-fold and was generally more profound in $CD8^+$ T-cell clones. It is presently unclear whether the observed reduction in mRNA levels, and presumably the levels of hIL-10R expression, would significantly impair the ability of activated T cells to respond to IL-10, but the loss of IL-10R expression by activated T cells may be responsible for the fact that these cells, in contrast to resting T cells, become refractory to inhibition by IL-10. This possibility should be taken into account in planning in vivo studies with IL-10 as an immunosuppressant for T-cell responses.

Murine IL-10R and hIL-10R exhibit no primary sequence homology with other genes, but structural analysis of the predicted protein sequences showed that they are novel members of the interferon receptor (IFNR) family. The structural relationship between the IL-10R and the IFNR is intriguing, because IL-10 and IFN-γ antagonize each other's functions and secretion in several systems. These findings suggest the possibility of interaction between the signaling pathways of IL-10R and IFNR. Further studies on the complete structure of IL-10R and the mechanisms by which binding of IL-10 to IL-10R transduces a signal to T cells will help to address this question and to better understand the mechanisms of action of IL-10.

III. IL-10-PRODUCING CELLS

IL-10 is produced by a variety of cells including T lymphocytes and monocytes (for review, see Ref. 19). In the mouse, IL-10 is secreted by activated Th2 cell clones, fetal thymocytes, and T-cell lines. In addition, IL-10 is synthesized by mast-cell lines, activated macrophages, keratinocytes, B-cell lymphomas, and both activated $CD5^+$ and $CD5^-$ peritoneal B cells (18). In humans, IL-10 is produced by activated T cells, monocytes, and B cells. Peripheral blood T cells can produce significant amounts of IL-10, depending on the mode of activation. Both $CD4^+$ and $CD8^+$ T cells secrete IL-10, although the levels of production by $CD4^+$ T cells are significantly higher. Among the $CD4^+$ T cells, the $CD45RA^-$ memory cells produce 5 to 20 times higher levels of IL-10 compared to the $CD45RA^+$ naive cells. Interestingly, in contrast to murine IL-10, which is produced exclusively by Th2 cells, human IL-10 is produced by Th0, Th1, and Th2 cell clones, although the levels of IL-10 production by human Th2 cells are generally higher than those of the Th0 or Th1 subsets (26). Kinetic studies have indicated that IL-10 is produced relatively late after activation of T cells and is preceded by the production of other cytokines such as IL-2 and IL-4, suggesting a regulatory role of IL-10 in later phases of the immune response. CsA inhibits IL-10 production by activated human T cells in vitro (R. de Waal Malefyt, manuscript in preparation) and by activated murine T cells in vivo (27), whereas FK506 has no significant effect on IL-10 production by murine Th2 cells (28).

Human monocytes produce large amounts of IL-10 after activation with lipopolysaccharide (LPS). As with T cells, the production of IL-10 by monocytes occurs late, as compared to synthesis of proinflammatory cytokines—such as IL-1α, IL-1β, TNF-α, and granulocyte-macrophage colony stimulating factor (GM-CSF)—and is positively or negatively affected by several cytokines (29). IL-2 and TNF-α have been shown to induce the synthesis of IL-10 by human peripheral blood monocytes (30) (M. G. Roncarolo, unpublished observation). More importantly, anti-TNF-α antibodies block IL-10 production induced by either IL-2 or TNF-α, indicating that the production of TNF-α positively regulates IL-10 expression. In contrast, IL-4, IL-13, and IFN-γ inhibit the IL-10 production by activated monocytes (31,32). Furthermore, IL-10 itself downregulates IL-10 mRNA expression in activated monocytes, indicating that it has negative autoregulatory feedback activity (29).

Interestingly, CsA induces significant levels of IL-10 synthesis in resting human monocytes, whereas both CsA and steroids inhibit IL-10 production by LPS-activated monocytes (R. de Waal Malefyt, manuscript in preparation; M. G. Roncarolo, unpublished observation). The underlying mechanisms responsible for the different effects of CsA on resting versus activated monocytes remain to be determined.

$CD5^+$ and $CD5^-$ human B lymphocytes can release IL-10 after activation through their receptor or through the CD40 molecule. EBV-transformed B-cell lines also produce large amounts of hIL-10. In contrast, vIL-10 can be detected in the supernatants of only a minority of EBV-transformed B-cell lines (19,33). Finally, various tumor cell lines—including B-cell lymphoma, ovarian and colon carcinomas—and certain melanoma cell lines have been shown to release IL-10 in vitro. In addition, IL-10 protein has been detected in the serum of patients with ovarian and other intra-abdominal cancers (for review, see Ref. 19).

IV. IN VITRO BIOLOGICAL PROPERTIES OF IL-10

Like all cytokines, IL-10 is pleiotropic. It modulates the function of lymphocytes, natural killer (NK) cells, monocytes/macrophages, dendritic cells, and thymocytes (16–18). In addition, it acts on myeloid and erythroid progenitors and stimulates the growth of mast cells (16–18). The major immunosuppressive and anti-inflammatory effects of IL-10, with particular emphasis on the effects on human cells, are summarized below.

A. Effects of IL-10 on Antigen-Presenting Cells

IL-10 strongly inhibits antigen-specific proliferative responses of murine and human T cells. In addition, similar strong inhibitory effects of IL-10 have been observed on the proliferation of human T-cell clones belonging to the Th0, Th1, and Th2 subsets to soluble protein antigens presented by monocytes. These inhibitory activities are mainly due to an indirect effect of IL-10 on the APC (34,35). Although the exact mechanism of action of IL-10 on APC has not been completely elucidated, it is clear that IL-10 prevents T-cell activation by downregulating the antigen-presenting capacity or accessory cell functions (or both) of APC. Optimal activation of T cells by antigens requires interaction of T-cell receptor (TCR) with antigenic peptide and class II major histocompatibility complexes (MHC). Additionally, costimulatory signals mediated through interactions between adhesion and costimulatory molecules—such as CD28/CTLA-4, LFA-1, or CD2 molecules expressed on T cells and CD80 or CD86, ICAM-1,2,3, or CD58 expressed on APC—are essential for T-cell activation (36). Interactions between CD28 and its ligands CD86 and CD80 are particularly important for initiating activation of resting T cells and for enhancing T-cell cytokine production and T-cell proliferation (37).

IL-10 downregulates the expression of these molecules on APC, such as monocytes and Langerhans cells (31,34,38). IL-10 strongly downregulates not only constitutive, but also IL-4, IL-13, or IFN-γ—induced class II MHC expression on human monocytes (31,34). Diminished expression of class II MHC antigens on the cell surface of human monocytes and Langerhans cells (LC) is thought to play an important role in the inhibitory effects of IL-10 on the antigen-specific activation of human T-cell clones. IL-10 also downregulates the constitutive and IFN-γ–induced expression of the adhesion molecule ICAM-1 (CD54) and the costimulatory molecules CD80 and of CD86 on monocytes and dendritic cells (19,39,40). Furthermore, IL-10 strongly inhibits the production of various cytokines such as IL-1, IL-6, TNF-α, and GM-CSF by monocytes, which act as costimulatory factors for T-cell proliferation and expansion (29).

Taken together, these effects of IL-10 may strongly interfere with the processes required for optimal T-cell activation. However, since resting T cells and T-cell clones reactive to soluble antigens have different activation requirements, the importance of each of these mechanisms for IL-10–mediated inhibition may vary, depending on the type of antigen and on the differentiation state of the T cells. In addition, it is possible that other, yet to be defined, costimulatory cytokines or cell surface molecules also play a role in the mechanisms responsible for IL-10–mediated inhibition of T-cell activation and proliferation.

B. Effects of IL-10 on Human T Cells

In addition to its effects on APC, IL-10 also has direct specific inhibitory effects on the survival, proliferation, cytokine production, and chemotaxis of human T cells. A direct effect of IL-10 on T cells was initially suggested by the fact that IL-10 inhibits the proliferation of human Th0, Th1, and Th2 T-cell clones induced by stimulation with cross-linked anti-CD3 or anti-CD2 monoclonal antibodies (mAbs) in the absence of APC. The observation that these inhibitory effects could be reversed by low concentrations of IL-2 led to the finding that IL-10 specifically inhibits IL-2 production by T cells at the transcriptional level, whereas the synthesis of IL-4, IL-5, GM-CSF, and IFN-γ was not affected (41). Similar results have been reported for resting T cells activated by anti-CD3 (41,42). In these experiments, IL-10 inhibited both IL-2 production and the proliferation of peripheral blood T cells. In addition, it was shown that IL-10 inhibits TNF-α production by T cells (R. de Waal Malefyt, unpublished observation). Thus, direct interactions of IL-10 with the IL-10R on T cells result in specific suppression of IL-2 and TNF-α production and inhibition of T-cell expansion. The relevance of these findings for T-cell stimulation in vivo is uncertain, but they suggest that IL-10 inhibits T-cell expansion in two ways: indirectly by inhibition of APC function and directly through inhibition of IL-2 gene transcription.

IL-10 has also a direct protective effect on T cells starved for IL-2 (43). Activated human T cells and T-cell clones are dependent on IL-2 for growth and survival. Deprivation of IL-2 leads to rapid cell death by apoptosis, which involves loss of cell volume, chromatin condensation, and DNA fragmentation. Incubation of these T cells with IL-10 significantly reduced apoptotic cell death. This effect was not due to an indirect effect on IL-2 production and could not be reversed by anti-IL-2 or anti-IL-2R mAbs. A comparable protective effect of IL-10 was observed with T lymphocytes from patients with acute EBV-induced infectious mononucleosis. IL-10 promoted the survival of these T cells, which are otherwise destined to die by apoptosis (44).

Finally, IL-10 has chemotactic activity on human $CD8^+$ T cells isolated from peripheral blood (45). This chemotactic activity is subset specific, since IL-10 was not chemotactic for $CD4^+$ T cells, monocytes, or neutrophils. However, IL-10 did inhibit IL-8-mediated chemotactic responses of $CD4^+$ T cells but not those of $CD8^+$ T cells. This differential response of $CD4^+$ and $CD8^+$ T-cell subsets is not due to differential IL-10R expression, because both $CD4^+$ and $CD8^+$ T-cell clones express high levels of IL-10R (25).

C. Effects of IL-10 on the Production of Proinflammatory Cytokines and Chemokines by Monocytes and Neutrophils

In addition to its inhibitory effects on T-cell activation and proliferation, IL-10 has potent anti-inflammatory effects. IL-10 inhibits the induction of nitric oxide synthase and the production of nitric oxide (NO) by murine macrophages (46,47). NO plays an important role in the elimination of intracellular and extracellular parasites, because inhibition of NO production significantly affects the cytotoxic potential of macrophages. There are no reports on the effects of IL-10 on NO production by human monocytes. However, the ability of human monocytes to produce superoxide anion, which is another agent involved in the oxidative burst and monocyte cytotoxicity, is inhibited by vIL-10 (48). In addition, IL-10 suppresses the production of pro-inflammatory cytokines, such as TNF-α, IL-1α, IL-1β, IL-6, and chemokines such as IL-8 and MIP-1α by activated human monocytes, polymorphonuclear leukocytes (PMN), and eosinophils (29,31,49–51). These soluble factors play an important role in the activation of granulocytes, monocytes/macrophages, NK cells, T cells, and B cells and in their recruitment to sites of inflammation. The inhibitory effects of IL-10 on the production of these proinflammatory cytokines and chemokines occur at the level of steady-state mRNA expression. IL-10 also inhibits the secretion of hematopoietic growth factors—such as G-CSF, M-CSF and GM-CSF—by activated human monocytes. Although the primary function of these cytokines is to promote the growth of early hematopoietic progenitor cells, these growth factors activate monocyte/macrophages and enhance the production of proinflammatory cytokines by these cells. Therefore they have a strong proinflammatory component. The endogenous secretion of IL-10 has important biological effects, because activation of human monocytes in the presence of neutralizing anti-IL-10 mAbs considerably enhances the production of proinflammatory cytokines and chemokines (29).

IL-10 also inhibits the production of IL-12 and IFN-α, and both these cytokines have been shown to direct Th1-cell development. Based on these observations, it can be speculated that IL-10 may favor the development of Th2 cells by blocking Th1 development (52,53).

Similar inhibitory effects of IL-10 on the production of cytokines have been described using resting and periodate- or thyoglycolate-induced peritoneal mouse macrophages (46,54).

Interestingly, IL-10 does not have general inhibitory effects on cytokine production by monocytes and neutrophils, since it enhances the production of the IL-1 receptor antagonist (IL-1ra) (31,55,56). IL-1ra binds with high affinity to type I and type II IL-1 receptors, without receptor activation, and it has been shown to have anti-inflammatory activity on its own (57). Collectively, these in vitro results indicate that IL-10 has not only potent anti-inflammatory activities—by inhibiting the effector functions of monocytes, PMN, eosinophils and T cells—but that it may also prevent these cells from migrating to or accumulating at the sites of inflammation.

V. EFFECTS OF IL-10 ON ALLOGENEIC RESPONSES IN VITRO

Similar to its inhibitory effects on T-cell responses to soluble antigens, IL-10 was found to strongly reduce the proliferation of human alloreactive T cells in classic one-way primary mixed lymphocyte reaction (MLR) in which peripheral blood mononuclear cells (PBMC) from two unrelated, HLA-mismatched individuals are used as stimulator and responder cells (58). Inhibitory effects were also observed when purified CD3$^+$ T cells were used as responder cells and purified allogeneic monocytes or B cells as stimulator cells. Interestingly, increased proliferation of the responder T cells was observed when primary MLR were carried out in the presence of neutralizing anti-IL-10 mAbs, indicating that endogenous IL-10 suppresses proliferative responses in these cultures (58).

The levels of cytokines (IL-2, TNF-α, GM-CSF, IFN-γ) produced in MLR, using unfractionated allogeneic PBMC as responder and stimulator cells, were reduced two- to threefold in the presence of exogenous IL-10. Furthermore, the proportions of T cells expressing the activation molecules CD25 and HLA-DR were lower in cultures containing IL-10 as compared to control cultures. Therefore, IL-10 suppresses proliferative T-cell responses toward alloantigens not only by inhibiting cytokine production but also by preventing T-cell activation (58).

IL-10 also inhibits the generation of allospecific cytotoxic T cells in primary MLR (58). The levels of cytotoxic activity against the allogeneic targets were significantly reduced in the IL-10–containing cultures and enhanced in cultures carried out in the presence of anti-IL-10 mAbs. Whether these results are due to direct inhibitory effects of IL-10 on the differentiation and activation of human $CD8^+$ cytotoxic T-cell precursors or to indirect effects of IL-10 on the activation of $CD4^+$ T cells that provide help for the generation of mature cytotoxic T cells remains to be determined. However, the observation that IL-10 was able to reduce the proliferation of purified $CD8^+$ T cells in response to T-cell–depleted allogeneic PBMC argues in favor of an inhibitory effect of IL-10 on $CD8^+$ T cells, which is independent of the presence of $CD4^+$ T cells but requires the presence of APC.

T-cell proliferation in primary MLR in which human dendritic cells, either freshly isolated from tonsils or generated from $CD34^+$ hematopoietic progenitors cultured in the presence of GM-CSF, were used as stimulators, was also inhibited by IL-10 (59). In addition, IL-10 suppresses the proliferative responses of purified $CD4^+$ and $CD8^+$ T cells to alloantigens presented by LC derived from human skin (38). In this study, IL-10 was found to act by reducing the antigen-presenting capacity of freshly isolated or cultured LC. The inhibitory effects of IL-10 could be partially overcome by exogenous IL-1, suggesting that suppression of IL-1 production by LC, at least in part, accounts for the inhibitory effects of IL-10 (38). Thus, IL-10 inhibits the proliferative response and cytokine production of human peripheral blood $CD4^+$ and $CD8^+$ T cells to alloantigens presented by professional APC. Interestingly, IL-10 did not affect the proliferation of T cells induced by allogeneic EBV-transformed B-cell lines, consistent with previous findings indicating that IL-10 did not inhibit the proliferative responses of T cells or T-cell clones toward soluble antigens, when EBV-transformed B-cell lines were used as APC (34).

More recent data suggest that IL-10 not only suppresses the proliferative responses of $CD4^+$ allogeneic T cells in primary MLR but also renders these allogeneic T cells unresponsive to secondary stimulation (M. G. Roncarolo, unpublished observation). Whether this induction of antigen-specific T-cell unresponsiveness by IL-10 is restricted to $CD4^+$ peripheral blood T cells or may occur also in $CD8^+$ T cells is presently under investigation.

The proliferative responses of human $CD4^+$ allogeneic T cell clones and the production of IL-2, IL-5, GM-CSF, and IFN-γ were also strongly suppressed by exogenous IL-10 when monocytes were used as stimulators. Although significant amounts of IL-10 produced by monocytes were detected in these cultures, incubation with anti-IL-10 mAbs did not significantly increase proliferative responses or cytokine synthesis by these T-cell clones (M. G. Roncarolo, unpublished observation) (60). This may be due to the fact that IL-10 production by both T cells and monocytes occurs late as compared to IL-2 production by activated T-cell clones. On the other hand, it cannot be ruled out that IL-2 produced by the T-cell clones counteracts the effects of monocyte-derived IL-10.

The cytotoxic activity of $CD8^+$ T-cell clones against allogeneic targets is not suppressed by IL-10. However, recent data suggest that IL-10 inhibits IL-2 production by allospecific $CD8^+$ T-cell clones (M. G. Roncarolo, unpublished observation). Furthermore, a recent study showed that pre-incubation of target cells such as melanoma cells or EBV-transformed B-cell lines with IL-10 protects these cells from lysis by tumor-specific or allospecific cytotoxic T-cell lines and T-cell clones (61). The inhibition of cytotoxic activity of $CD8^+$ T lymphocytes was associated with a moderate decrease in the expression of HLA class I on the target cells. This finding, which indicates that IL-10 protects target cells from allospecific cytotoxic T lymphocytes, might have important implications for tolerance induction toward HLA-mismatched allografts. These studies also imply that long-term IL-10 treatment may possibly have negative effects on potential anti-tumor responses.

The effects of IL-10 on primary MLR with murine T cells are comparable to those observed with human cells. IL-10 inhibits the allogeneic responses of murine T cells to minor and major histocompatibility antigens. Addition of IL-10 to MLR partially reduces the proliferation and IL-2 production of B10.BR splenocytes to MHC-incompatible B6 stimulators (62). In addition, IL-10 completely abrogates the growth and IL-2 secretion of B10.BR responder cells when stimulated with CBA cells, which express different minor histocompatibility antigens (62). IL-10 also strongly suppresses the proliferation of $CD4^+$ T cells obtained from spleens of naive CBA/J mice after stimulation with GM-CSF treated macrophages obtained from the bone marrow of BALB/c mice (63). In this study, no inhibition of IL-2 production and T-cell proliferation was observed when purified dendritic cells were used as stimulators, in contrast to results obtained using human dendritic cells. However, IL-10 significantly inhibited dendritic-cell–induced IFN-γ production by $CD4^+$ and $CD8^+$ T cells in primary MLR (63). Furthermore, it has been reported that proliferation of $CD4^+$ T cells obtained from the lymph nodes of BALB/C mice to allogeneic LC cells derived from C3H or CB/BL6 mice was not inhibited by pretreatment of the APC with IL-10, but IL-2 and IFN-γ production was strongly reduced at the transcriptional level (64). It is presently not clear why the results obtained with murine dendritic cells are different from those observed with their human counterparts, but one possibility is that they are related to the different sources of responder and stimulator cells used.

The effects of IL-10 on allogeneic responses by murine $CD8^+$ T cells may also be different from those observed with human $CD8^+$ T cells. IL-10 enhances the growth of mouse $CD8^+$ T cells in response to IL-2 and augments the cytolytic activity of effector cytotoxic T lymphocytes generated from Con A–activated spleen $CD8^+$ T cells (65). Furthermore, limiting dilution analysis (LDA) showed that IL-10, in combination with IL-2, substantially increased the frequencies of cytotoxic T-cell precursors. These results suggest that IL-10 functions as a cytotoxic T-cell differentiation factor, which promotes the proliferation and maturation of murine cytotoxic $CD8^+$ T-cell precursors.

This notion is supported by preliminary data obtained with alloreactive $CD8^+$

T cells in LDA performed in the presence of IL-2 and IL-10. In this study, the frequencies of murine $CD8^+$ T cells proliferating in response to allogeneic stimulation were significantly higher compared to those observed in LDA with IL-2 alone (B. Blazar, personal communication). However, comparable experiments carried out with human $CD8^+$ T cells failed to show similar results. The frequencies of human alloreactive $CD8^+$ cytotoxic T cells generated in the presence of IL-2 and IL-10 were either comparable to or lower than those observed with IL-2 alone (M. G. Roncarolo, unpublished observation).

VI. IN VIVO BIOLOGICAL PROPERTIES OF IL-10 IN MICE

A. Effects of IL-10 on Lethal Shock

IL-10 also has potent anti-inflammatory effects in vivo. In animal models of sepsis, administration of IL-10 was very effective in preventing lethal toxic shock. At very low concentrations of 1 μg/mouse, IL-10 prevents LPS-induced toxic shock, which would result in the death of the mice (66,67). IL-10 still had protective effects when administered up to 30 min after LPS injection (66). Measurement of macrophage-derived TNF-α, which is the main mediator of toxic shock in this model, showed that the circulating levels of TNF-α in the IL-10–treated mice were strongly reduced as compared to those of untreated control mice (66,67). IL-10 also inhibits lethal shock induced by the superantigen staphylococcal enterotoxin B (SEB) (68). In contrast to the LPS model, where the target is the macrophage, superantigen-induced lethal shock depends on massive T-cell activation and cytokine production by these cells in vivo (69). In particular, T-cell–derived TNF-α has been shown to be the most important mediator of SEB-induced lethal toxic shock (70). Therefore, these data suggest that IL-10 exerts a protective effect by direct inhibition of T cells. Interestingly, it has been shown that the drug chlorpromazine, which has the ability to prevent SEB-induced lethal septic shock in mice, significantly increased IL-10 production by phagocytic cells in vivo (71).

B. Role of IL-10 in Chronic Inflammatory Bowel Disease

IL-10–deficient mice have normal lymphocyte development and antibody responses. However, most of the animals were growth retarded and anemic, developing chronic enterocolitis and uncontrolled inflammatory processes at other locations (72). These symptoms could be prevented or dramatically improved when the mice were treated with exogenous IL-10 prior to the onset or during the course of the disease, respectively (72). These observations suggest that IL-10 plays an important role in controlling inflammatory processes and that its absence leads to chronic inflammatory responses, particularly in the gut, probably in response to normal enteric antigens.

IL-10 also inhibits inflammatory bowel diseases in another mouse model. IL-10 protects CB-17 SCID mice from colitis induced by transfer of $CD4^+$ $CD45RB^{high}$ cells from BALB/c mice (73). In this animal model, treatment with IL-10 results in lower levels of IFN-γ and TNF-α mRNA in the colon, suggesting that IL-10 may prevent development of colitis via inhibition of IFN-γ and TNF-α produced by Th1 cells (73).

These in vivo data indicate that IL-10 has potential therapeutic value in the treatment of chronic inflammatory bowel disease and Crohn's disease in humans.

C. Role of IL-10 in Autoimmune Diabetes

Systemic administration of IL-10 to nonobese diabetic (NOD) mice significantly delayed the onset and reduced the incidence of diabetes. This protective effect of IL-10 was also observed several weeks after termination of the treatment, suggesting that IL-10 had long-term effects (74). In addition, a significant increase in IL-10 mRNA expression, together with a decrease in IL-2 and IFN-γ mRNA levels, has been observed in NOD mice transplanted with syngeneic pancreatic islets in which the onset of autoimmune diabetes was prevented by injection of complete Freund's adjuvant. These findings suggest that the protective effect of complete Freund's adjuvant may result from the induction of endogenous IL-10 production (75,76). Expression of IL-10 under the rat insulin promoter led to leukocyte infiltration but not to destruction of insulin-producing β cells (77). However, expression of IL-10 transgene on a NOD background led to an accelerated onset and an increased incidence of diabetes (78). Similarly, in transgenic NOD mice in which IL-10 expression was targeted to islet α cells, an acceleration in the onset of the diabetes with enhanced severity of the autoimmune insulitis was observed (79). These conflicting results of the effects of IL-10 on autoimmune diabetes may be related to differences in the efficacy of IL-10 in preventing inflammatory responses, depending on the mode of delivery and its local concentration.

VII. IN VIVO BIOLOGICAL PROPERTIES OF IL-10 IN ANIMAL MODELS OF TRANSPLANTATION

A. Effects of IL-10 in Allograft Rejection

Conflicting results have been obtained in studies to determine the role of IL-10 in allograft rejection. Peripheral tolerance induction in a murine allogeneic heart transplant model has been associated with differential activation of CD4$^+$ Th2 cells, which release IL-4 and IL-10 and block activation and cytokine production by proinflammatory CD4$^+$ and CD8$^+$ effector cells (80). IL-4 and IL-10 transcripts were generally enhanced in the heart allografts and spleens of these mice, which had been rendered tolerant by donor-specific blood transfusions, anti-CD40 mAb pretreatment, and CsA administration. Similarly, preferential activation of Th2-type cells correlated with the delayed rejection of B10.BR skin grafts observed in C3H/HEJ mice who received pretransplant immunization with B10.BR cells (81). This delayed rejection was abolished by in vivo injection of anti-IL-10 mAbs, suggesting that endogenous IL-10 was responsible for increased graft survival in vivo.

High endogenous IL-10 production was also associated with prolonged survival in a mouse heart allograft model after therapy with anti-CD4 or anti-CD8 mAbs (82). In this model, transplantation of BALB/c hearts into CBA recipients, accompanied by a short treatment with anti-CD4 or anti-CD8 mAbs, resulted in prolonged cardiac allograft survival. In these tolerant animals, the graft-infiltrating cells showed a distinct cytokine profile with high levels of IL-4 and IL-10 but no IL-2 or IFN-γ expression.

In addition, allogeneic neonatal hearts from C57BL/6 mice injected with a retrovirus vector containing the viral IL-10 gene showed significant prolongation of graft survival when transplanted into allogeneic CBA recipients (83), suggesting that low levels of vIL-10 expression within the graft can generate local immunosuppression and graft acceptance. In contrast, no inhibition or delay in rejection was observed when fetal pancreases or adult islets producing IL-10 under control of an insulin promoter were transplanted into MHC-incompatible recipients (84). These contrasting effects of IL-10 in different models of organ transplant rejection are presently difficult to explain, but they may be due to different concentrations of IL-10 present in different microenvironments.

B. Effects of IL-10 in GVHD

The role of IL-10 in murine models of GVHD is still unclear and controversial. Endogenous IL-10 production has been detected in murine models of both tolerance and GVHD. Abramowicz et al. reported that injection of semiallogeneic spleen cells into neonatal Balb/c mice results in a state of tolerance, which is associated with expression of IL-4 and IL-10 mRNA in vivo (85). In addition, recent data suggest that Th2 cells are capable of modifying GVHD (86). In this murine parent-into-F_1 GVHR model that utilizes LPS to induce lethality, coinjection of Th2 cells together with the donor B6 spleen cells protected the B6C3FI recipient. These $CD4^+$ Th2 cells were obtained from donor B6 mice treated in vivo with large doses of IL-2 or combinations of IL-2 and IL-4 and were shown to secrete enhanced levels of IL-4 and IL-10 (86). Taken together, these studies strongly suggest a protective role of IL-4 and IL-10 in GVHD. However, IL-10 does not always protect mice from GVHD. High levels of IL-10 mRNA have been detected in spleens of mice undergoing acute or chronic GVHD (87–89). Whether these relatively high local levels of endogenous IL-10 play a role in the pathogenesis of the GVHD or result from the inflammatory process remains to be determined.

Murine studies aimed at investigating the in vivo effects of IL-10 administration in GVHD have also generated controversial and discordant results. Preliminary experiments in GVHD models, in which the disease is induced by transplantation of $CD4^+$ MHC class II mismatched T cells into irradiated hosts, indicated that administration of IL-10 prior to, or in the first days following, transplantation increased the survival rate, but did not significantly reduce GVHD symptoms such as weight loss (E. Holler and R. Korngold, personal communication). On the other hand, IL-10 had no clear protective effects in models of minor MHC disparity mediated by $CD4^+$ or $CD8^+$ T cells (62; N. Chao, personal communication). In CBA recipient mice transplanted with bone marrow and purified T cells from B10.BR donor mice, treatment with recombinant hIL-10 was not sufficient to alter significantly the clinical course of the disease as assessed by survival rate, splenomegaly, and weight loss. However, in this study, the expansion of $CD4^+$ and $CD8^+$ donor cells was significantly inhibited by IL-10, with a more profound effect on the $CD4^+$ subset. In addition, the in vitro IFN-γ production by T cells obtained from the treated animals was strongly inhibited, and the suppression of lymphocyte proliferation could be reversed with significantly less anti-IFN-γ antibody as compared to the saline-treated controls (62). One reason why IL-10 was unable to prevent systemic GVHD in this model may be that IL-10 was administered after transplantation, when the cascade of events leading to allogeneic T-cell activation had already been initiated and could not be stopped by IL-10. It is noteworthy that IL-10 is ineffective once T cells are activated. Therefore, it would be interesting to investigate whether IL-10 treatment prior to the transplant would prevent activation of alloreactive donor T cells, resulting in GVHD protection.

Injection of IL-10 in a fully allogeneic bone marrow transplantation model system, in which $CD4^+$ T cells drive $CD8^+$ T-cell–mediated acute GVHD, also failed to show any protection (90). In contrast, in this study it was shown that IL-10 treatment accelerates the GVHD and that in vivo infusion of anti-IL-10 mAbs diminished the GVHD (90). The mechanisms by which IL-10 exacerbated GVHD in this murine model are presently under investigation. One hypothesis is that IL-10 augmented the immune response of the donor cells by increasing the proportion or function of donor T cells with antihost activity. This effect would be directed mainly at donor cytotoxic T cells.

Based on these data, it is difficult to draw any definitive conclusions about the role of IL-10 in murine GVHD. Further studies are required to understand the mechanisms and the conditions which result in prevention or exacerbation of GVHD by IL-10. In particular, it is important to understand whether (a) IL-10 has a protective role only when administered prior to the transplant, since it may not act on already activated T cells; (b) only a short period of IL-10 treatment is required in order to prevent GVHD without inducing a general immunosuppression of the recipient; (c) IL-10 has a suppressive effect on $CD4^+$, but not $CD8^+$ murine T cells and, therefore, is not protective in models in which both T cell subsets mediate GVHD; (d) IL-10 inhibits the proliferative responses but not the effector cytotoxic function of murine T cells and therefore is ineffective in GVHD models mediated by cytotoxic T cells, which do not require helper T cells.

The role of irradiation in this experimental models of GVHD deserves attention, because it has been shown that ionizing radiation results in significant increases in IL-10 mRNA levels in the spleen and kidney of normal mice (91), suggesting that endogenous IL-10 production may vary depending on the doses of irradiation. Finally, it would be interesting to explore the effects of IL-10 in combination with other immunosuppressive drugs, such as FK506 and CsA, on GVHD, since several experimental data suggest that these compounds may either enhance or inhibit endogenous IL-10 production by different cell types (27,28).

VIII. IL-10 AND HUMAN DISEASES

In humans, resistance or susceptibility to certain diseases has been correlated with relatively high or low levels of endogenous IL-10 production. For example, elevated levels of IL-10 transcripts are present in bone marrow aspirates from patients with active visceral leishmaniasis, whereas low levels of IL-10 transcription correlated with a resolution of the disease (92). Similarly, in patients infected with *Mycobacterium leprae*, high levels of IL-10 are present in the multibacillary form of the disease, in contrast to the low levels observed in patients suffering from the tuberculoid, resistant form of the disease (93). In contrast, in patients with lymphatic filariasis, high levels of IL-10 correlate with an asymptomatic state of the disease

(94). High levels of IL-10 have also been detected in patients with gram-negative or gram-positive septicemia, suggesting that this cytokine might be involved in the control of the inflammatory response induced by bacterial products (95).

A. Role of IL-10 in Patients Transplanted with Hematopoietic Stem Cells

Patients with severe combined immunodeficiency (SCID) can be successfully transplanted with fetal hematopoietic stem cells derived from HLA-mismatched donors. After immunological reconstitution, these children developed a split chimerism, in which the T cells were of donor origin and the B cells and monocytes were of host origin (96). Despite the HLA incompatibility between the donor-derived T cells and the host cells, tolerance toward the donor and the host was established after transplantation in the absence of any immunosuppressive treatment. These patients had no signs of GVHD. In addition, the donor-derived T cells were specifically unresponsive to the host HLA antigens in primary MLR (96). However, extensive studies performed with T-cell clones established from different transplanted patients showed that the donor-derived T cells that recognize host HLA antigens were not deleted from the repertoire (96–98). Both $CD4^+$ and $CD8^+$ T cells specific for the host class II and class I HLA antigens, respectively, could be isolated with high frequencies from the peripheral blood of these patients several years after transplantation, indicating that these cells are not operational but are suppressed in vivo. In general, the $CD4^+$ T cells displayed low proliferative capacity and produced low levels of IL-2 after specific stimulation with host antigens. In contrast, high levels of IL-10 production were detected, particularly in one patient (60). These high levels of IL-10 synthesis were observed only after stimulation via the TcR and were a specific property of the host-reactive T-cell clones. Alloreactive T-cell clones isolated from the same patient produced significantly lower levels of IL-10, which were in the normal range and comparable to those detected using alloreactive T-cell clones isolated from normal donors. Kinetic studies indicated that T-cell clones isolated from normal donors produce IL-10 late after activation; no differences in these kinetics were observed between T-cell clones belonging to the Th0, Th1, or Th2 subsets (26). In contrast, the host-reactive T-cell clones produced IL-10 very early after activation. In addition, blocking experiments using neutralizing anti-IL-10 mAbs showed that this endogenously produced IL-10 was able to suppress the proliferation of these T-cell clones in an autocrine fashion (60). In addition to the high IL-10 production by the host-reactive T-cell clones, high levels of IL-10 were also detected in the supernatants of PBMC of these patients cultured in vitro in the absence of any stimuli. These findings correlated with the high levels of IL-10 mRNA detected by semiquantitative PCR analysis of freshly isolated PBMC from SCID patients transplanted with fetal liver or with haploidentical bone marrow. Cell fractionation experiments indicated that, in addition to the donor-derived T cells, freshly isolated monocytes of host origin constitutively produced high levels of IL-10 in vivo (60). This phenomenon was not observed with freshly isolated T cells or monocytes from normal donors. These data indicate that high levels of IL-10, produced by both host monocytes and donor-derived T cells, are present in patients in whom tolerance has been achieved after HLA-incompatible transplantation. The in vivo IL-10 production seems to be of biological relevance, since

HLA-DR expression on monocytes of one of these patients was significantly lower compared to its expression on monocytes isolated from normal donors. Furthermore, HLA-DR expression on the patient's monocytes could be partially upregulated by short-term incubation of these cells with neutralizing anti-IL-10 mAbs. However, despite the high IL-10 levels in vivo, these patients are able to mediate normal primary and secondary immune responses to exogenous antigens (60,99).

Collectively, these data indicate that endogenous IL-10 production is associated with tolerance in SCID patients transplanted with allogeneic stem cells and suggest that IL-10 may play an important role in maintaining transplantation tolerance and preventing GVHD.

Although the mechanism of induction of endogenous IL-10 production remains to be determined, recent data indicated that high levels of spontaneous IL-10 production are a preexisting condition in a subset of patients receiving stem-cell transplants. Preliminary analysis of spontaneous IL-10 production in vitro by PBMC of 63 patients with hematological malignancies, prior to conditioning and bone marrow transplantation, showed that PBMC of patients with stable engraftment and high survival rates produced higher levels of IL-10, as compared to the group of patients in whom severe GVHD or major complications developed after transplantation (100). None of the 14 patients producing IL-10 at >1000 pg/mL died from transplant-related complications. In addition, sequential TNF-α serum levels failed to increase during conditioning in patients with high IL-10 levels, in contrast to what was observed in patients with low IL-10 production. These data indicate that IL-10 is involved in downregulation of proinflammatory cytokines in allogeneic bone marrow transplantation. In addition, they suggest that high levels of endogenous IL-10 prior to the transplant may set the stage for induction of tolerance, which would result in a favorable outcome. On the other hand, IL-10 is not responsible for the delay in immune reconstitution following autologous stem-cell transplantation, because IL-10 production was found to be lower in these patients (101).

B. Role of IL-10 in Patients Transplanted with Allogeneic Organs

The role of IL-10 in preventing or suppressing rejection after solid organ transplantation is still under investigation. The presence of IL-10 has been analyzed in biopsies of patients who underwent heart or kidney transplantation (102,103) (P. Merville et al., manuscript submitted). The levels of IL-2, IL-4, and IL-10 mRNA in biopsies taken from hearts of patients with transplant rejection were higher than those found in biopsies from hearts with no evidence of rejection. However, in contrast to IL-2, IL-10 was present only in heart biopsies of patients with mild rejections and not in biopsies of patients with grade 3 rejection (102). The conclusion of this study was that none of the cytokines evaluated, including IL-10, was predictive of rejection. Similarly, IL-10-secreting $CD4^+$ T cells have been detected at high frequencies among graft-infiltrating lymphocytes obtained from biopsies of patients with acute rejection of kidney allografts. In contrast, low frequencies of $CD4^+$ IL-10 producing cells were observed in biopsies of patients with chronic rejection (103) (P. Merville et al., manuscript submitted). The major question that remains to be answered is whether endogenous IL-10 production contributed to the pathogenesis of the rejection or whether it merely reflected an attempt of the immune system to counteract the high levels of IL-2, TNF-α, and IL-1 produced by activated T cells and monocytes present at the site of rejection. Sequential analysis of in situ cytokine profiles during organ rejection in transplanted patients could help to address this question. Furthermore, it is important to elucidate the effect of immunosuppressive therapy on IL-10 production in these transplanted patients, particularly since it has recently been shown that CsA markedly enhances LPS-induced IL-10 release in vivo (27). Therefore, it cannot be ruled out that CsA treatment was responsible for the high levels of endogenous IL-10 production in some of these kidney- and heart-transplanted patients.

No information is presently available on the use of exogenous IL-10 to prevent or suppress organ rejection in transplanted patients. Based on the observation that IL-10 was able to prevent the massive release of TNF-α and IFN-γ but not IL-6 and IL-10 in mice treated with anti-CD3 mAbs in vivo (104), the use of IL-10 has been recently proposed for the prevention of shock syndrome, which occurs in kidney transplanted patients receiving the OKT3 mAb (105).

IX. A PHASE I STUDY OF IL-10 IN HEALTHY INDIVIDUALS

Based on its immunosuppressive and anti-inflammatory effects in vitro and in vivo as described above, clinical studies using IL-10 will be started in the near future in a number of inflammatory and Th1 cell-mediated diseases. At present, a phase I study of IL-10 in healthy individuals has shown very promising results. Intravenous single-bolus injections of escalating doses of IL-10 given to healthy male volunteers revealed no adverse effects, even at doses of up to 25 μg/kg (106). No clinically relevant differences were observed in blood chemistry, urinalysis, hemoglobin concentrations, platelet counts, coagulation parameters, complement components, or electrocardiograms of IL-10–treated and placebo-injected volunteers. Although IL-10 can stimulate B-cell growth and Ig production in vitro in the presence of anti-CD40 mAbs (19), no changes in serum Ig levels were observed in IL-10 treated volunteers 96 hr after IL-10 administration. PBMC of IL-10 treated volunteers, stimulated ex vivo with LPS, produced considerably less IL-1, IL-6, and TNF-α than control cultures from placebo-treated individuals. These reduced levels of pro-inflammatory cytokine production persisted for 48 hr after injection. Collectively, these data indicate that a single injection of recombinant IL-10 in healthy humans is safe and well tolerated. In addition, the fact that the suppressive effects on pro-inflammatory cytokine production are relatively long-lasting indicates that daily treatment will not be required in the future use of IL-10 for therapy.

X. CONCLUDING REMARKS

Alloreactive T cells initiate the immune responses that lead to GVHD. Furthermore, these processes have a strong inflammatory component, in which proinflammatory cytokines and chemokines produced by alloreactive T cells and monocytes/macrophages play an important role. IL-10 has strong anti-inflammatory activity. It inhibits the production of proinflammatory cytokines and chemokines, which are responsible for attracting inflammatory cells to the rejection site. Moreover, IL-10 enhances the production of IL-1ra by monocytes, which by itself is an anti-inflammatory cytokine, because it blocks the activities of IL-1α and IL-β. Furthermore, IL-10 inhibits antigen-specific T-cell activation, either directly by suppressing IL-2 production or indirectly by reducing the antigen-presenting and costimulatory function of APC. Based on these properties, it has been proposed that IL-10 may function as a natural dampener of immune and inflammatory responses. In addition, as discussed here, IL-10 may have potential clinical utility as an immunosuppressive agent for preventing or reducing GVHD and establishing transplantation tolerance. Although it is still too early to draw firm conclusions, it is tempting to speculate that the high levels of endogenous IL-10 production observed in successfully transplanted SCID patients contribute to the tolerance achieved. It is possible that these high levels of endogenous IL-10 in the transplanted SCID patients were already present before transplantation. In fact, the presence of relatively high levels of endogenous IL-10 before transplant seems to be critical for successful allogeneic bone marrow transplantation in patients with hematological diseases, since these patients have survival rates that are much higher than those of patients who had low levels of endogenous IL-10 production.

Taken together, these data suggest that the levels of endogenous IL-10 may determine the outcome of GVHD. Preliminary data suggesting that GVHD in mice can be prevented by starting IL-10 administration prior to the transplant also point in this direction. It has to be noted, however, that IL-10 was not effective in other transplantation models. In some cases, exacerbation of GVHD was even observed. In these situations, IL-10 was given either at the same time or after the transplant, which may be too late to be effective, since IL-10 does not act on already activated T cells. Therefore, the use of IL-10 prior to transplantation, to prevent activation of alloreactive T cells, deserves further investigation. It is also clear that more information is required, not only about the route of administration of IL-10 but also about the optimal doses and the duration of IL-10 therapy. It is possible that the endogenous IL-10 produced at low levels in transplanted patients generates local immunosuppression, which allows survival and differention of allogeneic donor cells, without systemic immunosuppression. In contrast, prolonged administration of exogenous IL-10, as applied in several of the experimental models of GVHD described here, may cause a profound systemic immunosuppression, which ultimately would be detrimental for the outcome of the transplant and the survival of the recipient. In addition, it should be taken into account that prolonged treatment with IL-10 could suppress the antitumor responses mediated by donor cells, which are essential for disease-free survival in transplanted patients. On the other hand, administration of IL-10 for a short period of time pre- and posttransplantation may be beneficial only if this cytokine is able to induce antigen-specific tolerance. Preliminary in vitro data, showing the induction of a long-lasting state of unresponsiveness in alloreactive T cells treated with IL-10, support this hypothesis. However, it remains to be proven that exogenous IL-10 is not required for the maintenance of tolerance in vivo. In this regard, it would be particularly interesting to test the effects of exogenous IL-10 in combination with CsA and FK506, which have been shown to selectively preserve or even enhance endogenous IL-10 production in vivo. In conclusion, further studies in transplanted patients and experimental models of GVHD addressing these questions are required to better understand the role of

IL-10 in transplantation and GVHD and to define whether this cytokine may have a future as an immunosuppressive drug to improve the outcome of hematopoietic stem-cell transplants.

REFERENCES

1. Parkman R. Graft-versus-host disease. Annu Rev Med 1991; 42:189–197.
2. Ferrara JLM, Deeg HJ. Graft-versus-host disease. N Engl J Med 1991; 324:667–674.
3. Korngold R. Biology of graft-vs.-host disease. Am J Pediatr Hematol Oncol 1993; 15: 18–27.
4. Antin JH, Ferrara JLM. Cytokine dysregulation and acute graft-versus-host disease. Blood 1992; 12:2964–2968.
5. Champlin R. T cell depletion for allogenic bone marrow transplantation: Impact on graft-versus-host disease, engraftment and graft-versus-leukemia. J Hematother 1993; 2:27–42.
6. Waldmann H, Cobbold S, Hale G. What can be done to prevent graft-versus-host disease? Curr Opin Immunol 1994; 6:777–783.
7. Siekierka JJ, Sigal NH. FK-506 and cyclosporin A: Immunosuppressive mechanism of action and beyond. Curr Opin Immunol 1992; 4:548–552.
8. Sharma VK, Li B, Khanna A, Sehajpal P, Suthanthiran M. Which way for drug-mediated immunosuppression? Curr Opin Immunol 1994; 6:784–790.
9. Lenschow DJ, Bluestone JA. T cell co-stimulation and in vivo tolerance. Curr Opin Immunol 1993; 5:747–752.
10. Charlton B, Auchincloss H Jr, Fathman CG. Mechanisms of transplantation tolerance. Annu Rev Immunol 1994; 12:707–734.
11. Dallman MJ. Cytokines as mediators of organ graft rejection and tolerance. Curr Opin Immunol 1993; 5:788–793.
12. Anasetti C, Martin PM, Hansen JA, et al. A phase I-II study evaluating the murine anti-IL-2 receptor antibody 2A3 for treatment of acute graft-versus-host disease. Transplantation 1990; 50:49–54.
13. McCarthy PL, Abhyankar S, Neben S, et al. Inhibition of interleukin-1 by and interleukin-1 receptor antagonist prevents graft-versus-host disease. Blood 1992; 78:1915–1918.
14. Holler E, Kolb HJ, Mittermüller J, et al. Modulation of acute GVHD after allogeneic bone marrow transplantation by TNF-α release in the course of pretransplant conditioning: role of conditioning regimens and prophylactic application of a monoclonal antibody neutralizing human TNF-α (MAk 195F). Blood 1995; 86:890–899.
15. Fiorentino DF, Bond MW, Mosmann TR. Two types of mouse T helper cell: IV. Th2 clones secrete a factor that inhibits cytokine production by Th1 clones. J Exp Med 1989; 170:2081–2085.
16. de Waal Malefyt R, Yssel H, et al. Interleukin-10. Curr Opin Immunol 1992; 4:314–320.
17. Moore KW, O'Garra A, de Waal Malefyt R, et al. Interleukin 10. Annu Rev Immunol 1993; 11:165–190.
18. Howard M, O'Garra A, Ishida H, et al. Biological properties of interleukin-10. J Clin Immunol 1992; 12:239–247.
19. de Vries JE, de Waal Malefyt R. Interleukin-10. Austin, TX: Landes, 1995.
20. Moore KW, Vieira P, Fiorentino DF, et al. Homology of the cytokine synthesis inhibitory factor (IL-10) to the Epstein-Barr virus gene BCRF1. Science 1990; 248:1230–1234.

21. Vieira P, de Waal Malefyt R, Dang MN, et al. Isolation and expression of human cytokine synthesis inhibitory factor cDNA clones: Homology to Epstein-Barr virus open reading frame BCRFI. Proc Natl Acad Sci USA 1991; 88:1172–1176.
22. Ho ASY, Moore KW. Interleukin-10 and its receptor. Ther Immunol 1994; 1:173–185.
23. Kim JM, Brannan CI, Copeland NG, et al. Structure of the mouse IL-10 gene and chromosomal localization of the mouse and human genes. J Immunol 1992; 148:3618–3623.
24. Ho AS, Liu Y, Khan TA, et al. A receptor for interleukin 10 is related to interferon receptors. Proc Natl Acad Sci USA 1993; 90:11267–11271.
25. Liu Y, Wei SH, Ho AS, et al. Expression cloning and characterization of a human IL-10 receptor. J Immunol 1994; 152:1821–1829.
26. Yssel H, de Waal Malefyt R, Roncarolo MG, et al. IL-10 produced by subsets of human $CD4^+$ T cell clones and peripheral blood T cells. J Immunol 1992; 149:2378–2384.
27. Durez P, Abramowicz D, Gérard C, et al. In vivo induction of interleukin-10 by anti-CD3 monoclonal antibody or bacterial lipopolysaccharide: Differential modulation by cyclosporin A. J Exp Med 1993; 177:551–555.
28. Wang SC, Morel PA, Wang Q, et al. A dual mechanism of immunosuppression by FK-506. Differential suppression of IL-4 and IL-10 levels in T helper 2 cells. Transplantation 1993; 56:978–985.
29. de Waal Malefyt R, Abrams J, Bennett B, et al. Interleukin-10 (IL-10) inhibits cytokine synthesis by human monocytes: An autoregulatory role of IL-10 produced by monocytes. J Exp Med 1991; 174:1209–1220.
30. Wanidworanun C, Strober W. Predominant role of tumor necrosis factor-α in human monocyte IL-10 synthesis. J Immunol 1993; 151:6853–6861.
31. de Waal Malefyt R, Figdor C, Huijbens R, et al. Effects of IL-13 on phenotype, cytokine production, and cytotoxic function of human monocytes: Comparison to IL-4 and modulation by IFN-γ or IL-10. J Immunol 1993; 151:6370–6381.
32. Chomarat P, Rissoan M-C, Banchereau J, Miossec P. Interferon γ inhibits interleukin 10 production by monocytes. J Exp Med 1993; 177:523–527.
33. Burdin N, Peronne C, Banchereau J, Rousset F. Epstein-Barr virus transformation induces B lymphocytes to produce human interleukin 10. J Exp Med 1993; 177:295–304.
34. de Waal Malefyt R, Haanen J, Spits H, et al. Interleukin-10 (IL-10) and viral IL-10 strongly reduced antigen-specific human T cell proliferation by diminishing the antigen-presenting capacity of monocytes via down-regulation of class II major histocompatibility complex expression. J Exp Med 1991; 174:915–924.
35. Fiorentino DF, Zlotnik A, Vieira P, et al. IL-10 acts on the antigen-presenting cell to inhibit cytokine production by Th1 cells. J Immunol 1991; 146:3444–3451.
36. June CH, Bluestone JA, Nadler LM, Thompson CB. The B7 and CD28 receptor families. Immunol Today 1994; 15:321–331.
37. Azuma M, Ito D, Yagita H, et al. B70 antigen is a second ligand for CTLA-4 and CD28. Nature 1993; 366:76–78.
38. Peguet-Navarro J, Moulon C, Caux C, et al. Interleukin-10 inhibits the primary allogeneic T cell response to human epidermal Langerhans cells. Eur J Immunol 1994; 24: 884–891.
39. Willems F, Marchant A, Delville JP, et al. Interleukin-10 inhibits B7 and intercellular adhesion molecule-1 expression on human monocytes. Eur J Immunol 1994; 24:1007–1009.
40. Ding L, Linsley PS, Huang LY, et al. IL-10 inhibits macrophage costimulatory activity by selectively inhibiting the up-regulation of B7 expression. J Immunol 1993; 151: 1224–1234.

41. de Waal Malefyt R, Yssel H, de Vries JE. Direct effects of IL-10 on subsets of human CD4$^+$ T cell clones and resting T cells. J Immunol 1993; 150:4754–4765.
42. Taga K, Mostowski H, Tosato G. Human interleukin-10 can directly inhibit T-cell growth. Blood 1993; 81:2964–2961.
43. Taga K, Cherney B, Tosato G. IL-10 inhibits apoptotic cell death in human T cells starved of IL-2. Int Immunol 1993; 5:1599–1608.
44. Taga K, Chretien J, Cherney B, et al. Interleukin-10 inhibits apoptotic cell death in infectious mononucleosis T cells. J Clin Invest 1994; 94:251-260.
45. Jinquan T, Larsen G, Gesser B, et al. Human IL-10 is a chemoattractant for CD8$^+$ T lymphocytes and an inhibitor of IL-8-induced CD4$^+$ T lymphocyte migration. J Immunol 1993; 151:4545–4551.
46. Bogdan C, Vodovotz Y, Nathan C. Macrophage deactivation by interleukin 10. J Exp Med 1991; 174:1549–1555.
47. Wu J, Cunha FQ, Liew FY, Weiser WY. IL-10 inhibits the synthesis of migration inhibitory factor and migration inhibitory factor-mediated macrophage activation. J Immunol 1993; 151:4325–4332.
48. Niiro H, Otsuka T, Abe M, et al. Epstein-Barr virus BCRF1 gene product (viral interleukin-10) inhibits superoxide anion production by human monocytes. Lymphokine Cytokine Res 1992; 11:209–214.
49. Ralph P, Nakoinz I, Sampson-Johannes A, et al. IL-10, T lymphocyte inhibitor of human blood cell production of IL-1 and tumor necrosis factor. J Immunol 1992; 148: 808–814.
50. Cassatella MA, Meda L, Bonora S, et al. Interleukin-10 (IL-10) inhibits the release of proinflammatory cytokines from human polymorphonuclear leukocytes: Evidence for an autocrine role of tumor necrosis factor and IL-1 beta in mediating the production of IL-8 triggered by lipopolysaccharide. J Exp Med 1993; 178:2207–2211.
51. Takanaski S, Nonaka R, Xing Z, et al. Interleukin-10 inhibits lipopolysaccharide-induced survival and cytokines production by human peripheral blood eosinophils. J Exp Med 1994; 180:711–715.
52. Parronchi P, De CM, Manetti R, et al. IL-4 and IFN-$\alpha\gamma$ exert opposite regulatory effects on the development of cytolytic potential by Th1 or Th2 human T cell clones. J Immunol 1992; 149:2977–2983.
53. Hsieh C-S, Macatonia SE, Tripp CS, et al. Development of Th1 CD4$^+$ T cells through IL-12 produced by *Listeria*-induced macrophages. Science 1993; 260:547–554.
54. Fiorentino DF, Zlotnik A, Mosmann TR, et al. IL-10 inhibits cytokine production by activated macrophages. J Immunol 1991; 147:3815–3822.
55. Jenkins JK, Malyak M, Arend WP. The effects of interleukin-10 on interleukin-1 receptor antagonist and interleukin-1 beta production in human monocytes and neutrophils. Lymphokine Cytokine Res 1994; 13:47–54.
56. Cassatella MA, Meda L, Gasperini S, et al. Interleukin-10 (IL-10) upregulates IL-1 receptor antagonist production from lipopolysaccharide-stimulated human polymorphonuclear leukocytes by delaying mRNA degradation. J Exp Med 1994; 179:1695–1699.
57. Dinarello CA. The interleukin-1 family: 10 years of discovery. FASEB J 1994; 8:1314–1325.
58. Bejarano MT, de Waal Malefyt R, Abrams JS, et al. Interleukin 10 inhibits allogeneic proliferative and cytotoxic T cell responses generated in primary lymphocyte cultures. Int Immunol 1992; 4:1389–1397.
59. Caux C, Massacrier C, Vandervliet B, et al. Interleukin 10 inhibits T cell alloreaction induced by human dendritic cells. Int Immunol 1994; 6:1177–1185.
60. Bacchetta R, Bigler M, Touraine J-L, et al. High levels of IL-10 production in vivo

are associated with tolerance in a SCID patient transplanted with HLA mismatched hematopoietic stem cells. J Exp Med 1994; 179:493–502.
61. Matsuda M, Salazar F, Petersson M, et al. Interleukin-10 pretreatment protects target cells from tumor- and allo-specific cytotoxic T cells and downregulates HLA class I expression. J Exp Med 1994; 180:2371–2376.
62. Krenger W, Snyder K, Smith S, Ferrara JLM. Effects of exogenous interleukin-10 in a murine model of graft-versus-host disease to minor histocompatibility antigens. Transplantation 1994; 58:1251–1257.
63. Macatonia SE, Doherty TM, Knight SC, O'Garra A. Differential effect of IL-10 on dendritic cell-induced T cell proliferation and IFN-γ production. J Immunol 1993; 150:3755–3765.
64. Enk AH, Angeloni VL, Udey MC, Katz SI. Inhibition of Langerhans cell antigen-presenting function by IL-10. J Immunol 1993; 151:2390–2398.
65. Chen W-F, Zlotnik A. IL-10: A novel cytotoxic T cell differentiation factor. J Immunol 1991; 147:528–534.
66. Howard M, Muchamuel T, Andrade S, Menon S. Interleukin-10 protects mice from lethal endotoxemia. J Exp Med 1993; 177:1205–1208.
67. Gerard C, Bruyns C, Marchant A, et al. Interleukin-10 reduces the release of tumor necrosis factor and prevents lethality in experimental endotoxemia. J Exp Med 1993; 177:547–550.
68. Bean AG, Freiberg RA, Andrade S, et al. Interleukin-10 protects mice against staphylococcal enterotoxin B-induced lethal shock. Infect Immunol 1993; 61:4937–4939.
69. Drake CG, Kotzin BL. Superantigens: Biology, immunology and potential role in disease. J Clin Immunol 1992; 12:149–162.
70. Miethke T, Wahl C, Heeg K, et al. T cell-mediated lethal shock triggered in mice by the superantigen staphylococcal enterotoxin B: Critical role of tumor necrosis factor. J Exp Med 1992; 175:91–98.
71. Tarazona R, González-García A, Zamzami N, et al. Chlorpromazine amplifies macrophage-dependent IL-10 production in vivo. J Immunol 1995; 154:861–870.
72. Kuhn R, Lohler J, Rennick D, et al. Interleukin-10-deficient mice develop chronic enterocolitis. Cell 1993; 75:263–274.
73. Powrie F, Leach MW, Mauze S, et al. Inhibition of Th1 responses prevents inflammatory bowel disease in SCID mice reconstituted with cd45rb^{hi} CD4^{+} T cells. Immunity 1994; 1:553–562.
74. Pennline KJ, Roque-Gaffney E, Monahan M. Recombinant human IL-10 prevents the onset of diabetes in the nonobese diabetic mouse. Clin Immunol Immunopathol USA 1994; 71:169–175.
75. Rabinovitch A, Sorensen O, Suarez-Pinzon WL, et al. Analysis of cytokine mRNA expression in syngeneic islet grafts of NOD mice: Interleukin-2 and interferon gamma mRNA expression correlate with graft rejection and interleukin-10 with graft survival. Diabetologia 1994; 37:833–887.
76. Calcinaro F, Shehadeh NN, Lafferty KJ. CFA-mediated regulation of diabetes in the NOD mouse: A role for IL-4 and IL-10. 30th Annual Meeting of the European Association for the Study of Diabetes, Dusesseldorf, Germany, September 27–October 1, 1994.
77. Wogensen L, Huang X, Sarvetnick N. Leukocyte extravasation into the pancreatic tissue in transgenic mice expressing interleukin-10 in the islets of Langerhans. J Exp Med 1993; 178:175–185.
78. Wogensen L, Lee M-S, Sarvetnick N. Production of interleukin 10 by islet cells accelerates immune-mediated destruction of β cells in nonobese diabetic mice. J Exp Med 1994; 179:1379–1384.

79. Moritani M, Yoshimto K, Tashiro F, et al. Transgenic expression of IL-10 in pancreatic islet A cells accelerates autoimmune insulitis and diabetes in non-obese diabetic mice. Int Immunol 1994; 6:1927–1936.
80. Takeuchi T, Lowry RP, Konieczny B. Heart allografts in murine systems. Transplantation 1992; 53:1281–1294.
81. Gorczynski RM, Wojcik D. A role for nonspecific (cyclosporin A) or specific (monoclonal antibodies to ICAM-1, LFA-1 and IL-10) immunomodulation in the prolongation of skin allografts after antigen-specific pretransplant immunization or transfusion. J Immunol 1994; 152:2011–2019.
82. Hancock W, Mottram PL, Purcell LJ, et al. Prolonged survival of mouse cardiac allografts after CD4 or CD8 monoclonal antibody therapy is associated with selective intragraft cytokine protein expression: Interleukin (IL)-4 and IL-10 but not IL-2 or interferon-γ. Transplant Proc 1993; 25:2937–2938.
83. Chavin KD, Qin L, Tahara H, et al. Gene transfer of TGF-β and viral IL-10 prolong cardiac allograft survival. Surg Forum 1993; 44:407–409.
84. Lee M-S, Wogensen L, Shizuru J, et al. Pancreatic islet production of murine interleukin-10 does not inhibit immune-mediated tissue destruction. J Clin Invest 1994; 93: 1332–1338.
85. Abramowicz D, Durez P, Donckier V, et al. Neonatal induction of transplantation tolerance in mice is associated with in vivo expression of IL-4 and -10 mRNA. Transplant Proc 1993; 25:312–313.
86. Fowler DH, Kurasawa K, Husebekk A, et al. Cells of Th2 cytokine phenotype prevent LPS-induced lethality during murine graft-versus-host reaction. J Immunol 1994; 152: 1004–1013.
87. Allen RD, Staley TA, Sidman CL. Differential cytokine expression in acute and chronic murine graft-versus-host disease. Eur J Immunol 1993; 23:333–337.
88. Garlisi CG, Pennline KJ, Smith SR, et al. Cytokine gene expression in mice undergoing chronic graft-versus-host disease. Mol Immunol (England) 1993; 30:669–677.
89. De Wit D, Van Mechelen M, Zanin C, et al. Preferential activation of Th2 cells in chronic graft-versus-host reaction. J Immunol 1993; 150:361–366.
90. Blazar BR, Taylor PA, Smith S, Vallera DA. Interleukin-10 administration decrease survival in murine recipients of major histocompatibility complex disparate donor bone marrow grafts. Blood 1995; 85:842–851.
91. Broski AP, Halloran PF. Tissue distribution of IL-10 mRNA in normal mice: Evidence that a component of IL-10 expression is T and B cell-independent and increased by irradiation. Transplantation 1994; 57:582–592.
92. Karp CL, El-Safi SH, Wynn TA, et al. In vivo cytokine profiles in patients with kala azar: Marked elevation of both interleukin-10 and interferon-gamma. J Clin Invest 1993; 91:1644–1648.
93. Yamamura M, Uyemura K, Deans RJ, et al. Defining protective responses to pathogens: Cytokine profiles in leprosy lesions. Science 1992; 254:277–279.
94. King CL, Mahanty S, Kumaraswami V, et al. Cytokine control of parasite-specific anergy in human lymphatic filariasis: Preferential induction of a regulatory T helper type 2 lymphocyte subset. J Clin Invest 1993; 92:1667–1673.
95. Marchant A, Debiére J, Byl B, et al. Interleukin 10 production during septicemia. Lancet 1994; 343:707–708.
96. Bacchetta R, Vandekerckhove BAE, Touraine JL, et al. Chimerism and tolerance to host and donor in severe combined immunodeficiencies transplanted with fetal liver stem cells. J Clin Invest 1993; 91:1067–1078.
97. Roncarolo MG, Yssel H, Touraine JL, et al. Autoreactive T cell clones specific for class I and class II HLA antigens isolated from human chimera. J Exp Med 1988; 167: 1523–1534.

98. Bacchetta R, Parkman R, McMahon M, et al. Dysfunctional cytokine production by host-reactive T-cell clones isolated from a chimeric SCID patient transplanted with haploidentical bone marrow. Blood 1995; 85:1944–1953.
99. Roncarolo MG, Yssel H, Touraine JL, et al. Antigen recognition by MHC-incompatible cells of a human mismatched chimera. J Exp Med 1988; 168:2139–2152.
100. Holler E, Roncarolo MG, Hintermeier-Knable R, et al. Low incidence of transplanted related complications in patients with high spontaneous cellular IL-10 production prior to conditioning: Evidence for a protective role of IL-10 in allogeneic BMT (abstr). 21st Annual Meeting of the EBMT, Davos, Switzerland, March 19–23, 1994.
101. Guillaume T, Sekhavat M, Rubinstein DB, et al. Defective cytokine production following autologous stem cell transplantation for solid tumors and hematologic malignancies regardless of bone marrow or peripheral origin and lack of evidence for a role for interleukin-10 in delayed immune reconstitution. Cancer Res 1994; 54:3800–3807.
102. Cunningham DA, Dunn MJ, Yacoub MH, Rose ML. Local production of cytokines in the human cardiac allograft. Transplantation 1994; 57:1333–1337.
103. Merville P, Pouteil-Noble C, Wijdenes J, et al. Detection of single cells secreting IFN-gamma, IL-6 and IL-10 in irreversibly rejected human kidney allografts and their modulation of IL-2 and IL-4. Transplantation 1993; 55:639–646.
104. Donckier V, Flament V, Gérard C, et al. Modulation of the release of cytokines and reduction of the shock syndrome induced by anti-CD3 monoclonal antibody in mice by interleukin-10. Transplantation 1994; 57:1436–1439.
105. Abramowicz D, Schandene L, Goldman M, et al. Release of tumor necrosis factor, interleukin-2 and gamma-interferon in serum after injection of OKT3 monoclonal antibody in kidney transplant recipients. Transplantation 1989; 47:606–608.
106. Chernoff AE, Granowitz EV, Shapiro L, et al. A phase I study of interleukin-10 in healthy humans: Safety and effects on cytokine production. In: de Vries JE, de Waal Malefyt R, eds. Interleukin 10. Austin, TX: Landes, 1995.

27

Positive Stem-Cell Selection for Hematopoietic Transplantation

Stephen J. Noga
Johns Hopkins Oncology Center
Johns Hopkins University School of Medicine
Baltimore, Maryland

Curt I. Civin
Johns Hopkins University School of Medicine
Baltimore, Maryland

I. DEFINING THE HEMATOPOIETIC STEM/ PROGENITOR-CELL POPULATION

The CD34 antigen defines a small population of cells comprising the stem and progenitor cell compartment (1–3). Hematopoietic cells giving rise to the most primitive colony-forming units possess the highest concentration of CD34 antigen on their surface (4,5). Outside of the blood system, the CD34 antigen is expressed by certain vascular endothelial cells, some neuronal elements, and a few specialized cells of mesodermal origin (6,7).

The human CD34 gene is localized at the q32 region of chromosome 1 and encodes a unique 40-kDa polypeptide without identity to known molecules (8). Most of the CD34 transmembrane protein molecule is extracellular and heavily glycosylated. The heavy glycosylation of the CD34 protein results in its anomalous electrophoretic mobility, resulting in an anomalous molecular weight of approximately 115 kDa by SDS PAGE analysis, instead of the much lower weight predicted by the cDNA sequence (8,9). There is a short intracytoplasmic tail which is phosphorylated on intracellular serines by protein kinase C, suggesting a role for CD34 in signal transduction (10). A second CD34 molecule, created by alternative RNA splicing, lacks most of this intracytoplasmic tail (9). Despite extensive characterization of the CD34 protein and gene, the function of the CD34 molecule remains elusive. The similarities between CD34 and several of the sialomucins (especially CD43/leukosialin) suggests that CD34 functions as an adhesion molecule (11).

The CD34 membrane phosphoglycoprotein is the marker of choice for human stem and progenitor cells because of its exquisitely specific expression on only the most immature cells within the lymphohematopoietic system (1–3,9,12–14). Additional properties of CD34 facilitate its wide use as a target antigen in research and clinical applications requiring identification and purification of stem and progenitor cells. First, CD34 expression is not downmodulated by antibody binding (9,12); endocytosis or shedding of targeted CD34 molecules would, of course, reduce cell labeling. Second, antibody binding to CD34 does not affect the major functions of stem and progenitor cells: survival, proliferation, and differentiation. Third, multiple, well-characterized CD34 monoclonal antibodies are widely available. By the time of the most recent International Leukocyte Differentiation Workshop, over 30 CD34 monoclonal antibodies had been reported (2). Fourth, these antibodies bind to at least three distinct extracellular domains (epitopes) (2,3,9,13). Antigen-antibody binding in one domain of the CD34 molecules does not block binding to another CD34 epitope(s). Likewise, enzymatic cleavage or alteration of a given molecular domain still allows the identification of other CD34 epitopes by antibodies specific for those unaltered epitopes. This provides a powerful resource for enumeration (or repeat purification) of positively selected hematopoietic stem/progenitor cells (14).

II. CLINICAL USE OF PURIFIED CD34$^+$ CELLS

Several methods for clinical scale CD34$^+$ hematopoietic stem cell selection have been designed and are in clinical trials using bone marrow (BM), cord, and peripheral blood stem cells (PBSC) as sources for stem-cell grafts (14). Certain devices are already marketed in Europe or Canada, although no device is yet licensed by the U.S. Food and Drug Administration. CD34 antibody can be directly (or indirectly) coupled to an affinity matrix, which will then capture the CD34$^+$ cells (immunoaffinity purification). The capture matrices can be either fluid/suspension (immunomagnetic beads, ferric colloids, flow cytometry) or solid (columns, tissue culture surfaces) (12–14). Clinical results to date for CD34$^+$ cell purities range from 40 to 95%, with overall CD34$^+$ cell recoveries (yields) of 25 to 70% (13). Recent clinical trials have established that isolated, autologous CD34$^+$ cells can readily reestablish hematopoietic engraftment following myeloablative transplant therapy (15,16,26). What advantage might these purified CD34$^+$ cells provide?

A. Autologous BMT

Relapse remains the major cause of treatment failure in autologous transplantation (17). It is now apparent that even many early-stage solid tumors (e.g., stage 2 breast cancer) metastasize to the marrow space (18). Tumor cells can be detected in a significant proportion of BM and PBSC harvests and have been shown to at least contribute to relapse (19). Thus, investigative treatments aimed at maximizing eventual cure rate must provide a cancer-free hematopoietic graft. Most tumor "purging" strategies rely on tumor-selective/specific drugs such as 4-hydroperoxycyclophosphamide (4-HC) or anti-tumor monoclonal antibodies (20,21). However, 4-HC eliminates nearly all (>90%) normal committed progenitor cells, leading to delayed engraftment (22). Antitumor antibody purging methods may also result in delayed engraftment, possibly due to nonspecific damage to or loss of stem/progenitor cells. On the other hand, antitumor drugs or antibodies may not purge all the tumor cells, due to drug resistance or tumor heterogeneity (13,23). In contrast, CD34$^+$ selection provides a "reverse purge" of CD34$^-$ cancer cells without these limitations. Of course, this approach is not useful for patients whose cancers express the CD34 antigen, such as many of the acute leukemias (1–3). The use of further cell purification steps after CD34$^+$ cell selection, involving additional monoclonal antibodies to remove cancer cells or to isolate nonneoplastic, pluripotent stem cells may eventually be possible (24). At present, it is not yet known which subpopulations of CD34$^+$ cells are required for short versus long-term lymphohematopoietic reconstitution. Ultimately, this will have to be determined by transplantation of CD34$^+$ cell subsets in patients. It is also clear that residual cancer elsewhere in the body of the patient contributes to relapse. This is substantiated clinically in that relapses of tumors after autologous or allogeneic BMT frequently occur at sites of prior disease (25). Thus, parallel studies must address residual host tumor burden.

Studies by Berenson (15), Shpall (16), and Civin (26) reported that CD34$^+$ selected autologous BM engrafted in patients who had received myeloablative preparative transplant chemo(radio)therapy for lymphoma, breast cancer, and pediatric solid tumors. Depletion of 2 to 4 logs of tumor cells has been reported (12,13,16). The optimal CD34$^+$ cell dose for prompt engraftment after autologous marrow transplant is not yet determined. In addition, the effects of hematopoietic growth factors (e.g., G-CSF, GM-CSF, SCF, IL3/GM-CSF fusion protein, FLT3 ligand, thrombopoietin) in shortening time to hematopoietic reconstitution are incompletely characterized.

B. Related, Allogeneic BMT

As discussed in the previous chapters, GVHD remains the major complication of allogeneic BMT. Although lymphocyte depletion of donor grafts significantly reduces GVHD, other complications such as graft failure, relapse, and secondary B-cell malignancies may obviate any survival advantage (27). Retrospective studies now show that many lymphocyte-depletion techniques resulted in the nonspecific loss of (or damage to) large numbers of clonogenic (progenitor) cells during the purging procedure (27). Animal studies also suggested that immunocompetent donor lymphocytes may actually facilitate engraftment by overcoming host-versus-graft resistance: a host immune response that is not extinguished by myeloablative therapy (28).

Use of marrow-depleted of lymphocytes by elutriation is also associated with delayed granulocyte and platelet engraftment kinetics (29). It was initially unclear why this occurred, since surrogate measures of graft adequacy (in vitro clonogenic assays for CFU-GM, CFU-MIX, BFU-E) showed high retention of progenitor cells in the elutriated "large cell" graft preparations (30). Recently, Jones et al. demonstrated that the long-term murine repopulating "stem" cell resides in the small-cell (lymphocyte-rich) elutriation fraction, whereas the committed progenitors (characterized by their ability to form 14 day colonies in vitro) are mainly in the lymphocyte-depleted large-cell fraction (31). It was found that two-thirds of the human CD34$^+$ cells reside in the small-cell elutriation fractions (32). In the past, small CD34$^+$ cells were almost totally excluded from the lymphocyte-depleted graft (only large cells, containing $\geq 90\%$ of the colony-forming cells, were used for the grafts) (29). This small-cell fraction has also been shown to contain the majority of high proliferative colony forming cells (HPP-CFC), which are believed to be more representative of long-term repopulating stem cells than those detected by routine clonogenic assays (33). The physical loss of this subset of smaller-sized hematopoietic cells might explain the delayed engraftment kinetics and high rates of mixed chimerism seen following transplant with elutriated marrow (27,34).

In the initial elutriation studies, the readdition of only low numbers of the cells (1 to 2 × 10^6/kg) from the previously discarded small-cell elutriation fractions to the marrow grafts resulted in GVHD, presumably due to the predominance (50 to 90%) of lymphocytes among the small cells (35). Therefore our group explored purifying the CD34$^+$ cells from the small-cell fractions and adding only these purified CD34$^+$ cells (putatively stem-cell–enriched) back to the lymphocyte-depleted, progenitor-enriched large-cell elutriation fraction to form the modified graft (Fig. 1). This small-cell fraction appears to be a favorable population for further manipulation, since CD34$^+$ cells were obtained in high yield and purity (Table 1). By adding back the resulting 80% pure CD34$^+$ small cells (only 6% T cells), the graft's CD34$^+$ cell content was doubled while only adding a small number (≤ 10^5/kg) of T lymphocytes. The patients in this phase I study engrafted rapidly, reaching 500 granulocytes/μL by day 19; 50,000 platelets/μL by day 24; and leaving the hospital by day 22 after transplant (medians) (56). This compares with median days of 23,

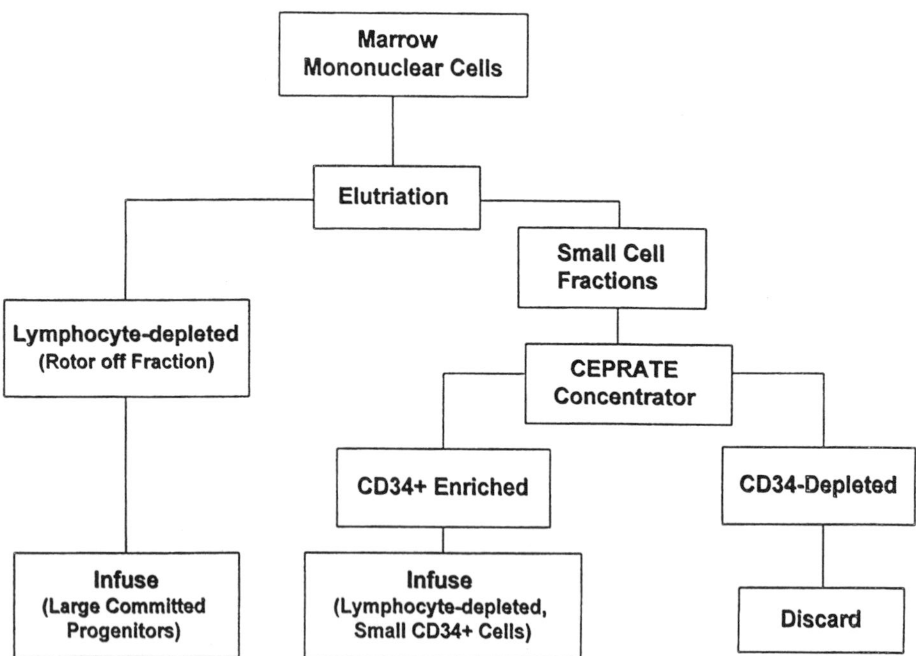

Figure 1 Schema for CD34$^+$ augmentation of elutriated bone marrow. Normal donor bone marrow is harvested and the mononuclear cells are isolated by apheresis. Lymphocyte depletion is accomplished by elutriation. The large-sized (committed progenitor–rich), lymphocyte-depleted fraction is infused immediately. The lymphocyte-predominant fractions containing small (and presumably less differentiated) CD34$^+$ cells are pooled, incubated, with biotinylated anti-CD34 monoclonal antibody, and the CD34$^+$ cells enriched over a biotin-avidin column (33). Following morphological verification, enumeration, and viability testing, this fraction is also reinfused in its entirety.

Table 1 Characteristics of the CD34$^+$ Augmented, Elutriated Allograft[a]

Fraction	Nuc Cells/ kg ($\times 10^7$)	Graft (%)	CD34$^+$/ kg ($\times 10^6$)	CD34$^+$ purity (%)	CFU-GM/ kg ($\times 10^4$)	CD3$^+$ (%)	CD3$^+$/ kg ($\times 10^5$)
Unseparated bone marrow	50.0 (7.7)	–	3.8 (1.0)	0.8 (1.0)	12	28 (6.0)	1400 (500)
Large (R/O)	2.8 (0.4)	94.1 (1.0)	1.8 (0.2)	6.4 (1.8)	9.0 (1.3)	1.7 (1.0)	4.8 (1.0)
Small(CD34$^+$)	0.2 (0.1)	5.9 (1.0)	1.7 (0.5)	79.0 (2.2)	1.2 (0.4)	5.9 (0.9)	1.2 (0.3)
Engineered graft	3.1 (0.4)	100	3.4 (0.5)	11.0 (2.0)	10.2 (1.3)	1.9 (1.0)	6.0 (1.1)

[a]Data ($N=10$) are reported as the mean ± SEM (parentheses) for the T-cell-depleted, large-cell elutriated fraction (rotor-off; R/O), the purified, small-sized CD34$^+$ stem cell fraction and the infused, composite graft. Cell doses are reported as cell/kg recipient IBW.

44, and 34, respectively in transplants of grafts processed by elutriation without CD34$^+$ augmentation (Fig. 2). The median days post-BMT for granulocyte/platelet engraftment and hospital discharge for patients receiving an unmanipulated graft during the same time period but using only cyclosporine A (CSA) and methotrexate as GVHD prophylaxis were 25, 28, and 32, respectively. When compared to patients receiving unmanipulated donor grafts, patients receiving CD34$^+$ augmented/elutriated grafts showed a 40% reduction in hospitalization charges, due in part to their early discharge, rapid engraftment, low blood product and antibiotic requirements, and low incidence of GVHD (36,37). Only 2 of these initial 10 patients developed minimal acute GVHD, which resolved with corticosteroids. None have developed chronic GVHD at a median follow up of 30 months.

In the development of such combined-modality approaches, seemingly small changes in therapeutic management can result in significant differences in clinical outcome. In the above phase I trial of CD34 augmentation/elutriation, CSA was used as additional GVHD prophylaxis for 6 months post-BMT, because functional T cells were intentionally included in the allograft. Cyclosporine A prophylaxis had been used in previous elutriation trials. In a prior study using elutriation alone, omission of CSA prophylaxis led to inordinately high (75%) graft failure rates (27). To determine whether an increased stem-cell dose would permit a significant CSA reduction, patients received a CD34$^+$ augmented graft with only a 30-day course of CSA. In 31 patients treated in this manner, there were no differences in engraftment kinetics or day of hospital discharge when compared to those receiving 180 days of CSA (38). Therefore, increasing the stem-cell dose appears to overcome allogeneic immune rejection mechanisms, so that minimal post-BMT immunosuppression is necessary to prevent graft rejection. However, 65% of these reduced CSA dose patients developed acute GVHD during the final CSA taper or within 2 weeks of discontinuation, with 25% progressing to chronic GVHD. While only 1 patient died from direct complications of GVHD (30% had grade II, 0% grade III/IV disease), there was considerable morbidity associated with its treatment (i.e., the immuno-

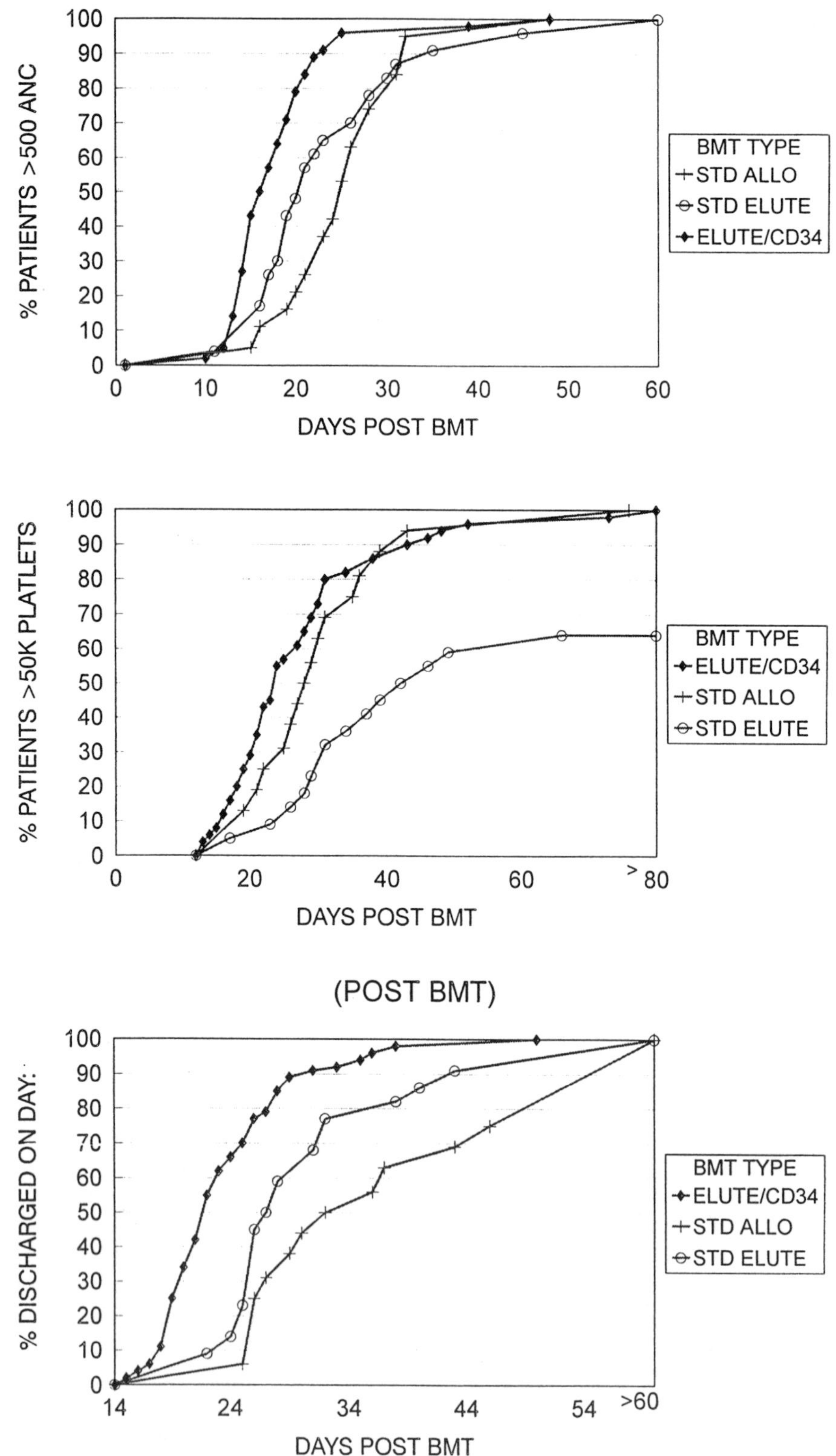

Figure 2 Engraftment kinetics and hospital stay of patients receiving a $CD34^+$ augmented/elutriated allograft. The data are from 56 patients receiving a $CD34^+$-augmented/elutriated

Table 2 Modeling Efficacy of T-Cell Depletion Using CD34⁺ Selection[a]

CD34⁺ selection of the unseparated marrow preparation								
Unseparated BM					Selected CD34⁺ fraction			
Marrow Cells/kg	T Cells (%)	T Cells /kg	CD34 (%)	CD34 /kg	Cells/kg	CD34 (%)	CD34 /kg	T Cells /kg
4×10^8	40	1.6×10^8	1	4×10^6	8×10^6	60	4.8×10^6	1.3×10^6
2×10^8	20	4×10^7	1	2×10^6	4×10^6	60	2.4×10^6	3.2×10^5
2×10^8	20	4×10^7	2	4×10^6	4×10^6	80	3.2×10^6	1.6×10^5
2×10^8	10	2×10^7	2	4×10^6	4×10^6	80	3.2×10^6	8.0×10^4
CD34⁺ selection of only the elutriated lymhocyte-rich fractions								
Elutriated lymphocyte-rich fractions					CD34⁺ Selected lymphocyte-rich fraction			
4.5×10^7	50	2.3×10^7	10	4.5×10^6	9×10^5	80	7.2×10^5	9.2×10^4
9×10^7	50	4.5×10^7	5	4.5×10^6	1.8×10^6	50	9.0×10^5	4.5×10^5

[a]A normal marrow collection for allogeneic BMT is $1\text{-}3\times10^{10}$ nucleated marrow cells, approx. $2\text{-}4\times10^8$ cells/kg recipient ideal body weight (IBW). Unlike small diagnostic marrow aspirates, large BM harvests are heavily contaminated with peripheral blood, which can increase the T-cell content to as high as 40%. Cell recovery following CD34⁺ selection assumes a standard 2% recovery of input cells (common to both avidin/biotin column and immunomagnetic bead separation). Various marrow percentages of nucleated cells, T cells, and CD34⁺ stem/progenitor cells are modeled to portray a predicted CD34⁺ cell recovery and a predicted T-cell content of the selected product, assuming that T cells behave as "innocent bystanders" during the CD34⁺ cell purification.

suppressive therapy). Upon these observations, we changed to 80 days of CSA prophylaxis. Thirty patients treated with 80-day CSA prophylaxis showed minimal (<10%) or no acute or chronic GVHD; rapid engraftment has been maintained (39). Thus, engineering of the allograft can influence other treatment modalities needed in conjunction with BMT.

An obvious question is whether CD34⁺ selection of the allograft is sufficient in itself for T cell depletion (TCD) without using the added step of elutriation. The moderately low incidence of graft failure in our previous elutriation trials suggests that a high level of safety was maintained in this initial study by employing the large cell, rotor-off (R/O) fraction, unaltered. Future trials will have to address whether there is a stringent requirement for elutriation in conjunction with CD34⁺ selection. However, elutriation is an integral part of our current clinical protocol. From a technical standpoint, it provides a useful preselection method for stem-cell isolation by removing a large number of non-targeted cells, platelets, and cellular debris, which may limit the purification and yield of CD34⁺ cells. Since graft T-cell content is determined by both the percentage and total number of T cells remaining after positive selection, this approach further reduces total graft T cells because the entire

---

graft. For comparison, 22 previously published patients receiving only elutriated marrow and 19 patients (with diagnoses of CML-chronic phase and aplastic anemia) who received unmanipulated marrow during the same period as the CD34 augmentation trial are depicted. A. Granulocyte engraftment. B. Platelet engraftment C. Day of hospital discharge (post-BMT).

$CD34^+$ selected fraction represents only 0.4% of the initial harvest (32). For this example, one applies the assumption that T-cell contamination of the $CD34^+$ product is non-specific and mirrors the T-cell content of the initial harvest. Thus, total T-cell contamination of the $CD34^+$ graft is the product of the initial percentage of unselected T cells multiplied by the percentage of cells recovered in the selected fraction (Table 2). The total percentage of T cells present in the $CD34^+$ selected graft equals this product (T-cell contamination) divided by the number of total cells comprising this fraction times 100. $CD34^+$ selection results in a 1.5- or 2-log reduction in total cell numbers (1 to 2% cell recovery following separation), which consequently reduces the total number of cells by 98%. Although this results in a substantial depletion of T cells, the variability in BM-harvest T-cell contamination can result in a wide range of final T-cell content in the $CD34^+$ selected product. However, if advances in immunoaffinity technology were to ensure higher $CD34^+$ purities, this would consequently result in lower final T-cell burdens, since T-cell contamination is assumed to be nonspecific. Alternatively, the lymphocyte-rich triation fractions contain only 10 to 20% of the initial marrow cells and and are partially enriched for $CD34^+$ cells; positive selection results in higher $CD34^+$ cell purities with T cells accounting for a smaller percentage of the total selected cells. It is possible that a sequential second or third $CD34^+$ selection of an unmanipulated graft or a further "negative" depletion step using anti-T-cell reagents could result in a similar degree of TCD to that obtained with CD34 augmentation/elutriation. This awaits further investigation. Another argument against using only $CD34^+$ selected cells is that allogeneic engraftment may be dependent upon the number of total cells in the graft; allogeneic grafts consisting solely of $CD34^+$ cells may be predisposed to immunological rejection because of the small number of cells (about 10^8) transplanted (40). The lymphocyte-depleted large cell elutriation fraction provides not only a significant number of committed progenitors but also a large number of total nucleated cells (10^{10}) that may be protective against immune rejection.

C. Unrelated and HLA-Mismatched Allogeneic BMT

The problems encountered in using HLA-matched donor marrow are amplified in mismatched or unrelated donor settings. Even without graft manipulation, there is an inherently high graft failure rate, and almost all patients develop significant acute and chronic GVHD (41). While the use of T-cell depletion and augmented immunosuppression can decrease the incidence of GVHD and appears to be associated with low relapse rates, this may be at the cost of higher rates of graft failure, life-threatening opportunistic infections, and development of B-cell neoplasms.

Using a similar graft-engineering approach to that of HLA-related BMT, donor grafts have been lymphocyte-depleted using elutriation and then augmented with purified small-sized $CD34^+$ cells recovered from the lymphocyte-rich elutriation fractions. This approach, currently used in phase I trials at Johns Hopkins University and the University of Minnesota, has resulted in durable engraftment in unrelated matched, and 1- and 2-antigen mismatched related BMT with a decreased incidence of clinically relevant GVHD (42). In contrast to HLA-matched BMT, intensified immunosuppression (longer CSA course and corticosteroids with or without anti-thymocyte globulin) is used for both engraftment and GVHD prophylaxis. The opportunity for further improving these engineering procedures is discussed below.

D. Peripheral Blood Stem-Cell (PBSC) Transplantation

Several recent developments have led to an increased use of PBSC grafts as a source of stem-cell rescue. Increased numbers of stem cells circulate in the blood following the use of cytotoxic drugs or hematopoietic growth factors, (or both), such that large numbers of $CD34^+$ cells can be harvested by leukapheresis (43). High flow apheresis can yield enough stem cells in one harvest procedure to ensure rapid, sustained engraftment (44). Although there is concern regarding the comobilization of cancer cells, several recent studies have suggested that there are fewer tumor cells in these PBSC products than in harvested marrow (45,46). There are now several studies evaluating the use of $CD34^+$ selected PBSC stem cells for transplantation (43).

Many PBSC transplant studies have identified a minimum $CD34^+$ cell dose above which engraftment is rapid and durable. Most of these studies have utilized non-CD34 selected ("unpurified"), mobilized PBSC grafts, followed by posttransplant administration of growth factors to these patients (47,48). These studies report that a threshold dose, ranging in various studies from approximately 0.5 to 5×10^6 $CD34^+$ cells/kg, will result in rapid and sustained tri-lineage hematopoiesis (49). Depending on the preparative regimen, it has been possible to reduce the period of significant neutropenia (granulocytes $< 500/\mu L$) to a few days (53). Shpall and colleagues have shown that administration of purified $CD34^+$ stem/progenitor cells results in approximately the same engraftment kinetics as found with unpurified PBSC preparations (54). There appear to be two reasons for the relatively wide variation in reported thresholds for optimal $CD34^+$ cell dose. First, in most studies, investigators have given their patients relatively high $CD34^+$ cell doses, such that only a few patients received subthreshold or near-threshold $CD34^+$ cell doses (50). Second, $CD34^+$ cell enumeration is not uniform or quantitatively comparable across institutions, although major standardization efforts are in progress (51,52).

Until recently, PBSC rescue was used only for autologous transplantation (55,56). There are now studies using normal, related donor PBSC grafts for allogeneic transplantation. Donors are mobilized with hematopoietic growth factors and harvested over several days. Engraftment is rapid and appears sustained. These PBSC products can contain 5 to 10 times more T cells than normal donor marrow harvests. Despite this high T-cell burden, investigators are reporting only minimal acute GVHD with the use of unmanipulated PBSC products. Most unmanipulated PBSC trials having adequate follow up suggest a high incidence of chronic GVHD, however (55,56). If these products trigger less GVHD than their marrow counterparts, would $CD34^+$ selection or other forms of specific T-cell depletion further decrease the incidence of GVHD? Studies using $CD34^+$ selection have recently started, but follow-up is short at present. For example T-cell-depleted PBSC along with similarly depleted BM have been used to improve engraftment following haplomismatched pediatric transplantation (57). In this case, increased stem-cell dose was used to overcome the allogeneic immune response of the recipient. While acute

GVHD was decreased, longer follow up is required to assess chronic GVHD and other long-term complications. This approach may also be applicable to unrelated BMT.

E. Cord Blood: In Utero Transplantation

Umbilical cord blood can serve as an alternative source of hematopoietic stem cells for transplantation. Many of the initial problems (adequate sample collection, sample manipulation, cryopreservation) have been minimized, and cord blood cell banks are now being established. Allogeneic transplants have demonstrated that cord blood has sufficient hematopoietic precursors for long-term engraftment and that the incidence of GVHD is low (58). Use of cord blood for unrelated donor BMT is currently under investigation (59). Since to date the recipients have been children, it is unclear whether sufficient progenitor cells can be obtained for use in adult transplantation (i.e., especially to increase the unrelated donor pool for allogeneic transplantation).

F. Transplantation for Inherited Diseases: in Utero Transplantation

The first gene therapy trials were actually performed via allogeneic BMT. Patients with inherited metabolic disorders lacking enzymes that can be supplied by normal hematopoietic precursors have had successful enzyme replacement and an arrest in their disease progression following transplantation (60). Unfortunately, many of these disorders result in early neurological impairment, including irreversible mental retardation.

Animal data suggest that stable donor chimerism can be established by in utero transplantation (61). Since the gravid uterus represents a protected immunological site, parental, mismatched stem cells may serve as an acceptable source of normal cells to correct the enzyme deficiency early in fetal development. Animal studies suggest that GHVD will be minimized in this setting. However, stem-cell dose (especially in the mismatched setting) and the small volumes that can be introduced before 12 weeks gestation raise significant problems. Positive selection of $CD34^+$ cells is currently being investigated for in utero transplantation, since it significantly reduces total cell numbers, T cells, and the inoculum volume (62). The high donor stem-cell dose in relation to the fetal hematopoietic pool may facilitate long-term donor chimerism and a continuous supply of the gene product.

III. FUTURE DIRECTIONS

A. Induction of Autologous GVHD

In terms of curative potential, the anti-tumor effect conferred by allogeneic transplant may exceed that offered by autologous BMT (63). It is unclear whether this allogeneic advantage is mediated by a graft-versus-host response. Whatever the mechanism, it appears that additional immunotherapeutic interventions are required to eliminate residual host leukemia or tumor cells. An autoimmune syndrome can be induced following a short course of immunosuppression. This "autologous GVHD" is MHC class II restricted and similar in clinical appearance and pathological morphology to GVHD (64). Autologous GVHD responses can be intensified by upregulating the target antigen (MHC class II) on residual tumor cells with interferon (65). The tempo of the immune response is further augmented by using IL-2 following BMT (66). Preliminary data suggest that improved disease-free survival has been achieved with this approach in breast cancer and lymphoma. Marrow purged with 4-HC is capable of generating an autologous GVHD response. Autologous GVHD can also be induced with cytokine-mobilized PBSC products; progression-free survival is longer for patients transplanted for stage three or four breast cancer using PBSCs and autologous GVHD induction (67). Can $CD34^+$ marrow or PBSC grafts be used to induce autologous GVHD? Since both 4-HC purged marrow grafts (which essentially contain only viable stem cells) and PBSC grafts can induce autologous GVHD, it is probable that a $CD34^+$ selected graft would generate autologous GVHD while providing a tumor-depleted stem cell source. These studies have yet to be conducted.

B. Augmenting $CD34^+$ Grafts with Ancillary Cell Populations

As previously discussed, other cell populations present in the hematopoietic graft may play key roles in engraftment, antitumor activity, immune reconstitution, and—in the case of autologous transplant—GVHD induction. Over the last 5 years, efforts in graft manipulation have concentrated on isolating the stem/progenitor cell population ($CD34^+$ cells) and demonstrating engraftment. Since this is well established, the contribution of other graft-cell populations can now be explored. This would involve their deliberate isolation, characterization, and infusion distinct from the $CD34^+$ stem-cell component. For example, graft lymphoid subpopulations could be depleted of $CD8^+$ cells (or, alternatively, positively selected for $CD4^+$ cells), cryopreserved and reinfused at selected time intervals after allogeneic BMT to augment anti-leukemic activity or else used therapeutically at the development of cytogenetic or molecular relapse (68,69). Champlin et al. have shown that CD8 depleted buffy-coat cells are capable of inducing remission in relapsed CML patients without graft failure or the development of clinically significant GVHD (70). Preliminary work also shows that following $CD34^+$ selection, the $CD34^+$ cell-depleted fraction can be incubated with a second monoclonal antibody, and further graft subpopulations can be purified. Preliminary data show that using this approach results, for example, in the isolation of $CD56^+$ NK cells in large quantities (71). These cells have high NK activity against both NK-sensitive and NK-resistant targets following isolation or when activated with IL-2 in culture (72). These cells could be cryopreserved and incorporated into a GVL strategy similar to that described for CD8-depleted cells. In fact, sequential cell populations could be obtained in this manner for immediate or delayed use, depending on their intended function.

IV. SUMMARY

While some aspects of this discussion are speculative, other points are less controversial.

1. Cells identified and purified by CD34 monoclonal antibody contain hematopoietic stem/progenitor cells capable of mediating prompt, sustained multilineage engraftment.
2. There is a "threshold" number of autologous $CD34^+$ PBSC cells that are

required for rapid, sustained engraftment. Several factors (including the stem-cell source, use of post-BMT cytokines, and the "relatedness" of the transplant) may affect this threshold value.

3. The CD34$^+$ cells do not directly cause GVHD.
4. Even small changes in the host therapeutic regimen or the hematopoietic graft product can have a profound influence on long-term transplant outcome and quality of life. This must be incorporated into the study design and long-term management of patients receiving engineered grafts.

REFERENCES

1. Civin CI, Strauss LC, Brovall C, et al. Antigenic analysis of hematopoiesis: III. A hematopoietic progenitor cell surface antigen defined by a monoclonal antibody raised against KG-1a cells. J Immunol 1984; 133:157–165.
2. Greaves MF, Titley I, Colman SM, et al. M10 CD34 cluster workshop report. In: Leukocyte Typing V. Oxford, England: Oxford University Press, 1995; Vol 1:840–849.
3. Civin CI, Trischmann TM, Fackler MJ, et al. Summary of CD34 cluster workshop section. In: Knapp W, Dorken B, Gilks WR, et al., eds. Leukocyte Typing IV. Oxford, England: Oxford University Press, 1990:818–825.
4. Civin CI, Banquerigo LC, Strauss LC, et al. Antigenic analysis of hematopoiesis: VI. Flow cytometric characterization of My-10 positive progenitor cells in normal human bone marrow. Exp Hematol 1987; 15:10–17.
5. Civin CI, Loken MR. Cell surface antigens on human marrow cells: Dissection of hematopoietic development using monoclonal antibodies and multiparameter flow cytometry. Int J Cell Cloning 1987; 5:1–13.
6. Beschorner WE, Civin CI, Strauss LC. Localization of hematopoietic progenitor cells in tissue with the anit-My10 monoclonal antibody. Am J Pathol 1985; 119:1–4.
7. Fina L, Molgaard HV, Robertson D, et al. Expression of The CD34 gene in vascular endothelial cells. Blood 1990; 75:2417–2426.
8. Simmons DL, Satterthwaite AB, Tenan DG, et al. Molecular cloning of a cDNA encoding CD34, a sialomucin of human hematopoietic stem cells. J Immunol 1992; 148:267–271.
9. Sutherland DR, Keating A. The CD34 antigen: Structure, biology, and potential clinical applications. J Hematother 1992; 1:115–129.
10. Fackler MJ, Civin CI, May WS. Up-regulation of surface CD34 is associated with protein kinase C-mediated hyperphosphorylation of CD34. J Biol Chem 1992; 267: 17540–17546.
11. Greaves MF, Brown J, Molgaard HV, et al. Molecular features of CD34: A hemopoietic progenitor cell-associated molecule. Leukemia 1992; 6(1):31–36.
12. Civin CI, Small D. Purification and expansion of human hematopoietic stem/progenitor cells. In: Sackstein R, Janssen WE, Eltenbein GJ, eds. Annals of the NY Academy of Sciences, 1995; Vol 770:91–98.
13. Champagne MA, Civin CI. CD34$^+$ progenitor/stem cells for transplantation. Hematol Rev 1994; 8:15–25.
14. Civin CI. Identification and positive selection of human progenitor/stem cells for bone marrow transplantation. In: Gee AP, Gross S, Worthington-White DA, eds. Advances in Bone Marrow Purging and Processing. New York: Wiley-Liss, 1992:461–473.
15. Berenson RJ, Bensinger WI, Hill RS, et al. Engraftment after infusion of CD34$^+$ marrow cells in patients with breast cancer or neuroblastoma. Blood 1991; 77:1717–1722.
16. Shpall EJ, Jones RB, Johnston C, et al. Purified CD34 positive marrow progenitor cells provide effective reconstitution for breast cancer and non-Hodgkin's lymphoma pa-

tients receiving high dose chemotherapy with autologous bone marrow support: Recombinant granulocyte colony stimulating factor accelerates hematopoietic recovery (abstr). J Clin Oncol 1992; 11:59.
17. Noga SF. Graft engineering: The evolution of hematopoietic transplantation. J Hematother 1992; 1:3–18.
18. Datta YH, Adams PT, Drobyski WR, et al. Sensitive detection of occult breast cancer by the reverse-transcriptase polymerase chain reaction. J Clin Oncol 1994; 12:475–484.
19. Vaughan WP, Weisenburger DD, Sanger W, et al. Early leukemic recurrence of non-Hodgkin's lymphoma after high-dose anti-neoplastic therapy with autologous marrow rescue. Bone Marrow Transplant 1987; 1:373–378.
20. Rowley SD, Davis JM. The use of 4-HC in autologous purging. In: Gee AP, ed. Bone Marrow Processing and Purging. Boca Raton, FL: CRC Press, 1991:247–262.
21. Dillman R. Monoclonal antibodies for treating cancer. Ann Intern Med 1989; 111:592–598.
22. Rowley S, Zuehlsdorf M, Braine H, et al. CFU-GM content of bone marrow graft correlates with time to hematologic reconstitution following autologous bone marrow transplantation with 4-hydroperoxycyclo-phosphamide-purged bone marrow. Blood 1987; 70:271–275.
23. LeBien TW, Stepan DE, Bartholomew RM, et al. Utilization of a colony assay to assess the variables influencing elimination of leukemic cells from complement. Blood 1985; 65:945–950.
24. Baum CM, Weissman IL, Tsukamoto AS, et al. Isolation of a candidate human hematopoietic stem-cell population. Proc Natl Acad Sci USA 1992; 89:2804–2808.
25. Jones RJ, Ambinder RF, Piantadosi S, et al. Evidence of a graft-versus-lymphoma effect associated with allogeneic bone marrow transplantation. Blood 1991; 77:649–653.
26. Civin C, Trischmann T, Davis J, et al. Highly purified $CD34^+$ cells reconstitute hematopoiesis (abstr). J Clin Oncol 1995; 14:437.
27. Noga SJ, Hess AD. Lymphocyte depletion in bone marrow transplantation: Will modulation of graft-versus-host disease prove to be superior to prevention? Semin Oncol 1993; 20:28–33.
28. Sykes M, Sachs DH, Strober S. Mechanisms of tolerance. In: Forman SJ, Blume KG, Thomas ED, eds. Bone Marrow Transplantation, Oxford, England: Blackwell Scientific, 1994:204–219.
29. Wagner JE, Santos GW, Noga SJ, et al. Lymphocyte depletion of donor bone marrow by counterflow centrifugal elutriation: Results of a phase I-II clinical trial. Blood 1990; 75:1370–1377.
30. Noga SJ, Donnenberg AD, Schwartz CL, et al. Development of a simplified counterflow centrifugation-elutriation procedure for depletion of lymphocytes from human bone marrow. Transplantation 1986; 41:220–229.
31. Jones RJ, Wagner JE, Celano P, et al. Separation of pluripotent hematopoietic stem cells from spleen colony-forming cells. Nature 1990; 347:188–189.
32. Noga SJ, Davis JM, Schepers K, et al. The clinical use of elutriation and positive stem cell selection columns to engineer the lymphocyte and stem cell composition of the allograft. Prog Clin Biol Res 1994; 392:317–324.
33. Chang Q, Harvey K, Akard LP, et al. Differences in $CD34^+$ subpopulations between bone marrow and "mobilized" peripheral blood as detected with elutriation (abstr). Blood 1994; 84:103.
34. Noga SJ, Wagner JE, Santos GW, et al. Allograft lymphocyte-dose modification with counterflow centrifugal elutriation (CCE): Effects on chronic GVHD and survival in a case/control study (abstr). Blood 1991; 78:227.
35. Wagner JE, Donnenberg AD, Noga SJ, et al. Lymphocyte depletion of donor bone marrow by counterflow centrifugal elutriation: Results of a phase I clinical trial. Blood 1988; 72:1168–1176.

36. Noga S, Miller C, Berenson R, et al. Combined use of $CD34^+$ stem cell augmentation and elutriation reduces the morbidity and cost of allogeneic bone marrow transplantation (abstr). J Clin Oncol 1994; 13:309.
37. Noga SJ, Jones RJ, Davis JM, et al. Graft engineering: II. augmenting lymphocyte depleted bone marrow with small CD34pos progenitors to improve engraftment kinetics (abstr). Blood 1993; 82:428
38. Noga S, Vogelsang G, Miller C, et al. Elutriation and $CD34^+$ augmentation improves allogeneic engraftment and decreases hospitalization: a phase I/II study (abstr). J Clin Oncol 1995; 14:75.
39. Noga SJ, Vogelsang GB, Seber A, et al. The incidence of GVHD, but not engraftment is affected by cyclosporine A (CSA) duration following transplantation with $CD34^+$ augmented/elutriated (A/E) marrow. Blood 1995; 86:(10):395a.
40. Reisner Y, Martelli MF, Lustig E. Stem cell dose increase offers new possibilities for BMT across major histocompatibility barriers in lethally and sublethally irradiated recipients (abstr). Blood 1994; 84:346.
41. Vogelsang GB. Acute and chronic graft-vs-host disease. Curr Opin Oncol 1993; 5:276–281.
42. Noga SJ, Vogelsang GB, Horn T, et al. Combination elutriation plus GVHD prophylaxis using cyclosporine in high risk mismatched and unrelated transplants. Protocol approved under FDA BB IDE 5538.
43. Shpall EJ, Jones RB. Mobilization and collection of peripheral blood progenitor cells for support of high-dose cancer therapy. In: Forman SJ, Blume KG, Thomas ED, eds. Bone Marrow Transplantation. Cambridge, MA: Blackwell Scientific, 1994:913–918.
44. Passos-Coelho JL, Braine HG, Wright SK, et al. Safety and efficacy of a single large volume 6-hour leukapheresis using regional citrate anticoagulation to collect peripheral blood progenitor cells (PBPC). J Hematother 1995; 4:11–20.
45. Passos-Coelho JL, Ross AA, Moss TJ, et al. Absence of breast cancer cells in a single day peripheral blood progenitor cell (PBPC) collection following priming with cyclophosphamide and granulocyte-macrophage colony-stimulating factor (GM-CSF). Blood 1995; 85:1138–1143.
46. Schiller G, Vescio R, Freytes C, et al. Transplantation of $CD34^+$ peripheral blood progenitor cells after high-dose chemotherapy for patients with advanced multiple myeloma. Blood 1995; 86:390–397.
47. Gianni A, Siena S, Gregni M, et al. Granulocyte-macrophage colony-stimulating factor to harvest circulating hematopoietic stem cells for autotransplantation. Lancet 1989; 2: 580–585.
48. Ho AD, Gluck S, Gremond G, et al. Optimal timing for collections of blood progenitor cells following induction chemotherapy and granulocyte-macrophage colony-stimulating factor for autologous transplantation in advanced breast cancer. Leukemia 1993; 7:1738–1746.
49. Siena S, Gregni M, Brando B, et al. Flow cytometry for clinical estimation of circulating hematopoietic progenitors for autologous transplantation in cancer patients. Blood 1991; 77:400–409.
50. Passos-Coelho JL, Braine HG, Davis JM, et al. Predictive factors for peripheral-blood progenitor-cell collections using a single large-volume leukapheresis after cyclophosphamide and granulocyte-macrophage colony-stimulating factor mobilization. J Clin Oncol 1995; 13:705–714.
51. Sovalat H, Wunder E, Zimmermann R, et al. Multicentric determination of $CD34^+$ cells. In: Wunder E, Sovalat H, Henon PR, Serke S, eds. Hematopoietic Stem Cells: the Mulhouse Manual. Dayton, OH: AlphaMed Press, 1994:61–66.
52. Sims L, Brecher M, Schmitz J, et al. Interinstitutional study of hematopoietic pluropotential immunoexpression by cytometry (abstr). J Hematother 1995; 4:239.
53. Peters WP, Kurzberg J, Romber G, et al. Comparative effects of G-CSF and GM-CSF

on priming peripheral blood progenitor cells for use with autologous bone marrow after high-dose chemotherapy. Blood 1993; 81:1709–1719.
54. Shpall EJ, Jones RB, Bearman SI, et al. Transplantation of enriched CD34-positive autologous marrow into breast cancer patients following high-dose chemotherapy: Influence of CD34-positive peripheral blood progenitors and growth factors on engraftment. J Clin Oncol 1994; 12:28.
55. Link H, Arseniev L, Bahre O, et al. Transplantation of allogeneic peripheral blood and bone marrow $CD34^+$ cells after immunoselection (abstr). Exp Hematol 1995; 23:855.
56. Korbling M, Przepiorka D, Engel H, et al. Allogeneic blood stem cell transplantation (allo-PBSCT) in 9 patients with refractory leukemia and lymphoma: Potential advantage of blood over marrow allografts (abstr). Blood 1994; 84:396.
57. Friedrich W, Muller S, Schreiner T, et al. The combined use of positively selected, T-cell depleted blood and bone marrow stem cells in HLA non-identical bone marrow transplantation in childhood leukemia (abstr). Exp Hematol 1995; 23:854.
58. Broxmeyer HE, Douglas GW, Hangoc G, et al. Human umbilical cord blood as a potential source of transplantable stem/progenitor cells. Proc Natl Acad Sci USA 1989; 86:3828–3832.
59. Rubinstein P, Migliaccio AR, Adamson JW, et al. Unrelated placental/umbilical cord blood (PCB) transplantation: Methods and early results of the New York blood center's PCB program (abstr). Exp Hematol 1995; 23:942.
60. Krivit W, Shapiro EG. Bone marrow transplantation for storage diseases. In: Forman SJ, Blume KG, Thomas ED, eds. Bone Marrow Transplantation. Oxford, England: Blackwell Scientific, 1994:883–893.
61. Zanjani ED, Mackintosh FR, Harrison MR. Hematopoietic chimerism in sheep and nonhuman primates by in utero transplantation of fetal hematopoietic stem cells. Blood Cells 1991; 17:349–363.
62. Bambach BJ, Moser HW, Blakemore K, et al. Engraftment following in utero bone marrow transplantation for globoid leukodystrophy. Lancet 1996. Submitted.
63. Fefer A. Graft-vs-tumor responses: adoptive cellular therapy in bone marrow transplantation. In: Forman SJ, Blume KG, Thomas ED, eds. Bone Marrow Transplantation. Oxford, England: Blackwell Scientific, 1994:231–241.
64. Hess AD, Jones RJ, Morris LE, et al. Autologous graft-vs-host disease: A new frontier in immunotherapy. Bone Marrow Transplant 1992; 10:16–21.
65. Noga SJ, Horwitz L, Kim H, et al. Gamma interferon potentiates the anti-tumor effect of cyclosporine-induced autoimmunity. J Hematother 1992; 1:75–84.
66. Hess AD, Kennedy MJ, Ruvolo PP, et al. Antitumor activity of syngeneic/autologous graft-vs-host disease. Ann New York Acad Sci 1995; 770:189–202.
67. Klingemann HG. Introducing graft-versus-leukemia into autologous stem cell transplantation. J Hematother 1995; 4:261–268.
68. Champlin R, Giralt S, Przepiorka D, et al. Selective depletion of CD8-positive T-lymphocytes for allogeneic bone marrow transplantation. Engraftment, graft-versus-host disease, and graft-versus-leukemia. Prog Clin Biol Res 1992; 377:385–398.
69. Canals C, Picon M, Torrico C, et al. GVHD Prophylaxis in CML: Complete depletion of CD4 cells and controlled numbers of CD8 lymphocyte in the donor BM (abstr). Exp Hematol 1994; 22:695.
70. Champlin R, Giralt S, Gajewski J, et al. CD8 depleted donor lymphocytes for CML relapsing post BMT (abstr). Exp Hematol 1995; 23:939.
71. Turner CE, Davis JM, Harris DP, et al. Graft engineering: IV. $CD56^+$ selection following elutriation and $CD34^+$ selection (abstr). J Hematother 1995; 4:213.
72. Turner CE, Davis JM, Harris DP, et al. Graft engineering: V. Isolation, cryopreservation, and activation of $CD56^+$ cells recovered after $CD34^+$ selection of elutriated bone marrow. Blood 1995; 86(10):117a.

28

Adoptive Immunotherapy in Bone Marrow Transplantation

David L. Porter
University of Pennsylvania School of Medicine
Philadelphia, Pennsylvania

Joseph H. Antin
Brigham and Women's Hospital and Harvard Medical School
Boston, Massachusetts

I. INTRODUCTION

The success of allogeneic bone marrow transplantation (BMT) for patients with hematological malignancies is limited primarily by leukemic relapse and by treatment-related complications such as organ toxicity from the conditioning regimen, graft-versus-host disease (GVHD), and infections. Successful conditioning regimens currently in use are already administered at near maximally tolerated doses, and because both chemotherapy and radiation kill cells via first order kinetics, these regimens are unlikely to eliminate every leukemia cell. Subtle changes in the myeloablative therapy, therefore, are unlikely to result in significant improvements in relapse rates or survival. Newer innovative approaches must be taken that will minimize both relapse rates and toxicity.

These new treatment strategies will be based on an understanding of the mechanisms underlying successful allogeneic BMT. These mechanisms can be divided into a cytotoxic component and an immunological component. High-dose cytotoxic therapy can be administered because allogeneic bone marrow provides a source of normal donor stem cells necessary for hematopoietic reconstitution. However, since it is unlikely that the conditioning regimen eliminates every leukemic cell, a high relapse rate is anticipated unless other mechanisms contribute to the antileukemic effect of BMT. A second component of successful BMT involves the transfer of alloreactive donor immune cells present in the marrow graft that may recognize residual leukemia cells surviving the ablative regimen; this immunological component is the "graft-versus-leukemia" (GVL) effect; hence allogeneic BMT can be viewed as a successful method of adoptive immunotherapy.

The importance of the GVL effect has been suspected since the earliest studies on BMT. Barnes and colleagues first noted that leukemic mice treated with a subtherapeutic dose of radiation and transplanted with syngeneic marrow were more likely to relapse than mice transplanted with allogeneic marrow (1,2). They hypothesized that an allogeneic graft contained cells with immune reactivity necessary for eradicating residual leukemic cells. They also noted that recipients of allogeneic grafts, though less likely to relapse, died of a "wasting syndrome" now recognized as GVHD. Thus, in addition to describing GVL, these experiments highlighted for the first time the intricate relationship between GVL and GVHD.

It is now well known that donor immune cells can react against disparate MHC antigens in the host, resulting in GVHD. In addition, the marrow graft contains cells that may react against residual host leukemic cells. This GVL reaction is vital to successful transplantation for many patients; therapeutic maneuvers designed to attenuate alloreactivity of the donor graft often result in higher relapse rates, presumably due to loss of the GVL effect. GVL reactivity has now been extensively demonstrated and defined in detail in animal models of BMT and is reviewed in Chap. 14. However, the evidence for the existence and significance of the GVL effect in clinical transplantation has been, until recently, largely indirect and circumstantial. This chapter focuses on efforts that have been made to enhance the "immunotherapeutic" potential of an allogeneic graft. It reviews the indirect evidence demonstrating a GVL component in clinical BMT, and discusses some of the innovative approaches that have been designed to manipulate the GVL reaction. Recently, the administration of donor mononuclear cells (MNC) to patients who have relapsed after allogeneic BMT has provided a direct demonstration of GVL in the clinical setting, and these studies are reviewed in detail. Finally, there is a discussion of the potential mechanisms underlying the GVL effects, as ultimately the ability to harness the GVL reactivity of the donor immune system may permit allogeneic BMT to be performed as a safer, more effective method of adoptive immunotherapy.

II. GVL IN CLINICAL TRANSPLANTATION

Since the work of Barnes and colleagues, several investigators have used murine models to dissect out the possible mechanisms underlying both GVHD and GVL; these studies are described in detail elsewhere in this volume. It has been more difficult to identify a clinically significant GVL reaction in human transplantation; until recently, the evidence has been circumstantial and based on several important but indirect clinical observations (Table 1). These observations not only provide important clinical evidence for GVL but begin to suggest potential mechanisms

Table 1 Indirect Evidence for a GVL Reaction in Clinical BMT

- Abrupt withdrawal of immunosuppression, or a flare of GVHD may result in complete remission in some patients with relapsed leukemia after BMT (anecdotal).
- Syngeneic BMT is associated with a higher risk of relapse than allogeneic BMT.
- GVHD disease after BMT results is a lower risk of relapse.
- T-cell depletion of the donor marrow graft results in an increased risk of relapse, especially for patients with CML.

underlying GVL reactivity; they also provide the basis for the development of rational approaches designed to enhance and manipulate GVL for clinical benefit.

A. Remission Induced by a Flare of GVHD or Withdrawal of Immune Suppression

There are several anecdotal reports describing patients with relapsed leukemia after BMT who have reentered complete remission associated with a flare of acute GVHD (3) or after discontinuation of immunosuppressive therapy (4–6). While these reports are intriguing, undoubtedly many more relapsed patients have had immunosuppressive therapy rapidly discontinued without an effect, and these cases are not likely to be reported. Discontinuation of immunosuppression is simple and is likely to be the first attempt at restoring GVL for relapsed patients on immunosuppressive therapy; unfortunately, only occasional responses should be anticipated.

B. Syngeneic Marrow Grafts Are Associated with Increased Relapse Rates

Consistent with early murine experiments in BMT, relapse rates after human syngeneic marrow transplantation are higher when compared to BMT with matched sibling allogeneic grafts. This effect was first suggested by the Seattle group in 1979 (7) and later confirmed in an update that analyzed over 800 patients transplanted with advanced leukemia—acute lymphocytic leukemia (ALL) or acute nonlymphocytic leukemia (ANLL)—in second or greater complete remission or relapse (8). The relapse rate was 62% for 785 recipients of allogeneic grafts compared to a relapse rate of 75% for 53 recipients of syngeneic grafts ($p < 0.0001$). A more dramatic difference in relapse rates was noted by Gale and Champlin for patients transplanted for acute myelocytic leukemia (AML) in first remission (9). In this multicenter review, 31 recipients of syngeneic marrow grafts had an almost threefold increase in relapse rate when compared with 339 recipients of allogeneic grafts (actuarial probability of relapse 59 ± 20% versus 18 ± 4%).

Large retrospective analyses from the International Bone Marrow Transplant Registry (IBMTR) have confirmed these findings (10,11) (Fig. 1). The IBMTR data further suggest that syngeneic transplantation is associated with a higher relapse rate when compared to allogeneic transplantation independent of GVHD, implying that the GVL effect associated with an allogeneic graft may be separate from GVHD (10,11). These findings have been noted both in standard risk patients (AML in first remission or CML in chronic phase) (9,11), and for patients at high risk for relapse (BMT performed for AML or ALL in second or greater remission or at relapse) (8). The magnitude of the GVL effect associated with allogeneic BMT may depend on both the diagnosis and disease activity at the time of BMT and still remains ill defined. For instance, although syngeneic transplantation results in higher relapse rates for patients with CML and AML, a recent update from the IBMTR found no significant increase in the relapse rate for patients with ALL in first remissions (10).

There has been some concern that the higher relapse rate after syngeneic BMT may be exaggerated due to other confounding factors. For instance, while the conditioning regimens for syngeneic and allogeneic BMT tend to be similar, recipients of non-T-cell–depleted allogeneic marrow grafts typically receive GVHD prophylaxis that includes methotrexate, while recipients of syngeneic grafts receive no

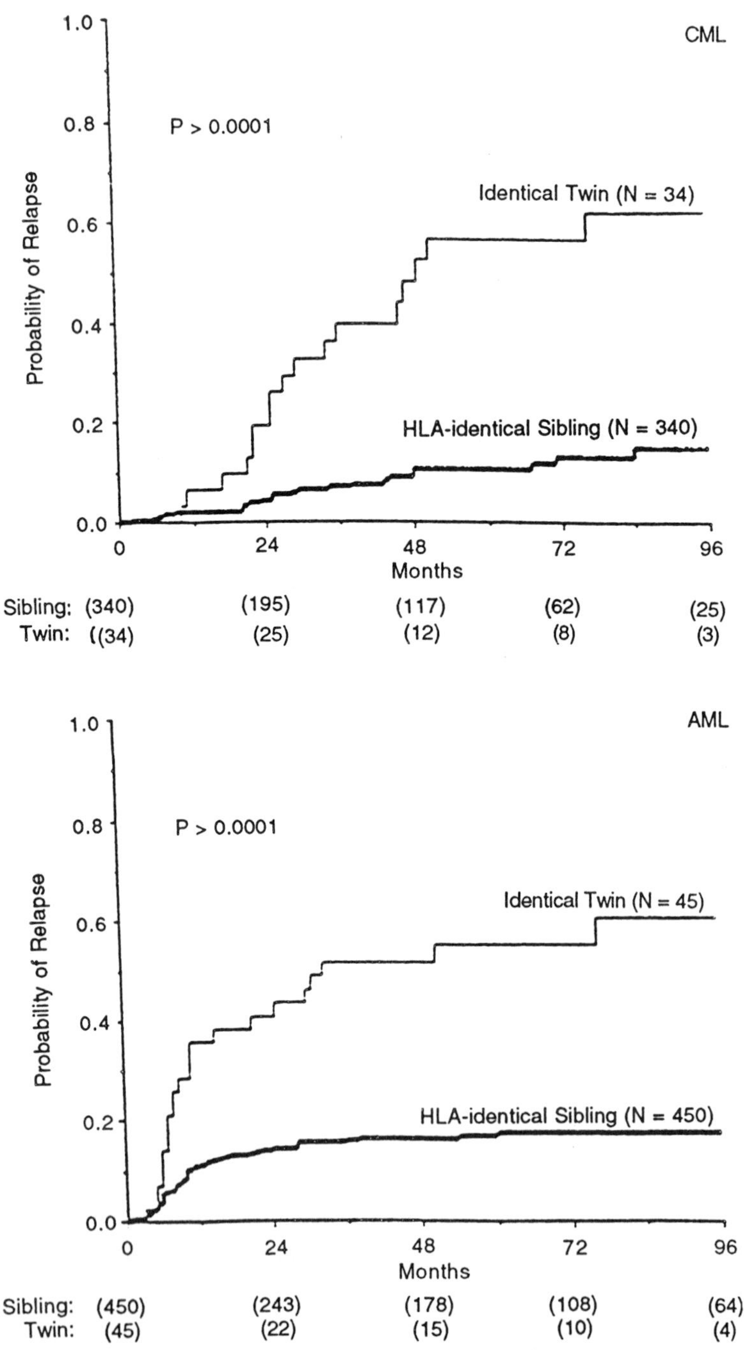

Figure 1 Probability of relapse after syngeneic (identical twin) versus allogeneic (HLA-identical sibling) bone marrow transplantation. Recipients of syngeneic grafts have a higher actuarial probability of relapse when transplantation is performed for CML (upper panel) and AML (lower panel). (From Ref. 10.)

GVHD prophylaxis. However, the total dose of methotrexate is relatively low, and while it is difficult to exclude the possibility that the GVHD prophylaxis contributes to the antileukemic effect of allogeneic BMT, this explanation is unlikely. Another improbable concern is that recurrent leukemia could arise from donor cells; these cells would be impossible to distinguish from the recipients' original leukemia in syngeneic twins.

C. GVHD Is Protective Against Relapse

There is now considerable evidence that patients who develop GVHD after allogeneic BMT have a lower risk of relapse when compared to similar patients who do not experience GVHD. Acute and chronic GVHD were both shown to be protective against relapse for patients transplanted with advanced leukemia (AML or ALL in relapse, CML in accelerated phase or blast crisis, or patients in remission but at high risk of relapse), (7,12,13), as well as for patients transplanted earlier in the disease course (11,14). In the largest review, the IBMTR analyzed the risk of relapse after BMT for over 2200 patients transplanted with "early leukemia" (AML or ALL in first remission or CML in chronic phase) (11); patients who had acute and chronic GVHD had a lower risk of relapse compared to patients who developed no GVHD (Fig. 2). For unclear reasons, the magnitude of this effect appears to be disease-dependent. For instance, the IBMTR concluded that for recipients of unmanipulated donor marrow grafts, acute GVHD protected against relapse of ALL, while the combination of acute and chronic GVHD was protective against relapse for patients with ALL, AML, and CML (Table 2).

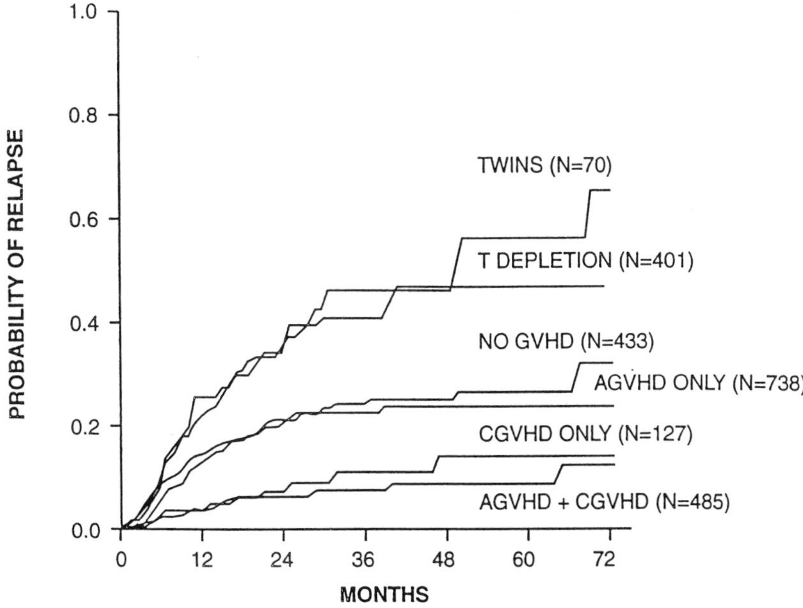

Figure 2 Probability of relapse after allogeneic bone marrow transplantation for 2254 patients from the International Bone Marrow Transplant Registry. (From Ref. 11.)

Table 2 GVHD is Associated with a Reduced Risk of Relapse after Allogeneic BMT

Patient Group (Allogeneic, Non-T-Cell Depleted)	ALL (p)		AML (p)		CML (p)		All Patients (p)	
• No GVHD	1.00		1.00		1.00		1.00	
• Acute GVHD only	0.36	(0.004)	0.78	(0.26)	1.15	(0.75)	0.68	(0.03)
• Chronic GVHD only	0.44	(0.16)	0.48	(0.12)	0.28	(0.16)	0.43	(0.01)
• Acute and chronic GVHD	0.38	(0.02)	0.34	(0.0003)	0.24	(0.03)	0.33	(0.0001)

Source: Ref. 11.

D. T-Cell Depletion of the Donor Marrow Graft Results in Increased Relapse Rates

It is generally accepted that GVHD is in large part mediated by alloreactive donor lymphocytes contained in the marrow graft. T-cell depletion of the donor marrow by a variety of methods has been one of the most successful means of limiting the incidence and severity of GVHD after allogeneic BMT (15–21). It was hoped that T-cell depletion would minimize transplant-related mortality and translate into improved survival rates. Unfortunately, several studies show that while the incidence and severity of GVHD is low, overall survival is not improved after T-cell-depleted BMT (14,20,22–24). This has been due in large part to a reciprocal increase in the rate of relapse and graft failure. The increase in relapse rate after T-cell-depleted BMT has been most dramatic in patients transplanted for CML, where the incidence of relapse is as high as 50% (11,14,24); the IBMTR analysis has found that compared to recipients of unmanipulated marrow grafts who develop no GVHD, patients with CML receiving T-cell-depleted marrow have a relative risk of relapse of 6.91 (11). These results provide strong but still indirect evidence that donor T cells possess important antileukemic properties that significantly influence the success of marrow transplantation.

It is clear that the immunological properties of the donor graft as well as the intrinsic properties of the specific leukemia subtype influence the susceptibility to the GVL effects of BMT. In clinical BMT, it has not been possible to separate GVL from GVHD, and it remains unclear if these are distinct rather than overlapping processes. Despite the many recent advances in immunology and supportive care, the ability to control GVHD without sacrificing critical GVL effects remains a difficult and central challenge for successful BMT.

III. MANIPULATION OF THE GVL REACTION WITH ADOPTIVE IMMUNOTHERAPY

Relapse after allogeneic BMT remains a significant cause of treatment failure. Although second transplants may be curative for a minority of patients, they are associated with very high morbidity and mortality rates (25–27); safer, more effective therapies to treat, or preferably, prevent relapse are clearly needed. Since it is unlikely that subtle changes in conditioning therapy will have a dramatic impact on relapse, innovative approaches designed to enhance the GVL effects of allogeneic donor cells are being explored. Different strategies have been developed to enhance GVL either (a) at the time of relapse, (b) at the time of BMT in order to irradicate minimal residual disease, or (c) shortly after BMT but prior to relapse.

A. GVL Induction to Treat Leukemic Relapse

Since donor T cells are vital for the GVL activity of allogeneic BMT, particularly for patients with CML, it was logical to test the use of donor mononuclear cell infusions to treat patients with relapsed CML after BMT. Kolb and coworkers first reported that three patients with relapsed CML experienced complete cytogenetic remissions after receiving interferon-alpha (IFN-α) and infusions of donor buffy-coat cells (28). Two of these patients developed acute GVHD that was controlled with immunosuppressive therapy. These initial findings have since been confirmed and expanded by other investigators (29–34); over 100 patients have received similar therapy worldwide and results from 66 patients reported in the literature are summarized in Table 3. Many of the patients treated with donor mononuclear cells (MNC) have been concurrently treated with a short course of IFN-α but receive no other cytoreductive therapy or GVHD prophylaxis. The antileukemic effects of donor MNC, with or without IFN-α, are quite dramatic in patients with chronic phase CML. Up to 70% of these patients achieve a complete molecular remission, defined as the absence of cells containing detectable *bcr/abl* mRNA transcripts assayed by reverse transcriptase and polymerase chain reaction (PCR). This technique is capable of identifying one leukemic cell in 10^5-10^6 normal cells (35). Assuming that patients with chronic-phase CML have a leukemic cell burden of approximately 10^{12} cells, a molecular remission using donor MNC infusions represents at least a 6-log cell kill (36).

Although many patients with relapsed CML treated with donor MNC infusions have also received IFN-α, it remains uncertain if this contributes to remission induction. At the Brigham and Women's Hospital, all patients initially receive IFN-α for 6 to 12 weeks prior to donor MNC infusions, for 4 weeks during MNC infusions, and for 4 weeks after the final MNC infusion, as diagrammed in Fig. 3. However, it is unlikely that IFN-α alone accounts for the 60 to 80% complete molecular remission rate. Although IFN-α can successfully induce complete cytogenetic remissions in a minority of patients with untreated CML (37) or with relapsed CML after BMT (38,39), these remissions usually require a prolonged and sustained course of IFN-α. In addition, IFN-α has not resulted in molecular remissions, even when cytogenetics appear normal (39,40). Several investigators have successfully administered donor MNC to patients with relapsed CML without IFN-α (30,32,34); a summary of European experiences did not find a correlation between response to donor MNC infusions and the use of IFN-α (41).

These findings do not preclude a beneficial effect of IFN-α, however. This cytokine possesses many important biological properties that make it a logical adjunct to adoptive immunotherapy. It has antiproliferative properties and can result in cytoreduction prior to cellular therapy. In addition, IFN-α can enhance and induce the expression of important cell surface antigens, such as HLA class I and II molecules (42) and the adhesion molecule LFA-3 (43), on the surface of CML cells. The expression of these antigens could enhance cell-mediated cytotoxicity. IFN-α

Table 3 Adoptive Immunotherapy for Relapsed CML

Reference	*N*	Disease Status	IFN-α	MNC Dose (10^8 /kg)	Complete Cytogenetic Response	Complete Molecular Response
Kolb (28)	3	CP: 3	3	4.4–7.4	3/3	ND
Bar (29)	6	CP: 6[a]	4	0.34–5.2	5/6	4/6
Drobyski (30)	8	CP: 6[b]	3	2.6–4.0[e]	6/6	5/6
		AP/BC: 2	1		1/2	0/2
Helg (31)	3	CP: 3[c]	3	3.8–12.3	3/3	2/2
Hertenstein (32)	8	CP: 6	0	3.0–5.5	3/6	3/6
		AP/BC: 2			0/2	0/2
van Rhee (48)	14	CP: 12[d]	0	0.6–10.0	10/12[f]	8/12
		AP/BC: 2			0/2	0/2
Porter (33)	18[g]	CP: 13	14	0.9–8.4	9/13	9/13
		AP/BC: 5			0/5	0/3
Collins (81)	6	CP: 4	ns	1.2–16.4	3/4	3/4
		AP/BC: 2			0/2	0/2
TOTAL	66	CP: 53	28/66	0.34–16.4	43/53 (81%)	30/49 (60%)
		AP/BC: 13			1/13 (8%)	0/11 (0%)

Abbreviations: AP, accelerated phase; BC, blast crisis; CP, chronic phase; MNC, mononuclear cell; IFN, interferon; nd, not done; ns, not stated, CR, cytogenetic release; MR, molecular relapse.

[a]One patient had CR only.

[b]These patients were clinically in chronic phase, although the authors classified them as "accelerated phase" due to complex chromosomal abnormalities. Because the majority of patients who relapse after allogeneic BMT have complex chromosomal abnormalities (personal observation), we have classified these patients as chronic phase unless other criteria are present.

[c]One patient had CR only.

[d]Of the total, 7 patients had hematological relapse, 5 had CR only, and 2 had MR only.

[e]This number refers to number of T lymphocytes infused.

[f]Of 10 CRs, 7 occurred in patients with CR or MR only. Of 7 patients in hematological relapse, 3 achieved cytogenetic remission.

[g]Seventeen of these patients have been reported in abstract form as referenced. One patient is previously unreported.

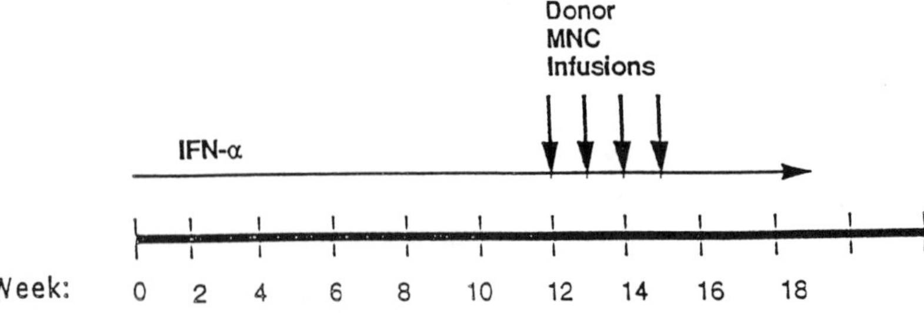

Figure 3 Treatment scheme used for adoptive immunotherapy for relapsed CML at the Brigham and Women's Hospital. Abbreviations: IFN, interferon; MNC, mononuclear cells. (From Ref. 33.)

Table 4 Association of GVHD with Clinical Response to Adoptive Immunotherapy for Patients with Relapsed CML[a]

$N = 60$	Response: 44/60	No Response: 16/60
GVHD	39/44 (89%)	6/16 (37%)
No GVHD	5/44 (11%)	10/16 (63%)

[a]Data is compiled from seven reports where the association of GVHD and response could be determined (28–33,48). Seven patients are included from our unpublished data. The majority of patients responding had complete cytogenetic and/or molecular remissions after donor mononuclear cell infusions, although several patients classified as responders for the purpose of this analysis died before remission could be documented.

may also influence the expression or induction of various other cytokines or effector cells (or both) that may be important for the GVL response. The data suggest that IFN-α may not be required for the GVL reaction; however, it may have other important influences on the magnitude of GVL or possibly on the tempo of the antileukemic response, but this will only be determined in comparative trials.

The majority of patients responding to donor MNC infusions experience both acute and chronic GVHD, and the development of GVHD correlates with response (Table 4 and Ref. 41). While the toxicity from GVHD may be significant, it has generally been mild to moderate (Table 5) and perhaps less severe than one might anticipate considering that the dose of T cells administered is up to 10 times higher than that typically contained in an unmanipulated allogeneic marrow graft (15). It is notable, however, that several patients treated for relapse with donor MNC

Table 5 GVHD Occurring After Donor Mononuclear Cell Infusions[a]

Disease	N	Acute GVHD Grade 0	Acute GVHD Grade I	Acute GVHD Grade II–IV	Chronic GVHD Limited/Extensive
CML	67	17 (25%)	26 (39%)	23 (34%)	Limited: 12/44 Extensive: 9/44
Acute Leukemia, MDS, MM, NHL, HD	50	18 (36%)	7 (14%)	25 (51%)	Most not reported
Total	117	35 (30%)	33 (28%)	48 (41%)	

[a]Data for CML patients is compiled from eight reports where details on GVHD were available (28–32,45,48,82). Data for patients with diseases other than CML is compiled from eight reports where details on GVHD were available (51,81,83–88).

Abbreviations: CML, chronic myelogenous leukemia; GVHD, graft-versus-host disease; HD, Hodgkin's disease; MDS, myelodysplasia; MM, multiple myeloma; NHL, non-Hodgkin's lymphoma.

infusions have entered remission without developing clinical GVHD (28,32,34), suggesting that at least in some cases, GVL and clinical GVHD may be dissociated.

In addition to GVHD, pancytopenia with marrow aplasia has been a major toxicity following donor MNC infusions. This phenomenon is reminiscent of transfusion-associated GVHD (TA-GVHD) (44) and is presumably due to destruction of the host leukemic cells prior to recovery of normal donor hematopoiesis. However, unlike TA-GVHD, marrow aplasia is usually transient, although many patients experience absolute neutropenia and require platelet and blood transfusions. Several patients have developed persistent marrow aplasia (30,33,45); while this has contributed to the death of some patients, aplasia has been successfully reversed with the infusion of donor bone marrow in others (30,33) (Fig. 4). It is unknown why some patients spontaneously recover hematopoiesis and others do not, since donor marrow should not be a target for donor lymphocytes. Marrow aplasia is not simply related to an absolute lack of normal donor stem cells. The patient whose response is diagrammed in Fig. 4 had detectable normal donor hematopoiesis prior to donor-cell infusions but was not protected against aplasia; following the GVL response, the limited hematopoiesis was completely of donor origin, although the patient remained markedly pancytopenic. Bone marrow recovery did not occur until the infusion of additional bone marrow, suggesting that the number of donor stem cells may have been insufficient to sustain normal hematopoietic function. Furthermore, the stem cells contained in the peripheral blood leukapheresis product were similarly inadequate to sustain hematopoiesis.

Despite the dramatic antileukemic potential of donor MNC infusions, the mortality from treatment-related complications has been relatively high (~20%) (Table

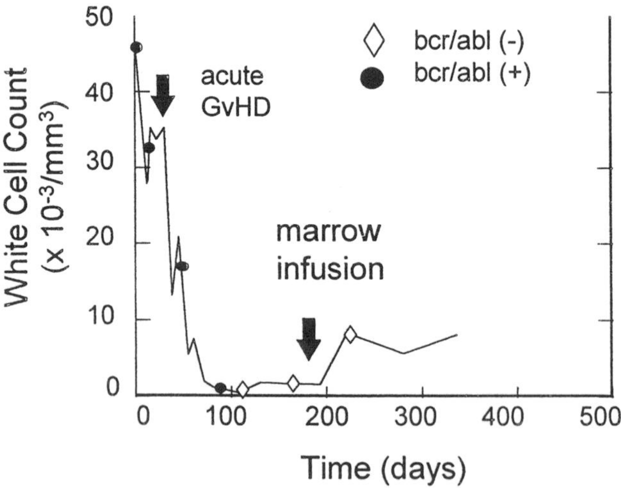

Figure 4 Response to adoptive immunotherapy for a patient with relapsed CML. The development of acute GVHD is associated with a decline in WBC (solid arrow). This patient remained pancytopenic until additional donor bone marrow was given on day 186, which resulted in prompt hematopoietic reconstitution (open arrow). Open circles denote a positive test by reverse transcription and PCR for the bcr/abl mRNA transcript. Closed circles denote a negative PCR test. (From Ref. 33.)

Table 6 Mortality Associated with Adoptive Immunotherapy for Relapsed CML[a]

Deaths	16/60	(27%)
• Therapy related	10/60	(17%)
GVHD	5	(8%)
CML CP	3/48	
Advanced CML[b]	2/12	
Marrow aplasia and/or infection	4	(7%)
CML CP	3/48	
Advanced CML	1/12	
Other	1	(2%)
CML CP	1/48	
• Disease progression	6	(10%)
CML CP	0/44	
Advanced CML	6/12	

[a]This data represents a compilation of patients from seven centers that have reported outcome and cause of death in patients donor MNC infusions for relapsed CML (28–31,33,48,89) and includes several previously unpublished cases treated at our institution.
[b]Advanced CML refers to patients with accelerated-phase or blast crisis CML (30,33) or greater than second chronic phase (32).
Abbreviations: CML, chronic myelogenous leukemia; CP, chronic phase.

6). The major causes of mortality have been related to GVHD or infections associated with either marrow aplasia or the use of immunosuppressive therapy to treat GVHD. The early administration of donor bone marrow may limit toxicity from prolonged marrow aplasia. In addition, several innovative approaches to limit toxicity from GVHD are currently under study. One approach is to administer lower doses of donor MNC in hopes of retaining the GVL effect while minimizing GVHD. After T-cell-depleted BMT, the dose of residual donor T cells included in the marrow graft may correlate with the severity of GVHD (46). No such correlation between MNC dose and GVHD or GVL has yet been noted using donor MNC to treat relapse; however, it is possible that doses currently used are already over a potential "threshold" (which may explain why no correlation between T-cell number and GVHD has been noted after BMT with unmanipulated marrow grafts); lower MNC doses may result in GVL without severe GVHD. A recent report suggests that a lower MNC dose (as low as 10^7 cells/kg) may retain the anti-leukemic properties without resulting in clinically evident GVHD in some patients (47). It is likely that an important relationship exists between the number of effector and target cells, such that patients with only minimal disease (i.e., *bcr/abl* detection by PCR with normal cytogenetics) will achieve remission with fewer donor cells than patients with a larger leukemic cell burden. Fewer numbers of effector cells in these patients may not result in clinically apparent GVHD. If these findings are confirmed, a logical strategy would be to administer donor MNC to patients at high risk for clinical relapse, as defined by sequential positive PCR tests for *bcr/abl* mRNA transcripts (35), but before hematological relapse. This is also logical in view of data suggesting that patients with lower leukemia cell burdens (molecular or cytogenetic relapses) are more likely to respond to donor MNC infusions than patients treated at the time of hematological relapse (48).

Another approach designed to limit toxicity is to deplete the donor MNC of effector cells suspected of causing GVHD. Studies using $CD8^+$-depleted donor MNC infusions are currently under way and suggest that GVHD can be minimized; conclusions regarding the GVL effects await further follow-up (49).

Donor MNC infusions appear to be less effective for patients who relapse with hematological diseases other than CML. Less than half of the patients treated for relapse of acute leukemia or myelodysplasia reenter remission, although occasional responses are noted (Table 7). Some responses have been noted in patients with non-Hodgkin's lymphoma (50) and multiple myeloma (51). However, many patients have been pretreated with chemotherapy prior to administration of donor MNC, and some responses have been reported as "transient." It is also likely that individual cases of negative results have not been reported, and the actual response rate may be lower than suggested. The less apparent GVL effect in this group of patients compared to patients with CML is in keeping with large retrospective analysis of BMT that demonstrate GVL is most significant against CML (11). This further implies that the immunological properties of the tumor cells strongly influence the GVL effects. For some patients with acute leukemia, myelodysplasia, or other hematological neoplasms, a definitive GVL effect can be induced and sustained remissions achieved. The toxicity of donor MNC in this group of patients is similar to that seen in patients treated with CML. Given the poor outcome anticipated for relapsed patients undergoing a second BMT (25–27), an initial trial of adoptive immunotherapy is a reasonable alternative for these patients.

Table 7 Adoptive Immunotherapy for Diseases Other Than CML[a]

Disease	*N*	Response
AML	28	9
ALL	6	2
MDS	4	2
Biphenotypic acute leukemia	1	0
MM	7	3
NHL	3	0
HD	1	0
Total	50	16 (32%)

[a]Data are compiled from published reports and abstracts where details of diagnosis and response have been given (51,81,83–88). An abstract by Kolb et al.(50) provides a similar summary for 31 patients which includes some but not all of the patients described above.

Abbreviations: ALL, acute lymphocytic leukemia; AML, acute myelocytic leukemia; CML, chronic myelogenous leukemia; HD, Hodgkin's disease; MDS, myelodysplasia; MM, multiple myeloma; NHL, non-Hodgkin's lymphoma.

B. GVL Induction During BMT to Prevent Relapse

Ultimately, the best approach to relapse is prevention. Unfortunately, strategies designed to augment GVL at the time of BMT have not been effective. One approach designed to enhance GVL taken by the Seattle group was to withhold GVHD prophylaxis at the time of BMT for patients transplanted for acute leukemia. They found that this increased the incidence of significant acute GVHD, as anticipated. Unfortunately, there was no improvement in subsequent relapse rates (52,53). However, preliminary data from a similar trial did report that withholding GVHD prophylaxis resulted in lower relapse rates and improved survival (54), but further follow-up is required; it is possible this approach may have some benefit in a small subset of patients. An analogous study undertaken by the Seattle group attempted to enhance GVL by augmenting GVHD (55). Patients with advanced leukemia undergoing allogeneic BMT were assigned to receive one of three regimens: standard GVHD prophylaxis with a long course of methotrexate (control arm), an abbreviated course of methotrexate, or the abbreviated methotrexate plus the addition of donor buffy-coat cells given at the time of BMT. The results are shown in Fig. 5 and demonstrate that by either limiting GVHD prophylaxis or by adding donor buffy coat, the incidence of significant GVHD was increased. Unfortunately, there was no impact on relapse or overall survival, in part due to the increase in nonrelapse mortality seen in the experimental arms of the study. Although these studies have not demonstrated improved outcomes, they do not exclude the possibility that the GVL potential of the donor marrow graft can still be manipulated for clinical efficacy. For instance, the patient population and the timing of the immune manipulation may be critical. In the Seattle study, patients were transplanted with advanced leukemia and had a very high risk of relapse. Similar manipulations may be more effective in patients transplanted with "early" leukemia (e.g., AML or ALL in first remission or CML in chronic phase).

C. "Delayed" GVL Induction After BMT to Prevent Relapse

The induction of GVHD and GVL to prevent relapse may still be a useful approach, but the timing in relation to BMT may be critical. For instance, no benefit could be demonstrated in the Seattle study described above, in part due to the increased toxicity of GVHD induction; too few patient may survive to note an improvement in relapse rates. While it may not yet be possible to dissociate the beneficial GVL effects from the toxic GVHD reaction, it is likely that patients would tolerate the toxicity from enhanced GVHD if it is separated from the other acute toxicities associated with the transplant (e.g., toxicities related to chemotherapy, radiation, or infections) (56). This phenomenon occurs in animal models where the administration of donor lymphocytes results in severe GVHD if given at the time of BMT; donor cells administered 21 days after the conditioning therapy results in a significant GVL effect without severe GVHD (57). In dogs, allogeneic lymphocytes can be administered safely after chimerism has been established (58). This limited toxicity may be due to the separation of the cytokine phases that occur after BMT (58,59). Therefore, it is still possible that strategies will be developed to enhance GVL without the untoward toxicity of GVHD.

The approach of delayed GVL induction is now being tested clinically. Slavin

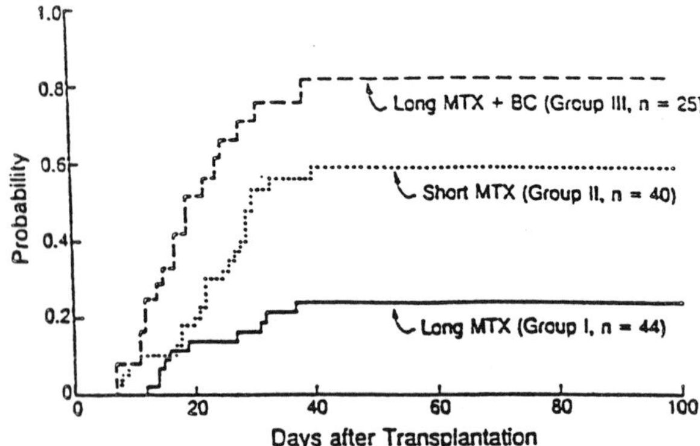

Kaplan–Meier Estimates of the Probability of the Development of Grade II to IV Acute GVHD, According to Treatment Group.

MTX denotes methotrexate, and BC buffy-coat cells (all groups, P = 0.0001; I vs. II, P = 0.0016; I vs. III, P = 0.0001; and II vs. III, P = 0.016).

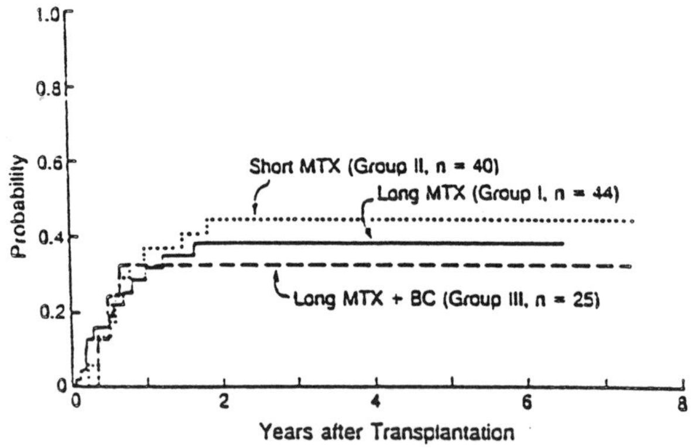

Probability of Relapse of Hematologic Neoplasm.

The differences between the groups were not statistically significant.

Figure 5 Response to manipulation of GVHD at the time of BMT for patients with advanced leukemia. Upper panel: Probability of developing GVHD grade II–IV according to treatment group. Lower panel: Probability of relapse according to treatment group. There is a significant difference in the risk of GVHD among treatment groups with no statistically significant difference in relapse rate. For explanation of treatment groups, see text. Abbreviations: BC, buffy-coat cells; MTX, methotrexate. (From Ref. 55.)

and colleagues have treated patients at high risk for relapse after T-cell-depleted allogeneic BMT with incremental doses of donor lymphocytes beginning 8 weeks after BMT (59). Preliminary data on a small number of patients suggest that 10^6-10^7 T cells/kg can be given safely, resulting in only mild to moderate GVHD. A similar study has recently been initiated at the National Institutes of Health with incremental doses of donor T cells administered beginning 30 days after BMT (60). Significant acute GVHD has not occurred in 5 patients reported to date. Both trials await longer follow-up to determine the ultimate effect on GVL and relapse.

The Hadassah group has taken this type of approach in efforts to control minimal residual disease after autologous BMT by administering partially matched allogeneic lymphocytes after autologous reengraftment has occurred (61,62). These patients should be markedly immunosuppressed immediately after autologous BMT, but interestingly, severe GVHD does not seem to occur, even though the donor cells are partially mismatched. It is unknown if these cells actually "engraft," and the benefit in terms of relapse and survival will be determined only with longer follow-up.

IV. CYTOKINE-MEDIATED IMMUNOTHERAPY

It is becoming increasingly clear that GVHD results from a complex interaction of effector cells and cytokines (56), and it is likely that cytokines are an important component of the GVL reaction. There have been several trials investigating the use of cytokines as a method to control minimal residual disease after transplantation. Interleukin-2 (IL-2) has been the most extensively studied due to its ability to activate lymphocytes and enhance natural killer (NK) cell number and function. Several observations suggest that these functions will provide useful antileukemic effects, including (a) lymphocytes obtained from patients early after autologous or allogeneic BMT are "activated"; they express cell surface activation antigens, and possess the ability to lyse NK resistant targets (63,64); (b) NK cells will lyse the CML-derived cell line K562 cells in vitro; (c) NK cell number and activity is increased in the peripheral blood of patients after BMT (64,65); (d) NK cells isolated from some patients after BMT are capable of lysing cryopreserved host leukemic cells (65,66) and inhibiting leukemic progenitor colony growth (67); (e) IL-2 exposure in vitro may induce the ability of peripheral blood MNC to lyse cryopreserved autologous leukemic cells (65,67); and (f) the risk of relapse for recipients of T-cell-depleted allografts for CML may correlate with the ability of IL-2–stimulated peripheral blood MNC to lyse leukemic targets (65).

It has therefore been logical to test the ability of IL-2 to enhance or induce GVL after BMT (16,68–70). The administration of low doses of IL-2 (200,000 to 600,000 Units/M^2) by continuous infusion after BMT has been given with minimal toxicity (62,71) and may result in up to a 10-fold increase in the number of circulating NK cells; GVHD is not exacerbated, presumably because low-dose IL-2 selectively activates NK cells without T-cell stimulation (71). However, it should be noted that use of IL-2 early after BMT may also alter the cytokine patterns secreted by donor T-cells (72). Initial reports suggest that low dose IL-2 after allogeneic T-cell-depleted BMT may at least partially restore the GVL activity of the marrow graft, resulting in lower relapse rates compared to similar patients who did not receive immunotherapy (71). IL-2 at varying doses has also been given to patients after autologous BMT with encouraging results (62,68,73). The optimal timing and dose of administration after BMT may be critical to achieve the maximal effect of IL-2, but the current results seem sufficiently promising to warrant the next step of a randomized controlled trial.

V. DONOR LYMPHOCYTE INFUSIONS TO TREAT OTHER TRANSPLANTATION-RELATED COMPLICATIONS

Adoptive immunotherapy with donor lymphocyte infusions has been used successfully to treat patients with Epstein-Barr virus (EBV)-related B-cell lymphoproliferative disorders (BLPD) occurring after allogeneic BMT. Posttransplantation BLPD typically are aggressive lymphomas of donor-cell origin that are unresponsive to standard therapy and are most often fatal (74). These disorders develop due to the uncontrolled proliferation of EBV-infected B cells in the absence of appropriate viral-specific cellular immunity; MNC infusions from a donor with poor viral exposure would be expected to restore antiviral cellular immunity. Several patients with posttransplantation BLPD who received donor MNC infusions have achieved sustained complete remissions (75,76). Unfortunately, acute and chronic GVHD may complicate therapy, as it does when donor MNC are used to treat leukemic relapse.

In order to further minimize the toxicity of cellular immunotherapy, genetically modified donor cells engineered to contain a "suicide gene" have been used to treat patients with posttransplantation BLPD. In an elegant strategy first reported by Servida et al. (77), donor MNC were transduced with a retroviral vector expressing two genes; a nonfunctional nerve growth factor receptor (NGFR) and the herpes simplex thymidine kinase (TK) gene. NGFR expression on the cell surface allowed for the immunoselection of an essentially pure population of virally transduced cells. The TK gene confers sensitivity of these cells to the drug gancyclovir. An infusion of genetically modified donor cells to a patient with BLPD resulted in complete remission; acute GVHD developed several weeks later and resolved after the administration of gancyclovir. It has subsequently been demonstrated that gancyclovir rapidly results in the elimination of marked lymphocytes from the circulation (78). Since only dividing cells are transduced with the retroviral vector, the exposure of donor cells in vitro to EBV antigens may further enhance the specificity of donor cells selected. This strategy has been effectively used to select EBV-specific CTL and restore cellular immunity against EBV-associated antigens after BMT (79).

It should be noted that the response of BLPD to donor MNC infusions is likely to be qualitatively and quantitatively different than the GVL response. Since these lymphomas arise from EBV-infected donor cells, this reaction represents an *autologous* rather than an allogeneic response that is necessary for GVL. In addition, the effective cell dose used to treat BLPD is likely to be significantly lower than that used to treat leukemic relapse (76), since the frequency of precursor cytotoxic T lymphocytes (pCTL) with antiviral specificity will be much higher in a previously exposed individual than the frequency of pCTLs with antileukemic specificity. Toxicity may be minimal because the frequency of pCTLs with antihost specificity should also be low. Therefore, it is anticipated that an effective cell dose required to restore anti-EBV-specific immunity would be lower than the cell dose required for a GVL response, and this lower cell dose may limit toxicity from GVHD.

In addition to treating relapse and BLPD after BMT, donor MNC infusions have been effective in reversing a life-threatening adenovirus infection (80). In the future, it is likely that adoptive immunotherapy with donor cells will have a wide range of clinical applications to treat both malignant and infectious complications of transplantation.

VI. SUMMARY

There is substantial indirect evidence that allogeneic BMT supplies a GVL effect for patients with leukemia. The use of donor MNC infusions as adoptive immunotherapy for patients who relapse after BMT now provides a direct demonstration of GVL in the clinical setting. The potent antileukemic reaction induced by donor MNC is associated with acceptable toxicity and may be preferable to a second allogenic BMT. Most responding patients develop mild to moderate GVHD, and it has not yet been possible to reliably dissociate GVHD from GVL. The mechanisms underlying GVL reactivity remain unclear but are likely influenced by the activity of the donor effector cells, by the immunological properties of the target cells, and by the production of various cytokines. Future studies are required to better define these mechanisms, and strategies will likely be employed to manipulate the immunological properties of the donor graft, to influence target-cell reactivity to GVL effectors, and to enhance GVL reactivity both during and after BMT. Ultimately the ability to harness the GVL potential of allogeneic donor cells without GVHD will lead to the safer, more effective applications of BMT and to the development of novel treatment strategies for leukemia.

ACKNOWLEDGMENTS

This work was supported in part by NIH grant CA58661 (JHA). DLP is a Fellow of the Leukemia Society of America.

REFERENCES

1. Barnes D, Corp M, Loutit J, Neal F. Treatment of murine leukaemia with x-rays and homologous bone marrow: Preliminary communication. Br Med J 1956; 2:626–630.
2. Barnes D, Loutit J. Treatment of murine leukaemia with x-rays and homologous bone marrow. Br J Haematol 1957; 3:241–252.
3. Odom L, August C, Githens J, et al. Remission of relapsed leukaemia during a graft-versus-host reaction. A "graft-versus-leukaemia reaction" in man? Lancet 1978; 2:537–540.
4. Collins R, Rogers Z, Bennett M, et al. Hematologic relapse of chronic myelogenous leukemia following allogeneic bone marrow transplantation: Apparent graft-versus-leukemia effect following abrupt discontinuation of immunosuppression. Bone Marrow Transplant 1992; 10:391–395.
5. Higano C, Brixey M, Bryant E, et al. Durable complete remission of acute nonlymphocytic leukemia associated with discontinuation of immunosuppression following relapse after allogeneic bone marrow transplantation: A case report of a probable graft-versus-leukemia effect. Transplantation 1990; 50:175–177.

6. Sullivan K, Shulman H. Chronic graft-versus-host disease, obliterative bronchiolitis, and graft-versus-leukemia effect: Case histories. Transplant Proc 1989; 21:51–62.
7. Weiden P, Flournoy N, Donnall Thomas E, et al. Antileukemic effect of graft-versus-host disease in human recipients of allogeneic-marrow grafts. N Engl J Med 1979; 300: 1068–1073.
8. Fefer A, Sullivan K, Weiden P, et al. Graft versus leukemia effect in man: The relapse rate of acute leukemia is lower after allogeneic than after syngeneic marrow transplantation. In: Truitt R, Gale R, Bortin M, eds. Cellular Immunotherapy of Cancer. New York: Liss, 1987:401–408.
9. Gale R, Champlin R. How does bone-marrow transplantation cure leukaemia? Lancet 1984; 2:28–30.
10. Gale R, Horowitz M, Ash R, et al. Identical-twin bone marrow transplants for leukemia. Ann Intern Med 1994; 120:646–652.
11. Horowitz M, Gale R, Sondel P, et al. Graft-versus-leukemia reactions after bone marrow transplantation. Blood 1990; 75:555–562.
12. Sullivan K, Weiden P, Storb R, et al. Influence of acute and chronic graft-versus-host disease on relapse and survival after bone marrow transplantation from HLA-identical siblings as treatment of acute and chronic leukemia. Blood 1989; 73:1720–1728.
13. Weiden P, Sullivan K, Flournoy N, et al. Antileukemic effect of chronic graft-versus-host disease: Contribution to improved survival after allogeneic marrow transplantation. N Engl J Med 1981; 304:1529–1533.
14. Goldman J, Gale R, Horowitz M, et al. Bone marrow transplantation for chronic myelogenous leukemia in chronic phase. Ann Intern Med 1988; 108:806–814.
15. Antin J, Bierer B, Smith B, et al. Selective depletion of bone marrow T lymphocytes with anti-CD5 monoclonal antibodies: Effective prophylaxis for graft-versus-host disease in patients with hematologic malignancies. Blood 1991; 78:2139–2149.
16. Soiffer R, Murray C, Mauch P, et al. Prevention of graft-versus-host disease by selective depletion of CD6-positive T lymphocytes from donor bone marrow. J Clin Oncol 1992; 10:1191–1200.
17. Wagner J, Santos G, Noga S, et al. Bone marrow graft engineering by counterflow centrifugal elutriation. Results of a phase I-II clinical trial. Blood 1990; 75:1370–1377.
18. Waldmann H, Polliak A, Hale G, et al. Elimination of GVHD by in-vitro depletion of alloreactive lymphocytes with a monoclonal rat anti-human lymphocyte antibody (Campath-1). Lancet 1984; 2:483–486.
19. Martin P, Hansen J, Buckner C, et al. Effects of in vitro depletion of T cells in HLA-identical allogeneic marrow grafts. Blood 1985; 66:664–672.
20. Mitsuyasu R, Champlin R, Gale R, et al. Treatment of donor bone marrow with monoclonal anti-T-cell antibody and complement for the prevention of graft-versus-host disease. Ann Intern Med 1986; 105:20–26.
21. Young J, Papadopoulos E, Cunningham I, et al. T-cell depleted allogeneic bone marrow transplantation in adults with acute nonlymphocytic leukemia in first remission. Blood 1992; 79:3380–3387.
22. Goldman J, Apperley J, Jones L, et al. Bone marrow transplantation for patients with chronic myeloid leukemia. N Engl J Med 1986; 314:202–207.
23. Marmont A, Horowitz M, Gale R, et al. T-cell depletion of HLA-identical transplants in leukemia. Blood 1991; 78:2120–2130.
24. Apperley J, Mauro F, Goldman J, et al. Bone marrow transplantation for chronic myeloid leukaemia in first chronic phase: Importance of a graft-versus-leukaemia effect. Br J Haematol 1988; 69:239–245.
25. Arcese W, Goldman J, D'Arcangelo E, et al. Outcome for patients who relapse after allogeneic bone marrow transplantation for chronic myeloid leukemia. Blood 1993; 82: 3211–3219.

26. Mrsic M, Horowitz M, Atkinson K, et al. Second HLA-identical sibling transplants for leukemia recurrence. Bone Marrow Transplant 1992; 9:269–275.
27. Radich J, Sanders J, Buckner C, et al. Second allogeneic marrow transplantation for patients with recurrent leukemia after initial transplant with total-body irradiation-containing regimens. J Clin Oncol 1993; 11:304–313.
28. Kolb H, Mittermuller J, Clemm C, et al. Donor leukocyte transfusions for treatment of recurrent chronic myelogenous leukemia in marrow transplant patients. Blood 1990; 76: 2462–2465.
29. Bär B, Schattenberg A, Mensink E, et al. Donor leukocyte infusions for chronic myeloid leukemia relapsed after allogeneic bone marrow transplantation. J Clin Oncol 1993; 11: 513–519.
30. Drobyski W, Keever C, Roth M, et al. Salvage immunotherapy using donor leukocyte infusions as treatment for relapsed chronic myelogenous leukemia after allogeneic bone marrow transplantation: Efficacy and toxicity of a defined T-cell dose. Blood 1993; 82: 2310–2318.
31. Helg C, Roux E, Beris P, et al. Adoptive immunotherapy for recurrent CML after BMT. Bone Marrow Transplant 1993; 12:125–129.
32. Hertenstein B, Wiesneth M, Novotny J, et al. Interferon-α and donor buffy coat transfusions for treatment of relapsed chronic myeloid leukemia after allogeneic bone marrow transplantation. Transplantation 1993; 56:1114–1118.
33. Porter D, Roth M, McGarigle C, et al. Induction of graft-versus-host disease as immunotherapy for relapsed chronic myeloid leukemia. N Engl J Med 1994; 330:100–106.
34. van Rhee F, Cullis J, Feng L, et al. Donor leukocyte transfusions (DLT) for relapse of chronic myeloid leukemia after allogeneic bone marrow transplant. Blood 1993; 82(suppl 1):416a.
35. Roth M, Antin J, Ash R, et al. Prognostic significance of Philadelphia chromosome-positive cells detected by the polymerase chain reaction after allogeneic bone marrow transplant for chronic myelogenous leukemia. Blood 1992; 79:276–282.
36. Antin J. Graft-versus-Leukemia: No longer an epiphenomenon. Blood 1993; 82:2273–2277.
37. Talpaz M, Kantarjian H, Kurzrock R, et al. Interferon-alpha produces sustained cytogenetic responses in chronic myelogenous leukemia: Philadelphia chromosome-positive patients. Ann Intern Med 1991; 114:532–538.
38. Higano C, Raskind W, Flowers M. Alpha Interferon (IFN) results in high complete cytogenetic response rate in patients with cytogenetic-only relapse of chronic myelogenous leukemia (CML) after marrow transplantation (BMT). Blood 1993; 82(suppl): 661a.
39. Higano C, Raskind W, Singer J. Use of alpha interferon for the treatment of relapse of chronic myelogenous leukemia in chronic phase after allogeneic bone marrow transplantation. Blood 1992; 80:1437–1442.
40. Opalka B, Wandl U, Becher R, et al. Minimal residual disease in patients with chronic myelogenous leukemia undergoing long-term treatment with recombinant interferon a-2b alone or in combination with Interferon-gamma. Blood 1991; 78:2188–2193.
41. Kolb H, Mittermuller J, Hertenstein H, et al. Adoptive immunotherapy in human and canine chimeras—The role of interferon alpha. Semin Hematol 1993; 30(3):37–39.
42. Balkwill F. Interferons. New York: Oxford University Press, 1989:8–53.
43. Upadhyaya G, Gupta S, Sih S, et al. Interferon-alpha restores the deficient expression of the cytoadhesion molecule lymphocyte function antigen-3 by chronic myelogenous leukemia progenitor cells. J Clin Invest 1991; 88:2131.
44. Anderson K, Weinstein H. Transfusion-associated graft-versus-host disease. N Engl J Med 1990; 323:315–321.
45. Frassoni F, Fagioli F, Sessarego M, et al. The effect of donor leukocyte infusion in

patients with leukemia following allogeneic bone marrow transplantation. Exp Hematol 1992; 20:712.
46. Kernan N, Collins N, Juliano L, et al. Lymphocytes in T cell-depleted bone marrow transplants correlate with development of graft-v-host disease. Blood 1986; 68:770–773.
47. Mackinnon S, Papadopoulos E, Carabasi M, et al. Adoptive immunotherapy using escalating doses of donor leukocytes for relapsed chronic myeloid leukemia following allogeneic bone marrow transplantation. Blood 1994; 84:538a.
48. van Rhee F, Lin F, Cullis J, et al. Relapse of chronic myeloid leukemia after allogeneic bone marrow transplant: The case for giving donor leukocyte transfusions before the onset of hematologic relapse. Blood 1994; 83:3377–3383.
49. Giralt S, Hester J, Huh Y, et al. $CD8^+$ depleted donor lymphocyte infusions as treatment for relapsed chronic myelogenous leukemia (CML) after allogeneic bone marrow transplantation (BMT): Graft vs leukemia without graft vs host disease (GVHD). Blood 1994; 84:538a.
50. Kolb H, deWitte T, Mittermuller J, et al. Graft-versus-leukemia effect of donor buffy coat transfusions on recurrent leukemia after marrow transplantation. Blood 1993; 82(suppl):840a.
51. Vesole D, Tricot G, Jagannath S, Barlogie B. Induction of graft-versus-myeloma (GVM) effect following allogeneic bone marrow transplantation. Blood 1994; 84:331a.
52. Sullivan K, Deeg H, Sanders J, et al. Hyperacute graft-v-host disease in patients not given immunosuppression after allogeneic marrow transplantation. Blood 1986; 67: 1172–1175.
53. Sullivan K, Storb R, Witherspoon R, et al. Deletion of immunosuppressive prophylaxis after marrow transplantation increased hyperacute graft-versus-host disease but does influence chronic graft-versus-host disease or relapse in patients with advanced leukemia. Clin Transplant 1989; 3:5–11.
54. Elfenbein G, Graham-Pole J, Weiner R, et al. Consequences of no prophylaxis for acute graft-versus-host disease after HLA-identical bone marrow transplantation (abstr). Blood 1987; 70(suppl 1):305a.
55. Sullivan K, Storb R, Buckner D, et al. Graft-versus-host disease as adoptive immunotherapy in patients with advanced hematologic neoplasms. N Engl J Med 1989; 320: 828–834.
56. Antin J, Ferrara J. Cytokine dysregulation and acute graft-versus-host disease. Blood 1991; 80:2964–2968.
57. Johnson B, Drobyski W, Truitt R. Delayed infusion of normal donor cells after MHC-matched bone marrow transplantation provides an antileukemia reaction without graft-versus-host disease. Bone Marrow Transplant 1993; 11:329–336.
58. Weiden P, Storb R, Tsoi M, et al. Infusion of donor lymphocytes into stable canine radiation chimeras: Implications for mechanism of transplantation tolerance. J Immunol 1978; 116:1212–1219.
59. Slavin S, Naparstek E, Nagler A, et al. Graft vs leukemia (GVL) effects with controlled GVHD by cell mediated immunotherapy (CMI) following allogeneic bone marrow transplantation (BMT). Blood 1993; 82:423a.
60. Couriel D, Cottler-Fox M, Burt R, et al. T-cell depleted marrow transplants with delayed lymphocyte add-back to prevent relapse in patients with leukemia and MDS. Blood 1994; 84:334a.
61. Slavin S, Naparstek E, Nagler A, et al. Cell mediated immunotherapy (CMI) for the treatment of malignant hematological diseases in conjunction with autologous bone marrow transplantation (ABMT). Blood 1993; 82a:292a.
62. Slavin S, Ackerstein A, Weiss L, et al. Immunotherapy of minimal residual disease by immunocompetent lymphocytes and their activation by cytokines. Cancer Invest 1992; 10:221–227.

63. Ikinciogullari A, Oblakowski P, Hamon M, et al. Activation marker expression on the peripheral blood lymphocytes of normal volunteers, recipients of interleukin-2 and patients undergoing bone marrow transplantation. Exp Hematol 1992; 20:819a.
64. Reittie J, Gottlieb D, Heslop H, et al. Endogenously generated activated killer cells circulate after autologous and allogeneic marrow transplantation but not after chemotherapy. Blood 1989; 73:1351–1358.
65. Hauch M, Gazzola M, Small T, et al. Anti-leukemia potential of interleukin-2 activated natural killer cells after bone marrow transplantation for chronic myelogenous leukemia. Blood 1990; 75:2250–2262.
66. Jiang Y, Cullis J, Kanfer E, et al. T cell and NK cell mediated graft-versus-leukaemia reactivity following donor buffy coat transfusion to treat relapse after marrow transplantation for chronic myeloid leukaemia. Bone Marrow Transplant 1993; 11:133–138.
67. Mackinnon S, Hows J, Goldman J. Induction of in vitro graft-versus-leukemia activity following bone marrow transplantation for chronic myeloid leukemia. Blood 1990; 76: 2037–2045.
68. Benyunes M, Massumoto C, York A, et al. Interleukin-2 with or without lymphokine-activated killer cells are consolidative immunotherapy after autologous bone marrow transplantation for acute myelogenous leukemia. Bone Marrow Transplant 1993; 12: 159–163.
69. Slavin S, Eckerstein A, Weiss L. Adoptive immunotherapy in conjunction with bone marrow transplantation-amplification of natural host defense mechanisms against cancer by recombinant IL-2. Natl Immunol Cell Growth Reg 1988; 7:180–184.
70. Verdonck L, van Heugten H, Giltay J, Franks C. Amplification of the graft-versus-leukemia effect in man by interleukin-2. Transplantation 1991; 51:1120–1124.
71. Soiffer R, Murray C, Gonin R, Ritz J. Effect of low-dose interleukin-2 on disease relapse after T-cell-depleted allogeneic bone marrow transplantation. Blood 1994; 84: 964–971.
72. Sykes M, Harty M, Szot G, Pearson D. Interleukin-2 inhibits graft-versus-host disease-promoting activity of $CD4^+$ cells while preserving CD4- and CD8-mediated graft-versus-leukemia effects. Blood 1994; 83:2560–2569.
73. Hamon M, Prentice H, Gottlieb D, et al. Immunotherapy with interleukin-2 after ABMT in AML. Bone Marrow Transplant 1993; 11:399–401.
74. Shapiro R, McClain K, Frizzera G, et al. Epstein-Barr virus associated B cell lymphoproliferative disorders following bone marrow transplantation. Blood 1988; 71:1234–1243.
75. Porter D, Orloff G, Antin J. Donor mononuclear cell infusions as therapy for B-cell lymphoproliferative disorder following allogeneic bone marrow transplant. Transplant Science 1994; 4:11–15.
76. Papadopoulos E, Ladanyi M, Emanuel D, et al. Infusions of donor leukocytes to treat Epstein-Barr virus–associated lymphoproliferative disorders after allogeneic bone marrow transplantation. N Engl J Med 1994; 330:1185–1191.
77. Servida P, Rossini S, Traversari C, et al. Gene transfer into peripheral blood lymphocytes for in vivo immunomodulation of donor anti-tumor immunity in a patient affected by EBV-induced lymphoma. Blood 1993; 82:214a.
78. Bonini C, Verzeletti S, Servida P, et al. Transfer of the HSV-TK gene into donor peripheral blood lymphocytes for in vivo immunomodulation of donor anti-tumor immunity after allo-BMT. Blood 1994; 84:110a.
79. Heslop H, Smith C, Ng C, et al. Use of genetically marked virus specific cytotoxic T lymphocytes to control Epstein-Barr virus related lymphoproliferation. Blood 1994; 84:110a.
80. Hroma R, Cornetta K, Srour E. Donor leukocyte infusion as therapy of life-threatening adenoviral infections after T-cell-depleted bone marrow transplantation (letter). Blood 1994; 84:1690–1691.

81. Collins R, Wolff S, List A, et al. Prospective multicenter trial of donor buffy coat infusion for relapsed hematologic malignancy post-allogeneic bone marrow transplantation (BMT). Blood 1994; 84:333a.
82. Porter D, Roth M, McGarigle C, et al. Induction of graft-vs-leukemia (GVL) reaction as therapy for relapsed leukemia after allogeneic bone marrow transplantation (BMT). J Cell Biochem 1994; 18B:94a.
83. Ferster A, Bujan W, Mouraux T, et al. Complete remission following donor leukocyte infusion in ALL relapsing after haploidentical bone marrow transplantation. Bone Marrow Transplant 1994; 14:331–332.
84. Pati A, Godder K, Lamb L, et al. Donor leukocyte infusions (DLI) to treat relapsed acute myeloid leukemia (AML) following partially mismatched related donor (PMRD) bone marrow transplantation (BMT). Blood 1994; 84:339a.
85. Porter D, Roth M, McGarigle C, et al. The graft-vs-leukemia (GVL) effect of donor mononuclear cell (MNC) infusions for patients with relapsed acute leukemia and myelodysplasia (MDS) after allogeneic bone marrow transplantation. Blood 1994; 84:338a.
86. Szer J, Grigg A, Phillipos G, Sheridan W. Donor leucocyte infusions after chemotherapy for patients relapsing with acute leukaemia following allogeneic BMT. Bone Marrow Transplant 1993; 11:109–111.
87. Verfaillie C, Weisdorf D, McGlave P, et al. High dose donor mononuclear cell infusion in post-transplant relapsed AML/MDS. Blood 1994; 84:333a.
88. Takahashi S, Nagayama H, Nagamura F, et al. Graft versus leukemia (GVL) effect with fatal graft versus host disease (GVHD) by donor leukocyte transfusion (DLT) in posttransplantation acute leukemia relapse: Reports of two cases. Blood 1994; 84:338a.
89. Heberman R, Ortaldo J, Rjubinstein M, Pestka S. Augmentation of natural and antibody-dependent cell-mediated cytotoxicity by pure human leukocyte interferon. J Clin Immunol 1981; 1:149–153.

29

Gene Therapy

Helen E. Heslop
St. Jude Children's Research Hospital and University of Tennessee
Memphis, Tennessee

John M. Cunningham
St. Jude Children's Research Hospital
Memphis, Tennessee

Stephen M. Jane
Royal Melbourne Hospital
Parkville, Victoria, Australia

I. INTRODUCTION

Although still in its early development stages, gene therapy will considerably affect bone marrow transplantation (BMT) procedures in the next few years. In some diseases, such as immunodeficiencies, hemoglobinopathies, and metabolic storage diseases, where BMT is the only current curative therapy, gene transfer into autologous stem cells or fibroblasts may eliminate the need for allogeneic BMT altogether and therefore abolish the risk of graft-versus-host disease (GVHD). In patients who receive allogeneic BMT for malignancy, gene transfer may provide a means for ablating alloreactive T cells in the event of GVHD. Furthermore, gene transfer could be used to exploit the beneficial aspects of alloreactivity by augmenting the antileukemic effectors that produce graft-versus-leukemia (GVL) effects. An obvious prerequisite for gene transfer is an effective delivery system, and we begin by reviewing current delivery systems for gene transfer into marrow derived cells as well as strategies to optimize gene transfer and the selection of transduced cells.

II. DELIVERY SYSTEMS

The replacement of a defective gene by targeting correct sequences to the site of the defect by homologous recombination is many years from realization in human diseases. Instead, current methods introduce genetic material via transforming viruses or by physical methods (1–3). The clinical applicability of any gene transfer system is dependent on several parameters: (a) a high frequency of infection of the target cells (usually the hematopoietic stem cell) with efficient integration and a selective advantage over nontransduced cells, (b) sufficient expression of the transgene to reverse the phenotype (except in the case of marking studies), (c) stable regulatable expression in the desired cell type, and (d) a genetically neutral event.

At present no single vector fulfills these requirements; therefore different vectors are being developed for specific therapeutic uses.

A. Retroviruses

Retroviruses have been used extensively as a gene delivery vector system. They are derived from the murine leukemia viruses (MuLV), particularly the Moloney murine leukemia virus (MoMuLV) (4,5). Retroviral particles contain two single-stranded RNA molecules that are converted to DNA by reverse transcriptase carried by the virus particle. The subsequent production and integration of duplex DNA into the host genome produces a proviral DNA template with all the information necessary for particle formation and subsequent productive infection. The wild-type replication-competent virus, like many retroviruses of this class, is oncogenic due to the risk of insertional mutagenesis. Figure 1A shows the two long-terminal repeats (LTR) flanking the coding sequence of the virus; these are involved in transcriptional control, polyadenylation, replication, and integration. The coding sequence contains three sets of structural genes: *gag*, which encodes structural proteins and confers high packaging efficiency: *pol*, which codes for replicative polymerases and integrase; and *env* which codes for envelope proteins. Upstream of the gag coding sequence lies a 35-nucleotide packaging signal (ψ), which is essential for retroviral RNA packaging into capsids (4–6).

MoMuLV viruses, like all murine leukemia viruses, display a variable host range that is dependent upon the gp70 envelope protein, which interacts with the retroviral receptor. Two major types of gp70 enveloped virus have been used: ecotropic, which infect murine cells only, and amphotropic, which have a broader range that includes human cells. They interact with recently defined cellular receptors, which are normally involved in ion transport (7,8). Pseudotyping the virus—for example, placing VSV-G protein (9) or erythropoietin (10) domains in the viral membrane, may allow concentration of the retrovirus and even specific targeting.

Retroviruses used for clinical gene transfer are engineered to be replication-defective by replacing the *gag*, *pol*, and *env* genes with the desired therapeutic genes, together with any necessary regulatory elements and polyadenylation signal (Fig. 1B) (4,6). Murine fibroblast packaging cell lines provide structural genes in *trans* to package the recombinant virus, which is subsequently secreted into the culture median (Fig. 1B). The replication-defective viral vector can then infect a target cell and integrate the therapeutic gene into the host genome, but it lacks the ability to reinfect. To improve the safety of viral vectors, packaging cell lines have been refined such that the *gag* and *pol* genes are carried on one plasmid and the *env* gene on another (11). Three separate recombination events would then be required to produce a replication-competent retrovirus. The method of vector introduction into the packaging cell line, the length of passage, and the confluency of the fibroblast layer all affect the number of infectious viral particles, or titer, in the supernatant. Optimal gene transfer is achieved with 10^6 to 10^7 particles per milliliter. Replication-defective retroviral producing cell lines are screened for titer, rearrangement, and often expression before further use.

Retroviruses such as MoMuLV can accommodate 8 to 9 kb of exogenous DNA, and the effects of the flanking viral sequences required for transduction are unpredictable and may be deleterious (12). The type of construct used is determined by

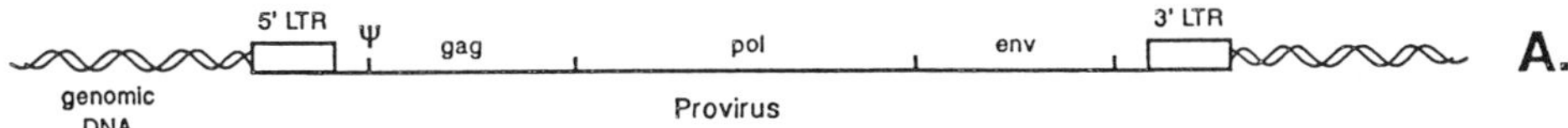

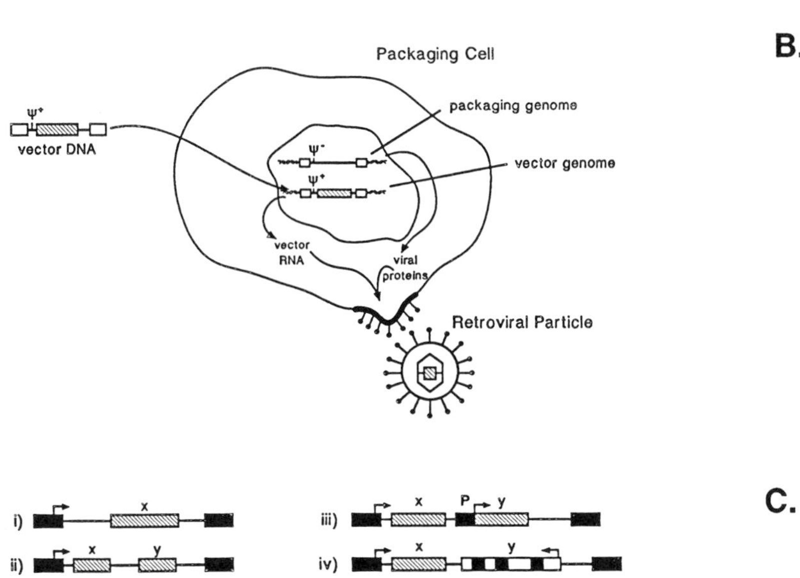

Figure 1 A. Diagrammatic representation of integrated retroviral genome. The virus is divided into regions consisting of (i) 5′ and 3′ long-terminal repeats (LTR), which contain promoter, enhancer, and polyadenylation sequences as well as inverted repeats; (ii) a packaging signal (Ψ); and (iii) three structural genes *gag*, *pol*, and *env*, which are required in *trans* for replication and packaging. B. Generation of helper-free retroviral particles. A retroviral vector is introduced by transfection into the packaging cell line. This vector is capable of being packaged but lacks the structural proteins necessary for infectious particle formation. This packaging genome provides these proteins, *gag*, *pol*, and *env*. The retroviral RNA transcripts complex with these proteins to form infectious particles. The supernatant from these cells thus contains replication-defective retroviruses, which are free of wild-type virus termed helper-free. C. Basic types of recombinant retroviral vector. (i) Simple type used in marking studies where single gene X is regulated by the LTR. (ii) Retroviral vector containing two genes each regulated by the LTR in which viral transcripts are spliced prior to translation to give two transcripts, X and Y. A similar construct in which splicing is prevented is termed a polycistronic vector. (iii) A dual promoter construct in which the Y gene is driven by an external promoter and the X gene is regulated by the LTR. (iv) A construct where regulatory sequences of the genomic structure of one gene (Y) are used. This design has been used for β-globin constructs to prevent inappropriate splicing of intronic variants during the viral life cycle.

the required therapeutic outcome and the size of the exogenous DNA used. Exogenous gene expression is dependent largely upon the regulatory sequences present in the viral construct (4,6). Several possibilities exist, as illustrated in Fig. 1C, including regulation of a single exogenous gene by the LTR promoter/enhancer or expression of two genes using splicing or polycistronic variants, where one gene is regulated by the LTR and one by an exogenous promoter.

Retroviruses require active mitosis for integration. As most hematopoietic stem cells are quiescent, this has limited the use of these vectors for therapeutic gene transfer. The use of cytokines and bone marrow stroma has improved transduction efficiency in mice to 20 to 30% (2,13–15). Reconstitution experiments have shown long-term expression of the transferred gene, an observation that suggests targeting to hematopoietic stem cells. Nonhuman primate (16) and human studies (17) are disappointing in comparison, with transduction efficiencies of 1 to 10%. However, selection of particular types of progenitors—such as peripheral blood or cord blood progenitors, which may have greater expansion potential—offers possibilities for further improvement (18,19). A higher transduction frequency has been obtained in mitogen-stimulated lymphocytes, but it is difficult to obtain stable long-term expression of many genes in these cells.

The major advantages of recombinant retroviral particle production are the homogeneity of vector particles in the supernatant, the high titer, and the lack of helper contamination. It is, however, crucial to test each batch for helper contamination, as supernatant containing replication-competent retroviruses induced thymic lymphomas in nonhuman primates (20). Problems of retroviral vector usage still exist, such as low hematopoietic stem-cell transduction efficiency, lack of sufficient expression of the therapeutic gene, and sometimes the lack of long-term expression. This is exemplified by our experience with globin-based vectors (see below). The availability of an adeno-associated virus-based delivery system may circumvent some of these problems.

B. Adeno-Associated Viruses

Adeno-associated virus (AAV), a defective parvovirus, is a single-stranded 4675-nt DNA virus. The genome is bordered by inverted terminal repeat (ITR) sequences of 145 nt (Fig. 2A). Two sets of structural genes, *rep* and *cap*, provide replicative and capsid proteins, respectively. *Rep* has also been implicated in the integration of the virus into host DNA. Wild-type AAV is a dependovirus requiring adenoviral gene products, provided by a coinfecting adenovirus, for packaging. The virus integrates preferentially into chromosome 19 and establishes a latent state (21). Thereafter infection of the cell with adenovirus or herpes simplex virus results in viral reactivation and cell lysis. The virus has a broad host range but is not associated with any disease state. Five stereotypes have been identified, the most studied being AAV-2 (2).

The ability of recombinant AAV (rAAV) to infect cells was first demonstrated

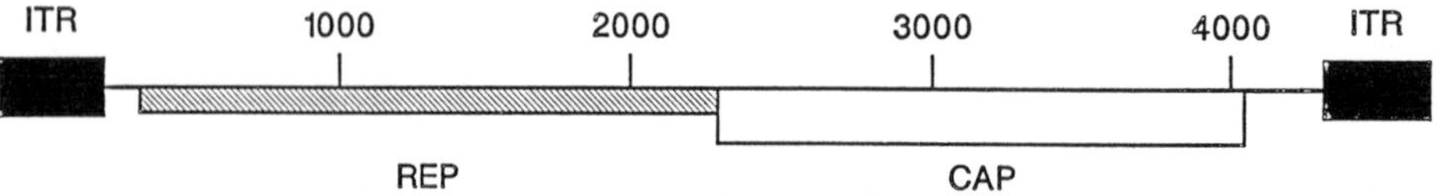

Figure 2 The wild-type adeno-associated virus genome. The virus is flanked by inverted terminal repeats (ITR), which are single-stranded hairpin structures. These are all that is required for recombinant vector production. The structural *rep* and *cap* genes are regulated by internal promoters.

by replacing the *cap* genes with a selectable marker (22). Transduction efficiencies of 80% were observed in tissue culture lines. Since then, the system has been refined (23). The *rep* and *cap* genes are removed and an exogenous gene with its own regulatory sequences is placed between the AAV ITRs, which provide integration, replication, and packaging signals. The construct is cotransfected with a second plasmid containing the *rep* and *cap* genes regulated by the adenoviral ITRs into a human kidney 293 cell line. This cell line constitutively expresses the adenoviral proteins required for packaging but is also infected with wild-type adenovirus 6 hr before cotransfection. In principle, this procedure allows up to 5 kb of DNA to be packaged without AAV helper contamination, while adenoviral contamination can be avoided by using differential heat inactivation of the viral supernatant at 56°C. Initial titers of 10^4 to 10^5 particles can be obtained and subsequent concentration of the viral supernatant can give titers exceeding 10^9 particles per milliliter. As more efficient packaging cell lines are developed, this approach should become less cumbersome.

Transduction of tissue culture cells with rAAV vectors—including constructs encoding neo^R for marking, β-globin for thalassemia and sickle cell disease (24,25), and glucocerebrosidase for Gaucher disease (26)—have shown the efficiency of this approach. Primary cells including murine (27) and human hematopoietic progenitors (28) and cord blood progenitors (29) have also been transduced with rAAV. Goodman and colleagues have shown that $CD34^+$ selected rhesus or human cells can be transduced with a β-galactosidase-containing virus (28). These cells showed high levels of expression of the transgene, suggesting that AAV vectors may be useful for hematopoietic stem-cell-targeted gene transfer. Unlike wild type AAV, the recombinant form of the virus appears to integrate randomly as 3 to 5 tandemly arranged copies (28).

This viral system has the advantages of lack of pathogenicity, the ability to transduce and integrate into quiescent hematopoietic stem cells (28), and the apparent lack of interference from flanking viral sequences. However, significant disadvantages, including lack of an efficient packaging system and the relatively small amount of DNA that can be packaged, have limited its use.

C. Other Viruses/Nonviral Technologies

Adenoviruses and herpes simplex viruses are being developed as vectors for use in pulmonary, hepatic, and CNS gene therapy, and some approaches have been approved for clinical trial (2). They are attractive in view of the large amount of DNA that can be packaged. Although adenoviral vectors can infect nondividing and dividing cells, current vectors do not integrate efficiently into recipient-cell nuclear DNA; thus their therapeutic gene is expressed transiently.

Nonviral DNA delivery methods involve the use of liposomes, DNA-coated particles, or macromolecular conjugates (polylysine, asialoglycoprotein) to facilitate entry into the target cell, often via normal physiological uptake mechanisms (30). This approach, although in its infancy compared to viral vectors, has the potential advantages of safety and a lack of size limitation. The addition of adenoviral proteins or fusogenic influenza hemagglutinin proteins in the liposome membrane correctly targets the exogenous DNA and prevents its degradation, suggesting that this approach warrants further study.

III. GENE TRANSFER TO HEMATOPOIETIC PROGENITORS

Hematopoietic progenitor cells are ideal targets for gene transfer; they are readily obtained and manipulated and their genetic modification could correct many single gene defects currently treated by allogeneic BMT. The disadvantages of using hematopoietic progenitors are that the transduction efficiency with current vectors is low and the biology of the true hematopoietic stem cell is not yet well defined. Thus clinical studies using hematopoietic progenitors as the target were originally confined to settings where useful information or therapeutic benefit may be obtained despite these limitations. One such situation is in gene marking studies that have aimed to answer biological questions about autologous BMT.

A. Gene Marking of Hemopoietic Progenitors

The rationale for initial marking studies was to determine whether residual malignant cells in autologous marrow contribute to subsequent relapse following autologous BMT. One approach to resolving this issue was to transfer marker genes into residual malignant cells in the marrow prior to reinfusion. If gene-marked malignant cells subsequently became detectable in the marrow or peripheral blood of patients who relapsed following autologous transplant, this would be definitive evidence that the harvested marrow contributed to disease recurrence. Studies at St. Jude addressed this issue in patients with neuroblastoma or acute myelogenous leukemia (AML) (31). Of 12 patients with AML, 4 have relapsed and gene-marked malignant cells have been identified in 2 of 3 cases evaluated so far (32). In the neuroblastoma study, 5 of the 9 patients have relapsed and marked malignant cells have been detected in 4 cases (33). Similar observations have been made at the MD Anderson Cancer Center, where marked malignant cells were found in two patients with chronic myelogenous leukemia (CML) who relapsed after autologous bone marrow transplant (BMT) (34).

While the primary aim of these studies was to determine the source of relapse, they also allowed assessment of the efficiency of gene transfer to normal progenitors in humans. In the St. Jude studies, semiquantitative PCR analysis for the neomycin resistance gene and clonogenic assays to quantitate G418-resistant colonies showed that the infused marrow clearly contributed to short- and long-term hematopoietic recovery (35). The marker gene was detected and expressed for up to 3 years in the mature progeny of marrow precursor cells, including peripheral blood T and B cells and neutrophils, and was also detected in lymphoblastoid cell lines and in cytotoxic T-cell lines derived from these patients. The long-term detection of the transferred gene may have been facilitated because these patients were harvested after recovery from intensive chemotherapy, when many early hemopoietic progenitor cells are in cycle.

Second-generation studies using this genetic marker technique have been designed to compare the regenerative potential of marrow to that of peripheral blood–derived progenitor cells. Genetic marking is also being used to determine which ex vivo or in vivo combination of cytokines will promote cell-cycle entry of long-term marrow-repopulating cells and thereby increase transduction efficiency. The results of these studies will influence the design of future gene therapy protocols (Sec. IV).

B. Use of In Vivo Selectable Markers

Because of the rather low efficiency of current gene transfer techniques in hematopoietic progenitor cells, it would be advantageous to be able to select in vivo for the transduced cell populations. The neomycin resistance gene used to select retroviral producer clones cannot be used for in vivo selection and may be deleterious to expression of a linked therapeutic gene (12). The identification of the genes involved in the metabolism of several cytotoxic agents has led to the design of strategies for in vivo hematopoietic stem cell selection/protection. These genes, often referred to as dominant selectable markers, may also allow dose escalation of chemotherapeutic regimens by protecting normal progenitors from the toxic effects of these compounds. This is the basis of several recently approved clinical trials. Other selectable markers include mutated surface antigens, such as CD24 (36), or a truncated version of the low-molecular-weight growth-factor receptor (37).

The dihydrofolate reductase gene (DHFR), which is involved in methotrexate (MTX) metabolism, was the first gene evaluated for its potential use as a dominant selectable marker. Mice transplanted with marrow previously transduced with a DHFR-containing retrovirus were protected from subsequent MTX-induced myelosuppression (38). Subsequently, the multidrug resistance-1 gene (MDR-1), which is involved in the efflux of several naturally occurring cytotoxic agents such as the vinca alkaloids, taxol, and anthracycline-based compounds, has been evaluated in murine and human studies. MDR-1–transduced marrow, when transplanted into mice, protected them from the effects of taxol (39). Recently, the work of Pastan and colleagues suggested that a bicistronic vector (see Fig. 1C), containing a MDR-1 gene and a therapeutic glucocerebrosidase gene allows high-level coexpression of both transcripts in tissue culture and selection of transduced cells (40). Studies of human hematopoietic progenitors have confirmed the results seen in mice, but with a lower transduction efficiency (41). Clinical trials, now under way, will help to validate this selection strategy. The approach is, however, currently limited by inefficient gene transfer as well as poor transient gene expression in hematopoietic stem cells.

IV. GENE THERAPY FOR SINGLE GENE DEFECTS

Single gene defects treated by allogeneic BMT and amenable to correction by modified hematopoietic progenitors include immunodeficiencies, hemoglobinopathies, and metabolic storage disorders. Prerequisites for gene therapy include availability of the cloned gene and knowledge of requirements for regulated expression. To illustrate some of the problems, gene transfer for ADA deficiency, hemoglobinopathies, and metabolic storage disorders is discussed.

A. ADA Deficiency

Adenosine deaminase (ADA) deficiency causes one form of severe combined immunodeficiency where T cells are the main cell type susceptible to accumulation of toxic metabolites. This immunodeficiency is a good model for gene therapy, as the gene is not subject to complex regulation, there should be a growth advantage for transduced cells, and clinical benefit may occur with correction of only a small number of T cells. Clinical protocols have evaluated transfer of ADA into peripheral blood lymphocytes, bone marrow, and umbilical cord blood cells which have been transduced ex vivo and returned to the patient (see Chap. 30). None of the patients have received ablation prior to return of transduced cells. In the first ADA gene therapy protocol at the National Institutes of Health (NIH) (42), two patients underwent leucaphereses to obtain peripheral blood mononuclear cells. After activation with OKT3 and IL-2, cells were transduced with a retroviral construct encoding the ADA gene. Transduction efficiencies varied from 1 to 10%. Following infusions, an increase in T-cell numbers and function as well as increased ADA activity and decreased incidence of infections was noted (42). One potential problem with this strategy is that repeated leucaphereses are necessary and multiple transduction procedures increase the risk of insertional mutagenesis. This protocol has now been modified so that patients receive transduced hemopoietic progenitors.

B. Hemoglobinopathies

The challenges of the hemoglobinopathies mirror those of many gene defects that may be amenable to hematopoietic progenitor targeted gene therapy. As a group, the hemoglobinopathies constitute one of the most prevalent human genetic disorders worldwide. Therapeutic options are limited and, with the exception of allogeneic bone marrow transplantation, are noncurative (43,44). Allogeneic BMT is an option only for patients who have a suitable donor, and the procedure is associated with morbidity and some mortality (45,46). Gene therapy for these diseases requires the replacement of the defective β-globin gene. For thalassemia, replacement should be with a normal functional β-globin gene. Although the same may be true for sickle cell disease (SCD), transfer of a functional γ-globin gene, which can prevent sickle hemoglobin polymerization (44), may be preferable. Significant amelioration of the disease phenotype requires at least 20% expression of a transduced γ- or β-globin gene relative to the endogenous levels (44,47). To achieve these therapeutic levels, we must understand the normal regulation of the human β-globin genes, develop more efficient gene delivery systems, and ensure that the expression of the transduced gene is both tissue-specific and maintained at high levels by erythroid progenitors.

The β-globin locus, located on chromosome 11, consists of the embryonic ϵ gene, the two fetal ${}^{G}\gamma$ and ${}^{A}\gamma$ genes, and the adult β and δ genes (48). Coding sequences for these genes are arranged over a 70-kb interval and coordinately regulated at the level of gene transcription (48). Studies in transgenic mice have shown that *cis*-acting regulatory sequences positioned directly adjacent to these genes—that is, the ϵ, ${}^{G}\gamma$, ${}^{A}\gamma$, and β promoters and the β and ${}^{A}\gamma$ enhancer—contain all the necessary elements to allow correct developmental and tissue-specific expression of the globin genes, albeit at low levels (49). More recently, a dominant regulatory region, approximately 15 kb long, termed the locus control region (LCR), which is required for high-level expression in transgenic models, has been identified (50,51). Four active sites in the LCR, termed HS1-4, contain the elements necessary for increased expression. Individual HS linked to the β-globin gene induce an expression level almost equivalent to that of the endogenous murine gene in transgenic mice (52).

The ability of retroviruses to transduce hematopoietic progenitor cells (53) stimulated the evaluation of β- or γ-globin gene-bearing retroviral vectors. Initially an ecotropic retrovirus, containing a neomycin resistance gene (Neo^R) and a 3-kb genomic fragment containing the β gene and its adjacent *cis*-acting regulatory sequences, was used to infect murine erythroleukemia (MEL) cells (54). Only retroviral constructs containing the globin gene in the reverse orientation were functional and allowed normal viral production. Single-copy proviral integration and expression levels of less than 0.1% of the endogenous β-globin level were obtained. Using amphotropic vectors containing a $\gamma\beta$ hybrid and a Neo^R, gene expression of the transgene reached 10% of endogenous levels (55). In these experiments, viral titer was low and the producer lines were prone to rearrangement. Subsequent experiments targeting erythroid progenitors with β-globin constructs showed low levels of infectivity (<0.1%) and 5% expression of the transgene with respect to endogenous levels (55). Similar transgene expression was observed in a bone marrow transplant (BMT) model. Although infectivity was low (less than 20% of reconstituted animals), all transduced animals showed long-term trilineage engraftment (56). Greatly enhanced transduction efficiency was later achieved using improved stem-cell isolation and higher viral titer (14,57). However, globin transgene expression remained unchanged. The identification of the LCR and its role in high-level expression prompted experiments with fragments of the individual and linked LCR-HSs coupled to the β or γ gene. Although MEL cell-bearing constructs that comprise HS2, the β gene, and NeoR show relatively high-level expression (58), it has been extremely difficult to consistently manufacture high-titer unrearranged producer cell lines. Indeed, less than 1% expression relative to endogenous levels is achieved in animals transduced with these constructs. In recent studies, retroviral constructs containing the HS1-4 or HS2-4 of the LCR and a human β-globin gene altered to reduce recombination were reported to induce transgene expression of up to 70% in MEL cells and relatively high expression in mice (59). Although encouraging, these results must be reproduced in nonhuman primates and human bone marrow.

In view of the difficulties with the retroviral approach, other viral vectors, particularly rAAV, have been investigated. The major potential advantage of AAV is its ability to stably integrate in a relatively site-specific manner in quiescent cells. Experiments with a $HS2^A\gamma Neo^R$ gene construct yielded expression levels 40 to 110% of the endogenous gene in K562 erythroleukemia cells (24). Genomic analysis revealed a randomly integrated single copy of unrearranged provirus per cell. These encouraging results have led several laboratories to investigate the expression of similar constructs in erythroid progenitors (27). Recently a construct containing core fragments of HS2, 3, and 4 coupled to the $^A\gamma$ gene ($v432^A\gamma$) without a selectable marker has given high-level expression in human burst-forming units–erythroid (BFU-E) (60).

In general, further advancement in gene transfer to correct hemoglobinopathies requires improved vector technology, a broader understanding of the role of the *cis*- and *trans*-acting elements in globin gene regulation, and improved stem-cell transduction.

C. Metabolic Storage Diseases

Gene therapy for metabolic storage diseases has been the focus of much interest. Many of these diseases are amenable to allogeneic BMT, but lack of donors and significant morbidity secondary to GVHD has limited its use (61). Problems related to stem-cell transduction and long-term expression, similar to those described for the hemoglobinopathies, have been encountered (62). Recent work in this area is reviewed briefly.

Gaucher disease is the most prevalent autosomal recessive lysosomal storage disease. It is due to glucocerebrosidase deficiency, which predominantly affects macrophage metabolism. Three clinical forms (types I–III) have been identified, all of which are associated with significant morbidity and mortality. Although recombinant enzyme replacement is available, a less expensive form of therapy is required (63). Correction of this enzyme deficiency by gene transfer was first demonstrated in skin fibroblasts, human lymphoblastoid cell lines, and bone marrow culture (62,64). Long-term reconstitution of mice with hematopoietic stem cells containing glucocerebrosidase expressing retroviral constructs was subsequently achieved (62). However, long-term expression in all lineages has been reported by only some groups. The neurological damage caused by this disease necessitates correction of the defect both in circulating macrophages and CNS microglia. Recently, expression in both cell types was documented in mice receiving glucocerebrosidase-transduced hematopoietic progenitors (65). This is important, not only for Gaucher disease but also for other diseases in which enzyme delivery to the CNS is crucial. The required level of gene expression to reverse the disease phenotype in these diseases will require further study.

The in vitro correction of the enzyme defect in human hematopoietic cells from patients with Gaucher disease and transduction of human long-term repopulating cells has been recently reported (66). Clinical trials using this construct are due to begin soon. Preliminary studies with variant retroviral backbones and the AAV system suggest that these systems may provide alternate approaches to this problem (26).

Other single-gene-defect syndromes—including the other lipidoses, mucopolysaccharidoses, chronic granulomatous disease, inborn errors of metabolism, and leukocyte adhesion abnormalities—have been corrected, at least in part, in tissue culture cell lines or in murine models (26,62). Of particular note is the correction of a subset of Fanconi anemia phenotypes by both retroviral and AAV vectors containing a correct copy of the defective DNA repair enzyme (67). This is particularly important in view of the high risk of both regimen-related toxicity and GVHD when allogeneic BMT is undertaken in such patients.

V. MODIFICATION OF T LYMPHOCYTES

A considerable body of evidence supports a role for T cells in eradicating residual leukemia following BMT. Initial evidence came from studies showing that the risk of relapse was reduced in patients with chronic GVHD (68) and increased in CML patients who had received T-cell-depleted marrow from matched siblings (69). Further support came from observations that donor leukocytes can both induce remission in patients who relapse after BMT (70,71) and control Epstein-Barr virus (EBV) lymphoproliferation (72,73) (see Chap. 28, "Adoptive Immunotherapy"). Although such adoptive immunotherapy approaches have produced clinical benefit, they are complicated by the frequent development of GVHD. In addition, it has been unclear whether GVL is merely a manifestation of GVHD or whether some T-cell clones recognize tumor-specific antigens rather than alloantigens expressed on a variety of recipient cells. Candidate antigens for specific recognition include peptides derived from proteins unique to the malignant cell (74,75) or minor histocompatibility antigens selectively expressed on hematopoietic cells that differed between donor and recipient [see Chap. 14, "Malignancy (GVL)"].

One strategy to harness the GVL effects of T cells while avoiding GVHD is to administer T cells that have been transduced with a suicide gene so that they are ablated if GVHD occurs. Another approach is to administer antigen-specific cytotoxic T lymphocytes (CTL) to reconstitute antiviral and antileukemia responses while avoiding GVHD. Gene transfer is being used to track infused CTL and to monitor efficacy. Finally, preclinical studies using gene-transfer strategies to improve CTL generation, enhance T-cell activity, and confer novel recognition properties are under way.

A. Gene Transfer to Confer Drug Sensitivity

Infusing donor-derived T cells following BMT can lead to GVHD initiated by alloreactive T cells. Even if CTL clones are used, cross-reaction with MHC polymorphisms may cause GVHD in an allogeneic setting (76). In addition, therapy of established disease with T cells can result in tissue damage, probably due to a hypersensitivity reaction (72). A possible solution to this problem is to transduce infused T cells with a "suicide" gene that confers drug sensitivity; if adverse effects ensue, the drug can be administered and infused T cells destroyed. The most widely used suicide gene is herpes simplex virus thymidine kinase, which renders transduced cells sensitive to ganciclovir. Although this strategy is theoretically attractive, there are several potential problems. All infused T cells must contain the gene conferring drug sensitivity, so a selectable marker must be included in the construct. Expression of the drug-sensitivity gene must be maintained in vivo. Finally although alloreactive T cells initiate GVHD, the process is maintained by cytokines and other immune system effectors that are recruited to the site, so that even if infused T cells are destroyed when GVHD or inflammatory reactions occur, the process may not necessarily be abrogated.

Suicide genes are currently being evaluated in two clinical trials of adoptive immunotherapy posttransplant. Bordignon and colleagues, who are using donor T cells to treat relapse or EBV lymphoma following BMT (77), transfect lymphocytes, after a brief 24- to 48-hr primary stimulation with antigen, with a construct containing a suicide gene and a truncated version of the low-molecular-weight nerve-growth-factor gene to serve as a selectable marker (37). Transduced T cells expressing the nerve-growth-factor receptor are harvested with magnetic beads and then infused to the patient. Should GVHD occur, the cells can theoretically be killed with ganciclovir. This approach is somewhat problematic in that alloreactive T cells will invariably remain after the brief primary stimulation. Furthermore, studies with tumor-infiltrating lymphocytes have shown that prolonged expression of transferred genes in T cells is difficult to obtain (78). Indeed, when a patient who developed GVHD was treated with ganciclovir, the percentage of thymidine kinase (Tk) containing cells fell only from 10 to 3% (77). For the suicide strategy to be successful, this problem must be overcome. Riddell and colleagues have initiated a protocol where *gag*-specific CTLs are administered to patients infected with the human immunodeficiency virus (HIV) receiving allogeneic BMT for lymphoma (79). Because of concerns that such HIV-specific CTL may cause tissue damage, the cells are transduced with the Tk gene, so that cell death can be induced if adverse effects occur (see Chap. 30).

Drug sensitivity genes could also be inserted into donor T cells administered at the time of BMT to preserve their beneficial effects on engraftment and GVL while allowing destruction if GVHD occurs. In preclinical studies, donor T cells stimulated with mitogen or with recipient cells are transduced with a construct containing both the neomycin resistance gene and a suicide gene (80) and then selected in G418. These cells can then be administered to recipients to produce GVL or killed if GVHD occurs. This approach is likewise feasible only if all transduced cells can be killed. Despite the uncertainty of whether the short-term presence of T cells will ensure engraftment and produce a GVL effect, clinical trials using this strategy will soon begin.

B. Evaluation Of Adoptive Transfer Strategies

An alternative means of reconstituting antiviral and antileukemic responses while avoiding GVHD is to administer antigen-specific CTL. At St. Jude, we are evaluating whether adoptive transfer of donor-derived EBV-specific cytotoxic T lymphocytes is effective prophylaxis for EBV lymphomas that arise after BMT (81). The pathogenesis of EBV lymphoproliferation is outgrowth of EBV-infected B cells that express a number of EBV-encoded antigens and are highly immunogenic. Normally, outgrowth is prevented by EBV-specific CTL and will occur only in severely immunosuppressed individuals. The incidence of EBV lymphoproliferation is particularly high (5 to 30%) in patients receiving T-cell–depleted allogeneic bone marrow from HLA-mismatched or HLA-matched unrelated donors (72) and almost always occurs in cells of donor origin. In recent reports, patients suffering from EBV lymphoproliferation were successfully treated with donor-derived peripheral blood leukocytes (72,73), suggesting that virus-specific T cells within the leukocyte population mediated these positive responses. Unselected leukocytes can, however, produce severe GVHD due to the presence of alloreactive T cells (73), while treatment of established disease can lead to fatal toxicity from tumor-cell lysis or inflammatory responses to virus-infected cells in the lung (72).

One solution to these problems is to reconstitute antiviral immunity with antigen-specific CTL. This strategy was first used at the Fred Hutchinson Research Institute in Seattle, where CMV-specific CTL clones were given to recipients of matched sibling marrow transplants (82). Administration resulted in no GVHD, and CMV-specific responses were detected following infusion. At our institution, we treated patients at high risk of developing EBV-lymphoproliferative disease after receiving T-cell depleted transplant from a mismatched family member or matched unrelated donor with donor-derived EBV-specific CTL. CTL were genetically marked prior to infusion, allowing us to determine whether adoptively transferred CTL persist long enough to confer significant protection and if they contributed to adverse effects, such as GVHD.

Ten patients have received CTL lines and no immediate adverse effects from infusion have been seen. The maker gene was detected by the polymerase chain reaction (PCR) for up to 16 weeks in peripheral blood mononuclear cells and for up to 9 months in EBV-specific CTL lines derived from patient cells. Semiquantitative

PCR analysis showed that between 1 in 100 and 1 in 5000 circulating lymphocytes were likely to have been derived from the infused line. There was also evidence of therapeutic benefit in three patients with evidence of EBV reactivation, where administration of EBV-specific CTL was followed by a 1000-fold fall in EBV DNA levels in peripheral blood within 3 to 4 weeks of infusion. One patient with a biopsy-proven immunoblastic lymphoma attained a complete remission after receiving 1.2×10^8 EBV-specific CTL (83). Hence, a limited number of infusions of T cells may be adequate to establish and maintain cellular immunity against EBV and BMT (83). By marking transferred T cells, we could also assess the contribution of infused cells to GVHD. One of our patients with preexisting chronic GVHD had persistence of this condition after therapy, but analysis of a biopsy specimen from a GVHD site showed no evidence for selective accumulation of gene-marked lymphocytes. One other patient developed a mild skin rash, which rapidly settled following a short course of steroids. Although biopsy showed appearance of mild GVHD, the market gene was not detected.

C. Gene Transfer to Enhance Graft Versus Leukemia

GVL activity may be enhanced by using gene transfer to amplify CTL generation, to augment effector function, or to modify receptor specificity. With increasing knowledge of the requirements for antigen presentation and for costimulation in induction of CTL responses (see Chap. 4, "Costimulation and Anergy," and Chap. 8, "Cytolytic T Lymphocytes") the use of gene transfer to optimize specific CTL generation for adoptive immunotherapy is being explored. Antigen presentation can be enhanced either by improved presentation of peptide by MHC or by enhanced costimulation. Several studies have shown that transduction of MHC molecules increases tumor immunogenicity. Moreover, studies involving costimulatory molecules such as B7 family members, which are constitutively expressed on professional antigen presenting cells, have shown that transfection of B7 either alone or together with a tumor antigen or MHC molecule results in increased immunogenicity of tumors (84–86). An alternative strategy could be to circumvent the requirement for T-cell help by transducing tumor cells with cytokines. In a number of animal models using different cytokines, transfection has resulted in increased immunogenicity, such that local injection of transduced tumor cells has led to the recruitment of immune system effector cells and tumor rejection (87,88). This strategy is currently being evaluated in leukemia cells with the aim of generating more specific CTL that could potentially be administered following BMT.

The antitumor activity of T cells may also be enhanced by increasing the levels of cytotoxic cytokines they produce at local tumor sites. Preclinical studies are evaluating the effects of transducing CMV-specific CTL with either the interleukin-2 (IL-2) gene or with a chimeric receptor comprising GMCSF receptor extracellular domain and IL-2 receptor cytoplasmic domain (89). Cells transduced with this construct bind GMCSF secreted by activated CD8-positive CTL and transduce the signal to produce an autocrine growth loop.

Studies are also underway to evaluate the effect of transducing CTL with appropriate antigen-specific T-cell receptors to confer novel tumor recognition properties. Many tumors express surface antigens that may be recognized by specific antibodies. If a cytotoxic T cell is transduced with a construct encoding a chimeric gene that contains a single-chain variable-region antibody linked with the gamma or zeta chain of the immunoglobulin receptor or the T-cell receptor (90), that CTL will recognize the tumor cell via the chimeric receptor. On binding to a tumor-specific antigen on the tumor-cell surface, the effector function of these modified CTL could be triggered. Unlike conventional CTL, which recognize antigen in the context of one MHC polymorphism, these modified lymphocytes would recognize a tumor-specific antigen in a MHC-unrestricted fashion. In vitro studies (91) have shown that tumor infiltrating lymphocyte lines transduced with a construct containing an antiovarian cancer antibody specifically recognized and lysed ovarian cancer cell lines. If CTL targeted to leukemic cells could be generated, their administration post BMT may produce GVL without GVHD.

VI. CONCLUSION

Gene transfer may have a significant impact on the incidence of GVHD in several ways. First, it may provide alternate therapies for genetic disorders due to single-gene defects currently treated by allogeneic BMT. For therapy of most single-gene defects to be effective, better delivery systems are required, as well as more precise knowledge of the optimal conditions for hematopoietic stem-cell transduction. For patients with leukemia who will still require allogeneic BMT, genetic modification of infused T cells may provide a means of ablating alloreactive T cells and preventing GVHD. Finally, gene transfer to antigen-specific CTL may allow separation of GVHD and GVL, with enhancement of antileukemia effects.

ACKNOWLEDGMENTS

This work was supported in part by NIH Cancer Center Support CORE Grant P30 CA21765, CA 61384 (HEH), Hl 55703 (HEH), PO1 HL53749 (JMC), the American Lebanese Syrian Associated Charities (ALSAC), the Assissi Foundation of Memphis (HEH, JMC), the Wellcome Trust (SMJ), and NHMRC grant 940573 (SMJ).

REFERENCES

1. Miller AD. Human gene therapy comes of age. Nature 1992; 357:455–460.
2. Nienhuis AW, Walsh CE, Liu J. Viruses as therapeutic gene transfer vectors. In: Young NS, ed. Viruses and Bone Marrow. New York: Marcel Decker, 1993:353–414.
3. Morgan RA, Anderson WF. Human gene therapy. Annu Rev Biochem 1993; 62:191–217.
4. Miller AD, Rosman GJ. Improved retroviral vectors for gene transfer and expression. Biotechniques 1989; 7:980–990.
5. Miller AD. Retroviral vectors. Curr Top Microbiol Immunol 1992; 158:1–24.
6. Armentano D, Yu S, Kantoff PW, et al. Effects of internal virus sequences on the utility of retroviral vectors. J Virol 1987; 61:1747–1750.
7. Miller DG, Edwards RH, Miller AD. Cloning of the cellular receptor for amphotropic murine retroviruses reveals homology to that for gibbon ape leukemia virus. Proc Natl Acad Sci USA 1994; 91:78–82.
8. Albritton LM, Tseng L, Scadden D, Cunningham JM. A putative murine ecotropic retrovirus receptor gene encodes a multiple membrane-spanning protein and confers susceptibility to viral infection. Cell 1989; 57:659–666.
9. Yee JK, Miyanohara A, LaPorte P, et al. A general method for the generation of high

titer, pantropic retroviral vectors: Highly efficient infection of primary hepatocytes. Proc Natl Acad Sci USA 1994; 91:9564–9568.
10. Kasahara N, Dozy AM, Kan YW. Tissue-specific targeting of retroviral vectors through ligand-receptor interactions. Science 1994; 266:1373–1376.
11. Danos O, Mulligan RC. Safe and effective generation of recombinant retroviruses with amphotropic and ecotropic host ranges. Proc Natl Acad Sci USA 1988; 85:6460–6464.
12. Apperley JF, Williams DA. Gene therapy: Current status and future directions. Br J Haematol 1990; 75:148–155.
13. Lim B, Apperley JF, Orkin SH, Williams DA. Long-term expression of human adenosine deaminase in mice transplanted with retrovirus-infected hematopoietic stem cells. Proc Natl Acad Sci USA 1989; 86:8892–8896.
14. Bodine DM, Karlsson S, Nienhuis AW. Combination of interleukins 3 and 6 preserves stem cell function in culture and enhances retrovirus-mediated gene transfer into hematopoietic stem cells. Proc Natl Acad Sci USA 1989; 86:8897–8901.
15. Moritz T, Patel VP, Williams DA. Bone marrow extracellular matrix molecules improve gene transfer into human hematopoietic cells via retroviral vectors. J Clin Invest 1994; 93:1451–1457.
16. Bodine DM, Moritz T, Donahue RE, et al. Long-term in vivo expression of a murine adenosine deaminase gene in rhesus monkey hematopoietic cells of multiple lineages after retroviral mediated gene transfer into $CD34^+$ bone marrow cells. Blood 1993; 82: 1975–1980.
17. Dunbar CE, Bodine DM, Sorrentino B, et al. Gene transfer into hematopoietic cells: Implications for cancer therapy. Ann NY Acad Sci 1994; 716:216–224.
18. Moritz T, Keller DC, Williams DA. Human cord blood cells as targets for gene transfer: Potential use in genetic therapies of severe combined immunodeficiency disease. J Exp Med 1993; 178:529–536.
19. Cassel A, Cottler-Fox M, Doren S, Dunbar CE. Retroviral-mediated gene transfer into CD34-enriched human peripheral blood stem cells. Exp Hematol 1993; 21:585–591.
20. Donahue RE, Kessler SW, Bodine D, et al. Helper virus induced T cell lymphoma in nonhuman primates after retroviral mediated gene transfer. J Exp Med 1992; 176:1125–1135.
21. Samulski RJ, Zhu X, Xiao X, et al. Targeted integration of adeno-associated virus (AAV) into human chromosome 19. EMBO J 1991; 10:3941–3950.
22. Hermonat P, Muzyczka N. Use of adeno-associated virus as a mammalian DNA cloning vector: Transduction of neomycin resistance into mammalian tissue culture cells. Proc Natl Acad Sci USA 1984; 81:6466–6470.
23. Samulski RJ, Chang LS, Shenk T. Helper-free stocks of recombinant adeno-associated viruses: Normal integration does not require viral gene expression. J Virol 1989; 63: 3822–3828.
24. Walsh CE, Liu JM, Xiao X, et al. Regulated high level expression of a human gamma-globin gene introduced into erythroid cells by an adeno-associated virus vector. Proc Natl Acad Sci USA 1992; 89:7257–7261.
25. Miller JL, Walsh CE, Ney PA, et al. Single-copy transduction and expression of human gamma-globin in K562 erythroleukemia cells using recombinant adeno-associated virus vectors: The effect of mutations in NF-E2 and GATA-1 binding motifs within the hypersensitivity site 2 enhancer. Blood 1993; 82:1900–1906.
26. Wei FF, Wei F, Samulski RJ, Barranger JA. Expression of the human glucocerebridase and arylsulfatase genes in murine and patient primary fibroblasts transduced by an adeno-associated virus vector. Gene Ther 1994; 1:261–268.
27. Zhou SZ, Li O, Stamatoyannopoulos G, Srivastava A. Adeno-associated virus 2-mediatd gene transfer in murine hematopoietic progenitor cells. Exp Hematol 1993; 21: 928–933.

28. Goodman S, Xiao X, Donaheu RE, et al. Recombinant adeno-associated virus-mediated gene transfer into hematopoietic progenitor cells. Blood 1994; 84:1492–1500.
29. Zhou SZ, Cooper S, Kang LY, et al. Adeno-associated virus 2-mediated high efficiency gene transfer into immature and mature subsets of hematopoietic progenitor cells in human umbilical cord blood. J Exp Med 1994; 179:1867–1875.
30. Nabel GJ, Nabel EG, Yang ZY, et al. Direct gene transfer with DNA-liposome complexes in melanoma: Expression, biologic activity, and lack of toxicity in humans. Proc Natl Acad Sci USA 1993; 90:11307–11311.
31. Brenner MK, Rill DR, Heslop HE, et al. Gene marking after bone marrow transplantation. Eur J Cancer 1994; 30A:1171–1176.
32. Brenner MK, Rill DR, Moen RC, et al. Gene-marking to trace origin of relapse after autologous bone marrow transplantation. Lancet 1993; 341:85–86.
33. Rill DR, Santana VM, Roberts WM, et al. Direct demonstration that autologous bone marrow transplantation for solid tumors can return a multiplicity of tumorigenic cells. Blood 1994; 84:380–383.
34. Deisseroth AB, Zu Z, Claxton D, et al. Genetic marking shows that Ph+ cells present in autologous transplants of chronic myelogenous leukemia (CML) contribute to relapse after autologous bone marrow in CML. Blood 1994; 83:3068–3076.
35. Brenner MK, Rill DR, Holladay MS, et al. Gene marking to determine whether autologous marrow infusion restores long-term haemopoiesis in cancer patients. Lancet 1993; 342:1134–1137.
36. Pawliuk R, Kay R, Lansdorp P, Humphries RK. Selection of retrovirally transduced hematopoietic progenitor cells using CD24 as a marker of gene transfer. Blood 1994; 84:2868–2877.
37. Mavilio F, Ferrari G, Rossini S, et al. Peripheral blood lymphocytes as target cells of retroviral vector-mediated gene transfer. Blood 1994; 83:1988–1997.
38. Williams DA, Hsieh K, DeSilva A, Mulligan RC. Protection of bone marrow transplant recipients from lethal doses of methotrexate by the generation of methotrexate-resistant bone marrow. J Exp Med 1987; 166:210.
39. Sorrentino BP, Brandt SJ, Bodine D, et al. Selection of drug-resistant bone marrow cells in vivo after retroviral transfer of human MDR1. Science 1992; 257:99–103.
40. Aran JM, Gottesman MM, Pastan I. Drug-selected coexpression of human glucocerebrosidase and P-glycoprotein using a bicistronic vector. Proc Natl Acad Sci USA 1994; 91:3176–3180.
41. Ward M, Richardson C, Pioli P, et al. Transfer and expression of the human multiple drug resistance gene in human $CD34^+$ cells. Blood 1994; 84:1408–1414.
42. Blaese RM. Development of gene therapy for immunodeficiency: Adenosine deaminase deficiency. Pediatr Res 1993; 33(1 suppl):S49–S53.
43. McDonagh K, Nienhuis AW. The thalassemias. In: Nathan DG, Oski FA, eds. Hematology of Infancy and Childhood. Philadelphia: Saunders, 1992:783–897.
44. Bunn HF. Sickle hemoglobin and other hemoglobin mutants. In: Stamatoyannopoulos G, Nienhuis AW, Majerus PJ, Varmus H, editors. The Molecular Basis of Blood Diseases. Philadelphia: Saunders, 1994:207–256.
45. Lucarelli G, Galimberti M, Polchi P, et al. Marrow transplantation in patients with advanced thalassemia. N Engl J Med 1987; 316:1050–1056.
46. Ferster A, De Valck C, Azzi N, et al. Bone marrow transplantation for severe sickle cell anaemia. Br J Haematol 1992; 80:102–105.
47. Rodgers GP, Dover GJ, Noguchi CT, et al. Hematologic responses of patients with sickle cell disease to treatment with hydroxyurea. N Engl J Med 1990; 322:1037–1045.
48. Stamatoyannopoulos G, Nienhuis AW. Hemoglobin switching. In: Stamatoyannopoulos G, Nienhuis AW, eds. The Molecular Basis of Blood Diseases. Philadelphia: Saunders, 1994:107–156.

49. Kollias G, Wrighton N, Hurst J, Grosveld F. Regulated expression of human gamma-, beta- and hybrid gamma beta-blogin genes in transgenic mice: Manipulation of the developmental expression patterns. Cell 1986; 46:89–94.
50. Orkin SH. Globin gene regulation and switching: Circa 1990. Cell 1990; 63:665–672.
51. Grosveld F, van Assenfeldt B, Greaves DR, Kollias G. Position independent high level expression of the human β-globin gene in transgenic mice. Cell 1987; 51:975–985.
52. Fraser P, Hurst J, Collis P, Grosveld F. DNase I hypersensitive sites 1, 2 and 3 of the human β-globin dominant control region direct position-independent expression. Nucleic Acids Res 1990; 18:3503–3508.
53. Williams DA, Orkin SH, Mulligan RC. Retrovirus-mediated transfer of human adenosine deaminase gene sequences into cells in culture and into muring hematopoietic cells in vitro. Proc Natl Acad Sci USA 1986; 83:2566–2570.
54. Cone RD, Weber-Benarous A, Baorto D, Mulligan RC. Regulated expression of a complete human beta-globin gene encoded by a transmissible retrovirus vector. Mol Cell Biol 1987; 7:887–897.
55. Karlsson S, Papayannopoulo T, Schweiger SG, et al. Retroviral-mediated transfer of genomic globin genes leads to regulated production of RNA and protein. Proc Natl Acad Sci USA 1987; 84:2411–2415.
56. Dzierzak EA, Papayannopoulou T, Mulligan RC. Lineage-specific expression of a human beta-globin gene in murine bone marrow transplant recipients reconstituted with retrovirus-transduced stem cells. Nature 1988; 331:35–41.
57. Bender MA, Gelinas RE, Miller AD. A majority of mice show long-term expression of a human β-globin gene after retrovirus transfer into hematopoietic stem cells. Mol Cell Biol 1989; 9:1426–1434.
58. Novak U, Harris EAS, Forrester W, et al. High-level β-globin expression after retroviral transfer of locus activation region-containing human β-globin gene derivatives into murine erythroleukemia cells. Proc Natl Acad Sci USA 1990; 87:3386–3390.
59. Plavec I, Papayannopoulou T, Maury C, Meyer F. A human β-globin gene fused to the human β-globin locus control region is expressed at high levels in erythroid cells of mice engrafted with retrovirus-transduced hematopoietic stem cells. Blood 1993; 81:1384–1392.
60. Miller JL, Donahue RE, Seller SE, et al. Recombinant adeno-associated virus (rAAV) mediated expression of a human gamma-globin gene in human progenitor derived erythroid cells. Proc Natl Acad Sci USA 1994: 91:10183–10187.
61. Krivit W, Shapiro E, Hoogerbrugge PM, Moser HW. Bone marrow transplantation treatment for storage diseases. Bone Marrow Transplant 1993; 11(suppl):87–101.
62. Karlsson S. Treatment of genetic defects in hematopoietic cell function by gene transfer. Blood 1991; 78:2481–2492.
63. Beutler E. Gaucher disease as a paradigm of current issues regarding single gene mutations of humans. Proc Natl Acad Sci USA 1993; 90:5384–5390.
64. Correll PH, Fink JK, Brady RO, et al. Production of human glucocerebrosidase in mice after retroviral gene transfer into multipotential hematopoietic progenitor cells. Proc Natl Acad Sci USA 1989; 86:8912–8916.
65. Krall WJ, Challita PM, Perlmutter LS, et al. Cells expressing human glucocerebrosidase from a retroviral vector repopulate macrophages and central nervous system microglia after murine bone marrow transplantation. Blood 1994; 83:2737–2748.
66. Xu L, Stahl SK, Dave HP, et al. Correction of the enzyme deficiency in hematopoietic cells of Gaucher patients using a clinically acceptable retroviral supernatant transduction protocol. Exp Hematol 1994; 22:223–230.
67. Walsh CE, Grompe M, Vanin E, et al. A functionally active retrovirus vector for gene therapy in Fanconi anemia group C. Blood 1994; 84:453–459.
68. Weiden PL, Flournoy N, Thomas ED, et al. Antileukemic effect of graft-versus-host

disease in human recipients of allogeneic-marrow grafts. N Engl J Med 1979; 300:1068–1073.

69. Goldman JM, Gale RP, Horowitz MM, et al. Bone marrow transplantation for chronic myelogenous leukemia in chronic phase: Increased risk for relapse associated with T-cell depletion. Ann Intern Med 1988; 108:806–814.
70. Kolb HJ, Mittermuller J, Clemm C, et al. Donor leukocyte transfusions for treatment of recurrent chronic myelogenous leukemia in marrow transplant patients. Blood 1990; 76:2462–2465.
71. van Rhee F, Lin F, Cullis JO, et al. Relapse of chronic myeloid leukemia after allogeneic bone marrow transplant: The case for giving donor leukocyte transfusions before the onset of hematologic relapse. Blood 1994; 83:3377–3383.
72. Papadopoulos EB, Ladanyi M, Emanuel D, et al. Infusions of donor leukocytes to treat Epstein-Barr virus–associated lymphoproliferative disorders after allogeneic bone marrow transplantation. N Engl J Med 1994; 330:1185–1191.
73. Heslop HE, Brenner MK, Rooney CM. Donor T cells to treat EBV-associated lymphoma. N Engl J Med 1994; 331:679–680.
74. Brenner MK, Heslop HE. Graft-versus-host reactions and bone marrow transplantation. Curr Opin Immunol 1991; 3:752–757.
75. Melief CJ, Kast WM. Potential immunogenicity of oncogene and tumor suppressor gene products. Curr Opin Immunol 1993; 5:709–713.
76. Burrows SR, Khanna R, Burrows JM, Moss DJ. An alloresponse in humans is dominated by cytotoxic T lymphocytes (CTL) cross-reactive with a single Epstein-Barr virus CTL epitope: Implications for graft-versus-host disease. J Exp Med 1994; 179:1155–1161.
77. Servida P, Rossini S, Traversari C, et al. Gene transfer into peripheral blood lymphocytes for in vivo immunomodulation of donor anti-tumor immunity in a patient affected by EBV-induced lymphoma. Blood 1993; 10(suppl 1):214a.
78. Kasid A, Morecki S, Aebersold P, et al. Human gene transfer: Characterization of human tumor infiltrating lymphocytes as vehicles for retroviral-mediated gene transfer in man. Proc Natl Acad Sci USA 1990; 87:473–477.
79. Riddell SR, Greenberg PD, Overall RW, et al. Phase I study of cellular adoptive immunotherapy using genetically modified CD8$^+$ HIV-specific T cells for HIV seropositive patients undergoing allogeneic bone marrow transplant. Hum Gene Ther 1992; 3: 319–338.
80. Tiberghien P, Reynolds CW, Keller J, et al. Ganciclovir treatment of herpes simplex thymidine kinase-transduced primary T lymphocytes: An approach for specific in vivo donor T-cell depletion after bone marrow transplantation? Blood 1994; 84:1333–1341.
81. Heslop HE, Brenner MK, Rooney CM, et al. Administration of neomycin-resistance-gene-marked EBV-specific cytotoxic T lymphocytes to recipients of mismatched-related or phenotypically similar unrelated donor marrow grafts. Hum Gene Ther 1994; 5:381–397.
82. Riddell SR, Watanabe KS, Goodrich JM, et al. Restoration of viral immunity in immunodeficient humans by the adoptive transfer of T cell clones. Science 1992; 257:238–241.
83. Rooney CM, Smith CA, Ng C, et al. Use of virus-specific cytotoxic T lymphocytes to control Epstein-Barr virus–related lymphoproliferation. Lancet 1995; 345, 9–13.
84. Chen L, Ashe S, Brady WA, et al. Costimulation of antitumor immunity by the B7 counterreceptor for the T lymphocyte molecules CD28 and CTLA-4. Cell 1992; 71: 1093–1102.
85. Townsend SE, Allison JP. Tumor rejection after direct costimulation of CD8$^+$ T cells by B7-transfected melanoma cells. Science 1993; 259:368–370.
86. Baskar S, Ostrand-Rosenberg S, Nabavi N, et al. Constitutive expression of B7 restores

immunogenicity of tumor cells expressing truncated major histocompatibility complex class II molecules. Proc Natl Acad Sci USA 1993; 90:5687–5690.

87. Colombo MP, Forni G. Cytokine gene transfer in tumor inhibition and tumor therapy: Where are we now? Immunol Today 1994; 15:48–51.
88. Pardoll DM. New strategies for engineering the immunogenicity of tumors. Curr Opin Immunol 1993; 5:719–725.
89. Greenberg P, Gilbert M, Nelson B, Riddell S. Adoptive therapy of infectious diseases in immunocompromised hosts by adoptive transfer of gene-modified T cell clones (abstr). Cancer Gene Ther 1994; 1:144.
90. Eshhar Z, Waks T, Gross G, Schindler DG. Specific activation and targeting of cytotoxic lymphocytes through chimeric single chains consisting of antibody-binding domains and the gamma or zeta subunits of the immunoglobulin and T-cell receptors. Proc Natl Acad Sci USA 1993; 90:720–724.
91. Hwu P, Shafer GE, Treisman J, et al. Lysis of ovarian cancer cells by human lymphocytes redirected with a chimeric gene composed of an antibody variable region and the Fc receptor gamma chain. J Exp Med 1993; 178:361–366.

30

Recent Advances and Future Directions

James L. M. Ferrara, Werner Krenger, Kenneth R. Cooke, and Lu Ying Pan
Dana–Farber Cancer Institute and Children's Hospital, Boston, Massachusetts

Bruce R. Blazar
University of Minnesota, Minneapolis, Minnesota

Robert Korngold and Robert M. Townsend
Kimmel Cancer Institute, Jefferson Medical College, Philadelphia, Pennsylvania

Robert B. Levy and Matthew Baker
University of Miami School of Medicine, Miami, Florida

Megan Sykes, Bimalangshu Dey, and Yong-Guang Yang
Massachusetts General Hospital, Boston, Massachusetts

Nelson J. Chao
Stanford University Medical Center, Stanford, California

H. Joachim Deeg and Effie Petersdorf
Fred Hutchinson Research Center, Seattle, Washington

Olle Ringdén
Karolinska Institute, Huddinge Hospital, Stockholm, Sweden

Ernst Holler
Klinikum Grosshadern der Universitat, Munich, Germany

Helen E. Heslop
St. Jude Children's Research Hospital and University of Tennessee, Memphis, Tennessee

Dietger Niederwieser
University Hospital, Innsbruck, Austria

George Murphy
University of Pennsylvania School of Medicine, Philadelphia, Pennsylvania

James M. Crawford
Brigham and Women's Hospital, Boston, Massachusetts

I. INTRODUCTION

The final chapter of this book has been compiled with the intention of bringing together the most recent advances and perspectives in our understanding of graft-versus-host disease (GVHD). First, there is a discussion of modulation of T-cell function by diverse strategies and the effects of such modulation in mouse models of GVHD. Studies involving the blockade of B7/CD28 costimulatory pathways are summarized, with perspectives for generation of antigen-specific tolerance. A different activation pathway is blocked by a peptide that mimics the three-dimensional configuration of a critical epitope on the CD4 molecule: it binds a public domain of MHC class II molecules thereby preventing T-cell activation; the next three summaries document advances that have been made in the manipulation of cytokines in GVHD. The first strategy is to polarize T cells toward type 2 responses (reviewed in Chapter 17), which can prevent acute GVHD but which does not inhibit all reactivity to host antigens, thus preserving a GVL effect. A second method involves the surprising effects of G-CSF on donor T cells, a partial polarization toward type 2 responses that is accompanied by a diminution in GVHD when G-CSF-mobilized progenitor cells are transplanted. Next is a review of IL-12 administration to recipients for the reduction of GVHD and the preservation of a GVL effect, again surprising because of the induction of INF-γ by IL-12 in vitro. This section concludes with a summary of important observations regarding the contributing of perforin- and Fas-mediated cytotoxicity to GVHD.

The third section focuses on advances in GVHD target organ pathophysiology. The elucidation of nitric-oxide-dependent and independent pathways of immunosuppression during GVHD, the apoptotic nature of keratinocyte death, advances in cytotoxic-mediated hepatic damage, and a quantitative examination of idiopathic pneumonitis in a murine model are all summarized. The role of endotoxin in pneumonitis has generated a hypothesis of a "gut-liver-lung" axis in GVHD similar to what has been observed in sepsis.

The chapter concludes with important recent observations that have been made in clinical bone marrow transplantation (BMT). Risk factors that predict for clinical GVHD, including cytokine release and cross-regulation during the conditioning regimen, are summarized from recent studies. Although the relevance of HLA-C typing as a risk factor for GVHD is not yet known, its identification as a factor in graft rejection is now recognized. Next is an overview from several studies confirming the relationship between clinical GVHD and graft-versus-leukemia effects, including the first reports of allogeneic BMT as successful (immuno)therapy for multiple myeloma and for breast cancer. The surprising and disappointing results of a randomized trial of thalidomide as prophylaxis for chronic GVHD are also included. A final contribution summarizes steady progress in the field of gene therapy, with strategies both to control T cells responsible for GVHD and to eventually eliminate the need for allogeneic transplantation in certain genetic diseases.

II. MODULATION OF THE DONOR T-CELL FUNCTION

A. Blockade of CD28/B7 Costimulation in GVHD

While rigorous in vitro T-cell depletion approaches can reduce the incidence and severity of GVHD by limiting the number of donor T cells available for expansion,

T cells may also mediate such beneficial effects as the facilitation of alloengraftment, improved antiviral immune responses, and antileukemia effects. Because few (<0.1% by limiting-dilution analysis) donor T cells have antihost specificities, an alternative approach would be to deplete selectively or to alter functionally the host-specific donor T cells that initiate GVHD.

Antigen-specific T-cell proliferation requires two distinct signals (reviewed in Chapter 4). The first signal is provided by antigen or peptide binding to the antigen-specific TCR, which sets off a cascade of signaling events culminating in cytokine mRNA transcription and subsequent translation. The continued production of cytokines is a prerequisite for T-cell proliferation. A second or costimulatory signal, typically provided by antigen-presenting cells, (APCs), stabilizes cytokine mRNA, thereby ensuring ongoing T-cell expansion. In the absence of costimulation, T cells are unable to enter a highly proliferative phase but instead become specifically nonresponsive to initial antigen or peptide presented to the TCR (1–3). Strategies that preclude effective T-cell costimulation may thus render donor T cells specifically nonresponsive to host antigens/peptides, especially in the early post-BMT period when cell surface proteins involved in T-cell costimulation are abundantly expressed during a period of intense tissue inflammation.

Although a number of cell surface determinants situated on APC have now been identified that fulfill the definition of costimulatory molecules, arguably the best studied to date are members of the CD28/B7 family (see Chapter 4). Using a soluble fusion protein termed CTLA4-Ig that consists of the extracellular domain of CTLA4 (a B7 counter receptor) and an immunoglobulin moiety that prolongs its half-life, Linsley and his collaborators demonstrated that in vitro and in vivo responses to foreign antigens were specifically diminished during CTLA4-Ig exposure (4,5). Blazar et al. and Wallace et al. (6,7) independently demonstrated that the in vivo infusion of large quantities of CTLA4-Ig for a period of up to 1 month post-BMT could lead to a reduction in GVHD lethality induced by fully or semiallogeneic donor T cells in heavily irradiated recipients. Although the GVHD lethality was reduced in these studies, both the clinical and subclinical manifestations of GVHD were not ameliorated.

In a canine model of DLA nonidentical unrelated marrow transplantation, CTLA4-Ig, when given by itself immediately after transplantation, interfered with engraftment. However, when dogs were given a standard regimen of methotrexate and cyclosporin immediately after transplant and CTLA4-Ig administration was begun on day +7, dogs achieved engraftment, and the development of GVHD was prevented in about 50% of dogs and 6/11 dogs are surviving (R. Storb, personal communication).

Why was GVHD lethality not completely prevented? One possibility is that a subset of donor T cells "escaped" CTLA4-Ig mediated inhibition. Apparently, some T cells (e.g., a subset of mature CD8+ T cells) do not require CD28/B7 costimulation. Costimulation also appears to be less essential when APC are not limited in number. Blazar and colleagues have observed that both CD4+ and CD8+ alloreactive T cells are at least partially susceptible to interference with CD28/B7 interaction (6).

Another possibility is that the CD28/B7 interaction was inadequately inhibited by CTLA4-Ig. In that regard, most investigators have typically reported results with human CTLA4-Ig (which does bind to mouse B7). However, because of disassociation rates and clearance, it is possible that murine CTLA4-Ig might have better efficacy than human CTLA4-Ig. Data by Linsley and colleagues suggest that the murine protein is superior to the human protein for mouse GVHD experiments, although it should be noted that murine CTLA4-Ig infusions were not completely effective in preventing lethality. Data in a different model system also do not support the hypothesis that the rate-limiting factor in preventing GVHD is species specificity (6). Recently, an in vivo infusion of large amounts of monoclonal antibodies directed against two murine B7 ligands (B7.1, B7.2), which also bind CTLA4-Ig with high affinity, was able to virtually eliminate GVHD mortality caused by a uniformly lethal dose of CD4+ or CD8+ T cells given to lightly irradiated MHC class II or I only disparate recipients (B. R. Blazar, unpublished data). Since direct comparison studies of anti-B7 antibodies to murine CTLA4-Ig have not been reported, no conclusions as to the relative efficacy of anti-B7 monoclonal antibodies versus fusion protein can yet be made.

An additional reason for the incomplete GVHD protection by CTLA4-Ig may relate to the fact that there are other pathways of T-cell activation. For example, proinflammatory and immunomodulatory cytokines released from damaged fibroblasts and stromal cells (e.g., IL-1 and IL-7) may serve as competence factors for T-cell proliferation and thereby create conditions where tolerance induction is prevented or even reversed. Moreover, a number of other pathways (e.g., CD40 ligand: CD40) exist that can provide T-cell costimulation, as discussed in Chapter 4. Therefore, even if the CD28/B7 pathway is limiting, sufficient expression of other molecules involved in costimulation may bypass the requirement for CD28/B7. Blockade of two or more pathways capable of conferring costimulatory signals may therefore be advantageous in the production of antigen-specific tolerance.

The expression of many cell surface properties occurs only under activation conditions (e.g., after chemoradiotherapy damage), and this regulated expression may make the blockade of the requisite costimulatory pathways in vivo considerably more difficult. In that regard, Hakim et al. have shown that CTLA4-Ig virtually abolished donor T-cell expansion in a system in which parental cells are infused into nonirradiated recipients (8). From this perspective, an alternative approach is to tolerize donor T cells to host alloantigens in vitro prior to infusion into conditioned recipients. An advantage to this approach is the possibility of specific inhibition of only those donor T cells capable of responding to normal, host alloantigenic stimulators, thereby avoiding tolerization to leukemia-specific antigens that would be expressed in vivo. Another advantage is the fact that an entirely in vitro approach precludes the possibility of in vivo side effects from injection of the tolerizing agents. Tolerization of human T cells to MHC identical or disparate host stimulators in vitro has been reported by several groups by blocking CD28/B7 interactions with CTLA4-Ig or anti-B7 antibodies (9–11).

Blazar and colleagues have recently attempted to render donor T cells specifically nonresponsive to host alloantigens by CD28/B7 blockade in vitro. Using a 3-4-day MLR culture of donor splenocytes and irradiated fully allogeneic host stimulator cells, the donor antihost response was markedly inhibited by incubation with CTLA4-Ig (12). However, the infusion of these manipulated donor cells did not alleviate GVHD lethality. A more profound degree of inhibition was observed when CTLA4-Ig was combined with blockade of the LFA1 : ICAM pathway (12). Unfortunately, GVHD lethality was once again not changed. Explanations for these findings, in addition to those described above, include the possibility that tolerance induction was incomplete, that each relevant histocompatibility antigen was either not sufficiently expressed on host stimulator cells or was expressed only in a tissue-specific fashion in vivo, or that only a subclass of T cells with the highest TCR affinity for host antigens was tolerized. Nontolerized cells with low affinities for host histocompatibility antigens may be expandable in vivo under conditions where APC are abundant, alloantigen density is high, and cytokines can act to costimulate T cells. Additional experiments were therefore performed in which both CTLA4-Ig and anti-LFA-1 antibody were infused in vivo after the in vitro tolerization period. With this combined approach, GVHD lethality was significantly reduced. Importantly, long-term chimeras were not globally immunosuppressed as measured by in vitro T-cell proliferative responses to third-party alloantigens (12).

In conclusion, there are several reasons to pursue the prevention of the morbidity and mortality of GVHD by specifically and selectively inhibiting donor antihost alloreactivity. The conceptual advantage of a selective, functional depletion over pan-T-cell or even T-cell subset depletion is that the remaining 99.9% or more of the donor T cells that do not efficiently bind host antigens/peptides should remain functionally intact. Much work needs to be done to determine whether antigen-specific nonresponsiveness is obtainable in vitro and whether it can be translated into a reduction of GVHD in vivo. If this is successful, additional experiments will need to address the potential impact of tolerance induction on alloengraftment, graft-versus-leukemia, and antiviral immune surveillance. Despite current obstacles, tolerance induction holds the promise of solving several critical issues that limit the efficacy of allogeneic BMT in humans.

B. GVHD Inhibition by CD4-CDR3 Peptide Analog

The CD4 molecule on helper T cells interacts with nonpolymorphic sites on MHC class II molecules and thereby increases the stability of the T-cell-receptor-complex recognition of specific antigen presented by those MHC class II molecules (see Chapter 3 and Refs. 13–15). In addition to those adhesion properties, CD4 plays a critical role in signaling pathways required for T-cell activation (16–18). It has been well established in murine models that CD4+ T cells alone are capable of mediating GVHD, across both MHC class II (19,20) and some minor histocompatibility barriers (21,22). Treatment of mice with monoclonal antibodies (MAb) directed against CD4 has effectively decreased the incidence of GVHD following BMT (23–25). However, MAb therapy has several limitations for potential clinical use, including but not limited to immunogenicity of the MAb and total subset depletion (26–28).

Jameson et al. and McDonnell et al. (29,30) have previously described the design and production of a peptide that specifically mimics a portion of the CDR3-like region in domain 1 of the murine CD4 molecule (rD-mPGPtide). The rD-mPGPtide is neither immunogenic nor T-cell-subset depletive and appears to affect only activated T cells. Experimental results have indicated that rD-mPGPtide is a potent inhibitor of CD4+ T-cell-mediated immune responses, both in vitro and in vivo (29). Townsend and Korngold have recently investigated whether the rD-mPGPtide could also inhibit the in vivo alloreactive responses associated with the onset of GVHD in a MHC-haploidentical murine BMT model (B6 × DBA/2)F_1 → (B6 × CBA)F_1(950 cGy). Injection of irradiated (B6 × CBA)F_1 mice with a donor T-cell-depleted bone marrow (ATBM) innoculum supplemented with 5 × 10^6 unseparated T cells exhibited 90% fatality by day 20 post-BMT with a MST of 10 days (Table 1). Treatment of mice with 0.5 mg rD-mPGPtide given i.v. every third day (days 0, 3, 6) significantly increased the MST to 28 days ($p = 0.005$), but was unable to produce any long-term survivors. Because the donor and recipient mice differ at both class I and class II MHC loci, both CD8+ and CD4+ T cells were likely to play a role in the development of GVHD. It has previously been established that CD4-independent CD8+ T cells are capable of mediating GVHD across a MHC class I barrier (20). The rD-mPGPtide would therefore be expected to have limited effect against the CD8+ T-cell-mediated component of GVHD.

To evaluate the effect of rD-mPGPtide specifically on CD4+ T cells during induction of GVHD, an acute form of the disease was induced by administration of 1×10^6 donor CD4+ T cells along with donor ATBM. The MST for those mice left untreated was 13 days, as shown in Table 1. Mice treated with 0.5 mg rD-mPGPtide on days 0, 3, 6 exhibited a dramatic increase in the MST to greater than 60 days ($p < 0.001$). Seventy percent of the mice treated with rD-mPGPtide survived for the duration of the experiment (60 days), as compared to 14% of the untreated GVHD mice and 85% of the control mice transplanted with only ATBM ($p < 0.001$). A single injection of rD-mPGPtide on day 0 resulted in the same increase in the MST with 70% of the mice surviving past 60 days. A control scrambled peptide (Scr-PGPtide), which is composed of the same amino acids but in a different sequence, was also tested to demonstrate the specificity of the rD-mPGPtide. This control peptide did not significantly affect survival as compared to the untreated mice, with only 30% surviving past 60 days. The rD-mPGPtide was therefore able to prevent GVHD induced by purified CD4+ T cells even though it was much less effective in preventing GVHD from unseparated donor T cells.

Table 1 Effect of rD-mPGPtide on Lethal GVHD Across MHC Barriers $(B6xD2)F_1 \rightarrow (B6CB)F_1$

		60-day Mortality			
Donor cells[a]	Treatment[b]	*n*	% Survival	MST Days	*p* value[c]
Experiment 1					
$(B6xD2)F_1$ ATBM	Untreated	10	90	>60	<0.001
$(B6xD2)F_1$ ATBM + T cells	Untreated	11	0	10	1.00
$(B6xD2)F_1$ ATBM + T cells	rD-mPGPtide Days 0,3,6	10	0	28	0.005
Experiment 2					
$(B6xD2)F_1$ ATMB		20	85	>60	<0.001
$(B6xD2)F_1$ ATMB + CD4	Untreated	21	14	13	1.000
$(B6xD2)F_1$ ATMB + CD4	rD-mPGPtide Days 0,3,6	20	70	>60	<0.001
$(B6xD2)F_1$ ATMB + CD4	rD-mPGPtide Day 0	10	70	>60	0.005
$(B6xD2)F_1$ ATMB + CD4	Scr-PGPtide Days 0,3,6	10	30	12	>0.040

[a]Donor $(B6xD2)F_1$ T-cell-depleted bone marrow (2×10^6) along with either 5×10^6 T-cells or 1×10^6 CD4+ T cells isolated from the spleens and lymph nodes of donor mice were injected i.v. as indicated into $(B6xD2)F_1$ (950 cGy) recipient mice 4–6 hr after irradiation.

[b]Mice were injected i.v. with 0.5 mg/mouse of peptide as indicated.

[c]Statistical comparisons between experimental groups were performed by the nonparametic Wilcoxon signed rank analysis, utilizing SYSTAT 5.2 software.

Treatment of donors with rD-mPGPtide most likely renders antihost-specific T cells dysfunctional in their ability to respond to alloantigen. This hypothesis is supported by several observations, including the reduction of specific in vitro alloreactivity to host antigens and reduced expression of activation antigens by positively selected T cells collected (4 days posttransplant) from the thoracic duct of mice treated with rD-mPGPtide (data not shown). This reduced proliferative capacity could be due to either deletion and/or inhibition of T-cell expansion. Several recent reports propose that alterations in the immune response can be induced that generate a protective effect against various immunologically based disorders. These mechanisms include inhibition of T-cell trafficking to target organs (31–34), a polarization in cytokine production from Th1 to Th2 phenotypes (35,36), potentiation of other specific cytokines (e.g., TGF-β) (37,38), or the generation of nonlethal regulatory cells in vivo (39,40).

Preliminary data indicate that the half-life retention of peptide in serum in mice is roughly 30 min; responsiveness to any type of antigen is significantly inhibited for up to 6 hr after administration, but is almost completely restored by 12 hr. It is therefore possible that administration of peptide only during the first week after transplant could leave the remaining non-host-reactive CD4+ T-cell population intact for subsequent development of responses to opportunistic infections or to counteract potential leukemic relapse. Investigations are ongoing to ascertain the precise mechanism by which the peptide regulates T-cell responses and to determine whether GVHD can be prevented while preserving other beneficial elements of T-cell function.

C. Polarization of T-Cell Function by IL-4 In Vitro

Krenger and colleagues have recently demonstrated that long-term survival of transplanted hosts is substantially improved after infusion of allogeneic bone marrow (minor HA mismatched) together with donor T cells that had been polarized toward a type 2 cytokine phenotype prior to BMT (41). Decreased mortality was associated with decreased weight loss (Fig. 1) and also with decreased LPS-induced TNF-α secretion by 2 weeks post BMT. These data are consistent with the observations that the induction of a systemic inflammatory response (e.g., TNF-α) early after allogeneic BMT mediates GVHD both experimentally (36,42) and clinically (43–46).

This study confirms and extends an earlier report that demonstrated that infusion of MHC-disparate, polarized type 2 T cells downregulates IFN-γ and TNF-α secretion in transplanted mice (36). Type 1 and type 2 cytokines are known to have antagonistic effects on the activation and function of monoclonal phagocytes (see Chapter 7). The data in this study suggest that changes in donor T-cell number and function most likely contribute to the reduction in TNF-α secretion to LPS and the subsequent improved survival. The CD8+ cell subset is the dominant cell type responsible for alloreactivity to minor H antigens in this and other GVHD models (reviewed in Ref. 47), and it is well established that murine CD8+ cells as well as CD4+ T cells can acquire a type 2 cytokine profile (48–51). Examination of T-cell subsets in this BMT model, however, revealed that T-cell populations were not polarized into "classic" type 1 or type 2 cytokine phenotypes at 2 weeks post BMT. Intermediate cytokine profiles of both CD8+ and CD4+ T-cell subsets appear to

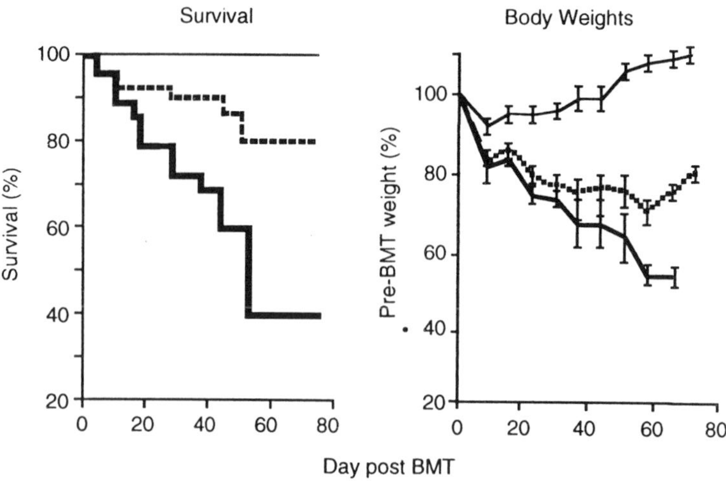

Figure 1 Reduction of systemic GVHD by polarized type 2 donor T cells. Irradiated (1100 cGy) CBA mice were transplanted with 5 × 10^6 bone marrow and 1 × 10^6 naive (▬) or polarized type 2 T cells (----) from B10.BR mice. Control mice received bone marrow only (——). (Apapted from Ref. 41.)

have developed similar to the emergence of incompletely polarized T-cell populations in other systems (52). The overall decrease of IFN-γ secretion appeared to be due to a combination of decreased numbers of CD8+ cells and less IFN-γ production by CD4+ T cells. These observations are consistent with a recent study documenting the differential changes in cytokine profiles among CD4+ cells that have been stimulated under sequential and opposite polarizing conditions (53).

This study also demonstrates that although systemic GVHD is substantially decreased, clinical signs of GVHD are still present in surviving mice and target organ pathology persists after infusion with type 2 donor T cells (Fig. 2). This dichotomy may be explained by distinct downstream effector mechanisms induced by T cells which secrete different cytokine patterns. Because systemic GVHD (mortality, weight loss) may be a direct cause of increased systemic inflammation mediated by TNF-α, the infusion of polarized type 2 donor T cells may decrease mortality by virtue of its inhibitory effect on inflammatory cytokine secretion. On the other hand, the effector mechanisms that directly lead to tissue damage may not be affected by type 2 cytokines or may even be enhanced. IL-4 is vigorously secreted by mitogen-activated splenocytes isolated 7 weeks post BMT from mice receiving type 2, but not type 1, donor T cells (W. Krenger and J. L. M. Ferrara, unpublished data). Since it has been suggested that IL-4 can amplify CTL responses (54,55), exposure to IL-4 after BMT may be important in the enhancement of cytotoxic activity after BMT, which has been linked to destruction of GVHD target tissues (56–58). Moreover, IL-4 has strong proinflammatory activities in other in vitro systems (59,60). It is therefore possible that IL-4 secreted by infused type 2 T cells contributes to the inflammatory lesions of transplanted animals.

The fact that donor-T-cell reactivity to minor H antigens is not eliminated suggests that beneficial consequences of T-cell alloreactivity, such as engraftment

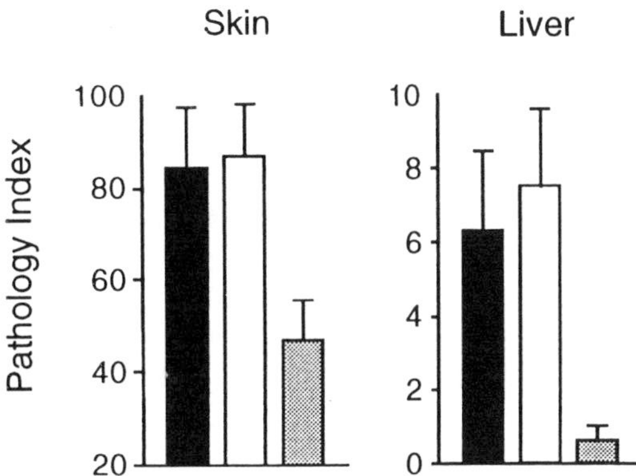

Figure 2 Semiquantitative analysis of tissue pathology 7 weeks post BMT. CBA recipient mice were transplanted with cells from B10.BR donor mice as in Figure 1 (■, naïve T cells; □, polarized type 2 T cells; ▨, no T cells). The skin index represents the total number of lymphocytes per high-powered field in oral mucosa (average of four to five fields); the liver index is the sum of the hepatic pathological score for 14 separate parameters as previously described (174). (Adpated from Ref. 41.)

and graft-versus-leukemic effects (61–63), may also be preserved with the transplantation of type 2 cells. This question has recently been examined in a murine BMT model across a single MHC class I difference (Krenger et al., manuscript in preparation). B6 mice were injected with 500 EL-4 host-type (H-2^b) tumor cells together with T-cell-depleted bone marrow (5×10^6) containing 2×10^5 naïve or type 2 T cells from donor bm1 mice. Figure 3A shows that mice receiving tumor cells but no T cells all died within 2 weeks after transplantation. In contrast, the inclusion of donor T cells (naïve or polarized) in the inoculum conferred partial protection from mortality. Recipients of polarized cells had little GVHD, with greater than 80% survival at day 70, whereas the majority of recipients of naïve T cells died of their GVHD. Polarized type 2 donor T cells thus were able to mediate an antitumor effect in vivo after allogeneic BMT as well as provide protection against the development of acute GVHD. Antileukemic efficacy of donor lymphocytes was also tested in an in vitro CTL assay (Fig. 3B). Polarized type 2 T cells lysed EL-4 tumor target cells with a comparable efficiency to polarized type 1 T cells. These encouraging data are consistent with the recent demonstration that subsets of IL-4-producing CD8+ T cells can maintain cytotoxic activity (64). Finally, it will be of interest to determine whether the infusion of type 2 donor T cells results in the development of a "chronic" GVHD syndrome, characterized by induction of type 2 cytokines and IgE secretion (65–69). Whether long-term survival can be significantly improved by such approaches, in the absence of histopathological evidence of GVHD after allogeneic BMT, remains to be determined.

D. G-CSF Mobilization of Donor PBPC

An unexpected dimension of cytokine networks has recently been observed with administration of G-CSF to donors that resulted in a long-lasting polarization of T-cell function toward an anti-inflammatory type 2 cytokine response; this polarization was associated with a reduction in the severity of acute GVHD after transplantation of G-CSF-mobilized peripheral blood progenitor cells (PBPC) into allogeneic recipients in an experimental model of GVHD to both minor H and MHC antigen (70) (Figure 4).

These results were surprising because G-CSF receptors are rarely detectable on T cells (71,72). G-CSF administration has been observed to temporarily increase the number of T lymphocytes in humans without significantly changing the ratio of CD4+/CD8+ cells (73). In the study by Pan et al., however, no change in splenic T-cell number or phenotype was observed after administration of G-CSF, including the expression of CD3, CD25 (IL-2 receptor, α chain), and CD69 (a very early activation antigen). G-CSF treatment therefore does not appear to alter the activation status of T cells in vivo.

It has been reported that the cytokine profile of a T-cell population can shift toward either type 1 or type 2 response depending on the type of stimulation and on the local microenvironment (49,52,74–76). Unseparated T cells and CD4+ and CD8+ T-cell subsets obtained from G-CSF-treated mice showed a persistent polarization toward type 2 cytokine production during both primary and secondary stimulation in vitro. Such polarization occurred despite the absence of G-CSF in the culture media. Although IL-4 production was below the limit of detection during primary stimulation, a marked increase of IL-4 production was observed during secondary stimulation, particularly by CD4+ T cells (70).

The anti-inflammatory effects of G-CSF have been well documented (71,72,77). G-CSF has been shown to enhance anti-inflammatory function of effector cells by increasing expression of CR1, CR3, and FcγRIII on monocytes (78,79). The cascade of inflammatory cytokines produced by these effector cells may also be regulated by G-CSF. In a murine model of sepsis induced by endotoxin, G-CSF administration suppressed serum TNF-α concentrations and TNF-α release by macrophages on ex vivo LPS challenge (79). Injection of G-CSF into normal volunteers also affected their monocyte responses to LPS challenge by upregulating two important cytokine antagonists, soluble TNF receptor and IL-1 receptor antagonist (80). Such antagonists have been shown to be important in reducing the severity of GVHD, both in experimental models and in clinical trials (see Chapter 25). Thus, modulation of cytokine production from both T cells and monocytes by G-CSF may help to explain the low incidence of clinical GVHD observed after transplantation of G-CSF-mobilized PBPCs (81–87).

E. IL-12 Effects on GVHD and GVL

IL-12 is a potent immunostimulatory cytokine that induces Th1 activity and enhances CTL and NK cell function (88–92) (see Chapter 7). Paradoxically, administration of a single injection of 4900 IU of recombinant murine IL-12 inhibits acute GVHD in lethally irradiated mice receiving fully MHC plus multiple HA antigen-mismatched bone marrow transplants (93) (Fig. 5). Even more marked protection has been observed in a haploidentical, full haplotype-mismatched strain combination (94). The protective effect of IL-12 is enhanced by administration of T cell-depleted host-type bone marrow cells. The host-type marrow is rapidly destroyed, however, and complete lymphohematopoietic reconstitution by donor cells is observed within approximately 1 week following transplantation (93).

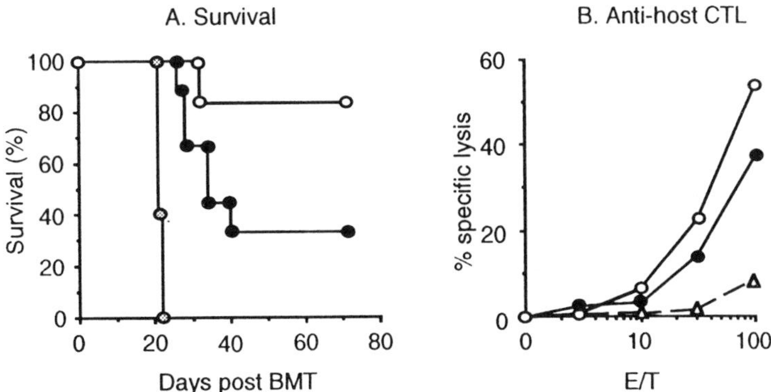

Figure 3 Graft-versus-leukemia activity of polarized type 2 donor T cells. (A): B6 recipients (H-2^b) were transplanted with T-cell depleted bone marrow (5×10^6 cells) and T cells (2×10^6) from bm 1 donor mice (●, naïve T cells; ○, polarized type 2 T cells; ⊘, no T cells). Survival was monitored for 75 days after BMT. (B): In vitro cytotoxic T lymphocyte (CTL) activity of polarized T cells. Responder bm 1 T cells were primed for 7 days with IL-2 alone (●) or in the presence of IL-2 and IL-4 (○). CTL activity of primed T cells was measured using tumor targets EL-4 (H-2^b) at different effector to target (E/T) ratios. An irrelevant tumor cell line (P815; H-2^d) was used (△) as a control.

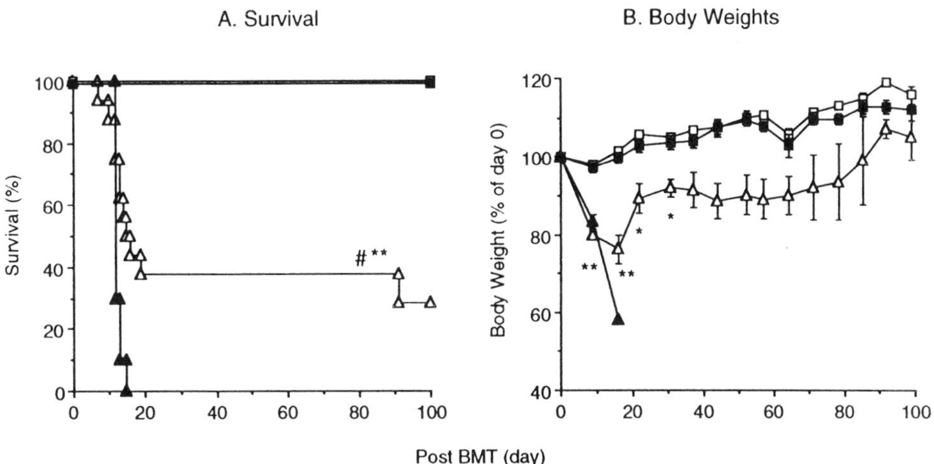

Figure 4 Survival and weight loss after allogeneic transplant of splenocytes from G-CSF or diluent-treated donors (B6 → $B6D2F_1$). B6 donors were injected with diluent or G-CSF for 6 days. Total-body-irradiated $B6D2F_1$ recipients received 5×10^6 splenocytes from G-CSF (△, $n = 16$) or diluent (▲, $n = 10$) treated donors, or 5×10^6 TCD splenocytes from G-CSF (■, $n = 10$) or diluent (□, $n = 10$) treated donors. Survival (A) and body weights (B) were measured to day 100 after BMT. The results represent mean ± SEM from two experiments. #$p < 0.0001$ versus recipients of diluent-treated donor splenocytes. **$p < 0.0001$, *$p < 0.02$ versus recipients transplanted with TCD splenocytes from either G-CSF or diluent treated donors.

The mechanism of IL-12-induced GVHD protection is currently being investigated. This treatment leads to increased serum IFN-γ levels compared to GVHD controls in the first 3 days post BMT. A large portion of this IFN-γ burst induced by IL-12 is produced by host-type NK cells. However, this pattern is reversed by day 4 or 5 post BMT, when a GVHD-associated increase in serum IFN-γ levels, produced predominantly by CD4+ cells, is observed in control mice. This increase is markedly inhibited in IL-12-protected mice (93). The early induction of IFN-γ by IL-12 appears to be critical to its protective effect against GVHD, because early administration of a high dose of neutralizing anti-IFN-γ antibody eliminates the protective effect of IL-12 (94).

IL-12 treatment induces marked alterations in the kinetics of donor T-cell expansion in GVHD. Reductions in donor CD4+ and CD8+ T cells are observed in the spleens of IL-12-protected compared to GVHD control mice on day 4 post BMT, when there is a marked inhibition of expression of the CD25 (IL-2 R α chain) and VLA-4 activation markers on donor T cells. CD25 is never markedly upregulated on T cells of IL-12 mice, but VLA-4 expression is increased to a similar extent as that observed for GVHD controls by day 7 (94), when a marked increase in donor CD8+ cells is also observed (93). It seems likely that this altered pattern of T-cell activation and suppressed early expansion of donor T cells is a manifestation of the protective effect of IL-12 against GVHD and may be related to the activation of host NK cells by IL-12. Studies are in progress to address this hypothesis.

Unlike broadly immunosuppressive methods for inhibiting GVHD, which are associated with loss of antileukemic efficacy, IL-12 has anti-tumor effects of its own (95–98), for which it is currently under clinical evaluation. This cytokine therefore has the potential to mediate antileukemic effects while inhibiting GVHD. We have begun to evaluate the GVL effect of donor T cells in IL-12-treated mice, using the EL4 $H\text{-}2^b$ leukemic/lymphoma model. Leukemic death was observed in all syngeneic BMT recipients of EL4, even if IL-12 treatment was given, with median survival times of 18–24 days. Allogeneic spleen cells mediated a marked GVL effect in mice protected from GVHD by IL-12, resulting in median survival times of 50 to >100 days, with a cure of leukemia (>100-day survival and absence of leukemia in syngeneic secondary recipients of spleens from long-term survivors) in 44–78% of animals (94). The GVL effect of allogeneic spleen cells in IL-12-treated mice was dependent on donor CD8+ cells (94). Preliminary data support a role for IFN-γ in the GVL effect of donor T cells, in addition to its role in the anti-GVHD effect. CD4+ cells do not normally play a role in the GVL effect of allogeneic T cells against EL4 leukemia, and because IL-12 may act predominantly on alloreactive CD4+ cells, it will be of interest to evaluate GVL effects in leukemic models in which CD4+ cells also play a role in suppressing leukemic growth.

F. Distinct Roles of Perforin and Fas-Dependent Donor Antihost Cytotoxicity in Acute GVHD

Cell-mediated cytotoxicity has historically been considered an immune-mediated effector mechanism essential for the development of acute GVHD. For two decades, observations from both clinical and experimental studies that were consistent with a role for cytotoxicity in GVHD have been reported, including morphological evidence suggestive of apoptotic cell death as well as the identification of lytic molecules in affected tissue (99–102). Despite the attractiveness of this hypothesis, it has been difficult to establish a consistent correlation between the presence of antihost cytotoxicity and the occurrence of GVHD in both mice and humans (22,103–105).

The functional redundancy in immune cell populations makes it virtually impossible to determine precisely the contribution of any singular effector modality in GVHD—including cytotoxicity—using donor inoculum containing enriched cell populations. Moreover, the elimination of a cell population concomitantly removes its total functional capacity, further complicating assessment of any individual effector mechanism (103,105). Recent studies have identified the perforin and Fas-dependent cytotoxic pathways together as being responsible for the majority of short-term cell-mediated cytotoxicity (106,107). Therefore, the inability of genetically engineered and naturally occurring mutant mouse strains to mediate perforin and Fas- dependent cytotoxicity in allogeneic BMT models offers a new approach to investigate the role of cytotoxicity in GVHD. Utilizing this type of approach, several laboratories have recently begun to dissect the individual roles of these two cytotoxic pathways in mouse models of GVHD (108–112).

Levy and colleagues have transplanted lethal numbers of T cells from perforin-deficient (B6-Perforin-0/0), Fas ligand(L)-defective (B6-*gld*), or wild-type normal B6 (H-2^b) mice together with T-cell-depleted normal marrow into lethally irradiated MHC-matched allogeneic recipients to evaluate the ability of these cytotoxically impaired T cells to induce GVHD (Fig. 6). In contrast to recipients of normal or Fas L-defective T cells, in which weight loss ensued shortly following BMT, the recipients of perforin-deficient T cells always exhibited a significant delay in the onset of weight loss. Notably, the absence of perforin in the donor inoculum did

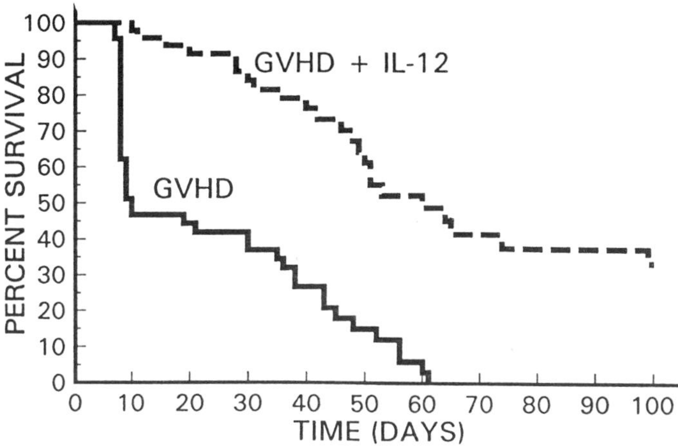

Figure 5 Delayed GVHD mortality in recipients of 4900 IU rmIL-12 on the day of BMT. Data are combined for six similar experiments ($n = 45$ GVHD control, 48 IL-12 treated; $p < 0.001$). Survival is shown for irradiated B10 (H-2^b) recipients of TCD B10 BMC plus A/J (H-2^a) BMC and spleen cells with no further treatment (——); or with IL-12 treatment (----).

Table 2 GVHD Histopathology After Allogeneic BMT as a Function of Donor Cytotoxic Capacity

Donor		Recipient	Skin	Liver
C3H.SW	→	C3H.SW	−	−
C57BL/6	→	C3H.SW	+ + +	+ + +
B6-PKO	→	C3H.SW	+ + +	+ + +
B6-*gld*	→	C3H.SW	±	±

The severity of GVHD histological lesions was graded as follows: −, unremarkable; ±, minimal; + +, moderate; + + +, severe.

not prevent the occurrence of mortality in these BMT recipients; however, the MST of these recipients was markedly increased. In contrast, the kinetics of mortality were not delayed in recipients on Fas L–defective T cells compared to recipients of normal B6 donor inoculum. Similar findings were previously observed in BMT across MHC class I and II disparities utilizing perforin-deficient donor inoculum (108). The results from these types of studies demonstrate that the presence of perforin-dependent cytotoxicity in the donor inoculum accelerated the kinetics of weight loss and mortality. Polymerization of perforin results in membrane lesions that enables access into the target cell cytoplasm by a number of granzymes (serine proteases) that contribute to target cell lysis. Consistent with the above findings, the use of granzyme B–deficient donors by Graubert and colleagues was found to result in prolonged recipient survival in acute GVHD models mediated by CD8+ but not CD4+ T cells after BMT across MHC class I or I and II disparities (110). Thus, non-perforin-dependent mechanisms are sufficient to induce weight loss and mortality following allogeneic BMT. Accordingly, increasing the numbers of transplanted perforin-deficient donor T cells results in kinetics equivalent to lower numbers of normal allogeneic donor T cells (111). Similarly, by decreasing the numbers of transplanted T cells, a number can be defined in which normal—but not perforin-deficient—T cells induce clinical GVHD (109).

The involvement of perforin and Fas L–mediated killing in the efferent phase of GVHD has been investigated by analyzing histopathological changes in target tissue (111). The tissues from mice that received normal allogeneic T cells exhibited alterations indicative of severe cutaneous and hepatic GVHD (Table 2). Recipients of perforin-deficient allogeneic T cells also ultimately exhibited severe GVHD in these target tissues that were virtually indistinguishable from the changes observed in the recipients of normal allogeneic T cells. In contrast, livers from recipients of Fas L–defective T cells were strikingly normal and the skin exhibited only minimal inflammation. The lack of cutaneous GVHD was consistent with the absence of clinically apparent desquamative dermatitis in recipients of Fas L–defective T cells (111). Thus severe hepatic and cutaneous GVHD occurred following transplant of T cells derived from normal or perforin-deficient allogeneic donors, which are capable of mediating Fas L–dependent donor and antihost cytotoxicity. In contrast, tissue damage was not observed following transplant of T cells derived from Fas L–defective allogeneic donors, which were capable of mediating perforin-dependent

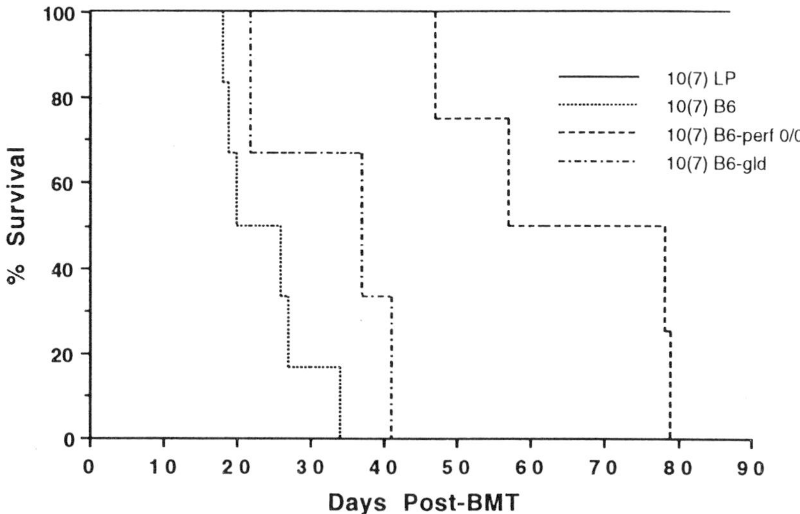

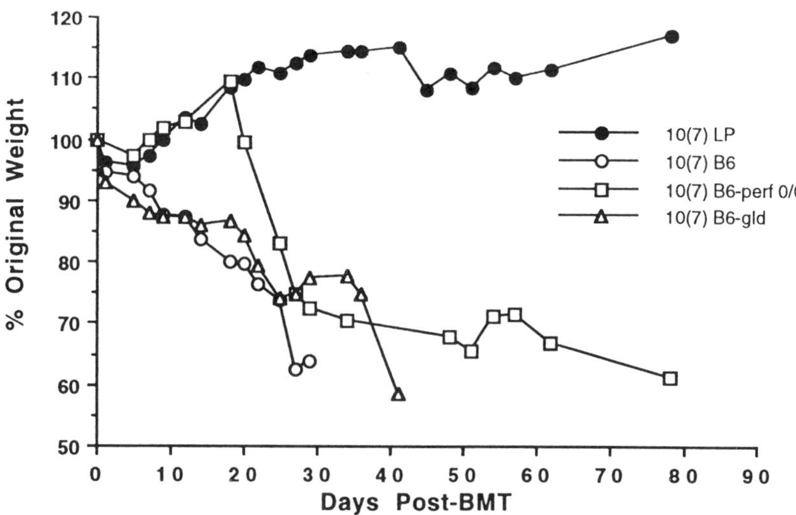

Figure 6 Survival (top) and body weight (bottom) during acute GVHD following allogeneic bone marrow transplantation of cytotoxically defective T cells. Lethally irradiated LP (H-2^b) recipients (7/group) were transplanted with 5×10^6 marrow cells from normal B6 (H-2^b) mice together with 1×10^7 T cells from either syngeneic (LP, ●), normal allogeneic (B6, ○), perforin-deficient allogeneic (B6-perf 0/0, □), or Fas L–defective allogeneic (B6-*gld*, △) donor mice. Recipients of syngeneic T cells survived and rapidly gained normal body weight. Mice receiving normal or B6-*gld* T cells developed acute GVHD associated with weight loss with 100% mortality. Recipients of B6-perf 0/0 T cells developed acute GVHD with 100% mortality after a significant delay. (Reprinted from Ref. 111.)

donor antihost cytotoxicity. These findings demonstrate a requirement for Fas-dependent cytotoxicity in the pathophysiology of hepatic and cutaneous GVHD.

To date, the findings reported demonstrate that both perforin and Fas L–mediated donor antihost cytotoxicity can contribute to acute GVHD, but each pathway in a distinctive manner. How might perforin-dependent cell-mediated cytotoxicity accelerate or amplify the onset of GVHD? Levy and colleagues have proposed that the killing of host cells early post BMT is an important contributory event to the amplification of the GVH reaction. Such cytotoxicity might be especially important in the intestine, where damage to the mucosa and subsequent systemic translocation of endotoxin may be a critical trigger to the effector phase of GVHD (see Chapter 18). Increased cytotoxicity could occur as a consequence of the release of host antigens and/or inflammatory mediators during or following death of host cells. Additionally, under circumstances when elements of host resistance are present, the absence of perforin-mediated antihost cytotoxicity might result in diminishing the overall GVH alloaggressive capacity of the donor inoculum. Fas L–mediated donor antihost cytotoxicity is apparently required at certain local sites of GVHD-induced tissue damage. Findings thus far suggest that Fas L-Fas-induced apoptosis of discrete cells in certain target tissues occurs prior to the emergence of GVHD lesions. Inflammatory cytokines including IFN-γ play a critical role in target tissue damage in GVHD, and such cytokines may enhance susceptibility of Fas L–mediated killing by upregulating expression of Fas on host target cells. Moreover, these inflammatory cytokines could play a critical role in the induction of GVHD-associated cachexia, consistent with the findings that weight loss and mortality were observed in the absence of either pathway. Finally, it has been difficult to reconcile the ability of either CD4+ or CD8+ T cells alone to mediate virtually identical GVHD pathology. It may therefore be worthwhile to consider the ability of both populations to mediate Fas L–dependent cytotoxicity in the development of tissue damage.

III. ADVANCES IN GVHD PATHOPHYSIOLOGY

A. Nitric Oxide, Cytokines, and the Immunosuppression of GVHD

The development of GVHD is associated with long-lasting and profound deficits in immune function that lead to increased morbidity and mortality after BMT (reviewed in Chapter 10). The immunodeficiency affects both T cells and B cells and is not specific to the response against host alloantigens (see Fig. 5, p. 269). Recent experimental studies have furthered our understanding of the interactions between nitric oxide (NO), which is an important predictor of GVHD (see below), and this immunosuppression. In a paper by Falzarano and colleagues, the mechanism of B-cell immunodeficiency was investigated in murine a model of GVHD to minor H antigens (113). NO was produced together with TNF-α in culture and was associated with dramatically reduced responses to the B-cell mitogen LPS. Specific inhibition of NO synthesis with L^{G}-monomethyl-arginine (NMMA) reduced NO and restored splenocyte response but did not significantly reduce TNF-α levels (Fig. 7). Neutralization of TNF-α with anti-TNF-α antibody also abrogated NO production and restored LPS-induced proliferation. Because NMMA did not reduce TNF-α levels,

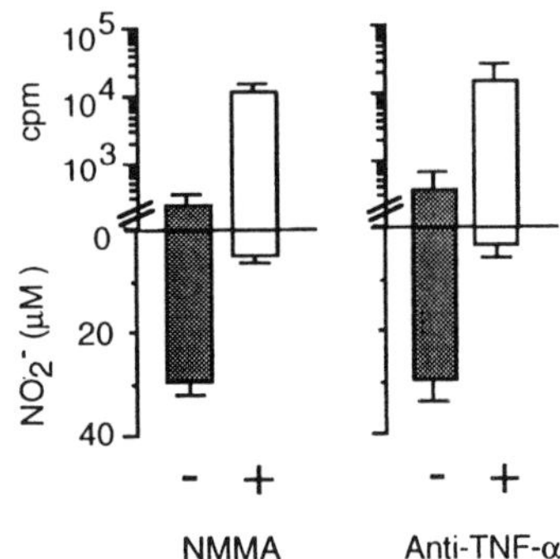

Figure 7 Suppression of splenocyte proliferation of lipopolysaccharide (LPS) during GVHD is associated with TNF-α and nitric oxide production. Irradiated (1100 cGy) CBA mice were transplanted with bone marrow (5×10^6) and T cells (1×10^6) from B10.BR mice. Splenocytes from recipient mice were analyzed 2 weeks post BMT for proliferation (cpm) and nitrite production (NO_2-) to the B-cell mitogen LPS in the absence (■) or presence (□) of *N*-monomethyl-arginine (NMMA) or a polyclonal antibody to murine TNF-α. (Adapted from Ref. 113.)

the authors concluded that TNF-α is critical to the induction of NO, which mediates B cell immunosuppression, but TNF-α per se is not responsible for NO generation, which must involve another factor(s).

One such candidate factor is IFN-γ. A second study from the Ferrara laboratory identified both NO-dependent and independent mechanisms of T-cell immunosuppression (114). In that study, splenocytes from mice with GVHD did not proliferate either to the T-cell mitogen concanavalin A (ConA) or to host alloantigens, but only mitogen-activated cultures produced increased levels of NO. The abrogation of NO synthesis with NMMA restored mitogen-induced proliferation but not the response to host antigens. The mechanism of impaired proliferation to mitogen was dependent on IFN-γ because blockade of this cytokine in culture inhibited NO production and restored proliferation to ConA to levels similar to transplanted control mice without GVHD (Fig. 8). NMMA did not substantially reduce IFN-γ levels, demonstrating that NO acted distally to IFN-γ in this immunosuppressive pathway. Furthermore, the prevention of IFN-γ production in vivo after allogeneic BMT by transplantation of polarized type 2 donor T cells also prevented NO production and restored splenocyte responses to mitogen (114).

IFN-γ alone did not appear to mediate the suppression of T-cell proliferation to mitogen in this study. First, the presence of IFN-γ per se did not affect the response to mitogen in control cultures: naive donor splenocytes secreted high levels of IFN-γ (>100 U/ml) when stimulated with ConA, but they did not produce detectable NO and they proliferated vigorously to ConA. Second, proliferation was not changed by the addition of IFN-γ (or anti-IFN-γMAb) to any culture where only background levels of NO were generated. Third, even though the addition of NMMA to cultures of GVHD splenocytes restored proliferation to ConA to control levels, it did not substantially affect IFN-γ production, ruling out the possibility

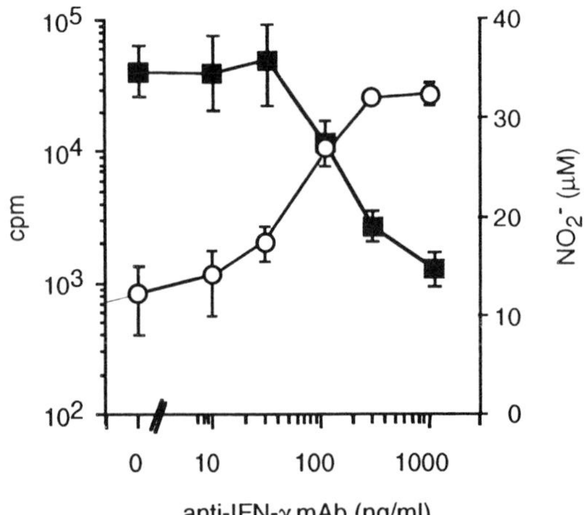

Figure 8 IFN-γ induces nitric oxide and suppresses T-cell proliferation to Concanavalin A during GVHD. Irradiated (1100 cGy) C57BL/6 mice were transplanted with T-cell-depleted bone marrow (5 × 10^6) and T cells (5 × 10^5) from bm12 mice. Splenocytes were isolated from recipients 2 weeks post BMT and cultured in the presence of increasing concentrations of anti-IFN-γ MAb. Proliferation (○, cpm) and nitrite production (■, NO_2-, μM) were measured after 48 hr of culture. (Adapted from Ref. 114.)

that NMMA mediated its effects via inhibition of cytokine synthesis. Taken together, these data confirm and extend the evidence that a type 1 cytokine response during acute GVHD regulates T-cell immunosuppression in response to mitogen through the induction of NO. Given the effect of TNF-α on NO induction in the first study, we postulate a unifying hypothesis in which IFN-γ primes mononuclear cells during acute GVHD to produce TNF-α and NO. This process may be initiated by LPS, a mechanism that has already been proposed for the cytokine cascade of acute GHVD (42) and which may be relevant to the process of idiopathic pneumonitis (see below).

B. Cutaneous GHVD

Target cell damage with epithelium has been a key feature in assessing pathological alterations in acute and chronic forms of GVHD. The mechanism of injury to cutaneous and mucosal epithelial cells has remained enigmatic, although damaged cells may be recognized and quantified as a consequence of characteristic cytological alterations (115). In a murine BMT model to minor H antigens, it now has been demonstrated that apoptosis, as determined by the terminal uridine deoxynucleotidyl transferase and ligation technique, is the predominant form of epithelial injury in acute GVHD (116,117). Apoptosis appears to preferentially involve subpopulations of lingual mucosa where stem cells have been shown to reside (118), providing further evidence that target cell injury in GVHD may involve recognition of epitopes on specific epithelial subsets (119). This observation, in addition to providing and additional tool for monitoring target cell injury in GVHD, may also provide insight into pathogenesis, because apoptosis is mediated by a number of mechanisms, including perforins, granzymes, inflammatory cytokines, and Fas ligand interactions (see above and Refs. 120–122).

With regard to models to study access and migration of lymphocytic cells into epithelial target sites, the SCID mouse has now been established as a system for reproduction and therapeutic manipulation of cytotoxic dermatitis mimicking human chronic lichen planus–like GVHD (123). Allogeneic (but not syngeneic) human peripheral blood mononuclear cells microinjected into human skin xenografted onto SCID mice produce GVHD-like epidermal injury via selective intraepidermal migration of CD8-positive cells containing the TIA-1 cytotoxic granule antigen (124). Epidermotropic migration of these effector cells is associated with epithelial expression of ICAM-1 and may be facilitated by graft priming with IFN-γ, which induces this adhesion molecule. The importance of ICAM-1 expression in mediating epidermotropic migration necessary for target cell injury is emphasized by the ability of antisense oligonucleotides to ICAM-1 to partially abrogate effector cell influx into the epidermis and attendant cellular damage. This advance provides the first in vivo model for exploration and therapeutic manipulation of human cytotoxic dermatitis relevant to GVHD.

C. Hepatic GVHD

Recent studies have documented that elevated levels of circulating TNF-α at the time of BMT induction are strongly predictive of the development of GVHD following transplantation (see Chapter 25 and Refs. 125,126). TNF-α has been found to play a key role in hepatic injury during inflammation. These effects are best examined from the standpoint of the hepatic sinusoid, hepatocytes, and the bile duct epithelium.

Within the sinusoid an interplay between epithelial cells, resident Kupffer cells, and neutrophils appears to be important in causing hepatocellular injury. The recruitment of neutrophils to the hepatic parenchyma in the setting of inflammation is promoted by their adhesion molecule-1 (ICAM-1) on the sinusoidal endothelium. ICAM-1 expression is enhanced in the setting of inflammation, as is expression of its complementary ligand, Mac-1, on neutrophils (127,128). The Kupffer cell is central to hepatic inflammation, through its release of TNF-α and IL-6 in response to a variety of inflammatory stimuli, including endotoxemia and elevated levels of IL-1 (129). IL-1β, through its promotion of TNF-α release, figures directly in parenchymal inflammation. TNF-α induces neutrophils to release noxious agents such as superoxide radicals and elastase (130). Both activated Kupffer cells and hepatocytes produce a potent neutrophil chemoattractant [cytokine-induced neutrophil chemoattractant (CINC) in rats and IL-8 in humans] (131), further promoting neutrophil accumulation in the hepatic parenchyma. The presence of neutrophils within the liver greatly potentiates the hepatotoxic effects of TNF-α (132); these effects are similar to the process observed in the lung (see below). TNF-α can also induce the expression of class II MHC molecules and ICAM-1 on bile duct epithelia, and the latter events play a key role in the bile duct damage of hepatic GVHD. Cholestatic levels of bile salts will ameliorate some of these events through their inhibition of TNF-α release by Kupffer cells (133). This added information points to the key role of TNF-α release from Kupffer cells in causing both the bile duct and hepatocellular damage characteristic of acute GVHD.

Hepatocytes are exceedingly sensitive to TNF-α and IL-6. TNF-α induces hepatocyte apoptosis (134,135) and at lower doses causes a substantive increase (>20%) in hepatocyte volume and liver size (136). Both cytokines downregulate bile salt uptake and biliary secretion of bile salts, thereby causing cholestasis through the inhibition of bile salt–dependent bile flow (137,138). IL-6 and TNF-α also are important inducers of the acute-phase response in hepatocytes (139). Thus, a proinflammatory cytokine environment will either cause outright hepatocyte destruction or, short of that, marked derangement of hepatocyte function.

The bile duct epithelium is a particularly interesting contributor to the "cytokine storm." As reviewed in Chapter 12, increased MHC class II expression occurs in temporal association with the onset of immunological damage to the bile ducts and appears to be mediated by inflammatory cytokines (including TNF-α and IFN-γ). MHC class II restricted–antigen presentation to T cells promotes subsequent immune-mediated bile duct damage. As ICAM-1 expression on interlobular bile duct is induced by proinflammatory cytokines such as TNF-α and IL-1 (140,141), neutrophils will be recruited for release of their destructive chemicals. Two recent findings are of particular interest. First, donor T cells recruited to portal tracts in murine GVHD enhance expression of both ICAM-1 and class II MHC molecules on bile duct epithelial cells (142). Second, bile duct epithelial cells themselves are capable of releasing cytokines, particularly IL-6, in response to IL-1 and TNF-α exposure (143,144). Thus, the activated bile duct epithelium in GVHD is likely to promote its own destruction through the aberrant expression of class II MHC molecules and increased expression of ICAM-1 and will promote hepatocellular cholestasis through the release of IL-6.

In this context, an innovation in the development of animal models of bile duct disease is the immunization of rats with bile duct epithelial cells (145). These animals develop a nonsuppurative cholangitis with a predominantly T-cell infiltrate and distortion and tortuosity of the entire intrahepatic biliary tree. This model may also prove useful in future studies of immune-mediated bile duct destruction of the type that occurs during GVHD.

D. Idiopathic Pneumonitis

The roles of LPS and inflammatory cytokines in idiopathic pneumonitis (IP) have recently been investigated in the B10.BR → CBA murine BMT model of GVHD to minor H antigenic differences (146). Lung pathology and bronchoalveolar lavage (BAL) fluid were analyzed in transplant recipients before and after both syngeneic and allogeneic BMT. At 2 weeks after BMT, no specific pathological abnormalities were noted in either group; at 6 weeks, pneumonitis and infiltration around vessels and bronchioles were observed in allogeneic recipients. This histopathology was associated with significant changes in BAL fluid composition, including increased neutrophils, endotoxin, and TNF-α levels (Table 3). Challenging transplanted mice with endotoxin exacerbated pulmonary damage only in animals with moderate GVHD (>10% weight loss), which was again reflected in BAL fluid changes and produced a qualitative histopathological change (alveolar hemorrhage) in a significant percentage of this group.

This study supports the hypothesis that both LPS and TNF-α, which are central to the pathophysiology of GVHD (reviewed in Chapter 18), are also important

Table 3 Lung Pathology, BAL Fluid Characteristics, and Serum Endotoxin Levels of CBA Mice Before and After BMT

LPS	Group	Pathology index	BAL polys $\times 10^5$	BAL TNF-α (pg/ml)	BAL LPS (pg/ml)	Serum LPS (pg/ml)
	Naïve CBA	0.10 ± 0.01	0.09 ± 0.04	10 ± 3	<2	<20
−	Syngeneic	0.96 ± 0.28	0.11 ± 0.04	14 ± 6	4 ± 2	<20
	Allogeneic (mild GVHD)	4.4 ± 1.2*	1.3 ± 0.1*	88 ± 35*	11 ± 2*	133 ± 49*
	Allogeneic (mod GVHD)	5.9 ± 1.0*	4.3 ± 2.4*	153 ± 22*	21 ± 3*	227 ± 87*
	Syngeneic	1.2 ± 0.2	0.12 ± 0.05	15 ± 6	ND	ND
+	Allogeneic (mild GVHD)	3.8 ± 0.9	3.7 ± 1.4	131 ± 42	ND	ND
	Allogeneic (mod GVHD)	10.2 ± 0.5**	26.1 ± 4.3**	422 ± 71**	ND	ND

CBA mice received syngeneic or allogeneic BMT and allogeneic recipients were categorized as having mild GVHD (weight loss < 10%) or moderate GVHD (weight loss > 10%). In some experiments, transplanted animals also received exogenous intravenous LPS (bottom). At the time of sacrifice, lung tissue, bronchoalveolar lavage (BAL) fluid, and serum were harvested and evaluated for degree of pulmonary histological damage (pathology index), polymorphonuclear cells (polys), TNF-α and LPS in the BAL fluid as well as LPS in the serum. Data are expressed as mean ± SEM. *$p < 0.05$, recipients of allogeneic BMT vs. syngeneic BMT; **$p < 0.05$, −LPS vs. +LPS.

mediators in the development of IP (see Chapter 15). The results of Cooke et al. suggest that parenchymal pneumonitis represents primarily a response to LPS because only this inflammatory process (and not the periluminal infiltrates) increased after LPS injection. Enhanced lung injury, along with increased neutrophils and TNF-α in BAL fluid, was noted after LPS challenge only in animals with more extensive GVHD; in fact, an important pathological finding (alveolar hemorrhage) was observed exclusively in that group. Endotoxin challenge had no effect in animals when GVHD was absent or mild, changing neither the pathology, the BAL fluid cellularity, nor the TNF-α concentration. These findings might be explained in two ways. First, increased cellularity in the lungs of mice with more extensive GVHD might provide an additional vector for amplifying the effects of endotoxin and the subsequent secretion of inflammatory cytokines and recruitment of neutrophils. Second, the ability of systemic endotoxin to reach the alveolar space might be directly related to the consequences of GVHD in other target organs. Animals with acute GVHD have reduced ability to neutralize endotoxin, and the appearance of circulating endotoxin during GVHD has been directly correlated to subsequent mortality (42). Interestingly, a recent study proposed a similar mechanism for endothelial damage after BMT with the demonstration that endotoxin enhances the endothelial cell apoptosis induced by irradiation via TNF-α (147). With respect to pulmonary damage, it is possible that early endothelial injury caused by irradiation may be self-limited in the setting of syngeneic BMT but subsequently enhanced by a systemic GVHD, driven by endotoxin and TNF-α.

The findings of Cooke et al. also suggest that the liver is a critical GVHD target organ in the pathway of LPS-mediated IP. Pivotally located immediately downstream (via the splanchnic circulation) of the intestinal reservoir of gram-negative bacteria and their toxic byproducts, liver macrophages produce and export inflammatory cytokines when confronted with a sudden endotoxin surge. If endotoxin surpasses the hepatic capacity for its clearance, both inflammatory cytokines and unprocessed endotoxin "spill over" into the systemic circulation. Several experimental studies have demonstrated that the presence of preexisting hepatic injury decreases the threshold at which the liver can effectively handle endotoxin (148–150). In the setting of acute GVHD, the endotoxin surge arises from increased LPS translocation across damaged intestinal mucosa. Underlying damage from hepatic GVHD could then serve to decrease the liver's capacity for LPS uptake and clearance. The administration of endotoxin to animals with no or mild GHVD had minimal effect on the lung because the liver was able to neutralize the LPS challenge. By contrast, the same amount of endotoxin could not be neutralized by livers of animals with moderate GVHD (demonstrated by a significant increase in hepatocellular damage); as a consequence, lung injury and mortality were observed only in the group with more extensive GVHD. In these animals, LPS remained in the systemic circulation for prolonged periods, triggering pulmonary mononuclear cell populations to secrete additional inflammatory cytokines and enhancing tissue damage. These experiments are consistent with a "gut-liver-lung" axis described in septic pathophysiology (149–151) and suggest that any process or combination of events early after BMT that allows large amounts of endotoxin into the pulmonary circulation and/or TNF-α into the alveolar space could promote the development of lung injury.

IV. CLINICAL ADVANCES

A. Risk Factors for Acute GVHD

A recent multivariate analysis in 291 consecutive recipients of HLA-identical sibling marrow revealed the following risk factors for acute GVHD: prophylaxis with monotherapy, methotrexate, or cyclosporin ($p = 0.015$), seropositivity for 3–4 herpes viruses versus 0–2 in the donor ($p = 0.015$), seropositivity for cytomegalovirus in the recipient ($p = 0.037$), and early engraftment ($p = 0.016$) (152). A high serum TNF-α level during conditioning therapy was also a significant risk factor for acute GVHD. The risk of grades II–IV acute GVHD increased with the number of risk factors. Factors previously reported to correlate with acute GVHD, such as age, female donor to male recipient, relative responses and donor-responding capacity in mixed lymphocyte culture, MNS blood group antigen, splenectomy, and bone marrow cell dose, were not associated with acute GVHD in this study.

As described above in the section pertaining to the immunosuppression of GVHD, NO has been shown to be an important inflammatory mediator of the disease in animal models. A recent analysis has shown that the stable end products of NO, nitrite/nitrate (NO_2^-/NO_3^-), are significantly elevated in patients with acute GVHD, after preceding the onset of clinical symptoms by 2 or 3 days (153). NO_2^-/NO_3^- levels were elevated neither during infection nor after autologous BMT, as is the case with other indices of macrophage activation such as neopterin. This study confirms the importance of NO in clinical GVHD and supports the approach of cytokine manipulation that may prevent its synthesis. Additional studies are needed to determine whether specific inhibitors of NO synthesis will be useful therapies in the prevention or treatment of acute GVHD.

The animal studies quoted have shown that IFN-γ is one of the cytokines that play a critical role in the induction of NO. A recent study has reexamined the levels of IFN-γ in clinical BMT and determined that IFN-γ levels, which increase after allogeneic BMT, are a function of mature T cells in the bone marrow inoculum (154). These results confirm and extend an earlier study by the Innsbruck group showing that increased serum IFN-γ levels precede the clinical onset of acute GVHD by several days (155). Interestingly, it was the cyclophosphamide component of the conditioning regimen that was associated with release of IFN-γ. TNF-α, on the other hand, was elevated after both cyclophosphamide and TBI in several experimental and clinical studies (see Chapter 25). Preliminary evidence from Holler and colleagues suggests that cross-regulation of cytokines during conditioning is an important factor in determining overall cytotoxicity (156). Analysis of peripheral blood for cytokines was conducted in patients with either placebo ($n = 8$) or anti-TNF-α ($n = 8$) during the conditioning regimen. These data (Table 4) show that treatment with anti-TNF-α significantly reduced serum IL-6 levels and intracytoplasmic IL-1β; there was borderline significance for intracytoplasmic TNF-α and IL-6. This observation confirms the first clinical report of cross-regulation of inflammatory cytokines in patients receiving IL-1 receptor antagonist for steroid-resistant GVHD (157). Further analysis of cytokine release early after BMT is likely to provide additional information on risk factors for the development of acute GVHD.

B. The Importance of HLA-C Alleles

HLA-C alleles have generally not been considered when selecting optimally matched donors for transplantation. Recent analyses, however, suggest that antigens encoded by these genes are relevant in transplant outcome (158). Petersdorf et al.

Table 4 Maximal Cytokine Production During Pretransplant Conditioning in Patients Receiving Prophylaxis with Anti-TNF Antibody or Placebo

	Prior to conditioning		Maximum during conditioning	
Cytokine levels	Anti-TNF-α	Placebo	Anti-TNF-α	Placebo
% TNF-α-positive cells	2.7 (0.8)	2.1 (0.9)	1.4 (0.6)	4.5 (1.9)
% IL-1β-positive cells	4.2 (1.4)	3.4 (1.2)	2.9 (1.2)	8.7 (2.2)
% IL-6-positive cells	2.7 (2.1)	5.0 (5.8)	1.2 (0.6)	7.1 (3.7)
IL-6 serum (pg/ml)	13 (5)	10 (2)	44 (19)	148 (78)

Intracytoplasmatic cytokines wer analyzed in 400 PBMC by saponin permeabilization and staining with specific antibodies against TNF-α, IL-1β, and IL-6 followed by detection with peroxidase-conjugated secondary antibodies; IL-6 serum levels were analyzed by specific ELISA (results of eight patients per group are shown). Analyses were performed prior to conditioning and every other day for intracytoplasmic cytokines and daily for IL-6 serum levels. Results are presented as mean (SEM). Differences between anti-TNF-α- and placebo-treated patients were significant for intracytoplasmic IL-1β and IL-6 serum levels ($p < 0.05$) and of borderline significance for intracytoplasmic TNF-α and IL-6 ($p < 0.10$).

carried out a matched case-control study based on 20 patients (19 CML, one aplastic anemia) who experienced graft failure after an initial graft from an unrelated donor; all were serologically HLA-A and B matched, 13 were DRB1 matched, and seven one locus mismatched. For each case two controls with sustained engraftment were selected. HLA-A, B, C, DRB1, and DQB1 alleles were determined by molecular methods. HLA-C allele mismatches were present in 15 (75%) of the 20 cases and in 12 (30%) of the controls. Therefore, the odds ratio of graft failure with an HLA-C mismatch was 8.3 (95% CI: 1.8, 18; $p < 0.01$). The difference was significant even after accounting for differences at other loci ($p = 0.02$). Clearly, therefore, HLA-C antigens impact on graft failure; an effect on GVHD remains to be investigated.

C. Graft-Versus-Malignancy Effects

A study from the European Blood and Marrow Transplant Group (EBMT) showed that the best leukemia-free survival after allogeneic bone marrow transplantation was seen in patients with grade I acute GVHD (159). The 5-year leukemia-free survival was 57 ± 2%, 63 ± 2%, 55 ± 3%, 32 ± 4%, 8 ± 3% in patients with acute GVHD grades 0, I, II, III, and IV, respectively. This confirms an earlier EMBT analysis that was restricted to chronic myelogenous leukemia and which showed the greatest survival for patients with grade I GVHD (160). The lower incidence of relapse (and hence greater survival) in patients with grade I GVHD confirms the clinical importance of graft-versus-leukemia effects associated with even limited GVHD.

A recent report suggests a graft-versus-breast cancer effect (161). A patient with metastatic breast cancer received an allogeneic BMT from her HLA identical sibling. Liver and bone metastases disappeared concurrently with onset of grade II acute GVHD. At the same time, minor H-antigen-specific CTL appeared in the patient's peripheral blood. These MHC class I restricted CTL lysed a number of breast carcinoma cell lines, and lysis was increased by pretreatment of the targets by TNF-α but not by IFN-γ. This study offers proof of principal of a graft- versus-carcinoma effect and further suggests that inflammatory cytokine production may play an important role in such an effect. Two recent articles have also reported a graft-versus-myeloma effect (162,163). Although laboratory studies showing lymphocyte reactivity against myeloma targets were not reported, several patients with recurrent multiple myeloma who received leukocyte infusions from the original donors achieved complete remission concurrent with the development of GVHD. Further studies will be needed to determine the optimal strategies to exploit immunological therapy in these diseases.

D. Thalidomide and Chronic GVHD

Thalidomide has been reported to be an effective agent for the treatment of chronic GVHD. Eighty patients who had failed to respond to prednisone and cyclosporin were treated with thalidomide (164). Sixteen patients (20%) achieved a sustained response (nine complete, seven partial). Twenty-nine patients (36%) had thalidomide discontinued due to side effects, which included sedation, constipation, neuritis, skin rash, and neutropenia. Based on these results, a prospective, randomized, double-blind study was performed to determine the efficacy of thalidomide as a prophylactic agent for chronic GVHD. A total of 59 patients were randomized to receive either placebo or thalidomide (200 mg po bid) beginning on day 80 after allogeneic BMT. Fifty-four patients, 26 given placebo and 28 on thalidomide, were evaluable. The first interim analysis showed there was a significant difference in the incidence of chronic GVHD, with patients receiving thalidomide developing chronic GVHD *more often* than patients receiving placebo ($p = 0.06$). Moreover, there was an overall survival advantage for patients on placebo compared to those receiving thalidomide ($p = 0.006$). Adjustment for possible confounding factors did not eliminate the negative effects of thalidomide. These results demonstrate that while thalidomide is an effective agent for the therapy of chronic GVHD, its use for the prophylaxis of chronic GVHD cannot be recommended.

E. Advances in Gene Therapy

1. Gene Therapy for ADA Deficiency

Results of three studies for gene therapy of ADA deficiency have recently been reported (165–167). Marrow or cord blood CD34+ selected cells and peripheral blood T cells were used as the target cells for gene transfer. In all three studies there was an increase in numbers of circulating T cells and ADA levels in conjunction with reconstruction of immune function. All the children also received PEG ADA, however, and therefore these results must be interpreted with caution. Nevertheless, the observation that the percentage of ADA-transduced T cells increases by 10- to 100-fold when PEG ADA is tapered (165) suggests that the transduced cells may have a selective advantage that will allow them to contribute to long-term reversal of phenotype.

2. Gene-Marking Studies

It has become clear that animal and human preclinical studies are not ideal surrogates to analyze the behavior of the human hematopoietic stem cells after clinical transplantation. Gene-marking studies can provide information on the optimal conditions for transduction of genes into hematopoietic stem cells that will influence the design of future gene therapy protocols. An update of the St. Jude studies described in Chapter 29 shows continued persistence of the marker gene for 4 years (168), albeit at low levels. The Toronto group has obtained high levels of gene transfer in a canine model where transduction was carried out in long-term bone marrow culture (169). The same approach is currently being evaluated in a human clinical trial (170).

In second-generation studies double-marking techniques using two distinguishable vectors allow intrapatient comparison of long-term reconstruction from different sources of differentially treated aliquots of hematopoietic stem cells. In a study at the National Institutes of Health, the reconstitution of CD34+ cells derived from blood and marrow has been compared in patients receiving autologous stem cell rescue as therapy for breast cancer of myeloma (170). The marker gene derived from blood cells has been detected for up to 12 months showing that peripheral blood derived stem cells can contribute to long-term recovery and are suitable targets for gene therapy. Similar studies are underway to compare the reconstitution of unmanipulated CD34+ cells with ex vivo expanded cells and to compare the contribution of lineage-positive and negative CD34+ subsets to short- and long-term reconstitution (168).

3. Gene Transfer into T Cells

Marking studies have also been used to demonstrate long-term persistence of infused T cells in immunotherapy protocols. Infused tumor-infiltrating lymphocytes persist up to 9 months (171) and EBV-specific CTL up to 23 months (172). The use of T cells as vehicles for transferred genes may, however, be limited by the immunogenicity of the transferred gene. In an adoptive transfer study, a construct encoding Tk and a selectable marker, hygromycin phosphotransferase, was transduced into gag-specific CTL and given to HIV+ patients so infused cells could be destroyed if adverse events occurred (173). Five of six patients enrolled on the study developed an immune response specific for the Tk or hygromycin gene product (173). The ability of immunosuppressed HIV+ patients to mount an immune response capable of destroying Tk-transduced cells may limit the utility of this suicide gene strategy; this approach is also being evaluated as a means of ablating T cells in the event of GVHD (see Chapter 29). This experience also illustrated a potential obstacle to long-term survival of any genetically modified cell when the transgene is a protein that the immune system can recognize as foreign.

V. CONCLUSIONS AND FUTURE DIRECTIONS

The first half of this decade has seen extraordinary progress in several areas of research that impact both directly and indirectly on BMT immunology. The efforts of dozens of outstanding research groups throughout the world have deepened our appreciation of the complexity and interdependence of many of the cellular and molecular mechanisms that control both specific and natural immune responses. Insights from the last several years have included the identification of many new proteins, both intracellular and extracellular, that control the immune system's specific functions: the transduction pathways of intracytoplasmic signals of lymphocytes, the interactions of the cell surface proteins that direct the flow and migration of white blood cells throughout the body, the cascades of soluble proteins that drive cellular differentiation and effector functions. One theme among these advances with particular relevance to GVHD is the variety of ways in which the immune system has developed its own internal controls for modifying or limiting inflammatory responses, apparently ensuring that no single cytokine will completely dominate any specific response. Much future therapy will likely exploit these systems of checks and balances in attempts to modify the complex set of interactions that comprises a GVH response.

Future advances will come from at least two areas. The first will be the production of mutant mouse strains that either overproduce or lack individual gene products and have begun to define the specific roles of these proteins during development and in steady-state physiology. The use of these mutant strains, as well as the relevant recombinant gene products, in well-defined BMT systems will be central to clarifying biological processes in complex systems where overlapping effects of proteins can often produce unexpected and even opposite results from the predictions of in vitro models. The second area will be to bring together advances in cell biology, such as insights into apoptosis, with increased sophistication in the effector functions of the immune system. The synergy inherent in such joining should lead to a more molecular understanding of GVHD target pathology and suggest further ways to enhance differences between GVL and GVHD, particularly chronic GVHD.

These studies should promote a far greater ability to model human GVHD in vitro. It is hoped that these advances will eventually translate into strategies that permit BMT across greater histocompatibility barriers in the early years of the twenty-first century.

REFERENCES

1. Guinan EC, Gribben JG, Boussiotis VA, Freeman GJ, Nadler LM. Pivotal role of the B7 : CD28 pathway in transplantation tolerance and tumor immunity. Blood 1994; 84: 3261.
2. June CH, Bluestone JA, Nadler LM, Thompson CB. The B7 and CD28 receptor families. Immunol Today 1994; 15:321.
3. Jenkins MK, Schwartz RH. Antigen presentation by chemically modified splenocytes induces antigen specific T cell unresponsiveness in vitro and in vivo. J Exp Med 1987; 165:302.
4. Linsley PS, Wallace PM, Johnson J, Gibson MG, Greene JL, Ledbetter JA, Singh C, Topper MA. Immunosuppression in vivo by a soluble form of the CTLA-4 T cell activation molecule. Science 1992; 257:792.
5. Lenschow DJ, Zeng Y, Thistlethwaite JR, Montag A, Brady W, Gibson MG, Linsley PS, Bluestone JA. Long-term survival of xenogeneic pancreatic islet grafts induced by CTLA4Ig. Science 1992; 257:789.
6. Blazar BR, Taylor PA, Linsley PS, Vallera DA. In vivo blockade of CD28/CTLA4: B7/BB1 interaction with CTLA4-Ig reduces lethal murine graft-versus-host disease across the major histocompatibility complex barrier in mice. Blood 1994; 83:3815.
7. Wallace PM, Johnson JS, MacMaster JF, Kennedy KA, Gladtone P, Linsley PS. CTLA4Ig treatment ameliorates the lethality of murine graft-versus-host disease across major histocompatibility complex barriers. Transplantation 1994; 58:602.
8. Hakim FT, Cepeda R, Gray GS, June CH, Abe R. Acute graft-vs.-host reaction can be aborted by blockade of costimulatory molecules. J Immunol 1995; 155:1757.
9. Tan P, Anasetti C, Hansen JA, Melrose J, Brunvand M, Bradshaw J, Ledbetter JA, Linsley PS. Induction of alloantigen-specific hyporesponsiveness in human T lymphocytes by blocking interaction of CD28 with its natural ligand B7/BB1. J Exp Med 1993; 177:165.
10. Van Gool SW, deBoer M, Ceuppens JL. The combination of anti-B7 monoclonal antibody and cyclosporin A induces alloantigen-specific anergy during a primary mixed lymphocyte reaction. J Exp Med 1994:179.
11. Gribben JG, Boussiotis VA, Freeman GJ, Rennert P, Jellis CL, Greenfield E, Grey GS, Nadler LM. Alloantigen and concomitant CTLA4 signaling induces clonal deletion of alloreactive T cells: A novel method to prevent GVHD. Blood 1994; 84:397.
12. Blazar BR, Taylor PA, Panaskoltsis-Mortari A, Gray GS, Vallera DA. Co-blockade of the LFA1 : ICAM and CD28/B7 pathways is a highly effective means of preventing acute lethal graft-versus-host disease induced by fully MHC disparate donor grafts. Blood 1995; 83:3815.
13. Doyle C, Strominger JL. Interaction between CD4 and class II MHC molecules mediates cell adhesion. Nature 1987; 330:256.
14. Gay D, Maddon P, Sekaly R, et al. Functional interaction between T-cell protein CD4 and the major histocompatibility complex HLA-DR antigen. 1987; 328:626.
15. Konig R, Huang L-Y, Germain RN. MHC class II interaction with CD4 mediated by a region analogous to the MHC class binding site for CD8. Nature 1992; 356:796.
16. Veillette A, Bookman MA, Horak EM, et al. The CD4 and CD8 T cell surface antigens

are associated with internal membrane tyrosine-protein kinase p56^{lck}. Cell 1988; 55: 301.

17. Barber EK, Dasgupta JD, S. F. et al. The CD4 and CD8 antigens are coupled to a protein-tyrosine kinase (p56^{lck}) that phosphorylates the CD3 complex. Proc Natl Acad Sci USA 1989; 86:3277.
18. Turner JM, Brodsky MH, Irving BA, et al. Interaction of the unique N-terminal region of tyrosine kinase p56^{lck} with cytoplasmic domains of CD4 and CD8 is mediated by cysteine motifs. Cell 1990; 60:755.
19. Korngold R, Sprent J. Surface markers of T cells causing lethal graft-vs-host disease to class I vs class II H-2 differences. J Immunol 1985; 135:3004.
20. Sprent J, Schaefer M, Lo D, Korngold R. Properties of purified T cell subsets: II. In vivo responses to class I vs. class II H-2 differences. J Exp Med 1986; 163:998.
21. Korngold R, Sprent J. Variable capacity of L3T4+ T cells to cause lethal graft-versus-host disease across minor histocompatibility barriers in mice. J Exp Med 1987; 165: 1552.
22. Hamilton BL. L3T4-positive T cells participate in the induction of graft-vs-host disease in response to minor histocompatibility antigens. J Immunol 1987; 139:2511.
23. Cobbold S, Martin G, Waldmann H. Monoclonal antibodies for the prevention of graft-vs-host disease and marrow graft rejection. The depletion of T cell subsets in vitro and in vivo. Transplantation 1986; 42:239.
24. Knulst AC, Tibbe GJ, Noort Wa, et al. Prevention of lethal graft-vs-host disease in mice by monoclonal antibodies directed against T cells or their subsets. I. Evidence for the induction of a state of tolerance based on suppression. Bone Marrow Transplant 1994; 13:293.
25. Reinecke K, Mysliwietz J, Thierfelder S. Single as well as pairs of synergistic anti-CD4 + CD8 antibodies prevent graft-vs-host disease in fully mismatched mice. Transplantation 1995; 57:458.
26. Hafler DA, Ritz J, Schlossman SF, et al. Anti-CD4 and anti-CD2 monoclonal antibody infusions on subjects with multiple sclerosis. Immunosuppressive effects and human anti-mouse responses. J Immunol 1988; 141:131.
27. Racadot E, Rumbach L, Bataillard M, et al. Treatment of multiple sclerosis with anti-CD4 monoclonal antibody: a preliminary report of B-F5 in 21 patients. J Autoimmun 1993; 6:771.
28. Lindsey JW, Hodgkinson S, Mehta R, et al. Repeated treatment with chimeric anti-CD4 antibody in multiple sclerosis. Ann Neurol 1994; 36:183.
29. Jameson BA, McDonnell JM, Marini JC, Korngold R. A rationally designed CD4 analogue inhibits experimental allergic encephalomyelitis. Nature 1994; 368:744.
30. McDonnell JM, Varnum JM, Mayo KH, et al. Rational design of a peptide analog of the L3T4 CDR3-like region. Immunomethods 1992; 1:33.
31. Schlegel PG, Vaysburd M, Chen Y, et al. Inhibition of T cell costimulation by VCAM-1 prevents murine graft-versus-host disease across minor histocompatibility barriers. J Immunol 1995; 155:3856.
32. Haug CE, Colvin RB, Delmonico FL, et al. A phase I trial of immunosuppression with anti-ICAM-1 (CD54) mAb in renal allograft recipients. Transplantation 1993; 55: 766.
33. Archelos JJ, Jung S, Maurer M, et al. Inhibition of experimental autoimmune encephalomyelitis by an antibody to the intercellular adhesion molecule ICAM-1. Ann Neuro 1993; 34:145.
34. Gorcyznski RM, Chung S, Fu XM, et al. Manipulation of skin graft rejection on alloimmune mice by anti-VCAM-1 : VLA-4 but not anti-ICAM-1 : LFA-1 monoclonal antibodies. Transplant Immunol 1995; 3:55.
35. Fowler DH, Kurasawa K, Husebekk A, Cohen PA, Gress RE. Cells of the Th2 cyto-

kine phenotype prevent LPS-induced lethality during murine graft-versus-host reaction. J Immunol 1994; 152: 1004.
36. Krenger W, Snyder KM, Byon CH, Falzarano G, Ferrara JLM. Polarized type 2 alloreactive CD4+ and CD8+ donor T cells fail to induce experimental acute graft-versus-host disease. J Immunol 1995; 155:585.
37. Racke MK, Dhib-Jalbut S, Cannella B, et al. Prevention and treatment of chronic relapsing experimental allergic encephalomyelitis by transforming growth factor-β_1. J Immunol 1991; 146:3012.
38. Johns LD, Flanders KC, Ranges GE, et al. Successful treatment of experimental allergic encephalomyelitis with transforming growth factor-β_1. J Immunol 1991; 147: 1792.
39. Lider O, Miller A, Miron S, et al. Nonencephalitogenic CD4-CD8-V alpha 2V beta 8.2+ anti-myelin basic protein rat T lymphocytes inhibit disease induction. J Immunol 1991; 147:1208.
40. Miller A, Lider O, Roberts AB, et al. Suppressor T cells generated by oral tolerization to myelin basic protein suppress both in vitro and in vivo immune responses by the release of transforming growth factor beta after antigen-specific triggering. Proc Natl Acad Sci USA 1992; 89:421.
41. Krenger W, Cooke KR, Sonis ST, Crawford J, Simmons R, Pan L, Kobzik L, Delmonte J, Karandikar M, Ferrara JLM. Transplantation of polarized type 2 donor T cells reduces systemic graft-versus-host disease induced by minor histocompatibility antigens. Transplantation. In press, 1996.
42. Nestel FP, Price KS, Seemayer TA, Lapp WS. Macrophage priming and lipopolysaccharide-triggered release of tumor necrosis factor alpha during graft-versus-host disease. J Exp Med 1992; 175:405.
43. Jadus MR, Wepsic HT. The role of cytokines in graft-versus-host reactions and disease. Bone Marrow Transplant 1992; 10:1.
44. Piguet PF. Tumor necrosis factor and graft-versus-host disease, in Burakoff SJ, Deeg HJ, Ferrara JLM, Atkinson K (eds): Graft-vs.-Host Disease: New York: Marcel Dekker, 1990; 258.
45. Holler E, Kolb HJ, Hintermeier-Knabe R, Mittermueller J, Thierfelde S, Kaul M, Wilmanns W. The role of tumor necrosis factor alpha in acute graft-versus-host disease and complications following allogeneic bone marrow transplantation. Transplant Proc 1993; 25:1234.
46. Holler E, Kolb HJ, Mittermueller J, Kaul M, Ledderose G, Duell T, Seeber B, Schleuning M, Hintermeier-Knabe R, Ertl B, Kempeni J, Wilmanns W. Modulation of acute graft-versus-host disease after allogeneic bone marrow transplantation by tumor necrosis factor α (TNFα) release in the course of pretransplant conditioning: role of conditioning regimens and prophylactic application of a monoclonal antibody neutralizing human TNFα (MAK 195F). Blood 1995; 86:890.
47. Korngold R, Sprent J. T cell subsets in graft-vs.-host disease, in Burakoff SJ, Deeg HJ, Ferrara J, Atkinson K (eds): Graft-vs.-Host Disease: Immunology, Pathophysiology, and Treatment. New York: Marcel Dekker, 1990; 31.
48. Mosmann TR, Sad S. The expanding universe of T-cell subsets: Th1, Th2 and more. Immunol Today 1996; 17:138.
49. Croft M, Carter L, Swain SL, Dutton RW. Generation of antigen-specific CD8 effector populations: Reciprocal action of interleukin (IL)-4 and IL-12 in promoting type 2 versus type 1 cytokine profiles. J Exp Med 1994; 180:1715.
50. Seder RA. The functional role of CD8+ T helper type 2 cells. J Exp Med 1995; 181:5.
51. Le Gros G, Erard F. Non-cytotoxic, IL-4, IL-5, IL-10 producing CD8+ T cells: their activation and effector functions. Curr Opin Immunol 1994; 6:453.
52. Kelso A. Th1 and Th2 subsets: paradigms lost? Immunol Today 1995; 16:374.

53. Murphy E, Shibuya K, Hosken N, Openshaw P, Maino V, Davis K, Murphy K, O'Garra A. Reversibility of T helper 1 and 2 populations is lost after long-term stimulation. J Exp Med 1996; 183:901.
54. Kawakami Y, Haas GP, Lotze MT. Expansion of tumor-infiltrating lymphocytes from human tumors using the T-cell growth factors interleukin-2 and interleukin-4. J Immunother 1993; 14:336.
55. Spits H, Yssel H, Paliard X, Kastelein R, Figdor C, DeVries JE. IL-4 inhibits IL-2 mediated induction of human lymphokine-activated killer cells, but not the generation of antigen-specific cytotoxic T lymphocytes in mixed leukocyte cultures. J Immunol 1988; 141:29.
56. Hakim FT, Sharrow SO, Payne S, Shearer GM. Repopulation of host lympohematopoietic systems by donor cells during graft-versus-host reaction in unirradiated adult F1 mice injected with parental lymphocytes. J Immunol 1991; 146:2108.
57. Knobloch C, Dennert G. Asialo-GM1-positive T killer cells are generated in F1 mice injected with parental spleen cells. J Immunol 1988; 140:744.
58. Korngold R. Lethal graft-versus-host disease in mice directed to multiple minor histocompatibility antigens: features of CD8+ and CD4+ T cell responses. Bone Marrow Transplant 1992; 9:355.
59. Mueller KM, Jaunin F, Masouye I, Saurat JH, Hauser C. Th2 cells mediated IL-4-dependent local tissue inflammation. J Immunol 1993; 150:5576.
60. Thornhill MH, Wellicome SM, Mahiouz DL, Lanchbury JSS, Kyan-Aung U, Haskard DO. Tumor necrosis factor combines with IL-4 or IFN-γ to selectively enhance endothelial cell adhesiveness for T cells. J Immunol 1991; 146:592.
61. Martin PJ, Kernan NA. T-cell depletion for the prevention of graft-versus-host disease, in Burakoff SJ, Deeg HJ, Ferrara JLM, Atkinson K (eds). Graft-vs.-Host Disease. New York: Marcel Dekker, 1985; 371.
62. Truitt RL, LeFever AV, Shih CCY, Jeske JM, Martin TM. Graft-vs.-leukemia effect, in Burakoff SJ, Deeg HJ, Ferrara J, Atkinson K (eds). Graft-vs.-Host Disease: Immunology, Pathophysiology, and Treatment. New York. Marcel Dekker, 1990; 177.
63. Keever CA, Small TN, Flomenberg N, Keller G, Pekle K, Black P, Pecora A, Gillio A, Kernan NA, O'Reilly RJ. Immune reconstitution following bone marrow transplantation: Comparison of recipients of T-cell depleted marrow with recipients of conventional marrow grafts. Blood 1989; 73:1340.
64. Sad S, Marcotte R, Mosmann TR. Cytokine-induced differentiation of precursor mouse CD8+ T cells into cytotoxic CD8+ T cells secreting TH1 or Th2 cytokines. Immunity 1995; 2:271.
65. Allen RD, Staley TA, Sidman CL. Differential cytokine expression acute and chronic murine graft-versus-host disease. Eur J Immunol 1993; 23:333.
66. Doutrelepont JM, Moser M, Leo O, Abramowicz D, Vanderhaegen ML, Urbain J, Goldman M. Hyper IgE in stimulatory graft-versus-host disease: role of Interleukin-4. Clin Exp Immunol 1991; 83:133.
67. Umland SP, Razac S, Nahrebne DK, Seymour BW. Effects of in vivo administration of interferon (IFN)-gamma, anti-IFN-gamma, or anti-interleukin-4 monoclonal antibodies in chronic autoimmune graft-versus-host disease. Clin Immunol Immunopathol 1992; 63:66.
68. DeWit D, Van Mechelen M, Zanin C, Doutrelepont J-M, Velu T, Gerard C, Abramowicz D, Scheerlinck J-P, De Baetselier P, Urbain J, Leo O, Goldman M, Moser M. Preferential activation of Th2 cells in chronic graft-versus-host disease. J Immunol 1993; 150:361.
69. Garlisi CG, Pennline KJ, Smith SR, Siegel MT, Umland SP. Cytokine gene expression in mice undergoing chronic graft-versus-host disease. Mol Immunol 1993; 30:669.
70. Pan L, Delmonte J, Jalonen CK, Ferrara JLM. Pretreatment of donors with granulocyte colony-stimulating factor polarizes donor T lymphocytes toward type 2 cytokine

production and reduces severity of experimental graft versus host disease. Blood 1995; 86:4422.
71. Demetri GD, Griffin JD. Granulocyte colony-stimulating factor and its receptor. Blood 1991; 78:2791.
72. Tkatch LS, Tweardy DJ. Human granulocyte colony-stimulating factor (G-CSF), the premier granulopoietin: biology, clinical utility, and receptor structure and function. Lymphokine Cytokine Res 1993; 12:477.
73. Weaver, CH, Longin K, Buckner CD, Bensinger W. Lymphocyte content in peripheral blood mononuclear cells collected after the administration of recombinant human granulocyte colony-stimulating factor. Bone Marrow Transplant 1994; 13:411.
74. Mosmann TR, Coffman RL. TH1 and TH2 cells: different patterns of lymphokine secretion lead to different functional properties. Annu Rev Immunol 1989; 7:145.
75. Swain SL, Bradley LM, Croft M, Tonkonogy S, Atkins G, Weinberg AD, Duncan DD, Hedrick SM, Dutton RW, Huston G. Helper T-cell subsets: Phenotype, function and the role of lymphokines in regulating their development. Immunol Rev 1991; 123:115.
76. Finkelman FD. Relationships among antigen presentation, cytokines, immune deviation, and autoimmune disease. J Exp Med 1995; 182:279.
77. Bronchud MH. Recombinant human granulocyte colony-stimulating factor in the management of cancer patients: five years on. Oncology 1994; 51:189.
78. Ohsaka A, Saionji K, Kuwaki T, Takeshima T, Igari J. Granulocyte colony-stimulating factor administration modulates the surface expression of effector cell molecules on human monocytes. J Haematol 1995; 89:465.
79. Gorgen I, Hartung T, Leist M, Niehorster M, Tiegs G, Uhlig S, Weitzel F, Wendel A. Granulocyte colony-stimulating factor treatment protects rodents against lipopolysaccharide-induced toxicity via expression of systemic tumor necrosis-α. J Immunol 1992; 149:918.
80. Hartung T, Docke WD, Grabtner F, Krieger G, Sauer A, Stevens P, Volk HD, Wendel A. Effect of granulocyte colony-stimulating factor treatment on ex vivo blood cytokine response in human volunteers. Blood 1995; 85:2482.
81. Dreger P, Suttorp M, Haferlach T, Loffler H, Schmitz N. Allogeneic granulocyte colony-stimulating factor-mobilized peripheral blood progenitor cells for treatment of engraftment failure after bone marrow transplantation. Blood 1993; 81:1404.
82. Russell NH, Hunter A, Rogers S, Hanley J, Anderson D. Peripheral blood stem cells as an alterative to marrow for allogeneic transplantation. Lancet 1993; 341:1482.
83. Sasaki A, Tsukaguchi M, Hirai M, Ohira H, Nakao Y, Yamane T, Park K, Im T, Tatsumi N. Transplantation of allogeneic peripheral blood stem cells after myeloablative treatment of a patient in blastic crisis of chronic myelocytic leukemia. Am J Hematol 1994; 47:45.
84. Molina L, Chabannon C, Viret F, Moine A, Leger J, Nicolini F, Hollard D, Sotto J-J. Granulocyte colony-stimulating factor-mobilized allogeneic peripheral blood stem cells for rescue graft failure after allogeneic bone marrow transplantation in two patients with acute myeloblastic leukemia in first complete remission. Blood 1995; 85:1678.
85. Bensinger WI, Clift RA, Anasetti C, Appelbaum FA, Demirer T, Rowley S, Sandmaier BM, Torok-Storb B, Storb R, Buckner CD. Transplantation of allogeneic peripheral blood stem cells mobilized by recombinant human granulocyte colony stimulating factor. Stem Cells 1996; 14:90.
86. Korbling M, Przepiorka D, Huh YO, Engel H, Van Besien K, Giralt S, Andersson B, Kleine HD, Seong D, Deisseroth AB, Andreeff M, Champlin R. Allogeneic blood stem cell transplantation for refractory leukemia and lymphoma: potential advantage of blood over marrow allograft. Blood 1995; 85:1659.
87. Schmitz N, Dreger P, Suttorp M, Rohwedder EB, Haferlach T, Loffler H, Hunter A, Russell NH. Primary transplantation of allogeneic peripheral blood progenitor cells mobilized by Filgrastim (granulocyte colony-stimulating factor). Blood 1995; 85:1666.

88. Bloom ET, Horvath JA. Cellular and molecular mechanisms of the IL-12-induced increase in allospecific murine cytolytic T cell activity. J Immunol 1994; 152:4242.
89. Trinchieri G. Interleukin-12: a cytokine produced by antigen-presenting cells with immunoregulatory functions in the generation of T-helper cells type 1 and cytotoxic lymphocytes. Blood 1994; 84:4008.
90. Manetti R, Parronchi P, Guidizi MG, Piccinni MP, Maggi E, Trinchieri G, Romagnani S. Natural killer cell stimulatory factor (interleukin 12 [IL-12]) induces T helper type 1 (Th1)-specific immune responses and inhibits the development of IL-4-producing Th cells. J Exp Med 1993; 177:1199.
91. Manetti R, Gerosa F, Guidizi MG, Biagiotti R, Parronchi P, Piccinni M-P, Sampognaro S, Maggi E, Romagnani S, Trinchieri G. Interleukin 12 induces stable priming for interferon gamma (IFN-gamma) production during differentiation of human T helper (Th) cells and transient IFN-gamma production in established Th2 cell clones. J Exp Med 1994; 179:11273.
92. Chan SH, Perussia B, Gupta JW, Kobayashi M, Pospisil M, Young HA, Wolf SA, Young D, Clark SC, Trinchieri G. Induction of interferon gamma production by natural killer cell stimulatory factor: characterization of the responder cells and synergy with other inductors. J Exp Med 1991; 173:869.
93. Sykes M, Szot GL, Nguyen PL, Pearson DA. Interleukin-12 inhibits murine graft-versus-host disease. Blood 1995; 86:2429.
94. Yang YG, Sergio JJ, Pearson DA, Szot GL, Sykes M. Interleukin 12 preserves the graft-vs-leukemia effect of allogeneic T cells while inhibiting graft-vs-host disease. Manuscript submitted, 1996.
95. Soiffer RJ, Robertson MJ, Murray C, Cochran K, Ritz J. Interleukin-12 augments cytotoxic activity of peripheral blood lymphocytes from patients with hematologic and solid malignancies. Blood 1993; 82:2790.
96. Rossi AR, Pericle F, Rashleigh S, Janiec J, Djeu JY. Lysis of neuroblastoma cell lines by human natural killer cells activated by interleukin-2 and interleukin-12. Blood 1994; 83:1323.
97. Nastala CL, Edington HD, McKinney TG, Tahara H, Nalesnik MA, Brunda MJ, Gately MK, Wolf SF, Schreiber RD, Storkus WJ, Lotze MT. Recombinant IL-12 administration induces tumor regression in association with IFN-gamma production. J Immunol 1994; 153:1697.
98. Brunda MJ, Luistro L, Warrier RR, Wright RB, Hubbard BR, Murphy M, Wolf SF, Gately MK. Antitumor and antimetastatic activity of interleukin 12 against murine tumors. J Exp Med 1993; 178:1223.
99. Gallucci BB, Sale GE, McDonald GB, et al. The fine structure of human rectal epithelium in acute graft-versus-host disease. Am J Surg Pathol 1982; 6:293.
100. Sale GE, Anderson P, Browne M, Myerson D. Evidence of cytotoxic T cell destruction of epidermal cells in human graft-versus-host disease. Arch Pathol Lab Med 1992; 116:622.
101. Takata M. Immunohistochemical identification of perforin-positive cytotoxic lymphocytes in graft-versus-host disease. Am J Clin Pathol 1995; 103:324.
102. Suda T, Okazaki T, Naito Y, et al. Expression of the Fas ligand in cells of T cell lineage. J Immunol 1995; 154:3806.
103. Thiele DL, Bryde SE, Lipsky PE. Lethal graft-versus-host disease induced by a class II MHC antigen only disparity is not mediated by cytotoxic T cells. J Immunol 1988; 141:3377.
104. Fussell ST, Donnellan M, Cooley MA, et al. Cytotoxic T lymphocyte precursor frequency does not correlate with either the incidence of severity of graft-versus-host disease after matched unrelated donor bone marrow transplantation. Transplantation 1994; 57:673.

105. Korngold R. Biology of graft-versus-host disease. Am J Pediatr Hematol Oncol 1993; 15:18.
106. Kagi D, Vignaux F, Ledermann B, et al. Fas and perforin pathways as major mechanisms of T cell-mediated cytotoxicity. Science 1994; 265:528.
107. Lowin B, Hahne M, Mattmann C, Tschopp J. Cytolytic T-cell cytotoxicity is mediated through perforin and Fas lytic pathways. Nature 1994; 370:650.
108. Levy RB, Baker M, Podack ER. Perforin deficiency delays the onset of GVHD following bone marrow transplantation across major and minor histocompatibility barriers. Ann NY Acad Sci 1995; 770:366.
109. Selvaggi G, Inverardi L, Levy RB, et al. Abrogation of graft-versus-host disease following allotransplantation of cytotoxically deficient bone marrow across major histocompatibility barriers. Ann NY Acad Sci 1996; 770:339.
110. Graubert TA, Russell JH, Ley T. The role of granzyme B in murine models of acute graft-versus-host disease and graft rejection. Blood 1996; 87:1232.
111. Baker MB, Altman NH, Podack ER, et al. The role of cell-mediated cytotoxicity in acute GVHD after MHC-matched allogeneic bone marrow transplantation in mice. J Exp Med 1996; in press.
112. Braun YM, Lowin B, French L, et al. Cytotoxic T cells deficient in both functional Fas ligand and perforin show residual cytolytic activity yet lose their capacity to induce lethal acute graft-versus-host disease. J Exp Med 1996; 183:657.
113. Falzarano G, Krenger W, Snyder KM, Delmonte J, Karandikar M, Ferrara JLM. Suppression of B cell proliferation to lipopolysaccharide is mediated through induction of the nitric oxide pathway by tumor necrosis factor-α in mice with acute graft-versus-host disease. Blood 1996; 87:2853.
114. Krenger W, Falzarano G, Delmonte J, Snyder KM, Byon JCH, Ferrara JLM. Interferon-γ suppresses T-cell proliferation to mitogen via the nitric oxide pathway during experimental acute graft-versus-host disease. Blood 88 1996; in press.
115. Murphy GF, Whitaker D, Sprent J, Korngold R. Characterization of target injury of murine acute graft-versus-host disease directed to multiple minor histocompatibility antigens elicited by either CD4+ or CD8+ effector cells. Am J Pathol 1991; 138: 983.
116. Gilliam AC, Whitaker-Menezes D, Korngold R, Murphy GF. Apoptosis is a major form of cell injury in experimental acute graft-versus-host disease in skin and mucosa. J Invest Dermatol 1996; 106:927.
117. Gilliam AC, Whitaker-Menezes D, Korngold R, Murphy GF. Apoptosis is the predominant form of epithelial target cell injury in acute experimental graft-versus-host disease. J Invest Dermatol 1996; in press.
118. Bickenback JR. Identification and behavior of label-retaining cells in oral mucosa and skin. J Dent Res 1981; 60:1611.
119. Sale GE, Shulman HM, Gallucci BB, Thomas ED. Young rete ridge keratinocytes are preferred targets in cutaneous graft-vs-host disease. Am J Path 1985; 118:278.
120. Trapani JA, Smyth MJ. Killing by cytotoxic and natural killer cells: multiple granule serine proteases as inhibitors of DNA fragmentation. Immunol Cell Biol 1993; 71:201.
121. Liu C-C, Walsh CM, Young JD-E. Perforin: structure and function. Immunol Today 1995; 16:194.
122. Itoh N, Yonehara S, Ishii A, Yonehara M, Mizushima SI, Sameshima M, Hase A, Seto Y, Nagata S. The polypeptide encoded by the cDNA for human cell surface antigen Fas can mediate apoptosis. Cell 1991; 66:233.
123. Christofidou-Solomidou M, Bennett CF, Albelda SM, Murphy GF. Anti-sense oligonucleotide therapy for cutaneous inflammation: A model for induction and treatment of cytotoxic dermatitis. J Invest Dermatol 1996; 106:830.
124. Sale GE, Anderson P, Browne M, et al. T-cell destruction of epidermal cells in human

graft-versus-host disease: Immunohistology with monoclonal antibody TIA-1. Arch Path Lab Med 1992; 116:622.

125. Remberger M, Ringden O, Markling L. TNF-α levels are increased during bone marrow transplantation conditioning in patients who develop acute GVHD. Bone Marrow Transplant 1995; 15:99.
126. Barak V, Levi-Schaffer F, Nisman B, Nagler A. Cytokine dysregulation in chronic graft versus host disease. Leukemia Lymphoma 1995; 17:169.
127. Panes J, Perry MA, Anderson DC, Muzykantov VR, Carden DL, Miyasaka M, Granger DN. Portal hypertension enhances endotoxin-induced intercellular adhesion molecule 1 up-regulation in the rat. Gastroenterology 1996; 110:866.
128. Spitzer JA, Zhang P, Mayer AMS. Functional characterization of peripheral circulating and liver recruited neutrophils in endotoxic rats. J Leukocyte Biol 1994; 56:166.
129. Callery MP, Mangino MJ, Kamei T, Flye MW. Interleukin-6 production by endotoxin-stimulated Kupffer cells is regulated by prostaglandin E_2. J Surg Res 1990; 48:523.
130. Oka Y, Murata A, Nishijima J, Ogawa M, Mori T. The mechanism of hepatic cellular injury in sepsis: an in vitro study of the implications of cytokines and neutrophils in its pathogenesis. J Surg Res 1993; 55:1.
131. Maher JJ. Rat hepatocytes and Kupffer cells interact to produce interleukin-8 (CINC) in the setting of ethanol. Am J Physiol 1995; 269:G518.
132. Holman JJM, Saba TM. Hepatocyte injury during post-operative sepsis: activated neutrophils as potential mediators. J Leukocyte Biol 1988; 43:193.
133. Greve JW, Gouma DJ, Buurman WA. Bile acids inhibit endotoxin-induced release of tumor necrosis factor by monocytes: An in vitro study. Hepatology 1989; 10:454.
134. Arai T, Hiromatsu K, Kobayashi N, Takano M, Ishida H, Nimura Y, Yoshikai Y. IL-10 is involved in the protective effect of dibutyryl cyclic adenosine monophosphate on endotoxin-induced inflammatory liver injury. J. Immunol 1995; 155:5743.
135. Leist M, Gantner F, Bohlinger I, Germann PG, Tiegs G, Wendel A. Murine hepatocyte apoptosis induced in vitro and in vivo by TNF-α requires transcriptional arrest. J Immunol 1994; 153:1778.
136. Qian DL, Brosnan JT. Administration of Escherichia coli endotoxin to rat increases liver mass and hepatocyte volume in vivo. Biochem J 1996; 313:479.
137. Whiting JF, Green RM, Rosenbluth AB, Gollan JL. Tumor necrosis factor-α decreases hepatocyte bile salt uptake and mediates endotoxin-induced cholestasis. Hepatology 1995; 22:1273.
138. Green RM, Whiting JF, Rosenbluth AB, Beier D, Gollan JL. Interleukin-6 inhibits hepatocyte taurocholate uptake and sodium-potassium-adenosine triphosphatase activity. Am J Physiol 1994; 267:G1094.
139. Ballmer PE, Imoberdorf R, Zbaren J. Immunohistochemical demonstration of interleukin-1β induced changes in acute-phase proteins and albumin in rat liver. Acta Histochem 1995; 97:281.
140. Ayres RCS, Neuberger JM, Shaw J, Joplin R, Adams DH. Intercellular adhesion molecule-1 and MHC antigens on human intrahepatic bile duct cells: Effect of proinflammatory cytokines. Gut 1993; 34:1245.
141. Van de Water J, Gershwin ME. Primary biliary cirrhosis: Cells, sera, and soluble factors. Mayo Clin Proc 1993; 68:1128.
142. Howell CD, De Victor D, Li J, Stevens J, Giorno RC. Liver T cell subsets and adhesion molecules in murine graft-versus-host disease. Bone Marrow Transplant 1995; 16:139.
143. Paradis K, Le ONL, Russo P, St-Cyr M, Fournier H, Bu DW. Characterization and response to interleukin 1 and tumor necrosis factor of immortalized murine biliary epithelial cells. Gastroenterology 1995; 109:1308.
144. Matsumoto K, Fujii H, Michalopoulos G, Fung JJ, Demetris AJ. Human biliary

epithelial cells secrete and respond to cytokines and hepatocyte growth factors in vitro: Interleukin-6, hepatocyte growth factor and epidermal growth factor promote DNA synthesis in vitro. Hepatology 1994; 20:376.

145. Ueno Y, Phillips JO, Ludwig J, Lichtman SN, LaRusso NF. Development and characterization of a rodent model of immune-mediated cholangitis. Proc Natl Acad Sci USA 1996; 93:216.
146. Cooke KR, Kobzik L, Martin TR, Brewer J, Delmonte J, Crawford JM, Ferrara JLM. An experimental model of idiopathic pneumonia syndrome after bone marrow transplantation. I. The roles of minor H antigens and endotoxin. Blood. In press, 1996.
147. Eisser G, Kohluber F, Grell M, Ueffing M, Scheurich P, Hieke A, Multhoff G, Bornkamm GW, Holler E. Critical involvement of transmembrane tumor necrosis factor α in endothelial programmed cell death mediated by ionizing radiation and bacterial endotoxin. Blood 1995; 86:4184.
148. Katz M, Grosfeld J, Gross K. Impaired bacterial clearance and trapping in obstructive jaundice. Am J Surg 1984; 199.
149. Matuschak GM. Liver-lung interactions in critical illness. New Horizons 1994; 2:488.
150. Nakao A, Taki S, Yasui M, Kimura Y, Nonami T, Harada A, Takagi H. The fate of intravenously injected endotoxin in normal rats and in rats with liver failure. Hepatology 1994; 19:1251.
151. Pugin J, Chevrolet JC. The intestinal-liver-lung axis on septic syndrome. J Suisse Med 1991; 121:1538.
152. Hagglund H, Bostrom L, Remberger M, Ljungman P, Nilsson B, Ringden O. Risk factors for acute graft-versus-host disease in 291 consecutive HLA-identical bone marrow transplant recipients. Bone Marrow Transplant 1995; 16:747.
153. Weiss G, Schwaighoffer H, Herold M, Nachbaur D, Wachter H, Niederwieser D, Werner ER. Nitric oxide formation as predictive parameter for acute graft-versus-host disease after human allogeneic bone marrow transplantation. Transplantation 1995; 60:1239.
154. Schwaighofer H, Kernan NA, O'Reilly RJ, Brankova J, Nachbaur D, Herold M, Eibl B, Niederwieser D. Serum levels of cytokines and secondary messages after T-cell-depleted and non-T-cell-depleted BMT: influence of conditioning and hematopoietic reconstitution. Transplantation, 1996; in press.
155. Niederwieser D, Herold M, Woloszczuk W, Aulitsky W, Meister B, Tilg H, Gastl G, Bowden R, Huber C. Endogenous IFN-gamma during human bone marrow transplantation. Transplantation 1990; 50:620.
156. Holler E, Ertl B, Hintermeier-Knabe R, Roncarolo MG, Eissner G, Mayer F, Fraunberger P, Behrends U, Pfannes W, Kolb HJ, Wilmanns W. Inflammatory reactions induced by pretransplant conditioning—an alternative target for modulation of acute GVHD and complications following allogeneic bone marrow transplantation. Leukemia Lymphoma, 1996; in press.
157. Antin JH, Weinstein HJ, Guinan EC, McCarthy P, Bierer BE, Gilliland DG, Parsons SK, Ballen KK, Rimm IJ, Falzarano G, Bloedow DC, Abate L, Lebsack M, Burakoff SJ, Ferrara JLM. Recombinant human interleukin-1 receptor antagonist in the treatment of steroid-resistant graft-versus-host disease. Blood 1994; 84:1342.
158. Petersdorf EW, Longton G, Anasetti C, et al. Donor-recipient disparities for HLA-C genes is a risk factor for graft failure following marrow transplantation from unrelated donors. Blood 1995; 86, Suppl. 1:291.
159. Ringden O, Hermans J, Labopin M, et al. The highest leukemia-free survival after allogeneic bone marrow transplantation is seen in patients with grade I acute graft-versus-host disease. Leukemia and Lymphoma, 1996; in press.
160. Gratwohl A, Hermans J, Apperley J, et al. Acute graft-versus-host disease: Grade and outcome in patients with chronic myelogenous leukemia. Blood 1995; 86:813.

161. Eibl B, Schwaighofer H, Nachbaur D, Marth C, Gachter A, Knapp R, Bock G, Gassner C, Schiller L, Petersen F, Niederwieser D. Evidence for a graft-versus-tumor (GvT) effect in a patient treated with marrow ablative chemotherapy and allogeneic bone marrow transplantation for breast cancer. Blood, 1996; in press.
162. Tricot G, Vesole DH, Jagannath S, et al. Graft-versus-myeloma effect: Proof of principle. Blood 1996; 87:1196.
163. Verdonck LF, Lokhorst HM, Dekker AW, et al. Graft-versus-myeloma effect in two cases. Lancet 1996; 347:800.
164. Parker PM, Chao N, Nademanee A, et al. Thalidomide as salvage therapy for chronic graft-versus-host disease. Blood 1995; 86:3604.
165. Kohn DB, Weinberg KI, Nolta JA, et al. Engraftment of gene-modified umbilical cord blood in neonates with adenosine deaminase deficiency. Nature Medicine 1995; 1.
166. Blaese RM, Culver KW, Miller AD, et al. T lymphocyte-directed gene therapy for ADA-SCID: Initial results after 4 years. Science 1995; 270:475.
167. Bordignon C, Notatangelo LD, Nobili N, et al. Gene therapy in peripheral blood lymphocytes and bone marrow for ADA-immunodeficient patients. Science 1995; 270: 470.
168. Heslop HE, Rooney CM, Brenner MK. Gene-marking and haematopoietic stem–cell transplantation. Blood Rev 1995; 9:220.
169. Beinzle D, Abrams-Ogg ACG, SA K, et al. Gene transfer into hematopoietic stem cells: Long-term maintenance of in vitro activated progenitors without marrow ablation. Proc Natl Acad Sci USA 1994; 91:350.
170. Stewart AK, Dube ID, Kamel-Reid S, Keating A. A Phase 1 study of autologous bone marrow transplantation with stem cell gene marking in multiple myeloma. Human Gene Therapy 1995; 6:107.
171. Merrouche Y, Negrier S, Bain C, et al. Clinical application of retroviral gene transfer in oncology: Results of a French study with tumor-infiltrating lymphocytes transduced with the gene of resistance to neomycin. J Clin Onc 1995; 13:410.
172. Heslop HE, Ng CYC, Li C, et al. Long-term restoration of immunity against Epstein-Barr virus infection by adoptive transfer of gene-modified virus-specific T lymphocytes. Nature Medicine 1996; 2:545.
173. Riddell SR, Elliot M, Lewinsohn DA, et al. T-cell mediated rejection of gene-modified HIV-specific cytotoxic lymphocytes in HIV-infected patients. Nature Medicine 1996; 2:216.
174. Blatter DD, Crawford JM, Ferrara JLM. Nuclear magnetic resonance of hepatic graft-versus-host disease in mice. Transplantation 1990; 50:1011.

Index